Paediatric Exercise Science and Medicine

Also published by Oxford University Press

Oxford Dictionary of Sports Science and Medicine

Michael Kent

Oxford Handbook of Sport and Exercise Medicine

Domhnall MacAuley

Forthcoming titles by Oxford University Press

Sports Injuries 2e

Hutson and Speed

Contents

Preface

The first edition of *Paediatric Exercise Science and Medicine* was welcomed by international reviewers as a volume which offered 'state of the art' research evidence-based coverage of the topic by recognized leaders in the field. However, this material is now almost 10 years old and in a rapidly developing subject requires updating, refreshing, and re-appraising. In the Preface to the first edition we referred to 'this emerging discipline' and commented on the 'dramatic increase in published research focusing on the exercising child and adolescent'. Since publication of the first edition research activity and publication in the field has continued to grow at an ever increasing rate. Experimental techniques initially pioneered with adults and new non-invasive technologies have been successfully developed and modified for use with children therefore opening up new avenues of paediatric research. According to PubMed, there has been a 123% *increase* in the number of published research papers in the 10 years to 2008 compared with the 10 years to 2000 when the first edition was published.

The second edition of *Paediatric Exercise Science and Medicine* has generally retained the format of the first edition. Each comprehensively referenced chapter critically analyses the research literature and, where appropriate, examines how recently developed experimental techniques and methods of interpreting paediatric data have provided new insights into understanding the exercising child. All contributors are internationally recognized experts in the field covered by their chapter and they draw upon their own research to enrich the text and to inform and challenge readers. Chapters are cross-referenced to promote access to complementary material and each chapter ends with a bulleted summary to support the rapid identification of key issues. Chapters on nine new topics have been added to this edition and even where chapter titles remain the same or similar to the first edition the content has been updated and re-written, often by new contributors who have emerged as leading researchers in their field since the publication of the first edition.

Children and adolescents are not mini-adults and measurement techniques developed with adults are often neither ethical nor appropriate for use with young people. Children are growing and maturing at their own rate and their physiological responses to exercise are difficult to interpret as they progress through childhood and adolescence into adult life. The initial sections of the book address these issues. Part I debates the ethical issues surrounding the involvement of children in non-therapeutic research, critically examines the estimation of body composition and maturity, and analyses methods of assessing and interpreting performance during exercise. A new chapter focuses on field tests. Part II discusses developmental biomechanics and motor development and rigorously examines the physiological responses to exercise of various types, intensities, and durations in relation to growth, maturation, and sex. The section ends with a consideration of the physiological responses to exercise during thermal stress. New chapters address growth and maturation and exercise metabolism.

The beneficial effects of appropriate physical activity during adult life are well-documented but the potential of physical activity to confer health benefits during childhood and adolescence is controversial and not explored fully. Part III critically reviews the extant literature and explores young people's health behaviours and the role of physical activity in the promotion of health and well-being, with particular reference to cardiovascular health, bone health, and social, psychological, and emotional health. A new chapter is devoted to gene–physical activity interactions. Part IV addresses sports participation, physical activity, and exercise testing in the context of children and adolescents suffering from chronic health conditions. The section begins with an examination of exercise testing in congenital heart disease and then comprehensively reviews the role of exercise and physical activity in children with asthma, cystic fibrosis, eating and weight disorders, diabetes, cerebral palsy, and other neurological diseases.

Intensive training and participation in sports competitions may start at an early age and even prepubertal children may be engaged in several hours per week of strenuous exercise including competitive sport. The growing and maturing young athlete is inevitably at risk of injury. Part V focuses on the elite young athlete. The section begins with a chapter devoted to the development of the elite young athlete and subsequent chapters scrutinize the evidence underpinning current training regimens during youth. Hormonal adaptations to exercise during childhood and adolescence are discussed and the sports participation of both able and disabled young people is analysed. The aetiology and prevention of injuries during youth sport are discussed in detail and the diagnosis and management of common sports injuries to the upper extremity, the trunk, the lower limb, the head, and the cervical spine are examined. The section includes chapters on five new topics.

The aim of the first edition of *Paediatric Exercise Science and Medicine* was to provide a 'state of the art' reference work to support and challenge scientists involved in developmental exercise science and medicine. Our aim remains the same and if this edition stimulates further interest in the study of the exercising child and adolescent, encourages exercise scientists and paediatricians to initiate research programmes in paediatric exercise science and medicine, and thereby contributes to the promotion of young people's health and well-being it will have served its purpose.

Exeter and Amsterdam
June 2008

Neil Armstrong
Willem van Mechelen

Contributors

Neil Armstrong PhD, DSc, Professor, Executive Suite, Northcote House, The Queen's Drive, University of Exeter, Exeter, EX4 4QJ, UK.

Frank JG Backx PhD, MD, Professor, University Medical Centre, University of Utrecht, Utrecht NL-3508 GA, the Netherlands.

Adam DG Baxter-Jones PhD, Professor, College of Kinesiology, University of Saskatchewan, 87 Campus Drive, Saskatoon, SK S7N 5B2, Canada.

Gaston Beunen PhD, Professor, Department of Biomedical Kinesiology, Faculty of Kinesiology and Rehabilitation Sciences, Katholieke Universiteit Leuven, Leuven, Belgium.

Cameron JR Blimkie PhD, Professor, Department of Kinesiology, McMaster University, Hamilton, L8P 4N9, Canada.

Shannon SD Bredin PhD, Cognitive and Functional Learning Laboratory, University of British Columbia, Vancouver, British Columbia, V6T 1Z3, Canada.

Nuala M Byrne PhD, Institute of Health and Biomedical Innovation, Queensland University of Technology, 60 Musk Ave, Kelvin Grove, Queensland, Australia 4059.

Robert C Cantu MD, Professor, Neurosurgery Service, Service of Sports Medicine, Emerson Hospital, Concord, MA 01742, USA.

Robert V Cantu MD, Dartmouth Hitchcock Medical Center, One Medical Center Drive, Lebanon, NH 03755, USA.

Akin Cil MD, Department of Orthopedic Surgery, Division of Sports Medicine, Children's Hospital Boston, MA, USA.

Albrecht L Claessens PhD, Professor, Department of Biomedical Kinesiology, Faculty of Kinesiology and Rehabilitation Sciences, Katholieke Universiteit Leuven, Leuven, Belgium.

Revd Mark Cobb MA, Clinical Directorate of Professional Services, Sheffield Teaching Hospitals NHS Foundation Trust, Sheffield, UK.

Dorrine CM Collard MSc, Department of Public and Occupational Health and EMGO Institute, VU University Medical Center, Amsterdam NL-1081 BT, the Netherlands.

Kirsten Corder PhD, MRC Epidemiology Unit, Institute of Metabolic Science, Box 285, Addenbrooke's Hospital, Cambridge, CB2 0QQ, UK.

Sean P Cumming PhD, School for Health, University of Bath, Bath, BA2 7AY, UK.

Annet J Dallmeijer PhD, Department of Rehabilitation Medicine and EMGO Institute, VU University Medical Center, Amsterdam NL-10007 MB, the Netherlands.

Mark BA De Ste Croix PhD, Faculty of Sport, Health and Social Care, University of Gloucestershire, Oxstalls Campus, Gloucester, GL2 9HW, UK.

Raffy Dotan MSc, Faculty of Applied Health Sciences, Brock University, St Catharines, Ontario, LS2 3AI, Canada.

Kelli L Drenner MA, The University of Texas Health Science Center at Houston, School of Public Health, Michael and Susan Dell Center for Advancement of Healthy Living, Houston, TX, USA.

Ulf Ekelund PhD, MRC Epidemiology Unit, Institute of Metabolic Science, Box 285, Addenbrooke's Hospital, Cambridge, CB2 0QQ, UK.

Roger G Eston DPE, Professor, School of Sport and Health Sciences, University of Exeter, EX1 2LU, UK.

Bareket Falk PhD, Department of Physical Education and Kinesiology, Brock University, St Catharines, Ontario, LS2 3AI, Canada.

Nathalie Farpour-Lambert MD, Exercise Medicine Clinic, Unit of Pediatric Cardiology, Department of Child and Adolescent, University Hospital of Geneva, 1211 Geneva 14, Switzerland.

Samantha G Fawkner PhD, Sport and Exercise Science, School of Life Sciences, Heriot-Watt University, Riccarton, Edinburgh, EH14 4AS, UK.

Isabel Ferreira PhD, Department of Clinical Epidemiology and Medical Technology Assessment and Department of Internal Medicine, University Hospital Maastricht, Maastricht, the Netherlands.

Paul W Franks PhD, Genetic Epidemiology and Clinical Research Group, Department of Public Health and Clinical Medicine, Umeå University Hospital, Sweden.

Julie C Garza DrPH, University of Texas Health Science Center at Houston, School of Public Health, Michael and Susan Dell Center for Advancement of Healthy Living, Houston, TX, USA.

Marc Gewillig PhD, MD, Professor, Department of Pediatric Cardiology, University Hospital Gasthuisberg, Herestraat 3000, Leuven, Belgium.

Helge Hebestreit PhD, MD, Professor, Universitäts-Kinderklinik, Josef-Schneider-Str. 2, 97080 Würzburg, Germany.

Andrew P Hills PhD, Professor, Institute of Health and Biomedical Innovation, Queensland University of Technology, 60 Musk Avenue, Brisbane, Queensland, Australia 4059.

Jaak Jürimäe PhD, Professor, Faculty of Exercise and Sport Sciences, Centre of Behavioural and Health Sciences, University of Tartu, 18 Ülikooli St., Tartu 50090, Estonia.

Toivo Jürimäe PhD, Professor, Faculty of Exercise and Sport Sciences, Centre of Behavioural and Health Sciences, University of Tartu, 18 Ülikooli St., Tartu 50090, Estonia.

Han CG Kemper PhD, DUniv (Hon), Professor, EMGO Institute, VU University Medical Centre, Amsterdam NL-1081 BT, the Netherlands.

Mininder S Kocher MD, Children's Hospital Boston, Harvard Medical School, Boston, MA, USA

Gerjo J Kok PhD, Professor, Department of Work and Social Psychology, Faculty of Psychology, Maastricht University, Maastricht NL-6200 MD, the Netherlands.

Stef PJ Kremers PhD, Department of Health Education and Promotion, Faculty of Health, Medicine and Life Sciences, Maastricht University, Maastricht NL-6200 MD, the Netherlands.

Susi Kriemler MD, Institute of Exercise and Health Science, University of Basel, Switzerland

Kevin L Lamb PhD, Department of Sport and Exercise Sciences, University of Chester, Chester, CH1 4 BJ, UK.

Umile Giuseppe Longo MD, Department of Trauma and Orthopaedics, Campus Biomedico University, 00155 Rome, Italy.

Helen C Looker MB, Division of Endocrinology, Mount Sinai School of Medicine, New York, USA.

Nicola Maffulli PhD, MD, Professor, Department of Trauma and Orthopaedic Surgery, Keele University School of Medicine, Stoke on Trent, ST4 7QB, UK.

Per Bo Mahler MD, Service de santé de la jeunesse, CP 3682, 1211 Geneva 2, Switzerland.

Anthony D Mahon PhD, Professor, Human Performance Laboratory, Ball State University, Muncie, IN 47306, USA.

Robert M Malina PhD, Professor, University of Texas at Austin and Tarleton State University, Stephenville, TX, USA.

Ree Meertens PhD, Department of Health Education and Promotion, Faculty of Health, Medicine and Life Sciences, Maastricht University, Maastricht NL-6200 MD, the Netherlands.

K Ashlee McGuire MSc, Cognitive and Functional Learning Laboratory, University of British Columbia, Vancouver, British Columbia, V6T 1Z3, Canada.

Alison M McManus PhD, Institute of Human Performance, University of Hong Kong, Pokfulam, Hong Kong, China.

Lyle J Micheli MD, Professor, Children's Hospital and Harvard Medical School, Boston, MA, USA.

Don W Morgan PhD, Professor, Department of Health and Human Performance, Middle Tennessee State University, Murfreesboro, TN 37132, USA.

Nancy G Murray DrPH, University of Texas Health Science Center at Houston, School of Public Health, Michael and Susan Dell Center for Advancement of Healthy Living, Houston, TX, USA.

Shareef Mustapha MD, Department of Pediatrics and Child Health, Winnipeg Children's Hospital, University of Manitoba, CH102–840 Sherbrook Street, Winnipeg, Manitoba, R3A 1S1, Canada.

Lindsay Nettlefold MSc, Faculty of Medicine, University of British Columbia, Vancouver, British Columbia, V6T 1Z3, Canada.

Patricia A Nixon PhD, Department of Health and Exercise Science, Wake Forest University, Winston-Salem, NC 27109–7868, USA.

Timothy S Olds PhD, Professor, Nutritional Physiology Research Centre, School of Health Sciences, University of South Australia, Adelaide SA, Australia 5001.

Gaynor Parfitt PhD, School of Sport and Health Sciences, University of Exeter, Exeter, EX1 2LU, UK.

Tony Reybrouck PhD, Professor, Department of Cardiovascular Rehabilitation, University Hospital Gasthuisberg, Herestraat 3000, Leuven, Belgium.

Chris Riddoch PhD, Professor, School for Health, University of Bath, Bath, BA2 7AY, UK.

Thomas W Rowland MD, Professor, Department of Pediatrics, Baystate Medical Center, Springfield, MA 01106, USA and Children's Health and Exercise Research Centre, University of Exeter, Exeter, EX1 2LU, UK.

Herman Schaalma PhD, Professor, Department of Work and Social Psychology, Faculty of Psychology, Maastricht University, Maastricht NL-6200 MD, the Netherlands.

Jost Schnyder PhD, MD, Sports Medicine and Physio Rehabilitation Centre, Rue Jacques Grosselin 25, 1127 Carouge, Geneva, Switzerland.

Shreela Sharma PhD, University of Texas Health Science Center at Houston, School of Public Health, Michael and Susan Dell Center for Advancement of Healthy Living, Houston, TX, USA.

Helen C Soucie PhD, 23 Rue de la Chimerie, Gatineau, Quebec, J9A 3L5, Canada.

David Sugden PhD, Professor, School of Education, University of Leeds, Leeds, LS2 9JT, UK.

Wendell C Taylor PhD, University of Texas Health Science Center at Houston, School of Public Health, Center for Health Promotion and Prevention Research, Houston, TX, USA.

Keith Tolfrey PhD, School of Sport and Exercise Sciences, Loughborough University, Epinal Way, Loughborough, LE11 3TU, UK.

Grant R Tomkinson PhD, Nutritional Physiology Research Centre, School of Health Sciences, University of South Australia, Adelaide SA, Australia 5000.

Susan R Tortolero PhD, University of Texas Health Science Center at Houston, School of Public Health, Center for Health Promotion and Prevention Research, Houston, TX, USA.

Stewart G Trost PhD, Department of Nutrition and Exercise Sciences, Oregon State University, Corvallis, OR 97331, USA.

Jos Twisk PhD, Department of Methodology and Applied Biostatistics, Institute of Health Sciences, Vrije Universiteit, Amsterdam NL-1081 BT, the Netherlands.

Willem van Mechelen PhD, MD, Professor, Department of Public and Occupational Health and EMGO Institute, VU University Medical Centre, Amsterdam NL-1081 BT, the Netherlands.

Edgar GAH van Mil, PhD, MD, Department of Pediatrics, Jheronimus Bosch Medical Centre, PO Box 90153, 5200 ME 's-Hertogenbosch, the Netherlands.

Evert ALM Verhagen PhD, Department of Public and Occupational Health & EMGO Institute, VU University Medical Center, Amsterdam NL-1081 BT, the Netherlands.

Darren ER Warburton PhD, Cardiovascular Physiology and Rehabilitation Laboratory, University of British Columbia, Vancouver, V6T 1Z3, Canada.

James Watkins PhD, Professor, Department of Sports Science, School of Human Sciences, Swansea University, Singleton Park, Swansea, SA2 8PP, UK.

Joanne R Welsman PhD, School of Sport and Health Sciences, University of Exeter, Exeter, EX1 2LU, UK.

Craig A Williams PhD, Children's Health and Exercise Research Centre, University of Exeter, Exeter, EX1 2LU, UK.

Edward M Winter PhD, Professor, Centre for Sport and Exercise Science, Sheffield Hallam University, Sheffield S10 2BP, UK.

Rachel E Wood PhD, Institute of Health and Biomedical Innovation, Queensland University of Technology, 60 Musk Ave, Kelvin Grove, Queensland, Australia 4059.

Merrilee Zetaruk MD, Department of Pediatrics and Child Health, Winnipeg Children's Hospital, University of Manitoba, CH102–840 Sherbrook Street, Winnipeg, Manitoba, R3A 1S1, Canada.

PART I

Assessment in Paediatric Exercise Science

CHAPTER 1

Ethics in paediatric research: principles and processes

Edward M. Winter and Mark Cobb

Introduction

The pace of developments in research continues both in the number of studies that are published in peer review journals and texts such as this and in the complexity and detail of topic material. Characteristic of these complexities have been advances in molecular biology and, in particular, genomics—the study of an organism's entire genetic make-up—and related proteomics—the study of the structures and functions of proteins. Added to the challenges that researchers face have been increasingly stringent requirements for ethics approval of studies that comprise the process of research governance. While the history of such approvals is well established, the introduction of statutory and related requirements in the comparatively short period of time since the first edition of this volume was published has accentuated the need for the topic to be addressed formally. Moreover, there has been a marked increase in the number of texts and other publications that address this area.[1–5]

In essence, ethics approval for research attempts to ensure that the moral status of children is upheld and that there is adherence to ethical and legal requirements. Accordingly, good research practice is identified as that which avoids wronging or harming participants, in this case, children. Accordingly, research ethics concerns what we *ought* to do in paediatric research and is a way of deliberating on how we might do good research in moral terms. Such research has three requirements: first, respect for participants; second, beneficence (i.e. doing good); and third, justice. If these guiding principles are in place, an important practical consequence follows: protection for both parties (i.e. participants and investigators).

The purpose of this chapter is therefore two-fold, and it outlines, first, principles that underpin ethics approval and, second, processes by which ethics approval can be sought and granted. While the former is important, emphasis will be placed on the latter because it is the practicalities that are particularly challenging, and a key intention of this chapter is to help researchers chart their way through the tortuous and convoluted pathways that characterize research governance. Out of necessity, the approach will tend to take a United Kingdom-centric perspective, but much of current practice is determined by European Union legislation, and similar procedures are in place elsewhere in the world.

Care has to be taken to distinguish between the noun ethics and the adjective ethical. Ethics committees provide ethics approval. It is to be hoped that they do so ethically and that all committees, irrespective of their function, are ethical, but the fact of the matter is that it is ethics approval that these committees grant.

Principles

The term ethics implies a set of standards that regulate behaviour, enable us to recognize the difference between right and wrong and act accordingly. This sounds simple, but, of course, in practice matters are much more complicated. These complications are both theoretical and practical and apply especially when children are participants in research.

At the outset, the fundamental principle is remarkably simple: any study that has humans as participants should have ethics approval from an appropriate body. Indeed, it can be argued that 'should' should be 'must,' and that is the stance that is taken here. This presents a key question: how should such approval be obtained so as to ensure that the moral and legal interests of participants are upheld and that they and investigators are protected?

When taking part in research participants waive certain aspects of their rights that normally restrict ways in which others can behave towards them. In other circumstances, these behaviours would, similarly, be unacceptable. Waving these rights so as to allow researchers to perform actions that would normally be prohibited could be justifiable on the grounds that new knowledge could be obtained that could in turn be used to benefit others. However, the rights waived are particular and specific. For example, participants should still be treated as humans and not as guinea pigs. Consequently, conducting ethically acceptable research with the full consent of participants can be considered not to breach certain ethical and legal norms. Thus, the process provides a way to gain restricted permission to carry out actions that might otherwise be illegal or immoral. Consideration must also be given to the need for approval, and, regrettably, such need stems from episodes in the history of human kind that are both salutary and sombre.

In brief, ethical actions emanate from principles and values[1] that in turn are derived from ethical theories. Broadly, there are three such theories: virtue, utilitarian, and deontology, although it is acknowledged that this is a simplified approach to a more complex pattern. Virtue theory addresses the characteristics of a good person and their behaviours, that is, being fair, decent, and honest. Utilitarian theory, sometimes referred to as consequential theory, embodies the end and justifies the means approach to actions, whereas deontology—the study of the nature of duty and obligation—holds that an individual's rights, interests, and preferences should be respected and upheld. It is deontology that guides most practices in research governance because such governance is rules based.[1]

History

Prior to Nuremberg

Table 1.1 illustrates a simplified time line for major landmarks in the history of ethics in research. For a detailed consideration, interested readers might like to consult MacIntyre.[6] The first documented recognition of ethics stems from medicine and can be traced back to Hippocrates. It is enshrined in the Hippocratic oath that still guides medical practice and physicians' duties. The Greek theme continued through the work of Galen, but the late Renaissance period saw the first faltering footsteps of modern science and, with it, emerging principles of ethics in terms of the design of clinical studies and embryonic randomized controlled trials (RCTs). It was not until the early seventeenth century, however, that Sir Francis Bacon laid one of the founding stones of modern empiricism.

Sir Robert Talbor expressed concern at some unsavoury aspects of medicine that were appearing, which, in a literary sense, were highlighted by Jonathan Swift in *Gulliver's Travels*. De Branchini is perhaps the first to describe the placebo approach to clinical trials, although it is James Lind to whom the first RCT is attributed. Throughout the nineteenth century from Percival onwards, attempts were made by the likes of Bernard, Hansen, and Neisser to ally the technical aspects of experimentation to the rights of 'subjects' but it was the twentieth century that saw the keystones of current practice being laid and the edifices being erected.

The background was not always noble and based on philanthropy. Indeed far from it, some of the needs for ethics approval were chilling. The Tuskegee Syphilis Study of 1932 allowed inmates in penitentiaries to go untreated so that the path of the disease could be charted. Then, arising from atrocities committed by the Japanese and Nazis prior to and during the Second World War from 1939 to 1945, the Nuremberg War Trials tribunals were held in 1946 and 1947. It is often overlooked that there were two main trials: one for military staff such as Göering, Himmler, and Goebels, but another solely for medical personnel who had been involved in the mistreatment of prisoners of war or inmates of concentration camps. This mistreatment involved experimentation either with or without anaesthetization and without the approval of victims or their next of kin. It is sobering to reflect that our current procedures and processes are based largely on the outcome of these trials.

Table 1.1 Key developments in the history of research ethics

Date	Person or event	Notable feature
500 BC	Hippocrates	A medical oath that outlined physicians' duties
AD 130–210	Galen	A major influence on the theory and practice of medicine
1620	Sir Francis Bacon	His 'Great Instauration' was one of the founding stones of modern empiricism
1672	Sir Robert Talbor	Secrecy and deception in medicine
1724	Jonathan Swift	Gulliver's Travels an attack on the new 'Natural Philosophers'
1751	De Branchini	A description of experimentation and placebo
1798	Dr. E. Jenner	Experimentation using cow pox to protect against smallpox
1803	Dr. Thomas Percival	A description of medical ethics
1865	Claude Bernard	An introduction to the study of experimental medicine
1879	Dr. Armauer Hansen	Experimentation without consent
1898	Professor Neisser	Experimentation without consent
1932	Tuskegee Syphilis Study	An observational study continued after possible therapy was available
1947	Nuremberg code	Precepts against which war crime defendants were judged
1964	Helsinki Declaration	A code of practice for physicians involved in medical research
1966	The first Research Ethics Committee (REC) in the United Kingdom	Provides formal approvals for research projects
1991	Department of Health	Guidance for Local RECs
2000	Establishment of Central Office for Research Ethics Committees (COREC)	Coordination of Local RECs
2001	European Union Directive 2001/20/EC	Outlines requirements for Good Clinical Practice
2001	Department of Health	Governance Arrangements for Research Ethics Committees (GAfREC)
2004	UK Regulations	The Medicines for Human use (Clinical Trials) Regulations
2007	National Research Ethics Service (NRES) launched	New regulatory for NHS research in the United Kingdom

Adapted from the National Research Ethics Service website.[9]

Since Nuremberg

It took 17 years, but in 1964 a major event occurred that was based on the outcome of Nuremberg: the World Medical Association[7] that had been formed in 1945 adopted and published the Helsinki Declaration of Human Rights.[8] This Declaration laid out fundamental requirements for medical and scientific research that were firmly based on principles of ethics. Prior to Nuremberg, research was largely unregulated. This applies even to Edward Jenner's pioneering work into vaccines. Regulation had occurred in the use of cadavers in anatomy classes via the Anatomy Act of 1832. This Act was introduced to counter malpractice in the ways in which bodies were supplied to anatomists.

The year 1966 saw the first formal Research Ethics Committee established in the United Kingdom, and by 1991, the need for coordination of such committees that were proliferating was met by the Department of Health's document, Guidance for Research Ethics Committees.[9] This document was aimed at National Health Service (NHS) related research. In 2000, a further major development occurred: the Central Office for Research Ethics Committees (COREC) was established to oversee and harmonize the operation of Local Research Ethics Committees (LRECs) that dealt with all NHS-related research. These LRECs tended to reflect Local Health Authority boundaries, but the continual restructuring of the United Kingdom's NHS increased the complexities of managing LRECs. Furthermore, studies were not necessarily restricted to one LREC. Some were national and embraced several LRECs so Multi-Centre Research Ethics Committees (MRECs) and systems were introduced. The pattern was becoming increasingly complex, bureaucratic, and unwieldy. In parallel, RECs were emerging in universities and other institutes of higher education[10] because of the need to ensure that non-NHS research was also conducted according to strict principles of ethics as enshrined in the Helsinki Declaration,[8] although it should be noted that the Declaration itself has undergone six or so revisions.

These parallel systems began to create tensions. In addition to the proliferation of medical research for which LRECs had to provide approval, there was much non-NHS research taking place. In the context of sport and exercise science in particular, there has been a remarkable rise in this discipline both in the United Kingdom and elsewhere. For instance, since its introduction in the United Kingdom in mid-1970s, some 10,000 students now graduate annually with sport- or exercise-related degrees at undergraduate, masters, and doctoral levels. Students undertake dissertations and research projects with humans as participants. This includes those in which children participate. The sheer volume and variety of projects was creating severe challenges to the processes involved in research governance.

It should also be noted that another driver for these developments was the emergence in the 1960s of bioethics and its subsequent growth since.[11] This has arisen from the advances in the use of medical technology both in research and practice. Most notable was the introduction of organ transplantation characterized by Barnard's first recorded human heart transplant in December 1967. Since then, organ transplantation has become commonplace and, of course, human *in vitro* fertilization has raised concerns about aspects of its application. Bioethics now features prominently in medical schools, and academics, publications, and departments have evolved to meet the growing need.

Finally, another challenge that underscored the need for research governance arose from anxieties about researchers and pharmaceutical companies withholding negative results of trials.[12] This adds another dimension to the already complex array of considerations.

However, irrespective of the nature of committees (i.e. NHS-related RECs or institutional versions), their roles are essentially similar, and to protect participants and investigators they ensure that (i) beneficence will occur (i.e. studies aim to do positive good), (ii) non-malfeasance is central (i.e. no harm will arise from the research), (iii) informed consent has been obtained from participants, and (iv) confidentiality of information and anonymity of participants is upheld.

Statutory requirements

Elsewhere, in 2001 the European Union issued Directive 2001/20/EC that is concerned with 'the approximation of the laws, regulations and administrative provisions of the member States relating to the implementation of Good Clinical Practice in the conduct of clinical trials on medicinal products for human use'. This gave rise to the Medicine and Healthcare products Regulatory Agency (MHRA) that was established in 2003.[13] The year 2001 also saw the publication of the Department of Health's Governance Arrangements for Research Ethics Committees.[9]

Of concern was the continuation of malpractice in research exemplified by the Bristol doctors' case at Bristol Royal Infirmary in the early 1980s, Alder Hey in the 1990s, and fraud perpetrated in Korea in the 1990s and 2000s in connection with cloning. The retention of body parts and intact foetuses at Alder Hey Hospital near Liverpool without the approval or even knowledge of next of kin gave rise to the Human Tissue Act (2004)[14] and, in the same year, the establishment of the Act's regulatory body, the Human Tissue Authority (HTA).[15] The HTA laid down stringent requirements for the storage of human tissue. Such tissue can be stored only if (i) the study for which storage is required has LREC approval or (ii) if the premises on which storage occurs have an HTA licence. Contravention of these requirements is illegal, and a possible penalty is imprisonment.

Moreover, the Committee on Publication Ethics (COPE)[16] was established in 1997 to address increasing concern that fraudulent research was not being detected in the process of peer-review and was being published. Furthermore, in 2007, the UK Research Integrity Office[17] was established as a mechanism by which biomedical scientists could report suspected malpractice by colleagues. Finally, 2007 saw the launch of the National Research Ethics Service (NRES)[9] that replaced COREC.

Criminal Records Bureau (CRB) checks

While all this was taking place, alarming cases of sex abuse by coaches on young athletes had come to light. For instance, in 1996, Paul Hickson who had trained swimmers for the Seoul and Los Angeles Olympic Games in 1984 and 1988 was convicted of 17 offences, including rape. In 2001, Michael Drew—at the time one of the United Kingdom's leading swimming coaches—was convicted for sexual abuse against young boy swimmers and was sentenced to 8 years in prison. Such cases were not restricted to swimming nor were they solely UK based. Professor Celia Brackenridge has done much to alert all involved of the risk and steps that can be taken to counter paedophilia in sport.[18] Rightly, she deserves credit for so doing.

In 1999, the Protection of Children Act[19] was introduced and shortly after, in 2001, the Child Protection in Sport Unit (CPSU)[20] was inaugurated. Arising from the Protection of Children Act was the need for those intending to work with children to have a check on their suitability to do so by the CRB.[21] The CRB is an Executive Agency of the Home Office and was established in 2002 under Part V of the Police Act (1997).[22] The service allows organizations in the public, private, and voluntary sectors to make safer recruitment decisions by identifying candidates who might be unsuitable for certain work, especially that which involves children and vulnerable adults. According to the Criminal Justice and Court Services Act,[23] in the United Kingdom, a child is technically a minor and is defined as someone who is under 18 years of age. However, as regards the law, this definition is adjustable according to circumstances. A vulnerable adult is defined as a person who is 16 or over and who

i) is, or may be, in need of community care services by reason of mental or other disability, age or illness and
ii) is or may be unable to take care of him or her self, or unable to protect him or herself against significant harm or exploitation

(Paragraph 9.6)[24]

One of the authors (E.M.W.) has first-hand experience of acting as an expert witness for the prosecution in a case of child molestation under the guise of supposed sport science research perpetrated by a coach. There is much distress in such cases, especially for the victims. This is a serious and depressing issue.

Checks on an individual's criminal record are called disclosures, and there are two types: enhanced and standard.[21] Enhanced disclosure is required for those who will be working with children unsupervised as normal practice. Standard disclosure is provided for those who will probably be working under supervision or whose involvement with children is infrequent or brief.

It should be noted that there have been no prosecutions in the United Kingdom for sex abuse of minors by sport and exercise scientists. While this is reassuring, it should not lead to complacency. Denial was a major impediment to the introduction of measures that were designed to identify and deal accordingly with paedophile sport coaches and, better still, deny them the opportunities to become involved with children in the first place. Nevertheless, the need for CRB checks and the like causes resentment among innocent individuals who, understandably, feel aggrieved that their integrity is in question. Regrettably, the fact of the matter is that such checks are necessary.

Data Protection Act (1988)

This Act[25] was introduced to control the ways in which information about an individual was distributed to other parties. As a result, the privacy of an individual could be protected. In most cases few would perhaps disagree with the basic tenets of the Act, but in the context of CRB checks and work with minors, a particularly distressing precedent has occurred that impacts directly on those involved with children and has led to a fundamental review of the ways in which the CRB and the Data Protection Act interface. In 2005, Ian Huntley was convicted of the murder of two 10-year-old girls in Soham, Cambridgeshire and was sentenced to 40 years imprisonment. At the time of the murders, Huntley was employed in a community college immediately adjacent to the school his victims attended. His partner Maxine Carter, who was also convicted, was a teaching assistant at the school. In spite of several formal allegations in preceding years made to the police, Huntley had never been convicted of an offence against children. At the time, only convictions, not allegations, would show in CRB checks, so there was no apparent reason to deny him employment. At the time of his trials, the police claimed that the Data Protection Act prevented them from warning the authorities. Clearly, this is an extreme example, but the deaths of the two schoolgirls was a stark indication of the need for improved protection.

The ways in which the CRB and Data Protection Act align with each other was the subject of formal enquiry,[26] and the implications are still under consideration. Those charged with providing ethics approval have a precedent, not a hypothetical situation, to guide their deliberations.

Fraser guidelines

Normally, minors cannot consent to participate in studies or receive medical treatment; their parents, guardians, or carers do so on their behalf. However, following a ruling by Lord Fraser in the House of Lords in 1985,[27] minors aged 16 or 17 years can consent to medical care, even if that is counter to the wishes of their next of kin. The same applies to minors who are aged less than 16 years, provided they are deemed competent by medical staff to make decisions. These guidelines arose from the case of Gillick versus West Norfolk and Wisbech Area Health Authority and were originally known as Gillick competence. A parent took formal action against the Health Authority when one of its doctors prescribed contraception to one of the parent's daughters without telling the parent. The action was dismissed and the parent appealed to the House of Lords. It was Lord Fraser who presided and dismissed the appeal.

Since then, this therapeutically-related edict has been applied to research that is clinically oriented, but it can also be applied to research that is non-therapeutic. The justification for this extension into research resides partly in law, because here a 16 year old is deemed competent to consent to medical treatment without either the knowledge or approval of their parents, guardians, or carers. If a 16- or 17-year-old person is considered not to be competent (e.g. they are unconscious), a person with parental responsibility can consent for them. However, the parental right ends when they reach 18 years old. Those aged 12–15 years can provide consent if they are deemed sufficiently mature by the researcher. As a general rule, children under 12 years cannot provide individual consent, but they should provide assent and this assent should be noted formally. The issue is not so much about maturity in general but the competence and, now, capacity of the child to make a decision.

For non-therapeutic research, the situation is less clear, although, in principle, it is at least similar. The fundamental problem is the establishment of maturity for those aged 12–15 years. Researchers must 'accept the possibility of prosecution if their interpretation of a child's competence to consent is deemed unacceptable'.[28] At the time of writing, the authors are not aware of any prosecution in the United Kingdom that has arisen from this interpretation.

The authors have first-hand experience of the application of Fraser guidelines to research. A proposal was submitted to the ethics committee on which the authors sat to investigate mechanisms of cigarette smoking cessation. Participants included adolescents aged 16 and 17 years. If parental consent was required, it was likely that several potential participants would be dissuaded from taking part and this would undermine the study. After seeking legal advice, Fraser guidelines were invoked and the study proceeded.

Informed consent

It is apposite at this point to consider a central tenet both of medical care and research—informed consent. Such consent means that a participant has been able to make a reasoned decision about whether or not to take part in a study and that as a result, and where they have decided to participate, this decision is confirmed by their signing an informed consent form (ICF). The participant must be given a detailed description both verbally and in writing of what precisely is involved, and, normally, the literary form of this information is the participant information sheet (PIS). An example of an ICF and detailed guidelines for the content of a PIS are available on the NRES website.[9]

The PIS should contain the following:

1 A general statement of the background to the study and its objectives.

2 An explanation of the procedures, identifying experimental ones and describing inherent risks.

3 A description of any benefits that are anticipated.

4 An offer to answer any questions on procedures and other aspects of the study.

5 An instruction to the effect that each participant is free to withdraw consent and discontinue participation at any time without prejudice.

6 An instruction to the effect that in any questionnaire or interview each participant is free to refuse to answer specific questions or items.

7 An instruction to the effect that no disadvantage—in terms of associated services—will arise from any decision on whether or not to participate.

8 An explanation of the procedures that are to be used to ensure the confidentiality of all data and information that is to be derived from the participant. If participants are to be identified by name in a manuscript, then express permission for this should be included in the ICF.

Moreover, informed consent should not arise as a result of coercion. Researchers need to be aware of this because of the seniority they hold over minors and the likelihood of children feeling intimidated or otherwise pressurized to participate. However, while perhaps more serious, the issue of coercion and the possibility of the introduction of bias is similar to other nuisance variable factors that can influence results.[29] Skilled researchers should know techniques and designs to minimize such influences and so improve the strength of their proposed studies—but this now has to be verified independently.

A separate ICF should accompany the PIS, and each should be distributed at least a week before any procedures begin. This is to give potential participants a cooling-off period, that is, sufficient time to consider their involvement. That sufficient time was given is actually an item on the ICF. A copy of the PIS and ICF should be retained by the participant and principal investigator (PI).

In the case of children, the language used should be child-friendly and of a form that a child can understand. Where a parent, guardian, or carer gives the consent, the child should give their assent, and a space on the ICF should be made available and identified accordingly.

One aspect of informed consent forms is that they can be demanded by bodies that deal with suspected fraud or similar malpractice. Participants can then be traced for verification they did indeed participate.

Mental Capacity Act (2005)

This Act[30] applies in general to people aged 16 years and above who lack the capacity to make decisions for themselves, and it specifically protects them if they take part in research (other than clinical trials of medicines). For example, people with Down's syndrome might not have the capacity to consent to being involved with research about improving their health through physical exercise. Consequently, researchers should understand their duties under the Act and are required to have regard for the Code of Practice[31] that devotes separate chapters on how the Act applies to children and to research. The Act was fully implemented by October 2007; however, further specific guidance expected on research involving those under the age of 18 years was unavailable at the time of publication and readers should consult relevant authorities about this, including the Department of Constitutional Affairs.[32]

This Act[30] makes provision for those who are incapable of making a decision that affects their well-being and identifies individuals who can make decisions on their behalf. The implementation of the Act has been subject to several delays because of difficulties that include establishing nationwide provision. Researchers need to be aware of the Act's existence and its implications for their work. The Department of Health Code of Practice[31] for the Mental Capacity Act devotes separate chapters to how the Act applies to children and research.

Risk assessment

Alongside all of the other statutory and regulatory requirements that have been introduced and apply to research governance, there are those that address health and safety issues in occupational, health, and research settings. In the United Kingdom, the regulatory body for such matters is the Health and Safety Executive (HSE)[33] that stemmed from the Health and Safety at Work Act (1974).[34] The HSE deals with issues such as risk assessment of procedures and tasks and impacts directly on research governance.[35] Researchers have to undertake a formal assessment of the risk(s) inherent in intended procedures. Most institutions have mechanisms and processes for this as part of occupational activities with an individual who has overall responsibility to ensure that these processes are implemented.

Precisely how the assessment of risk should be undertaken varies. One way is to assign scores for the consequence of an incident occurring and the likelihood of that occurrence. The product of the two quantifies the severity of risk.[35] An alternative is to have a green–amber–red approach. Either way allows the identification of control measures that are required.

Researchers whose interests are children find themselves at the confluence of these regulatory and statutory bodies. They have to be aware of all the mechanisms that enable them to satisfy the requirements. This is a severe challenge. Similarly, chairs and members of ethics committees who make decisions on the worth of studies face stern challenges and they too have major responsibilities.

Indemnity

It is essential that appropriate indemnity is in place for public and professional liability. For most, if not all, major institutions, this will be provided to each employee by dint of their inclusion on the payroll. For clinicians and other practitioners, normally they would have to take additional insurance cover. For others not so covered, they should be insured by other means. The possibility of litigation has to be considered, although there is extensive debate about whether or not society in general is increasingly litigious.

Some institutions have special arrangements for high-risk clinical trials and have to pay extra premiums for additional indemnity. The extent of insurance cover required usually has to be decided at the outset, and precise details of indemnity must be stated in proposals. Similarly, the responsibility of each individual investigator has to be identified and stated at the outset. Examples of studies to which this applies are those that investigate the effectiveness of medicinal products, and have participants who are pregnant or for whom exercise challenges could be hazardous.

Codes of practice

Most learned and similar bodies such as the British Association of Sport and Exercise Sciences,[36] the British Psychological Society,[37] and the British Medical Association[38] have codes of practice by which their members are expected to abide. These bodies also have accreditation or registration schemes, and if members contravene codes, they can be disciplined or even expelled. Each has a website where both the codes and disciplinary procedures are laid out in detail. Most, if not all, researchers should be members of an appropriate professional body and, hence, should have access to the requirements for membership of that body to which they should adhere.

Similarly, institutions have HSE-related procedures that control working practices of staff. Many of these reflect learned and professional bodies' codes of practice. For instance, there should be two people in attendance when working with children. One acts as chaperone, either clandestinely or overtly, to guard against actual impropriety or act as a witness in cases where allegations might be made. Another reason, of course, is that if an accident occurs, one person can tend to the participant while the other summons further help. This also, of course, applies to laboratory- and field-based assessments, but consideration must also be given to interview- and questionnaire-based research. What are the chaperone arrangements for possible one-to-one interviews? On what premises will such interviews occur? Again, resorting to relevant codes of practice will help to ensure that the required twin protections are firmly in place.

That researchers are governed by appropriate learned or professional bodies or HSE-based institutional codes is yet something else that has to be verified for intending researchers.

Researchers whose interests are in paediatric exercise science and medicine find themselves at the confluence of all these statutory and regulatory bodies that flow into the ocean that is research governance. Charting and navigating the various waters is no easy task but is a task that must be undertaken. The next section will address this matter and explore the practicalities of seeking and gaining ethics approval for studies of mechanisms that influence children's abilities to perform exercise.

Processes

Suitable procedures

It is useful to start by confirming what is suitable for children because this might not be the same as for adults. First, the use of children in studies is entirely appropriate provided their interests are safeguarded as indicated by mechanisms for research governance. This is formally acknowledged by the Medical Research Council[39] and includes research that has therapeutic and non-therapeutic outcomes that do not necessarily benefit the child involved. However, such involvement must be with procedures that have 'negligible risk,' and such risk is defined as no greater than the risk of harm ordinarily encountered in daily life.[39] The following test procedures are examples of those that present negligible risk:

1. Observation of behaviour.
2. Non-invasive physiological monitoring.
3. Developmental assessments and physical examinations.
4. Changes in diet.
5. Obtaining blood and urine samples, the former by finger- or earlobe-prick.

With the provisos about chaperoning mentioned earlier, anthropometry is also acceptable, but there is one major potentially problematic area. Frequently, distinction has to be made between chronological and physiological (maturational) age[40] in attempts to log children's developmental progress. Radiography has been used[41] and occasionally is still used.[42] Usually radiographs of the left wrist are taken and stages of ossification are assessed. These tend not be used routinely, mainly because of the exposure to ionizing radiation. Similarly, computer-assisted tomography scanning is inadvisable. Conversely, magnetic resonance imaging in not contraindicated.

Perhaps the most well-known technique of assessing maturation is that described by Tanner.[40] This uses a five-point scale to ascribe biological maturity/pubertal stages by means of observation of the development stage of the secondary sexual characteristics. It requires trained health professionals such as paediatricians or school nurses. Morris and Udry[43] developed a self-assessment equivalent and reported that it was sufficiently precise for research use. With all the concerns about child protection, understandably but frustratingly, it has become increasingly difficult to secure ethics committee approval for studies that involve observational assessment of pubertal stage. To avoid these problems, Mirwald *et al.*[44] reported the use of simple anthropometry based on decimal age, body mass, stature, sitting height, and leg length to predict pubertal stage with acceptable precision.

At this point caution should be raised about assessments of body composition. Such assessments should be approached with care. While great interest in reported increases in childhood obesity has highlighted the need for suitable techniques to assess fat content of the body, there is similar concern about eating-related disorders. Paradoxically, such disorders could be triggered by insensitive or inappropriate management of assessments of body composition.

As regards exercise testing, provided they are suitably practised at the procedures, assessments such as those of maximal aerobic power that require tests to volitional exhaustion are well tolerated by children. This includes treadmill and cycle ergometer based exercises. Discontinuous protocols are preferred because encouragement and support can be given in rest periods[45] (see Chapter 8). Compared with those of adults, tests differ in that the traditional plateau of oxygen uptake is rarely if ever seen with children, so the term peak oxygen uptake should be used as opposed to maximal oxygen uptake[46] (see Chapter 8).

In the same way, assessments of maximal intensity (all-out) exercise are also well tolerated. Usually, cycle ergometry or isokinetic dynamometry are the modalities[45] (see Chapter 5).

Marked invasive procedures such as venepuncture, cannulation, and muscle biopsies are inadvisable for use with children because of the discomfort and distress they might cause.

Genomics and proteomics in children is a challenging area both for the biological and the ethical implications. The ability to identify at-risk individuals for whom appropriate therapy could then be planned or delivered before disease progression becomes marked and possibly refractory is laudable. More worrying perhaps are attempts to identify genetically advantaged athletes or genes that could be inserted into young athletes to enhance their abilities.[5] This is now an issue that is under serious debate about how best to proceed.[5]

Field-based procedures such as the 20-m shuttle run test and EUROFIT battery are also suitable, but care should be taken to ensure that they can expose children to mass testing and perhaps unwelcome competition and embarrassment (see Chapter 9). Suitable awareness of this possibility would have to be stated in an application for ethics approval.

Finally, assessments of physical activity are acceptable. These are either of the less robust recall-based questionnaire techniques or preferred direct measures based on accelerometry, pedometry, or heart rate telemetry[45] (see Chapter 10). The latter are unobtrusive and have acceptable although not necessarily fine precision.

Ethics applications

Mechanisms for ethics applications can be categorized under two deceptively simple rubrics: NHS and non-NHS. The deception is that the procedures can be demanding, especially for NHS-related research where they are tortuous and convoluted.

Non-NHS research

Most institutions have research ethics committees or institutional review boards that oversee research to ensure that research is conducted with due regard for ethics requirements. Implementation tends to be devolved to faculty or departmental committees. The membership of such committees should comprise those with specific discipline-based knowledge, expertise in statistical and other analytical techniques, and expertise in health-and-safety related issues, and at least one person with formal specific expertise in ethics and lay representation from the community. All should have at least some experience of undertaking research. The fundamental requirements are expertise, independence, and impartiality.

To minimize the bureaucratic load, procedures are often subdivided into major and minor categories.[10] This is especially important for taught courses in which annually hundreds, perhaps thousands, of dissertations and projects have to be managed. Minor procedures are comparatively risk free and are exemplified by assessments of submaximal exercise or non-controversial questionnaires. These procedures are managed at supervisory level and are not presented formally to the committee. Nevertheless, appropriate documentation should be completed, signed off, and included as an appendix in a dissertation or thesis.

Major categories involve, for instance, tests to volitional exhaustion, questionnaires, and interviews that might create distress because of the recall of troublesome episodes and, important here, studies that involve minors. Normally, proposals for these types of study are presented formally to the committee. Consideration can be by way of a rapporteur-type system or in which the committee meets regularly and frequently. The rapporteur system relies on well-trained personnel who can provide consistent, expert opinions, but it is flexible and provides a quicker response than the physically-meeting alternative. Where committees do meet, there is the advantage that all members have the opportunity to contribute to debate, and theoretically at least, consistency is more likely. The accompanying administrative load is severe and requires skilled administrative staff. The titles and Principal Investigators (PI) are usually logged centrally to demonstrate due process and, importantly, in the case of ensuing insurance claims. This is no trivial matter.

The process of consideration is based on principles of sound research. Is there a good research question the answer to which will add to knowledge, change practice, or, in some other way, benefit human kind? Is the proposed design likely to answer the question adequately? For instance, have there been calculations of sample size required to provide sufficient statistical power? Are processes for single or double blinding appropriate? Are proposed statistical or other analytical techniques sound? Are techniques acceptable? Other considerations are: Has the investigator undergone CRB disclosure and provided a copy of their certificate? Are arrangements for confidentiality and indemnity in place? Are there mechanisms for the referral of participants should some medical condition or psychological problem arise from the research? Clearly, this places considerable demands on personnel involved.

For reasons that become apparent in the next section, institutional ethics committees should have procedures that reflect those of LRECs, and, where possible, there should be formal or other good working relationships between the two.

NHS-related research

The NRES is the overseeing body that regulates NHS-related research and so determines the procedures for seeking and gaining ethics approval for such studies. These procedures provide the model for most, if not all, other UK-based approaches. The NHS system is also reflected elsewhere, for instance, in Europe, North America, and Australasia where Institutional Review Boards tend to characterize the process. The NRES system is involved, and is cumbersome, although major, largely successful efforts have been made to reduce the time it takes to manage proposals. Nevertheless, there are concerns that the sheer amount of work involved in the assembling of proposals might be acting more as a disincentive rather than facilitator for researchers.[47] A major change has been the abandonment of the distinction between LRECs and MRECs. Such committees are now, simply, RECs.

However, it is the route that must be taken for all researchers whose work involves NHS patients, premises, or staff. Initially, all studies had to have (L)REC approval, but not all were clear clinical trials that investigated the effectiveness, for instance, of therapeutic surgical, medical, psychological, and pharmacological strategies. Some, for example, were audits of service and related provision. These types of study have two categories and are termed Clinical Audit and Service Evaluation to distinguish them from Research as defined by NRES.

The bureaucratic and administrative loads on beleaguered (L)RECs were simply unsustainable. To counter this problem audits and service provision were removed from the procedures that had formally to be considered. Even so, this still left all the therapeutic- and mechanistic-based trials. Research governance is an immense operation. There are just under 200 RECs in the United Kingdom, and, in addition, most of the 150 or so Institutes of Higher Education also have committees and subcommittees that are outside the NHS system.

The complex process is illustrated in Fig. 1.1 from the NRES Quick Guide for Applicants.[9]

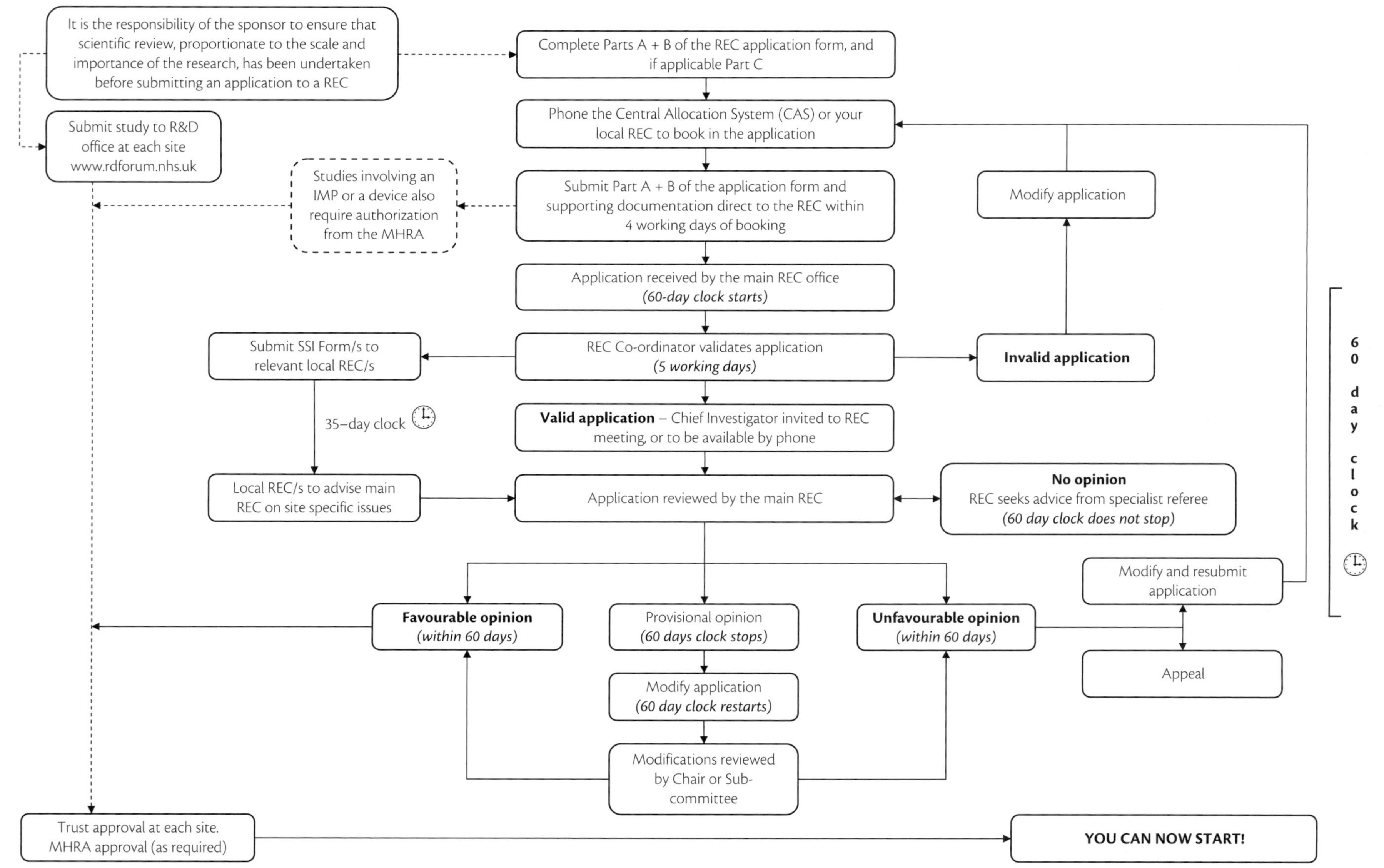

Fig. 1.1 Quick guide for applicants. Reproduced with permission of the National Research Ethics Service.[9]

It can be summarized as having four broad parts: first, the proposal; second, ISR; third, sponsorship; and fourth, consideration by the REC. The proposal is presented on a standardized application form that is available from the NRES website. It is a lengthy document and comprises 61 pages, although depending on the study not all have to be completed and there is automatic bypass of sections as appropriate. Prior to completion, an intended study has to be registered with the respective Strategic Health Authority research and development office, and a registration number is allotted. The proposal requires not only a broad outline in layperson's terms of the aim and intended outcomes of the study but also detailed information about all aspects of the study outlined in previous sections of this chapter.

A proposal has to be headed by what is termed the Chief Investigator (CI). If the research will be conducted on several sites, each site must have a lead person and he or she is termed a PI. Clearly, the CI could be one and the same as the PI. Individual sites could have to have site-specific assessments (SSI) to ensure that personnel, facilities, and processes are satisfactory. This adds another layer of possible inspection.

The veracity of the scientific or other epistemological technique(s) used in the study should have been determined previously in the process of independent scientific review (ISR), and, broadly, there are three ways in which this could occur. First, if the proposal is for a grant award that was secured by competitive tender, the associated review mechanism might be recognized as appropriate ISR. This can be checked by the investigator either through the awarder or the recipient REC. Such recognition avoids duplication of effort both on the part of applicants and reviewers. Second, the PI's institution might, through its research ethics approval mechanism, undertake ISR in a way that is recognized and approved by the recipient REC. Indeed, such recognition should be an aim for institutional RECs. Third, the Strategic Health Authority might undertake ISR as part of its organizational support for research. The ISR is essentially a technical though important process. It provides an opinion on the research question, that is, whether or not it is a good one in that the answer will either or both add to knowledge or change practice; the study in terms of its design, sample size, blinding procedures and the like are appropriate; the personnel are suitable in terms of their expertise and clearance of, say, CRB disclosure; and appropriate financial probity and indemnity are in place.

Sponsorship is not the same as funding. It is the mechanism by which indemnity is provided, and usually, although not always, it will be given by the PI's host institution.

Finally, consideration by the REC might involve the applicant being invited to attend the respective meeting either to clarify matters or, similarly, to answer questions posed by Committee members. It is advisable to make one's self available on such occasions.

The simplicity of this overview belies what is actually involved. For instance, the storage of tissues involves the HTA, if medication is to be administered the MHRA is involved and, germane here, if children are participants, the CRB is involved. Moreover, in addition to the proposal, all approvals and permissions, arrangements for indemnity, details of financial management and so on have to be obtained in writing and kept in a project site file. These site files can occupy two large ring files, but they are a requirement and, moreover, should be immediately available for inspection should the need arise. It is recommended that equivalents of site files should be used in all studies and not just those that fall under the aegis of the NHS.

Summary

- All studies in which children are participants should have formal ethics approval.
- The process for seeking and gaining ethics approval for NHS-related research is complex and the key challenge is to balance the need for such approvals with mechanisms that are manageable both for researchers and those charged with the responsibility for review.
- Few, if any, argue against the need for ethics approval, but many are anxious about the bureaucratic load that the process of approval imposes. This is especially the case when children are participants.
- Principles of research ethics have a long history but formally have their genesis in the Nuremburg war trials of 1946 and 1947.
- The Helsinki Human Rights agreement of 1964 and its iterations since then provide the framework for processes.
- The principle of informed consent is fundamental to the conduct of research.
- The National Research Ethics Service regulates NHS-related research in the United Kingdom.

References

1. Olivier S (2007). Ethics and physiological testing. In: Winter EM, Jones AM, Davison RCR, Bromley PD, Mercer TH (eds.), *Sport and exercise physiology testing guidelines. Volume 1 Sport testing* (4th ed.), pp. 30–7. Routledge, Abingdon.
2. McNamee MJ, Olivier S, Wainwright P (2006). *Research ethics in exercise, health and sport sciences.* Routledge, Abingdon.
3. Loland S, Skirstad B, Waddington I (eds.) (2006). *Pain and injury analysis in sport.* Routledge, Abingdon.
4. McNamee MJ (ed.) (2005). *Philosophy and the sciences of exercise, health and sport.* Routledge, Abingdon.
5. Miah A (2004). *Genetically modified athletes.* Routledge, Abingdon.
6. MacIntyre A (2002). *A short history of ethics.* Routledge, Abingdon.
7. World Medical Association. Available at http://www.wma.net/e/
8. Helsinki Declaration of Human Rights. Available at http://www.wma.net/e/policy/b3.htm
9. National Research Ethics Service. Available at http://www.nres.npsa.nhs.uk/
10. George A (ed.) (1989). *Establishing and running an ethics committee.* Liverpool Polytechnic, Liverpool.
11. Ramsay P (2002). *Explorations in medical ethics* (2nd ed.). Yale University Press, Yale.
12. Dickersin K, Rennie D (2003). Registering clinical trials. *JAMA* **290**, 516–23.
13. Medicines and Healthcare Products Regulatory Agency. Available at http://www.mhra.gov.uk/home/idcplg?IdcService=SS_GET_PAGE&nodeId=5
14. Human Tissue Act (2004). Available at http://www.opsi.gov.uk/acts/acts2004/20040030.htm
15. Human Tissue Authority. Available at http://www.hta.gov.uk/
16. Committee on Publication Ethics. Available at http://www.publicationethics.org.uk/
17. UK Research Integrity Office. Available at http://www.ukrio.org/home/index.cfm
18. Brackenridge C (2001). *Understanding and preventing sexual exploitation in sport.* Routledge, Abingdon.

19. Protection of Children Act (1999). Available at http://www.opsi.gov.uk/acts/acts1999/19990014.htm
20. Child Protection in Sport Unit. Available at http://www.thecpsu.org.uk/Scripts/content/Default.asp
21. Criminal Records Bureau. Available at http://www.crb.gov.uk/
22. Police Act (1997). Available at http://www.opsi.gov.uk/acts/acts1997/1997050.htm
23. Criminal Justice and Court Services Act (2000). Available at http://www.opsi.gov.uk/acts/acts2000/20000043.htm
24. Law Commission Report 231 (1995). *Mental Incapacity*. Law Commission, London.
25. Data Protection Act. Available at http://www.opsi.gov.uk/ACTS/acts1998/19980029.htm
26. The Bichard Inquiry (2004). Available at http://www.bichardinquiry.org.uk/
27. Fraser Guidelines (1986). http://statguidance.ipcc.gov.uk/docs/Gillick%20v%20West%20Norfolk%20&%20Wisbech%20HA%20(1986)%20AC112.doc
28. Jago R, Bailey R (2001). Ethics and paediatric exercise science: Issues and making a submission to a local ethics and research committee. *J Sports Sci* **19**, 527–35.
29. Thomas JR, Nelson JK, Silverman SJ (2005). *Research methods in physical activity* (5th ed.). Human Kinetics, Champaign, IL.
30. Mental Capacity Act (2005). Available at http://www.opsi.gov.uk/acts/acts2005/20050009.htm
31. Department of Health Code of Practice (2007). Available at http://www.opsi.gov.uk/acts/en2005/ukpgaen_20050009_en_cop.pdf
32. Department of Constitutional Affairs. Available at http://www.dca. gov.uk
33. Health and Safety Executive. Available at http://www.hse.gov.uk/
34. Health and Safety at Work Act (1974). Available at http://www.opsi.gov.uk/SI/si2001/20012127.htm
35. Jarman G (2007). Health and Safety. In: Winter EM, Jones AM, Davison RCR, Bromley PD, Mercer TH (eds.), *Sport and exercise physiology testing guidelines. Volume 1 Sport testing* (4th ed.), pp. 11–17. Routledge, Abingdon.
36. British Association of Sport and Exercise Sciences. Available at http://www.bases.org.uk/newsite/home.asp
37. British Psychological Society. Available at http://www.bps.org.uk/
38. British Medical Association. Available at http://www.bma.org.uk/ap.nsf/content/splashpage
39. Medical Research Council. Available at http://www.mrc.ac.uk/index.htm
40. Tanner JM (1962). *Growth at adolescence* (2nd ed.). Blackwell Scientific, CA. Oxford.
41. Greulich WW, Pyle SI (1959). *Radiographic atlas of skeletal development of the hand and wrist* (2nd ed.). Stanford University Press, Stanford.
42. Roche AF, Chumlea WC, Thissen D (1988). *Assessing the skeletal maturity of the hand-wrist: Fels method.* Charles Thomas, Springfield, IL.
43. Morris NM, Udry JR (1980). Validation of a self-administered instrument to assess stage of adolescent development. *J Youth Adolesc* **9**, 271–80.
44. Mirwald RL, Baxter-Jones AD, Bailey DA, Beunen GP (2002). An assessment of maturity from anthropometric measurement. *Med Sci Sports Exerc* **34**, 689–94.
45. Stratton G, Williams CA (2007). Children and fitness testing. In: Winter EM, Jones AM, Davison RCR, Bromley PD, Mercer TH (eds.). *Sport and exercise physiology testing guidelines. Volume 1 Sport testing* (4th ed.), pp. 321–33. Routledge, Abingdon.
46. Armstrong N, Welsman J, Winsley R (1996). Is peak $\dot{V}O_2$ a maximal index of children's aerobic fitness? *Int J Sports Med* **17**, 356–9.
47. Tysome T (2007). Red tape ties up health service studies. *The Times Higher Education Supplement* 25 May 2007, 6–7.

CHAPTER 2

Interpreting exercise performance data in relation to body size

Joanne R. Welsman and Neil Armstrong

Introduction

The appropriate normalization of exercise performance data for differences in body size underpins the clarification of growth and maturational influences on physiological function. Therefore, scaling is an issue of fundamental importance for all paediatric exercise scientists. The selection and application of a scaling method appropriate for the data and research question being addressed is at least as important as ensuring that the methodology used to collect the data is valid, reliable, and appropriate for use with young people. Several scaling methods are available and some methods can be applied in different ways. Unfortunately, taken as a whole, the extant literature presents a confusing picture as to which of these techniques is preferable, how they should be applied, and the meaning of the results obtained. The aim of this chapter is to clarify these issues through a description of the techniques available for analysing both cross-sectional and longitudinal data sets, highlighting their statistical and theoretical derivations. Where appropriate, brief examples are included to illustrate how the application of appropriate scaling has produced new insights into the interpretation of growth- and maturation-related exercise performance previously obscured by traditional scaling methods.

It is important to emphasize from the outset that all methods described below are valid and useful in certain applications. But equally, all techniques are constrained by underlying statistical assumptions which, if ignored, may invalidate findings or confuse interpretations based on them. The technique of choice will depend on the research question being addressed or context within which it is being applied. Confusions will arise not only when an inappropriate technique is applied, but also when a more suitable method is applied incorrectly or indiscriminately.

Scaling for body size differences in cross-sectional data sets

Ratio scaling

Conventional scaling consists of constructing the simple ratio Y/X where Y is the size-dependent exercise performance measure and X is the body size variable, usually body mass, for example, peak oxygen uptake (peak $\dot{V}O_2$) expressed as $mL \cdot kg^{-1} \cdot min^{-1}$. Stature, body surface area or lean body mass are also, if less commonly, used as denominators but the accuracy with which the latter two measures can be obtained in children and adolescents raises questions as to their validity as dependent variables.[1]

This ratio will produce appropriately size-adjusted values only when the data conform to the mathematical expression of a simple linear model,

$$Y = b \cdot X + \varepsilon$$

This equation describes a straight line which passes through the origin (zero), where b is the linear coefficient (the slope of the line describing the bivariate relationship) and ε is the additive, or constant, error term.

It has long been recognized that, where the aim of scaling is to remove the influence of body size, that is, to create a size-free variable, the simple per body mass ratio is frequently deficient in achieving this goal.[2–4]

Albrecht *et al.*[4] list three criteria by which the effectiveness of the per body mass ratio to produce a size-free performance variable can be judged. Of these, perhaps the simplest and most revealing is the statistical criterion which requires a product-moment correlation coefficient between Y/X and X, which is not significantly different from zero. However, significant negative correlations (ranging from $r = -0.35$ to -0.41) have been observed between mass-adjusted peak $\dot{V}O_2$ and body mass in adults.[5–7] The data summarized in Fig. 2.1, representing 245 12 years old, confirm the inability of the simple ratio to remove the influence of body mass from peak $\dot{V}O_2$ in young people with significant negative coefficients of $r = -0.48$ and $r = -0.64$ obtained for boys and girls, respectively. The practical implication of this tendency to 'overscale'[6] is to artefactually penalize heavier individuals whilst advantaging those of light body mass.[8] This can lead to statistical difficulties when ratio standards are incorporated into subsequent correlation or regression analyses leading to potentially spurious results.[5] This was recently demonstrated by Bloxham *et al.*[9] who examined the effects of scaling technique upon the relationship between cycle ergometer derived peak $\dot{V}O_2$ and Wingate anaerobic test 1s peak power (PP). In the 28 boys tested the correlation between the respective power values

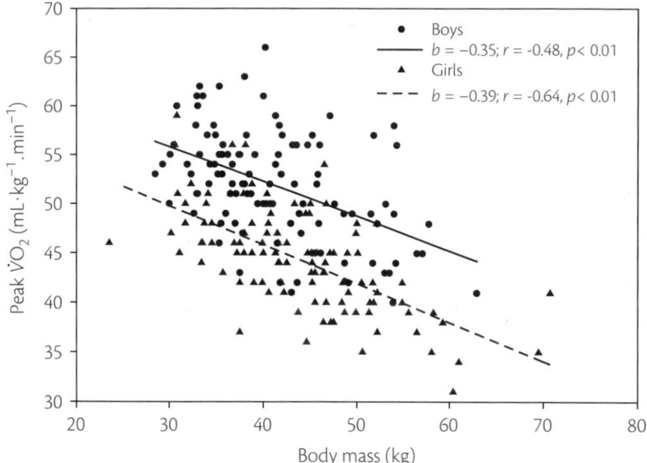

Fig. 2.1 The relationship between ratio scaled peak $\dot{V}O_2$ (mL·kg^{-1}·min^{-1}) and body mass in 12 year olds. Redrawn from Welsman and Armstrong[52] used with permission from The American Physiological Society.

expressed as ratio standards was $r = 0.48$ ($p < 0.05$). Expressed using allometrically adjusted power function ratios (see below) the correlation was reduced to a non-significant value of $r = 0.37$.

Despite longstanding concerns with their validity, much of our current understanding of developmental exercise science is based on data interpreted via ratio standards and they continue to be widely used in studies with young people. However, 'continued usage does not confer validity when the application is inappropriate'[10] and unless it can be demonstrated that a data set truly conforms to a simple linear model (as, for example, has been shown for sprint running performance in adults[6]), and the computed ratio is uncorrelated with the body size variable, an alternative method should be considered.

Linear regression scaling (regression standards)

In recognition of the limitations of ratio standards, several authors[3,5] have proposed a scaling method based on a least squares linear regression model which incorporates an intercept term,

$$Y = a + b{\cdot}X + \varepsilon$$

Here a is the intercept, that is, the point at which the regression line joins the Y axis, b is the slope of the line, and ε is the error term (residual) which, as with the simple ratio model, is assumed to be constant (additive) throughout the range of X.

This scaling technique may be used to construct 'regression-adjusted scores' or 'regression standards', that is, where the individual's residual error (predicted minus observed score) is added to the group's arithmetic mean score.[4,5] Katch and Katch[5] demonstrated, within the same data set, a significant correlation of $r = -0.460$ ($p < 0.05$) between body mass and $\dot{V}O_2$ max expressed in mL·kg^{-1}·min^{-1} (i.e. the ratio standard) reduced to non-significance ($r = -0.002$, $p > 0.05$) for the regression adjusted scores, these latter values therefore representing a size-free variable.

An alternative approach suitable for group comparisons is to use analysis of covariance (a statistical technique which combines linear regression and analysis of variance) to compare the slopes and intercepts of regression lines generated for different subject groups.[6,11–13] Where the slopes (b values) are shown to be parallel (i.e. not significantly different) differences in the intercept and computed adjusted means reflect differences of magnitude between groups. In one of the first studies to challenge the accepted practice of scaling children's exercise data using simple ratios Williams *et al.*[11] demonstrated a significantly higher peak $\dot{V}O_2$ in 15-year-old boys compared to 10-year-old boys—a finding which contrasted with the non-significantly different values of 50 and 49 mL·kg^{-1}·min^{-1}, respectively, identified by the conventional ratio standard method. Similarly, Eston *et al.*[14] demonstrated how differences between young boys and men in ratio scaled submaximal running economy ($\dot{V}O_2$ in mL·kg^{-1}·min^{-1}) disappeared when linear regression modelling was used to interpret the data. The principles behind these findings are presented in Fig. 2.2 in which both the simple ratio and linear regression lines are illustrated for groups of 11- and 17-year-old boys.[15] According to simple ratio scaling the boys share the same linear relationship between body mass and peak $\dot{V}O_2$. However, when linear regression is applied separately to each age group, the differentiation in the relationship between body mass and peak $\dot{V}O_2$ is immediately apparent: although sharing a common slope (b), the intercept value a is clearly significantly higher for the older boys indicating their higher fitness relative to body mass compared to the younger boys.

The improved statistical fit provided by linear adjustment scaling demonstrated by a reduction in residual sum of squares compared with the simple ratio method[6] has given rise to the recommendation that this should be the scaling technique of choice.[12] However, authors have cautioned that this is not appropriate given the limitations of the technique.[16] Although it may be more appropriate to model data with an intercept term rather than forcing the relationship through the origin (as is the case for simple ratio scaling) the incongruity of a model which, through the finding of a positive intercept term, implies a physiological response for zero body size has long been noted.[17] Furthermore, statistical assumptions underlying the use of linear regression techniques require the residuals to have constant variance with a mean of zero. Residuals should also be mutually independent, independent of the body size variable and, in order to carry out parametric tests of significance, these residuals should be normally distributed.[18–20] Unfortunately, these conditions are rarely met by body-size related performance vari-

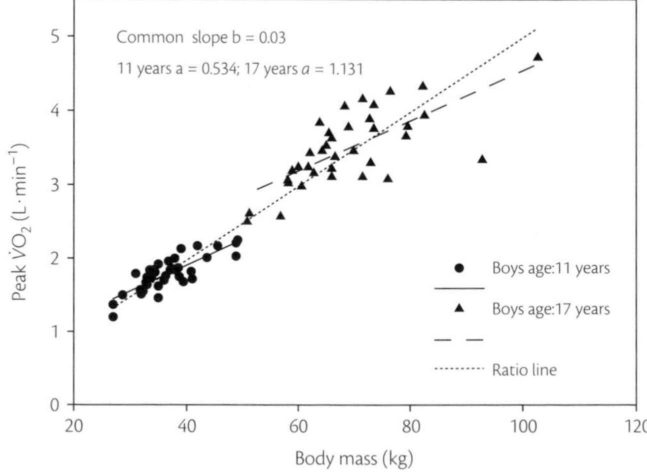

Fig. 2.2 The linear relationship between peak $\dot{V}O_2$ and body mass in 11- and 17-year-old boys. Redrawn from Welsman and Armstrong[52] with permission from the American Physiological Society.

ables in which the data are frequently skewed with heteroscedastic (multiplicative) residuals.[21–23] The data presented in Fig. 2.2 provide an indication of these limitations. For example, a close examination of the individual data points for the older male subjects reveals that the data points for the heavier individuals tend to lie further from the regression line than for the lighter subjects, that is, the residual or error terms demonstrate heteroscedasticity.

Allometric (log-linear) scaling and power function ratios

Where the relationship between the body size and performance variable is proportional but not necessarily linear, a scaling technique based upon the allometric or power function model[24] may be appropriate,

$$Y = a \cdot X^b \cdot \varepsilon$$

This equation describes a curvilinear relationship in which the value of the b exponent describes the curvature of the line and the influence of the body size variable upon the performance measure. Where the dependent variable (Y) increases at a slower rate than the independent variable (X) the b exponent will be less than 1.0, for example, peak $\dot{V}O_2$ in prepubertal children scales to mass$^{0.65}$.[25] Conversely, a mass exponent greater than 1.0 indicates that the dependent variable (Y) is increasing faster than the independent variable (X)—for example, PP in children has been reported as proportional to mass$^{1.2}$.[26] A slope exponent of 1.0 indicates direct proportionality in which the relationship is not curvilinear but described by the straight line of the simple linear model (ratio standard) described above and illustrated in Fig. 2.2.

The multiplicative error termed assumed by the allometric/log-linear model is an important feature of this scaling technique as it accommodates the heteroscedasticity frequently observed in size-related performance measures.[6,22] Log-linearization of data will also correct skewness and, although the effect of outliers and their possible exclusion should always be carefully considered, their effect will be minimized in allometric scaling.[19,27]

Parameters a and b of the allometric relationship are usually solved by applying standard least squares regression (LSR) to logarithmically transformed data, the linear form of the allometric equation being,

$$\log_e Y = \log_e a + b \cdot \log_e X \cdot \log \varepsilon$$

This is appropriate providing, as previously mentioned, the log of the error term is independent and has a normal distribution with constant variance.[20,27]

Frequently in the biological sciences[4,28] and also in the longitudinal interpretation of paediatric exercise performance[29] reduced major axis regression (RMAR) or major axis regression (MAR) of logarithmically transformed data have been used to solve for the terms to be used in allometrically adjusted ratios. Albrecht *et al.*[4] caution against this procedure where the intended purpose is to derive a size-adjusted variable which is uncorrelated with body size. Unless data are collinear (i.e. $r = 1.0$), using parameters derived from RMAR rather than LSR will introduce systematic bias causing the adjusted variables to remain correlated with X, with the magnitude of this residual correlation increasing as the correlation between $\log_e X$ and $\log_e Y$ decreases.

Logarithmic transformation of data also facilitates intergroup comparisons using analysis of covariance as described for the linear model above. The derived values of parameter a (its antilog corresponding to the constant multiplier a of the allometric equation) describe differences in magnitude of the Y variable between groups which can be demonstrated to share a common b exponent, that is, the slopes of the regression lines are not significantly different between groups. Thus, although its significance is often overlooked in preference for solving for the b exponent (see discussion below), the key to understanding differences in size-related performance between, for example, different sex or maturity groups often lies within the parameter a.[6,22,25,30] Although this analysis is, in itself, sufficient to examine group differences, where an appropriately constructed size-free ratio is required for subsequent correlational or regression analyses the derived slope statistic may be used to compute power function ratios by dividing the Y variable by body size raised to the value of b identified (i.e. Y/X^b). The resultant ratios should retain no residual correlation with size although, as for the simple ratio standard, the distributional properties of the allometrically adjusted ratios may be altered.[4]

Echoing concerns expressed in the comparative biology literature,[4,19] several authors have noted the importance of modelling physiological data sets with regard for the assumptions underlying least squares linear regression[20,31] and cautioned against indiscriminate application of allometric scaling techniques. As mentioned above, it is essential to examine whether residual errors display homoscedasticity (constant error variance) following log transformation, for example, by checking for lack of correlation between the residuals and log body mass[20,22,31] and the assumption of normally distributed errors should be statistically verified.[20,31] However, even where these criteria are fulfilled there may be circumstances where allometric modelling yields a power function ratio which does not represent a dimensionless variable, that is, the derived ratio is not independent of body size. Batterham and George[31] demonstrated in adult maximal muscle power data that, although the allometrically derived ratio Y/mass^b was not significantly correlated with body mass, visual inspection of the data suggested a quadratic curvature indicative of poor initial model specification and residual mass-dependence. In this data set the incorporation of a second-order polynomial term (mass^2) into the allometric equation was necessary to appropriately describe the power–mass relationship in this subject sample.

Solving for the b exponent and theoretical alternatives to $b = 1.0$

It has been stated that 'the objective of allometric scaling is to solve for the exponent of the scaling variable'.[7] Indeed there are numerous examples in both the adult and paediatric exercise science literature where allometric scaling is used solely to identify the mass exponent which describes the relationship between exercise performance (usually peak $\dot{V}O_2$) and body size variables in various subject groups.[29,32–35] Intrinsic to many of these studies has been the aim of supporting or refuting one of the theoretically justified exponents (discussed below) in order to provide a universal alternative to the commonly accepted value of $b = 1.0$, that is, the ratio standard.

This approach is understandable given that the roots of allometric scaling lie in the biological sciences where allometry, more specifically the b exponent, is frequently used to interpret interspecific structure–function relationships in animals ranging vastly in both body size and shape.[24,36] However, it is important to realize that this is only one facet of allometric scaling which, in application to human developmental exercise science (i.e. intraspecific allometry), is of limited utility, and underestimates the true potential of allometric scaling to elucidate key issues regarding sex, maturation, and age effects upon exercise performance.

To illustrate this point consider the results from our laboratory in which allometric scaling was applied to the interpretation of peak $\dot{V}O_2$ data derived from subjects ranging in maturation age. An initial analysis identified separate b exponents for prepubertal, pubertal, and adult males and females yielding values ranging from 0.647 to 0.917. Subsequently, log-linear analysis of covariance demonstrated that these exponents were not significantly different and that the relationship between body mass and aerobic power in all groups could be adequately described by a common mass exponent of 0.798.[22] Significant differences were apparent however in the adjusted means derived from the intercept (parameter a) terms demonstrating significant increases in peak $\dot{V}O_2$ across male groups (contrasting to the non-significant change indicated by the ratio standard) whilst in females, peak $\dot{V}O_2$ increased significantly from prepuberty to puberty in females with no decline evident into adulthood as suggested by traditional scaling techniques (see Chapter 20 for a physiological interpretation of these findings). Thus, the former analysis which simply solved separate mass exponents for the six groups provided limited meaningful information—different mass exponents preclude comparisons amongst groups as a different denominator would be used in the derived power function ratios for each sex and maturity group. In contrast, appropriate allometric (log-linear) scaling demonstrated, first through identification of a common exponent of 0.80, that the ratio standard would not enable valid comparisons among groups independent of body mass and second, through comparison of the derived constant multipliers (or log-linear intercept terms) demonstrated patterns of change in aerobic fitness which were masked by conventional ratio scaling. Thus appropriate allometric scaling provided important insights into the growth and maturation of peak $\dot{V}O_2$ which have subsequently been confirmed[30] whereas ostensibly the same scaling technique applied differently simply provided descriptive data of little interpretative value.

Similarly, in one of the earliest studies to interpret aerobic power using allometric techniques, McMiken[32] re-analysed data from classic studies of trained[37,38] and untrained[39] subjects and concluded that observed differences in mass exponents differentiated the trained ($b = 1.0$) from the untrained subjects ($b = 0.88$). However, this analysis ignored the possibility that the differences in fitness among groups were simply one of magnitude, that is, reflected by differences in the intercept with trained and untrained groups sharing a common b exponent.

Appropriate normalization of exercise performance data is fundamental to understanding aspects of developmental exercise performance free from the confounding influence of body size. Thus, where comparisons in exercise performance amongst groups are made using allometric scaling an important first step is to examine, for example, using log-linear analysis of covariance, whether the groups can be described by a common slope (b exponent) with the magnitude of intergroup differences then described by differences in the constant multiplier. Data should only be modelled allowing separate exponents when this is demonstrated to be statistically justifiable.[6]

Dimensionality theory

Despite the continued and almost universal application of the ratio standard to partition body size effects from exercise performance it has been suggested, even within the paediatric exercise science literature[32,33] that there are scaling exponents for exercise performance measures such as peak $\dot{V}O_2$ derived from theoretical principles which may represent plausible alternatives.

Assuming geometric similarity (isometry) amongst individuals, that is, that proportions of body components are constant regardless of size, all linear measurements of the body such as stature, breadths, and skinfolds have the dimension L; all areas, including body surface area and muscle cross-sectional area, have the dimension L^2, and body mass and volumes (e.g. of lungs and heart etc.) the dimension L^3. From Newton's second law, time has the dimension L in physiological systems. Thus, peak $\dot{V}O_2$ measured as a volume per unit time should be proportional to $L^3 – L = L^2$. In other words, in order to dissociate peak $\dot{V}O_2$ from body size values should be expressed as $mL{\cdot}min^{-1}{\cdot}m^{-2}$. Alternatively, as stature^2 is analogous to mass raised to the 2/3 power in geometrically similar bodies, an alternative, equivalent denominator for peak $\dot{V}O_2$ would be mass$^{0.67}$.[40] It is important to note that others have suggested that this is theoretically simplistic[41] and demonstrated that simple dimensionality theory does not necessarily predict a mass exponent of 2/3.

Other authors have advocated a scaling exponent of mass raised to the power 3/4 (analogous to stature$^{2.25}$) based on empirical observations[42,43] that metabolic rate in many species of homeotherms does not appear to conform to the expected surface law—mass$^{0.67}$ but rather increases proportional to mass$^{0.75}$. To provide a rationale for this apparent departure from theoretical predictions, McMahon[44] proposed a model of elastic similarity based on engineering principles whereby biological proportions and metabolic rates are limited by the elastic properties of the animal, properties which ensure that bending and buckling forces during locomotion do not impair the structural integrity of the limbs and joints. However, the concept of elastic similarity has been questioned[45] and the exponent of 3/4 explained as a statistical artefact caused by fitting a single allometric model to data obtained from a number of different species[46] which, when analysed separately, have intraspecific slopes of $b = 0.67$.[47] Other authors maintain that there is no biologically meaningful explanation for the 3/4 power[48] or question the validity of extrapolating an exponent for resting oxygen consumption to describe maximal oxygen uptake[33] but, nevertheless, both theoretical values have been, and continue to be, explored as possibilities of representing a universal alternative to 1.0 for the expression of size-independent peak $\dot{V}O_2$.

Empirical findings

Several studies modelling adult peak $\dot{V}O_2$ data have identified mass exponents close to or equal to 0.67[6,49,50] which have been interpreted as providing support for more general application of the 2/3 power suggested by geometric similarity and empirical intraspecific allometry. Other authors modelling a broader age range (up to 79 years) have provided data to support the preferential application of the 3/4 power when mass is included as the sole covariate, but demonstrated that this reduces to a value not significantly different from 0.67 when other known covariates are partitioned out.[51]

Empirical data from studies with young people present an inconsistent picture. A recent review[52] summarizing mass exponents for peak $\dot{V}O_2$ identified in cross-sectional studies with young people reports values which, although typically less than the 1.0 of the ratio standard, range from 0.37 to 1.07 with virtually no two studies yielding the same values. Given this variability in results it is not surprising that some authors have commented that there is no sound reason to abandon general application of the simple ratio standard.[53,54]

What reasons can be offered in explanation for the diversity of exponents reported? One possibility is that the assumption of isometry is untenable during growth and maturation. Although, overall, geometric similarity appears to be a reasonable supposition in children and adults at least from the age of 7 years[55] differential rates of individual growth during puberty may distort the proportional relationship. However, it has been suggested that as children follow a common rhythm of growth, deviations from geometric similarity during growth should themselves be systematic.[56] The range of reported exponents suggests that this is not the case.

Much of the variation in reported mass exponents is likely to be explained by differences in factors such as sample size and heterogeneity. It has been suggested that meaningful exponents will only be observed in large subject groups encompassing a wide range of body size[57] but homogeneity with respect to other confounding covariates may also be important. In adults, Heil[51] has suggested that an exponent of 0.67 will be identified in groups homogeneous for covariates such as stature, training status, and body composition, whereas a value of 0.75 may be a more appropriate descriptor for heterogeneous subject groups.

Such factors are likely to influence mass exponents identified in young people. For example, we reported a mass exponent of 0.65 in a sample of 164 prepubertal children,[25] but this value was reduced to 0.52 in another sample of only 32 prepubescents.[58] Similarly, exponents close to 1.0 have tended to derive from studies where a large age range (and hence body size and maturational age range) is represented.[59–61] In these cases, the mass exponent may be inflated if other confounding variables are not concurrently covaried out. For example, it has been postulated[62] that the theoretical 0.75 exponent is an artefact caused by failing to account for the disproportionate increase in muscle mass which accompanies increasing body size.[63,64] Nevill[62] demonstrated in heterogeneous subject groups how extension of the allometric equation to include stature as an additional covariate reduced the mass exponent to values closer to the theoretically anticipated 0.67. A similar reduction in the mass exponent from 0.80 to 0.71 has been demonstrated in the comparison of peak $\dot{V}O_2$ in prepubertal, pubertal, and adult subjects following the incorporation of stature as an additional covariate in the allometric analysis.[22]

Although Nevill's hypothesis has been dismissed as statistical artefact resulting from collinearity between stature and mass in a LSR analysis,[65] studies with adults[51] and young people[22,66] have demonstrated a significant, independent contribution of stature to peak $\dot{V}O_2$. Although the significance of the stature exponent remains contentious, and recent work has demonstrated the redundancy of the term once a measure of body fatness is included,[67] these studies do demonstrate the flexibility of the allometric approach and the need to incorporate several covariates into an analysis. The independent effect of mass on the performance variable will be observed only once other covariates, which may include age, stature, and skinfold thickness, have been investigated and statistically accounted for.

It is important to emphasize that the lack of concordance between empirically derived values and theoretical exponents when scaling peak aerobic performance no more invalidates allometry as an effective tool for elucidating group differences in a variety of size-dependent exercise performance measures than does continued usage of ratio standards confer validity upon their use as a scaling technique. As illustrated above, the *b* exponent obtained is often of secondary importance in comparative studies and is evidently sample-specific and influenced by other known covariates.

Scaling for body size differences in longitudinal data sets

Ontogenetic allometry

The interpretation of size-dependent performance measures in longitudinal data sets represents a formidable challenge to the paediatric exercise scientist. As discussed above there is considerable evidence to suggest that the simple ratio approach will fail to produce a size-free variable and thus is unlikely to provide a satisfactory picture of developmental trends. An analysis based on allometric interpretation is likely to be more revealing. Various approaches to partitioning body size effects from longitudinal data sets based on allometric principles have been applied to studies of peak aerobic fitness in young people and these will serve to illustrate their relative merits and disadvantages.

Several studies have adopted an ontogenetic allometric approach,[36] ontogenetic allometry referring to the examination of differential growth rates within the individual growth process. This technique involves the computation of a body size exponent for each subject from the slope of the log-linear regression line describing the individual's longitudinal data set.[29,61,68] This process is illustrated in Fig. 2.3 which summarizes the longitudinal measurements of peak $\dot{V}O_2$ in five individual subjects. These individual exponents can be subsequently averaged to describe, for example, sex or maturity groups.[29,68,69]

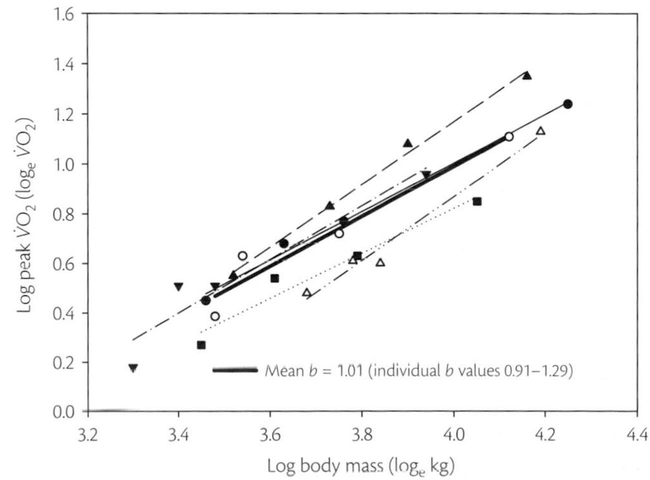

Fig. 2.3 Longitudinal relationships between peak $\dot{V}O_2$ and body mass in five individual children.
Redrawn from Welsman and Armstrong[52] with permission.

The range of mean ontogenetic exponents observed in these studies is broadly comparable to that demonstrated in cross-sectional studies. In several of these studies a stated aim has been to compare the empirically derived mean exponents against the theoretically predicted values (0.67 and 0.75) in order to recommend a universal exponent. However, a common feature of these studies has been an extremely broad interindividual range in mass exponents: Rowland *et al.*[68] reported values ranging from $b = 0.18$ to 1.74 in 20 children measured annually for 5 years from the mean age of 9.2 years. Similarly Beunen *et al.*[69] reported values ranging from $b = 0.56$ to 1.18 with an average of 0.87 in boys measured between the ages of 8 and 16 years.

Thus, the application of a single theoretical value of 0.67 to assess longitudinal tracking of aerobic fitness[70] is not recommended as, although likely to provide more plausible results than the ratio standard, it is unlikely to provide an exact sample-specific exponent.

One limitation of the ontogenetic approach is its focus upon deriving exponents for individuals or discrete groups making it difficult to examine key questions such as the interactive effect of sex, maturation, and body size upon the development of aerobic power. Furthermore, from a statistical viewpoint this approach is inefficient as statistics from the individual analyses (the slope and intercept parameters) can only be partially accommodated in a subsequent between group analysis.[66]

Multilevel modelling

Multilevel modelling[71] is essentially an extension of multiple regression which is appropriate for analysing hierarchically structured or nested data. In simple longitudinal studies, for example, where children are tested annually for peak $\dot{V}O_2$ this hierarchy can be seen to occur at two levels. As illustrated in Fig. 2.3, the repeated data points represent level 1 and these are grouped or 'nested' within the individual subject who represents the level 2 unit. Multilevel modelling is preferable to conventional analytical approaches for longitudinal data as, in addition to describing the population mean response, random variation around this mean at both levels is recognized and statistically described. For example at level 2, individuals have their own growth rates which are allowed to vary randomly around the underlying mean group response (e.g. the distance of the individual regression lines from the regression line describing the total population in Fig. 2.3 represents the level 2 variation). Similarly, at level 1, each individual's observed measurements vary around their own underlying growth trajectory, particularly where the testing occasions are not equally spaced. Furthermore, unlike traditional methods based on repeated measures analysis of variance which require a complete longitudinal data set, this method is able to handle unbalanced data, for example, where one or more measurement occasions has been missed. Similarly, as individual growth trajectories can be modelled, differing intervals between measurement occasions can be accommodated. The procedure is statistically efficient and easily adaptable to a multivariate approach, allowing the effects, and relative importance of a variety of explanatory variables or combinations of explanatory variables to be investigated and quantified.[71,72]

As with the scaling of cross-sectional data the same problems and issues regarding the use of an additive linear (polynomial) versus a multiplicative allometric approach apply when using multilevel regression modelling with the latter demonstrated to be theoretically and statistically superior for longitudinal analyses.[66,73]

The technique is being used with increasing frequency to interpret aspects of young people's physiological performance including strength,[74] short-term power,[26,75–77] submaximal cardiovascular performance,[78,79] and aerobic fitness[67,80] with some of these studies detailed elsewhere in this volume (see Chapters 15, 19 and 20). To illustrate how multilevel modelling can be used to tease out which factors affect the growth of physiological performance, Table 2.1 illustrates the results of a multilevel regression analysis for peak $\dot{V}O_2$ derived from a longitudinal study of 11-year-old children (119 boys and 115 girls in year 1) tested on three occasions at approximately yearly intervals.[67]

Two models are presented to demonstrate how the progressive modelling process allows a parsimonious solution to be formulated and highlights the effects of adding and removing various explanatory variables. The model initially explored (model 1) was based on that derived by Nevill and Holder[21] following careful evaluation of several alternative model formulations and can be written as follows:

$$\text{Peak } \dot{V}O_2(Y) = \text{mass}^{k1} \cdot \text{stature}^{k2} \cdot \exp(\alpha_i + b_j \cdot \text{age}) \cdot \varepsilon_{ij}$$

Where all parameters are fixed with the exception of the constant (α, intercept term) and age parameters which are allowed to vary randomly at level 2 (between individuals), and the multiplicative error ratio ε_{ij} that also varies randomly at level 1, describing the error variance between occasions. The subscripts i and j denote

Table 2.1 Longiudinal multilevel regression analyses for peak aerobic power in 11–13 year olds

Parameter	Model 1 estimate (SE)	Model 2 estimate (SE)
Fixed		
Constant	−1.2526 (0.0978)	−1.8735 (0.0945)
$\log_e$ mass	0.4765 (0.0320)	0.8629 (0.0317)
$\log_e$ stature	0.8105 (0.1172)	NS
$\log_e$ skinfolds		−0.1704 (0.0134)
Age	0.0428 (0.0116)	0.0450 (0.0108)
Age^2	−0.0073 (0.0035)	NS
Sex	−0.1495 (0.0094)	−0.1340 (0.0084)
Age·sex	−0.0177 (0.0068)	−0.0177 (0.0065)
Maturity stage 2	0.0382 (0.0090)	0.0301 (0.0086)
Maturity stage 3	0.0548 (0.0106)	0.0372 (0.0105)
Maturity stage 4	0.0902 (0.0140)	0.0571 (0.0138)
Maturity stage 5	0.0892 (0.0221)	0.0435 (0.0212)
Random		
Level 2		
Constant	0.0042 (0.0005)	0.0029 (0.0004)
Age	0.0008 (0.0003)	0.0006 (0.0003)
Covariance	0.0004 (0.0003)	0.0003 (0.0002)
Level 1		
Constant	0.0024 (0.0003)	0.0025 (0.0003)
−2·log-likelihood	−1359.6730	−1432.6730

Redrawn from Armstrong *et al*[67] with permission.

this random variation at levels 1 and 2, respectively. To ensure the model is correctly formulated within the data set the age term is centred on the average age of the participants.

In order to allow the unknown parameters to be solved using multilevel regression the model is linearised by logarithmic transformation. Once transformed, the equation above becomes

$$\text{Log}_e \text{ peak } \dot{V}O_2 (\log_e y) = k_1 \cdot \log_e \text{mass} + k_2 \cdot \log_e \text{stature} + \alpha_j + b_j \cdot \text{age} + \log_e (\varepsilon_{ij})$$

From this baseline model additional explanatory variables were investigated including sum of triceps and subscapular skinfold thicknesses, sex, and stage of maturity. Categorical variables such as sex and stage of pubertal development are introduced into the model in such a way that sets the constant value to a baseline, that is, boys, maturity stage 1, from which the parameters for differing maturity groups or for girls are allowed to deviate. Interaction terms may also be constructed to investigate interactions between explanatory variables. In this example, the interaction term 'age by sex' was constructed to investigate differential growth in boys and girls.

For each model, fixed parameters are presented along with random effects specified at levels 1 and 2 of the analysis. The fixed effects describe the underlying population mean response. As age was centred on the group mean age, and sex and maturity were included as categorical variables, the intercept term represents the mean peak $\dot{V}O_2$ for a prepubertal boy of average age. The remaining parameter estimates therefore represent deviations from this baseline. The statistical significance of a parameter estimate is judged by dividing the value of the parameter estimate by its standard error. If this ratio exceeds ±2.0, the estimate may be considered significantly different from zero at $p < 0.05$.[72]

The results of model 1 show that longitudinal changes in peak $\dot{V}O_2$ in this group were related to the overall increase in body size, with both stature and mass making significant, independent contributions. The negative coefficient for sex would be deducted from the model for girls only, and thus reflects a lower peak $\dot{V}O_2$ for girls once body size effects have been controlled for. The model also indicates a positive and incremental effect of maturity, with significant coefficients obtained for stages 2 through 5, which is over and above the independent positive effect of age. However, the age by sex interaction term (deducted from the age term for girls only) indicates that the magnitude of this age effect is greater for boys than for girls. In this model a small, but significant, non-linear effect of age was also identified as indicated by the term age^2. This model suggests, therefore, that longitudinal increases in peak $\dot{V}O_2$ cannot be interpreted solely with reference to changes in body size as age and maturation exert additional independent effects for both boys and girls.

Model 2 summarizes the results of including sum of two skinfolds (triceps and subscapular) as an explanatory variable. The positive effect for body mass combined with the negative effect for sum of skinfolds suggest that peak $\dot{V}O_2$ increased in relation to lean body mass. Adding a measure of body fatness rendered the terms for stature and age^2 non-significant and also reduced the value of the coefficients for maturation identified in model 1 (by almost half) and explained part of the difference originally attributed to sex.

The value of the deviance statistic ($-2 \cdot$ log-likelihood) reflects the model's goodness of fit. In nested models such as presented here, that is, where explanatory variables are added to an existing model, the smaller the number the better the model fit. The change in the deviance statistic must be considered relative to the change in the number of fitted parameters. Thus in model 2, there is a deviance of 73.046 for two fewer fitted parameters—stature and age—(which represent 2 degrees of freedom) compared with model 1. This exceeds the chi-squared critical value of 5.99 for significance at $p < 0.05$.

The random parameters reflect the error associated with specified terms at both levels of the analysis, that is, they represent the part of the model unexplained by the fixed parameter estimates. The random structure of the models presented in Table 2.1 was comparatively simple. In models 1 and 2 the random variation associated with the intercept (constant) reflects the degree of variation from the mean intercept both between (level 2) and within (level 1) individuals. Age varied randomly at level 2 (between individuals) allowing each child to have their own growth trajectory. The variation associated with the slope parameter for age was significant in both models but the covariance between the slope and intercept parameters was not thus indicating that the magnitude of peak $\dot{V}O_2$ in year 1 did not influence the predicted increase with age.

Summary

- Conventional ratio scaling rarely represents an appropriate means of enabling size-adjusted group comparisons in measures of exercise performance. Simple per body mass ratios (e.g. mL·kg^{-1}·min^{-1}) often remain size dependent thus confounding interpretations based on them.
- Although offering some advantages, linear regression scaling is limited by its assumption of an additive error term, as exercise performance data are typified by heteroscedastic (multiplicative) error terms, and positive intercept.
- Cross-sectional group comparisons are most effectively achieved using allometric (log-linear) scaling techniques that not only control for heteroscedasticity but also facilitate the construction of appropriately size-adjusted ratios for use in subsequent analyses.
- The application of allometry to longitudinal data is more complex. Given the sample-specificity of the b exponent, the application of a theoretically derived value, such as 0.67, cannot be recommended.
- Ontogenetic allometry describes the individual growth process but cannot quantify the magnitude of changes in performance or fully describe group or population responses.
- For interpreting longitudinal data multilevel regression modelling offers many advantages. Working within an allometric framework, underlying group trends can be modelled whilst concurrently investigating individual growth trajectories. This process thus enables the effects of body size and other explanatory variables upon the performance measure to be examined in a sensitive and flexible manner.

References

1. Rowland TW (2005). *Children's exercise physiology* (2nd ed.), pp. 15–16. Human Kinetics, Champaign, IL.
2. DuBois PH (1948). On the statistics of ratios. *Am J Psychol* **3**, 309–15.
3. Tanner JM (1949). Fallacy of per-weight and per-surface area standards and their relation to spurious correlation. *J Appl Physiol* **2**, 1–15.
4. Albrecht GH, Gelvin BR, Hartman SE (1993). Ratios as a size adjustment in morphometrics. *Am J Phys Anthropol* **91**, 441–68.

5. Katch VL, Katch FI (1974). Use of weight-adjusted oxygen uptake scores that avoid spurious correlation. *Res Q* **45**, 447–51.
6. Nevill A, Ramsbottom R, Williams C (1992). Scaling physiological measurements for individuals of different body size. *Eur J Appl Physiol* **65**, 110–7.
7. Davies MJ, Dalsky GP, Vanderburgh PM (1995). Allometric scaling of $\dot{V}O_2$ max and lean body mass in older men. *J Age Phys Activ* **3**, 324–31.
8. Winter EM (1992). Scaling: Partitioning out differences in size. *Pediatr Exerc Sci* **4**, 296–301.
9. Bloxham SR, Welsman JR, Armstrong N (2005). Ergometer-specific relationships between peak oxygen uptake and peak power output in children. *Pediatr Exerc Sci* **17**, 136–48.
10. Cotes JE, Reed JW (1995). Ratios and regressions in body size and function: A commentary. *J Appl Physiol* **78**, 2328–9.
11. Williams JR, Armstrong N, Winter EM, Crichton N (1992). Changes in peak oxygen uptake with age and sexual maturation in boys: Physiological fact or statistical anomaly? In: Coudert J, Van Praagh E (eds.), *Children and exercise XVI*, pp. 35–7. Masson, Paris.
12. Toth MJ, Goran MI, Ades PA, Howard DB, Poehlman ET (1993). Examination of data normalization procedures for expressing peak $\dot{V}O_2$ data. *J Appl Physiol* **75**, 2288–92.
13. Nindl BC, Mahar MT, Harman E, Patton JF (1995). Lower and upper body anaerobic performance in male and female adolescent athletes. *Med Sci Sports Exerc* **27**, 235–41.
14. Eston RG, Robson S, Winter E (1993). A comparison of oxygen uptake during running in children and adults. In Duquet W, Day J (eds.), *Kinanthropometry IV*, pp. 236–41. E and FN Spon, London.
15. Welsman J, Armstrong N (2007). Interpreting performance in relation to body size. In Armstrong N (ed.), *Paediatric exercise physiology*, pp. 27–46. Churchill Livingstone, Edinburgh.
16. Cooper DM, Berman N (1995). Ratios and regressions in body size and function: A commentary. *J Appl Physiol* **77**, 2015–17.
17. Kleiber M (1950). Physiological meaning of regression equations. *J Appl Physiol* **2**, 417–23.
18. Manaster BJ, Manaster S (1975). Techniques for estimating allometric equations. *J Morphol* **147**, 299–308.
19. Smith RJ (1984). Allometric scaling in comparative biology: Problems of concept and method. *Am J Physiol* **246**, R152–60.
20. Nevill AM, Holder RL (1995). Scaling, normalizing and per ratio standards: An allometric modelling approach. *J Appl Physiol* **79**, 1027–31.
21. Nevill AM, Holder RL (1994). Modelling maximum oxygen uptake—a case-study in non-linear regression model formulation and comparison. *Appl Stat* **43**, 653–66.
22. Welsman J, Armstrong N, Kirby BJ, Nevill AM, Winter E (1996). Scaling peak oxygen uptake for differences in body size. *Med Sci Sports Exerc* **28**, 259–65.
23. Nevill AM (1997). The appropriate use of scaling techniques in exercise physiology. *Pediatr Exerc Sci* **9**, 295–8.
24. Huxley J (1932). *Problems of relative growth*. Methuen, London.
25. Armstrong N, Kirby B, McManus A, Welsman J (1995). Aerobic fitness of pre-pubescent children. *Ann Hum Biol* **22**, 427–41.
26. Armstrong N, Welsman JR, Chia MYH (2001). Short term power output in relation to growth and maturation. *Br J Sports Med* **35**, 118–24.
27. Jolicoeur P, Heusner AA (1971). The allometry equation in the analysis of the standard oxygen consumption and body weight of the white rat. *Biometrics* **27**, 841–55.
28. Corruccini RS (1986). Multivariate morphometric data transformations. *J Hum Evol* **15**, 139–41.
29. Beunen GP, Rogers DM, Woynarowska B, Malina RM (1997). Longitudinal study of ontogenetic allometry of oxygen uptake in boys and girls grouped by maturity status. *Ann Hum Biol* **24**, 33–43.
30. Armstrong N, Welsman JR, Kirby BJ (1998). Peak $\dot{V}O_2$ and maturation in 12-yr olds. *Med Sci Sports Exerc* **30**, 165–9.
31. Batterham AM, George KP (1997). Allometric modelling does not determine a dimensionless power function ratio for maximal muscular function. *J Appl Physiol* **83**, 2158–66.
32. McMiken DF (1976). Maximum aerobic power and physical dimensions of children. *Ann Hum Biol* **3**, 141–7.
33. Bailey DA, Ross WD, Mirwald RL, Weese C (1978). Size dissociation of maximal aerobic power during growth in boys. *Med Sport* **11**, 140–51.
34. Rogers DM, Olson B, Wilmore JH (1995). Scaling for the $\dot{V}O_2$-to-body size relationship among children and adults. *J Appl Physiol* **9**, 958–67.
35. Zakeri I, Puyau MR, Adolph AL, Vohra FA, Butte NF (2006). Normalization of energy expenditure data for differences in body mass or composition in children and adolescents. *J Nutr* **136**, 1371–6.
36. Gould SJ (1966). Allometry and size in ontogeny and phylogeny. *Biol Rev* **41**, 587–640.
37. Astrand PO, Engstrom L, Eriksson BO, Karlberg P, Nylander I, Saltin B, Thoren C (1963). Girl swimmers. *Acta Paediatr* **47**, 3–75.
38. Daniels JT, Oldridge N (1971). Oxygen consumption and growth of young boys during running training. *Med Sci Sports* **3**, 161–5.
39. Klissouras V (1971). Heritability of adaptive variation. *J Appl Physiol* **31**, 338–44.
40. Astrand PO, Rodahl K (1986) *Textbook of work physiology*. McGraw-Hill, New York.
41. Butler JP, Feldman HA, Fredberg JF (1987). Dimensional analysis does not determine a mass exponent for metabolic scaling. *Am J Physiol* **253**, R195–9.
42. Brody S, Proctor RC, Ashworth US (1934). Basal metabolism, endogenous nitrogen, creatine and neutral sulphur excretions as functions of body weight. *Univ Missouri Agr Exp Sta Res Bull* **220**, 1–40.
43. Kleiber M (1932). Body size and metabolism. *Hilgardia* **6**, 315–53.
44. McMahon T (1973). Size and shape in biology. *Science* **174**, 1201–4.
45. Cooper DM (1989). Development of the oxygen transport system in normal children. In Bar-Or O (ed.), *Advances in paediatric sports sciences vol. 3*, pp. 67–100. Human Kinetics, Champaign, IL.
46. Heusner AA (1982). Energy metabolism and body size. Is the 0.75 mass exponent of Kleiber's equation a statistical artefact? *Respir Physiol* **48**, 1–12.
47. Schmidt-Nielsen K (1984). *Scaling: Why is animal size so important?* Cambridge University Press, Cambridge.
48. Heusner AA (1987). What does the power function reveal about structure and function in animals of different size? *Ann Rev Physiol* **49**, 121–33.
49. Bergh U, Sjodin B, Forsberg A, Svedenhag J (1991). The relationship between body mass and oxygen uptake during running in humans. *Med Sci Sport Exerc* **23**, 205–11.
50. Nevill AM, Lakomy HKA, Lakomy J (1992). Rowing ergometer performance and maximum oxygen uptake of the 1992 Cambridge University boat crews. *J Sports Sci* **10**, 574.
51. Heil DP (1998). Body mass scaling of peak oxygen uptake in 20- to 79-yr-old adults. *Med Sci Sports Exerc* **29**, 1602–8.
52. Welsman J, Armstrong N (2008). Scaling for size: Relevance to understanding effects of growth on performance. In Hebestreit H, Bar-Or O (eds.), *The young athlete: Encyclopaedia of sports medicine*, pp. 50–62. Blackwell, London.
53. Bar-Or O (1983). *Pediatric sports medicine for the practitioner.* Springer-Verlag, New York.
54. Shephard RJ (1994). *Aerobic fitness and health*. Human Kinetics, Champaign, IL.
55. Asmussen E, Heeboll-Nielsen KA (1955). A dimensional analysis of physical performance and growth in boys. *J Appl Physiol* **7**, 593–603.
56. Ross WD, Bailey DA, Mirwald RL, Faulkner RA, Rasmussen R, Kerr DA, Stini WA (1991). Allometric relationship of estimated muscle mass and maximal oxygen uptake in boys studied longitudinally age 8 to 16 years. In Frenkl R, Szmodis I (eds.), *Children and exercise,*

paediatric work physiology XV, pp. 135–42. National Institute for Health Promotion, Budapest.

57. Calder WA III (1987). Scaling energetics of homeothermic vertebrates: An operational allometry. *Ann Rev Physiol* **49**, 107–20.
58. Welsman JR, Armstrong N, Kirby BJ, Winsley RJ, Parsons G, Sharpe P (1997). Exercise performance and MRI determined muscle volume in children. *Eur J Appl Physiol* **76**, 92–7.
59. Cooper DM, Weiler-Ravell D, Whipp BJ, Wasserman K (1984). Aerobic parameters of exercise as a function of body size during growth. *J Appl Physiol* **56**, 628–34.
60. Paterson DH, McLellan TM, Stella RS, Cunningham DA (1987). Longitudinal study of ventilation threshold and maximal O_2 uptake in athletic boys. *J Appl Physiol* **62**, 2051–7.
61. Sjodin B, Svedenhag J (1992). Oxygen uptake during running as related to body mass in circumpubertal boys: A longitudinal study. *Eur J Appl Physiol* **65**, 150–7.
62. Nevill A (1994). The need to scale for differences in body size and mass: An explanation of Kleiber's 0.75 mass exponent. *J Appl Physiol* **77**, 2870–3.
63. Alexander RM, Jayes AS, Maloiy GMO, Wathuta EM (1981). Allometry of the leg muscles of mammals. *J Zool* **194**, 539–52.
64. Nevill AM (1994). Evidence of an increasing proportion of leg muscle mass to body mass in male adolescents and its implication for performance. *J Sports Sci* **12**, 163–4.
65. Batterham AM, Tolfrey K, George KP (1997). Nevill's explanation of Kleiber's 0.75 mass exponent: An artefact of collinearity problems in least squares model? *J Appl Physiol* **82**, 693–7.
66. Nevill AM, Holder RL, Baxter-Jones A, Round JM, Jones DA (1998). Modelling developmental changes in strength and aerobic power in children. *J Appl Physiol* **84**, 963–70.
67. Armstrong N, Welsman JR, Nevill AM, Kirby BJ (1999). Modeling growth and maturation changes in peak oxygen uptake in 11-13-year olds. *J Appl Physiol* **87**, 2230–6.
68. Rowland T, Vanderburgh P, Cunningham L (1997). Body size and the growth of maximal aerobic power in children: A longitudinal analysis. *Pediatr Exerc Sci* **9**, 262–74.
69. Beunen G, Baxter-Jones ADG, Mirwald RL, Thomis M, Lefevre J, Malina RM, Bailey DA (2002). Intraindividual allometric development of aerobic power in 8- to 16-year-old boys. *Med Sci Sports Exerc* **33**, 503–10.
70. Janz KF, Mahoney LT (1997). Three-year follow-up of changes in aerobic fitness during puberty: The Muscatine study. *Res Q Exerc Sport* **68**, 1–9.
71. Goldstein H, Rasbash J, Plewis I, Draper D, Browne W, Yang M, Woodhouse G, Healy M (1998). *A user's guide to MlwiN*. University of London, Institute of Education, London.
72. Duncan C, Jones K, Moon G (1996). Health-related behaviour in context: A multilevel modelling approach. *Soc Sci Med* **42**, 817–30.
73. Baxter-Jones A, Goldstein H, Helms P (1993). The development of aerobic power in young athletes. *J Appl Physiol* **75**, 1160–7.
74. De Ste Croix MBA, Armstrong N, Welsman JR, Sharpe P (2002). Longitudinal changes in isokinetic leg strength in 10–14 year olds. *Ann Hum Biol* **29**, 50–62.
75. Armstrong N, Welsman JR, Kirby BJ, Williams CA (2000). Longitudinal changes in young people's short term power output. *Med Sci Sport Exerc* **32**, 1140–5.
76. De Ste Croix MBA, Armstrong N, Chia MYH, Welsman JR, Parsons G, Sharpe P (2001). Changes in short term power output in 10–12 year olds. *J Sports Sci* **19**, 141–8.
77. Santos AMC, Armstrong N, De Ste Croix MBA, Welsman JR (2003). Optimal peak power in relation to age, body size, gender and thigh muscle volume. *Pediatr Exerc Sci* **15**, 405–17.
78. Armstrong N, Welsman J (2002). Cardiovascular responses to submaximal treadmill running in 11 to 13 year olds. *Acta Paediatr* **91**, 125–31.
79. Welsman JR, Armstrong N (2000). Longitudinal changes in submaximal oxygen uptake in 11–13 year olds. *J Sports Sci* **18**, 183–9.
80. Armstrong N, Welsman JR (2001). Peak oxygen uptake in relation to growth and maturation in 11–17 year olds. *Eur J Appl Physiol* **85**, 546–51.

CHAPTER 3

Anthropometry, physique, body composition, and maturity

Albrecht L. Claessens, Gaston Beunen, and Robert M. Malina

Introduction

Body size, physique, composition, and biological maturity status are central to the many domains of the paediatric exercise sciences. In the context of the school age population, approximately 6–18 years, this chapter describes a series of anthropometric dimensions and several ratios, discusses somatotype methodology and methods of body composition assessment, and reviews methods for assessing the biological maturity status of children and adolescents. It is a revision and update of the chapter published in the first edition of *Paediatric Exercise Science and Medicine.*[1]

Anthropometry in assessing size and proportional characteristics

Anthropometry (anthropos = man; metry = measure) refers to a series of standardized techniques used to quantify external dimensions of the body and its parts. It is also used increasingly to estimate body composition. Anthropometry is often viewed as the traditional and perhaps basic tool of physical or biological anthropology,[2–4] but it also has a long tradition in physical education and sport[5] and biomedical sciences, especially monitoring growth status, physique, and the prevalence of overweight and obesity.[6]

Choice of measurements and standardized procedures

The number of measurements that can be taken on an individual is almost limitless. A key issue is the selection of measurements, which depends on the purpose of a study and the specific questions under consideration. Measurements should be selected to provide specific information within the context of a study design. Thus, no single battery of measurements will meet the needs of every study.[3]

Choice of measurements depends on several criteria: relevance, accuracy and reliability, equipment, convenience, and cost.[7] Relevance refers to the selection of measurements that will most accurately test the research hypothesis. Only measurements that can be made with a high degree of accuracy and reliability should be selected. Appropriate equipment, if correctly handled and regularly checked and calibrated, is essential and will help reduce error. Other factors being equal, the convenience of a particular measurement may give it preference over another. Cost is a major consideration and may lead to the use of cheaper, perhaps less accurate, instruments. Time investment is a related factor. Only those measurements that are absolutely essential to the purposes of a study should be included. It makes no sense to take an extensive battery of dimensions simply because one has the opportunity to do so.

Measurements should be made in a 'standardized' manner, following accepted procedures. Although several 'standardized' protocols are available,[7–9] similarly labelled techniques and perhaps measurement sites are not always identical. As noted, selected dimensions should be consistent with the purpose of a study or survey. The following describes a series of dimensions relevant to the paediatric exercise sciences.

Measuring body size

Overall body size

Body mass (weight) and height (stature) are estimates of body size that are incorporated into almost every study/survey protocol. *Body mass* (kg) should be measured on an accurately calibrated balance and recorded to the nearest 0.1 kg. Ideally, the subject should be nude (but this is usually impractical), or with minimal (indoor) clothing (e.g. gym shorts and T-shirt) and without shoes. If this is not possible, the subject should be weighed in light weight clothing, which should be noted so that a correction can be applied. *Stature* (cm) can be measured in several ways: (i) free standing, (ii) standing against a wall or fixed stadiometer (with or without stretch), and (iii) in a recumbent position (for subjects who cannot stand upright). The method described subsequently is standing against a fixed stadiometer, without stretch, but the subject is instructed 'to stand as erect as possible'. The subject without shoes stands upright against the stadiometer so that the heels, buttocks, and scapulae are in contact with the backboard, and the feet are together. The head should be positioned in the Frankfort horizontal plane, and the headboard of the instrument should be moved down to make contact with sufficient pressure to compress the hair on to the vertex of the skull. Stature is recorded to the last completed unit (mm) and expressed in centimetres.

Mass and stature are affected by diurnal variation, that is, variation during the course of a day. This is of special interest for short-term longitudinal studies, in which observed 'change' may not reflect 'real' change, but may simply reflect the time of day at which the measurements were taken. On average, an individual is lightest in the morning and body mass increases gradually during the course of the day. Mass is also affected by diet and physical activity. Daily changes, which may reach about 1 kg, are most likely to be due to variation in body water and/or gastrointestinal contents.[10] Variation in the phase of the menstrual cycle is another factor.[6]

Stature is also affected by time of the day. It is greatest in the morning and decreases gradually during the day. This 'shrinking' is limited to the vertebral column (and thus to sitting height) and is related to the compression of the intervertebral cartilages. As a result, stature diminishes by a centimetre or more, depending on measurement technique. These changes should not be ignored since, on average, the diurnal variation in stature is greater than measurement error.[11] Diurnal change in stature may also be influenced by vigorous high impact activity. Stature is ordinarily regained by having the individual lie still for ~30 min on a flat surface.[6]

Segment lengths

Although many segment lengths can be measured (directly or indirectly as projected lengths) two measurements, sitting height and leg length are often used in paediatric exercise, and more specifically in growth studies. *Sitting height* (cm) is measured with an anthropometer (or with a sitting height stadiometer) as the distance from the sitting surface to the top of the head. The subject sits on a bench or table and is positioned with the head in the Frankfort plane, shoulders relaxed, back straight, and legs at right angles into the knees. The subject is instructed to sit as erect as possible (as described for stature). *Leg length* (cm), more appropriately subischial length, is estimated as the difference between stature and sitting height.

Skeletal breadths

Robustness of the skeleton is estimated by breadths (widths) across specific landmarks on a bone or bones. Measurements can be taken with the upper end of an anthropometer used as a sliding calliper, a spreading calliper, a sliding calliper *per se*, or a Vernier calliper. Four breadths are often taken: biacromial and bicristal breadths on the trunk, and distal humerus and femur breadths on the extremities.

Biacromial breadth (cm) is the distance between the tips of the acromial processes. It is measured from the rear. The position of the lateral tips of the acromial processes is slightly different in each subject; it is recommended that the landmarks are marked before applying the instrument. The subject stands with relaxed shoulders; the military posture with shoulders thrust backward is not normal. The instrument is applied to the lateral margins of the acromial processes with firm pressure so that the thickness of the overlying tissues is minimized. The measurement is read to the nearest millimetre and expressed in centimetres.

Bicristal breadth (cm) is the distance between the most lateral points of the iliac crests. The subject stands in a relaxed position, with the arms somewhat away to ensure access to the iliac crests. The anthropometer is held horizontally and the blades are applied to the most lateral points of the crests. The blades must be pressed firmly against the crests so that the overlying soft tissues are compressed and minimized. The measurement is read to the nearest millimetre and expressed in centimetres.

Biepicondylar breadth is the distance between the most lateral points of the epicondyles of the humerus. Either a broad-blade or a small sliding spreading calliper, accurate to 1 mm, is used. The subject stands facing the technician with the arm raised to the horizontal and the elbow flexed to 90°. The calliper is applied to the medial and lateral epicondyles of the humerus with some pressure to compress the soft tissue.

Bicondylar breadth is the distance between the most lateral points of the condyles of the femur and is best measured with a small spreading calliper. The subject stands facing the technician with the foot on a small bench so that there is a right angle in the knee. The subject may also sit on a chair or table with the legs flexed 90° at the knees and the feet on the floor. The calliper is applied to the medial and lateral condyles of the femur with sufficient pressure to compress the soft tissue.

Circumferences

Circumference or girth measurements are ordinarily taken on the limbs and trunk. Upper arm, both relaxed and flexed, forearm, calf, and thigh circumferences are often taken as indicators of relative muscularity. Two trunk girths, waist and hip circumferences, are increasingly used as indicators of relative subcutaneous fat distribution.

A flexible, non-stretchable tape, accurate to 1 mm, is required. The tape is applied at the appropriate site at a right angle to the long axis of the segment measured. Contact with the skin should be continuous along the tape but without compressing the underlying soft tissues.

For *upper arm circumference relaxed* (cm), the subject stands relaxed with his/her side to the technician, the arm hanging freely at the side and the palm facing the thigh. The tape is passed around the arm at the level of the midpoint of the upper arm. This landmark is the point on the lateral side of the upper arm, midway between the lateral border of the acromial process and the tip of the olecranon process when the arm is flexed at 90°. The measurement is performed with the arm relaxed and hanging beside the body.

For *upper arm circumference flexed* (sometimes referred to as *biceps circumference*) (cm) the subject stands upright and maximally contracts the biceps brachii muscle. The tape is passed around the arm so that it touches the skin surrounding the maximum circumference.

Forearm circumference (cm) is measured at the maximum level immediately distal to the elbow joint. The subject stands relaxed, facing the technician, with the arm fully stretched and held in supination, slighty elevated in front of the subject. The tape is passed around the forearm at the maximum horizontal level.

Calf circumference (cm) is measured with the subject in a standing position (preferable on a small bench) with the feet slightly apart and body mass distributed equally on both feet. The tape is positioned horizontally around the calf (perpendicular to its long axis) and moved up and down to locate the maximum circumference.

If a calf skinfold is measured later, this level should be marked on the medial side of the calf.

Thigh circumference can be measured at three levels: proximal, mid-thigh, and distal.[8]

Proximal thigh circumference is measured just below the gluteal fold and perpendicular to the long axis. The subject stands erect with the feet slightly apart and body mass evenly distributed between both legs. For practical reasons, the subject may stand on a small bench, so that the technician can be close to eye level with the upper thigh. *Mid-thigh circumference* is measured at the level midway between the centre of the inguinal crease and the proximal border of the patella. This level is marked while the subject is seated (and will also serve as the landmark for measuring the front thigh skinfold). The circumference is taken with the subject standing and body mass evenly distributed between the legs. For *distal thigh circumference,* the tape is placed around the thigh just proximal to the femoral epicondyles, while the subject stands in an erect position, preferably on a bench.

The recommended technique for measuring *waist circumference* is at the level of the natural waist, that is, at the narrowest part of the torso.[8] This level is approximately one-half the distance between the costal border and iliac crest. The subject stands erect with the abdomen relaxed and arms hanging slightly away from the body. Three other anatomic body sites for measuring waist circumference are also used: immediately below the lowest ribs; at the midpoint between the lowest rib and the iliac crest; and immediately above the iliac crest.[12] Waist circumference values at the four sites differ considerably in adults, which has implications for clinical practice in which the measurement is used as a risk factor for disease. Corresponding variation in waist circumference measurements by level in children and adolescents has not been reported.

Hip circumference (sometimes labelled *buttocks circumference*) is taken at the level of maximum protrusion of the buttocks. The subject stands erect, with the body mass distributed equally on both feet. In most cases, hip circumference is taken with the subject wearing light clothing. In this case, pressure needs to be applied to compress the clothing. The measurement is taken from the side as a front approach may be invasive to the subject. The level of maximum extension of the buttocks can be more easily seen from a side view.

Skinfold thicknesses

Skinfold thicknesses (in short skinfolds) are thicknesses of double folds of skin and underlying soft tissues, including adipose tissue, at specific sites. The utility of skinfolds is two-fold: (i) they provide a relatively simple and non-invasive method of estimating general fatness (adiposity), and (ii) they characterize to some extent the distribution of subcutaneous adipose tissue. The following general description of techniques is independent of the type of calliper used and is based on the assumption that the technician is right-handed. After the site is located and marked, the thumb and index finger of the left hand are used to raise a skinfold about 1 cm above the site at which the skinfold is to be measured. The fold is grasped firmly and held throughout the measurement. The calliper is then applied at the site for approximately 3 s. Skinfold thicknesses are measured to the nearest 0.1 mm, and expressed in millimetres. The skinfold sites often used in paediatric exercise and sport sciences are the triceps, biceps, subscapular, suprailiac, front thigh, and medial calf.

The *triceps skinfold* is measured at the marked level midway between the acromial and the olecranon processes (the same level as upper arm circumference relaxed) over the posterior surface of the triceps brachii muscle. The *biceps skinfold* is measured on the anterior aspect of the arm, over the biceps brachii muscle at the same level as described for the triceps skinfold. For both measurements, the subject stands facing the technician and with the arm hanging relaxed and palm facing forward.

The site of the *subscapular skinfold* is immediately below the inferior angle of the scapula. The subject stands with the back to the measurer with shoulders relaxed and arms hanging loosely at the sides. The skinfold is picked up at an angle laterally and downward, following the natural cleavage line of the skin.

The *suprailiac skinfold* is measured approximately 1 cm above the iliac crest in the midaxillary line. The skinfold used in estimating endomorphy in the Heath–Carter anthropometric protocol is measured over the anterior superior iliac spine. It is called the '*supraspinale skinfold*' (see below).

The *front thigh skinfold* is located in the midline of the anterior aspect of the thigh, midway between the inguinal crease and proximal border of the patella. The subject is seated on a bench for locating the measuring point. The thickness of a vertical fold is measured on the thigh while the subject is standing and body mass shifted to the non-measured leg; the measured leg is relaxed with the knee slightly flexed and the foot flat on the floor.

The *medial calf skinfold* is measured as a vertical fold on the medial aspect of the calf at the level of maximum calf circumference with the subject sitting on a bench and the knee at a right angle.

Left or right side to be measured?

Although the human body is bilaterally symmetrical, there are asymmetries in morphology that are apparent in comparisons of the preferred and non-preferred limbs, especially of non-athletes and athletes engaged in extreme unilateral activities.[13–15] Asymmetries are generally more pronounced in the upper than in the lower extremities, and tend to be right-side oriented, that is, the right side tends to be larger than the left. Asymmetries tend to be more pronounced in adults than in children,[13,14] but are also observed in mentally retarded subjects[13] and undernourished children.[16] Nevertheless, within a reference group the bias associated with side of measurement is generally less than measurement error.[14] Although it would be advisable, simply on the grounds of greater scientific uniformity, to recommend one side for measurement, consensus would be difficult to achieve. As such, it is best to leave the choice of side to the discretion of investigators. Once the choice is taken, it is understood that all bilateral measurements should be taken on the selected side.[14] Note, however, that bilateral measurements used in prediction equations must be measured on the side on which the measurements were originally taken.

Measurement error

Measurements should taken by trained individuals in an accurate and reliable manner following standardized techniques. Estimates of measurement variability, for example, technical errors of measurement within and between technicians (quality control) should also be reported. It is not sufficient to simply note that measurements were taken by a trained technician. This is especially important in short (e.g. training studies, activity interventions) and long-term (e.g. longitudinal growth studies) serial designs.[6] In epidemiologic studies, 'in-field' reliability, that is, the reliability of observers during the course of the study, should be systematically evaluated.[17]

Body proportions

Measurements provide specific information about absolute dimensions. They can also be related to each other as indices or ratios, and provide information on body proportions. Ratios are derived variables that simply express one dimension relative to another in the form of a single number that can be expressed as a quotient or percentage. At times the term index is used but often in the restricted sense of the ratio of one dimension divided by the larger, standard dimension of the anatomical unit.[18,19] The most commonly used ratio of this type is the ratio of sitting height to stature. Measurements of different anatomical elements are also expressed as ratios, for example, the ratio of biacromial to bicristal breadths. These are ratios of analogous dimensions[19], that is, breadth versus breadth.

Ratios provide information that is not ordinarily available in the original measurements. They are, however, influenced by the relationship between the measurements and assume that the two dimensions change in a linear manner during growth. Ratios may not have a normal distribution and do not indicate the form of the relationship between the two dimensions expressed in the ratio.[18] Ratios are affected by the measurement variability associated with each dimension and have limitations for statistical analysis.[20]

Mass-for-stature ratios express body mass relative to height (length). They are often used in the context of underweight, overweight, and obesity. The most commonly used mass-for-stature ratio at present is the Quetelet index or *body mass index* (BMI), mass (in kg) divided by stature (in m^2). Another 'mass/stature' relationship is the so-called reciprocal ponderal index or *somatotype ponderal index* (see below), in which stature (cm) is divided by the cube root of mass (kg).[21]

The *sitting height/stature* ratio provides an estimate of head, neck, and trunk length relative to stature, or conversely, relative leg length. It is calculated as sitting height (cm) × 100 / height (cm).

A very widely used ratio in sports science, especially in surveys of young athletes, is the bicristal/biacromial ratio, expressing the breadth of the hips relative to that of the shoulders. It is calculated as bicristal diameter (cm) × 100 / biacromial diameter (cm). Shoulder–hip relationships vary among young athletes in a number of sports and among athletes compared to non-athletes[6].

The ratio of *waist-to-hip circumferences* is often used as an indicator of relative fat distribution, that is, waist circumference is an indicator of adipose tissue in the waist and abdominal region, while hip circumference is an indicator of adipose tissue over the hips and buttocks. The ratio has limited validity as an indicator of relative adipose tissue distribution in children and adolescents.[6,22]

Estimating physique by somatotyping

General concepts

Somatotyping is a method for describing the human physique as it refers to an individual's body form as a whole, the configuration of the entire body rather than of specific features. The concept of *somatotype* (soma = body) was introduced by William Sheldon and co-workers.[21] It is the most commonly used conceptual approach to physique at present.

An individual's somatotype is a composite of the contributions of three more or less independent components: endomorphy, mesomorphy, and ectomorphy. The three components are always recorded in this order. *Endomorphy,* the first component, describes the relative degree of fatness of the body, regardless of where the fat tissue is distributed. It also characterizes a predominance of digestive organs, softness and roundness of the body, and relative volume of the abdominal trunk and distal tapering of the limbs. The second component, *mesomorphy,* is characterized by the predominance of muscle, bone, and connective tissue. It also describes corresponding physical aspects such as the 'robustness' of the body and the relative volume of the thoracic trunk. *Ectomorphy,* the third component, is characterized by linearity, slenderness, and fragility of build, with poor muscular development, and a predominance of surface area over body mass.

Sheldon's method is basically photoscopic or anthroposcopic, based on the visual observation and evaluation of the configuration of the body as 'Gestalt'. In this concept, an evaluation is made of the shape of the body as a whole; size is not a factor, although height and weight are used in the reciprocal ponderal index. Each component is evaluated individually on a 7-point scale from a standardized somatotype photograph (front, side, and back views), with 1 representing the least expression and 7 representing the fullest expression. The three ratings together comprise the somatotype; they should be treated as a unit and not individually. Based on this system, the three extreme somatotypes are 7–1–1 (extreme endomorph), 1–7–1 (extreme mesomorph), and 1–1–7 (extreme ectomorph). Sheldon initially viewed the somatotype as an estimate of the 'genotype'.[21,23] This provoked a stream of criticism; modification of somatotype, especially by extreme dieting and training, was noted by many. Modifications of the method for estimating somatotype followed, although not the concept. The modifications of Parnell[24] and Heath and Carter[25] incorporate anthropometry, but view somatotype as a *phenotype,* based on body measurements at a given point in time. Nevertheless, there is substantial genetic influence on somatotype, though estimates of heritability vary with age and between the sexes.[26–29]

Estimation of somatotype with the anthropometric protocol of Heath and Carter appears to be worldwide in application, given international interest in elite athletes, both youth and adult,[6,30] and in the context of talent identification and development.[31–33] The protocol has also been applied in the context of constitutional medicine,[34] specifically somatotype and risk factors for disease in youth and young adults.[35–38]

The Heath–Carter somatotype method

As initially described, the Heath–Carter method combines photoscopic and anthropometric procedures.[30,39] In practice, however, the technique is used primarily in its anthropometric form for the reasons that (i) anthropometry is more objective and accessible, and (ii) more importantly, obtaining standardized somatotype photographs (front, side, back views) is quite difficult and costly.[6] The Heath–Carter anthropometric somatotype is calculated from 10 dimensions: body mass, stature, four skinfolds, two bone breadths, and two limb girths. *Endomorphy* is derived from the sum of three skinfolds: the triceps, subscapular, and supraspinale, adjusted for stature. *Mesomorphy* is derived from biepicondylar (humerus) and bicondylor (femur) breadths, flexed-arm and calf circumferences corrected for the triceps and medial calf skinfolds, respectively, and stature. The four limb measurements are adjusted for stature. *Ectomorphy* is based on the somatotype ponderal index (stature, cm, divided by the cube root of mass, kg).[21]

To estimate the Heath–Carter anthropometric somatotype, two methods are available: (i) the traditional approach that uses the Heath–Carter Somatotype Rating Form (i.e. the step-by-step procedure), and (ii) specific algorithms for each component (see Carter and Heath[30] and Duquet and Carter[39] for details).

Application of the Heath–Carter anthropometric protocol to children requires special attention. The rating forms for anthropometric somatotypes, as originally designed by Heath and Carter,[25] provide mesomorphy and ectomorphy scales adjusted for height, but no similar adjustments for endomorphy and the sum of three skinfolds. However, on the assumption that skinfolds diminish during growth in proportion to an increase in height, it was suggested that the sum of three skinfolds be multiplied by 170.18/height (cm) before rating endomorphy in children.[30] In addition, the algorithms are developed from data gathered on adult samples, and their applicability to children and perhaps early adolescents needs evaluation.[6]

Endomorphy and mesomorphy in the Heath–Carter somatotype method are described as related to specific body composition concepts. Endomorphy is defined as relative fatness (or leanness), whereas mesomorphy is described as relative musculoskeletal development adjusted for stature, expressing the relative amount of fat free mass (FFM) in the body. However, results of several studies do not support these notions, especially for children and young adults.[40–45] Correlations between endomorphy and percentage fat are moderate, but those between mesomorphy and FFM are low. Recent observations in adult males indicate higher significant correlations between 'Heath–Carter' mesomorphy and the size-corrected FFM (relative to stature) as determined by dual-energy x-ray absorptiometry (DXA) and bioelectrical impedance analysis (BIA).[46] However, mesomorphy is primarily related to muscular and, to a much lesser degree, to bone development, questioning the validity of referring to mesomorphy as FFM in the context of body composition.[47]

The dimensions for estimating mesomorphy with the Heath–Carter method are limited to the limbs to the exclusion of the trunk so that an estimate of mesomorphy that does not include a measurement on the trunk does not appear to make biological sense.[6,47,48] The trunk is a major component of physique as highlighted in the original Sheldonian photoscopic methodology.

Of particular relevance, the definition of somatotype and procedures for estimating somatotype with the Heath–Carter anthropometric method are not identical to those as described by Sheldon, although the same terms are used. In the original Sheldonian concept, somatotype refers only to the individual's body shape and not to body composition. Although the term somatotype is generically used, it has a different meaning in each method.[6,47,48]

As noted, somatotype is a 'Gestalt' and must be treated as a unit for statistical analysis.[49] Most studies relating somatotype to growth, performance, and other aspects of the paediatric exercise and health sciences, however, ordinarily treat each component as an independent variable. Principles of quality control in anthropometry also apply to the estimate of somatotype, and the influence of measurement variability associated with each of the 10 dimensions used to derive the Heath–Carter anthropometric somatotype must be considered. Errors less than 0.5 somatotype units have been reported when dimensions are measured by experienced technicians.[6]

Body composition assessment: models, methodological aspects, and techniques

The study of body composition attempts to partition and quantify body weight/mass into its basic components. It has a long tradition, which has been driven/limited by the availability of assessment techniques. During the past decade, there has been significant progress in theoretical frameworks and technology.[50–54] A good deal of early body composition research was limited to adults; at present, youth in general[6,55–57] and adolescent and young adult athletes[6,58,59] are a primary focus.

Five levels of body composition

Body mass can be viewed as the sum of all components at the atomic, molecular, cellular, tissue-system, and whole body levels.[50]

The atomic level includes the basic chemical elements and is the 'basic' level of analysis. About 50 of the 106 elements that exist in nature are found in the human body and can be measured in the living subject, but approximately 95% of body mass is composed of four elements: oxygen, carbon, hydrogen, and nitrogen.

The molecular level includes primarily water, lipid, protein, and minerals. Carbohydrate, in the form of glycogen found in the cytoplasm of most cells, is also a molecular component but is not usually considered in estimates of body composition. The molecular level is the conceptual foundation for most studies of body composition and associated technologies.

At the cellular level, body mass is composed of cells and substances outside of cells—extracellular fluids and extracellular solids. At present, methods are not available to measure solids within cells *in vivo*. The body cell mass is the metabolically active component of the body and therefore important in body composition research. Nevertheless, relatively little research has been directed at this level, perhaps because of the difficulty in quantifying some of the components.

The tissue-system level of body composition focuses on skeletal muscle, adipose, bone, blood, viscera, and brain tissues. This level is very complex and interfaces with several branches of human biology. Although several indirect techniques estimate major tissue compartments, only few *in vivo* direct methods are available.

The whole body level of body composition concerns size, shape, proportions, and exterior physical characteristics. Anthropometry is the basic tool for estimating body size and configuration, while the BMI and skinfolds are perhaps the most widely used anthropometric indicators at this level of body composition. Other whole-body properties that are important in the study of body composition are body volume, body density, and body resistance, which are described in more detail subsequently.

Models of body composition

Several models have been used to partition body mass into meaningful components or compartments. The traditional two-component model has evolved into more complex models with three, four, or more compartments. The models are described briefly; more detailed discussions of each and associated methods are available.[52–54,57,60,61]

The two-component model partitions body mass into *fat mass* (FM) and FFM. This model has the widest application in the study of body composition. A shortcoming of this model is the heterogenous composition of the FFM, including water, protein, minerals, and glycogen.

The three-component model includes FM but divides the FFM component into *total-body water* (TBW) and *fat-free dry mass* (FFDM), which includes protein, glycogen, and minerals (bone and soft tissue mineral).

The four-component model is a logical extension of the three-component model since bone mineral (BM) can now be easily measured. The FFDM now is thus partitioned into BM and the residual, which is mainly protein and glycogen.

Body composition methods used in the paediatric population

The variety of methods for measuring or estimating body composition is quite numerous and at times complex. Detailed discussions of the specific methods are available and are beyond the scope of this chapter.[52] Note, however, that many of the methods have been developed on adults or in some cases only young adult males.[6] The biological uniqueness of children and adolescents make the selection and application of body composition methods different from those of adults.[6,55] Although a variety of methods is available, this discussion highlights several used with children and adolescents in the laboratory and the field. Changes in body composition with age, and variation associated with sex, maturation, and ethnicity, are discussed in detail elsewhere.[6,62]

Densitometry

Densitometry refers to the measurement of body density, the ratio of body mass to body volume. Body volume is commonly measured by underwater (or hydrostatic) weighing, but air displacement plethysmography (ADP) is also used.[63]

Densitometry by the underwater weighing technique

Body mass is determined by weighing the subject in the air in the usual manner. Body volume is measured under water using the Archimedean principle that a body immersed in a fluid is acted upon by a buoyancy force that is evidenced by a loss of mass equal to the mass of the displaced fluid. Weight is thus measured with the subject fully submerged in the water. The difference between weight in the air and that fully submerged in the water is the weight of the displaced volume of water, corrected for the density of the water at the time of measurement. Two other volumes affect the accurate measurement of body weight under water: residual lung volume, which is the air remaining in the lungs after full expiration, and *the amount of gas in the gastrointestinal tract.* Residual volume has to be measured independently; it varies during growth and is related to stature, sex, and age. The amount of gastrointestinal gas is usually estimated at 100 mL.

Although the underwater technique is often used, it has several limitations with children. The technique requires a high degree of subject cooperation; the subject must be able to exhale completely and hold their breath under water for at least 10 s; and the process must be repeated several times.

Densitometry by air displacement plethysmography

ADP has overcome many of the practical problems associated with the measurement of body volume by underwater weighing.[64] With ADP, air displacement instead of water displacement is used to measure body volume. At present, one commercial system, the BOD POD Body Composition System, is available for measuring body density by ADP.[65] The BOD POD is a large, egg-shaped fibreglass chamber that uses air displacement and pressure–volume relationships to derive body volume. This equipment consists of a test chamber large enough (450 L) to hold an adult subject, separated by a diaphragm from a reference chamber. Vibration of the diaphragm induces pressure changes that allow determination of the test chamber volume, first with, then without, the subject, permitting the measurement of the subject's volume. The raw body volume must be corrected for body surface area, clothing, and thoracic gas volume (TGV), which is similar to but not identical with residual volume. Body surface area is calculated from height and weight based on the—quite old—equations developed by Du Bois and Du Bois.[66] TGV is either directly measured or estimated by the BOD POD system using equations developed for adults, 17–91 years of age. The adult TGV estimating equations do not work well with children; hence, child-specific TGV prediction equations for use with ADP were recently developed.[67]

Although ADP is a promising method, its validity needs further clarification.[64,68,69] Research on the sensitivity of ADP for detecting changes in body composition in individuals over time is limited.[70]

Converting body density to percentage body fat

Although body density can be measured with a high degree of precision, the derivation of estimated body composition varies with models and equations used. The two-component model has the longest tradition of use in the paediatric sport sciences. The equations of Brozek *et al.*[71] and Siri[72] for converting density to percentage fat (%BF), developed on adult males, have been used most often, but application to children ordinarily gives elevated fat estimates. The model assumes that the composition of FM and FFM is constant, with density values of 0.900 and 1.100 $g \cdot cm^{-3}$, respectively. However, estimated composition of the FFM changes with growth and maturation and differs between the sexes, and mature composition (chemical maturity) is not attained until young adulthood.[6,73] The equations have been modified for sex-, growth-, and maturity-related differences in composition of the FFM based on multi-component estimates.[74,75]

Dual-energy x-ray absorpiometry

The relatively recent development of dual-energy x-ray absorpiometry (DXA) technology permits measures of BM content and soft tissue composition of the body, but the use of DXA as a 'gold standard' for body composition is not justified at this stage.[53] The theoretical and physical principles of DXA are beyond the scope of this chapter (see Lohman and Chen[76]). Briefly, DXA requires a low-dose radiation exposure (0.02–1.5 mrem); an x-ray tube with a filter to convert the polychromatic beam into low- and high-energy peaks permits differentiation of bone, non-bone lean and fat tissues.

Several types of commercially available DXA instruments are presently used. Each type has its own computer algorithms for deriving estimates of body composition, with the consequence that estimates vary by manufacturer, data collection mode, and software version.[76,77] The DXA technique is reliable, reasonably rapid (5–30 min), and requires minimal subject cooperation. Of specific relevance, DXA provides a measure of BM content and density.[53,76] The validity of DXA with children and adolescents may need further study[77]; the ethics of using ionizing radiation, though in very low amounts, also needs consideration[53,76] (see Chapter 1).

Body composition assessment by anthropometry

By far the most common technique for estimating body composition by anthropometry involves skinfold thicknesses. Details of skinfold measurement techniques were described earlier. Individual skinfolds or a sum of several skinfolds are entered into a regression equation to predict either body density (from which %BF is subsequently derived) and/or %BF. Several skinfold equations have been developed for use in the paediatric population (see Heyward and Wagner,[53] p. 113). A major concern is the accuracy of the equations, which limits their use with samples other than those upon which they were derived, for example, young athletes and the obese.[58,78] In a cross-validation study, for example, the limits of agreement (±2 standard deviations) for the triceps + calf and triceps + subscapular equations developed by Slaughter *et al.*[79] for children and adolescents relative to %BF determined with a four-component model were 8.1 %BF and 9.9 %BF, respectively.[80] The triceps + calf equation did not predict well when %BF > 30% and over-predicted %BF more so in boys than in girls. The triceps + subscapular equation tended to under-predict fat in girls and to over-predict fat in boys. Accordingly, the widely used equations[79] have major limitations and require further refinement.[80,81] Errors associated with measurement *per se* and with specific prediction equations should be noted but are rarely considered.[82,83]

The BMI is widely used in epidemiologic surveys of weight status, specifically overweight and obesity.[6,84] Nevertheless, its validity as a measure of body composition in the paediatric population can be questioned. The BMI is about equally correlated with FM and FFM[6] and is not a direct measure of adiposity.[55] Although several studies show good correlations between BMI and body fat in samples, it is of limited utility in individuals.[84]

Bioelectrical impedance analysis

Bioelectrical impedance analysis (BIA) is a non-invasive, rapid, and relatively easy technique for estimating body composition. The equipment is inexpensive and portable. As such, BIA has potential for use with individuals across a broad age spectrum and in a variety of settings.[53,85] The fundamental theory and principles of BIA are discussed in detail elsewhere.[85–87] Briefly, BIA is based on the principle that biological tissues act as conductors or insulators and that the flow of current through the body follows the path of least resistance. Because bone-free lean tissue has a greater electrolyte and water content and greater conductivity than adipose and bone tissues, an estimate of FFM from the magnitude of electrical conductivity of the body can be made. BIA uses an imperceptible electrical current. Impedance (Z) to the flow of current is directly related to the length (L) of the conductor and inversely related to its cross-sectional area, assuming that the specific resistivity of bodily tissues is constant. Impedance yields a measure of resistance that is used with stature to estimate TBW.[53,85] TBW is then converted to an estimate of FFM from which FM is derived.

BIA is a reasonable technique for estimating body composition in the paediatric population because measurements are fast, non-invasive, inexpensive, painless, require little subject cooperation, do not require a high level of technical skill, and can be used in obese individuals[53]. However, as with other methods of estimating body composition, BIA is based on a number of underlying assumptions related to extremity proportions and tissue composition that need to be verified for children and adolescents[6,85]. Its application also requires prediction equations specific to age, sex, and stage of puberty.[55,88] Although several BIA equations for children and adolescents have been reported[53,55], cross-validation studies against accepted reference methods give generally unacceptable results.[55,89] Further study is needed before the value of BIA with paediatric samples is fully established. BIA is useful for describing the body composition of groups, but estimates have large errors in individuals, up to more than 25% systematic bias compared with multi-compartment analyses, which limits its application.[89] In addition, a number of factors can influence BIA, including the level of hydration, nutritional status, posture, measurement protocol and/or skin temperature, age, gender, athletic status, body composition status, and ethnicity.[6,85,90–92] These and other factors (e.g. timing and content of last ingested meal, skin temperature, phase of menstrual cycle) need careful consideration before BIA is used in short- or long-term longitudinal studies.[85]

Assessing biological maturity

The concept of biological maturation

Growth and maturation are concepts that are often used together and sometimes considered as synonymous. Growth refers to the increase in size of the whole body or the size attained by different parts of the body. The changes in size are outcomes of the increase in cell number or hyperplasia, increase in cell size or hypertrophy, or increase in intercellular material or accretion. Growth is a dominant biological activity during the first two decades of life. It starts at conception and continues until the late teens or early twenties in some individuals. Maturation is a process that marks progress towards the adult (mature) state. Maturation is a process, whereas maturity is a state. All tissues, organs, and organ systems of the body mature but do so at different times and rates. As a result, assessment of biological maturity status varies with the bodily system considered. Of necessity, therefore, the concept of maturation is operational.

Maturation of different systems proceeds independently of chronological (calendar) age (CA) so that CA is not a good indicator of biological maturity. Nevertheless, the growth and maturity status of an individual or sample of individuals is routinely placed in the context of CA. The processes of growth and maturation are related, and both influence physical performance. Those engaged with youth are certainly familiar with the following scenario: John has a CA of 13.5 years, with a stature of 171 cm, body mass 60 kg, and arm pull strength of 65 kg, while Jim also has a CA of 13.5 years but with a stature of 150 cm, body mass 40 kg, and arm pull strength of 32 kg. These boys are often required to compete against each other in many sports and are compared on fitness tests.[93,94]

In constructing objective, reliable, and valid markers of biological maturity status, selected indicators should (i) reflect the maturation of a biological system; (ii) be to some degree independent of growth; (iii) be applicable from birth to adulthood; (iv) reach the same end point in all individuals, that is, the mature or adult state; and (v) show a continuous increase over the entire process.[6,93–97]

The first condition is obvious. The second condition implies that the system does not measure growth *per se* (size attained or changes in size attained, i.e. growth velocity), although it is related to growth, since there normally is harmony between growth and maturation. The system should be applicable throughout the period of growth and maturation from birth (perhaps from conception) to adulthood, though some indicators of maturity appear only during puberty/adolescence. The fourth condition reflects the essence of maturation: all individuals should ultimately reach the same end point, that is, maturity and this end point should be the same for all individuals. By definition maturity is progress towards the adult/mature state; hence, the system of choice should show continuous progress towards maturity.

Since Boas[98] first realized that CA is not an adequate timescale for identifying tempo and timing of changes in biological characteristics and milestones, considerable effort has been made to develop techniques of assessment of biological maturation, a process that varies in tempo (rate) and timing. Four biological systems have been and are still used to estimate biological maturity: reproductive, skeletal, somatic (morphological), and dental. Both growth and maturation are dependent on specific hypothalamic–pituitary–end organ axes, but these biochemical and hormonal control mechanisms are not considered here (see Beunen *et al.*[99]).

Indicators of biological maturation

Sexual maturity

Sexual maturation is a process that extends from early embryonic differentiation of sex organs to full maturity of the organs and fertility. Puberty is a transitional period between childhood and adulthood during which the reproductive system matures and the growth spurt occurs. Major psychological, behavioural, cognitive, and emotional changes also occur during puberty. Inter-individual and intra-individual differences in timing and tempo of pubertal events are considerable.

Assessment of sexual maturation is based on secondary sex characteristics—breasts and age at menarche in girls, genitalia (penis and testes) in boys, and pubic hair in both sexes. Development of the breasts, genitals, and pubic hair is most often rated on 5-point scales described by Tanner,[96] though similar stages have been previously described by others. The stages should not be identified as 'Tanner stages', but as stages of sexual maturation, with identification of the specific characteristic(s) assessed. The stages of each characteristic are neither equivalent nor inter-changeable. Stage 1 of each characteristic indicates the prepubertal state—absence of development—and stage 2 indicates the initial, overt development of each characteristic that marks the transition into puberty. Stages 3 and 4 mark the progress in maturation and stage 5 indicates the adult (mature) state. Detailed descriptions are provided by Tanner[96] and Malina *et al.*[6]

Ratings of secondary sex characteristics are ordinarily made by direct clinical examination, or sometimes from standardized, nude photographs.[100,101] In non-medical settings, self-assessments by youth are increasingly used.[6] There is obviously a need for quality control (intra- and inter-observer reliability), and in the case of self-assessment concordance with experienced assessors should be verified. Overall reproducibility by experienced assessors is generally good, about 80% of agreement in assigning stages, although some studies report a percentage of agreement as low as 40%.[6]

Menarche, the first menstruation, is perhaps the most widely monitored secondary sex characteristic in females. It can be obtained in three different ways: (i) prospectively (longitudinal design) by interrogating the same girls at regular intervals, 3–6 months, (ii) retrospectively by interrogating post-menarcheal girls or women, and asking them to recall when they experienced their first menstruation, and (iii) *status quo*, by interrogating large samples of girls approximately 9–16 years of age about their menarcheal status (i.e. pre- or post-menarcheal; see below). The first two methods provide ages at menarche for individuals, while the *status quo* method provides an estimated age at menarche for a sample and does not apply to individuals.

Other secondary sex characteristics include axillary hair in both sexes and facial hair and voice change in boys. As a rule, these are late developing indicators during puberty and are not widely used in studies of biological maturation. A more direct estimate of genital maturity in boys is provided by testicular volume. The method is used primarily in the clinical setting and requires a series of ellipsoid models of known volume, which have the shape of the testes (Prader orchidometer).[102,103]

Ages at which specific stages of sexual maturity are reached are ordinarily derived from longitudinal studies in which children are examined at regular intervals, preferably every 3 months, starting in late childhood (prepuberty) and continuing through puberty into early adulthood. Data obtained from prospective studies provide estimates of the age at initiation of a stage and duration of a stage. Mean ages and associated standard deviations can be calculated. Such longitudinal studies require, of course, long examination periods and are most often restricted in sample size and representativeness of the sample. Cross-sectional designs (*status quo*) provide ages of 'being in a particular stage'. The percentages of children in a particular stage at each age are used with probits or logits to obtain sample statistics (median, means, and standard deviations) for each stage of a characteristic or for menarche.

Secondary sex characteristics are reasonably easy to obtain, reflect an important biological system, and are closely related to underlying hormonal axes. Though useful, stages of puberty have several limitations. The method of assessment is invasive in non-clinical settings, though this is not necessarily true for self-assessment. Of more relevance, the stages are somewhat arbitrary and discrete and are limited to the pubertal period only. They are also specific, that is, G3 is not equivalent to PH3, or B3 is not equivalent with PH3. Moreover, it is not biologically correct to average ratings to come up with a single sexual maturity score, that is, there is no such stage as 1.5 or 3.5. When a youngster is examined in a study, he/she is in a particular stage of puberty. Being in a stage indicates nothing about age at entry into this stage and duration of the stage. The prepubertal state (G1, B1, PH1) simply indicates the lack of overt development of the respective indicators. However, prepubertal children, though uniform in sexual maturity status as assessed, do in fact vary in hormones associated with the hypothalamic–pituitary–gonadal axis and in skeletal maturity.[6,99] It is common in the paediatric exercise sciences to group youth of the same stage of puberty and then to make comparisons across stages independent of CA. This is an erroneous approach. This overlooks CA *per se* as a source of variation in size, body composition, and performance capacity; a 12-year-old boy in G4 is very different from a 16-year-old boy in G4, and this difference in CA would be reflected in measures of size and performance.

Somatic or morphological maturity

Body size *per se* is not a valid indicator of biological maturity status since the adult state is not the same for all individuals. As such, it is not appropriate as an indicator of biological maturity status. Concepts such as morphological age or height age, that is, the corresponding CA at which a specific stature is, on average, attained in a given population, are not useful maturity estimates. However, if longitudinal height data that span late childhood through adolescence are available, the characteristics of the adolescent growth spurt provide two useful indicators of somatic maturity status: age at the onset of the growth spurt (first inflection point of the adolescent growth curve, take-off) and age at maximum velocity (second inflection point of the adolescent growth curve, peak height velocity). Corresponding parameters of the growth spurt can also be derived for other linear measurements, for example, sitting height and leg length. To accurately estimate the parameters of the growth curve, careful measurements that span adolescence and that are taken at regular intervals, at least two times per year (preferably three or four times a year) are needed. Curve fitting techniques, based on structural and non-structural models, have facilitated estimation of the parameters.[104–106]

The assessment of somatic maturity based on the parameters of the growth curve (age at onset, age at maximum velocity) is limited to the adolescent period, and only one or two biological events are considered. Although derivation requires longitudinal measurements of individual children over a relatively long age span, they provide an accurate estimate for a major event in the pubertal period.

If adult height is available (as in longitudinal studies), percentage of adult height attained at a given CA or the CA at which a specific percentage of adult height is attained serve as potential maturity indicators. Adult height is ordinarily measured in longitudinal studies. It can also be estimated at younger ages. Prediction formulae are available for European and American samples, but have not been validated on other populations.[107–114] Most height prediction protocols require an estimate of skeletal age (SA). However, efforts have also been made to predict adult stature without SA.[115,116] These predictions have not been used extensively, and validation is generally lacking. Recently, the Khamis–Roche[115] equation to predict adult height without SA and in turn percentage of predicted adult height attained at a given CA has been validated against SA (Fels method; see below) in a sample of 143 youth American football players.[117] The concordance between the two maturity classifications was 62%, indicating moderate agreement.

Percentage of predicted adult height attained at a given age is an indirect estimate of somatic maturity, which may have application during childhood and early adolescence. In later adolescence, it has limitations as the majority of youth are approaching adult height.

Another non-invasive estimate of somatic maturity utilizes time before or after PHV, labelled as maturity offset, as a maturity indicator.[118] The protocol requires age, height, weight, sitting height, and estimated leg length in sex-specific equations. The method has been validated in a sample of elite female gymnasts. Mean predicted age at PHV deviated linearly from the criterion age at PHV. There also was a systematic bias between the prediction and criterion; correlations between the two varied between −0.13 and +0.76. Care is therefore warranted in utilizing maturity offset *per se* and predicted age at PHV based on maturity offset as an indicator of biological maturity timing in female gymnasts and probably also in short late maturing females in general.[119]

Skeletal maturity

The maturation of the skeleton is widely recognized as the best single indicator of maturity status.[97] All children start with a skeleton of cartilage and progress towards the fully ossified, adult, axial skeleton. In the case of the tubular bones (long and short bones), maturity is attained when epiphyses are fused with their corresponding diaphyses; in the case of round or irregularly shaped bones, maturity is defined by adult morphology (shape). The bones comprising the craniofacial skeleton differ in embryonic origin and their growth and maturation are approached differently, and these are not considered in this discussion of skeletal maturation.

The bones of the hand and wrist provide the primary basis for assessing maturity status, although the knee, hip, and foot have also been used. Maturation of the skeleton is ordinarily monitored with standardized radiographs upon which changes occurring from initial ossification to adult morphology of individual bones can be evaluated. Criteria for individual bones are labelled maturity indicators—specific features of individual bones that are universal and occur regularly in a definite, irreversible order. Three methods for the assessment of skeletal maturity—the Greulich–Pyle, the Tanner–Whitehouse (TW), and the Fels methods—are commonly used at present.

Greulich–Pyle method

The method[120] is based on the original work of Todd,[121] and it is sometimes called the atlas or the inspectional technique. The atlas consists of sex-specific radiographs representative of the maturity status at a given CA from birth to 19 years. The radiograph that was most typical for the skeletal maturity state for each sex at each age level was selected as the reference plate. The skeletal maturity of a child is obtained by comparing his/her hand-wrist skeleton to the standard plates of the atlas. Skeletal maturity is expressed as an SA. The most adequate procedure is to assign for each bone separately the SA of the plate with which the individual bone most closely coincides, and the SA assigned to the child is the median value of the SAs of all bones.[107]

Tanner–Whitehouse method

The TW method is sometimes called the bone-specific approach.[108,109] Maturity indicators were defined and described for each bone. Each indicator is expressed as a stage from initial ossification to union (radius, ulna, metacarpals, and phalanges) or adult morphology (carpals) and a point score is assigned to each stage. Twenty bones are used: radius, ulna, seven carpals (excluding the pisiform), and metacarpals and phalanges of the first, third, and fifth digits (rays). The scores are summed and can be expressed either as a maturity score or as an SA. The maturity scale (0–1000) was constructed to minimize the overall disagreement between the bones of the hand and wrist.

The first version of the method (TWI)[108,109] provided an SA based on the sum of maturity scores for 20 bones. The second version (TWII)[108,109] provided three different scales and SAs: (i) a 20-bone scale; (ii) an RUS scale for the radius, ulna, and short bones (13 bones); and (iii) a CARP scale for the seven carpal or round bones. Both TWI and TWII skeletal maturity references are based on a sample of about 3000 healthy British children. In the second version, the final stage of a number of bones was no longer assessed, and the scoring system was modified, but the maturity indicators were not changed. The third version of the method (TWIII)[111] considers only the RUS and carpal bones (no longer includes a 20-bone SA), and the reference values are now based on samples of British, Belgian, Italian, Spanish, Argentinean, United States (a well-off sample from the suburbs of Houston, Texas), and Japanese children.

Fels Method

The Fels method is bone-specific and is based on a sample of middle-class children from south-central Ohio enrolled in the Fels Longitudinal Study.[122] The authors defined an extensive series of maturity indicators for all bones of the hand-wrist skeleton;[122] ratios between linear measurements of epiphyseal and diaphyseal widths for individual long bones were included among the indicators. The potential of each indicator was tested on its ability to differentiate between individual children of the same CA, universal appearance, reliability, validity, and completeness. The resulting Fels method is based on the final grading of 85 grade maturity indicators for the radius, ulna, carpals, metacarpals, and phalanges, and 13 measured ratios of epiphyseal and diaphyseal diameters of the radius, ulna, metacarpals, and phalanges. The CA and sex of the child, and ratings and ratios are entered into a microcomputer that calculates a SA and associated standard error of estimate.

Other methods for the assessment of skeletal maturity have been proposed. Some are of historical interest and others are less commonly used.[6,96] At present, several computer-based protocols have been applied to the TWII method, and experimental results are reasonably consistent with ratings of expert assessors.[111,123,124]

The three currently used methods for the assessment of skeletal maturity are similar in principle, but differ in maturity indicators, scales of maturity (scores, SA), and reference samples. The Greulich–Pyle and Fels methods provide a single SA, while the TW method provides several SAs. A SA corresponds to the level of skeletal maturity attained by a child relative to the reference sample for each method. Given differences in the methods and in the reference samples for each, SAs derived from each are not equivalent. In fact, the skeletal maturity status of a child rated by all three methods may be quite different.[6,93,95,96,125] Recently the TWIII and Fels methods were used to assess skeletal maturity in a sample of 40 elite youth soccer players. The Fels and TWIII yield different SAs. Among 14 players over 15 years of age, two were skeletally mature with the Fels and 11 with the TWIII method.[126] The authors argued that these discrepancies are largely due to the less precise definition of the final maturity stages in the TWIII method, although maturity differences in the samples upon which the two methods are based cannot be ruled out. Regardless of the method used, quality control in assessment is essential. Variation within and between assessors can be considerable and should be reported.

Skeletal age has limited utility by itself, but SA relative to CA is a valuable maturity indicator. SA may simply be compared to CA, may be expressed as the difference between SA and CA (SA minus CA), or may be expressed as a ratio of SA/CA. There is considerable variation in SA at each CA. Standard deviations of RUS SA (TWIII) are ~1 year from 5 to 14 years in girls and 5 to 16 years in boys[111]; corresponding standard deviations with the Fels method from 5 to 16 years vary from 0.82 to 1.26 years in boys and 0.83 to 1.12 years in girls.[122]

Advantages of skeletal maturity assessment as an indicator of biological maturity include the following: (i) methods of assessment are reasonably precise and provide reliable estimates; (ii) methods are applicable from birth to young adulthood; and (iii) assessments reflect maturation of an important biological system. Disadvantages include (i) exposure to low-level radiation, and (ii) somewhat arbitrary nature of stages or maturity indicators that suggest discrete steps in a continuous process.[6,93,95,96] Like all methods of assessment, the protocols require specific training and quality control for accurate application.

Skeletal age and more recently magnetic resonance imaging (MRI) stages of radial fusion have been suggested as estimates of passport age in international age-group international soccer competitions.[126,127] Given the normal range of variation in SA within relatively narrow CA groups, which approximates 2 years or more in adolescents,[111,122] CA cannot be accurately estimated from SA.[128,129] In addition, accelerated skeletal maturation among adolescent athletes, specifically males, guarantees a high likelihood of a relatively large number of false negatives (SA is estimated older then the true CA).[126,128,129]

Dental maturity

Dental maturity has been traditionally estimated from ages of eruption of deciduous and/or permanent teeth, the number of teeth erupted at a specific CA, or the age at which a specific number of teeth have erupted.[130] Note, however, that definitions of eruptions vary from a tooth simply piercing the gum line to full eruption. Dental calcification as evaluated on radiographs also provides an indicator of maturity status. Demirjian *et al.*[131] developed a scale of dental maturity based on the principles of the TW method for assessment of SA.[108] Age-at-attainment of the dental stages shows no major differences in children from Australia, Belgium, Canada, England, Finland, France, South-Korea, and Sweden.[132] It has been suggested, however, that reference values for the Demirjian method may not be applicable to British (English, Welsh, Scottish) and Bangladeshi children resident in London.[133] In addition, dental maturation does not correlate very well with the other maturity indicators.[134,135]

Interrelationships among maturity indicators

Indicators of sexual, morphological, and skeletal maturation are highly interrelated during puberty but not to the extent that maturity status in one system can be used to predict maturity status in another system, for example, predict skeletal maturity from secondary sex characteristics or vice versa.[135–137] There is some evidence that indicators of prepubertal status cluster somewhat independently from pubertal indicators.[135,136] This suggests that different hormonal and related growth factors are the driving forces that underlie these events. In general, the hypothalamic–pituitary GH/IGF-I and the hypothalamic–pituitary–gonadal axes, and their interactions drive adolescent growth and maturation, given adequate thyroid status.[99]

Summary

This chapter has four discrete, though related, sections:

1 *Anthropometry* comprises a series of measurement techniques for describing the size and proportions of the body and also for estimating physique and body composition. A battery of measurements commonly used in the exercise and sport sciences and their application is presented. The need for quality control and an estimate of measurement variability is highlighted. Special attention is given to the BMI and its use with children and adolescents.

2 *Physique* is most commonly described through somatotype, a term that has different meanings within methods of assessment currently available. Focus is on the Heath–Carter

anthropometric protocol given its wide use, though the method has limitations.

3 The section on *body composition* reviews theoretical models and models currently in use. Although densitometry is widely used in the paediatric population, it has major shortcomings, given the assumption of a constant density of the FFM during growth and maturation. DXA, though promising as a potential 'gold standard', requires further refinement for use with children and adolescents.

4 The final section reviews methods for the assessment of the *biological maturation*, specifically sexual, skeletal, somatic, and dental maturity. There is a need for more attention to the refinement of 'non-invasive' methods for maturity assessment of maturity.

References

1. Claessens AL, Beunen G, Malina RM (2000). Anthropometry, physique, body composition and maturity. In: Armstrong N, van Mechelen W (eds.), *Paediatric exercise science and medicine,* pp. 11–22. Oxford University Press, Oxford.
2. Lasker GW (1994). The place of anthropometry in human biology. In: Ulijaszek SJ, Mascie-Taylor CGN (eds.), *Anthropometry: The individual and the population*, pp. 1–6. Cambridge University Press, Cambridge.
3. Malina RM (1988). Physical anthropology. In: Lohman TG, Roche AF, Martorell R (eds.), *Anthropometric standardization reference manual,* pp. 99–102. Human Kinetics Books, Champaign, IL.
4. Malina RM (1995). Anthropometry. In: Maud PJ Foster C (eds.), *Physiological assessment of human fitness*, pp. 205–19. Human Kinetics, Champaign, IL.
5. Malina RM (1997). Anthropometry in physical education and sport sciences. In: Spencer F (ed.), *History of physical anthropology*, Vol. 1. A-L, pp. 90–4. Garland Publishing, New York.
6. Malina RM, Bouchard C, Bar-Or O (2004). *Growth, maturation, and physical activity* (2nd ed.). Human Kinetics Books, Champaign, IL.
7. Cameron N (1984). *The measurement of human growth.* Croom Helm, London.
8. Lohman TG, Roche AF, Martorell R (eds.) (1988). *Anthropometric standardization reference manual.* Human Kinetics Books, Champaign, IL.
9. Norton K, Olds T (ed.) (1996). *Antropometrica.* University of New South Wales Press, Sydney.
10. Jones PRM, Norgan NG (1994). Anthropometry and the assessment of body composition. In: Harries M, Williams C, Stanish WD, Micheli LJ (eds.), *Oxford textbook of sports medicine*, pp. 149–60. Oxford University Press, New York.
11. Lampl M (1992). Further observations on diurnal variation in standing height. *Ann Hum Biol* **19**, 87–90.
12. Wang J, Thornton JC, Bari S, Williamson B, Gallacher D, Heymsfield SB, Orlick M, Kotler D, Laferrère B, Mayer L, Pi-Sunyer FX, Pierson RN Jr (2003). Comparisons of waist circumferences measured at 4 sites. *Am J Clin Nutr* **77**, 379–84.
13. Malina RM, Buschang PH (1984). Anthropometric asymmetry in normal and mentally retarded males. *Ann Hum Biol* **11**, 515–31.
14. Martorell R, Mendoza F, Mueller WH, Pawson IG (1988). Which side to measure: Right or left? In: Lohman TG, Roche AF, Martorell R (eds.), *Anthropometric standardization reference manual*, pp. 87–91. Human Kinetics Books, Champaign, IL.
15. Tomkinson GR, Popovic N, Martin M (2003). Bilateral symmetry and the competitive standard attained in elite and sub-elite sport. *J Sport Sci* **21**, 201–11.
16. Little BB, Buschang PH, Malina RM (2002). Anthropometric asymmetry in chronically undernourished children from southern Mexico. *Ann Hum Biol* **29**, 526–37.
17. Lefevre JAV, Beunen GP, Wellens R (1990). Data input and quality control. In: Simons J, Beunen GP, Renson R, Claessens ALM, Vanreusel B, Lefevre JAV (eds.), *Growth and fitness of Flemish girls. The Leuven Growth Study*, pp. 47–56. Human Kinetics Books, Champaign, IL.
18. Sokal RR, Rohlf FJ (1981). *Biometry: The principles and practice of statistics in biological research* (2nd ed.). Freeman, San Francisco, CA.
19. Simpson GG, Roe A, Lewontin RC (1960). *Quantitative zoology, revised edition.* Harcourt, Brace and World, New York.
20. Malina RM (1991). Ratios and derived indicators in the assessment of nutritional status. In: Himes JH (ed.), *Anthropometric assessment of nutritional status,* pp. 151–71. Wiley-Liss, New York.
21. Sheldon WH, Stevens SS, Tucker WB (1970). *The varieties of human physique.* An introduction to constitutional psychology. Hafner, Darien, CT.
22. Taylor RW, Jones IE, Williams SM, Goulding A (2000). Evaluation of waist circumference, waist-to-hip ratio, and the conicity index as screening tools for high trunk fat mass, as measured by dual-energy X-ray absorptiometry, in children ages 3–19 y. *Am J Clin Nutr* **72**, 490–5.
23. Sheldon WH, Dupertuis CW, McDermott E (1954). *Atlas of men.* A guide for somatotyping the adult male at all ages. Hafner, Darien, Connecticut.
24. Parnell WH (1958). *Behaviour and physique. An introduction to practical and applied somatometry.* Greenwood, Westport, CT
25. Heath BH, Carter JEL (1967). A modified somatotype method. *Am J Phys Anthropol* **27**, 57–74.
26. Peeters MW, Thomis MA, Claessens AL, Loos RJF, Maes HHM, Lysens R, Vanden Eynde B, Vlietinck R, Beunen G (2003). Heritability of somatotype components from early adolescence into young adulthood: A multivariate analysis on a longitudinal twin study. *Ann Hum Biol* **30**, 402–18.
27. Katzmarzyk PT, Malina RM, Perusse L, Rice T, Province MA, Rao DC, Bouchard C (2000). Familial resemblance for physique: Heritabilities for somatotype components. *Ann Hum Biol* **27**, 467–77.
28. Bouchard C, Malina RM, Perusse L (1997). *Genetics of fitness and physical performance.* Human Kinetics, Champaign, IL.
29. Peeters MW, Thomis MA, Loos RJF, Derom CA, Fagard R, Claessens AL, Vlietinck RF, Beunen GP (2007). Heritability of somatotype components: A multivariate analysis. *Int J Obes* **31**, 1295–1301.
30. Carter JEL, Heath BH (1990). *Somatotyping. Development and applications.* Cambridge University Press, Cambridge.
31. Beunen GP, Claessens AL (2003). Auxological issues in youth sports. In: Malina RM, Clark MA (eds.), *Youth sports—perspectives for a new Century*, pp. 26–39. Coaches Choice, Monterey, CA.
32. Chaouachi M, Chaouachi A, Chamari K, Chtara M, Feki Y, Amri M, Trudeau F (2005). Effects of dominant somatotype on aerobic capacity trainability. *Br J Sport Med* **39**, 954–9.
33. Claessens AL (2001). Kinanthropometric issues in sports performance: The case of talent identification and talent development. In: Fu F, Ruskin H (eds.), *Physical fitness and activity in the context of leisure education*, pp. 45–76. Glory Printing and Productions, Hong Kong.
34. Damon A (1970). Constitutional medicine. In: Von Mering O and Kasdan L (eds.), *Anthropology and the behavioral and health sciences*, pp. 179–205. University of Pittsburgh Press, Pittsburgh.
35. Katzmarzyk PT, Malina RM, Song TMK, Theriault G, Bouchard C (1998). Physique and echocardiographic dimensions in children, adolescents and young adults. *Ann Hum Biol* **25**, 145–57.
36. Katzmarzyk PT, Malina RM, Song TMK, Bouchard C (1998). Somatotype and indicators of metabolic fitness in youth. *Am J Hum Biol* **10**, 341–50.
37. Katzmarzyk PT, Malina RM, Song TMK, Bouchard C (1999). Physique, subcutaneous fat, adipose tissue distribution, and risk factors in the Quebec Family Study. *Int J Obes* **23**, 476–84.

38. Malina RM, Katzmarzyk PT, Song TMK, Theriault G, Bouchard C (1997). Somatotype and cardiovascular risk factors in healthy adults. *Am J Hum Biol* **9**, 11–9.
39. Duquet W, Carter JEL (2001). Somatotyping. In: Eston R, Reilly T (eds.), *Kinanthropometry and exercise physiology laboratory manual* (2nd ed.), pp. 47–64. Routledge, London.
40. Bolonchuk WW, Hall CB, Lukaski HC, Siders WA (1989). Relationship between body composition and the components of somatotype. *Am J Hum Biol* **1**, 239–48.
41. Lohman TG, Slaughter MH, Selinger A, Boileau RA (1978). Relationship of body composition to somatotype in college men. *Ann Hum Biol* **5**, 147–57.
42. Slaughter MH, Lohman TG (1976). Relationship of body composition to somatotype. *Am J Phys Anthropol* **44**, 237–44.
43. Slaughter MH, Lohman TG (1977). Relationship of body composition to somatotype in boys ages 7 to 12 years. *Res Q* **48**, 750–8.
44. Slaughter MH, Lohman TG, Boileau RA (1977). Relationship of Heath and Carter's second component to lean body mass and height in college women. *Res Q* **48**, 759–68.
45. Wilmore JH (1970). Validation of the first and second components of the Heath-Carter modified somatotype method. *Am J Phys Anthropol* **32**, 369–72.
46. Claessens AL, Lefevre J, Philippaerts R, Thomis M, Beunen G (2004). Relation between body composition and Heath-Carter somatotype in adult males. In: Bodzsár EB, Susanne C (eds.), *Variability and sources of variations. Physique and body composition.* (Biennal Books of EAA—Vol. 3), pp 41–51. Eötvös University Press, Budapest.
47. Claessens A, Beunen G, Simons J (1986). Stability of anthroposcopic and anthropometric estimates of physique in Belgian boys followed longitudinally from 13 to 18 years of age. *Ann Hum Biol* **13**, 235–44.
48. Claessens A, Beunen G, Simons J (1985). Anthropometric principal components and somatotype in boys followed individually from 13 to 18 years of age. *Humanbiologia Budapestinensis* **16**, 23–36.
49. Cressie NAC, Withers AT, Craig NP (1986). The statistical analysis of somatotype data. *Phys Anthropol* **29**, 197–208.
50. Wang ZM, Pierson RNJ, Heymsfield SB (1992). The five-level model: A new approach to organizing body composition research. *Am J Clin Nutr* **56**, 19–28.
51. Wang ZM, Heshka S, Pierson RN, Heymsfield SB (1995). Systematic organization of body composition methodology: An overview with emphasis on component-based methods. *Am J Clin Nutr* **61**, 457–65.
52. Heymsfield SB, Lohman TG, Wang ZM, Going SB (eds.) (2005). *Human body composition* (2nd ed.). Human Kinetics, Champaign, IL.
53. Heyward VH, Wagner DR (2004). *Applied body composition assessment.* (2nd edn.). Human Kinetics, Champaign, IL.
54. Roche AF, Heymsfield SB, Lohman TG (eds.) (1996). *Human body composition.* Human Kinetics, Champaign, IL.
55. Sopher A, Shen W, Pietrobelli A (2005). Pediatric body composition methods. In: Heymsfield SB, Lohman TG, Wang ZM, Going SB (eds.), *Human body composition* (2nd ed.), pp 129–39. Human Kinetics, Champaign, IL.
56. Pietrobelli A, Heo M, Faith MS (2001). Assessment of childhood and adolescents' body composition: A practical guide. In: Dasgupta P, Hauspie R (eds.), *Perspectives in human growth, development and maturation*, pp. 67–75. Kluwer Academic Publishers, Dordrecht.
57. Wells JCK, Fuller NJ, Dewit O, Fewtrell MS, Elia M, Cole TJ (1999). Four-component model of body composition in children: Density and hydration of fat-free mass and comparison with simpler models. *Am J Clin Nutr* **69**, 904–12.
58. Malina RM (2007). Body composition in athletes: Assessment and estimated fatness. *Clin Sport Med* **26**, 37–68.
59. Kohrt WM (2000). Body composition. In: Drinkwater BL (ed.), *Women in sport*, pp. 353–63. Blackwell Science, Oxford.
60. Shen Wei, St-Onge MP, Wang ZM, Heymsfield SB (2005). Study of body composition: An overview. In: Heymsfield SB, Lohman TG, Wang ZM, Going SB (eds.), *Human body composition* (2nd ed.), pp 3–14. Human Kinetics, Champaign, IL.
61. Wang ZM, Shen W, Withers RT, Heymsfield SB (2005). Multicomponent molecular-level models of body composition analysis. In: Heymsfield SB, Lohman TG, Wang ZM, Going SB (eds.), *Human body composition* (2nd ed.), pp. 163–76. Human Kinetics, Champaign, IL.
62. Malina RM (2005). Variation in body composition associated with sex and ethnicity. In: Heymsfield SB, Lohman TG, Wang ZM, Going SB (eds.), *Human body composition* (2nd ed.), pp. 271–98, 473–6. Human Kinetics, Champaign, IL.
63. Going SB (2005). Hydrodensitometry and air displacement plethysmography. In: Heymsfield SB, Lohman TG, Wang ZM, Going SB (eds.). *Human body composition* (2nd ed.), pp. 17–33. Human Kinetics, Champaign, IL.
64. Fields DA, Goran MI, McCrory MA (2002). Body composition assessment via air-displacement plethysmography in adults and children: A review. *Am J Clin Nutr* **75**, 453–67.
65. Dempster P, Aitkens S (1995). A new air displacement method for the determination of human body composition. *Med Sci Sport Exer* **27**, 1692–7.
66. Du Bois D, Du Bois E (1916). A formula to estimate the approximate surface area if height and weight be known. *Arch Intern Med* **17**, 863–71.
67. Fields DA, Hull HR, Cheline AJ, Yao M, Higgins PB (2004). Child-specific thoracic gas volume prediction equations for air-displacement plethysmography. *Obes Res* **12**, 1797–804.
68. Ittenbach RF, Buison AM, Stallings VAa, Zemel BS (2006). Statistical validation of air-displacement plethysmography for body composition assessment in children. *Ann Hum Biol* **33**, 187–201.
69. Buison AM, Ittenbach RF, Stallings VA, Zemel BS (2006). Methodological agreement between two-compartment body-composition methods in children. *Am J Hum Biol* **18**, 470–80.
70. Secchiutti A, Fagour C, Perlemoine C, Gin H, Durrieu J, Rigalleau V (2007). Air displacement plethysmography can detect moderate changes in body composition. *Eur J Clin Nutr* **61**, 25–9.
71. Brozek J, Grande F, Anderson JT, Keys A (1963). Densitometric analysis of body composition, revision of some quantitative assumptions. *Ann NY Acad Sci* **110**, 113–40.
72. Siri WE (1961). Body composition from fluid spaces and density: Analysis of methods. In: Brozek J, Henschel A (eds.), *Techniques for measuring body composition*, pp. 223–44. National Academy of Sciences, Washington, D.C.
73. Boileau RA (1996). Body composition assessment in children and youths. In: Bar-Or O (ed.), *The child and adolescent athlete,* pp. 523–37. Blackwell, Oxford.
74. Lohman TG (1986). Applicability of body composition techniques and constants for children and youth. *Exerc Sport Sci Rev* **14**, 325–57.
75. Lohman TG (1989). Assessment of body composition in children. *Pediatr Exerc Sci* **1**, 19–30.
76. Lohman TG, Chen Z (2005). Dual-energy X-ray absorptiometry. In: Heymsfield SB, Lohman TG, Wang ZM, Going SB (eds.), *Human body composition* (2nd ed.), pp. 63–77. Human Kinetics, Champaign, IL.
77. Lee H, Wang J, Gallagher D, Heshka S, Shen W, Chambers E, Heymsfield SB, Wang ZM (2006). Dual-energy X-ray absorptiometry: Validity of the Lunar Prodigy fan-beam system for body composition measurement in pediatrics. *Int J Body Comp Res* **4**, 81–6.
78. Claessens AL, Delbroek W, Lefevre J (2001). The use of different prediction equations for the assessment of body composition in young female gymnasts—Is there a best equation? In: Jürimäe T, Hills AP (eds.), *Body composition assessment in children and adolescent*, pp. 139–54. Karger, Basel.
79. Slaughter MH, Lohman TG, Boileau RA, Horswill CA, Stillman RJ, Van Loan MD, Bemben DA (1988). Skinfold equations for estimation of body fatness in children and youth. *Hum Biol* **60**, 709–23.

80. Roemmich JN, Clark PA, Weltman A, Rogol AD (1997). Alterations in growth and body composition during puberty. I. Comparing multicompartment body composition models. *J Appl Physiol* **83**, 927–35.
81. Dezenberg CV, Nagy TR, Gower BA, Johnson R, Goran MI (1999). Predicting body composition from anthropometry in pre-adolescent children. *Int J Obesity* **23**, 253–9.
82. Bellisari A, Roche AF (2005). Anthropometry and ultrasound. In: Heymsfield SB, Lohman TG, Wang ZM, Going SB (eds.), *Human body composition* (2nd ed.), pp. 109–27. Human Kinetics, Champaign, IL.
83. Sun SS, Chumlea WC (2005). Statistical methods. In: Heymsfield SB, Lohman TG, Wang ZM, Going SB (eds.), *Human body composition* (2nd ed.), pp. 151–60. Human Kinetics, Champaign, IL.
84. Wells JCK (2001). A critique of the expression of paediatric body composition data. *Arch Dis Child* **85**, 67–72.
85. Chumlea WmC, Sun SS (2005). Bioelectrical Impedance Analysis. In: Heymsfield SB, Lohman TG, Wang ZM, Going SB (eds.), *Human body composition* (2nd ed.), pp. 79–88. Human Kinetics, Champaign, IL.
86. Chumlea WmC, Guo SS (1997). Bioelectrical impedance: A history, research issues, and recent consensus. In: Carlson-Newberry SJ, Costello RB (eds.), *Emerging technologies for nutrition research,* pp. 169–92. National Academy Press, Washington, D.C.
87. Patterson R (2000). Bioelectric impedance measurements. In: Bronzino JD (ed.), *The biomedical engineering handbook,* Vol. I (2nd ed.), pp. 73(1)–73(8). CRC Press LLC, Boca Raton, FL.
88. Going S, Davis R (2001). Body composition. In: American College of Sports Medicine (eds.), *ACSM's resource manual for guidelines for exercise testing and prescription* (4th ed.), pp. 391–400. Lippincott Williams and Wilkins, Philadelphia, PA.
89. Veldhuis JD, Roemmich JN, Richmond EJ, Rogol AD, Lovejoy JC, Sheffield-Moore M, Mauras N, Bowers CY (2005). Endocrine control of body composition in infancy, childhood, and puberty. *Endocr Rev* **26**, 114–46.
90. Andreacci JL, Dixon CB, Lagomarsine M, Ledezma C, Goss FL, Robertson RJ (2006). Effect of maximal treadmill test on percent body fat using leg-to-leg bioelectrical impedance analysis in children. *J Sport Med Phys Fitness* **46**, 454–7.
91. Goss FL, Robertson RJ, Dube J, Rutkowski J, Andreacci J, Lenz B, Ranalli J, Frazee K (2003). Does exercise testing affect the bioelectrical impedance assessment of body composition in children? *Pediatr Exerc Sci* **15**, 216–22.
92. Hills AP, Lyell L, Byrne NM (2001). An evaluation of the methodology for the assessment of body composition in children and adolescents. In: Jürimäe T, Hills AP (eds.), *Body composition assessment in children and adolescent,* pp. 1–13. Karger, Basel.
93. Beunen G (2001). Physical growth, maturation and performance. In: Eston R, Reilly T (eds.), *Kinanthropometry and exercise physiology laboratory manual, Vol. 1: Anthropometry. Tests, procedures and data,* pp. 65–90. Routledge, London.
94. Beunen G, Malina RM (1996). Growth and biological maturation: Relevance to athletic performance. In: Bar-Or O (ed.), *The child and adolescent athlete,* pp. 3–24. Blackwell, Oxford.
95. Roche AF (1986). Bone growth and maturation. In: Falkner F, Tanner JM (eds.) *Human growth. Volume 2. Postnatal growth, neurobiology,* pp. 25–60. Plenum, New York.
96. Tanner JM (1962). *Growth at adolescence* (2nd ed.). Blackwell, Oxford.
97. Acheson RM (1966). Maturation of the skeleton. In: Falkner F (ed.), *Human development,* pp. 465–502. Saunders, Philadelphia, PA.
98. Boas F (1893). The growth of children. *Science* **19/20**, 257–7; 281–2; 351–2.
99. Beunen GP, Rogol AD, Malina RM (2006). Indicators of biological maturation and secular changes in biological maturation. *Food Nutr Bull* **27**, S244–56.
100. Marshall WA, Tanner JM (1969). Variation in pattern of pubertal changes in girls. *Arch Dis Child* **44**, 291–303.
101. Marshall WA, Tanner JM (1970). Variations in the pattern of pubertal changes in boys. *Arch Dis Child* **45**, 13–23.
102. Prader A (1966). Testicular size: Assessment and clinical importance. *Triangle* **7**, 240–3.
103. Zachman M, Prader A, Kind HP, Hafliger H, Budliger H (1974). Testicular volume during adolescence: Cross-sectional and longitudinal studies. *Helv Paediatr Acta* **29**, 61–72.
104. Gasser T, Köhler W, Müller H-G, Kneip A, Largo R, Molinari L, Prader A (1984). Velocity and acceleration of height growth using kernel estimation. *Ann Hum Biol* **11**, 397–411.
105. Hauspie R, Chrzastek-Spruch H (1999). Growth models: Possibilities and limitations. In: Johnston FE, Eveleth PB, Zemel B (eds.), *Human growth in context,* pp. 15–24. Smith-Gordon, London.
106. Marubini E (1978). Mathematical handling of long-term longitudinal data. In: Falkner F, Tanner JM (eds.), *Human growth. Volume 1. Principles and prenatal growth,* pp. 209–25. Plenum, New York.
107. Roche AF, Wainer H, Thissen D (1975). *Skeletal maturity: The knee joint as a biological indicator.* Plenum Press, New York.
108. Tanner JM, Whitehouse RH, Healy MJR (1962). *A new system for estimating skeletal maturity from the hand and wrist, with standards derived from a study of 2,600 healthy British children.* International Children's Centre, Paris.
109. Tanner JM, Whitehouse RH, Marshall WA, Healy MJR, Goldstein H (1975). *Assessment of skeletal maturity and prediction of adult height (TW2 method).* Academic Press, New York.
110. Tanner JM, Whitehouse RH, Cameron N, Marshall WA, Healy MJR, Goldstein H (1983). *Assessment of skeletal maturity and prediction of adult height* (2nd ed.). Academic Press, New York.
111. Tanner JM, Healy MJR, Goldstein H, Cameron N (2001). *Assessment of skeletal maturity and prediction of adult height (TW3 method)* (3rd ed.). Saunders, London.
112. Bayley N, Pinneau SR (1952). Tables for predicting adult height from skeletal age: Revised for use with the Greulich-Pyle hand standards. *J Pediatr* **40**, 423–41.
113. Roche AF, Wainer H, Thissen D (1975). *Predicting adult stature for individuals. (Monographs in Paediatrics 3).* Karger, Basel.
114. Roche AF, Wainer H, Thissen D (1975). The RWT method for the prediction of adult stature. *Pediatrics* **56**, 1026–33.
115. Khamis HJ, Roche AF (1994). Predicting adult stature without using skeletal age: The Khamis-Roche method. *Pediatrics* **94**, 504–7 (see *Pediatrics* 1995; 95: 457, for the corrected version of the tables).
116. Beunen GP, Malina RM, Lefevre J, Claessens AL, Renson R, Simons J (1997). Prediction of adult stature and non-invasive assessment of biological maturation. *Med Sci Sport Exerc* **29**, 225–30.
117. Malina RM, Dompier TP, Powell JW, Barron MJ, Moore MT (2007). Validation of a non-invasive maturity estimate relative to skeletal age in youth football. *Clin J Sport Med* **17**, 362–8.
118. Mirwald RL, Baxter-Jones ADG, Bailey DA, Beunen GP (2002). An assessment of maturity from anthropometric measurements. *Med Sci Sport Exerc* **34**, 689–94.
119. Malina RM, Claessens AL, Van Aken K, Thomis M, Lefevre J, Philippaerts R, Beunen GP (2006). Maturity offset in gymnasts: Application of a prediction equation. *Med Sci Sport Exerc* **38**, 1342–7.
120. Greulich WW, Pyle SI(1959). *Radiographic atlas of skeletal development of the hand and wrist* (2nd ed.). Stanford University Press, Stanford, CA.
121. Todd TW (1937). *Atlas of skeletal maturation.* Mosby, St. Louis.
122. Roche AF, Chumlea WC, Thissen D (1988). *Assessing the skeletal maturity of the hand-wrist: Fels Method.* CC Thomas, Springfield, IL.
123. Tanner JM, Gibbons RD (1994). A computerized image analysis system for estimating Tanner-Whitehouse 2 bone age. *Horm Res* **42**, 282–7.
124. Tanner JM, Oshman D, Lindgren G, Grunbaum JA, Elsouki R, Labarthe D (1994). Reliability and validity of computer-assisted estimates of Tanner-Whitehouse skeletal maturity (CASAS): Comparison with the manual method. *Horm Res* **42**, 288–94.

125. Roemmich JN, Blizzard RM, Peddada SD, Malina RM, Roche AF, Tanner JM, Rogol AD (1997). Longitudinal assessment of hormonal and physical alterations during normal puberty in boys. IV: Prediction of adult height by the Bailey-Pinneau, Roche-Wainer-Thissen, and Tanner-Whitehouse methods compared. *Am J Hum Biol* **9**, 371–80.
126. Malina RM, Chamorro M, Serratosa L, Morate F (2007). TW3 and Fels skeletal ages in elite youth soccer players. *Ann Hum Biol* **34**, 265–72.
127. Dvorak J, George J, Junge A, Hodler J (2006). Age determination by magnetic resonance imaging of the wrist in adolescent male football players. *Br J Sports Med* **41**, 45–52.
128. Malina RM (2005). Estimating passport age from bone age: Fallacy. *Insight: The F.A. Coaches Assoc J (Autumn/Winter)* **8**, 23–7.
129. Malina RM, Beunen G (2007). Comment on age determination in adolescent male football players: It does not work! *Br J Sports Med*, (electronic letter http://bjsm.bmj.com/cgi/eletters/41/1/45).
130. Demirjian A (1986). Dentition. In: Falkner F, Tanner JM (eds.), *Human growth. Volume 2. Postnatal growth, neurobiology*, pp. 269–98. Plenum, New York.
131. Demirjian A, Goldstein H, Tanner JM (1973). A new system for dental age assessment. *Hum Biol* **45**, 211–27.
132. Liversidge HM, Chaillet N, Mörnstad H, Nyström M, Rowlings K, Taylor J, Willems G (2006). Timing of Demirijan's tooth formation stages. *Ann Hum Biol* **33**, 454–70.
133. Liversidge HM, Speechly T, Hector MP (1999). Dental maturation in British children: Are Demirjian's standards applicable? *Int J Paediatr Dent* **9**, 263–9.
134. Demirjian A, Buschang PH, Tanguay R, Patterson DK (1985). Interrelationships among measures of somatic, skeletal, dental, and sexual maturity. *Am J Orthodontics* **88**, 433–8.
135. Bielicki T, Koniarek J, Malina RM (1984). Interrelationships among certain measures of growth and maturation rate in boys during adolescence. *Ann Hum Biol* **11**, 201–10.
136. Bielicki T (1975). Interrelationships between various measures of maturation rate in girls during adolescence. *Studies Physl Anthropol* **1**, 51–64.
137. Nicolson AB, Hanley C (1953). Indices of physiological maturity: Deviation and interrelationships. *Child Dev* **24**, 3–38.

CHAPTER 4

Muscle strength

Nathalie J. Farpour-Lambert
and Cameron J.R. Blimkie

Introduction

This chapter focuses on laboratory-based strength assessment techniques and considerations for the paediatric population. The theoretical and practical considerations underlying strength assessment in adults[1,2] and children and adolescents[3–5] have been previously and thoroughly reviewed. This chapter will supplement, with emphasis on paediatric considerations, but not replicate, the material covered in these references. The topic of strength development and its correlates or determinants during childhood are beyond the scope of this chapter. These issues have been thoroughly reviewed elsewhere[5–9] and are elaborated in Chapter 15 of this volume. The reader is encouraged to refer to these previous works for a more complete understanding of the general issues pertaining to strength development and assessment in children.

Strength is a construct which is generally understood to represent the ability of muscles to exert force either for the purpose of resisting or moving external loads (including the body) or to propel objects (again including one's own body) against gravity. In youth sport, strength is recognized as a variable, but nonetheless it is an important determinant for performance success in many activities, especially during the adolescent years. Strength may exert its influence on sports performance in a permissive manner, for example, by increasing joint stability and thereby minimizing the risk of musculoskeletal injury, or it may have a more direct influence by providing the increased force required to differentiate successful from less successful performances in sports where strength is a factor. Strength is but one of numerous traits, however, which may influence success in sports. The relationship between strength and other fitness components, including anaerobic power, aerobic power, and speed, and their relative importance in determining success in sport remains to be satisfactorily determined in the paediatric population. Strength is also an important health-related fitness component, which, for example, may influence the timing of, and success of re-entry into sport after injury, or one's physical independence, for example, ability to move about freely without assistance, particularly in children with chronic paediatric diseases. Strength may also be an enabling factor which facilitates the development of persistent physical activity habits in youth and the establishment of positive attitudes towards exercise, which may carry over into adulthood. Again, the importance of strength, in relation to health status during childhood and adolescence, has not been addressed extensively. Given its potential importance in the realms of sport, rehabilitation medicine, and health, not surprisingly, then, strength assessment is a relevant and important issue for the paediatric population.

There are numerous rationales for strength assessment in the paediatric population, and many of these are exemplified in current practices of strength testing by various groups working with children. Strength testing may be used to describe developmental patterns of muscle function for the purpose of establishing normative values against which to compare muscle function of children with various paediatric diseases. Standardized strength testing may be used to examine secular trends among different cohorts of children, trends which may be predictive of future population health risk or which may influence the direction of public policy in the areas of health and fitness planning and programming. As muscle is a major storage site for body protein, strength testing may provide a useful and non-invasive means of assessing the adequacy of skeletal muscle function and protein nutritional status in at risk paediatric populations. Clinically, strength assessment may be used to describe functional profiles of specific neuromuscular diseases, to determine the level of residual function following injury or surgical intervention, and to assess the effectiveness of various rehabilitation procedures. In sport, strength assessment may be used to determine the relative importance of strength for performance success, and subsequently to assist in the process of talent identification, providing a better match between the strength profiles of young athletes and the strength requirements of specific sports or positions within sports. Strength assessment may also be used to identify specific areas of muscle weakness in athletes which are then targeted for remedial training. Finally, strength assessment may be used in paediatric research to examine any number of issues such as the effectiveness of resistance training on strength development and sports performance, or the functional adaptation of muscle to various other controlled interventions such as weight loss and re-feeding.

Terminology

From a scientific perspective, strength is a specific construct that refers to the ability of muscle (single or group) to produce measurable force, torque, or moment, about a single joint or multiple joints, under a defined set of controlled conditions. For the purpose of this chapter, a slightly modified version of the definition of strength provided by Knuttgen and Kraemer[10] will be used: strength is defined as 'the maximal force, torque or moment developed by a muscle or muscle groups during one maximal voluntary or evoked action of unlimited duration, at a specified velocity of movement'. This definition captures the essence of traditional approaches to strength assessment which incorporates maximal voluntary efforts, but also includes the assessment of strength under conditions of involuntary or electrically stimulated conditions; the latter is a less common, but nevertheless viable additional condition for assessment of muscle function in humans, including children. For the purposes of this chapter, strength assessment will be considered for both voluntary and electrically stimulated conditions.

In most laboratories, muscle strength is expressed in units of force, torque, and moment, terms which refer similarly to the measurable tension generated by muscle in its activated state. In certain situations, particularly with athletic populations, strength is still measured in the units of the external load, for example, pounds (lb) or kilograms (kg), which are lifted in the execution of a weightlifting manoeuvre. These units adequately reflect the muscle forces required and applied to overcome external loads and are legitimate expressions of strength in this context. For most other purposes, however, and for the sake of international standardization, strength results should be expressed in units defined by The Système d'Unités Internationales (SI system): force in Newtons (N), torque in Newton metres (N·m), and moment in Newton metres (N·m^2). Some of the earlier literature reported strength in foot pounds (ft·lb), and for purposes of comparison can be converted to the equivalent SI units simply by multiplying by 1.355818 N·m.

The term force typically refers to the level of active tension generated by isolated muscle preparations *in vitro*, or to *in vivo* measurements of muscle tension where force is measured directly at the site of load application, for example, dynamometer pad, rather than distally to the point of application such as the central axis of rotation of dynamometer. In isolated muscle preparations, the measured tension is largely determined by the underlying morphological (size), physiological (muscle fibre type distribution, size, length, and activation), and biochemical (enzyme profiles) characteristics of the muscle, with no regard to biomechanical influences such as the angle of muscle insertion on joint articulations that can influence external forces measured *in vivo* in humans. In contrast, *in vivo* measurements of strength in humans, measured at the site of load application, are also influenced by factors extrinsic to the muscle *per se*, such as muscle angle of insertion.

The terms force and torque are often used interchangeably in the strength assessment literature, although in the strictest sense, torque represents the product of both intrinsic (muscle) and extrinsic (anatomical, biomechanical, and mechanical) factors on muscle strength expression. Torque is an expression of the effective measurable tension, which will vary as a function of the intrinsic muscle characteristics as above, the distance of the point of muscle insertion on the skeletal lever from the axis of rotation of the involved joint, and the angle of insertion of the active muscle's tendon on the skeletal lever. This relationship is presented schematically in Fig. 4.1 and is described by the equation

$$\text{Torque (Tq)} = Td\sin\Phi$$

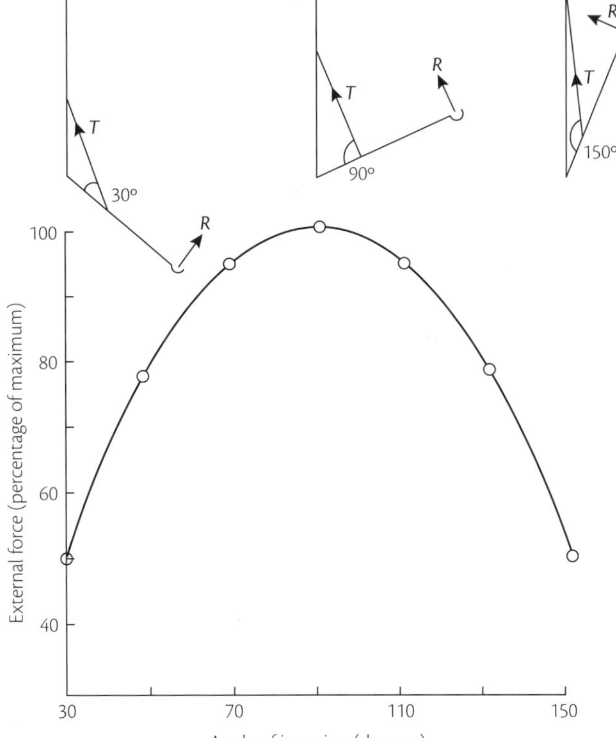

Fig. 4.1 The effect of angle of muscle insertion on the external torque produced by a muscle during a concentric shortening action. *T* is the direction of muscle contraction (shortening) and *R* is the external load or resistance. Adapted from Lakomy.[11]

where T is the intrinsically generated constant force or tension of the active muscle transmitted via the tendon to the bone, d is the distance from the point of tendon insertion on the bone to the axis of joint rotation, and Φ is the angle of tendon insertion on the bone.[11]

Static strength measured at discrete joint angles with the joint position fixed and the dynamometer axis of rotation distal to the point of application of the resistance, for example, during isometric testing using an isokinetic dynamometer, is typically expressed in terms of torque. If tension is measured directly at the source of application of the resistance such as with hand grip dynamometry or manometry, or with custom-built dynamometers, then strength is more appropriately expressed as force.

Finally, activated muscles may also cause continuous dynamic angular rotation of skeletal segments around joint axes: strength measured under these conditions is expressed more commonly as torque or joint moments. As with static torque measurements, the measured tension at any point throughout the range of motion is also dependent on the parameters T, d, and sin Φ. *In vivo*, statically determined torques and dynamically determined moments are also influenced by extrinsic mechanical factors such as the length of the moment arm, the distance between the point of attachment of the limb segment to the testing device, and the axis of joint rotation—not to be confused with the anatomical factor d, the distance from the point of tendon insertion on the bone to the axis of joint rotation. Although it is important conceptually to understand how muscle morphology and physiology, muscle–tendon anatomy, joint biomechanics, and the mechanics of dynamometry relate to the terminology used to describe muscle strength in children, it is even more important to understand and account for the potential influence of these myriad factors in the interpretation of strength assessment in the paediatric population. The significance of each of these factors in the interpretation of strength assessment in children will be addressed in a later section.

It is evident from above that both static and dynamic muscle strength, regardless of the terminology by which strength is expressed, are influenced not only by the intrinsic physiological characteristics of the active muscle, but also by the joint-specific musculoskeletal anatomical and biomechanical factors. Whereas the distance between the muscle insertion and the axis of joint rotation remains constant within individuals during any particular strength assessment manoeuvre, in many joint actions (such as elbow flexion), the angle of muscle insertion will change with varying limb position within its range of motion, resulting in variable measurable torques at different joint positions. In addition, differences in the distance of muscle insertion from the axis of joint rotation among individuals of varying size, for example, short and tall children of the same age, will influence external torque measurements and must be considered when assessing and comparing 'muscle function' *per se*, independent of biomechanical influences among heterogeneously sized children. It is important to understand how the various intrinsic and extrinsic factors described above can influence the outcome and interpretation of strength assessment results. For example, the reproducibility of repeated strength measurements (torques or moments) for a given individual made under varying conditions of moment arm length would be poor, if correction was not made for the differences in moment arm length between testing sessions. Similarly, higher measured torques or moments in a tall child compared to the torques or moments in a shorter child of the same age and with comparable muscle cross-sectional area (CSA) might be attributed falsely to a greater intrinsic force producing capacity of the taller boy's muscle, when in fact the difference might be wholly accounted for by the biomechanical advantage afforded to the taller boy by the greater distance of tendon insertion from the axis of joint rotation—assuming that the tendon insertion distance from the axis of rotation varies in proportion to the length of the skeletal segment being acted upon. Numerous other factors including age, gender, maturity, level of physical activity, and training status can also influence the expression of strength,[7,9] and similar biomechanical influences must be considered carefully in the interpretation of strength assessment data from children.

Skeletal muscle active states

For all practical purposes, whether strength is being measured under voluntary or involuntary conditions, muscle activation results in one of three different muscle action types: concentric, isometric, or eccentric actions. A schematic representation of these different types of muscle actions is presented in Fig. 4.2. It is important to understand the differences between these different types of muscle actions, because their differences dictate in large part, which is the most relevant type of action to incorporate during strength testing.

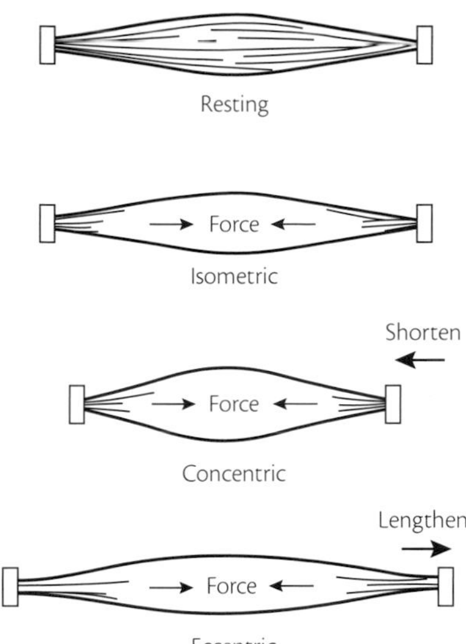

Fig. 4.2 Three basic types of muscle actions: isometric (no change in length with fixed attachments), concentric (force generation brings the bony attachments closer together), and eccentric (muscle is forcibly lengthened because external force is pulling the bony attachments further apart while the muscle is attempting to shorten). Adapted from Knuttgen and Kraemer.[10]

In a concentric action, the distance between the origin and insertion of the muscle becomes shorter (the muscle length shortens), and the generated muscle tension is greater than the opposing resistance. These types of actions result in dynamic limb or trunk movement of variable or constant external velocity. Concentric actions of variable velocity are more common in activities of daily living and sports than the more rarely occurring constant velocity or isokinetic actions; however, the latter are easily achievable now with sophisticated dynamometry, and are rapidly becoming the norm rather than the exception in strength testing in rehabilitation medicine, fitness testing, and exercise science research.

Confusion has arisen in the past regarding the proper usage of the terms, concentric and isotonic muscle actions. The term isotonic typically was used to describe dynamic muscle actions that were common manoeuvres in various sports, for example, knee extension in kicking a soccer ball or elbow flexion in single arm biceps curl strength training exercise. As the roots of the term suggest, isotonic actions imply that a constant (iso) force (tonic) is applied throughout the range of motion of a manoeuvre. Although the external resistance or load may remain constant in these situations (mass of the soccer ball or dumbbell), the intrinsic muscle tension is not constant during these actions and will vary as a function of muscle length (external joint angles) and contraction speed (external angular velocities), as described by the force–velocity–length relationship.[2,11] Truly isotonic muscle actions rarely occur in human performance and continued use of this term to describe 'muscle action type' in the strength assessment literature should be discouraged.[10] The term isotonic has nevertheless become solidly entrenched in the exercise science literature, and because of its familiarity may still be used legitimately to describe strength assessment techniques that incorporate constant external loading, for example, a weightlifting task, where the limb velocity and intrinsic muscle tension will vary as a function of joint angle

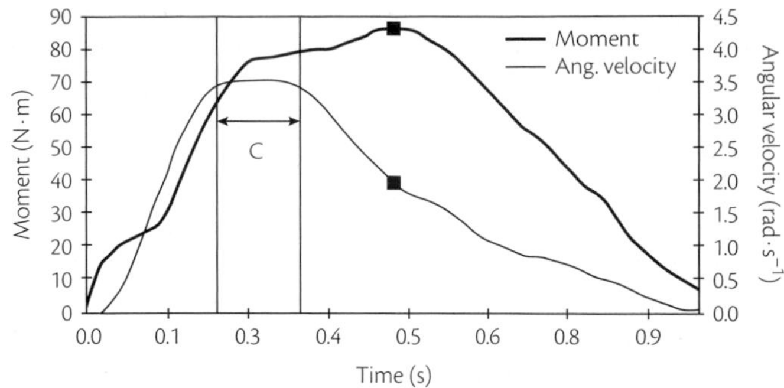

Fig. 4.3 Moment and angular velocity data during a knee extension test at a preset angular velocity of 3.15 rad·s^{-1}. Notice the shorter constant-velocity phase and the longer acceleration and deceleration periods. The maximum moment indicated by the square is clearly outside the isokinetic phase, and was recorded when angular velocity of the joint was decreasing and was approximately 2.0 rad·s^{-1}. Adapted from Baltzopoulos and Kellis.[3]

during the manoeuvre. The term isoinertial has recently been used to replace and describe traditional isokinetic strength tests.[1] This term provides a more accurate description of the mechanics of these types of manoeuvres, but perhaps at the expense of further terminological confusion.

A word of caution also about concentric isokinetic actions. The term implies that the movement velocity (kinetic) is constant (iso) throughout the range of movement. Although isokinetic movements are performed at a constant preset angular velocity selected by the test administrator, the proportion of the movement, which is actually performed under truly isokinetic conditions, is variable and dependent on the chosen angular velocity and the range of motion of the exercise.[3] Generally, the higher the preset angular velocity and the smaller the range of motion of the exercise, the smaller the isokinetic portion of the exercise (Fig. 4.3). Muscle moments reported from the non-isokinetic portion of a strength testing manoeuvre misrepresent the true isokinetic capability of the muscle and are problematic to the valid interpretation of strength results. This effect may be even more problematic in testing situations involving children with muscle weakness, where movements are composed solely of limb acceleration and deceleration without a plateau phase to the strength curve, or in situations where the joint range of motion is limited due to injury or chronic disease, for example, arthritis. In these situations, recorded moments from the non-isokinetic phase of the movement should be corrected,[12] or perhaps an alternative muscle action, for example, isometric, would provide a more valid measure of the strength capability of the muscle.

Eccentric muscle actions represent a second type of dynamic muscle activity. In eccentric muscle actions, the intrinsic muscle tension is less than the externally applied load or resistance, the muscle lengthens and the distance between limbs or the joint angular displacement increases. Eccentric muscle actions are quite common in activities of daily living, for example, walking down stairs, and in sports performance, for example, dipping action at the knee in preparation for jumping in volleyball, but compared to isometric and concentric muscle actions they have not been used as extensively in strength assessment, especially in the paediatric population.

In isometric muscle actions, the intrinsic muscle tension matches the external resistance, and although the muscle is in an active state, there is no visible or measurable change in the external length of the

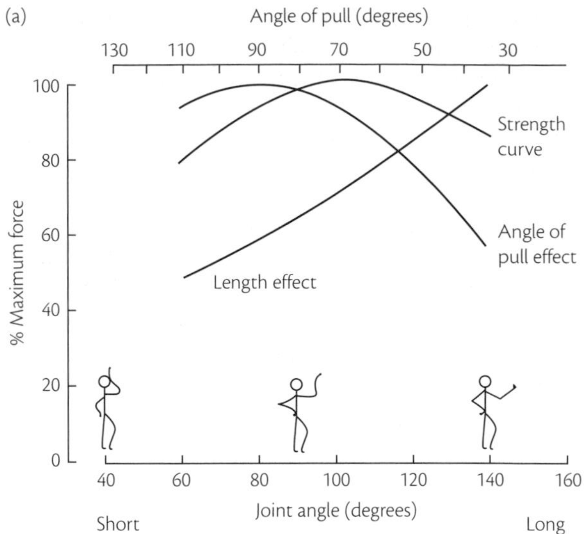

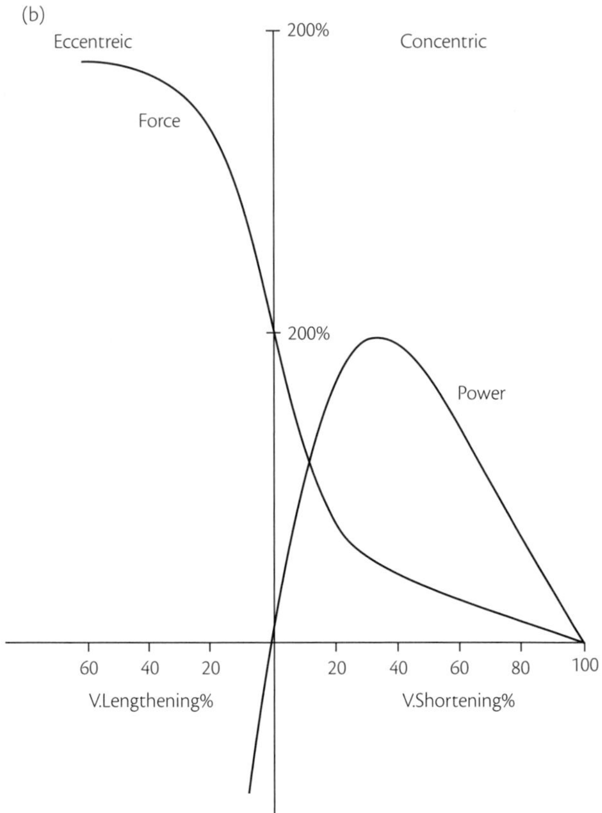

Fig. 4.4 (**a**) Effect of muscle length and angle of pull upon elbow flexion strength. The length–tension effect and the angle of pull effect interact to produce the strength curve for elbow flexion. The length effect acts to increase muscle tension from the shortest to longest muscle lengths, through the range of movement depicted. The longest length corresponds to an elbow joint angle (bottom horizontal axis) of 140°. In contrast, the optimum angle of pull (90°—top horizontal axis) occurs at a joint angle of 80°. Thus, the peak of the resultant strength curve, expressed as a per cent of maximum force, would be expected to occur somewhere between joint angles of 80° and 140°; in this example, it occurs at a joint angle of about 100°. Adapted from Sale and Norman.[13] (**b**) Schematic representation of the effect of velocity of contraction, expressed as a percentage of the maximum velocity, on force production (force–velocity relationship) in relation to isometric (0 velocity at the midpoint of the horizontal axis), concentric (shortening) velocity to right of the centre axis, and eccentric (lengthening) velocity to the left of the centre axis. Adapted from Sale and Norman.[13]

muscle and, therefore, no resultant movement. Isometric actions occur frequently in sport to stabilize joints, for example, during the neck-bridging manoeuvre in freestyle wrestling, and the drive swing in golf, as well as in activities of daily living, for example, trunk stabilization when lifting groceries or sneezing. Since there is no apparent joint movement, isometric muscle actions result in static muscle activity.

It should be evident that each of these three specific muscle actions will provide measures of strength which reflect muscle activation under specific testing conditions of variable muscle length (lengthened or shortened), joint position, and/or movement velocity. Comparison of the strength producing capacity of muscle during concentric, isometric, and eccentric actions, across the continuum of variable muscle lengths, joint positions, and shortening/lengthening velocities, has been extensively investigated *in vitro* (isolated muscle preparations) and *in vivo* in adults, and described by the classic muscle length–joint angle–tension[13] and force–velocity relationships.[10,13,14] These relationships are depicted schematically in Fig. 4.4(a) and (b).

In short, at a given joint angle or muscle length, isometric static strength is typically greater than concentric strength measured at the same joint angle during a dynamic shortening action, but is perhaps slightly less or not different *in vivo* from eccentric strength measured at the same joint angle during a dynamic lengthening action. During dynamic concentric muscle action, strength typically decreases with increasing joint angular velocity, whereas it may increase only slightly initially or not change with increasing dynamic eccentric muscle action, throughout a muscle's range of motion. During static isometric muscle action, peak strength occurs at an optimal muscle length or joint angle, which varies for different muscles or muscle groups; strength is typically (for most muscle groups) lower on either side of this optimal length and decreases progressively with increased shortening or lengthening beyond this point (Fig. 4.5). These classic relationships have been established mostly for adults, although limited studies in children suggest that the length–tension and force–velocity relationships generally also hold true for isometric, concentric, and eccentric muscle actions in the paediatric population.[15–19]

These relationships have a significant influence on strength outcome, and the accuracy of the interpretation of strength assessment is highly dependent on a full appreciation of the interaction between these relationships. The validity of strength comparisons among different children, within the same child at different times, or between children and adults requires first and foremost that similar muscle actions be contrasted, and that comparisons are made either at the same joint angle or muscle length for isometric actions, or identical angular velocities or limb movement speeds for dynamic concentric or eccentric muscle actions. Other factors besides these, which will

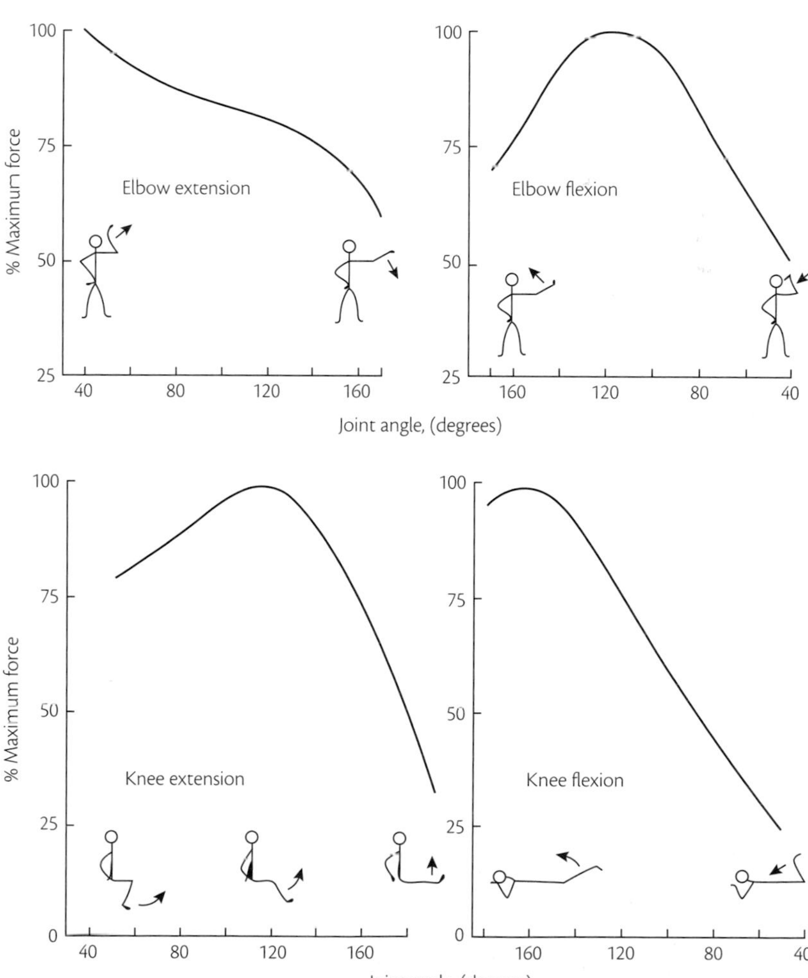

Fig. 4.5 Schematic representation of strength curves for selected muscle groups and exercise tests through given ranges of movement. Note that the shape of the strength curves varies for different movements. Adapted from Sale and Norman.[13]

be addressed later in the chapter, will particularly influence the validity and reliability of strength assessment results in children, but these are by far the most salient issues considered in assuring the validity of strength assessment procedures in children and adults.

Determinants of a strength assessment method

In keeping with the principle of specificity,[2,20] the strength assessment method should include the specific prime movers involved in the action of interest; isolate the type of muscle action, which is most characteristic of its involvement in sport, training, or rehabilitation; and include exercises that mimic the activity movement pattern of interest as closely as possible in terms of range of joint angle involvement and velocity or speed of limb movement. Selection of the most appropriate testing method depends first and foremost on identifying and isolating as closely as possible the specific muscle or muscle groups to be tested. A decision must then be made about the relevance of the different types of muscle actions in relation to the specific purpose of the test. Decisions regarding the joint angle of testing, the testing velocity, and the degree of replication of the movement pattern are then made, while trying to satisfy both the requirements of the specificity principle and individual constraints imposed by the peculiarities of various sports, injuries, rehabilitative exercises, or current medical status. Practical issues such as the availability of size-appropriate or disability-modified equipment will also influence the testing method to be selected. As a general principle, the more specific the strength testing method, the more valid the strength assessment results. At the very least, the selected method should satisfy the principle of muscle or muscle group specificity; muscle action type is perhaps not important to mimic since there is a moderate to strong positive correlation[21] between the three muscle action types (at least in adults), and although not ideal, strength results from one type of muscle action may serve as a surrogate for another type.

The validity of strength assessment results, and particularly the interpretation of these results, is also strongly influenced by the reliability or reproducibility of the test measurement. Reliability, which reflects the amount of variability in repeated measurements made at different intervals (short term or long term), is determined primarily by biological variation and experimental sources of error. Biological variability reflects the consistency with which an individual can perform a given task, and this is dependent primarily on intrinsic biological, physiological, and psychological factors. The main purpose of strength assessment is to isolate and detect biological sources of variation in strength performance, free of experimental sources of error. Experimental error is inevitable in any testing situation, but it should be kept to a minimum. Standard testing procedures for minimizing experimental error, with special considerations for children, which apply to strength testing for all muscle action types, will be provided later in the chapter. These testing procedures will improve the reliability of the strength assessment results and provide greater sensitivity to detect biological sources of variation in the child's ability to exert maximal muscle force.

The decision to incorporate a specific mode of muscle action or a specific type of test in strength assessment will depend in part on the level of required precision and the reliability of the selected strength method. If extremely precise measurements are required to detect subtle changes in strength, for example, short-term changes in twitch torque due to nutritional intervention, then the greater the importance of the reliability of the measurement. Reliability tolerances, although always important, are perhaps less critical, the larger the expected or anticipated difference in strength performance.

Isometric strength assessment

In the laboratory, isometric strength is usually assessed by cable tensiometry, dedicated isometric dynamometers, for example, hand grip dynamometer, or by custom-designed dynamometers consisting of a testing frame which is configured with a force transducer or strain gauge. The former provides greater versatility in terms of the number of muscle groups that can be tested, whereas the latter two approaches are usually a bit more constricting and limit testing only to a select number of muscles or muscle groups. Examples of custom-made dynamometers used to test isometric elbow flexion and ankle plantar and dorsiflexion strength in children are depicted in Fig. 4.6.[22,23] Because custom-designed dynamometers usually provide a greater degree of muscle or muscle group isolation and stability, these are often the dynamometers of choice when assessing muscle function using electrical stimulation protocols. In addition, most commercially available isokinetic dynamometers can also be used to test isometric muscle strength, simply by presetting the joint angular velocity control at 0 rad·s^{-1} or 0 deg·s^{-1} (1.0 rad·s^{-1} = 57.307 deg·s^{-1}).

Since muscle strength varies as a function of muscle length or joint angle, a complete assessment of the muscle's isometric force producing capacity requires multiple tests at various joint angles throughout the range of motion of interest. Repetitive testing of this nature is time consuming and fatiguing to both the subject and the test administrator. Multiple joint angle isometric testing protocols can also be very tedious, contributing to boredom and poor subject motivation. This may be of greater concern when testing children, who generally have shorter attention spans than adults, or children with chronic diseases that may predispose to early onset central (anaemias) or peripheral muscle (mitochondrial myopathies) fatigue. Nevertheless, isometric strength testing can be accomplished relatively inexpensively if cable tensiometry or dedicated isometric dynamometers, for example, hand grip or back lift dynamometers, are used, and cable tensiometry has the additional advantage of being more readily modifiable than commercially available isokinetic dynamometers for the extreme variations in body size experienced in paediatric exercise testing. An additional advantage of isometric strength testing, especially in a clinical setting, is that it can be used to measure strength safely, without risk of aggravation, within the residual functional range of an injured or pathological joint.

There is no agreed standard protocol for assessing isometric strength in children, or for that matter, adults. When performing isometric testing, adequate time must be provided to permit the development of peak force. In adults, this is usually achieved within 5 s from the initiation of the test. Similarly in children, voluntary peak isometric strength is usually achieved within 2–5 s of a given trial.[22–29] A minimum of 30 s is usually given between consecutive trials and subjects typically perform between 2 and 5 trials for a specific muscle group. The highest of all trials results, or the average of the most consistent results, when more than one trial is performed, may be used as the criterion measure of isometric strength.[28,30,31]

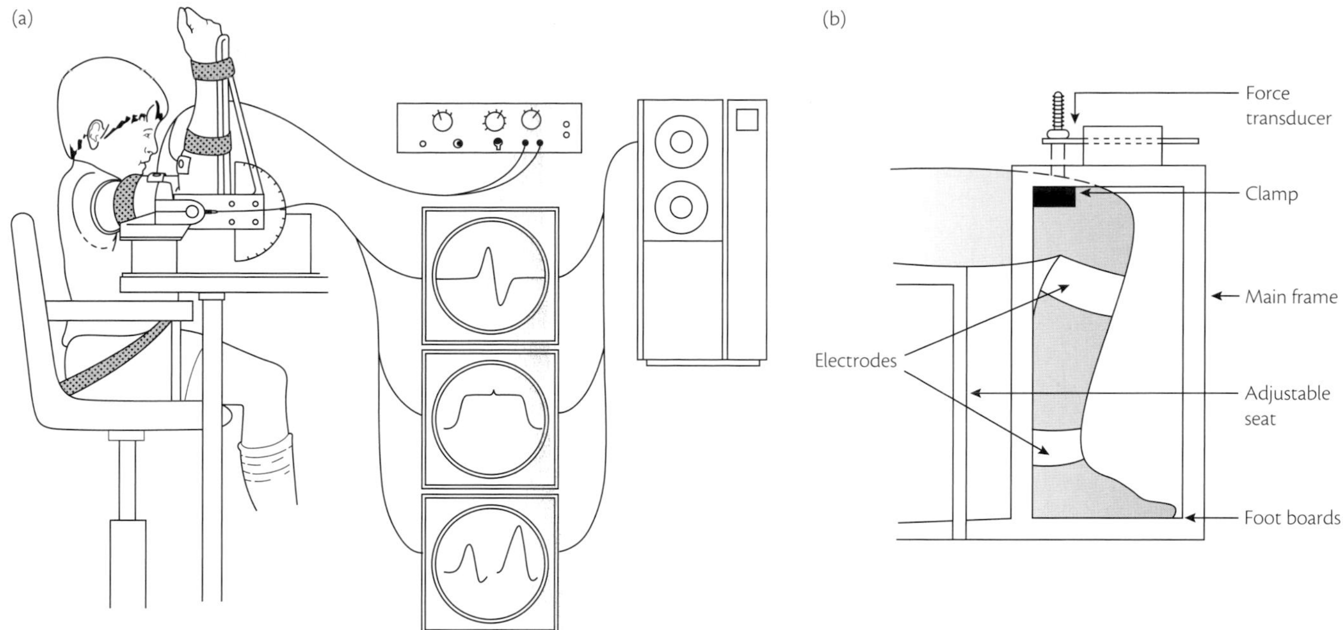

Fig. 4.6 (**a**) Schematic representation of the experimental procedures for the determination of voluntary strength, motor unit activation, and contractile properties of the elbow flexor muscle group in children. Adapted from Blimkie *et al.*[22] (**b**) Schematic representation of the dynamometer and experimental set-up for measuring maximal voluntary and electrically evoked ankle plantar flexor forces in children. Adapted from Davies.[23]

If only one joint angle is to be assessed, which represents the isometric peak force producing capacity of the muscle, then the test administrator must establish *a priori*, on the basis of the length–tension relationship, the optimal joint angle at which to perform the test. It is important to remember that the optimal joint angle varies across muscle groups. The isometric length–tension relationship has not been thoroughly described for all major muscle groups in children, and neither should this relationship be assumed to be constant across different developmental stages, disease conditions, or identical to adults. Ideally, if testing is to be done at only a single joint angle, then the selection should be based on individually determined muscle-specific length–tension relationships, akin to the procedure used to determine optimal breaking force for the assessment of peak anaerobic power from the force–velocity and force–power relationships during leg cycling[32] (see Chapter 5). In practice, however, and to reduce assessment time, isometric tests are usually carried out at one or several predetermined joint angles that are constant for all subjects. The preselected joint angle may be optimal for some, but certainly not for all, and testing expediency is gained at the price of compromised validity. In addition, the optimal joint angle might change with developmentally associated increases in muscle size and limb segment lengths, and these changes may compromise the validity of isometric strength comparisons (at both the individual and group levels) made at a constant joint angle, across different stages of development.

Although there are no supporting comparative data, habituation time to achieve consistent peak voluntary isometric force measures within the proscribed 5-s window may be greater in very young children compared to adolescents or adults. It may also be influenced by the level of prior testing or practice experience and the size of the muscle tested. In the authors' experience, younger children (under 8 years of age) are unfamiliar with the concept of rapid, almost instantaneous force development and the idea of force maintenance or plateau once the peak force is achieved. Consequently, there is a tendency for a slower rise phase to the peak and then oscillation between peak and suboptimal force production during the hold phase of the testing protocol. Consequently, longer habituation may be required for younger children first exposed to isometric strength testing. This process can be shortened by providing the child with visual feedback on an oscilloscope or computer screen, and as with adults, by offering verbal coaching to exert greater effort. Similarly, children seem to find it more difficult to elicit and consistently reproduce maximal voluntary isometric effort with larger than smaller muscle groups, for example, knee extension versus elbow flexion, and when the required action is unfamiliar, for example, maximal sustained dorsiflexion; slightly longer periods of habituation and more practice trials may also be required to improve the efficiency of isometric testing under these latter conditions.

The reliability of isometric strength measurements has not been examined extensively in children. Test–retest variations in the range of 3.7%–13.0% have been reported for several muscle groups in samples ranging from 10 to 18 years of age.[31,33–35] whereas slightly poorer reproducibility (15%) has been reported for a younger population (4–13 years of age) of both sexes, using myometry.[36] In 10-year-old boys, Wood and co-workers[35] reported test–retest variation of 6.6% (isometric elbow flexion at 90°) and 13.1% (isometric elbow extension at 27°). Test–retest correlations for isometric hand grip and leg strength were moderately high in boys between 7 and 12 years of age, ranging between 0.86 and 0.90, and reliability was slightly higher for simultaneous double ($r = 0.90$), compared to single right ($r = 0.86$) and left ($r = 0.88$) leg strength measures.[37] Another study examined the back extensor isometric strength in 6- to 10-year-old boys and girls[38] and observed test–retest correlation coefficients ranging from 0.55 to 0.79. High reliability has also been described for isometric strength measures in boys with muscular dystrophy.[39] Recently, normative reference data for maximal isometric grip strength in a population of 315 healthy children and adolescents from 6 to 19 years old have been established[40]; however, they did not report reliability indices. The variability reported in children lies within the range for adults, with a tendency towards the higher end of the range.[41] Clearly, more information is required regarding the effects of age, gender, disease, dynamometer type, muscle group, and exercise complexity (e.g. single joint vs. multiple joint, unilateral vs. bilateral) on the reliability of isometric strength measurements in the paediatric population.

Isokinetic concentric strength assessment

Today, isokinetic concentric muscle testing is more the norm, than the exception, in many research laboratories, orthopaedic clinics, and rehabilitation centres throughout the world. Although not yet used as extensively as with adults, isokinetic concentric strength testing is also being used more commonly with children. There are numerous commercially available dynamometers which provide an array of strength testing modalities, of which isokinetic concentric mode testing is one. The technical specifications and capabilities of these systems have been thoroughly reviewed elsewhere.[2,14]

Isokinetic assessment has several advantages over isometric testing. Most activities of daily living or actions in sport involve phases of dynamic concentric muscle action, and in this sense isokinetic testing may provide more specificity in terms of muscle action type than isometric or static testing. With isokinetic testing, the peak functional capacity of most major prime mover muscles can be assessed throughout their entire functional range of motion, in a single effort without the need for repositioning; this improves the efficiency of strength assessment, which may be especially important when assessing children. Perhaps most important, however, is the inherent safety of isokinetic actions, afforded by the mechanism of accommodating resistance. This, in addition to the preset velocity control, are the two primary features that distinguish isokinetic strength testing from most other modes. Accommodating resistance is a particularly important feature with naive subjects such as children, or in testing situations involving injured muscles, since the resistance mechanism will disengage when overexertion might otherwise initiate, or cause a reoccurrence of injury.

Isokinetic testing is not without its limitations, however. Human activities of daily living or actions in sport are rare if ever executed in an isokinetic mode, and often the joint angular velocity of movements of interest in youth sports, for example, pitching in baseball, far exceed the velocity capabilities of most commercially available dynamometers. In addition, reliable isokinetic measurements are possible only through the three cardinal planes of movement for the body, and most activities of humans are not constrained in such a manner. These limitations detract somewhat from the specificity principle, but no more so, than any of the other strength testing methods or modalities. Most commercially available isokinetic dynamometers have been designed for adults, necessitating equipment and procedural modifications when testing children.[4] Some authors place a back pad behind young children to allow their lower leg to hang freely from the edge of the seat[42,43]; however, one pad cannot accommodate all leg lengths. Others designed an adjustable seat[44,45] or employed the dynamometer's short arm usually used for upper extremity testing of adults in order to assess the knee strength of children.[43] Some dynamometers can now be ordered with paediatric specifications such as adjustable seat length and short attachments. Inconsistent equipment and procedural modifications within and between testing centres will have a negative impact on the reliability and reproducibility of isokinetic strength measures and compromise the validity of isokinetic strength comparisons.

When isokinetic testing comprising movement of a limb segment through a gravity-dependent position is performed, gravity correction procedures must be employed to ensure that forces against gravity are not underestimated and forces aided by gravity are not overestimated.[46] Current correction methods necessitate measurement of the gravitational moments of the limb lever arm system statically at a determined angular position. As children may have difficulty in relaxing completely, it is important to give sufficient time to the participants to obtain accurate measures. The investigator can check whether the subject loosens the muscles by shaking the foot or the hand before measurement. The validity of peak torque measurements rely on correct gravity correction procedures.

In addition, printed data reports from most of these isokinetic dynamometers will uncritically report the peak torque detected within the range of movement of the test, whether it occurs within or beyond the true isokinetic phase of a test manoeuvre. Particularly at high testing velocities and perhaps more so for children with relative muscle weakness, the highest peak torque will be caused by the impact artefact,[2] which is not a true measure of the isokinetic force producing capacity of the muscle (Fig. 4.7). These data would not provide a valid measure of isokinetic torque and should not be accepted as a representative of the maximal voluntary isokinetic torque producing capacity of the muscle. Windowing and filtering procedures should be used to account for the acceleration and deceleration artefacts and to select only constant velocity periods in the determination of the torque.[44,45]

Notwithstanding these largely mechanical considerations, perhaps the other most important potential limitation of isokinetic

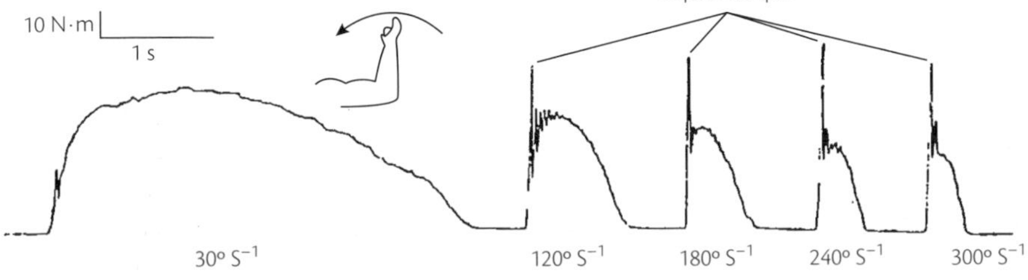

Fig. 4.7 Schematic representation of impact torque recordings during an isokinetic concentric elbow flexion exercise test at various joint angular velocities on a Cybex dynamometer. Note the predominance of the impact torque at the higher joint angular velocities, for example, from 120 deg·s^{-1} and above. Adapted from Sale.[2]

testing for children is the novelty of accommodating resistance action. Whereas the concept and feel of providing maximal voluntary effort against a resisting force throughout the full range of joint motion is foreign to children and adults alike, it is perhaps more difficult for children to grasp the idea and adapt to this type of action than adults. Either because of their immature motor control or simply the sheer novelty of the action, children seem to find it more difficult than adults to alternate continuously between reciprocal isokinetic concentric flexion and extension actions. Unfamiliarity with these testing modes and protocols may require either longer periods of habituation, or separate testing of the agonist and antagonist muscles in a reciprocal pair for younger children. Some authors report that concentric flexion and extension of the knee have to be separated by a time delay in 9- to 11-year-old children, in order to illicit maximal torque values.[47] The requirement for, sometimes, different testing protocols in children, depending on the age and level of motor development, confounds the interpretation of test results. Strength results obtained under the two conditions (continuous reciprocal vs. separate agonist and antagonist) may not be directly comparable since the physiological conditions (e.g. regional blood flow, muscle temperature, muscle prestretch, co-contraction, and inhibition) under which force is measured probably vary considerably between testing protocols. Further research is needed to examine the influence of these two conditions on muscle strength in children and adolescents.

As for isometric strength testing, there are no officially accepted testing protocols for concentric isokinetic strength testing for children. Testing guidelines and protocols are provided for each of the major muscle groups by most of the isokinetic manufacturers, but little, if any, consideration is ever given to potential modifications to these procedures, which might enhance the validity and reliability of isokinetic strength measurements in children. Since the primary purpose of isokinetic strength testing is to elicit maximal force production throughout the full range of joint motion, adequate warm-up is essential to minimize the risk of injury. There are no physiological reasons for providing a longer warm-up for children than for adults, but given the novelty of the isokinetic action a greater number of submaximal warm-up trials might be warranted to help facilitate habituation. Typically, children are provided a minimum of two and sometimes as many as eight submaximal trials at a given preset velocity, followed by two or three maximal efforts, a recovery period of at least 30 s and then the criterion test which may consist of a minimum of two and usually a maximum of six all-out efforts using either a continuous or interrupted protocol.[7,17,19,44,48,49] An alternative during the warm-up phase is to ask the subject to gradually increase the effort over the course of the practice trials so that maximal effort is achieved only during the last or penultimate effort.

Discounting the impact (Fig. 4.7) or overshoot torque,[2,50] the highest peak torque of all trails,[7,17,28,43,51] or the average peak torque of several trials at given angular velocities[48,49] have been used as the criterion measure of isokinetic concentric strength in children. Generally, during multiple velocity isokinetic testing, warm-up and criterion trials progress from lower to higher test velocities[42,43,48,51] as recommended by most manufacturers of commercial isokinetic dynamometers. Others[7,19,28] have randomized isokinetic testing velocity to eliminate ordering effects. This latter approach has proven safe with children, provided an adequate generalized and muscle-specific warm-up is given which incorporates all the preselected test velocities. Information regarding the effects of test protocol variability on the reliability and reproducibility of isokinetic concentric strength test results in children is sadly lacking. Standardization of isokinetic concentric test protocols for children is required.

The reliability and reproducibility of isokinetic concentric strength measures has not been investigated extensively in children. The mean score deviations in maximal isokinetic concentric strength of eight muscle groups (angular velocity unspecified) in 7- to 15-year-old boys and girls was 5.3%–5.8% for within-trial results and 7.9%–9.8% for trials conducted 7–10 days apart.[52] Isokinetic concentric hip flexion and extension peak torques were moderately reliable ($0.63 < r < 0.84$) at angular velocities of 30 and 90 deg·s^{-1} in boys of 6–10 years of age, whereas hip abduction and adduction measures were less reliable ($0.49 < r < 0.59$) at the same angular velocities, when retested 1–2 weeks apart.[48] More recently, isokinetic knee extension and flexion peak torques at an angular velocity of 100 deg·s^{-1} were shown to be highly reliable ($0.85 < r < 0.95$) and quite reproducible (8% and 12% coefficients of variation, respectively) in young boys, 6–8 years of age.[49] Similar results (coefficients of variation between 5% and 11%) have been reported for the reproducibility of between trial (same day) isokinetic elbow flexion and knee extension strength measures in 10-year-old boys,[31] the reproducibility worsened, however, when measurements were made on separate days (10.8%–16.2% coefficients of variation). Others observed that elbow extensor ($0.72 < r < 0.76$) and flexor peak torque ($0.79 < r < 0.84$) measures were moderately reliable in prepubertal males.[42] In 10-year-old boys, Wood and co-workers[35] reported coefficients of variation of 1.1% (arm length), 14.5% (concentric elbow flexion), and 15.2% (concentric elbow extension). However, the majority of isokinetic strength reliability studies report the correlation coefficient, a measure that assesses the strength of the relationship between variables, not their level of agreement which is better evaluated using the Bland and Altman[53] approach. One study has examined the reliability of isokinetic concentric knee extension and flexion measures[44] in adolescent males and females and observed limits of agreement ranging from −14.2 N·m for flexion peak torque to −20.5 N·m for extension peak torque, with repeatability coefficients of 21 N·m.

Reliability can also be influenced by the number of testers performing the isokinetic strength assessment. It stands to reason that the greater the number of testers used, the poorer the procedural standardization and the lower the reliability of the test results. Although not examined extensively, the between tester mean score deviations in one study[52] for shoulder and hip flexion and abduction, and knee and elbow flexion and extension ranged between 8.7% and 10.0%. The mean peak torques did not differ significantly when the assessment was done by different testers, but the magnitude of the differences was generally greater than those obtained with repeat testing by a single tester. These observations suggest that isokinetic concentric strength results may be more reliable when administered by a single rather than by multiple testers.

Reliability of isokinetic concentric strength measurements may also be influenced by limb dominance. Regrettably, there is little clear direction offered by the literature as to which limb might provide the most reproducible and reliable results. Several studies have reported no difference in bilateral isokinetic concentric strength results,[18,42,49,54,55] suggesting good reproducibility regardless of limb dominance. It has been speculated that strength differences in relation to the natural limb dominance may develop when children become more skilled in their activities.[54] Others, however, have reported significant and substantial differences between dominant and non-dominant limbs, implying poor reproducibility.[43,52,56] There are no data to our knowledge that can compare the reliability coefficients of repeated isokinetic concentric test results of dominant and non-dominant limbs, for example, test–retest correlations for the dominant compared to the non-dominant limb. Correlations for isokinetic concentric peak torque between dominant and non-dominant limbs for knee and elbow flexion and extension are moderately high and range between $r = 0.65$ and $r = 0.94$ in 6- to 8-year-old boys,[42,49] whereas at least in one study[42] the correlations for shoulder flexion and extension strength were considerably lower ($r = 0.37$–0.76). These bilateral limb comparisons provide no information about the reliability of strength measures in the dominant and non-dominant limbs, but rather suggest that there is considerable individual variability in the ability to produce peak isokinetic torque between limbs. On a practical basis and to ensure optimal testing reliability, these observations suggest that measurements should be made consistently on the same limb.

Finally, isokinetic concentric test reliability may also be influenced by the dynamometer type. Although each of the commercially available isokinetic dynamometers measures isokinetic peak torque, the absolute torques may vary considerably for essentially the same muscle action, across different dynamometers. One study[57] of adolescent male high school athletes reported no difference in peak torques at 60 deg·s^{-1} for knee flexion or extension among three different brand name dynamometers at a relatively slow angular velocity (60 deg·s^{-1}), but statistically significant and substantial differences at higher testing velocities of 180 and 300 deg·s^{-1}. Differences in isokinetic concentric peak torques across dynamometer types have also been reported for adults.[57,58] Although there are no comparable data on children, observations in adults suggest that differences in peak torque might also occur across different models of the same commercial dynamometer.[59] These observations suggest that the reliability of isokinetic peak torque assessments in children will be enhanced if measurements are made consistently with the same type and model of commercial dynamometer.

Isokinetic eccentric strength assessment

The advantages and disadvantages of isokinetic concentric dynamometry, as described above, generally also apply for isokinetic eccentric dynamometry. In contrast to concentric strength testing, however, isokinetic eccentric strength testing is a relatively underutilized testing modality in children, despite the availability of the eccentric testing mode on most models of commercially available isokinetic dynamometers.[2,14]

The paucity of information on eccentric muscle function in children may stem in part from the unsubstantiated concern that eccentric testing with its high peak torque producing capacity might predispose children to higher risk of muscle injury. This issue needs to be investigated more thoroughly, for there is no *a priori* reason to expect greater muscle injury with controlled isokinetic eccentric, compared to the other forms of testing, provided children are adequately instructed in the manoeuvre and given sufficient warm-up, familiarization, and recovery between trials. Perhaps the more important reason for the underutilization of this testing mode, however, is the novelty and complexity of performing isolated eccentric muscle actions for children. Children apparently find it more difficult to comprehend the nature of the manoeuvre and to exert the level of motor co-ordination required for smooth and consistent executions of eccentric muscle testing,[3,4] compared to adults. Whether it is due to limited attention span, lack of understanding, or immature motor control, these limitations will necessitate greater patience and more thorough explanations by the tester, and longer periods of familiarization for the subjects. Learning may be facilitated by providing simple, thorough, and non-technical instructions[3] relating the required action to actions that the child may be familiar with from sport or activities of daily living, and by providing actual demonstrations of the testing manoeuvre.

There are no accepted standardized protocols for eccentric muscle testing for children. In the few studies that have utilized this testing mode in children, the testing procedures and protocols have not been described thoroughly or differentiated from the concentric testing mode,[15,17,18] and the tests have been restricted to the elbow flexor[17] and knee extensor[15,18,19] muscle groups. The testing sequences used to date involve initiation of the manoeuvre with an isokinetic concentric action, followed by the eccentric action. In three of these studies, it is unclear whether the eccentric actions were tested immediately following concentric manoeuvres or whether they were assessed individually.[15,17,19] In the other study, the eccentric action followed immediately after and as a continuation of the concentric action.[18] Eccentric strength measurements are typically assessed at the same joint angular velocities as during concentric testing (between 0.21 and 3.14 rad·s^{-1} or 12 and 180 deg·s^{-1}) and the mean of two or three trials was used as the criterion measure. With the exception of the study by Mohtadi and co-workers,[18] information regarding warm-up procedures, instructions, and familiarization are sadly lacking.

Given the complexity and novelty of eccentric muscle actions, it may be advisable to perform concentric and eccentric muscle testing separately.[4] Testing of these actions separately removes the possible effect of potentiation from prior eccentric loading, on subsequent concentric actions, as would occur in the more common continuous combined concentric–eccentric testing protocols. Concentric–eccentric muscle strength ratios derived from the continuous and separate protocols are therefore not comparable across these different testing conditions. In addition, there are only a few reports to our knowledge of the reproducibility of eccentric thigh muscle strength in children and adolescents, and none of its reliability. In a small sample of 10- to 12-year-old boys, there were no significant test–retest (within a 2-week period) differences in eccentric knee extension torques, and the coefficients of variation were 4.0% and 9.9% for the non-dominant and dominant legs, respectively.[18] Reliability may also be improved by a familiarization session. In circumpubertal soccer players, Kellis and co-workers[60] included a separate familiarization session and observed test–retest correlation coefficients ranging from 0.89 to 0.98 in concentric and from 0.70 to 0.92 in eccentric conditions. In contrast, another study[61] assessed both concentric and eccentric average torques in preadolescent girls and observed considerable variability (concentric r of 0.41–0.77; eccentric r of 0.48–0.79), although they included a separate familiarization session. The authors highlighted that a minimum torque of 20 N·m is required to activate a Kin-Com dynamometer and this could account for some variability in their results. They also suggested that prepubertal girls may not have developed the neuromuscular skills necessary to perform these muscle actions. Clearly, the utility of eccentric strength testing in children cannot be established until issues of reliability and reproducibility are clarified and age-appropriate protocols are established and standardized. The agonist concentric–antagonist eccentric muscle action is common in many every day and sport activities, and the concentric-agonist to eccentric-antagonist peak strength ratio may be a useful index of functional muscle status in children.[3] The utility of this ratio, however, will depend on the yet to be established reliability and reproducibility of the peak eccentric strength component in children.

Isotonic strength testing

Isotonic or isoinertial testing has been used extensively in the past with adults, and especially with athlete groups to measure peak strength. These tests are often considered as field-based rather than laboratory-based tests, even though they have been, and legitimately can be, considered as a component of a thorough laboratory strength assessment battery. Isotonic testing is typically conducted using free weights (dumbbells or barbells), weight stack machines, and many commercially available isokinetic dynanometers.[2,14] Isotonic testing incorporates dynamic muscle actions which, depending on exercise sequencing, may activate the stretch-shortening cycle and more closely mimic actions in sport than isometric actions. Moreover, isotonic testing can incorporate multiple joint manoeuvres which may more closely mimic sport actions while perhaps also eliciting greater co-contraction of agonist muscles, thereby providing greater joint stability and protection against injury than other testing modes. Limitations of the isotonic testing mode, however, include the variability in joint angular velocity throughout the range of motion of a manoeuvre and the inability to control contributions from other ancillary muscle groups: these factors limit the validity of strength comparisons across muscles within individuals and for similar muscles amongst individuals. In addition, the actions executed in most isolated isotonic strength manoeuvres do not resemble very closely in pattern or speed, typical actions in sport or daily living. Finally, maximal isotonic strength testing, especially for multijoint exercises, for example, squat press, involve substantial skill and experience to be executed properly and safely.

Isotonic strength testing has been used less extensively in children than in adults, perhaps because of the putative increased risk of injury with this mode of testing compared to isometric and isokinetic modes. The one repetition maximum (1RM) lift, expressed in lb, kg, or N of weight lifted, has been the traditional method of determining peak isotonic strength in adults. This is the maximum external load or resistance that an individual can lift just once with proper technique throughout the entire range of motion of an action. In this sense, the 1RM qualifies as a true measure of maximal voluntary strength as defined earlier in the chapter. Because of the high skill requirement, and the potential for injury, the 1RM test is generally not recommended for prepubertal children.[62,63] The concern over the 1RM stems largely from injuries associated with training for, or execution of, maximal lifts in junior competitive weightlifting competitions.[64] There is no evidence that 1RM strength testing of fairly simple exercises, such as the bench press, double leg press, or arm curl, done in the laboratory, with modified weight stack machines and with proper adherence to lifting technique, exposes a child to higher risk of injury than isometric or isokinetic testing.

The 1RM approach has been used only sparingly, however, to assess maximal voluntary isotonic strength in prepubescent children[28,31,65] and adolescent girls.[66] With the exception of the study by Ozmun *et al.*,[65] which used free weights in the form of dumbbells, testing in these studies was always conducted on commercially available or custom-made weight stack machines. Typically, with these protocols, children are given proper technical instruction in the execution of each exercise, the technique is usually demonstrated by the tester, and then the subject attempts several repetitions of each lift, at minimal load, while receiving feedback. Novice subjects are usually given one session of habituation to the various isotonic exercises and the criterion 1RM test is usually performed the next day or within a couple of days. During the criterion test, subjects are given a warm-up consisting of 3–8 repetitions of the specific exercise at low-moderate load. The 1RM load is searched for by performing a graduated series of single repetitions of increasing load separated by 30–60 s of recovery, beginning with the warm-up load. Each increment in loading should be perceptively more difficult and the 1RM load should be reached between six and eight trials. Once the 1RM load is identified, the subject can be given a few moments rest and the 1RM load can be attempted again. This will confirm whether the true 1RM maximum load has been achieved.

There are no published data on the reliability and reproducibility of the 1RM approach in children. In one of the author's (CJB) own experiences, 1RM bench press, double leg press, and arm (biceps) curl were found to be highly reliable (test–retest correlation of $r > 0.90$) and reproducible (coefficient of variation of <8%) in children 9 years of age and older (unpublished observations). Improved accuracy of the 1RM load assessment can be achieved by modifying the weight machine such that smaller weight increments than those provided by the manufacturer can be added to the stack, without exceeding the subject's 1RM peak. It is the authors' opinion that relatively simple 1RM isotonic strength tests such as the bench press, double leg press, and arm curl exercises can be performed safely and effectively in the laboratory with children 9 years of age or older on weight stack type machines, provided subjects are properly instructed in the technique, given adequate familiarization, and the testing protocol includes adequate warm-up and incremental loading to maximum. If testing is not done on equipment especially designed for children, then special care is required to ensure that technical adjustments and the testing set-up permit biomechanically correct and safe execution of the exercises. Attempts at 1RM testing in the field, under less controlled conditions, and using free weights and multijoint manoeuvres may predispose the child to a higher risk of injury and should not be attempted with young children.

Several variations of multiple repetition submaximum load protocols, for example, 5RM, 6 RM, and 10 RM lifts, have also been used to test isotonic strength in children.[67,68] These are generally claimed as safer alternatives to the 1RM procedure. These protocols are similar to the 1RM in that they all require an initial series of trials with different loads to search for the target load that will lead to exhaustion at a predetermined number of repetitions. For example, the criterion strength measure for a 5RM test will be the load or resistance that brings the child to failure at five repetitions, for example, can lift the load only five times. This target load is usually identified within three to four sets or trials. Once the target load is determined, subjects should be given a rest period and then the criterion test load should be attempted again to verify that the true repetition maximum load has been identified. These multiple repetition submaximum protocols have been used to test isotonic strength for the squat, bench or chest press, overhead press, leg extension, leg curl, and arm curl exercises using free weights[68] and child sized dynamic constant resistance machines.[67,69] These protocols provide highly reliable measures of isotonic strength in children between 8 and 13 years of age with test–retest reliability coefficients ranging from 0.88 to 0.99;[67,68] there are no available published data on the reproducibility of these measures in children.

Although it seems to be an attractive alternative to the 1RM protocol, the multiple submaximum repetition protocols do not satisfy our earlier definition of maximal voluntary strength. While there is little doubt that these protocols measure at least in part, the functional strength of the child, they also measure the endurance capacity of the muscle or muscle group being tested; the greater the number of repetitions in the protocol, the more the test becomes a measure of muscle endurance rather than strength. In addition, although being lauded as safer than the 1RM protocols, there is no published information comparing the safety of the multiple submaximum versus 1RM protocols, or of the isotonic approaches generally, to isometric or isokinetic testing approaches. Finally, many of the commercially available isokinetic dynamometers also have isotonic testing capability.[2,14] There are, however, no published reports to our knowledge of maximal isotonic strength measures in children obtained on isokinetic dynamometers. Clearly, more work needs to be done in this area to establish the relationship between 1RM and multiple repetition submaximum isotonic strength measures, between isotonic strength measurements and peak isometric and isokinetic strength, and the relative risk of injury associated with these different strength testing approaches in children.

Electrically evoked muscle strength testing

The preceding sections have discussed various approaches that have been used to measure maximal voluntary strength in children. The validity of these approaches rests entirely on the assumption that the child is first, capable of, and second, willing to exert maximal effort during testing. Test results are dependent on the degree to which instructions are understood, the skill level in executing the manoeuvre, the degree of co-operation and motivation of the child during the test, and whether there is any underlying pathology that might directly or indirectly influence the force producing capacity of the muscle. These conditions may vary within an individual over time, among individuals within a given population, and between different populations, for example, younger versus older children, normal healthy children versus young athletes, and healthy children compared to children with various chronic paediatric diseases. These factors directly influence the validity, reliability, and reproducibility of strength results and ultimately their utility in research and clinical practice.

Various electrical stimulation protocols have been used in experimental studies and clinical practice to assess evoked (involuntary) measures of muscle force production in healthy children[23,24,26–29,70] and children with various paediatric diseases.[22,29,36,71] The advantage of evoked protocols is that strength measurements are independent of most of the factors mentioned above which can influence the validity, reliability, and reproducibility of maximal voluntary strength measures. Perhaps, most importantly, they are independent of skill and volition. Evoked protocols have been applied successfully to measure twitch torque or tetanic force production for the extensor hallucis brevis,[25] adductor pollicis,[27,70] elbow flexors,[22,29,71] plantar flexors,[24,71] dorsiflexors,[24] triceps surae,[23,26] and knee extensor[27–29,71,72] muscle groups in children as young as 4 years old,[27] but more typically from 9 years of age and older.

Ironically, there are no published data to our knowledge of the reliability and reproducibility of evoked twitch or tetanic strength measures in children. Unpublished observations (Blimkie *et al.*, unpublished results), however, indicate that evoked twitch torque measures for the elbow flexor and knee extensor muscle groups are just as reproducible as isometric and isokinetic strength measures in 10 year olds (coefficients of variation between 5.5% and 8.7%). The relationship between twitch torque and maximal voluntary isometric strength has not been extensively examined in children. Twitch torque of the triceps surae increases in concordance with maximal voluntary isometric strength in boys and girls between 9 and 21 years of age[23,26] and twitch torque and maximal voluntary strength are highly correlated ($r = 0.81$) in children and adolescents for the plantar flexors,[24] but only moderately correlated for the dorsiflexors ($r = 0.65$–0.67).

For evoked twitch protocols, the muscle group of interest is secured in a custom-made dynamometer which is configured with a sufficiently sensitive force transducer or strain gauge to record the resultant electrically stimulated isometric force. Since this procedure is basically measuring isometric force production, the measurable resultant force will be influenced not only by the intrinsic force producing capacity of the muscle, but also by the length of the muscle or joint angle position.[73] The optimal muscle length or joint angle will vary for different muscle groups and among individuals, and should not be presumed to be identical for children and adults. As for maximal voluntary isometric strength assessment, the joint angle and muscle length for optimal peak twitch torque determinations should be established on an individual and muscle-specific basis. This will provide the most valid measure of the peak twitch torque capacity of the muscle under investigation. If this procedure is not followed, then at the very least, measurements should be made consistently at the same muscle length or joint angle for all subjects.

Evoked protocols involve either percutaneous electrical stimulation applied directly over the motor end point of the muscle as is the case for the elbow flexors, or over a portion of the muscle belly in the case of larger muscle groups such as the quadriceps, plantar flexors, or triceps surae. Twitches can also be induced by direct stimulation of the main nerve serving the muscle group such as the femoral nerve for the quadriceps, the ulnar nerve for the adductor pollicis, and the tibial nerve for the tibialis anterior muscle. Whereas full muscle activation can only be assured during direct nervous stimulation of the muscle, there appears to be a fairly strong relationship between force production patterns of the percutaneous and directly stimulated quadriceps muscle,[29] suggesting that at least for this muscle group, the percutaneously evoked twitch measure is an acceptable surrogate of the true intrinsic force producing capacity of the muscle. Absolute twitch torques will differ, however, between techniques, and valid comparisons of twitch torques can only be made when measurements are obtained using the same technique.

Evoked twitch protocols typically involve the application of unidirectional square wave pulses of varying duration (depending on muscle size) and increasing voltage delivered via a stimulator through surface electrodes until maximal activation of the muscle is achieved. Maximal muscle activation is achieved when there is no further increase in twitch force production or when there is a plateau in the muscle electrical activity as measured by electromyography. To ensure that the peak twitch response has been obtained, the stimulation voltage is increased above that which elicited the peak twitch torque: if full activation is achieved the supramaximal stimulation will not elicit any further increase in twitch torque. Twitch torques can be substantially potentiated by prior voluntary muscle contractions,[29,73] so that these protocols are usually performed before tests of maximal or even submaximal voluntary effort, or after a recovery period of known sufficient duration to normalize the twitch response to its prepotentiated state (Fig. 4.8).

The technical preparation involved with these protocols, and the novelty of the evoked muscle isometric actions may cause apprehension and fear in some children and negatively influence compliance to the protocol. These tests are not suitable for all children and the tester must be sensitive to the situation and the feelings of the child. The child's comfort, welfare, and wishes should be upheld at all costs. Nevertheless, these protocols have been used successfully in several laboratories throughout the world with children of various ages, but mostly from 9 years of age and above. Twitch protocols are a valid and feasible means of assessing intrinsic muscle strength in children, but perhaps these techniques are most applicable for strength assessment in the clinical and research areas. More work is required to establish the reliability and reproducibility of twitch strength measurements for different muscle groups and with different stimulation procedures, and their relationship to maximal voluntary strength measured by isokinetic and isotonic techniques.

Electrically evoked tetanic protocols have been used less extensively in children than the evoked twitch protocols. Tetanic force is measured using the same dynamometers and testing set-up as for the twitch protocols. With these protocols, a series of stimulation trials of variable duration, increasing stimulation frequency (5–50 Hz), and sometimes increasing voltage, separated by a brief period of recovery between trials is applied until there is a plateau in tetanic tension. The peak torque is taken as the criterion measure of tetanic tension (Fig. 4.9). Tetanic force has been measured and reported for the elbow flexors,[29] adductor pollicis,[27,70] quadriceps,[27,29] and triceps surae[23,26] muscle groups. For the triceps surae muscle group,[23,26] the maximal voluntary isometric force always exceeded the peak tetanic force at the highest stimulation frequency of 50 Hz by ~15%. This difference could be due to either the additional contribution of synergistic muscles to the maximal voluntary force output or to suboptimal tetanic stimulation at 50 Hz.

There is little information regarding the relationship between maximal voluntary isometric strength and tetanic torque in children. For the triceps surae, tetanic force increases in concordance with maximal voluntary strength between 9 and 21 years of age in both sexes, and tetanic force at 50 Hz was highly positively correlated (r = 0.83) with maximal voluntary isometric force.[23,26] Similar concordance has also been observed between increases in tetanic force of the adductor pollicis and hand grip strength in both sexes between 9 and 15 years of age.[70] There is no information to our knowledge of the reliability and reproducibility of tetanic force measurements in children. Although tetanic protocols may provide the most valid index of intrinsic muscle or muscle groups isometric force producing capacity, forces produced under these conditions cannot be considered representative of maximal strength capability under voluntary effort or for more complex isokinetic and isotonic manoeuvres.

Whereas most children can tolerate twitch protocols, the level of compliance for tetanic protocols is substantially poorer. Only 25 out of 53 children successfully completed the 50-Hz tetanic stimulation of the triceps surae.[26] Fewer than 50% of the 9 year olds, but 69% of adolescent girls and 79% of adolescent boys, completed the 50-Hz tetanic protocol for the adductor pollicis.[70] Tetanic protocols at high stimulation frequencies are noxious and discomforting to many children. Children seem to have slightly greater tolerance of the tetanic protocol at lower stimulation frequencies (10 Hz vs. 50 Hz) and the correlation (r = 0.79) between tetanic forces at 10 Hz and 50 Hz is quite good,[23] suggesting that perhaps lower frequency stimulation protocols might be used instead of higher

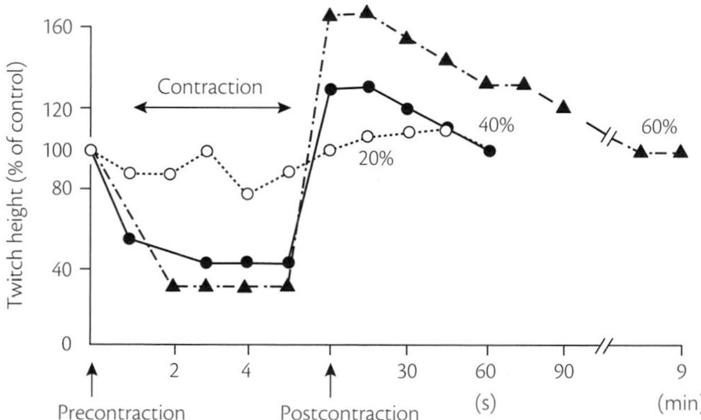

Fig. 4.8 Effect of prior muscle contraction on recorded twitch force production expressed as a percentage of the precontraction twitch height. Note that the twitch force (% height) decreases during the 5-s contraction in two subjects compared to the control in the open circles, but is augmented or potentiated immediately postcontraction in subjects who performed prior exercise. Adapted from Rutherford *et al.* [29]

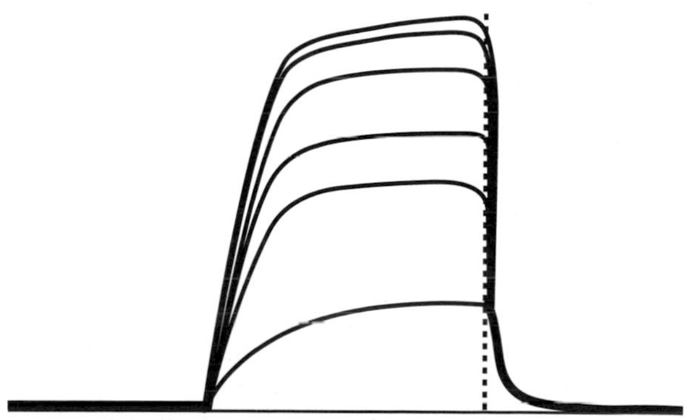

Fig. 4.9 Representation of tetanic force of the triceps surae muscle group with a stimulus frequency of 50 Hz and increasing voltage. Adapted from Davies.[23]

frequency protocols to improve compliance. The noxious nature of tetanic stimulation protocols raise an interesting question of ethics regarding the use of this technique in young children. The reliability and reproducibility of tetanic force measurements in children need to be established and these protocols should be reserved for research purposes and clinical applications in children with suspected or diagnosed neuromuscular disease.

Evoked isometric twitch torque measurements have also been used in combination with maximal voluntary isometric testing to determine the level of motor unit activation during volitional effort in children.[22,24,28,29,71,72] This procedure (the interpolated twitch technique) does not strictly measure maximal strength, but rather provides an estimate of the degree of activation of a muscle or muscle group at various levels of volitional effort. It is a useful technique to confirm the level of motivation during the execution of a manoeuvre in otherwise healthy individuals or the degree of inhibition associated with pathology or injury. More detailed descriptions of this procedure are provided by Belanger and McComas[24] and Rutherford *et al.*[29]

Interpretative considerations

Normalization of strength results

Isometric, isokinetic, and isotonic strength measures are all influenced to various degrees by intrinsic (muscle size and composition) and extrinsic (biomechanical and mechanical) factors that vary among individuals of a given age and within individuals over time, especially in growing children.

If strength comparisons are made between children of similar age and generally similar body composition, but different sizes, and the muscle in question is a large muscle important in weight-bearing and locomotion, then perhaps normalizing the strength score by body mass provides the most convenient and still valid basis of comparison. This may, however, underestimate the true force producing capacity of children with abnormal body composition, for example, obese children, and this may bias the interpretation of their test results. Recently, several studies have used allometric scaling principles[74] (see Chapter 2) to control for body size differences in strength assessments in paediatric populations.[44,45,75,76] These investigators suggest that suitable scaling factors should be derived from careful modelling of individual data sets and be sample specific, rather than incorporating theoretical scaling indices. Normalizing for fat-free mass (FFM) may also be considered in populations with abnormal body composition. During childhood and puberty, muscle strength increases and matches with augmentation of FFM.[76] Isokinetic studies have reported moderate to strong correlations between FFM and knee extension or flexion strength,[77,78] though there is an absence of data for other muscle groups. Further research is needed to determine the relationships between FFM and the age, and gender-associated development of strength across a broader number of muscle groups.

Normalizing by body mass is also problematic when strength comparisons are made across different age and maturity groups or between genders following puberty, since the ratio of muscle mass to body mass is inconstant and varies with age and gender during childhood. If, however, strength is considered for one of the smaller muscles, particularly of the upper body, then perhaps normalizing by the muscle size or estimated CSA, from anthropometry or medical imaging, is a more appropriate means of controlling for size differences. Since the maximum force a muscle can produce depends on its CSA, it is justifiable to use the size of the muscle or muscle group that produces the force as the independent variable in scaling procedures. The use of muscle size may overcome the confounding influence of varying body fat mass and its regional distribution during growth and maturation. However, a methodological problem is to establish the optimal site for the measurement of maximal muscle CSA within individuals and muscle groups.[45,79]

Since force output is also influenced by biomechanical factors such as moment arm lengths or mechanical advantage, these factors should also be considered in the normalization of strength scores. In a practical sense, it is difficult to measure precisely the distance of insertion of tendons from the axis of rotation about a joint, but if one assumes that these distances will vary in proportion to height or segment length, then crude adjustments on this basis can be made which will minimize the potential biomechanical advantage of taller compared to shorter children. This is perhaps a more important factor to consider when comparing strength results across different age groups and at different stages of growth and development. However, there are only limited data on the relationship between thigh strength per muscle CSA and mechanical advantage covering different age groups, both genders and different muscle groups. Young adults have significantly higher ratios of isokinetic knee extension peak torque per unit of CSA × thigh length than children, with the difference becoming greater with increasing velocity of movement.[7] Others found that peak concentric knee torque was significantly correlated ($r = 0.72$–0.83) to CSA × thigh length in both boys and girls[80] and sex differences in absolute peak torque remained statistically significant, although reduced, when expressed per unit CSA × thigh length. The persistence of sex and age differences after normalizing by CSA × stature or limb segment length in the thigh musculature suggests that neither muscle CSA nor biomechanical advantage can account for sex differences in peak torque, at least for the knee joint. To our knowledge, there are no data for other muscle groups.

Mechanical considerations

Considerable size differences exist between children of similar age and individual children change dramatically in size during the course of childhood. This variability in growth, if not accounted for, may impose mechanical constraints on the interpretation of strength test results. The external position of the mechanical load or resistance in relation to limb segment length can have a significant effect on measurable torques or forces in isometric and isokinetic strength testing, and confound data interpretation. Standard positioning of external loads in relation to limb segment length (specific proportion of limb length) under these testing conditions should be adhered to when testing children of similar age but different size, and perhaps more importantly when testing the same child at different stages of growth and development. Failure to account for this potential mechanical influence will lead to erroneous and biased interpretations of strength results.

Contralateral limb comparisons

In certain situations, and perhaps more so in clinical practice and rehabilitative medicine, strength of an injured muscle or limb is compared to that of the uninjured contralateral side. Acutely, this is a legitimate means of assessing the severity of injury. However, if there is a substantial lapse in time between reassessments and if the contralateral limb has increased its functional load to compensate for reduced function in the injured limb, then contralateral strength results may provide an inflated reference for the recovering limb. In this case, the strength of the contralateral limb at the time of injury would perhaps provide a more suitable baseline against which to assess degree of recovery in the injured limb.

In addition, when testing young athletes, and for the sake of testing efficiency, a decision must be made whether to test the dominant or non-dominant limb. The literature on the effects of limb dominance on voluntary strength is at best equivocal. In sports where there is clearly a limb preference and if only one limb is to be tested, then clearly the dominant limb for that activity should be selected. This may be a more important consideration in post- than prepubertal children, where a combination of increased training intensity, and more mature neuroendocrinological development may facilitate greater differentiation between dominant and non-dominant limbs. Whether to test dominant or non-dominant limbs or both will depend on the purpose of the test; regardless of purpose, however, consistency in limb selection should be adhered to when performing strength testing of children.

Test instructions

Similar to size, there is considerable variability in intelligence, attention span, and motivation among children of the same age and within children as they mature. The first priority in strength testing children is to ensure safety. This is achieved through instruction in the techniques to be used and by the adequacy of familiarization and warm-up procedures. The younger the child, the greater the need for simplicity in instructions, and generally the longer the familiarization procedure. This will depend also on the complexity of the movement required during testing and the child's familiarity with the movement pattern from life experience. Learning occurs fairly rapidly for simple manoeuvres such as isometric elbow flexion testing, but may take a bit longer for novel activities such as isokinetic concentric testing and even longer for eccentric testing or weightlifting exercises, especially for children. Motivation is a key factor to reliable testing and may be even more important for a young child who is unaccustomed to providing maximal effort on demand. To enhance reliability, standardized motivational procedures should be used consistently within and across different strength testing procedures and muscle action types.

Summary

- Strength testing serves numerous meaningful functions in paediatric populations.
- There is a substantial literature base on isometric strength testing of children but surprisingly little about isokinetic and isotonic strength testing. The reliability and reproducibility of various testing modes, especially isokinetic and isotonic testing, and their relative safety for children of different ages needs to be further elaborated.
- Biomechanical effects of musculoskeletal changes with growth and maturation on strength development have not been extensively studied. Research into muscle size and moment arms using magnetic resonance imaging may provide further insights into the age- and sex-associated development of strength.
- There is much more to learn about the relationships between muscle strength as assessed by these different testing modalities and health, injury prevention, and sports performance at different ages and for both genders during childhood.

References

1. Abernethy P, Wilson G, Logan P (1995). Strength and power assessment. Issues, controversies and challenges. *Sports Med* **19**, 401–17.
2. Sale DG (1991). Testing strength and power. In: MacDougall JD, Wenger HA, Green HJ (eds.), *Physiological testing of the high-performance athlete* (2nd ed.), pp. 21–106. Human Kinetics Publishers, Champaign, IL.
3. Baltzopoulos V, Kellis E (1998). Isokinetic strength during childhood and adolescence. In: Van Praagh E (ed.), *Pediatric anaerobic performance*, pp. 225–40. Human Kinetics, Champaign, IL.
4. Gaul CA (1996). Muscular strength and endurance. In: Docherty D (ed.), *Measurement in pediatric exercise science*, pp. 225–8. Human Kinetics, Champaign, IL.
5. De Ste Croix M, Deighan M, Armstrong N (2003). Assessment and interpretation of isokinetic muscle strength during growth and maturation. *Sports Med* **33**, 727–43.
6. Beunen G (1997). Muscular strength development in children and adolescents. In: Froberg K, Lammert O, St Hansen H, Blimkie CJR (eds.), *Exercise and fitness—benefits and risks*, pp. 193–207. Odense University Press, Odense, Denmark.
7. Blimkie CJR (1989). Age- and sex-associated variation in strength during childhood: Anthropometric, morphologic, neurologic, biomechanical, endocrinologic, genetic, and physical activity correlates. In: Gisolf CV, Lamb DR (eds.), *Perspectives in exercise science and medicine. Vol. 2. Youth exercise and sport*, pp. 66–163. Benchmark Press, Indianapolis, IN.
8. Blimkie CJR, Sale DG (1998). Strength development and trainability during childhood. In: Van Praagh E (ed.), *Pediatric anaerobic performance*, pp. 193–224. Human Kinetics, Champaign, IL.
9. Froberg K, Lammert O (1996). Development of muscle strength during childhood. In: Bar-Or O (ed.), *The child and adolescent athlete*, pp. 25–41. Blackwell Scientific, London.
10. Knuttgen HG, Kraemer WJ (1987). Terminology and measurement of exercise performance. *J Appl Sport Sci Res* **1**, 1–10.
11. Lakomy HKA (1994). Strength. In: Harries M, Williams C, Stanish WD, Micheli LJ (eds.), *Textbook of sports medicine*, pp. 112–7. Oxford University Press, Oxford.
12. Baltzopoulos V (1995). Muscular and tibiofemoral joint forces during isokinetic concentric knee extension. *Clin Biomech* **10**, 208–14.
13. Sale DG, Norman RW (1982). Testing strength and power. In: MacDougall JD, Wenger HA, Green HJ (eds.), *Physiological testing of the high-performance athlete* (1st ed.), pp. 7–37. Mutual Press, Ottawa.
14. Perrin DH (1993). *Isokinetic exercise and assessment*. Human Kinetics, Champaign, IL.
15. Abe T, Kawakami Y, Ikegawa S, Kanehisa H, Fukunaga T (1992). Isometric and isokinetic knee joint performance in Japanese alpine ski racers. *J Sports Med Phys Fitness* **32**, 353–7.
16. Calmers P, Borne I, Nellen M, Domenach M, Minaire P, Drost M (1995). A pilot study of knee isokinetic strength in young, highly trained, females gymnasts. *Iso Exerc Sci* **5**, 69–74.
17. 17. Kawakami Y, Kanehisa H, Ikegawa S, Fukunaga T (1993). Concentric and eccentric muscle strength before, during and after fatigue in 13 year-old boys. *Eur J Appl Physiol* **67**, 121–4.
18. Mohtadi NG, Kiefer GN, Tedford K, Watters S (1990). Concentric and eccentric quadriceps torque in pre-adolescent males. *Can J Sport Sci* **15**, 240–3.

19. Seger JY, Thorstensson A (1994). Muscle strength and myoelectric activity in prepubertal and adult males and females. *Eur J Appl Physiol* **69**, 81–7.
20. Hakkinen K, Komi PV, Kauhanen H (1986). Electromyographic and force production characteristics of leg extensor muscles of elite weight lifters during isometric, concentric, and various stretch-shortening cycle exercises. *Int J Sports Med* **7**, 144–51.
21. Knapick JJ, Wright JE, Mawdsley RH, Braun JM (1983). Isokinetic, isometric and isotonic strength relationships. *Arch Physiol Med Rehab* **64**, 77–80.
22. Blimkie CJ, Ebbesen B, MacDougall D, Bar-Or O, Sale D (1989). Voluntary and electrically evoked strength characteristics of obese and nonobese preadolescent boys. *Hum Biol* **61**, 515–32.
23. Davies CTM (1985). Strength and mechanical properties of muscle in children and young adults. *Scand J Sports Sci* **7**, 11–5.
24. Belanger AY, McComas AJ (1989). Contractile properties of human skeletal muscle in childhood and adolescence. *Eur J Appl Physiol* **58**, 563–7.
25. McComas AJ, Sica RE, Petito F (1973). Muscle strength in boys of different ages. *J Neurol Neurosurg Psychiatry* **36**, 171–3.
26. Davies CT, White MJ, Young K (1983). Muscle function in children. *Eur J Appl Physiol* **52**, 111–4.
27. Hosking GP, Young A, Dubowitz V, Edwards RH (1978). Tests of skeletal muscle function in children. *Arch Dis Child* **53**, 224–9.
28. Ramsay JA, Blimkie CJ, Smith K, Garner S, MacDougall JD, Sale DG (1990). Strength training effects in prepubescent boys. *Med Sci Sports Exerc* **22**, 605–14.
29. Rutherford OM, Jones DA, Newham DJ (1986). Clinical and experimental application of the percutaneous twitch superimposition technique for the study of human muscle activation. *J Neurol Neurosurg Psychiatry* **49**, 1288–91.
30. Andersen LB, Henckel P (1987). Maximal voluntary isometric strength in Danish adolescents 16–19 years of age. *Eur J Appl Physiol* **56**, 83–9.
31. Blimkie CJR, Ramsay J, Sale DG, McDougall JD, Smith K, Garner S (1989). Effects of 10 weeks of resistance training on strength development in prepubertal boys. In: Oseid S, Carlson KH (eds.), *Children and exercise XIII*, pp. 183–97. Human Kinetics Champaign, IL.
32. Van Praagh E, Franca NM (1998). Measuring maximal short-term power output during growth. In: Van Praagh E (ed.), *Pediatric anaerobic performance*, pp. 155–89. Human Kinetics Champaign, IL.
33. Asmussen E (1973). Growth in muscular strength and power. In: Rarick GL (ed.), *Physical activity human growth and development*, pp. 60–79. Academic Press, New York.
34. Edwards RH, Chapman SJ, Newham DJ, Jones DA (1987). Practical analysis of variability of muscle function measurements in Duchenne muscular dystrophy. *Muscle Nerve* **10**, 6–14.
35. Wood LE, Dixon S, Grant C, Armstrong N (2004). Elbow flexion and extension strength relative to body or muscle size in children. *Med Sci Sports Exerc* **36**, 1977–84.
36. Hosking JP, Bhat US, Dubowitz V, Edwards RH (1976). Measurements of muscle strength and performance in children with normal and diseased muscle. *Arch Dis Child* **51**, 957–63.
37. Teeple JB, Lohman TG, Misner JE, Boileau RA, Massey BH (1975). Contribution of physical development and muscular strength to the motor performance capacity of 7–12 year old boys. *Br J Sports Med* **9**, 122–9.
38. Woods GW, Elkousy HA, O'Connor DP (2006). Arthroscopic release of the vastus lateralis tendon for recurrent patellar dislocation. *Am J Sports Med* **34**, 824–31.
39. 39. Scott OM, Hyde SA, Goddard C, Dubowitz V (1982). Quantitation of muscle function in children: a prospective study in Duchenne muscular dystrophy. *Muscle Nerve* **5**, 291–301.
40. Rauch F, Neu CM, Wassmer G, Beck B, Rieger-Wettengl G, Rietschel E, Manz F, Schoenau E (2002). Muscle analysis by measurement of maximal isometric grip force: new reference data and clinical applications in pediatrics. *Pediatr Res* **51**, 505–10.
41. Tornvall G (1963). Assessment of physical capabilities with special reference to the evaluation of maximal working capacity. *Acta Physiol Scand* **58 (Suppl. 201)**, 1–101.
42. Weltman A, Tippett S, Janney C (1988). Measurement of isokinetic strength in prepubertal males. *J Orthop Sports Phys Ther* **9**, 345–51.
43. Henderson RC, Howes CL, Erickson KL, Heere LM, DeMasi RA (1993). Knee flexor-extensor strength in children. *J Orthop Sports Phys Ther* **18**, 559–63.
44. De Ste Croix MBA, Armstrong N, Welsman JR (1999). Concentric isokinetic leg strength in pre-teen, teenage and adult males and females. *Biol Sport* **16**, 75–86.
45. De Ste Croix MB, Armstrong N, Welsman JR, Sharpe P (2002). Longitudinal changes in isokinetic leg strength in 10–14-year-olds. *Ann Hum Biol* **29**, 50–62.
46. Osternig LR (1986). Isokinetic dynamometry: implications for muscle testing and rehabilitation. *Exerc Sport Sci Rev* **14**, 45–80.
47. Docherty D, Gaul CA (1991). Relationship of body size, physique, and composition to physical performance in young boys and girls. *Int J Sports Med* **12**, 525–32.
48. Burnett CN, Betts EF, King WM (1990). Reliability of isokinetic measurements of hip muscle torque in young boys. *Phys Ther* **70**, 244–9.
49. Merlini L, Dell'Accio D, Granata C (1995). Reliability of dynamic strength knee muscle testing in children. *J Orthop Sports Phys Ther* **22**, 73–6.
50. Baltzopoulos V, Brodie DA (1989). Isokinetic dynamometry. Applications and limitations. *Sports Med* **8**, 101–16.
51. Gilliam TB, Villanacci JF, Freedson PS, Sady SP (1979). Isokinetic torque in boys and girls ages 7–13: effect of age, height and weight. *Res Q* **50**, 599–609.
52. Molnar GE, Alexander J, Gutfeld N (1979). Reliability of quantitative strength measurements in children. *Arch Phys Med Rehabil* **60**, 218–21.
53. Bland JM, Altman DG (1986). Statistical methods for assessing agreement between two methods of clinical measurement. *Lancet* **i**, 307–310.
54. Burnie J, Brodie DA (1986). Isokinetic measurement in preadolescent males. *Int J Sports Med* **7**, 205–9.
55. Capranica L, Cama G, Fanton F, Tessitore A, Figura F (1992). Force and power of preferred and non-preferred leg in young soccer players. *J Sports Med Phys Fitness* **32**, 358–63.
56. Sunnegardh J, Bratteby LE, Nordesjo LO, Nordgren B (1988). Isometric and isokinetic muscle strength, anthropometry and physical activity in 8 and 13 year old Swedish children. *Eur J Appl Physiol* **58**, 291–7.
57. Wilk KE, Johnson RD, Levine BA (1987). A comparison of peak torque values of knee extension and flexor muscle groups using Biodex, Cybex and Kin-Com Isokinetic Dynamometers. *Phys Ther* **67**, 789–90.
58. Heinrichs, D.H., Perrin DH, Weltman A, Gieck GH, Ball DW (1995). Effect of protocol and assessment device on isokinetic peak torque of the quadriceps muscle group. *Iso Exerc Sci* **5**, 7–13.
59. Thigpen LK, Blanke D, Lang P (1990). The reliability of two different Cybex isokinetic systems. *J Sports Phys Ther* **12**, 157–62.
60. Kellis E, Kellis S, Gerodimos V (1999). Reliability of isokinetic concentric and eccentric strength in circumpubertal soccer players. *Pediatr Exerc Sci* **11**, 218–28.
61. Hildebrand KA, Mohtadi NG, Kiefer GN (1994). Thigh muscle strength in preadolescent girls. *Clin J Sports Med* **4**, 108–12.
62. Freedson PS, Ward A, Rippe JM (1990). Resistance training for youth. In: Grana WA, Lombardo JA, Sharkey BJ (eds.), *Advances in sports medicine and fitness*, pp. 57–63. Year Book Medical, Chicago, IL.
63. National Strength and Conditioning Association (NSCA) (1985). Position paper on prepubescent strength training. *Nat Strength Conditioning J* **7**, 27–31.
64. Brown EW, Kimball RG (1983). Medical history associated with adolescent powerlifting. *Pediatrics* **72**, 636–44.

65. Ozmun JC, Mikesky AE, Surburg PR (1994). Neuromuscular adaptations following prepubescent strength training. *Med Sci Sports Exerc* **26**, 510–14.
66. Rice S, Blimkie CJ, Webber CE, Levy D, Martin J, Parker D, Gordon CL (1993). Correlates and determinants of bone mineral content and density in healthy adolescent girls. *Can J Physiol Pharmacol* **71**, 923–30.
67. Faigenbaum AD, Zaichkowsky LD, Westcott WL, Micheli LJ, Fehlandt AF (1993). The effects of a twice-a-week strength training program on children. *Pediatr Exerc Sci* **5**, 339–46.
68. Sailors M, Berg K (1987). Comparison of responses to weight training in pubescent boys and men. *J Sports Med Phys Fitness* **27**, 30–7.
69. Faigenbaum AD, Westcott WL, Micheli LJ, Outerbridge AR, Long CJ, LaRosa-Loud R, Zaichkowsky LD (1996). The effects of strength training and detraining on children. *J Strength Conditioning Res* **10**, 109–14.
70. Backman E, Henriksson KG (1988). Skeletal muscle characteristics in children 9–15 years old: Force, relaxation rate and contraction time. *Clin Physiol* **8**, 521–7.
71. Hanning RM, Blimkie CJ, Bar-Or O, Lands LC, Moss LA, Wilson WM (1993). Relationships among nutritional status and skeletal and respiratory muscle function in cystic fibrosis: does early dietary supplementation make a difference? *Am J Clin Nutr* **57**, 580–7.
72. Blimkie CJ, Sale DG, Bar-Or O (1990). Voluntary strength, evoked twitch contractile properties and motor unit activation of knee extensors in obese and non-obese adolescent males. *Eur J Appl Physiol* **61**, 313–18.
73. Bulow PM, Norregaard J, Nneskiold-Samsoe B, Mehlsen J (1993). Twitch interpolation technique in testing of maximal muscle strength: influence of potentiation, force level, stimulus intensity and preload. *Eur J Appl Physiol* **67**, 462–6.
74. Welsman JR, Armstrong N. Statistical techniques for interpreting body size related exercise performance during growth. *Pediatr Exerc Sci* **12**, 112–27.
75. Kanehisa H, Yata H, Ikegawa S, Fukunaga T (1995). A cross-sectional study of the size and strength of the lower leg muscles during growth. *Eur J Appl Physiol* **72**, 150–6.
76. Nevill AM, Holder RL, Baxter-Jones A, Round JM, Jones DA (1998). Modeling developmental changes in strength and aerobic power in children. *J Appl Physiol* **84**, 963–70.
77. Housh TJ, Johnson GO, Housh DJ, Weir JP, Weir LL, Eckerson JM, Stout JR (1996). Age, fat-free weight, and isokinetic peak torque in high school female gymnasts. *Med Sci Sports Exerc* **28**, 610–13.
78. Weir JP (2000). Youth and isokinetic testing. In: Brown LE (ed.), *Isokinetics in human performance*, pp. 299–323. Human Kinetics Champaign, IL.
79. Deighan M, De Ste Croix M, Grant C, Armstrong N (2006). Measurement of maximal muscle cross-sectional area of the elbow extensors and flexors in children, teenagers and adults. *J Sports Sci* **24**, 543–6.
80. Kanehisa H, Ikegawa S, Tsunoda N, Fukunaga T (1994). Strength and cross-sectional area of knee extensor muscles in children. *Eur J Appl Physiol* **68**, 402–5.

CHAPTER 5

Maximal intensity exercise

Neil Armstrong, Joanne R. Welsman, and Craig A. Williams

Introduction

Maximal intensity exercise is often associated with maximal or peak oxygen uptake ($\dot{V}O_2$). However, this convention ignores the fact that, for short periods of time, anaerobic provision of adenosine triphosphate (ATP) can support exercise of much greater intensity than that at peak $\dot{V}O_2$. Therefore, for the purpose of this chapter, maximal intensity exercise is defined as that which is performed 'all-out' and is sustained by an anaerobic ATP yield which exceeds that of oxidative metabolism.

Energy pathways do not operate in isolation during exercise and the relative intensity and duration of exercise dictates which pathways are the predominant providers of ATP. In submaximal dynamic exercise, the anaerobic pathways provide the majority of energy during the initial stages of the activity but the aerobic pathway makes a gradually increasing contribution as the duration of the exercise increases. The overlapping provision of energy by the aerobic and anaerobic pathways makes it very difficult to determine the rate or capacity of ATP production by a single pathway and understanding of the underlying mechanisms of maximal intensity exercise is restricted by the ethical limitations of direct measurement, and the fact that several performance tests of 'anaerobic power' include a significant contribution of energy from aerobic sources[1,2] further clouds the issue.

An elegant study during maximal intensity exercise with adults has demonstrated that, using needle biopsy of muscle and venous and arterial catheterization, direct quantitative measurement of anaerobic energy turnover is possible.[3] However, the use of these techniques with children or adolescents is unethical and paediatric exercise scientists must normally rely upon non-invasive methodology[4,5] [see Chapter 1]. The recent application of phosphorus magnetic resonance spectroscopy (^{31}PMRS) to studies in paediatric exercise science offers a promising non-invasive technique of directly quantifying anaerobic energy yield which has been shown to be reliable with children,[6] and exploratory work with both children[7] and adolescents[8] has been reported. Research is, however, limited to single leg or arm exercise, as currently available magnets do not allow assessment of whole-body exercise. Further details on paediatric exercise science applications of ^{31}PMRS can be found in Chapter 16.

Indirect estimates of children's anaerobic metabolism during exercise have been made from determination of the accumulated oxygen deficit (AOD).[9,10] Accumulated oxygen deficit is measured as the difference between the actual $\dot{V}O_2$ during a maximal intensity exercise bout (i.e. 110% of peak $\dot{V}O_2$) and the oxygen demand predicted by extrapolation from the linear regression of exercise intensity and $\dot{V}O_2$ within a series of submaximal 'steady-state' $\dot{V}O_2$ exercise bouts (see ref. 11, p. 122, for a sample calculation). The security of the premises underlying the technique has been challenged[12] and estimates of young people's 'anaerobic capacity'[12] from AOD must be interpreted cautiously.

Post-maximal intensity exercise blood lactate has also been used to indirectly quantify the glycolytic contribution to exercise but the assessment and interpretation of blood lactate accumulation is complex. Lactate is produced in the muscles and diffuses into the blood, where it is removed by oxidation in the heart or skeletal muscles or is converted to glucose through gluconeogenesis in the liver. Consequently, the lactate measured in blood reflects all those processes by which lactate is produced and eliminated. Blood lactate therefore provides only a qualitative indication and not a precise measure of glycolytic activity. The methodological factors which can influence blood lactate accumulation and its interpretation are discussed in detail in Chapter 8.

Further development of technologies such as ^{31}PMRS may provide new insights into young people's anaerobic characteristics but direct measurement of children's and adolescents' anaerobic energy turnover is not presently possible. Indirect methods of assessment such as determination of post-exercise blood lactate accumulation only provide qualitative estimates of glycolytic activity. This chapter will therefore focus on the variety of performance tests that have been developed to investigate maximal intensity exercise.

Maximal intensity exercise tests

Although in the past decade there has been a dramatic increase in the number of published studies of paediatric anaerobic performance, by comparison to aerobic performance the mechanisms responsible for children's anaerobic metabolism during exercise are not well documented. This can be partly explained by the difficulty of measuring physiological variables during non-steady-state exercise and by the ethical restrictions of involving child participants in investigations using invasive techniques. The lack of scientific literature is still surprising, however, as most sports include maximal intensity exercise and the daily physical activity patterns of young children consist of sporadic bouts of high-intensity activity.[13]

The understanding of anaerobic performance has been clouded by the use of different terminology. Terms such as short-term muscle power, supramaximal intensity exercise, and maximal intensity exercise have all been used to describe anaerobic performance. Supramaximal exercise is often used to describe exercise intensities greater than those found at maximal aerobic power, but tautologically this implies that a system that is already at a maximum can be somehow surpassed. Clearly, this cannot be the case. If we accept the term maximal to mean 'all-out' effort, irrespective of which energy system supplies the demand, this expression more accurately describes the exercise. As outlined above, direct physiological measures of anaerobic exercise are not readily available but indirect measures of performance such as mechanical power, speed, or force allow the researcher of anaerobic performance clarity of thought if not precision of measurement. The difficulties in defining anaerobic performance indicate the problems in assessing maximal intensity exercise and the technical challenges which impact on the researcher's ability to infer physiological processes.

The two components of anaerobic performance of most interest are peak and mean power output. Peak power output (PP) is the maximum rate at which energy is transferred to the external system and mean power output (MP) is the total work done during the performance test divided by the time taken.[14] Young people's PP has been assessed using jumping, cycling, running, and, more recently, isokinetic dynamometry, but the validity of these tests is difficult to assess.

For a test to be valid it must also be reliable, and because of the widespread and inappropriate use of the correlation coefficient as a measure of test–retest reliability,[15,16] there is little information on the variation in repeated measurements by the same participant on the same anaerobic performance test. Even if anaerobic performance tests have acceptable reliability it is difficult to confirm their validity, as there is no 'gold standard' test against which to compare. Furthermore, as maximal intensity power output is predominantly dependent on energy supply intrinsic to the active muscles, performance test data are specific to the movement pattern used.[17] In other words, we cannot assume that power output in running tests will be similar to power output generated during cycling, as the contribution of the muscles involved may vary markedly between the two activities[17]

Jump tests

According to Van Praagh[18,19] the first scientific investigation of leg power was carried out by Marey[20] who recorded the simultaneous measurement of force (pneumatic force platform) and displacement during a vertical jump (VJ). Other jumps, such as the standing broad jump, have been proposed as tests of anaerobic power[21] and some investigators[22] have advocated the use of a repeated series of VJs but the simple VJ has proved the most popular of this type of test.

Vertical jump

Sargent[23] popularized the VJ as a measure of muscular power and a range of protocols have evolved from his original test. In most protocols, subjects are allowed counter-movements (e.g. momentary crouch, forward arm swing) to aid their performance,[24] but in others counter-movements are minimized.[25] Typically, subjects are required to jump vertically as high as they can and the highest point reached by the fingers, with the arms extended is compared to the height reached by the fingers when the subject is standing erect, with arms extended upwards.

VJ performance is highly dependent on protocol and the general lack of standardization across studies confounds inter-study comparisons.[26] Furthermore, with young people, growth and maturation and the resulting increase in neuromuscular activation and motor coordination must be considered. Only about 40% of 9- to 13-year-olds perform the VJ with a mature pattern.[27] VJ performance appears to improve linearly with age during childhood but during adolescence, VJ performances of girls reach a plateau while those for boys show evidence of an adolescent spurt.[28] Nevertheless, Bar-Or[29] compared VJ scores with PP in the Wingate anaerobic test (WAnT) and reported 'fair to good' validity.

The VJ as described by Sargent[23] has the dimension of work not power and several formulae have been proposed to add velocity to the body mass and vertical height components,[30,31] but the validity of these formulae is questionable[26]. Use of a force platform allows the calculation of instantaneous power from the product of instantaneous force exerted by the subject on the force platform and the acceleration of the subject's centre of mass.[32–34] Using this method with ten 11-year-old children (six boys and four girls) Davies and Young[35] reported PP in the VJ to be 45% lower than that obtained during the first 5 s of all-out cycling. Interestingly, the same study reported that externally loading the children (from 5% to 30% of body mass) resulted in a linear decrease in PP proportional to the added load. This finding indicates that body mass is not less than optimal for maximal PP output in a VJ.

Jumping is, however, an impulsive activity with the height jumped being a function of the product of force and time and not the product of force and velocity (see Chapter 13). The VJ has therefore been strongly criticized as a measure of power output[36] and although it remains a popular field test it is rarely used as a laboratory measure of young people's anaerobic performance (see Chapter 9 for the use of jump tests as field tests of maximal intensity exercise).

Monoarticular force–velocity tests

Torque during movement across a single joint can be measured using isokinetic dynamometers [37] and as the angular velocity can be preset it is possible to calculate power output. This approach enables the characteristics of single muscle groups to be measured under controlled conditions. There are, however, several potential problems associated with the use of commercially available isokinetic dynamometers, not the least of which is the necessity to modify appropriately for children equipment which was designed for use by adults. Isokinetic dynamometer readings are rarely generated under true constant angular velocity[38] and the difficulty of voluntarily accelerating a limb to optimal velocity for PP output has been noted.[17] Results are often difficult to interpret because of the range of angular velocities at which torque is reported. Van Praagh[18] commented that the force–velocity relationship is highly specific and the torque–velocity relationship cannot be simply evaluated by an isolated movement at a markedly different velocity. Adult data suggest that the maximal power measured during monoarticular exercises is less than half the maximal power measured during polyarticular exercise.[39] This is partly explained by the additional power produced by other joints, which act simultaneously during a polyarticular movement.[26]

Some studies have investigated total work output using monoarticular isokinetic techniques.[40,41] Bar-Or[29] described a test involving 25 maximal knee extensions and flexions at an angular velocity of 3.14 rad·s^{-1}, and he reported, in forty-eight 9- to 17-year-old boys, a correlation between total work of the extensors and total work in the WAnT of $r = 0.94$. With the subjects classified according to maturational status and body mass 'corrected for' (see Chapter 2 for a critique) by expressing the work output in ratio with mass (i.e. J·kg^{-1}) the correlation coefficients were 0.68, 0.80, and 0.21 for pre-, mid-, and late-pubescents, respectively.[41]

Monoarticular force–velocity data from children are sparse and focus on peak torque rather than power output.[42–47] Coefficients of repeatability[48] for peak torque do not appear to have been published, but research in our Centre (De Ste Croix and Armstrong, unpublished data) revealed, with twenty-three 10-year-old boys tested 1 week apart, repeatability coefficients varying from 12.4 to 21.8 N·m (mean torque values, 42.7–66.3 N·m) for extension and from 12.6 to 21.0 N·m (mean torque values, 33.7–48.2 N·m) for flexion, over velocities ranging from 0.52 to 3.14 rad·s^{-1}. Repeatability was more variable at slower velocities. In the only isokinetic reliability study to include girls, De Ste Croix *et al.*[49] investigated the reliability of an endurance test for extensor and flexor torque. Sixteen boys 12.2 ± 0.3 years and 14 girls 12.2 ± 0.3 years participated in the study. The reliabilities of the percentage fatigue of quadriceps and hamstrings extension and flexion torque using a Biodex dynamometer were found to be significantly different. Intra-class correlations indicated significant and positive correlations between test 1 and test 2 for extension torque $r = 0.90$ ($p < 0.05$) but not flexor torque $r = 0.36$ ($p > 0.05$). Coefficients of variation (CV) also varied, 0.4% for extensor torque compared to 0% for flexor torque. The repeatability coefficients and the limits of agreement using Bland and Altman plots[48] also confirmed that the endurance measures for the extensor torque were more reliable than the flexor torque.[49] Kellis *et al.*[50] found knee extensor moment measurements to be more reliable than knee flexor tests in a group of circumpubertal football players. The authors also concluded that for the reliable examination of moments of force for eccentric tests and fast velocities, extensive familiarization of the subjects prior to the tests were required. More research is clearly required before this technique of assessing young people's maximal intensity torque and power output can be recommended.

Cycle tests

At the Fourth International Symposium on Pediatric Work Physiology, Cumming[51] introduced a 30-s friction-braked cycle ergometer test which was further developed under the innovative leadership of Oded Bar-Or at the Wingate Institute in Israel.[52] As the WAnT, it has become the most widely used test of anaerobic performance providing measures of PP and MP.[53] Pirnay and his associates[54,55] focused specifically on PP and proposed a cycle test consisting of short maximal sprints (5–7 s) against several braking forces on a friction-braked ergometer. The highest recorded power output was assumed to correspond to PP. This protocol has been subsequently modified, and, as the force-velocity test (F-V test), it has gained popularity with adults[26,56] and children[57–60] and has been adapted for use with isokinetic cycle ergometers.[61–63]

Wingate anaerobic test

The WAnT involves pedalling a cycle ergometer against a constant braking force, with maximal effort for 30 s; the majority of data on young people's anaerobic performance have been generated in this manner.[7,8] The WAnT can be easily modified for upper body assessment and several studies of children's and adolescents' maximal intensity power output during arm cranking have been published.[64,65] The WAnT has been demonstrated to be highly related to young people's performance in a range of predominantly anaerobic tasks,[66] and it has been found to be both feasible and informative when used with children with a neuromuscular disability.[29] High test–retest correlation coefficients have been reported[66] but to date the only study to investigate the repeatability and validity of the WAnT is by Sutton *et al.*[67] Nineteen children (9 boys and 10 girls) aged 10.9 ± 0.3 years participated in the study. Repeatability coefficients in the range of 44–50 W for PP and 34–42 W for MP for WAnT test–retests 1 week apart were found for 18 of the children (one removed as an outlier). A significant correlation $r = 0.82$ ($p < 0.01$) was found between the WAnT PP and the PP generated during a 30-s non-motorized treadmill sprint test (see later in this chapter). A similar result was found for MP, $r = 0.88$ ($p < 0.01$).

The WAnT requires a cycle ergometer in which the braking force can be kept constant and a means of monitoring pedal or flywheel revolutions can be ensured. Most paediatric exercise science laboratories have developed and customized online automated data collection systems to retrieve the number of pedal (or flywheel) revolutions and calculate the performance indices, but several versions of appropriate software are commercially available. Monark or Fleisch friction-loaded cycle ergometers are the instruments of choice, and the use of toe clips has been demonstrated to improve power output by 5–12% in adults.[68] With small children, the cycle crank length may be problematic and if the crank length is inappropriate for the child's leg length the muscle length–tension relationship may adversely affect power output.[69] Bar-Or[70] has observed this effect to be small within the usual range of subject size, and he reported that a change in optimal crank length of 5 cm would be expected to alter PP by only 1.24%.

Several laboratories have modified the original Wingate protocol and the lack of standardization across studies makes it difficult to interpret data from different laboratories. The advantages of a pre-test warm-up have been demonstrated,[71] and, as changes in muscle temperature change the rate of cross-bridge detachment and therefore the maximal velocity of shortening,[72] it is advisable to carefully standardize the warm-up and build it into the test protocol.[71] With children, a rolling start is generally preferred and the ergometer seat and handlebars need to be adjusted appropriately for each subject. A typical protocol[73] following a 3–4-min standardized warm-up, which includes three or four short sprints, would be to commence the WAnT from a rolling start, at 60 rev·min^{-1} against minimal resistance (weight basket supported). When a constant pedal rate of 60 rev·min^{-1} is achieved, a countdown of '3-2-1-go' is given, the test braking force applied, and the online data collection system activated. Subjects must remain seated but they are verbally encouraged to pedal maximally throughout the test. Power output is conventionally calculated from the formula:

$$P(W) = \omega \cdot \mathrm{Tr}$$

where ω is the angular velocity of the flywheel in rad·s^{-1} and Tr is the resistive torque in N·m given by the product of the braking force and the radius of the flywheel.

This method of calculating power output in the WAnT does not take into account the work done in overcoming the inertia of the flywheel or the internal resistance of the cycle ergometer. Using a Monark 814E cycle ergometer, Chia *et al.*[74] factored in these components and calculated adjusted power output from the following equation:

$$P_{adj} = \omega\ [\mathrm{Ti} + \mathrm{Tr}] = \omega\ [I\ (d\omega/dt) + L_{\text{plus } 9\%}\ r]$$

where ω is the angular velocity of the flywheel; Tr is the resistive torque given by the product of $L_{\text{plus } 9\%}$ and r; $L_{\text{plus } 9\%}$ is the applied force plus the frictional loss in overcoming the internal force of the ergometer;[55,56] r is the radius of the flywheel; and Ti is the inertial torque given by the product of inertia [flywheel inertia[74] plus sprocket and crank inertia[75] and angular acceleration of the flywheel ($d\omega/dt$)].

Chia *et al.*[74] demonstrated that when the corrected method of calculation was applied to the PP of 9-year-old children, PP occurred earlier in the test and values were about 20% higher in both boys and girls. These findings are in accord with those for adults[14] but to date there are no similar data available from young people despite the simplicity of the technique.

In the traditional WAnT, the Wingate team initially recommended calculating PP over a 5-s time interval and assumed that this was a reflection of alactic anaerobic performance. However, subsequent research in adults demonstrated a dramatic surge in muscle lactate concentration during the first few seconds of the test,[76] and the convention was adopted that PP represented the highest mechanical power generated during a cycling or arm-cranking motion without reference to the energy pathways supporting the activity.[29] Experimenters have reported PP over 1-, 3-, or 5-s time segments, and it has been recommended that with the relative ease of computer-driven data collection systems PP over several time periods should be reported to facilitate cross-study comparisons.[74] The total work done over 30 s was originally referred to as 'anaerobic capacity'[77] but as protocols longer than 30 s have yielded more anaerobic work than the WAnT[78] the term MP has been adopted to describe the power output over the 30-s period.

The choice of a 30-s duration for the WAnT was influenced by the work of Cumming[51] and Margaria *et al.*[79] and by pilot work which indicated that some adult subjects were unable to complete longer all-out cycle tests.[70] The 30-s WAnT is, however, well tolerated by young people, and a recent study[80] demonstrated that children recover following a WAnT much faster than adults. Bar-Or[29] has suggested that if a WAnT needs to be repeated, a rest period for children need not exceed 5–10 min, but investigators following this advice should be wary of a possible cumulative temperature effect on cross-bridge cycling.

The 30-s duration of the WAnT guarantees a significant contribution from the aerobic energy pathway which, in children, may be as high as 40%[74] and investigators should be aware that MP is not an exclusively anaerobic variable. Some studies have indicated that during the WAnT children and adolescents attain about 70% of their peak $\dot{V}O_2$.[81] Nevertheless, blood lactate following a WAnT progressively rises as lactate diffuses from muscle and accumulates in blood. In children, peak blood lactate following a WAnT occurs at 2–3 min post-exercise,[58,74,82] which is somewhat earlier than in adults.[83] The interpretation of post-exercise blood lactates is complex and confounded by methodological problems related to sampling sites and assay techniques[84,85] [see Chapter 8]. The lack of longitudinal data makes it impossible to identify accurately the rate and timing of the progression of children's post-exercise lactates towards the higher values normally found in adults.[4,85] Table 5.1 presents typical data on post-WAnT lactates with the blood sampled from either the fingertip or earlobe, 2–3 min post-exercise, and with a whole blood assay used.

Power is the product of force and velocity and as each combination of braking force and pedal revolutions may produce a different power output, optimal performance on the WAnT is therefore dependent on the selection of an appropriate braking force for each subject. The prototype of the WAnT[51] used the same braking force for all subjects but subsequent versions of the test have related the braking force to body mass. Bar-Or[66] published tables of optimal braking forces for both boys and girls according to body mass, but there is some evidence to suggest that, at least with 6- to 12-year-olds, PP is independent of braking force on the Monark cycle ergometer, in the range 0.64–0.78 N·kg^{-1}.[86] A braking force of 0.74 N·kg^{-1} is commonly used with older children and adolescents.[73,87] However, as the WAnT progresses, fatigue will cause a decrease in pedalling rate, thus affecting the power/velocity ratio and consequently resulting in a further fall in power output in addition to that directly caused by fatigue. In other words, the braking force will not be optimal for both MP and PP. This problem has been addressed with the development of special isokinetic cycle ergometers, which maintain velocity at a constant level throughout the test.[62,88–90] Few studies with children have been reported and it appears that appropriately sophisticated isokinetic cycle ergometers are not commonly purchased due to the high financial cost.[61,91]

The limitations of setting a braking force in relation to body mass when performance is better related to muscle mass are readily apparent.[17,92] Identification of an appropriate braking force is particularly difficult during growth and maturation due to the complex changes in body composition, which occur at this time.[7,28] This was clearly illustrated in a study by Welsman *et al.*[93] that determined the thigh muscle volume of 9-year-old children using magnetic resonance imaging. A common braking force of 0.74 N·kg^{-1} was applied to both boys and girls but further analysis revealed that, despite their similar body mass, the girls were exercising against a braking force, which was, on average, 19% higher than that of the boys in relation to their thigh muscle volume. Individual differences varied by 49%. As many of the available data on young people's anaerobic performance are from the WAnT using body-mass-related braking forces, the calculated maximal power outputs may not have been optimal. As a consequence, these factors may have clouded our understanding of sex differences and changes in PP and MP in relation to growth and maturation.

Force–Velocity test

The F–V test focuses on optimized peak power (OPP) and overcomes the methodological problem, experienced by the WAnT, of selecting the appropriate braking force to elicit PP. The test consists of a series (typically four to eight) of maximal 5–8-s sprints by a seated subject, performed against a range of constant braking forces.

Table 5.1 Blood lactate in children and adolescents following a WAnT

Citation	Sex	Age (years)	*n*	Blood lactate (mmol·L^{-1})
Van Praagh *et al.*[82]	M	7.4 (0.3)	19	7.0 (3.2)
Falgairette *et al.*[100]	M	7.7 (0.4)	36	6.2 (2.1)
Falgairette *et al.*[100]	M	9.3 (0.7)	27	5.1 (1.8)
Armstrong and Welsman (unpublished)	F	9.9 (0.3)	17	5.2 (1.4)
Falgairette *et al.*[100]	M	11.3 (1.0)	26	8.0 (1.8)
Falgairette *et al.*[100]	M	11.6 (0.5)	34	7.7 (2.1)
Armstrong *et al.*[73]	M	12.2 (0.4)	100	6.2 (1.6)
Armstrong *et al.*[73]	F	12.2 (0.4)	100	6.0 (1.3)
Van Praagh *et al.*[58]	F	12.8 (0.4)	12	9.0 (1.8)
Van Praagh *et al.*[58]	M	12.9 (0.5)	15	10.0 (1.6)
Falgairette *et al.*[100]	M	13.1 (0.4)	29	8.4 (2.1)
Armstrong and Welsman (unpublished)	M	13.2 (0.4)	78	6.2 (1.7)
Armstrong and Welsman (unpublished)	F	13.1 (0.4)	67	6.1 (1.8)
Armstrong and Welsman (unpublished)	M	14.1 (0.3)	16	7.3 (1.3)
Falgairette *et al.*[100]	M	14.4 (0.4)	18	7.8 (1.6)

Note: Values are mean (standard deviation).

In contrast to the characteristic curvilinear relationship between force and velocity in the contracting muscle, quasi-linear braking force–velocity and parabolic braking force–power relationships have been widely observed during cycling at pedal rates between 50 and 150 rev·min^{-1}.[26,56] These relationships enable the optimal velocity and braking force for OPP to be clearly identified for each subject as illustrated in Fig. 5.1. According to Vandewalle *et al.*,[26] the force (F) and velocity (V), which elicit OPP, are about 50% of F_0 and V_0 respectively, where F_0 corresponds to the extrapolation of F for zero braking force and V_0 corresponds to the extrapolation of V for zero velocity. OPP is therefore equal to 25% of the product of F_0 and V_0. Winter[56,94] has provided details of the calculation of OPP from the relationship between pedalling rate and braking force and a simple computer program facilitates the process (Fig. 5.2).

Recent publications by Dore *et al.*[60,95,96] have utilized the protocol of 'all-out' sprint cycling. In one study using three different and randomized braking forces (0.245, 0.491, and 0.736 N·kg^{-1}) subjects pedalled as fast as possible until maximal velocity was reached.[95] Accounting for the flywheel inertia and the constant frictional force against the braking resistance applied to the flywheel, several variables were determined: cycling PP (maximal power value averaged per half revolution), optimal velocity, force which corresponds to the velocity, force at cycling PP, and the time to reach cycling PP. In another study with a large sample size (n = 520 males aged 8–20 years), Dore *et al.*[96] determined anthropometric characteristics and PP. In agreement with previous publications, PP increased with growth but slowed after 15–16 years of age. The highest correlations were found between cycling PP, fat-free mass, and lean leg volume. The authors argued that although it might make sense to standardize cycling measurements to lean muscle volume, age and fat-free mass can provide as consistent a prediction of cycling PP during growth. From a practical approach, fat-free mass estimations are easier to determine than leg volumes but other age-related qualitative characteristics should not be ignored.

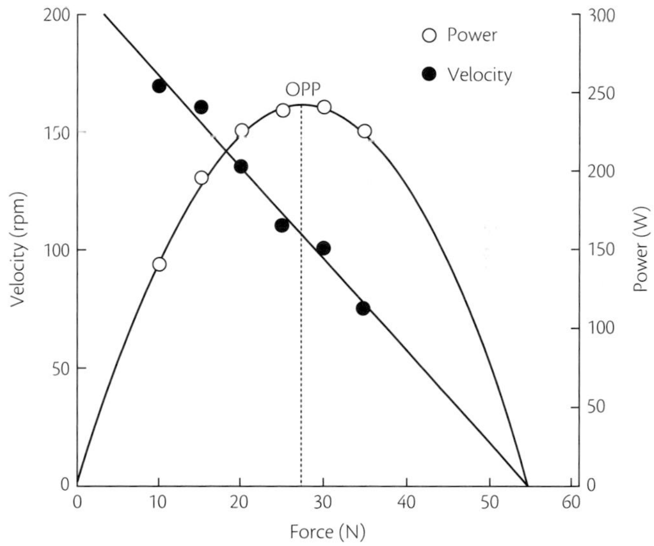

Fig. 5.1 The interpolation of optimal peak power for force–velocity and force–power relationships. Reprinted from Armstrong and Welsman[4] with permission.

Santos *et al.*[97] used the F–V test to examine OPP in 12- to 14-year-old boys and girls over four occasions at 6-month intervals. The longitudinal design of the study although relatively short was strengthened by its statistical analyses, a multi-level modelling procedure. In contrast to the findings of Dore *et al.*[96], who proposed a single braking force across a wide range of ages for boys (8–20 years) to determine cycling PP, this study found that the braking force increased with age and that a single braking force did not adequately estimate changes in power due to growth during adolescence. In addition, gender differences in OPP were not

The relationship between peak pedalling rate in rev·min^{-1} (R) and applied braking force (F) in Newtons is of the form:

$$R = a + bF$$

where a is the intercept and b is the slope.

On Monark ergometers, one revolution of the pedals moves a point on the flywheel a distance of 6 m. Consequently, an expression for power output (P) in watts can be produced:

$$P = \frac{R}{60} \times 6 \times F$$

$$\therefore P = \frac{(a + bF)}{60} \times 6 \times F$$

$$\therefore P = \frac{aF}{10} + \frac{bF^2}{10}$$

By differentiating this expression the gradient at any point on the power force curve can be identified:

$$\frac{dP}{dF} = a + 2bF$$

At the apex of the curve, the gradient is zero:

$$\therefore 0 = a + 2bF$$

$$\therefore F = \frac{-a}{2b}$$

Substituting this value of F in the original equation yields the peak value of power output (OPP)

$$\text{OPP} = \frac{a(-a/2b)}{10} + \frac{b(-a/2b)^2}{10} = \frac{-0.025a^2}{b}$$

As b is negative, OPP and the braking force and pedalling rate corresponding to OPP can be identified.

Fig. 5.2 Determination of OPP from pedalling rate and applied braking force. Adapted from Winter[94] and reproduced with Professor Winter's permission.

significant in contrast to previous investigations of power output measured during the WAnT.[98] This is most likely to be explained by the effects of a fixed braking force protocol in the WAnT compared to the optimized protocol of the F–V test (for further explanation see Chapter 17).

The F–V test is being increasingly used in studies of young people,[57,58,97,99–102] but the number of sprints employed, the rest period between sprints, the use of a rolling or standing start, the randomization and increments of braking forces applied, and the standardization of warm-ups all still need to be addressed before meaningful comparisons can be made between studies. Published studies with young people that have taken into account the inertia of the flywheel, the internal resistance of the cycle ergometer, and have used appropriate statistical procedures to assess reliability are sparse. In one reproducibility study, 27 pre-pubertal children (14 females and 13 males, mean age 9.8 ± 0.5 years) and 27 adult physical education students (9 females and 18 males, mean age 24.4 ± 4.3 years) completed five F–V tests over 15 days.[102] Braking forces between 1.5% and 7.5% of body mass for the children and 2.5% and 10% of body mass for the adults were applied. It was noted with some children that during tests 3, 4, and 5 markedly lower PPs were recorded compared to their results in test 1. Consequently, there was a bias in the mean differences between results in tests 3–5 and test 1 (−26.2 ± 27.3 W) confirming the decreased performance. If the children's reproducibility was assessed for only tests 1 and 2, the coefficient of variation was found to be less than 3%. Using the Bland and Altman method,[49] the non-significant bias between test 1 and 2 measurements was found to be −0.31% with upper and lower limits of agreement 7.72% (5.82; 9.61) and −8.34% (−10.23; −6.45), respectively. It was concluded that a habituation session with the full completion of the protocol is required and that higher levels of motivation by the children are needed if there are more than two tests in order to prevent decreases in cycling performance. This study confirmed an earlier study with prepubertal children which demonstrated that on a test–retest basis OPP and optimal velocity increased by 9.3% and 7.1%, respectively.[103]

The principal disadvantage of the F–V test is the total time required for completion in relation to other anaerobic tests and there is a possibility of lactate stacking over the series of sprints.[59] However, the F–V test deserves further attention because the OPP achieved is more likely to reflect the 'true' PP cycling than that measured by the WAnT or other cycling protocols and the interrelationship of optimal braking force and optimal velocity during growth and maturation is worthy of study. Some investigators have advocated the use of the F–V test to identify the optimal braking force for the WAnT[29,58] but this is contentious as the optimal braking force for a sprint of about 5 s is unlikely to also be optimal for a 30-s sprint. The F–V test provides a promising model for the investigation of young people's maximal intensity power output in its own right and not just as a prerequisite for another test.

Isokinetic cycle tests

Researchers in the early 1980s began to develop isokinetic cycle ergometers by maintaining a constant cadence and measuring force at the pedal cranks.[104,105] In the original isokinetic cycle ergometers, the braking forces used to maintain a constant cadence were achieved by driving the pedals at a constant speed.[104,105] Nowadays the braking forces are only engaged when the participant reaches the preset cadence. These early ergometers have been constantly refined resulting in commercially available but expensive cycle ergometers (e.g. SRM, Lode, and Biodex).

To overcome the financial expense of commercially constructed ergometers, Williams and Keen[63] developed a novel cycle mounted to a large treadmill. This purpose-built ergometer resolved two of the major disadvantages of a traditional friction-braked flywheel ergometer. First, the dynamometry allowed control of the cadence and therefore application of the fundamental muscle force–velocity characteristics. Second, as the ergometer measured force at the cranks and cadence was controlled to within ±1 rev·min^{-1}, issues related to problems of inertial load of the flywheel and variation in velocity due to acceleration and deceleration were resolved. This new type of ergometer incorporates a normal but strengthened cycle mounted on to a motorized treadmill. The power output is measured using a commercially available crank unit system (SRM powercrank, Julich, Germany). The unit measures and records the power output during cycling and can be integrated into any system that uses a chain drive and crank bearing set-up. The back wheel of the bicycle is in contact with the treadmill belt. The participant is able to free-wheel but is unable to overcome the resistance of the treadmill motor, therefore maximum pedal cadence is controlled by the speed of the treadmill belt. The transmitted torque between the crank axle and drive chain is measured by 20 strain gauges located in an aluminium disc attached to the crank axle in the chain wheel. The strain is processed within the crank unit and transmitted inductively as an analogue signal, the frequency being proportional to the produced torque. The forces exerted tangentially on the pedal cranks and the cadence data are directly sampled to a personal computer via a small data logger box fixed on the handlebars at a frequency of 250 Hz. Several studies using this device have measured maximal intensity exercise in both boys and girls.[90] Data generated using this ergometer have been found to be reliable.[88,106]

In the only published study of comparisons between different cycle ergometers, a commercially available isokinetic ergometer (SRM performance Ergo, Julich, Germany), a modified friction-braked Monark and a modified friction-braked Ergomeca cycle ergometer were compared.[89] Using a modified 20-s WanT, 14 boys aged 8.9 ± 0.3 years performed identical maximal sprint cycling on all three ergometers over three consecutive days. Common indices of PP, MP, and time to PP produced similar mean values. The calculation of the typical error, as described by Hopkins,[15] for PP varied from 34 W between the Ergomeca and the Monark ergometer, 32 W between the Ergomeca and the SRM ergometer, and 27 W between the Monark and the SRM ergometer. The typical error for the MP ranged from a low of 23 W to a high of 29 W. The error for the time to PP ranged from 1.2 to 2.5 s. Intra-class correlations were higher for PP indices ($r = 0.60–0.77$) than MP ($r = 0.45–0.66$) and time to PP (range of $r = 0.24–0.53$). Despite the contrasting instrumentation and measurement of power output, it was concluded that the typical errors were similar for all three ergometers.

In summary, if PP is to be measured during cycling then the external force should be optimally matched with the ability of the muscle groups exercised to operate at their optimal velocity. The F–V test is therefore the method of choice especially as it also provides information on the force and velocity components of power output. Data on young people, however, are sparse and the reliability of the test with this population requires further investigation. For a more sustained test of power output (i.e. >10 s) the WAnT is likely to retain its current popularity despite the well-documented problems associated with the selection of an appropriate braking force to determine PP and MP. Isokinetic cycle ergometers, which can maintain velocity at a constant level throughout the test, may eventually replace the WAnT but appropriate isokinetic cycle ergometers are not yet commercially available at a reasonable cost.

Running tests

A number of running tests have been used to estimate young people's anaerobic performance,[18,19] but the development of a running test which measures maximal intensity power output remained elusive until Margaria *et al.*[107] solved the problem by requiring subjects to run up a flight of stairs. From the the height ascended, the time taken, and the subject's body mass, external power output was calculated. The Margaria step test (MST) became the most popular test of anaerobic performance for two decades and it is still widely used as a field test of young people's maximal power.

In the laboratory, assessment of power output while running on a motorized treadmill is problematic[108] although some investigators have used the time subjects can maintain a set exercise intensity (fixed slope and constant belt velocity) as a measure of young people's anaerobic performance.[1] However, the non-motorized treadmill (NMT) has the greater potential to provide a running model for the assessment of both adults'[109,110] and children's[111,112] maximal power output.

Margaria step test

In the original MST protocol, subjects were invited to sprint up a flight of stairs, two steps of 17.5 cm each at a time, after a 2 m run on a flat surface. The time taken to climb an even number of stairs was measured with an electronic clock driven by two photoelectric cells. The reason for an even number of steps was to have the subject intercept the beam of light while in the same position and in the same phase of movement. Margaria *et al.*[107] reported that maximal speed was attained in 1.5–2 s and then maintained constant for at least 4–5 s. It was assumed that all the external work was done in raising the centre of mass of the body and that this rise was the same as the level difference between the steps. Power was then calculated from the formula:

$$\begin{aligned}\text{Power}\,(W) &= \text{force} \times \text{velocity}\\ &= \text{body weight}\,(N) \times \text{vertical speed}\,(\text{m}\cdot\text{s}^{-1})\\ &= [\text{body mass (kg)} \times 9.81\text{m}\cdot\text{s}^{-1}] \times \left[\frac{h(\text{m})}{t(\text{s})}\right]\end{aligned}$$

where h is the level difference between the steps where the cells are set, t is the time taken, and 9.81 is the acceleration due to gravity.

Margaria *et al.*[107] reported data on 131 subjects of both sexes, aged from 10 to 70 years. They claimed the data to be 'very reproducible' with repeated tests in the same session giving values that never exceeded ±4% of the average. Pressure-activated switch mats linked to an electronic timer superseded the use of photocells[111] and subsequent modifications of the original protocol have shown that variations in step height, length of run-up, and the use of external loading can markedly affect the external power recorded with both adults and children.[111–113]

With the realization that good motor coordination is essential for optimal performance and the likelihood of a considerable learning effect, especially with young children, the popularity of the MST waned. Although the MST has generally been replaced by the WAnT as the principal measure of young people's maximal intensity power output, Margaria's elegant work provided a methodology, which stimulated research into anaerobic performance and provided several insights into the topic. For example, the MST generated the first data to suggest that children's anaerobic performance may be inferior to that of adults.[107]

Non-motorized treadmill test

A 30-s maximal sprint on an NMT was proposed by Lakomy and his associates[109,110] as a useful way of investigating human responses to brief periods of high-intensity exercise. Van Praagh's research group used the test with trained and untrained 8- to 13-year-olds, but only for periods of less than 10 s. They reported, in abstract form, a correlation of $r = 0.94$ between PP on the NMT and PP during an F–V test.[111,116] Peak power during the F–V test was significantly higher than 'running power' on the NMT and Van Praagh and Franca[19] reported that, whereas no learning effects were observed during the F–V test, a significant learning effect was observed (test–retest) during running on the NMT. No further details on reliability were reported and, despite stressing the potential of NMT tests for the measurement of an individual's running power, this group do not appear to have published further research on this topic to date.

Falk *et al.*[117,118] tested 11- to 17-year-old athletes on an NMT and reported PP over 2.5 s. The young athletes were instructed to sprint 'all-out' for 30 s but as most subjects found this duration of exercise too difficult to complete MP was reported over a 20 s period. The PP and MP scores were compared to WAnT performances of similarly aged but untrained young people. The NMT scores were generally higher but as the WAnT PP and MP were calculated over 5-s and 30-s periods this was not unexpected. The subjects appear to have only experienced the test once and no habituation period was described in the reports. Test–retest reliability was determined with 29 males and females aged 10–31 years who performed the test twice. Nineteen of these subjects performed the test three times. Test–retest coefficients of 0.80 and 0.81 for PP and MP, respectively, were found between the second and third tests but the relationship between the first and second tests was found to be less consistent.[118] The findings of both Falk and Van Praagh emphasize the importance of a period of habituation prior to performance on an NMT.

Sutton *et al.*[112] refined Lakomy's model and developed a permanent anaerobic test station for children as illustrated in Fig. 5.3. A safety frame bolted to the floor with the harness clipped to the child provides a safe environment in which following habituation the children are confident to sprint maximally. The internal resistance of the NMT is standardized through an external motor fixed to the front drum of the NMT, which rotates the belt at a constant velocity for 5 min prior to each trial. A strain gauge, fixed to a wall bracket adjustable to the size of the child and an extensible tether, with the other end of the tether attached to a non-elastic belt around the child's waist, provides the horizontal force component. Power output is calculated from the product of the restraining force and the treadmill belt velocity, which is monitored online with an electronic sensor. The children are fully habituated to the test during a comprehensive habituation session conducted in the testing week. The recorded test is held on a subsequent day and the subjects warm-up and commence the test from a rolling start with the belt speed at 1.67 $\text{m}\cdot\text{s}^{-1}$. When a constant belt speed is attained, a countdown of '3-2-1-go' is given, the computerized online system is activated, and the child sprints maximally for a period of 30 s.

Sutton *et al.*[112] reported a study in which 19 well-habituated 10-year-olds completed two NMTs and two WAnTs counterbalanced over 2 days. The PP and MP for the NMT and WAnT were 212.7 ± 39.6 W, 150.2 ± 29.3 W and 256.8 ± 88.2 W, 226.1 ± 77.8 W, respectively. Significantly higher 2-min post-exercise blood lactates were reported following the NMT (7.1 ± 1.4 vs. 5.2 ± 1.2 $\text{mmol}\cdot\text{L}^{-1}$). The correlations between PP and MP on the NMT and WAnT were 0.82 and 0.88 ($p < 0.01$), respectively. The NMT demonstrated repeatability coefficients[48] of 26.6 W for PP and 15.3 W for MP. The corresponding values for the WAnT were 44.5 W for PP and 42.1 W for MP. The same authors[112] demonstrated that following habituation the NMT was appropriate for 8-year-olds and reported average PP over two tests of 207.9 W and average MP of 143.6 W. The repeatability coefficients were 28.4 W and 14.1 W for PP and MP, respectively.

Oliver *et al.*[119] tested 12 adolescent boys (15.3 ± 0.3 years) for the reliability of laboratory tests of repeated sprint ability (7 × 5-s sprints) using the NMT. In a well-controlled study, mean CVs calculated across all the trials were <2.9% for velocity and <8.4% for power output. This study also analysed the fatigue index (mean results over the first two and last two sprints) to represent the

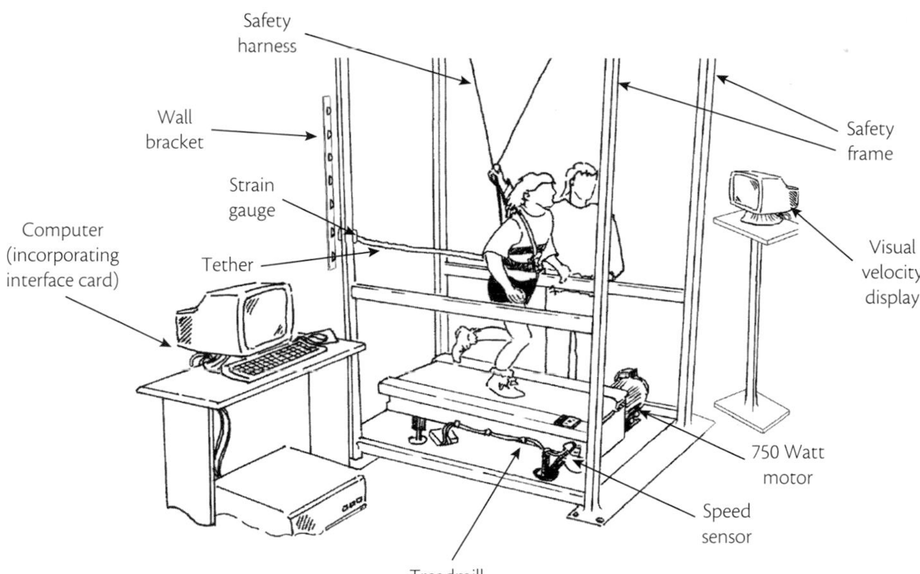

Fig. 5.3 The non-motorized treadmill test. Reproduced with permission of the Children's Health and Exercise Research Centre, University of Exeter.

drop-off but recommended that the resulting CV which was >46% did not support its use in future studies. These authors appear to be the first to differentiate the reliability of the resulting power output as a function of the force and velocity measurements. The measurement of power output during the laboratory test was found to be less reliable than velocity.

Sutton *et al.*[112] reported coefficients of repeatability of 26.6 W for PP and 15.3 W for MP, a recalculation of their data to present as mean CVs results in values of 6.3% and 5.1%, respectively. The variability of Sutton *et al.*'s MP is similar to the data of Oliver *et al.*[119] with the larger variability in PP a likely function of the subject starting each sprint from a rolling start and hence slightly different velocities each time. However, when the data are averaged to represent MP, the affect of this variation in the rolling start is reduced. These small changes in the reliability of PP and MP are important because the more reliable the measure, the greater the confidence an investigator will have to detect an observed difference between two groups or two time periods. To date these are the only studies that have reported the test–retest repeatability of an NMT test in young people.

One study has reported maximal intensity exercise using both the NMT and cycle ergometer[120] on the same group of children. A total of 28 boys and 28 girls aged 11–12 years completed two 30-s 'all-out' sprint tests, one running and one cycling. This study is discussed in detail in Chapter 17 but a clear advantage of assessing maximal intensity exercise with both ergometers is that any performance differences will be a reflection of the differing muscle recruitment, biochemical profiles, and fatigue profiles in cycling versus running. Similarly, in two subsequent papers by Ratel *et al.*[121,122] which are also analysed fully in Chapter 17, cycle and treadmill ergometry were utilized to investigate the fatigue and recovery profiles of young adolescent boys from multiple sprint trials.

In summary, the NMT test offers a promising laboratory model for research into young people's maximal power output during running but more research is required before its potential can be evaluated fully. The use of both cycling and running tests with the same children may provide further insights into maximal intensity exercise during growth and maturation.

Summary

- New technologies such as ^{31}PMRS have potential for the future but it is not presently possible to obtain direct measurements of children's anaerobic energy turnover during whole-body exercise.
- Difficulties in quantifying anaerobic performance have meant that the majority of studies of children's anaerobic performance have focused on the measurement of mechanical work or power output to reflect anaerobic metabolism.
- To simplify terminology the use of the term maximal intensity exercise to signify 'all-out effort' irrespective of which energy system is predominantly supplying the muscular activity seems appropriate.
- The majority of maximal intensity exercise studies with young people have used cycle ergometry and measured indices of peak and mean power, often in combination with post-exercise blood lactate accumulation.
- Cycle ergometry is a convenient, safe, and inexpensive method of measurement but it is not without inherent problems. Methodological issues include the duration of the test and appropriate braking force (a particular problem with growing and maturing children), and accounting for the inertia of the flywheel and the acceleration of the flywheel at the start of the test.
- Friction-braked ergometers using a constant resistance are constrained by the lack of application to F–V characteristics. Amendments to constant load tests by the use of F–V tests of short duration (<8 s) across a range of loads adhere more closely to muscle dynamics and are now becoming more commonly reported.

- Commercially available isokinetic cycle ergometers although expensive can control for some of the inertial and velocity-dependent factors which affect peak power. However, more paediatric data are needed to examine these factors.
- Studies using running on an NMT to investigate maximal intensity exercise during childhood and adolescence have recently been published. This methodology is as robust and reliable as cycle ergometry and offers a sound ecological validity for those sports that are running based. Further research is needed and studies involving both running and cycling tests may provide new insights into maximal intensity exercise during growth and maturation.

References

1. Paterson DH, Cunningham DA (1985). Development of anaerobic capacity in early and late maturing boys. In: Binkhorst RA, Kemper HCG, Saris WHM (eds.), *Children and exercise XI*, pp. 119–28. Human Kinetics, Champaign, IL.
2. De Bruyn-Prévost P, Sturbois X (1984). Physiological responses of girls to aerobic and anaerobic endurance tests. *J Sport Med Phys Fitness* **24**, 149–54.
3. Bangsbo J, Gollnick PD, Graham TE, Juel C, Kiens B, Mizuno M, Saltin B (1990). Anaerobic energy production and O_2 deficit–debt relationship during exhaustive exercise in man. *J Physiol* **422**, 539–59.
4. Armstrong N, Welsman JR (1997). *Young people and physical activity*. Oxford University Press, Oxford.
5. Rowland TW (1996). *Developmental exercise physiology*. Human Kinetics, Champaign, IL.
6. Barker A, Welsman J, Welford D, Fulford J, Williams CA, Armstrong N. (2006). Reliability of ^{31}P magnetic spectroscopy during an exhaustive incremental exercise test in children. *Eur J Appl Physiol* **98**, 556–65.
7. Zanconato S, Buchthal S, Barstow TJ, Cooper DM (1993). ^{31}P-magnetic resonance spectroscopy of leg muscle metabolism during exercise in children and adults. *J Appl Physiol* **74**, 2214–8.
8. Kuno S, Takahashi H, Fujimoto K, Akima H, Miyamaru M, Nemoto I, Itai Y, Katsuta S (1995). Muscle metabolism during exercise using phosphorus-^{31}nuclear magnetic resonance spectroscopy in adolescents. *Eur J Appl Physiol* **70**, 301–4.
9. Naughton GA, Carlson JS (1995). Anaerobic capacity assessment in male and female children with all-out isokinetic cycling exercise. *Aust J Sci Med Sport* **27**, 83–7.
10. Naughton GA, Carlson JS, Buttifant DC, Selig SE, Meldrum K, McKenna MJ, Snow RJ (1997). Accumulated oxygen deficit measurements during and after high-intensity exercise in trained male and female adolescents. *Eur J Appl Physiol* **76**, 525–31.
11. Carlson JS, Naughton GA (1998). Assessing accumulated oxygen deficit in children. In: Van Praagh E (ed.), *Pediatric anaerobic performance*, pp. 118–36. Human Kinetics, Champaign, IL.
12. Bangsbo J (1996). Oxygen deficit: A measure of the anaerobic energy production during intense exercise. *Can J Appl Physiol* **21**, 350–63.
13. Bailey RC, Olson J, Pepper SL, Porszasz J, Barstow TT, Cooper DM (1995). The level and tempo of children's physical activities: An observational study. *Med Sci Sport Exerc* **27**, 1033–41.
14. Lakomy HKA (1994). Assessment of anaerobic power. In: Harries M, Williams C, Stanish WD, Micheli LJ (eds.), *Oxford textbook of sports medicine*, pp. 180–7. Oxford University Press, Oxford.
15. Hopkins WG (2000). Measures of reliability in sports medicine and science. *Sports Med* **30**, 1–15.
16. Atkinson G, Nevill AM (1998). Statistical methods for assessing measurement error (reliability) in variables relevant to sports medicine. *Sports Med* **26**, 217–38.
17. Sargeant A (1989). Short-term muscle power in children and adolescents. In: Bar-Or O (ed.), *Advances in pediatric sports sciences, Vol. 3*, pp. 41–63. Human Kinetics, Champaign, IL.
18. Van Praagh E (1996). Testing of anaerobic performance. In: Bar-Or O (ed.), *The encyclopaedia of sports medicine. The child and adolescent athlete*, pp. 602–16. Blackwell Scientific, London.
19. Van Praagh E, Franca NM (1998). Measuring maximal short-term power output during growth. In: Van Praagh E (ed.), *Pediatric anaerobic performance*, pp. 155–89. Human Kinetics, Champaign, IL.
20. Marey EJ, Demeny G (1885). Locomotion humaine: Méchanisme du saut (Human locomotion: the jump mechanism). *Compte Rendu Séances Acad Sci* 489–94.
21. Baumgartner TA, Jackson AS (1991). *Measurement for evaluation in physical education and exercise science*. Brown, Dubuque, IA.
22. Bosco C, Luhtanen P, Komi PV (1983). A simple method for measurement of mechanical power in jumping. *Eur J Appl Physiol* **50**, 273–82.
23. Sargent LW (1921). The physical test of a man. *Am Phys Educ Rev* **26**, 188–94.
24. Kirby RF (1991). *Kirby's guide for fitness and motor performance tests*. Ben Oak, Cape Girardeau, MO.
25. Ferretti G, Gussoni M, di Prampero PE, Ceretelli P (1987). Effects of exercise on maximal instantaneous muscular power of humans. *J Appl Physiol* **62**, 2288–94.
26. Vandewalle H, Pérès G, Monad H (1987). Standard anaerobic exercise tests. *Sports Med* **4**, 268–89.
27. Martin JC, Malina RM (1998). Developmental variations in anaerobic performance associated with age and sex. In: Van Praagh E (ed.), *Pediatric anaerobic performance*, pp. 45–64. Human Kinetics, Champaign, IL.
28. Malina RM, Bouchard C (1991). *Growth, maturation and physical activity*. Human Kinetics, Champaign, IL.
29. Bar-Or O (1996). Anaerobic performance. In: Docherty D (ed.), *Measurement in pediatric exercise science*, pp. 161–82. Human Kinetics, Champaign, IL.
30. Gray RK, Start KB, Glencross DJ (1962). A test of leg power. *Res Q* **33**, 44–50.
31. Fox EL, Bowers R, Foss M (1993). *The physiological basis for exercise and sport*. Brown and Benchmark, Madison, WI.
32. Davies CTM (1971). Human power output in exercise of short duration in relation to body size and composition. *Ergonomics* **14**, 245–56.
33. Davies CTM, Rennie R (1968). Human power output. *Nature* **217**, 770.
34. Offenbacher EL (1970). Physics and the vertical jump. *Am J Physiol* **38**, 7.
35. Davies CTM, Young K (1984). Effects of external loading on short-term power output in children and young male adults. *Eur J Appl Physiol* **52**, 351–4.
36. Adamson GT, Whitney RJ (1971). Critical appraisal of jumping as a measure of human power. *Med Sport* **6**, 208–11.
37. Baltzopoulos V, Kellis E (1998). Isokinetic strength during childhood and adolescence. In: Van Praagh E (ed.), *Pediatric anaerobic performance*, pp. 225–40. Human Kinetics, Champaign, IL.
38. Murray DA, Harrison E (1986). Constant velocity dynamometer: An appraisal using mechanical loading. *Med Sci Sport Exerc* **6**, 612–24.
39. Avis FJ, Hoving A, Toussaint HM (1985). A dynamometer for the measurement of force, velocity, work and power during an explosive leg extension. *Eur J Appl Physiol* **54**, 210–5.
40. Saavedra C, Lagassé P, Bouchard C, Simoneau J-A (1991). Maximal anaerobic performance of the knee extensor muscles during growth. *Med Sci Sport Exerc* **23**, 1083–9.
41. Calvert RE, Bar-Or O, McGillis LA, Suei K (1993). Total work during an isokinetic and Wingate endurance tests in circumpubertal males. *Pediatr Exerc Sci* **5**, 398.

42. Faro A, Silva J, Santos A, Iglesias P, Ning Z (1997). A study of knee isokinetic strength in preadolescence. In: Armstrong N, Kirby BJ, Welsman JR (eds.), *Children and exercise XIX*, pp. 313–8. E and FN Spon, London.
43. De Ste Croix MBA, Armstrong N, Welsman JR, Winsley RJ, Parsons G, Sharpe P (1997). Relationship of muscle strength with muscle volume in young children. In: Armstrong N, Kirby BJ, Welsman JR (eds.), *Children and exercise XIX*, pp. 319–24. E and FN Spon, London.
44. Weltman A, Tippett S, Janney C, Strand K, Rians C, Cahill BR, Katch FI (1988). Measurement of isokinetic strength in prepubertal males. *J Orthop Sport Phys* **9**, 345–51.
45. Gilliam TB, Villanacci JF, Freedson PS (1979). Isokinetic torque in boys and girls ages 7 to 13: Effect of age, height and weight. *Res Quart* **50**, 599–609.
46. Burnie J, Brodie DA (1986). Isokinetic measurement in preadolescent males. *Int J Sports Med* **7**, 205–9.
47. Kanecisa H, Ikagawa S, Tsunoda N, Fukunaga T (1994). Strength and cross-sectional areas of knee extensor muscles in children. *Eur J Appl Physiol* **65**, 402–5.
48. Bland JM, Altman DG (1986). Statistical methods for assessing agreement between two methods of clinical measurement. *Lancet* **i**, 307–10.
49. De Ste Croix MBA, Armstrong N, Welsman JR (2003). The reliability of an isokinetic knee muscle endurance test in young children. *Pediatr Exerc Sci* **15**, 313–23.
50. Kellis E, Kellis S, Gerodimos V, Manou V (1999). Reliability of isokinetic concentric and eccentric strength in circumpubertal soccer players. *Pediatr Exerc Sci* **11**, 218–22.
51. Cumming GR (1973). Correlation of athletic performance and aerobic power in 12 17-year-old children with bone age, calf muscle, total body potassium, heart volume and two indices of anaerobic power. In: Bar-Or O (ed.), *Pediatric work physiology*, pp. 109–34. Wingate Institute, Netanya, Israel.
52. Ayalon A, Inbar O, Bar-Or O (1974). Relationships between measurements of explosive strength and anaerobic power. In: Nelson RC, Morehouse CA (eds.), *International series on sports sciences: Vol. 1, Biomechanics IV*, pp. 527–32. University Park Press, Baltimore, MD.
53. Inbar O, Bar-Or O, Skinner JS (1996). *The Wingate anaerobic test.* Human Kinetics, Champaign, IL.
54. Maréchal R, Pirnay F, Creilaard JM, Petit JM (1979). Influence de l'age sur la puissance anaerobie (Influence of age on anaerobic power). Economica, Paris.
55. Pirnay F, Creilaard JM (1979). Mesure de la puissance anaerobic alactique. *Med de Sports* **53**, 13–6.
56. Winter EM (1991). Cycle ergometry and maximal exercise. *Sports Med* **11**, 351–7.
57. Santos AMC, Welsman JR, De Ste Croix MBA, Armstrong N (2002). Age and sex-related differences in optimal peak power. *Pediatr Exerc Sci* **14**, 202–12.
58. Van Praagh E, Fellmann N, Bedu M, Falgariette G, Coudert J (1990). Gender difference in the relationship of anaerobic power output to body composition in children. *Pediatr Exerc Sci* **2**, 336–48.
59. Williams C, Armstrong N (1995). Optimized peak power output of adolescent children during maximal sprint pedalling. In: Ring FJ (ed.), *Children in sport*, pp. 40–4. University Press, Bath.
60. Dore E, Diallo O, Franca NM, Bedu M, Van Praagh E (2000). Dimensional changes cannot account for all differences in short-term cycling power during growth. *Int J Sports Med* **21**, 360–65.
61. Sargeant AJ, Dolan P (1986). Optimal velocity of muscle contraction for short-term (anaerobic) power output in children and adults. In: Rutenfranz J, Mocellin R, Klimt F (eds.), *Children and exercise XII*, pp. 39–42. Human Kinetics, Champaign, IL.
62. Sargeant AJ, Hoinville E, Young A (1981). Maximum leg force and power output during short-term dynamic exercise. *J Appl Physiol* **51**, 1175–82.
63. Williams CA, Keen P (1997). Test–retest reproducibility of a new isokinetic cycle ergometry. In: Armstrong N, Kirby B, Welsman JR (eds.), *Children and exercise XIX*, pp. 300–5. E & FN Spon, London.
64. Blimkie CJR, Roache P, Hay JT, Bar-Or O (1988). Anaerobic power of arms in teenage boys and girls: Relationship to lean tissue. *Eur J Appl Physiol* **57**, 677–83.
65. Nindle BC, Mahar MT, Harman EA, Patton JF (1995). Lower and upper body anaerobic performance in male and female adolescent athletes. *Med Sci Sport Exerc* **27**, 235–41.
66. Bar-Or O (1993). Noncardiopulmonary pediatric exercise tests. In: Rowland TW (ed.), *Pediatric laboratory exercise testing*, pp. 165–85. Human Kinetics, Champaign, IL.
67. Sutton NC, Childs DJ, Bar-Or O, Armstrong N (2000). A nonmotorized treadmill test to assess children's short-term power output. *Pediatr Exerc Sci* **12**, 91–100.
68. Lavoie N, Dallaier J, Brayne S, Barrett D (1984). Anaerobic testing using the Wingate and the Evans–Quinney protocols with and without toe stirrups. *Can J Appl Sport Sci* **9**, 1–5.
69. Sargeant AJ (1998). The determinants of anaerobic muscle function during growth. In: Van Praagh E (ed.), *Pediatric anaerobic performance*, pp. 97–117. Human Kinetics, Champaign, IL.
70. Bar-Or O (1987). The Wingate anaerobic test: An update on methodology, reliability and validity. *Sports Med* **4**, 381–94.
71. Inbar O, Bar-Or O (1975). The effects of intermittent warm-up on 7- to 9-year-old boys. *Eur J Appl Physiol* **34**, 81–9.
72. Sargeant AJ (1987). Effect of muscle temperature on leg extension force and short-term power output in humans. *Eur J Appl Physiol* **56**, 693–8.
73. Armstrong N, Welsman JR, Kirby BJ (1997). Performance on the Wingate anaerobic test and maturation. *Pediatr Exerc Sci* **9**, 253–61.
74. Chia M, Armstrong N, Childs D (1997). The assessment of children's anaerobic performance using modifications of the Wingate anaerobic test. *Pediatr Exerc Sci* **9**, 80–9.
75. Monger LS, Allchorn A, Doust J (1993). An automated bicycle ergometer system for the measurement of Wingate Test indices with allowance for inertial and accelerative influences. *J Sport Sci* **7**, 77–8.
76. Jacobs I, Tesch PA, Bar-Or O, Karlsson J, Dotan R (1983). Lactate in human skeletal muscle after 10 and 30 s of supramaximal exercise. *J Appl Physiol* **55**, 365–7.
77. Bar-Or O (1983). *Pediatric sports medicine for the practitioner.* Springer-Verlag, New York.
78. Katch V, Weltman A, Martin R, Gray L (1977). Optimal test characteristics for maximal anaerobic work on the bicycle ergometer. *Res Q* **48**, 319–27.
79. Margaria R, Oliva D, di Prampero PE, Ceretelli P (1969). Energy utilization in intermittent exercise of supramaximal intensity. *J Appl Physiol* **26**, 752–6.
80. Hebestreit H, Minura K-I, Bar-Or O (1994). Recovery of muscle power after high intensity short-term exercise: Comparing boys to men. *J Appl Physiol* **74**, 2875–80.
81. Van Praagh E, Bedu M, Falgairette G, Fellmann N, Coudert J (1991). Oxygen uptake during a 30 s supramaximal exercise in 7 to 15 year old boys. In: Frenkl R, Szmodis I (eds.), *Children and exercise: Pediatric work physiology XV*, pp. 281–7. National Institute for Health Promotion, Budapest.
82. Van Praagh E, Falgairette G, Bedu M, Fellmann N, Coudert J (1989). Laboratory and field tests in 7-year-old boys. In: Oseid S, Carlsen KH (eds.), *Children and exercise XIII*, pp. 11–7. Human Kinetics, Champaign, IL.
83. Creilaard JM, Franchimont P (1985). La mesure de la capacité anaérobie lactique: mise au point actuelle. *Med Sport* **59**, 150–2.
84. Williams J, Armstrong N, Kirby B (1992). The influence of site of sampling and assay medium upon the measurement and interpretation of blood lactate responses to exercise. *J Sport Sci* **10**, 95–107.

85. Welsman J, Armstrong N (1998). Assessing post-exercise lactates in children and adolescents. In: Van Praagh E (ed.), *Pediatric anaerobic performance*, pp. 137–54. Human Kinetics, Champaign, IL .
86. Carlson J, Naughton G (1994). Performance characteristics of children using various braking resistances on the Wingate anaerobic test. *J Sport Med Phys Fitness* **34**, 362–9.
87. Falk B, Bar-Or O (1993). Longitudinal changes in peak aerobic and anaerobic mechanical power of circumpubertal boys. *Pediatr Exerc Sci* **5**, 318–31.
88. Williams CA, Keen P (2001). Isokinetic measurement of maximal muscle power during leg cycling—a comparison of adolescent boys and adult men. *Pediatr Exerc Sci* **13**, 154–166.
89. Williams CA, Dore E, Albaan J, Van Praagh E (2003). Short term power output in 9 year old children: Typical error between ergometers and protocols. *Pediatr Exerc Sci* **15**, 302–312.
90. Williams CA, Hammond A, Doust JH (2003). Short term power output of females during isokinetic cycling. *Iso Exerc Sci* **11**, 123–131.
91. Sargeant AJ, Dolan P, Thorne A (1984). Optimal velocity of muscle contraction for short-term output in children and adults. In: Ilmarinen J, Valimaki I (eds.), *Children and sport*, pp. 93–8. Springer-Verlag, Berlin.
92. Sargeant AJ (1992). Problems in, and approaches to the measurement of short term power output in children and adolescents. In: Coudert J, Van Praagh E (eds.), *Children and exercise XVI, Pediatric work physiology*, pp. 11–7. Masson, Paris.
93. Welsman JR, Armstrong N, Kirby BJ, Winsley RJ, Parson G, Sharp P (1997). Exercise performance and magnetic resonance imaging determined thigh muscle volume in children. *Eur J Appl Physiol* **76**, 92–7.
94. Winter EM, Brown D, Roberts NKA, Brookes FBC, Swaine IL (1996). Optimized and corrected peak power output during friction-braked cycle ergometry. *J Sport Sci* **14**, 513–21.
95. Dore E, Bedu M, Franca NM, Van Praagh E (2001). Anaerobic cycling performance characteristics in prepubescent, adolescent and young adult females. *Eur J Appl Physiol* **84**, 476–81.
96. Dore E, Bedu M, Franca NM, Diallo O, Duche P, Van Praagh E (2000). Testing peak cycling performance: Effects of braking force during growth. *Med Sci Sport Exerc* **32**, 493–98.
97. Santos AMC, Armstrong N, De Ste Croix, Sharpe P, Welsman JR (2003). Optimal peak power in relation to age, body size, gender, and thigh muscle volume. *Pediatr Exerc Sci* **15**, 406–18.
98. Armstrong N, Welsman JR, Chia MYH (2001). Short term power output in relation to growth and maturation. *Brit J Sport Med* **35**, 118–124.
99. Duché P, Falgairette G, Bedu M, Fellman N, Lac G, Robert A, Coudert J (1992). Longitudinal approach of bio-energetic profile in boys before and during puberty. In: Coudert J, Van Praagh E (eds.), *Pediatric work physiology*, pp. 43–5. Masson, Paris.
100. Falgairette G, Bedu M, Fellmann N, Van Praagh E, Coudert J (1991). Bioenergetic profile in 144 boys aged from 6 to 15 years with special reference to sexual maturation. *Eur J Appl Physiol* **62**, 151–6.
101. Mercier B, Mercier J, Ganier P, La Gallais D, Préfaut C (1992). Maximal anaerobic power: Relationship to anthropometric characteristics during growth. *Int J Sports Med* **13**, 21–6.
102. Dore E, Duche P, Rouffer D, Ratel S, Bedu M, Van Praagh E (2003). Measurement error in short-term power testing in young people. *J Sport Sci* **21**, 135–42.
103. Lavorel M, Dore E, Bedu M, Van Praagh E, Duche P (1998). Motor learning affects the child's anaerobic performance. In: Sargeant AJ, Siddons H (eds.), *From community health to elite sport. Proceedings of the third annual congress of the European College of Sports Science*, pp. 266. Centre for Health Care Development, Liverpool.
104. McCartney N, Heigenauser GJF, Sargeant AJ, Jones NL (1983). A constant-velocity cycle ergometer for the study of dynamic muscle function. *J Appl Physiol* **55**, 212–7.
105. Sargeant AJ, Hoinville E, Young A (1981). Maximum leg force, and power output during the short-term dynamic exercise. *J Appl Physiol* **51**, 1175–82.
106. Jones SM, Passfield L (1998). The dynamic calibration of bicycle power measuring cranks. In: Haake SJ (ed.), *The engineering of sport*, pp. 265–74. Blackwell Science, Oxford.
107. Margaria R, Aghemo P, Rovelli E (1966). Measurement of muscular power (anaerobic) in man. *J Appl Physiol* **21**, 1662–4.
108. Asmussen E, Bonde-Petersen F (1974). Storage of elastic energy in skeletal muscle in man. *Acta Physiol Scand* **91**, 385–92.
109. Lakomy HKA (1987). The use of a non-motorized treadmill for analysing sprint performance. *Ergonomics* **30**, 627–37.
110. Cheetham MF, Williams C, Lakomy HKA (1985). A laboratory running test: metabolic responses of sprint and endurance trained athletes. *Br J Sport Med* **19**, 81–4.
111. Fargeas MA, Van Praagh E, Léger L, Fellmann N, Coudert J (1993). Comparison of cycling and running power outputs in trained children. *Pediatr Exerc Sci* **5**, 415.
112. Sutton NC, Childs DJ, Bar-Or O, Armstrong N (2000). A nonmotorized treadmill test to assess children's short-term power output. *Pediatr Exerc Sci* **12**, 91–100.
113. Armstrong N, Ellard R (1983). The measurement of alactacid anaerobic power in trained and untrained adolescent boys. *Phys Educ Rev* **7**, 73–9.
114. Davies CTM, Barnes C, Godfrey S (1972). Body composition and maximal exercise performance in children. *Hum Biol* **44**, 195–214.
115. Caiozzo VJ, Kyle CR (1980). The effect of external loading upon power output in stair climbing. *Eur J Appl Physiol* **51**, 750–4.
116. Van Praagh E, Fargeas MA, Léger L, Fellmann N, Coudert J (1993). Short-term power output in children measured on a computerized treadmill ergometer. *Pediatr Exerc Sci* **5**, 482.
117. Falk B, Weinstein Y, Epstein S, Karni Y, Yarom Y (1993). Measurement of anaerobic power among young athletes using a new treadmill test. *Pediatr Exerc Sci* **5**, 414.
118. Falk B, Weinstein Y, Dotan R, Abramson DA, Mann-Segal D, Hoffman JR (1996). A treadmill test of sprint running. *Scand J Med Sci Sport* **6**, 259–64.
119. Oliver JL, Williams CA, Armstrong N (2006). Reliability of a field and laboratory test of repeated sprint ability. *Pediatr Exerc Sci* **18**, 339–50.
120. Bloxham SR, Welsman JR, Armstrong N (2005). Ergometer-specific relationships between peak oxygen uptake and short-term power output in children. *Pediatr Exerc Sci* **17**, 136–48.
121. Ratel S, Williams CA, Oliver JL, Armstrong N (2005). Effects of age and recovery duration on performance during multiple treadmill sprints. *Int J Sports Med* **26**, 1–8.
122. Ratel S, Williams CA, Oliver J, Armstrong N (2004). Effects of age and mode of exercise on power output profiles during repeated sprints. *Eur J Appl Physiol* **92**, 204–10.

CHAPTER 6

Pulmonary function

Patricia A. Nixon

Introduction

At rest and during exercise, the pulmonary system is responsible for transporting air to and from the alveoli along the airways, and exchanging oxygen and carbon dioxide between the alveoli and the capillary blood. Together, these serve to maintain acid–base balance. In healthy children, the lungs are generally not thought to be limiting to exercise. However, children with cardiopulmonary and other disorders may exhibit abnormal pulmonary responses which may ultimately contribute to a limitation to exercise.

The focus of this chapter is the assessment and interpretation of pulmonary function during exercise in children, with emphasis on the parameters commonly measured in the paediatric setting. The measurements of resting pulmonary function (i.e. lung volumes and expiratory flow rates) are presented to provide the basic foundation for understanding changes that occur with exercise. Some measurements are more relevant to children with cardiopulmonary disorders, and examples of normal and abnormal responses are provided. In some instances, data on children are lacking, so responses of adults are presented. A more detailed discussion of the physiology and the changes in lung function that occur with growth and development in healthy children is provided in Chapter 18. In view of these changes throughout childhood and adolescence, normal reference values and prediction equations are not provided in this chapter, but they can be found in the extensive works of Polgar and Promadhat,[1] Zapletal,[2] the compilation by Quanjer *et al.*,[3] the analysis of NHANES III data by Hankinson *et al.*[4] for resting pulmonary function, and Godfrey[5] for exercise responses.

Assessment of pulmonary function at rest

The assessment of resting pulmonary function via spirometry and the measurement of lung volumes are not routinely carried out as part of the exercise evaluation of the healthy child. However, this information is useful for understanding the pulmonary responses to exercise, particularly in the child with a pulmonary disorder.

Lung volumes

Static lung volumes and capacities are presented schematically in Fig. 6.1.[6] Capacities are defined as the sum of two or more volumes. The spirographic tracing starts with resting breathing providing the tidal volume (V_T), that is, the volume of air that is breathed in or out during normal respiration (denoted by TV in Fig. 6.1). The subject then inhales maximally reaching maximal inspiratory level. The volume of air maximally inspired above V_T is the inspiratory reserve volume (IRV). The subject then exhales maximally reaching maximal expiratory level. The volume of air maximally expired beyond normal V_T is the expiratory reserve volume (ERV). Vital capacity (VC) is the sum of IRV, V_T, and ERV and reflects the volume exhaled from maximal inspiratory level to maximal expiratory level. The volume of air that remains in the lungs after a maximal expiration is the residual volume (RV). Functional residual capacity (FRC) is the sum of RV and ERV and reflects the volume of air that is left in the lungs after a normal expiration. Conversely, the sum of V_T and IRV equals the inspiratory capacity, and reflects the volume of air that is maximally inhaled after a normal expiration. Total lung capacity (TLC) is the volume of air that is in the lungs after a maximal inspiration, and is the sum of IRV, V_T, ERV, and RV.

TLC and RV are calculated from the measurement of FRC, generally by the nitrogen washout method, the helium-dilution technique, or plethysmography.[7] For the first two methods, lung

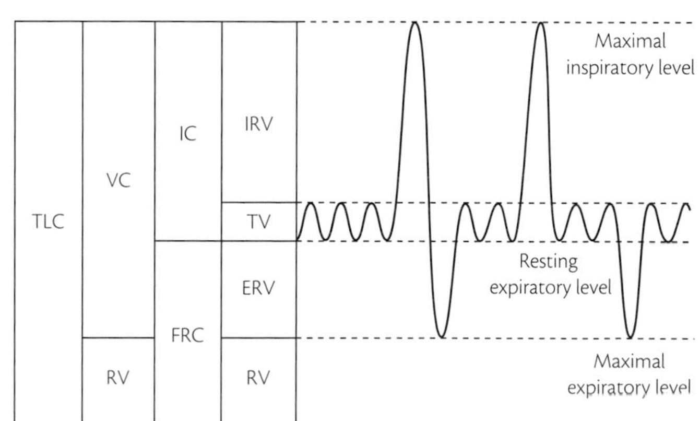

Fig. 6.1 Lung volumes as they appear on a spirographic tracing. TLC = total lung capacity, VC = vital capacity, RV = residual volume, IC = inspiratory capacity, FRC = functional residual capacity, IRV = inspiratory reserve volume, TV = tidal volume, ERV = expiratory reserve volume. From Comroe JH *et al.*,[6] p. 8.

volumes are determined from the measurement of expired gas volumes and concentrations, and known starting concentrations. These methods underestimate FRC in patients with airway obstruction who have poorly ventilated regions of the lung with trapped air. The last method, plethysmography, calculates FRC based on the theory of Boyle's law, which assumes that in a closed container such as the plethysmograph, or 'body box', changes in lung volumes can be calculated from changes in pressure under constant temperature.[7] This method is better suited for patients with poorly ventilated regions of the lung because it estimates virtually all of the gas volume in the lungs.

All of these static lung volumes and capacities increase non-linearly from childhood to adulthood, correlating with age, body surface, and most closely with height.[2]

Airway patency or flow

Airway patency is assessed by examining expiratory air flow rates and volumes, most commonly in the form of a flow/volume loop, measured via standard spirometric techniques.[8–10] The components of the flow/volume loop in a healthy child are shown in Fig. 6.2a. Forced vital capacity (FVC) is the maximal volume of air forcefully expired after a maximal inspiration. The maximal or peak expiratory flow rate (PEFR) occurs early in the forced expiratory manoeuvre. The amount of air expired during the first second of a forced maximal manoeuvre is the forced expiratory volume in one second (FEV_1). It provides a measure of larger airway function or patency. Smaller airway function or patency is provided by the forced expiratory flow rate between 25% and 75% of FVC (FEF_{25-75}). Smaller airway function is also reflected by the flow rate after 75% of FVC has been exhaled (FEF_{75}). In this example, the maximal inspiratory flow (MIF) loop (the curve below the *X*-axis) and the tidal volume loop during normal breathing are also provided. Measures of FVC, PEFR, FEV_1, and MIF are effort dependent, whereas FEF_{25-75} is considered to be relatively independent of effort.[2]

The flow/volume loop of a child with obstructive lung disease is presented in Fig. 6.2b. In obstructive disorders such as asthma or cystic fibrosis, there is limited airway patency and reduced expiratory flow. As shown, the FVC of the patient is normal, but there is evidence of both larger and smaller airway obstruction, as reflected in the concave appearance of the expiratory portion of the loop and reduced FEV_1, FEF_{25-75}, and FEF_{75}. In contrast, with restrictive lung disorders, such as scoliosis, the airway flow is normal (no concavity), but the amount of air that the lungs contain is decreased, as shown by the reduced FVC (Fig. 6.2c). As a consequence of all lung volumes being reduced, the absolute and percentage predicted values for FEV_1 and other flow rates will be reduced, suggesting airway obstruction. For this reason, the ratio of FEV_1/FVC is examined to obtain a more accurate measure of airway patency relative to lung volume. Children tend to have higher FEV_1/FVC values (~86%) than adults (~80%) with values inversely associated with age and height.[11,12] Furthermore, it is possible to have both restrictive and obstructive defects as may be present in a child with cystic fibrosis who has more advanced lung disease.

Maximal voluntary ventilation

The resting measure of maximal voluntary ventilation (MVV) is also often performed to provide an estimate of the mechanical capacity of the lungs. For this test, the child is instructed to breathe as deeply and quickly as he/she can for 12 s.[8] The volume of air breathed is then extrapolated to 1 min. Some investigators suggest that MVV in children can be estimated from the product of $FEV_1 \times 35$.[5,13]

Spirometic measurement

A variety of spirometers can be used to determine flow rates, FVC, and MVV.[14] The majority of spirometers operate either by measuring volume displacement or by directly measuring flow. The volume displacement spirometers include water-sealed spirometers, dry-rolling-seal spirometers, and bellows or wedge-bellows spirometers. With a closed system, the volume of air expired or inspired mechanically displaces a recording pen on a chart recorder or

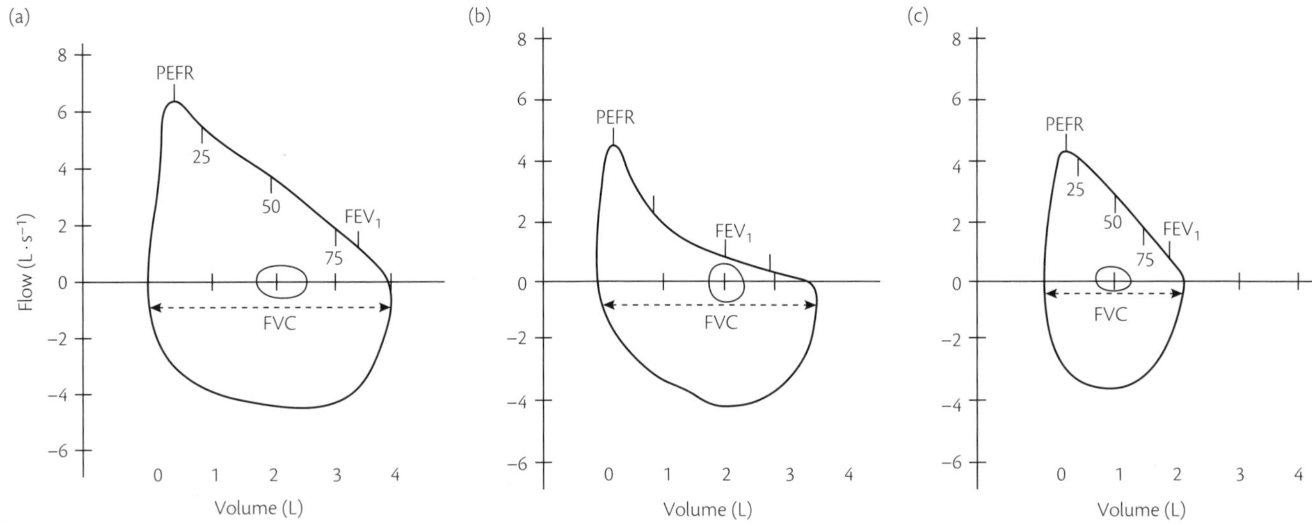

Fig. 6.2 The flow/volume loops of a healthy child (a), a child with obstructive lung disease (b), and a child with restrictive disease (c). Peak expiratory flow rate (PEFR), forced expiratory volume in 1 s (FEV_1), and forced vital capacity (FVC) are labelled. The values 25, 50, and 75 refer to the forced expiratory flow rates at 25%, 50%, and 75% of FVC. The curve below the *x*-axis reflects inspiration.

activates a potentiometer that measures the volume and flow rates. The advantage of these systems is that they provide a mechanical tracing of the flow/volume curve. The disadvantages are that some systems are not very mobile (water-sealed), the closed systems can become contaminated and are cumbersome to clean, and they may not be computerized.[14] Currently, most standard equipment utilizes flow sensing pneumotachometers, including pressure differential, heated wire, and turbine flow sensors, for performing spirometry. With pneumotachometers, the flow of gas produces a signal from which flow can be measured and gas volumes integrated. The most common type of flow sensor is the pressure differential pneumotachometer. On the basis of Poiseuille's law, gas flow and pressure drop are linearly related, assuming laminar (non-turbulent) flow. The change in air pressure across a resistive element (either capillary tubes or metal screens) is detected and measured by a pressure transducer from which flow and volume can be calculated. The heated wire pneumotachometer senses the change in temperature in a heated element (thermistor) with changes in gas flow. The gas flow is determined by the amount of current necessary to maintain a preset temperature of the thermistor, from which flow and volume can likewise be calculated. Both the pressure differential and heated wire pneumotachometers can be affected by debris and moisture collecting on the sensing elements. Furthermore, it is important that the pneumotachometer is the appropriate size and calibrated in the expected range of flow rates for the test subject to reduce measurement error.

The turbine flow sensor consists of a lightweight impeller or vane connected to a series of gears that move with and directly measure the volume of gas flow. The accuracy of the turbine may also be affected by moisture and saliva. In addition, the impeller may be slow to start up at the beginning of each breath and to slow down at the end of each breath due to inertia, leading to measurement error.[15]

Assessment of pulmonary function during exercise

Detailed information regarding indications, standardization, measurement, and interpretation for pulmonary exercise testing are beyond the scope of this chapter and can be found elsewhere.[16,17]

Minute ventilation

The pulmonary parameter most commonly measured during exercise is minute ventilation ($\dot{V}_E$), that is, the volume of air exhaled during 1 min and expressed as litres per minute [body temperature, pressure, saturated (BTPS)]. Minute ventilation is a required component for the calculation of oxygen uptake ($\dot{V}O_2$) using open-circuit spirometry. In earlier days, expired air was collected in Douglas bags or meteorological balloons, and the volume was measured as the bag was manually emptied into a dry gas meter or a large Tissot type water-sealed spirometer. The dry gas meter and the water-sealed spirometer could also be connected to the breathing circuit for direct measurements of minute ventilation.

Today, flow sensing pneumotachometers, as described previously, are popular devices for determining $\dot{V}_E$ during exercise. The potential error measurements, due to moisture, inertia, and so on, become exaggerated with the higher flow rates during exercise. In addition, the density and viscosity of different gases such as 100% oxygen can also affect the pressure–flow relationship. Consequently, calibration should be performed under the same conditions as the testing to reduce measurement error.[17]

During progressive exercise, $\dot{V}_E$ increases as a function of its components—V_T and f_R. In adults, the increase in $\dot{V}_E$ during progressive exercise is met initially by increases in V_T up to about 60%–70% of VC with f_R contributing more at higher exercise intensities.[18] As noted in Chapter 18, the healthy child may exhibit a similar response[5,19] or may rely more heavily on f_R initially, followed by greater reliance on V_T to increase $\dot{V}_E$ to meet increasing metabolic demands.[20,21] The child with restrictive lung disease has to compensate for a limited V_T by increasing f_R to meet the ventilatory demands of exercise, and by utilizing a greater fraction of vital capacity.[22–24] Minute ventilation is related to age, body size, fitness, and exercise intensity, and therefore has wide normal variation that limits its interpretation as a single measure of ventilatory function. However, examination of the increase in $\dot{V}_E$ relative to increases in $\dot{V}O_2$ and carbon dioxide production ($\dot{V}CO_2$) may provide information on ventilatory efficiency, as determined by ventilation-perfusion ($\dot{V}_A/\dot{Q}$) matching and chemoreceptor arterial carbon dioxide tension ($PaCO_2$) set point.[17] (More discussion of the physiology is presented in Chapter 18.)

Ventilatory efficiency

During progressive exercise, $\dot{V}_E$ increases linearly with increasing $\dot{V}O_2$ until a point at which the increase in $\dot{V}_E$ is accelerated due to the addition of anaerobic metabolism and resulting increase in CO_2 and lactic acid production (see section on ventilatory threshold). Consequently, the increase in $\dot{V}_E$ is more tightly coupled with increasing $\dot{V}CO_2$, with the correlation being fairly linear until the respiratory compensation point. At this point, $\dot{V}_E$ increases slightly faster in response to the decrease in pH associated with the buffering of lactic acid, and the need to expel excess CO_2 to maintain acid–base balance. Ventilatory efficiency can be examined by calculating the slope of the best-fit regression line of $\dot{V}_E$ versus $\dot{V}CO_2$ (slope = $\Delta\dot{V}_E/\Delta\dot{V}CO_2$). As noted in Chapter 18, $\Delta\dot{V}_E/\Delta\dot{V}CO_2$ is higher in children compared to adults indicating that children ventilate more for a given increase in metabolic rate (as reflected by $\Delta\dot{V}CO_2$) most likely due to a lower $PaCO_2$ set point.[25,26] Excessive ventilation relative to metabolic rate (high $\Delta\dot{V}_E/\Delta\dot{V}CO_2$) has been reported in children with cystic fibrosis (36.8 ± 1.3) compared to their healthy peers (23.4 ± 0.4) most likely to compensate for increased dead space, but also, perhaps, due to changes in chemoreceptor set point.[27] Similarly, children with congenital heart disease (CHD) who had undergone Fontan operation were shown to exhibit a higher mean $\Delta\dot{V}_E/\Delta\dot{V}CO_2$ (43 ± 12) than controls (33 ± 6).[28] At peak exercise, the children with CHD also had significantly greater dead space to tidal volume ratio (V_D/V_T), lower oxyhaemoglobin saturation (SaO_2), and lower $PaCO_2$ than control subjects. Furthermore, the $\Delta\dot{V}_E/\Delta\dot{V}CO_2$ was inversely correlated to resting $PaCO_2$ ($r = -0.53$) and SaO_2 ($r = -0.44$) suggesting that their ventilatory inefficiency was related to alveolar ventilation and pulmonary capillary perfusion ($\dot{V}_A/\dot{Q}$) mismatching, as well as altered chemosensitivity to $PaCO_2$. It should be noted that the slope of $\dot{V}_E$ versus $\dot{V}CO_2$ will be affected by early hyperventilation (as may occur in the anxious child). For this reason, some investigators prefer to examine ventilatory efficiency by determining the $\dot{V}_E/\dot{V}CO_2$ at, and, shortly after, the ventilatory threshold (T_{VENT}).[17,29]

Ventilatory threshold

The ventilatory threshold has been described as the point during progressive exercise where $\dot{V}_E$ increases disproportionately with the increase in $\dot{V}O_2$.[30] It is believed that the accelerated increase in $\dot{V}_E$ occurs in response to the increase in CO_2 and lactic acid production associated with anaerobic metabolism. While many studies have shown that the threshold for the accelerated increase in ventilation corresponds to the anaerobic threshold for increase in lactic acid (T_{Lact}),[31–35] controversy exists as to whether this represents a cause and effect relationship.[36,37] Despite this controversy, the non-invasive measurement of T_{VENT} is quite useful in the testing of paediatric populations for several reasons: (i) the measurement is non-invasive and therefore avoids the discomfort of blood sampling; (ii) it has been shown to correlate with maximal oxygen uptake ($\dot{V}O_2$ max) and endurance performance in adults,[38] and with tests of physical work capacity in children;[39] (iii) it does not require a maximal effort that is sometimes hard to obtain in children; (iv) it has good test–retest reliability;[40,41] (v) it can be used to prescribe exercise intensity, and (vi) it has been shown to increase with endurance training.[42] In general, the T_{VENT} of children occurs at a higher percentage of $\dot{V}O_2$ max than in adults,[31,43] decreases with age,[44,45] and is lower in girls than boys.[43]

There are several commonly used methods for determining T_{VENT}. In general, the T_{VENT} is more easily determined using breath-by-breath measurement of gas exchange and ramp or 1-min increments in work rate. The T_{VENT} is identified as the $\dot{V}O_2$ at which an accelerated nonlinear increase in $\dot{V}_E$ occurs as shown in Fig. 6.3.[32]

The threshold can also be identified by plotting $\dot{V}_E/\dot{V}CO_2$ and $\dot{V}_E/\dot{V}_{O2}$versus time on the *x*-axis and noting where the $\dot{V}_E/\dot{V}_{O2}$ inflects upward.17 The nadir of the $\dot{V}_E/\dot{V}CO_2$ curve denotes the beginning of respiratory compensation for lactic acidosis. An increase in end-tidal oxygen tension ($PetO_2$) will occur in conjunction with the increase in $\dot{V}_E/\dot{V}O_2$ at T_{VENT}, and a decrease in end-tidal CO_2 tension ($PetCO_2$) will occur with the increase in $\dot{V}_E/\dot{V}CO_2$ at the start of respiratory compensation.17

In patients with breathing irregularities, examination of the relationship between $\dot{V}CO_2$ and $\dot{V}O_2$, or the *V*-slope method, may help to identify the T_{VENT} independent of $\dot{V}_E$.[46] With this method, two slopes of $\dot{V}CO_2$ versus $\dot{V}O_2$ are determined by regression analysis, and the breakpoint or intercept of the two slopes indicates the T_{VENT}, or the point at which an accelerated increase in $\dot{V}CO_2$ occurs relative to $\dot{V}O_2$ (Fig. 6.4).

Normal T_{VENT} values for children range from 58% to 83% of $\dot{V}O_2$ max, and vary according to age, gender, and fitness level.[47] As previously mentioned, the measurement of T_{VENT} provides information on a child's aerobic fitness, and can be used to prescribe exercise, and follow changes that may occur with growth or training.

The T_{VENT} may also provide useful information in some children with chronic diseases, particularly when maximal exercise testing may be deemed too stressful or potentially unsafe. For instance, Reybrouck *et al.*[48] found the T_{VENT} to be more sensitive in detecting subnormal exercise performance in children with CHD than other estimates of exercise performance capacity, such as the $\dot{V}O_2$, at a given submaximal heart rate (e.g. $\dot{V}O_2$ 170). Twice as many children were found to have below normal values (<95% confidence interval) for T_{VENT} compared to below normal values for exercise capacity observed in only 28% of the children for the $\dot{V}O_2$170 test. More recently, Reybrouck and colleagues[49] suggested that a more sensitive and reproducible approach for detecting anaerobic threshold in children with impaired cardiovascular exercise function (e.g. CHD) may be achieved by calculating a third slope of $\dot{V}CO_2$ versus $\dot{V}O_2$ between the T_{VENT} and the exercise intensity at which a heart rate of 170 beats·min^{-1} was reached.

It should be noted that, the T_{VENT} may be difficult to detect in children who exhibit hyperventilation at very low levels of exercise,

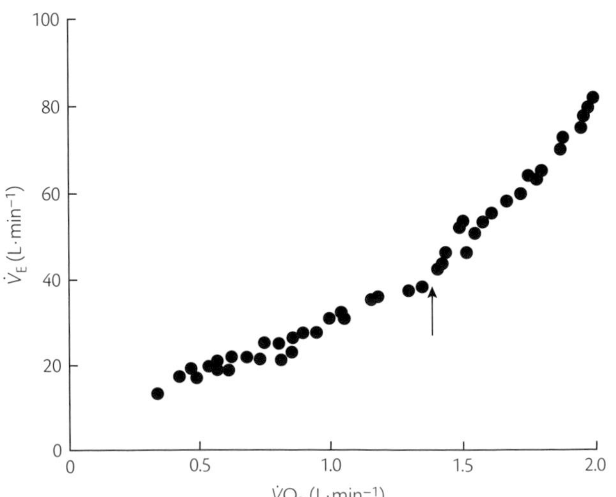

Fig. 6.3 The ventilatory threshold (T_{VENT}) is determined from the plot of minute ventilation ($\dot{V}_E$) versus oxygen uptake ($\dot{V}O_2$). The T_{VENT} (indicated by the arrow) occurs at the $\dot{V}O_2$ where there is an accelerated increase in $\dot{V}_E$ relative to $\dot{V}O_2$.

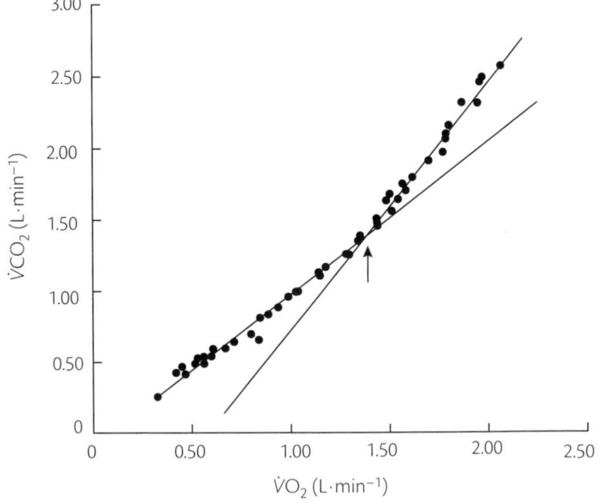

Fig. 6.4 The ventilatory threshold determined by the *V*-slope method occurs where the two slopes intersect (as indicated by the arrow).

are unable to increase ventilation sufficiently at higher work rates, or have very low fitness levels.[5]

Pulmonary gas exchange

Pulmonary gas exchange during exercise is most accurately determined by direct measurement of arterial O_2 and CO_2 tension (PaO_2 and $PaCO_2$). However, arterial sampling can be quite painful and therefore is not warranted in the healthy child, and is often refused by the sick child (see Chapter 1). Consequently, a number of investigators advocate the use of arterialized ear lobe blood samples as a less invasive alternative to direct arterial blood gas sampling[50–52]. With proper techniques,[50] the validity and reliability of arterialized ear lobe measurements have been supported by many studies[50–52], while a more recent investigation of a large sample of adults suggests that PaO_2 (measured at rest only) may be underestimated by the assessment of arterialized ear lobe blood.[53] However, differences between arterial and ear lobe measures of PCO_2 were negligible in the same study.[53] Despite the potential error with ear lobe measurements, this method appears to be superior to non-invasive indirect estimates of PaO_2 and $PaCO_2$ such as pulse oximetry and transcutaneous monitoring.

Transcutaneous measures of PO_2 and PCO_2 as indirect indices of PaO_2 and $PaCO_2$ during exercise have been discouraged due to error resulting from slow response times.[54,55] Better agreement between the direct and indirect measures has been shown with higher electrode temperatures (to enhance skin perfusion), gradual work load increments (to allow for slow response times), and calibration with an arterialized ear lobe capillary sample.[56] It should be noted that measurement drift and possible skin burn from the heated electrode may result from long-term recording.[57]

The measurement of oxyhaemoglobin saturation (SaO_2) via pulse oximetry should not be considered an indirect estimate of PaO_2. However, pulse oximetry measurement of SaO_2 is useful in the clinical setting for providing information about oxyhaemoglobin saturation. Pulse oximetry works by detecting differences in light wavelengths absorbed by oxygenated versus desaturated haemoglobin.[55] Measurement error may be introduced by poor finger or ear lobe perfusion, dark skin pigmentation, pierced ear holes, finger nail polish, movement, stray light, and increased levels of carboxy- and met-haemoglobin. True values of arterial SaO_2 have been shown to be overestimated as well as underestimated by pulse oximetry, with inaccuracy worsening during episodes of hypoxaemia ($SaO_2 < 90\%$) (58–60).

Oxyhaemoglobin saturation should be near >99% and generally not decrease during exercise in healthy children. Elite athletes have been shown to exhibit SaO_2 with very intense exercise.[61] As noted in Chapter 18, a recent study reported some evidence of exercise-induced hypoxaemia (indicated by a decrease in $SaO_2 \geq 4\%$) in healthy active prepubertal children as measured by pulse oximetry.[62] Further study is warranted to validate the results with direct measurements. In patients with cardiac defects and/or pulmonary disease, SaO_2 may be normal or decreased at rest, and may remain stable or decrease or even increase during exercise.[63] In patients with cystic fibrosis, it has been shown that resting pulmonary function could identify children at risk for desaturating during maximal exercise. No patient with an $FEV_1 \geq 50\%$ of predicted had an $SaO_2 < 91\%$ during exercise. In patients with FEV_1 values <50% of predicted, many, but not all, exhibited a fall in SaO_2 below 91%.[64]

The measurement of CO_2 tension in the expired air at the end of expiration ($PETCO_2$) should also not be used as an indirect estimate of $PaCO_2$, particularly in children with ventilation/perfusion abnormalities. However, some information about $PaCO_2$ can be obtained assuming (i) CO_2 equilibrium is achieved between end-capillary blood and alveolar gas; (ii) $PETCO_2$ approximates the time-weighted average of the ventilation-weighted alveolar CO_2 tension; (iii) the lung is sufficiently uniform in terms of ventilation to perfusion ratio ($\dot{V}_A/\dot{Q}$).[55] The difference between $PETCO_2$ and $PaCO_2$ varies with V_T, f_R and CO_2 output, thus limiting the usefulness of $PETCO_2$ as an index of $PaCO_2$ during exercise.[65] However, a general pattern of response can be observed during exercise. With progressive increments in work rate, $PETCO_2$ increases by several mm Hg above resting values because of increased CO_2 production and delivery to the lungs, until heavy exercise, when $PETCO_2$ begins to fall as the respiratory rate increases substantially to eliminate excess CO_2 and maintain acid–base balance. (Fig. 6.5) In patients with severe obstructive lung disease such as asthma or cystic fibrosis, $PETCO_2$ may continue to increase or fail to decrease suggesting hypoventilation or the inability to increase ventilation sufficiently to eliminate excess CO_2 and maintain acid–base balance. It is important to note that children are often apprehensive and may hyperventilate prior to exercise, resulting in a low 'resting' $PETCO_2$ for comparison with exercise.

Dead space

At rest, 25–35% of inspired air is wasted ventilation in the sense that it does not participate in gas exchange, creating physiological dead space. Physiologic dead space includes the conducting airways such as the mouth, nose, trachea, bronchi, and bronchioles (anatomic dead space) and the alveoli that are not adequately perfused by pulmonary capillary blood flow (alveolar dead space). The portion of inspired air that participates in gas exchange is $\dot{V}_A$. In the healthy child, physiologic dead space is about 33% of the V_T.[2] For a given level of $\dot{V}_E$, dead space (VD) will increase and $\dot{V}_A$ will decrease if V_T falls and f_R rises.

During exercise, VD increases as V_T increases but to a lesser extent. As exercise intensity increases, the ratio of dead space to

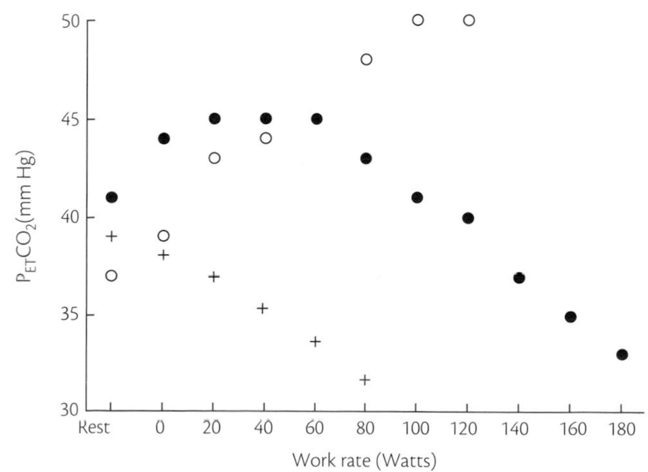

Fig. 6.5 The end-tidal carbon dioxide ($PETCO_2$) response to progressive exercise in a healthy child (•), a child with severe obstructive lung disease (O), and a child with a severe restrictive lung defect (+). In children with milder obstructive or restrictive defects, the $PETCO_2$ response pattern will be similar to the healthy child's response.

tidal volume (V_D/V_T) falls by about 33% reaching values in the range of 0.20–0.25 in both children and adults[66].

Measurement of V_D/V_T requires the measurement of arterial $PaCO_2$ for accuracy. Some automated testing systems estimate V_D/V_T from equations that use $P_{ET}CO_2$ as a substitute for $PaCO_2$.[67] However, this non-invasive method has been shown to overestimate $PaCO_2$ and thus V_D/V_T in healthy persons,[68] and also to be unreliable and inaccurate in patients with lung disease.[69,70] Consequently, these estimates should be viewed with caution.

For optimal gas exchange, the capillaries supplying the ventilated alveoli must be properly perfused; that is, there must be adequate ventilation to perfusion matching. Pulmonary blood flow and the perfusion of the pulmonary capillary bed are determined by $\dot{Q}$ pulmonary vascular resistance, and pulmonary arterial pressure. When many ventilated regions are underperfused, hypoxaemia (i.e. a drop in PaO_2) will occur. Conversely, when many perfused regions are underventilated, hypoventilation (i.e. an increase in $PaCO_2$) will occur.

Diffusing capacity

Gas exchange is also determined by the transfer or diffusion of gases across the alveolar–capillary membrane. The diffusing capacity of the lungs is dependent on (i) the gas pressure gradient between the alveoli and capillary, (ii) the transit time of the red blood cell, (iii) the solubility of the gases in the liquids and tissues, (iv) the permeability and thickness of the alveolar–capillary membrane, and (v) the amount and quality of haemoglobin.[2] The diffusing capacity of the lungs is most easily measured by determining the diffusion of carbon monoxide (DL_{CO}) using the single-breath technique.[71] Zapletal *et al.*[2] found DL_{CO} to increase with increasing body height and TLC and age, whereas the ratio of DL_{CO} to TLC decreased with increasing body height and age. Pulmonary diffusing capacity is decreased in patients with thickened alveolar–capillary membranes such as sarcoidosis, lupus, and pulmonary fibrosis as well as in persons with anaemia.[72] Resting diffusing capacity has been shown to be predictive of exercise oxyhaemoglobin desaturation in patients with obstructive pulmonary disease,[73,74] and with exercise $PaCO_2$ levels and dead space ventilation in patients with CHD.[75]

The measurement of gas diffusion during exercise is also possible. With exercise, DL_{CO} increases significantly, reaching values nearly three times greater than rest.[76] The increase in DL_{CO} correlates directly with $\dot{V}O_2$, and the slope of $DL_{CO}/\dot{V}O_2$ was found to be twice as high in children than adults.[77] Mitchell and Teague[78] found reduced DL_{CO} both at rest and during exercise in children born prematurely with bronchopulmonary dysplasia (BPD) compared to prematurely born peers without BPD and healthy, term-born controls, which may be due to reduced alveolar–capillary surface area or reduced pulmonary blood flow associated with right ventricular dysfunction.

Breathing reserve

The ratio of minute ventilation at peak exercise to the resting MVV ($\dot{V}_E$/MVV) has been used to give some indication of the proportion of mechanical ventilatory capacity used at peak exercise. The unused portion is considered to be the breathing reserve (1–MVV).[79] In the healthy child, the $\dot{V}_E$ at peak or maximal exercise is usually well below the MVV obtained at rest ($\dot{V}_E$/MVV = 60–70%), indicating sufficient mechanical reserve.[5] In contrast, the peak $\dot{V}_E$ of the child with obstructive lung disease may approach or even exceed the MVV, leaving little or no ventilatory reserve, and suggesting ventilatory limitation to exercise.[64] The fact that $\dot{V}_E$ can exceed MVV may be attributed to bronchodilation during exercise, but may also be due to the problem or limitation of comparing an effort-dependent resting voluntary manoeuvre (MVV) with an involuntary exercise measure. The forced MVV manoeuvre produces high expiratory pressures which may cause the airways to collapse somewhat. In contrast to exercise ventilation, the MVV is generally performed at higher end-expiratory lung volumes which increases the inspiratory elastic load and thus the work of breathing.[80] Consequently, the $\dot{V}_E$/MVV should be used cautiously in suggesting a ventilatory limitation to exercise.

Flow/volume loops with exercise

To provide additional insight into possible ventilatory constraints during exercise, more recent metabolic testing carts enable the examination of the exercise tidal flow-volume loop (extFVL) plotted within the resting maximal flow-volume loop (MFVL).

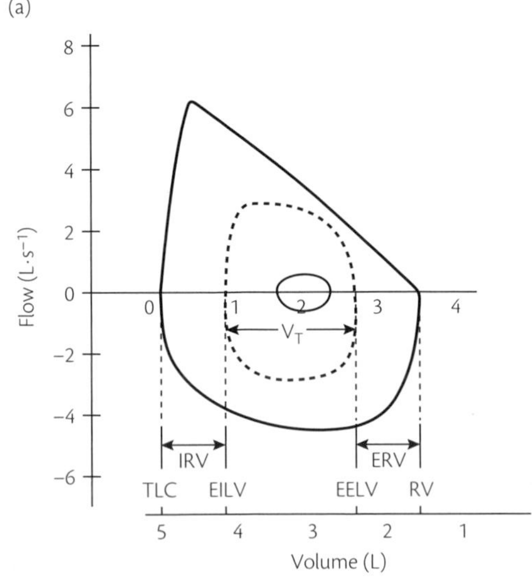

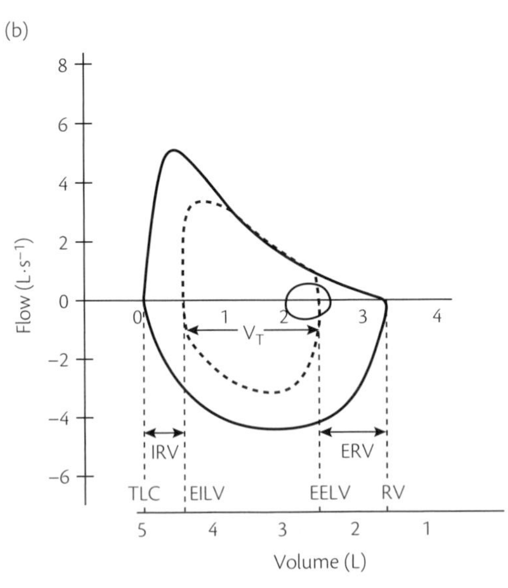

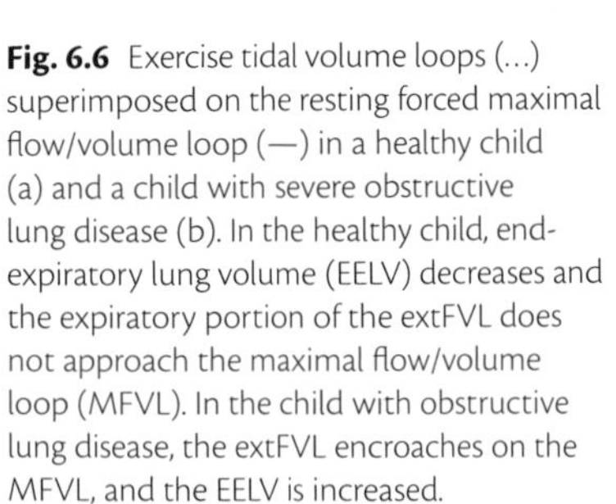
Fig. 6.6 Exercise tidal volume loops (...) superimposed on the resting forced maximal flow/volume loop (—) in a healthy child (a) and a child with severe obstructive lung disease (b). In the healthy child, end-expiratory lung volume (EELV) decreases and the expiratory portion of the extFVL does not approach the maximal flow/volume loop (MFVL). In the child with obstructive lung disease, the extFVL encroaches on the MFVL, and the EELV is increased.

As previously mentioned, $\dot{V}_E$ is increased by increases in both V_T and f_R. In the healthy child (Fig. 6.6a), the increase in V_T encroaches on both the IRV and ERV, and the end-expiratory lung volume (EELV) is reduced compared to rest, which optimizes inspiratory muscle length and reduces elastic load.[80] In addition, the extFVL does not approach the resting MFVL even at maximal exercise. In contrast, in the child with obstructive lung disease (expiratory flow limitation) (Fig. 6.6b), the extFVL encroaches upon the resting MFVL during exercise, and the EELV increases to take advantage of flow at higher lung volumes.[81] However, the increase in EELV will also increase the elastic load and the work of breathing as well as reduce inspiratory flow reserve. More detailed information about the measurement and interpretation of the extFVL can be found in excellent reviews by Johnson *et al.*.[80,81]

Exercise-induced bronchoconstriction

More commonly, measurements of the expiratory flow rates are performed before and after exercise, rather than during, to aid in the diagnosis of exercise-induced bronchoconstriction (EIB). Guidelines for exercise challenge testing have been developed by the American Thoracic Society.[82] Generally, the standard EIB testing protocol is performed on a motorized treadmill with the exercise intensity increasing rapidly to a level that can be sustained for 6–8 min and elicits a heart rate equal to 80–90% of age predicted maximum heart rate or a $\dot{V}_E$ that is 40–60% of MVV (82–84). Forced expiratory flow rates and volumes are measured pre-exercise, and approximately 2, 5, 10, and 15 min post-exercise, and then 20 min after the administration of an inhaled bronchodilator. A 10% decrease in FEV_1 (expressed as % change from pre-exercise values) following exercise is considered to be abnormal, and ≥15% is considered to be a positive diagnosis of EIB.[82] In the healthy child, the airways dilate during exercise (as a result of sympathetic stimulation). However, in the child with exercise-induced asthma, while bronchodilitation may occur initially, bronchoconstriction occurs during or, more commonly, after exercise.[5] As shown in Fig. 6.7, substantial decreases in larger airway flow rates from pre- to post-exercise are evident in a child with EIB.

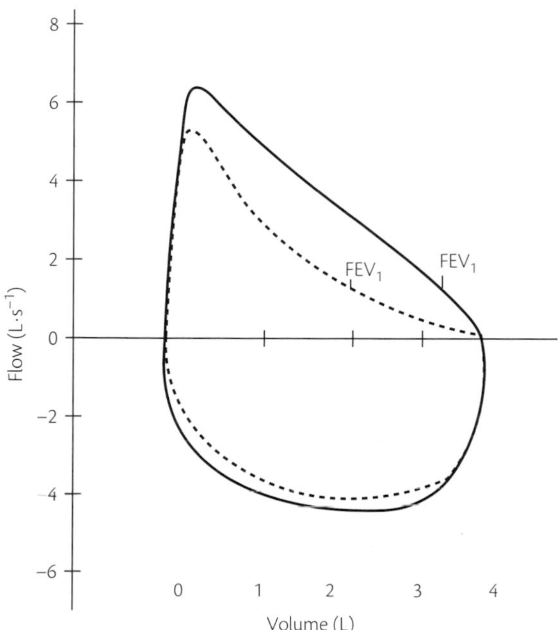

Fig. 6.7 Forced expiratory flow/volume loops measured before (—) and after (....) exercise in a child with exercise-induced asthma. Note the concavity of the expiratory loop and the lower FEV_1 following exercise compared to normal pre-exercise value.

The exercise challenge test is fairly good for correctly identifying persons without asthma (specificity ≥ 80–90%); however, its sensitivity or ability to identify persons with asthma is considerably lower (at 40%–70%).[85] Godfrey and colleagues[85] determined (from receiver operating characteristic curves) that the optimal cut-off point for decrease in FEV_1 was 13% which yielded the highest sum of specificity and sensitivity (at 94% and 63%, respectively). The sensitivity may be increased by having subjects inhale cold, dry air during exercise.[86] It should be noted, however, that the methacholine-inhalation challenge yields substantially greater sensitivity (93%) than exercise testing for making a diagnosis of asthma.[85]

Interpretation of pulmonary exercise testing

For proper interpretation, it is important to choose the appropriate testing protocol. For example, an EIB provocation testing protocol should be followed for the assessment of EIB. Submaximal exercise testing may provide sufficient information when maximal testing is deemed too stressful or unnecessary. Generally, most of the normative data are based on progressive maximal exercise testing, and comparisons to the normative data should be made using the same testing protocol.

The interpretation of exercise test results is ideally based on both numerical data and graphical displays. Different strategies for interpreting test results with emphasis on pulmonary disease are presented by Younes,[87] the European Respiratory Society Task Force,[54] and Wasserman *et al.*.[17] In children, the interpretation of tests is usually limited to non-invasive data and their graphical display. Suggestions for graphical displays include the following *x*–*y* plots: work rate (or time) on the *x*-axis versus separate plots of $\dot{V}O_2$, heart rate, $\dot{V}_E$, $\dot{V}_E/\dot{V}O_2$and $\dot{V}_E/\dot{V}CO_2$ combined, and $P_{ET}CO_2$ and $P_{ET}O_2$ combined on the *y*-axis; $\dot{V}O_2$ on the *x*-axis versus heart rate, $\dot{V}_E$, and $\dot{V}CO_2$ separately; and $\dot{V}CO_2$ on the *x*-axis versus $\dot{V}_E$ on the *y*-axis.

For accurate interpretation of progressive maximal exercise test results, it is important to determine if the child gave a maximal effort. A maximal effort may be determined by examining the respiratory exchange ratio (RER), heart rate, $\dot{V}_E$/MVV, and the subject's effort at peak exercise. General criteria for the healthy child are (i) the peak RER should be greater than 1.00 in younger children (increasing to ≥1.10 in post-pubescent adolescents); (ii) the peak heart rate should be near age predicted values; (iii) the peak $\dot{V}_E$/MVV should be at least 60%; and (iv) the subject should appear to have given a maximal effort. In some cases, the $\dot{V}O_2$ at near-maximal exercise may level off despite further increases in exercise intensity, although this may not always be seen in children or with specific testing protocols, and therefore may not be a useful criterion for determining a maximal effort (see Chapter 8).

In the child with a health problem, all of the criteria may not be met despite a maximal effort. It is important to realize that one parameter can appear to be submaximal or abnormal due to the effects of another parameter. For instance, peak heart rate may be reduced because the child has a ventilatory or peripheral limitation to exercise that prevents the cardiovascular system from reaching its maximum capacity. Similarly, the child with a cardiac defect may have a chronotropic limitation to exercise that prevents the ventilatory system from being stressed. Furthermore, the child may terminate exercise because of symptoms, and, as a result, may not meet any of the physiologic criteria for a maximal effort. Consequently, the examiner's subjective assessment of the child's effort plays an important role.

Once it has been determined that the child gave a maximal effort, then the child's physical work capacity and peak $\dot{V}O_2$ should be compared to reference values of healthy children (similar in age, race, and anthropometric characteristics) obtained using the same testing protocol. If subnormal, the explanation may lie in one, or a combination, of the other parameters measured. The other parameters should be examined for abnormalities even if the child's fitness level is normal or above normal.

The submaximal progressive data should also be examined for inappropriate responses or patterns of response. For instance, as previously mentioned, a high $\Delta \dot{V}_E/\Delta \dot{V}CO_2$ may reflect ventilatory compensation for increased dead space in a child with obstructive pulmonary disease, or an accelerated increase in $\dot{V}_E$ at a low $\dot{V}O_2$ may indicate a low T_{VENT} in an unfit child.

Finally, the results of the exercise test may not fully explain the child's exercise intolerance. It is possible that peripheral limitations to exercise exist, which are not reflected in the cardiorespiratory data. The child with a chronic disease may also be afraid or unwilling to exercise because of the usually false belief that it is unsafe for him/her to exercise which he/she has learned from the cues of parents, teachers and others.

Summary

- The evaluation of pulmonary function at rest and during exercise can provide useful information about the lungs' ability to provide sufficient volume and flow of air, as well as adequate exchange of oxygen and carbon dioxide.
- Examination of the ventilatory efficiency as reflected in $\Delta\dot{V}_E/\Delta\dot{V}CO_2$ during progressive exercise may provide information about excessive ventilation, $\dot{V}_A/\dot{Q}$ mismatching, and altered chemosensitivity to $PaCO_2$.
- Non-invasive determination of the T_{VENT} may provide information about aerobic fitness and impairment, particularly in the child with chronic disease.
- In the absence of arterial blood gas measurements, non-invasive measurements may provide some information about pulmonary gas exchange, and help to identify children who exhibit oxyhaemoglobin desaturation and/or CO_2 retention with exercise.
- Examination of the tidal flow-volume loop during exercise may provide information about ventilatory limitations and maladaptive responses to exercise beyond that obtained by $\dot{V}_E$/MVV alone.
- In the child with disease, exercise testing can help to identify abnormal responses which may contribute to exercise intolerance, and can be useful for following changes with disease progression and treatment.

References

1. Polgar G, Promadhat V (1971). *Pulmonary function testing in children. Techniques and standards.* W.B. Saunders Co., Philadelphia.
2. Zapletal A, Samanek M, Paul T (1987). *Lung function in children and adolescents.* Karger, Basel.
3. Quanjer PhH, Stocks J, Polgar G, Wise M, Kalberg J, Borsboom G (1989). Compilation of reference values for lung function measurements in children. *Eur Respir J* **2**, 184s-261s.
4. Hankinson JL, Odencrantz JR, Fedan KB (1999). Spirometric reference values from a sample of the general U.S. population. *Am J Respir Crit Care Med* **159**, 179–87.
5. Godfrey S (1974). *Exercise testing in children.* W.B. Saunders Co., London.
6. Comroe JH, Forster RE II, Dubois AB, Briscoe WA, Carlsen E (1962). *The lung. Clinical physiology and pulmonary function tests.* Year Book Medical Publishers, Inc., Chicago.
7. Wanger J, Clausen JL, Coates A, Pedersen OF, Brusasco V, Burgos F, Casaburi R, Crapo R, Enright P, van der Grinten CP, Gustafsson P, Hankinson J, Jensen R, Johnson D, Macintyre N, McKay R, Miller MR, Navajas D, Pellegrino R, Viegi G (2005). Standardisation of the measurement of lung volumes. *Eur Respir J* **26**, 511–22.
8. American Thoracic Society (1995). Standardization of spirometry—1994 update. *Am J Respir Crit Care Med* **152**, 1107–36.
9. Quanjer PhH, Helms P, Bjure J, Caultier C (1989). Standardisation of lung function tests in paediatrics. *Eur Resp J* **2**, 121S-264S.
10. Miller MR, Hankinson J, Brusasco V, Burgos F, Casaburi R, Coates A, Crapo R, Enright P, van der Grinten CP, Gustafsson P, Jensen R, Johnson DC, MacIntyre N, McKay R, Navajas D, Pedersen OF, Pellegrino R, Viegi G, Wanger J; *ATS/ERS Task Force* (2005). Standardisation of spirometery. *Eur Respir J* **26**, 319–38.
11. Schoenberg JB, Beck GJ, Bouhuys A (1978). Growth and decay of pulmonary function in healthy blacks and whites. *Respir Physiol* **33**, 367–93.
12. Zapletal A (1987). Lung function in children and adolescents. *Prog Respir Res* **22**, 1–220.
13. Fulton JE, Pivarnik JM, Taylor WC, Snider SA, Tate AL, Rankowski RF (1995). Prediction of maximum voluntary ventilation (MVV) in African-American adolescent girls. *Pediatr Pulmonol* **20**, 225–33.
14. Ruppel GE (1991). *Manual of pulmonary function testing.* Mosby, St. Louis.
15. Cooper CB, Harris ND, Howard P (1990). Evaluation of a turbine flow meter (Ventilometer Mark 2) in the measurement of ventilation. *Respiration* **57**, 243–7.
16. American Thoracic Society and American College of Chest Physicians (2003). ATS/ACCP Statement on cardiopulmonary exercise testing. *Am J Respir Crit Care Med* **167**, 211–77.
17. Wasserman K, Sue DY, Hansen JE (2005). *Principles of exercise testing and interpretation.* Lippincott, Williams & Wilkins, Philadelphia.
18. Jones NL, Makrides L, Hitchcock C, Chypchar T, McCartney N (1985). Normal standards for an incremental progressive cycle ergometer test. *Am Rev Respir Dis* **131**, 700–8.
19. Armstrong N, Kirby BJ, McManus AM, Welsman JR (1997). Prepubescents' ventilatory responses to exercise with reference to sex and body size. *Chest* **112**, 1554–60.
20. Boule M, Gaultier C, Girard F (1989). Breathing pattern during exercise in untrained children. *Respir Physiol* **75**, 225–33.
21. Rowland TW, Green GM (1990). The influence of biological maturation and aerobic fitness on ventilatory responses to treadmill exercise. In: Dotson CO, Humphrey JH (eds.), *Exercise physiology: Current selected research*, pp. 51–9. AMS Press, New York.
22. Barrios C, Perez-Encinas C, Maruenda JI, Laguia M (2005). Significant ventilatory functional restriction in adolescents with mild or moderate scoliosis during maximal exercise tolerance test. *Spine* **30**, 1610–5.
23. Smyth RJ, Chapman KR, Wright TA, Crawford JS, Rebuck AS (1986). Ventilatory patterns during hypoxia, hypercapnia, and exercise in adolescents with mild scoliosis. *Pediatrics* **77**, 692–7.

24. Schneerson JM (1980). Cardiac and respiratory responses to exercise in adolescent idiopathic scoliosis. *Thorax* **35**, 347–50.
25. Cooper DM, Springer C (2006). Pulmonary function assessment in the laboratory during exercise. In: Chernick V, Boat TF, Wilmott RW, Bush A (eds.), *Kendig's disorders of the respiratory tract in children*, pp. 186–204. Elsevier, New York.
26. NaganoY, Baba R, Kuraishi K, Yasuda, T, Ikoma M, Nishibata K, Yokota M, Nagashima M (1998). Ventilatory control during exercise in normal children. *Pediatr Res* **43**, 704–7.
27. Moser C, Tirakitsoontorn P, Nussbaum E, Newcomb R, Cooper DM (2000). Muscle size and cardiorespiratory response to exercise in cystic fibrosis. *Am J Respir Crit Care Med* **162**, 1823–7.
28. Ohuchi H, Ohashi H, Takasugi H, Yamada O, Yagihara T, Echigo S (2004). Restrictive ventilatory impairment and arterial oxygenation characterize rest and exercise ventilation in patients after Fontan operation. *Pediatr Cardiol* **25**, 513–21.
29. Sun X-G, Hansen JE, Garatachea N, Storer TW, Wasserman K (2002). Ventilatory efficiency during exercise in healthy subjects. *Am J Respir Crit Care Med* **166**, 1443–8.
30. Wasserman K, McIlroy MB (1964). Detecting the threshold of anaerobic metabolism in cardiac patients during exercise. *Am J Cardiol* **14**, 844–52.
31. Reybrouck TM (1989). The use of the anaerobic threshold in pediatric exercise testing. In: Bar-Or O (ed.), *Advances in pediatric sport sciences*, pp. 131–49. Human Kinetics, Champaign, IL.
32. Wasserman K, Whipp BJ, Koyal SN, Beaver WL (1973). Anaerobic threshold and respiratory gas exchange during exercise. *J Appl Physiol* **35**, 236–43.
33. Macek J and Vavra J (1985). Anaerobic threshold in children. In: Binkhort RA, Kemper HCG, Saris WHM (eds.), *Children and exercise*, pp. 110–3, Human Kinetics, Champaign, IL.
34. Eriksson BO (1972). Physical training, oxygen supply and muscle metabolism in 11–13 year old boys. *Acta Physiol Scand* **86**, 1–48.
35. Eriksson BO, Koch G (1973). Effects of physical training on haemodynamic response during submaximal and maximal exercise in 11–13 year old boys. *Acta Physiol Scand* **87**, 27–39.
36. Hughes E, Turner SC, Brooks GA (1982). Effects of glycogen depletion and pedalling speed on 'anaerobic threshold'. *J Appl Physiol* **52**, 1598–1607.
37. Brooks GA (1985). Anaerobic threshold: Review of the concept and directions for future research. *Med Sci Sports Exerc* **17**, 22–31.
38. Davis JA (1985). Anaerobic threshold: Review of the concept and directions for future research. *Med Sci Sports Exerc* **17**, 6–18.
39. Reybrouck T, Weymans M, Ghesquiere J, van Gerven D, Stijns H (1982). Ventilatory threshold during treadmill exercise in kindergarten children. *Eur J Appl Physiol* **50**, 79–86.
40. Mahon AD, Marsh ML (1992). Reliability of the rating of perceived exertion at ventilatory threshold in children. *Int J Sports Med* **13**, 567–71.
41. Weymans M, Reybrouck T (1989). Habitual level of physical activity and cardiorespiratory endurance capacity in children. *Eur J Appl Physiol* **58**, 803–7.
42. Mahon AD, Vaccaro P (1989). Ventilatory threshold and VO2 max changes in children following endurance training. *Med Sci Sports Exerc* **21**, 425–31.
43. Washington RL (1989). Anaerobic threshold in children. *Pediatr Exerc Sci* **1**, 244–56.
44. Cooper DM, Weiler-Ravell D, Whipp BJ, Wasserman K (1984). Aerobic parameters of exercise as a function of body size during growth in children. *J Appl Physiol* **5**, 628–34.
45. Reybrouck T, Weymans M, Stijns H, Knops J, Van der Hauwaert L (1985). Ventilatory anaerobic threshold in healthy children: Age and sex differences. *Eur J Appl Physiol* **54**, 278–84.
46. Sue DY, Wasserman K, Moricca RB, Casaburi R (1988). Metabolic acidosis during exercise in patients with chronic obstructive pulmonary disease. Use of the v-slope method for anaerobic threshold determination. *Chest* **94**, 931–8.
47. Washington RL, Van Gundy JC, Cohen C, Sondheimer H, Wolfe R (1988). Normal aerobic and anaerobic exercise data for North American school-age children. *J Pediatr* **112**, 223–33.
48. Reybrouck T, Weymans M, Stijns H, Van der Hauwaert LG (1986). Ventilatory anaerobic threshold for evaluating exercise performance in children with congenital left-to-right intracardiac shunt. *Pediatr Cardiol* **7**, 19–24.
49. Reybrouck T, Mertens L, Kalis N, Weymans M, Dumoulin M, Daenen W, Gewillig M (1996). Dynamics of respiratory gas exchange during exercise after correction of congenital heart disease. *J Appl Physiol* **80**, 458–63.
50. Godfrey S, Wozniak ER, Courtney Evans RJ, Samuels CS (1971). Ear lobe blood samples for blood gas analysis at rest and during exercise. *Br J Dis Chest* **65**, 58–63.
51. Christoforides C, Miller JM (1968). Clinical use and limitations of arterialized capillary blood for PO_2 determination. *Amer Rev Respir Dis* **98**, 653–7.
52. Spiro SG, Dowdeswell IRG (1976). Arterialized earlobe blood samples for blood gas tensions. *Br J Dis Chest* **70**, 263–8.
53. Sauty A, Uldry C, Debetaz L-F, Leuenberger P, Fitting J-W (1996). Differences in PO_2 and PCO_2 between arterial and arterialized earlobe samples. *Eur Respir J* **9**, 186–9.
54. European Respiratory Society Task Force (1997). Clinical exercise testing with reference to lung diseases: indications, standardization and interpretation strategies. *Eur Respir J* **10**, 2662–89.
55. Clark JS, Votteri B, Ariagno RL, Cheung P, Eichhorn JH, Fallat RJ, Lee SE, Newth CJ, Rotman H, Sue DY (1992) Noninvasive assessment of blood gases. *Amer Rev Respir Dis* **145**, 220–32.
56. Carter R, Banham SW (2000). Use of transcutaneous oxygen and carbon dioxide tensions for assessing indices of gas exchange during exercise testing. *Respir Med* **94**, 350–5.
57. Pradal U, Braggion C, Mastella G (1990). Transcutaneous blood gas analysis during sleep and exercise in cystic fibrosis. *Pediatr Pulmonol* **8**, 162–7.
58. Hansen JE, Casaburi R (1987). Validity of ear oximetry in clinical exercise testing. *Chest* **91**, 333–7.
59. Orenstein DM, Curtis SE, Nixon PA Hartigan ER (1993). Accuracy of three pulse oximeters during exercise and hypoxemia in patients with cystic fibrosis. *Chest* **104**, 1187–90.
60. Chapman K, D'Urzo A, Rebuck A (1983). The accuracy and response characteristics of a simplified ear oximeter. *Chest* **83**, 860–4.
61. Williams JH, Powers SK, Stuart MK (1986). Hemoglobin desaturation in highly trained athletes during heavy exercise. *Med Sci Sports Exerc* **18**, 168–73.
62. Nourry C, Fabre C, Bart F, Grosbois JM, Berthoin S, Mucci P (2004). Evidence of exercise-induced arterial hypoxemia in prepubescent trained children. *Pediatr Res* **55**, 674–81.
63. Nixon PA, Orenstein DM (1988). Exercise testing in children. *Pediatr Pulmonol* **5**, 107–22.
64. Nixon PA (1996). Role of exercise in the evaluation and management of pulmonary disease in children and youth. *Med Sci Sports Exerc* **28**, 414–20.
65. Jones HL, McHardy GJR, Naimark A, Campbell EJM (1966). Physiological dead space and alveolar–arterial gas pressure differences during exercise. *Clin Sci* **31**, 19–29.
66. Shephard RJ, Bar-Or O (1970). Alveolar ventilation in near maximum exercise. Data on pre-adolescent children and young adults *Med Sci Sports Exerc* **2**, 83–92.
67. Jones NL (1988). *Clinical exercise testing*. WB Saunders, Philadelphia.
68. Robbins PA, Conway J, Cunningham DA, Khamnei S, Paterson DJ (1990). A comparison of indirect methods for continuous estimation of arterial PCO_2 in men. *J Appl Physiol* **68**, 1727–31.
69. Lewis DA, Sietsema KE, Casaburi R, Sue DY (1994). Inaccuracy of non-invasive estimates of V_D/V_T in clinical exercise testing. *Chest* **106**, 1476–80.

70. Yamanaka MK, Sue DY (1987). Comparison of arterial-end-tidal PCO_2 difference and dead space/tidal volume ratio in respiratory failure. *Chest* **92**, 832–5.
71. American Thoracic Society (1996). Single-breath carbon monoxide diffusing capacity (transfer factor). Recommendations for a standard technique—1995 update. *Am J Respir Crit Care Med* **152**, 2185–98.
72. Hyatt RK, Scanlon PD, Nakamura M (1997). *Interpretation of pulmonary function tests: A practical guide.* W.B. Saunders, Philadelphia, PA
73. Lebecque P, Lapierre J-G, Lamarre A, Coates AL (1987). Diffusion capacity and oxygen desaturation effects on exercise in patients with cystic fibrosis. *Chest* **91**, 693–7.
74. Owens GR, Rogers RM, Pennock BE, Levin D (1984). The diffusing capacity as a predictor of arterial oxygen desaturation during exercise in patients with chronic obstructive pulmonary disease. *N Engl J Med* **310**, 1218–21.
75. Ohuchi H, Yasuda K, Suzuki H, Arakaki Y, Yagihara T, Echigo S (2000). Ventilatory response to exercise in patients with major aortopulmonary collateral arteries after definitive surgery. *Am J Cardiol* **85**, 1223–9.
76. Andersen SD, Godfrey S (1971). Transfer factor for CO_2 during exercise in children. *Thorax* **26**, 51–4.
77. Shephard RJ, Allen C, Bar-Or O, Davies CTM, Degre S, Hedman R, Ishi K (1969). The working capacity of Toronto schoolchildren. Part II. *Can Med Assoc J* **100**, 705–14.
78. Mitchell SH, Teague WG (1998). Reduced gas transfer at rest and during exercise in school-age survivors of bronchopulmonary dysplasia. *Am J Respir Crit Care Med* **157**, 1406–12.
79. Wasserman K, Whipp BJ (1975). Exercise physiology in health and disease. *Am Rev Respir Dis* **112**, 219–49.
80. Johnson BD, Weisman IM, Zeballos RJ, Beck KC (1999). Emerging concepts in the evaluation of ventilatory limitation during exercise. *Chest* **116**, 488–503.
81. Johnson BD, Beck KC, Zeballow RF, Weisman IM (1999). Advances in pulmonary laboratory testing. *Chest* **116**, 1377–87.
82. American Thoracic Society (2000). Guidelines for methacholine and exercise challenge testing—1999. *Am J Respir Crit Care Med* **161**, 309–29.
83. Cropp GJA (1979). The exercise bronchoprovocation test: Standardization of procedures and evaluation of response. *J Allerg Clin Immunol* **64**, 627–33.
84. NHLBI Expert Panel Report (1991). Guidelines for the diagnosis and management of asthma. *J Allerg Clinl Immunol* **88**, 425–534.
85. Godfrey S, Springer C, Bar-Yishay E, Avital E (1999). Cut-off points defining normal and asthmatic bronchial reactivity to exercise and inhalation challenges in children and young adults. *Eur Respir J* **14**, 659–68.
86. McFadden ER, jr (1988). Exercise-induced asthma. Recent approaches. *Chest* **93**, 1282–3.
87. Younes M (1984). Interpretation of clinical exercise testing in respiratory disease. *Clin Chest Med* **5**, 189–206.

CHAPTER 7

Cardiovascular function

Darren E.R. Warburton, Lindsay Nettlefold, K. Ashlee McGuire, and Shannon S.D. Bredin

Introduction

The physiological adaptations to exercise training have been evaluated extensively in children and youth. In particular, considerable research has examined the changes in cardiovascular function that occur with aerobic exercise training. Various indicators of cardiovascular function have been assessed at rest and during exercise. Many of these measures have important implications from performance and health-related perspectives. Owing to the importance of oxygen (O_2) transport for human performance and health, this chapter reviews comprehensively the varied non-invasive and invasive methods of assessing cardiac function including an in-depth evaluation of the limitations and strengths of each methodology. Specific reference is given to the applicability and ease of usage of each technology with young people. This chapter also deals extensively with the evaluation of cardiovascular regulation and vascular function owing to their role in optimal exercise performance and health.

Cardiac output

Cardiac output ($\dot{Q}$) is the product of heart rate (HR) and stroke volume (SV) and represents the volume of blood pumped by the heart per minute. The ability to increase $\dot{Q}$ reflects the body's ability to cope with and adapt to an increased metabolic demand.[1,2] Oxygen transport and human performance are intimately linked to $\dot{Q}$[3,4] and $\dot{Q}$ is often considered to be the primary limiting factor of exercise performance in healthy individuals.[5] Its accurate measurement is therefore essential in the assessment of cardiovascular function and cardiovascular responses to exercise, physical training, and the normal processes of growth and maturation.[1,2] The measurement of $\dot{Q}$ during exercise conditions, in particular maximal exercise conditions, is one of the most important and difficult measures in exercise and cardiovascular physiology.[1,2]

A number of methods capable of estimating $\dot{Q}$ have been developed and evaluated to determine their suitability for use in both resting and exercise conditions.[1,2] These techniques have been predominantly used in adults. This section will briefly review the techniques and the evidence, if any, supporting or opposing the use of these techniques in the paediatric population.

Invasive techniques

The accepted gold standard measures of $\dot{Q}$ during steady-state conditions (rest and submaximal exercise) are the direct Fick and dye-dilution methods. These methods are considered to be reliable and accurate during steady state; however, their validity during non-steady-state conditions is debatable.[1,2] Moreover, the invasive nature and inherent risks associated with these procedures limit their use during maximal exercise and with healthy individuals.[1] In youth, the majority of the studies (as evaluated in the following section) using catheterization were performed in ill children who required catheterization as part of their medical treatment. The invasiveness of these procedures also makes it difficult to mimic real world situations in both adults and children, thereby limiting the real world transferability (ecological validity) of these procedures. This appears to be of particular concern for healthy children, where it is neither practical nor warranted in most instances to use direct catheterization.

Direct Fick method

The direct Fick method calculates $\dot{Q}$ using measurements of O_2 [or carbon dioxide (CO_2)] content from arterial and mixed venous blood in combination with a measurement of oxygen uptake ($\dot{V}O_2$) [or CO_2 elimination ($\dot{V}CO_2$)] during steady-state conditions. An arterial blood sample is taken from a systemic arterial catheter while the mixed venous sample is drawn from a catheter placed in the pulmonary artery.[1] Analysis of expired air yields measures of $\dot{V}O_2$ (or $\dot{V}CO_2$).[1] The Fick equation is used to calculate $\dot{Q}$, where the CaO_2 refers to the arterial content of O_2, and the $C\bar{v}O_2$ refers to the mixed venous content of O_2:

$$\dot{Q} = \frac{\dot{V}O_2}{CaO_2 - C\bar{v}O_2}$$

The direct Fick method has a low margin of error at rest (~5%) that has been shown to decrease during submaximal, steady-state exercise. It provides reliable and accurate assessments of $\dot{Q}$ under steady-state conditions such as rest and moderate exercise. However, the direct Fick method is limited during maximal exercise as steady-state conditions are seldom achieved. Moreover, this method requires a series of highly trained medical personnel and often has lower reliability and validity than other procedures if it is not performed meticulously.[1] There are also several potential lethal complications associated with ventricular catheterization (e.g. ventricular arrhythmias and fibrillation, and perforation of the pulmonary artery or right ventricle);[1] however, the incidence of these complications is relatively low.

Although this technique has and continues to be used in healthy adult populations, it has several limitations that make it suboptimal for use during strenuous to maximal exercise conditions (particularly in children). With advances in non-invasive $\dot{Q}$ assessment technologies we would not advocate the use of direct Fick to assess $\dot{Q}$ in healthy individuals, particularly young people.

Dye-dilution method

Dye dilution (also called indicator dilution) is another invasive technique used in the assessment of $\dot{Q}$. This technique has been extensively compared against the direct Fick method with the same relative accuracy. A bolus of dye, typically 1 mL indocyanine green, is injected into the venous circulation (at the pulmonary artery or close to the right atrium) and arterial blood is sampled continuously downstream. A curve of concentration over time is generated, and $\dot{Q}$ is calculated by dividing the volume of dye injected by the area under the curve. A larger $\dot{Q}$ value will produce a dye-dilution curve that rises and falls more rapidly.[1]

The coefficients of variation reported at rest and during submaximal exercise range from 5% to 10%.[1] Although relatively few studies have reported coefficients of variation during maximal exercise,[1] some investigators have observed reliability values similar to those obtained during submaximal exercise.[6] Studies using dye dilution to assess $\dot{Q}$ have been predominantly conducted in adult populations with those in children limited to those who are critically ill.[1] This is largely due to the practical limitations and inherent risks associated with the procedure. As with the direct Fick method, we do not advocate the use of dye dilution with healthy children. This is particularly salient given the accuracy, reliability, and the relative ease of administration of various non-invasive procedures with children.[1]

Pulse dye densitometry is a modification of this procedure that is less invasive and thus might be more appropriate for use in healthy populations. Indicator dye is injected through a central or peripheral venous line and changes in dye concentration are detected using the principles of pulse oximetry (spectrophotometry).[7,8] A probe, often located over the finger or nose, is used to detect changes in the absorption of light of specific wavelengths [9] thus providing information about pulsatile changes in the arterial concentration ratios of dye and haemoglobin.[8] There is debate regarding the accuracy and reliability of pulse dye densitometry, especially at low $\dot{Q}$.[7,10] Preliminary research has shown adequate agreement when compared against thermodilution in adult patients;[11–13] however, limited research exists for youth. This method was recently used to calculate the blood volume of infants, and the obtained values compared favourably with invasive blood measurements.[14] Another recent study revealed marked difficulties in obtaining reliable pulse waveforms using a two-wavelength pulse dye densitometry system in small infant and neonate piglets. In comparison, a three-wavelength model was more effective in obtaining acceptable measures of $\dot{Q}$ in young piglets.[15] It has been postulated that this three-wavelength model may be appropriate for use with human children.[15]

It is clear that the pulse dye densitometry technology requires further investigation. To our knowledge, no investigation has examined this technology during incremental to maximal exercise (in adults or children). One study has compared this technology to another non-invasive technique (the Modelflow technique) during light stepping exercise.[16] However, it remains unclear whether movement artefact during strenuous exercise conditions will be a serious concern to this procedure. Owing to the invasiveness of the procedure, the paucity of information regarding its ability to assess $\dot{Q}$ during exercise conditions, and the current lack of supporting literature in children, we would not currently recommend using this technology for assessing $\dot{Q}$ in young people.

Thermodilution method

This technique follows the method of dye dilution except that a bolus of cold fluid is injected (into the right atrium) instead of dye.[1] Cardiac output is calculated by measuring the cooling of the blood using a thermistor (temperature probe) in the tip of the pulmonary artery catheter. A number of studies have reported that this technique overestimates $\dot{Q}$ in adults in comparison to other methods [as reviewed in ref. 1]; however, a comparison in children against the direct Fick technique yielded a correlation of $r = 0.92$ and no systematic differences between the two methods.[17] The invasive nature once again means that the only studies involving children are those examining critically ill children. Furthermore, repeated $\dot{Q}$ measurements by thermodilution may cause fluid overload in small subjects.[17] As reviewed by Warburton *et al.*[1] there are several limitations to the thermodilution technique that affect its reliability and validity, including unknown heat loss during the handling of the coolant before it enters the circulation, unknown coolant loss through the vessel wall, and physiological variations in the temperature of pulmonary blood. Although some consider thermodilution to be a good measure to compare other techniques against, concerns regarding its reliability and validity preclude it from being considered a 'gold standard' measure.[1]

The transpulmonary indicator dilution method injects cold saline through a central venous catheter and measures thermal dilution in the aorta (as opposed to in the pulmonary artery). This was developed owing to the risks associated with pulmonary artery catheters; however, this procedure remains invasive requiring central venous and aortic catheterization. This technology has been validated against the pulmonary artery catheter method in paediatric patients with a mean difference of 4.4%.[18] Pauli *et al.*[19] and Tibby *et al.*[20] have compared the transpulmonary indicator dilution method with the direct Fick method in infants and children receiving either heart surgery or catheterization and found that the two methods were equivalent in terms of $\dot{Q}$ measures.

Given the invasive nature of the thermodilution procedure (and its variations), and the questions surrounding the reliability and validity of the measure, we would not currently advocate the use of thermodilution for the determination of $\dot{Q}$ in healthy young people.

Lithium dilution method

Another dilution technique that has been evaluated in children is the lithium dilution technique.[21] This method requires catheterization of a peripheral vein and artery. In this method, an isotonic lithium chloride solution is injected intravenously and a curve demonstrating concentration over time is constructed by drawing arterial blood through a lithium sensor.[22] Very limited information exists on this topic; however, clinical evaluations have revealed strong correlations with transpulmonary thermodilution in paediatric patients.[21] A review of PubMed revealed that to date there are no published papers evaluating the reliability and validity of this procedure during exercise conditions in adults or young people. We would not currently advocate the lithium dilution procedure for use with healthy young people, given the limited information available regarding its reliability and validity at rest and during exercise conditions, and the invasiveness of the procedure.

Non-invasive techniques

Foreign gas rebreathing

Because of the risks associated with invasive measures of $\dot{Q}$, a variety of non-invasive measures have been developed and validated for use at rest, during exercise, and in healthy populations. Foreign gas techniques estimate pulmonary blood flow (which is equivalent to $\dot{Q}$ during equilibrium) by measuring the rate at which an inert, soluble gas enters and leaves the bloodstream via the lungs.[1] The rate of disappearance of the inert soluble gas is directly proportional to the flow of blood past the lungs, providing a valid and reliable measure of $\dot{Q}$. There are varied foreign gas methods to assess $\dot{Q}$,[1,2] including closed-circuit rebreathing,[23] open-circuit rebreathing, and single-breath constant exhalation methods.[24]

Nitrous oxide rebreathing method

This method permits an evaluation of $\dot{Q}$ in non-steady-state conditions but is affected by ventilatory abnormalities.[1] Overall, the method is thought to be more accurate and reliable during submaximal and maximal exercise than at rest. This is because the slight hyperventilation required (at rest) as part of the protocol may influence resting $\dot{Q}$.[1] A number of studies have examined the utility of the nitrous oxide (N_2O) rebreathing method at rest and during exercise in adults;[1] however, limited research exists in children. In one investigation,[25] 10 children (7–16-years old) were studied at rest and at two levels of submaximal exercise (1/3 and 2/3 of their $\dot{V}O_2$ max). Values obtained via N_2O rebreathing were compared with nearly simultaneous measures using an indirect Fick (CO_2) rebreathing method (plateau method; see below). The $\dot{Q}$ was within the expected range and, for a given $\dot{V}O_2$, $\dot{Q}$ was lower in children than in adults. Pulmonary recirculation time was longer in the children than in the adults, and this was attributed to a larger blood volume:weight ratio in comparison to adults. Overall, the simultaneous measures of N_2O and CO_2 showed 'reasonable agreement' in children [$r = 0.94$ for $\dot{Q}$ (CO_2) vs. $\dot{Q}$ (N_2O)]. Unfortunately, the N_2O method was not validated against a gold standard measure of $\dot{Q}$. In addition, repeat measures were not conducted in the children, so there is limited information regarding the variability of this method in children. In adults, the coefficients of variation were similar for the N_2O and CO_2 methods. Despite the limited use in children, the N_2O rebreathing procedure does hold promise for the evaluation of $\dot{Q}$ in young people (particularly during submaximal and maximal exercise conditions). The gas mixture is relatively easy to rebreathe and can be assessed using fast-response analysers (although mass spectrometry remains the preferred assessment tool). This technique is highly reliable during strenuous and non-steady-state conditions, making it particularly attractive for use during maximal exercise conditions.[1]

A recent non-invasive bedside device utilizing N_2O rebreathing and a photo-acoustic gas analyser has been created (Innocor, Innovision, Odense, Denmark). This device is portable and markedly cuts down on the start-up costs traditionally associated with foreign gas rebreathing (viz. a mass spectrometer). This device has been utilized during exercise conditions in adults, and it is likely that it will be increasingly utilized with children during exercise conditions.

Acetylene rebreathing method

The acetylene rebreathing method is utilized in several international exercise physiology and sport cardiology laboratories. Warburton *et al.*[1] concluded that 'many investigators consider it the most viable means of estimating $\dot{Q}$ during submaximal and/or maximal exercise'. There are various techniques that make use of acetylene to determine $\dot{Q}$, including open-circuit, closed-circuit rebreathing, and single breath.

Briefly, the closed-circuit acetylene procedure involves rebreathing a gas mixture containing 35–45% O_2, 0.5–1.0% acetylene, 5–10% helium, and a balance of N_2. The rebreathing frequency is set at a rate of approximately 1 breath every 1.5 s at rest and 1 breath·s^{-1} during maximal exercise, lasting for approximately 18 and 10 s, respectively. The gases within the system are generally sampled continuously by a mass spectrometer interfaced with a computer and customized software to calculate $\dot{Q}$. Adequate mixing of the lung-bag rebreathing system is confirmed via a constant level of helium. After the point of equilibration of acetylene, the rate of disappearance of acetylene is directly proportional to the flow of blood past the lungs, and hence, $\dot{Q}$. The detailed description of the mathematical formula used to calculate $\dot{Q}$ is provided elsewhere.[1]

Acetylene rebreathing has been shown to have relatively low coefficients of variation during exercise conditions (5–10%), with the reliability improving with increasing exercise intensity. The accuracy of the technique during exercise conditions has also been shown to be similar to that observed with the direct Fick and dye-dilution methods.[1]

The open-circuit acetylene technique is a non-rebreathing version of the foreign gas technique. This method involves the normal breathing of a gas mixture containing two inert gases (soluble acetylene and insoluble argon) in an open gas circuit. The technique requires a wash-in period of 6–10 breaths of the inert gases such that there is no alteration in breathing pattern.[2,26] Gledhill's laboratory (internationally renowned for its usage of the acetylene rebreathing procedure) was the first to use the open-circuit technique during incremental to maximal exercise conditions in healthy adults.[24] For instance, Card *et al.*[24] reported a high correlation ($r = 0.974$) between the open- and closed-circuit acetylene technique during incremental to maximal exercise in healthy adult males.[24] As pointed out at that time, this technique has several advantages over the closed-circuit technique. Card *et al.*[24] stated that the 'non-rebreathe is easily tolerated by all subjects, it imposes no alteration in the physiological condition (unlike the rebreathe technique) and represents a major advancement for exercise physiology laboratories' (p. S120). The major advantages of this technique are the ease of operation for both the evaluator and the participant, and the use of spontaneous breathing with no disturbance in the normal breathing pattern.[2] These advantages are particularly important for its use with young people at rest and during exercise conditions.

Recent work has demonstrated good agreement between the open-circuit acetylene technique and other established measures of $\dot{Q}$, including direct Fick and acetylene rebreathing methods.[26,27] Many investigations have been conducted in healthy adults during exercise conditions[26–28] reflecting the ease of administration of this procedure during exercise. The open-circuit acetylene technique has also been shown to have similar reliability (during exercise conditions) to that found with acetylene rebreathing.[27,28] It has been speculated that the open circuit may be better for use with children due to the freedom afforded to breathing patterns during the procedure.[29]

Acetylene-based techniques have numerous advantages that make them a preferred choice for the assessment of cardiac function during submaximal and maximal exercise conditions. The ability to accurately and reliably determine $\dot{Q}$ during strenuous and non-steady-state conditions make this technology a natural choice for use during maximal exercise in young people and adults alike.[1] The recent creation of fast-response acetylene gas analysers also markedly reduces the costs traditionally associated with this methodology.[1] With the increasing implementation of the open-circuit acetylene technology,[24] it is envisioned that more and more laboratories will use this technology to assess the $\dot{Q}$ of young people during exercise conditions. At this time, we would recommend the use of both the open- and closed-circuit acetylene systems for the determination of $\dot{Q}$ in young people.

Acetylene single-breath constant exhalation procedure

In recent years, rapid response infrared acetylene analysers have been integrated into commercially available metabolic carts (such as the Ergocard from Medisoft). These systems allow for the use of a single, prolonged constant expiration of acetylene to measure pulmonary blood flow and $\dot{Q}$.The participants are required to breathe a gas mixture that contains 0.3% methane, 0.3% acetylene, 21% O_2, 0.3% carbon monoxide (CO), and balance N_2.[2] Participants are asked to inhale the gas mixture to total lung volume and then hold their breath for approximately 2 s to allow for acetylene tissue absorption and gas distribution equilibration.[2,30] Participants then exhale at a constant rate of 200–500 $mL{\cdot}s^{-1}$.[2] Rapid response infrared sensors detect the changes in the respective gas concentrations during the manoeuvre allowing for the determination of $\dot{Q}$.[2] The specific details regarding the mathematical relationship between gas absorption and $\dot{Q}$ can be found elsewhere.[2,30]

As reviewed elsewhere, various studies have examined the reliability and/or validity of the single-breath constant exhalation procedure.[2] Good correlations have been shown between this technique and other more established measures of cardiac function in adult patient populations.[30] This technique has also been shown to be reliable during exercise conditions in healthy adults.[28,31] The reliability and the values attained during exercise conditions appear to be consistent with that obtained from both open- and closed-circuit acetylene rebreathing.[28,31] However, as pointed out by Zenger *et al.* [30] and Dibski *et al.*,[28] some participants are unable to exhale at a constant flow rate, particularly during maximal exercise conditions. Given this limitation, it may be difficult to obtain accurate and reliable measures in young people. Further research is clearly warranted to examine the reliability, validity, and feasibility of this procedure for assessing $\dot{Q}$ in young people.

Carbon dioxide rebreathing (indirect Fick) method

The CO_2 rebreathing method has been used frequently and with success in paediatric exercise studies.[1] It uses the same equation as the direct Fick to calculate $\dot{Q}$, but instead of measuring the CO_2 content of the blood, it is estimated by either the Collier method[32] or the Defares method.[33] The Collier method requires a participant to rebreathe a gas mixture containing 10–20% CO_2 until an equilibrium plateau is observed. At this point, there is no further exchange of CO_2 between the alveolar-capillary membrane and the rebreathing bag. It is assumed that the CO_2 at the point of equilibration represents the partial pressure of mixed venous CO_2 ($P\bar{v}O_2$). The partial pressure of mixed arterial CO_2 ($PaCO_2$) can either be measured from the blood (an arterial blood sample, a capillary blood sample from the fingertip or ear lobe, or an arterialized venous blood sample) or estimated non-invasively from end-tidal measures of CO_2 ($P_{ET}CO_2$) immediately prior to the start of rebreathing. Correction factors are sometimes applied to $PaCO_2$ to correct for alveolar-arterial differences and to $P\bar{v}O_2$ to correct for gas–blood differences.[1]

The Defares method involves the participant rebreathing from a bag containing a low concentration of CO_2 (i.e. 0–5%). During the rebreathe procedure, the CO_2 increases in an exponential fashion towards the $P\bar{v}O_2$. The exponential slope is used to extrapolate the point of equilibrium using the end-tidal CO_2 values allowing for the determination of $P\bar{v}O_2$. No correction is applied for gas to blood pCO_2 differences owing to the fact that this procedure does not require the attainment of an equilibrium pCO_2.

For both the Collier and Defares methods, the values for $P\bar{v}O_2$, or $PaCO_2$, are used with an appropriate CO_2 dissociation curve to estimate CO_2 content. A complete review of the strengths and limitations of these two methods can be found in Warburton *et al.*[1] Briefly, the CO_2 rebreathe method can be performed using fast-response CO_2 analysers and provides accurate and reliable estimations of submaximal exercise $\dot{Q}$ As such, it does not require the use of a costly mass spectrometer. There are several limitations of the procedure.[1] For instance, in using a standard dissociation curve for CO_2 (which eliminates the need for blood sampling) individual changes in pH, venous oxygen saturation, and temperature cannot be controlled for. It is assumed that these changes have a negligible effect on the determination of $\dot{Q}$, an assumption that may not be correct during exercise conditions.[1] Similar to the foreign gas rebreathing systems, the accuracy and reliability of the procedure is somewhat limited during resting conditions. Moreover, a major limitation of the technology is the requirement of steady-state conditions for the valid measurement of $\dot{Q}$.Most researchers who utilize the CO_2 rebreathe method do so at exercise intensities below 85% of maximum. However, it is important to note that the Defares method has been shown to provide somewhat accurate $\dot{Q}$ during maximal exercise in adults.[34] The Collier method is more difficult to use during high-intensity exercise owing to the relatively high concentration of CO_2.

Research utilizing the CO_2 rebreathe procedure in children has revealed several strengths and weaknesses. Similar to adults, it is more accurate during exercise than at rest.[25,35] Patterson and Cunningham[36] used the CO_2 rebreathing procedure in nine girls (aged 12–13 years) and six women (aged 20–24 years) during steady-state exercise at four intensities (25–80% of VO_2max) and found that $\dot{Q}$ varied up to 15–20% depending on which estimates of $P\bar{v}O_2$ and dead space were used.[36] Similarly, Sady *et al.*[37] found variations in $\dot{Q}$ of 9–21% depending on which dissociation curve was used and 0–19% depending on the dead-space calculation.

Paterson *et al.*[38] used the equilibrium method repeatedly over 4 months in a group of boys to evaluate the consistency of $\dot{Q}$ measures. While group mean data was reproducible, the day-to-day variability (7–8%) was higher than in adults. This was attributed to inaccuracy in the estimation of $PaCO_2$ and greater variation across children in measures such as HR. The authors concluded that the estimates of $\dot{Q}$ were stable enough for use in research and clinical settings but that more work is required to evaluate the relationship between end-tidal and arterial pCO_2 in children.

A validation of the Defares method against thermodilution was performed at rest and during exercise in 16 children with congenital heart disease.[35] The variable error associated with the measures of $\dot{Q}$ was ±19%. Despite this, the correlations were significant at $r = 0.65$ and 0.81 for rest and exercise, respectively. The high variability led the authors to suggest that the CO_2 rebreathing method may be more useful for group comparisons as opposed to measuring change on an individual level.

Pianosi and Hochman[39] evaluated the effect of different estimates of $PaCO_2$ on the calculation of $\dot{Q}$ using the indirect Fick CO_2 method in 23 healthy children during light to moderate exercise. They discovered that $PaCO_2$ values estimated from $P_{ET}CO_2$ and the Bohr equation over and underestimated $\dot{Q}$, respectively (in comparison to direct measures of $PaCO_2$). To remedy this, they set out to generate a new prediction equation for the estimation of $PaCO_2$. The equation was generated by regressing (in a stepwise fashion) measured $PaCO_2$ against $P_{ET}CO_2$, tidal volume, respiratory rate, and $\dot{V}O_2$. The resulting equation was as follows: $PaCO_2 = 0.647$ $P_{ET}CO_2 + 12.4$ mmHg ($r^2 = 0.625$). It is interesting to note that despite insignificant contributions from the other ventilatory parameters, their new equation produced more accurate and less variable measures of $\dot{Q}$ than other estimates. This study also contained a group of children with cystic fibrosis. Children with severe cases of cystic fibrosis had their $\dot{Q}$ underestimated when end-tidal CO_2 was used as an estimate instead of directly measured $PaCO_2$ and led the authors to conclude that using $P_{ET}CO_2$ to estimate $\dot{Q}$ is not a reliable method in patients with severe pulmonary disease.

To compare the exponential and equilibrium methods and tackle the question of whether the downstream correction factor was needed or not, Jacob *et al.*[40] studied a group of 23 children and 12 adults. Of these 23 children, 14 completed both methods while performing steady-state exercise on the cycle ergometer. After downstream correction, the equilibrium $P\bar{v}O_2$ was more closely associated with the exponential $P\bar{v}O_2$ and fell closer to the line of identity. The authors suggest that all studies involving the measurement of $\dot{Q}$ in children should apply the downstream correction factor to the values obtained through the equilibrium method.

The CO_2 rebreathing method has gained widespread acceptance for use during submaximal exercise in adults and youths alike. Its current use during maximal exercise appears to be limited. It also appears that special precautions must be taken when attempting to achieve valid and reliable measures of $\dot{Q}$ in children. If these precautions are not taken, the reliability and validity of the procedure appears to be lower in young people than that observed in adults.

Doppler echocardiography

Doppler echocardiography determines SV by measuring the velocity of blood in the aorta, pulmonary artery, or mitral valve and the diameter of the blood vessel through which it is flowing. The advantages and limitations of this procedure have been thoroughly reviewed elsewhere.[2,41] Briefly, Doppler echocardiography can be used to obtain non-invasive, beat-to-beat measurements of cardiac function. It can be used during maximal exercise as it does not require steady-state conditions. However, the equipment is expensive and requires a high level of training by the operator for accurate measurement.[42] Moreover, movement artefact can have a significant impact upon the reliability and validity of the procedure (particularly during strenuous exercise).[2]

According to the Doppler principle, an ultrasound wave is transmitted through blood flow passing through a vessel (often the aorta). The most common placement site for the Doppler transducer is the suprasternal notch which allows for the ultrasound signal to pass through the blood flowing through the ascending aorta.[2] The movement of blood cells causes a shift in the frequency (i.e. Doppler frequency shift) of the ultrasonic transmission which yields a measure of blood velocity according to the following formula:

$$V = \frac{\Delta f \cdot c}{2f \cdot \cos\theta}$$

where, Δf is the shift in frequency (Hz), f is the frequency of the original ultrasound wave (Hz), c is the velocity of sound in tissue (1540 m·s^{-1}), and θ is the angle between the blood flow and ultrasound signal.[2] SV is calculated as the product of the velocity time integral and the cross-sectional area of the blood vessel where the measurement was taken.[2,41]

There is considerable debate surrounding the accuracy and reliability of Doppler echocardiography during exercise conditions in adults and young people.[2] In a review of the literature, Warburton and colleagues[2] concluded that Doppler echocardiography provides reasonable estimates of resting $\dot{Q}$ in comparison to established invasive and non-invasive techniques. Moreover, it appeared that Doppler echocardiography could be used during submaximal exercise conditions to evaluate temporal changes in $\dot{Q}$. In addition, the reliability at rest and during exercise conditions is similar to many invasive and non-invasive procedures (approximating 10–15%). However, the authors did acknowledge that several investigations have reported an underestimation of $\dot{Q}$ (approximately 15–20%) with Doppler echocardiography in comparison to other non-invasive and invasive measures of $\dot{Q}$ during exercise conditions. In particular, one study reported that Doppler echocardiography underestimated $\dot{Q}$ (15%) during maximal exercise conditions (in healthy adults) in comparison to thermodilution.[43] In another study, Shaw *et al.*[44] reported that the SV and $\dot{Q}$ during maximal exercise were approximately 17% lower than previously reported values (calculated from regression equations from investigations using invasive procedures). Difficulties associated with elevated breathing frequency and movement artefact are thought to somewhat limit Doppler echocardiography during strenuous exercise conditions (along with a series of other technical issues as discussed later). However, Warburton *et al.*[2] did not discount the ability of Doppler echocardiography to assess $\dot{Q}$ during maximal exercise owing to the inherent limitations of the invasive criterion measures (particularly during maximal exercise conditions).

A 20-year review of the literature[45] observed that the precision of Doppler measurements was about 30% when compared to Fick methods, dye-dilution, or thermodilution methods. Inter- and intra-observer repeatability was similar and ranged from 2 to 22%. The authors concluded that Doppler measures were acceptable for use in children but were perhaps more suited for tracking change from baseline than for reporting absolute values.

A comprehensive review by Rowland and Obert[41] summarized the literature on the reliability of the Doppler echocardiography method during exercise and outlined its advantages and disadvantages. They stated that the Doppler technique provides limited risk or discomfort to the participant and can be used during maximal exercise but is limited by cost and skill requirements. As experts in the utilization of this technology, the authors were clearly aware of the relative strengths of Doppler echocardiography. They highlighted that the technique has shown strong construct and concurrent validity and similar reliability to other measures of $\dot{Q}$. In particular, they highlighted the ability of this technology to determine exercise $\dot{Q}$ in young children. Despite the obvious advantages for the assessment of $\dot{Q}$ in young people, the authors did acknowledge a series of limitations that need to be considered when implementing the technology. For instance, the authors acknowledged that most Doppler studies have been performed on a cycle ergometer rather than a treadmill.[41] This is owing to the fact that some form of stabilization is required for accurate and reliable Doppler measurements. Other factors that need to be considered include 'transducer angulation, change in aortic cross-sectional area during exercise, turbulence and alteration of a flat velocity profile in the aorta with increased $\dot{Q}$, and uncertainties regarding the proper location for measurement of aortic outflow area' (p. 973, 41).

Several studies have shown good reliability of Doppler echocardiography in young people during exercise conditions. For instance, Vinet *et al.*[46] examined the reproducibility of $\dot{Q}$ measures during exercise in children and adults.[46] There were no significant differences in SV or $\dot{Q}$ suggesting that Doppler echocardiography provided good test–retest reliability. Against the CO_2 rebreathing method, Doppler echocardiography showed better reproducibility with coefficients of variation of 7.5% at rest and 5.2% at maximal exercise.[47] Other findings were low coefficient of variation (<10%) for measures of $\dot{Q}$ and SV[48,49] and inter- and intra-observer variability.[50,51]

In summary, Doppler echocardiography has several advantages for use with young people, as reflected by its widespread usage. Its accuracy and reliability is similar to many invasive and non-invasive protocols, and it can be used to non-invasively determine $\dot{Q}$ on a beat-by-beat basis. It is also not reliant on steady-state conditions, which makes it suited for strenuous exercise conditions. Questions, however, remain regarding the accuracy of the technique during strenuous and maximal exercise.

Impedance cardiography

Impedance cardiography or transthoracic electric bioimpedance measures $\dot{Q}$ by passing a high-frequency (HF) (100 kHz), small (4 mA) alternating current through the chest.[2] Changes in electrical impedance, caused by pulsatile changes in aortic blood flow, are measured by recording electrodes placed at specific locations on the body. It is assumed that changes in thoracic impedance during systole are related to SV. There are several formulae used to calculate SV from impedance measures. A full description of the formulae and the assumptions of each formula is available in Warburton *et al.*[2]

There is considerable debate regarding the reliability and validity of impedance cardiography at rest and during exercise conditions.[2] In particular, the theoretical constructs of impedance cardiography have been questioned. On the basis of a review of predominantly adult literature at the time, Warburton and colleagues[2] observed how several early studies, which used impedance cardiography, reported low to moderate correlations with other techniques.[2] They also highlighted commentaries by various researchers outlining the inherent technical and theoretical limitations of impedance cardiography. This review also revealed how several authors have utilized exercise pauses and/or breath holding to minimize the problems associated with movement artefact during strenuous exercise conditions. Although these steps allow for the determination of $\dot{Q}$ during exercise conditions, both exercise pauses and breath holding are known to affect SV and $\dot{Q}$. These limitations led the authors to state that, 'Unless there are further improvements in performance which can allay doubts about its reliability, the use of impedance cardiography in exercise physiology and clinical setting will continue to be limited' (p. 251). It is, however, important to note that the authors did not discount impedance cardiography completely. The authors did acknowledge the growing body of literature that supported the utility of this technology during exercise conditions in healthy and clinical populations. This included supporting evidence of a moderate to high relationship between impedance cardiography-derived $\dot{Q}$ during exercise conditions and other more established measures. The authors also recognized the ability of this methodology to track relative changes in cardiac function (rather than providing accurate absolute measures). In addition, the authors reported how the reliability of impedance cardiography was often shown to be of the same order as that reported using other methods.

Since the systematic review of the literature by Warburton *et al.*,[2] there have been significant advances in impedance cardiography technology, in particular with reference to its administration during exercise conditions. For instance, there has been considerable recent research examining the temporal $\dot{Q}$ response to exercise in healthy individuals (predominantly adults) using impedance cardiography. This research has revealed similar findings to those observed with other technologies throughout incremental to maximal exercise[52,53] providing support for impedance cardiography's use during incremental exercise.

Owing to its ease of administration and non-invasiveness, impedance cardiography has been used in several studies with children. This includes comparative[53–56] and reliability[55,56] studies. Collectively, these studies support the adequacy of impedance cardiography for measuring $\dot{Q}$, particularly in terms of reliability. Similar to the research literature on adults, authors have stated that the major value of impedance cardiography was in observing changes from baseline rather than in determining absolute values.[54] Many of these authors also commented that, in addition to being non-invasive, impedance cardiography is desirable because it requires little in the way of cooperation from the participant.[55] In this regard, it may be a very useful method to use with young people.

It is important to note that a relatively new impedance cardiography system, PhysioFlow, has been developed, which may overcome some of the limitations of previous impedance cardiography measurements.[57,58] It does not require the measurement of baseline impedance (which is affected by hydration status, blood resistivity, and distance between electrodes). This technique has been shown to provide similar results to direct measures of cardiac function during resting and exercise (including maximal exercise) conditions.[57,58] The technique has also been shown to be reliable when used with children. For instance, Welsman *et al.*[42] studied 20 children (average 10.7 years) three times, each a week apart, and measured the reliability of PhysioFlow in the determination of $\dot{Q}$ and SV during a peak $\dot{V}O_2$ test on a cycle ergometer.[42] The coefficient of variation was 4.1% for peak $\dot{V}O_2$, 9.3% for $\dot{Q}$, and 9.3% for SV. The authors concluded that the PhysioFlow method is reasonable for use during maximal exercise in children and that the reliability falls in between Doppler echocardiography and CO_2 rebreathing.

In summary, despite widespread criticisms regarding its theoretical construct, recent research has shown the ability of impedance cardiography to be used during exercise conditions. The technique has many advantages for use with children, including being non-invasive, versatile, cost-effective, and suitable for beat-by-beat changes in cardiac function.[2]

Arterial pulse contour method

The potential for the arterial pulse contour to be used to indirectly assess $\dot{Q}$ was originally proposed in 1904.[59] In 1970, Kouchoukos *et al.*[60] examined SV from the area under the systolic peripheral arterial waveform. In recent years, several researchers have proposed that modifications of this technology may provide an adequate assessment of temporal changes in $\dot{Q}$.[61–64] The methodology (and various modifications) is described in detail elsewhere.[63,65,66]

This method permits a continuous, beat-to-beat evaluation of $\dot{Q}$ from arterial pressure waveform tracings. It is important to note that the pulse contour method provides measures of relative changes in SV, and as such, calibration against an established absolute method is required when absolute values are needed.[67] This technology has been shown to provide reasonable agreement with other methods in young adults,[61,66] pregnant women,[65] and various clinical populations.[63,66] To date there have been limited studies using pulse contour analyses (such as the Modelflow method) in children. It is, therefore, unknown whether this method provides an appropriate measurement technique in young people.

The continuous beat-to-beat nature of the measurement presents an advantage over other methods whose values for $\dot{Q}$ are averaged over several heart beats. A continuous, beat-to-beat measure of $\dot{Q}$ allows for the measurement of rapid changes such as at the onset of exercise or during postural changes.[68] Furthermore, Portapres is an ambulatory model of the Finapres that is commonly used in the measurement of beat-to-beat blood pressure; thus, if pulse contour analyses (e.g. Modelflow) proved to be an accurate mechanism of $\dot{Q}$ measurement, it may be possible to monitor $\dot{Q}$ continuously throughout activities of daily living. This would represent a significant contribution to the available literature. However, it should be noted that the determination of a reliable pulse contour during exercise conditions is extremely difficult. In our practice, it has been very difficult to use the Finapres, Finometer, or Portapres during strenuous exercise conditions with adults and children thereby limiting the utility of this procedure during exercise conditions. Movement artefact is a serious problem when attempting to utilize this technology. Moreover, the fact that absolute values can only be obtained after calibration against another method restricts the technology in terms of ease of usage and/or non-invasiveness, thus limiting its use with healthy children.

In summary, the arterial pulse contour analysis method shows promise in the non-invasive measurement of $\dot{Q}$ under resting conditions but appears to be somewhat limited during exercise conditions. Current methodology permits the tracking of changes in $\dot{Q}$ but requires an independent method for calibration if accurate absolute values are desired.[68] Research examining its validity in the paediatric population and during exercise conditions is required. At this time, we would not recommend this technology for the assessment of the cardiovascular response to strenuous exercise in children, especially as some researchers have reported difficulty in obtaining a reliable pulse contour for analysis in children.[69] This is particularly salient given the other non-invasive procedures that are currently available (including Doppler echocardiography and impedance cardiography) that can assess cardiac function on a beat-by-beat basis.

Cardiovascular regulation

Heart rate variability

The evaluation of spontaneous variations or modulation of HR [i.e. heart rate variability (HRV)] is a powerful non-invasive tool for the prediction of the risk for cardiovascular disease (CVD) and all cause mortality.[70] A healthy cardiovascular control system is thought to have high HRV.[71] An unfavourable autonomic profile balance (reflected by low HRV) indicates a greater sympathetic influence on control of HR. Low HRV has been related directly with obesity,[72] high visceral fat deposition,[73] lower aerobic fitness,[74,75] male gender,[76] and increasing age.[77] Moreover, HRV has been shown to be low in individuals with coronary artery disease,[78] myocardial infarction,[70] congestive heart failure,[79] hypertension, and left ventricular hypertrophy.[80]

Time and frequency domains of HRV calculated from either long 24-h or short 2–15-min electrocardiogram (ECG) recordings have been used to predict time to death after myocardial infarction.[81] Specifically in children, decreased components of HRV are used to predict the severity of insulin-dependent diabetes mellitus,[82] asthma,[83] and various heart conditions.[84,85] Indices of HRV have also been shown to reflect cardiovascular health and health-related physical fitness in children.[71]

HRV measurements are easy to perform, non-invasive, and have good reproducibility if standardized conditions are used. Standardization is required because HRV is influenced by factors such as respiratory rate and posture.[86] The analysis can be performed on either short ECG segments lasting from 0.5 to 5 min or on 24-h ECG recordings.[86] Short-term assessments are completed within controlled laboratory conditions with measurements at rest, before and after tilt, or other conditions that challenge the autonomic system (such as exercise).[87] With a short-term procedure, the frequency domain methods are preferred to the time domain methods (as outlined in the comprehensive review of the field).[88] The total variance of HRV increases with the length of the analysed recording; therefore, it is inappropriate to compare measures obtained from recordings of different durations.[88] Long-term assessments are made while subjects perform their usual daily activities. This type of assessment is useful for risk stratification or for quantifying autonomic dysfunction.[87] It has been suggested that sleep provides the ideal situation in which to record HRV because it is free of conditions, such as environmental conditions and daily physical activity that affect HRV.[89] Slow-wave sleep may provide the most optimal condition for HRV analysis and better discrimination between parasympathetic and sympathetic influences due to a more pronounced vagal tone, spontaneous regular respiratory patterns, and a high electrocardiographic stationarity during this stage.[90] Thus, some studies utilize only the data collected during sleep.[91,92]

The decline in HRV with age begins in childhood. Infants have high sympathetic activity that decreases rapidly between the ages of 5 and 10 years.[93] In support of this is evidence from Goto *et al.*[91] who documented that parasympathetic activity, as measured by analysis of power spectral density, increased from 3 to 6 years of age and then decreased from 6 to 15 years.[91] Furthermore, the influence of provocation on HRV is more pronounced at younger ages.[94] Developmental changes in the cardiac autonomic system in childhood can be described by using HRV analysis, and the non-invasive quantification of the relation between indices of HRV may be useful for assessing the influence of autonomic innervation of the heart in children, leading to a better understanding of cardiac disease in the paediatric population.[91] Girls have lower HRV than age-matched boys.[71,77]

There is a need to develop numerically robust techniques that are suitable for fully automatic measurement. The possibilities of being able to characterize and quantify the dynamics of the RR interval and the transient changes in HRV are still under mathematical development.[88] Longitudinal studies are necessary to establish normal HRV standards for the various age and sex groups.[88] There is currently no consensus on the best HRV assessment, and there are many different methods to calculate non-spectral HRV indices and numerous definitions of low- and high-frequency HR power.[86]

The assessment of HRV is straightforward, easy to administer, and non-invasive, which makes it particularly suitable and attractive for use with young people. The measures are highly reproducible when conducted in a standardized fashion. A growing body of literature supports the relationship between HRV and cardiovascular health in young people. These features warrant further investigation of HRV and its relationship to cardiovascular function and health in young people.

Baroreflex sensitivity

Baroreflex receptor sensitivity (BRS) is defined as the transfer function between changes in blood pressure and pulse interval and is an integrative measure for short-term sympathetic and parasympathetic cardiovascular regulation of HR and blood pressure.[95] One condition associated with diminished BRS is a reduction in vagal influences on the cardiovascular system. When assessed by HRV, diminished vagal control results in a loss of flexibility of cardiac control and is associated with increased mortality from sudden cardiac death.[96] Evidence indicates that both BRS and HRV provide significant prognostic value for various cardiovascular complications[97,98] and, in several pathological conditions, both BRS and HRV are impaired.[99,100]

Traditionally, pharmacological manipulations were used to elicit a response in HR and blood pressure to evaluate BRS; however, non-invasive methods have now been introduced and established in adults.[101–103] Bertinieri *et al.*[101] identified spontaneous sequences of cardiac cycles having either increasing or decreasing systolic blood pressure with concomitant reflexive changes in heart period. This sequence technique was then validated against the invasive pharmacological method in a group of adults. In this validation study, estimates of baroreflex control provided by the sequence method were significantly correlated with estimates derived from pharmacological manipulation of pressure; however, the sequence method was less sensitive than the pharmacological method.[104] It uses the regression coefficient between concomitant changes in systolic blood pressure and pulse interval in the time domain.[103] In this study, beat-to-beat systolic blood pressure and HR changes were measured continuously with the Finapres. Another technique, namely, the spectral technique, uses either the square roots between the spectral power of systolic blood pressure and pulse interval in the frequency domain[105] or the gain of the transfer function between changes of blood pressure and pulse interval in the frequency domain.[106] This latter technique has been used in several clinical studies in adults.[95] These techniques have also been increasingly used with young people. The following two sections will outline the use of the sequence technique and spectral analysis in young people.

Sequence technique

Allen *et al.* (2000) were the first group of researchers to utilize the non-invasive sequence technique in a group of prepubertal and adolescent youth.[96] Both systolic blood pressure (via the Finapres) and pulse interval were calculated for analysis. Customized software identified sequences of three or more beats in which systolic blood pressure increased or decreased at least 1 mmHg for consecutive cycles. If pulse interval sequentially increased by at least 2 ms, then the sequence was considered valid. The measure of BRS for each sequence was defined as the slope expressed in ms of pulse interval change per mmHg change in systolic blood pressure.[96] In addition, pulse interval measures were also obtained using impedance cardiography, derived from EKG. The average of the difference between successive pulse intervals for a given time period was defined as the mean-sqaured displacement (MSD) statistic.[96] MSD has previously been shown to effectively track pharmacologically manipulated cardiac vagal control.[107] The authors concluded that the sequence method worked well for both groups of youth. A very strong positive correlation was found between BRS and MSD despite differences in the measurement and how they were computed. The high correlations provide concurrent validity for the ability of the measures to index resting cardiac vagal tone in youth.[96]

Other researchers measured BRS in youth calculated in both the time and frequency domain. Using the sequence technique (time domain) BRS was calculated from baroreflex sequences (runs of three or four consecutive beats characterized by a progressive increase or decrease in systolic blood pressure with a minimal beat-to-beat change of 1 mmHg) as the slope of the regression line between systolic blood pressure and pulse interval.[95] In addition, sequences were estimated if the pulse interval response was shifted by one beat (lag 1), calculating BRS from the regression line between systolic blood pressure and pulse interval of the following beat. The correlation coefficient ($r > 0.7$) had to occur between sequences to be considered for analysis. The baroreflex effectiveness index (BEI) was calculated as the quotient of the numbers of baroreflex sequences divided by the number of blood pressure ramps. This index is suitable for examining the arterial baroreflex in a dynamic manner with a short time resolution.[108] Di Rienzo and colleagues[108] stated that the inclusion of both BRS and BEI provide a more comprehensive picture of reflex cardiovascular regulation since the two measures provide information on different aspects of the baroreflex control of the heart. Rudiger and Bald[95] used this method in children and concluded that the best estimates were achieved using three consecutive beats without lag and that BRS can be reliably calculated in young people using this method.

Spectral analysis in children

Spectral analysis (frequency domain) of pulse interval and systolic blood pressure has been done with the trigonometric regressive spectral analysis in youth. Oscillations are calculated with an optimal variance reduction at every frequency which reveals a continuous physiological frequency spectrum.[109] In youth, the calculation of the percentage of reduction of total variance in different spectral bands [low and high frequency (LF and HF)] has been used for spectral analysis so that BRS can be calculated separately for the LF and HF bands. Results from the calculation of total variance allow spectral power of systolic blood pressure and pulse interval to be calculated by multiplication of the reduction in percentage of total power with the total spectral variance for each spectral band.[103,105] Geritsen *et al.* [106] calculated further using the gain of the transfer function between changes of blood pressure and pulse interval at frequencies with proven coherence. The authors concluded that BRS can reliably be calculated from continuous blood pressure and pulse interval recordings in healthy children and adolescents, using frequency domain techniques.

Rudiger and Bald[95] demonstrated that the BRS estimated by the sequence technique was significantly higher than the BRS gain using all frequencies; however, the correlation was high between the methods in children.[95] Reproducibility coefficients were high for both methods. BRS calculated in the LF band was significantly lower than in the HF band. The importance of attaining reliable measures of BRS in youth is to obtain proper reference values in healthy children and adolescents, which can be used to compare with children and adolescents with various pathological conditions and the impact these conditions have on BRS.[95]

Age and maturation

Maturation of cardiovagal autonomic function has been assessed using the sequence method. Results indicated that spontaneous indices increased as age increased and attained maximum values during adolescence despite stiffening of the carotid artery.[110] Post-adolescence, spontaneous indices decreased. Since age-related changes in spontaneous indices and cardiovagal autonomic function were directly proportional, central parasympathetic signal processing may play a role in the maturation of cardiovagal autonomic function.[111]

Systolic and diastolic function

Cardiac morphology and functional properties (i.e. systolic and diastolic) constitute an integral part of the cardiovascular system.[112] Increasing research has examined the left ventricular function of young people and adults alike. Two-dimensional and Doppler echocardiography have proven increasingly useful as a non-invasive means for characterizing changes in left ventricular function, allowing for the assessment of left ventricular filling parameters, cardiac dimensions, wall thicknesses, wall motion velocities, and valve motion, to name a few.

At rest

The echocardiographic assessment of left ventricular function at rest in young people is straightforward, non-invasive, and accomplished in the majority of participants. To assess systolic and diastolic function at rest, participants lay in a supine position for approximately 15 min prior to and during testing.[112] In order to determine left ventricular internal dimension at end diastole (LVIDd) and end systole (LVIDs), posterior wall thickness at end diastole (PWT), interventricular septal thickness at end diastole (IVST), left ventricular shortening fraction (FS), and ejection fraction (EF), the M mode, short-axis and long-axis measurements can be used.[112] The American Society of Echocardiography recommends the leading-edge-to-leading-edge method for obtaining all measurements and calculations[113] using the M mode two-dimensional imaging system. Recordings can be obtained from the standard parasternal two-dimensional long-axis and short-axis planes, at the level of the cordea tendineae or just below the tips of the mitral valve leaflets. The clearest cardiac images are recorded with the transducer positioned in the intercostal space to the left of the sternum. The reference point for end-diastolic measurements is the peak of the R wave of a simultaneously recorded ECG and for end systole, the minimum separation of the posterior wall and septum during systole.[112] Left ventricular mass can be calculated from Devereux's formula.[114]

Left ventricular inflow, typically used to assess diastolic function, can be examined in the apical four-chamber view, with the sample volume placed between the mitral leaflet tips and the ultrasound beam placed parallel to the presumed flow of blood. The measurements and calculations made from this recording are as follows: peak-velocity and time-velocity integral of early diastolic rapid inflow (peak E, TVI-E) and of atrial contraction filling (peak A, TVE-A), time-velocity integral of the total diastolic filling period (TVI-T), ratio peak E/peak A, ratio TVI-E/TVI-A, ratio peak E/TVI-T, rapid filling fraction (RFF = TVI-E/TVI-T), atrial filling fraction (AFF = TVI-A/TVI-T).[112] Obert and colleagues[112] successfully utilized these techniques in prepubertal children.

Recent advancements in echocardiography are likely to lead to greater understanding of the effects of exercise training on the cardiovascular function of young people (similar to what has been seen in adults). For instance, the use of tissue Doppler imaging (TDI) will likely move the field forward greatly. The TDI technology provides the opportunity to assess systolic and diastolic myocardial function non-invasively by estimating mean velocity of ventricular wall excursion.[115] When measured from the base of the ventricle, a measurement of the velocity of myocardial excursion in systole is obtained. This corresponds closely to other markers of ventricular contractile function. In addition, early diastolic tissue velocity (E′) serves as an indicator of the rate of diastolic myocardial relaxation which is less dependent on preload than other echocardiographic measures.[116]

During static exercise

Although resting echocardiographic measures provide insight into left ventricular function, the major insights in the field of exercise physiology have been derived during exercise conditions. Both standard and novel measures (such as TDI) have been conducted recently in youth during exercise conditions. For instance, Rowland *et al.*[116] studied markers of systolic and diastolic function in pre-adolescent boys using Doppler echocardiographic techniques and TDI during bilateral static leg extension. Markers of both systolic and diastolic function increased significantly during exercise indicating enhanced function during exercise. TDI-S (indicative of systolic function) rose by 59% and TDI-E′ (marker of rate of diastolic relaxation) rose by 38%. There were no changes in left ventricular pressures, as measured by E:E′.[116] The cardiovascular responses observed are similar to those traditionally associated with static exercise in adults and children.[116]

During dynamic exercise

On an upright cycle ergometer, colour-coded TDI has proven to be a feasible technique for obtaining satisfactory group data for ventricular function.[117] An investigation measuring systolic and diastolic function in a group of healthy boys aged 7–12 years reported that both systolic and diastolic cardiac properties are enhanced during an acute bout of dynamic exercise. From rest to peak exercise, peak aortic velocity and systolic ejection rate rose significantly while systolic acceleration time and systolic ejection time declined indicating increased systolic function. Both average systolic tissue Doppler velocity (S) and E′ rose significantly from rest to peak exercise suggesting that diastolic function is enhanced during exercise.[117]

After-exercise training and detraining

Using resting measures of diastolic function in children (combined with measures of ventricular dimensions), taken before an endurance training programme, immediately after, and then again after 2 months of detraining, Obert *et al.*[112] discovered that left ventricular remodelling occurs in moderately trained prepubertal children. Specifically, LVIDs increased by 4.6% and both IVST and PWT decreased by approximately 10.7%. In addition, all measurements of left ventricular inflow (except Peak E) increased significantly after training. After 2 months of detraining, these values returned to pre-training values.[112] The findings of Obert and colleagues (2001) are consistent with those reported by others who employed intensive training programmes in children and observed significant changes in cardiac dimensions.[118,119] In an investigation prescribing exercise of a lower intensity in children, there was no change in LVID detected.[120]

It is important to acknowledge some of the inherent limitations of two-dimensional Doppler echocardiography. Pulsed-wave Doppler only measures the velocity at the sampled point;[121] however, flow-velocity profiles are not uniform, and it has been shown that there is a parabolic flow-velocity distribution. Maximal velocities occur near the centre and minimal velocities occur at the vessel periphery. This profile can be skewed with higher velocities at the septal and anterior wall.[122] In addition, two-dimensional volume calculations are error prone due to difficulties in defining left ventricular borders or abnormal ventricular geometry and valve area may be inaccurate due to changing shape and size over the cardiac cycle.[123]

Given the inherent assumptions of two-dimensional echocardiography, real-time three-dimensional Doppler echocardiography has been proposed as a superior method. This is most important for the imaging of the mitral and pulmonary valves as the cross-sectional area of these valves changes markedly throughout the cardiac cycle. Three-dimensional Doppler echocardiography captures all of the flow-velocity data over a valve as opposed to just a sample point as with the two-dimensional pulsed-wave velocity time interval (VTI).[123] It has been demonstrated that the three-dimensional echocardiography Doppler data can be used to calculate flow volumes in both adult and paediatric patients, and the results correlate well with reference to two-dimensional pulsed-wave Doppler VTI.[123] It is likely that three-dimensional Doppler echocardiography will be used increasingly in the assessment of cardiac function of children.

Peripheral blood flow

A major difficulty in measuring O_2 delivery to the local tissues in humans is methodological due to the emphasis on non-invasive experiments. Common non-invasive measurements of local blood flow are plethysmography and Doppler imaging which provide global measures of flow. Plethysmography measures changes in limb volume corresponding to total arterial inflow, and Doppler imaging corresponds to the volume flow in a large artery. Neither of these measures reflect the actual delivery and utilization of O_2 in skeletal muscle. By contrast, near-infrared spectroscopy (NIRS) is able to indicate the balance between local oxygen delivery and oxygen utilization.[124]

Pulse oximetry

Peripheral perfusion index (PFI) is derived from the photoelectric plethysmography signal of pulse oximetry and can be used as a non-invasive measure of peripheral perfusion.[125] Pulse oximetry is widely used for trauma, critically ill, and surgery patients. Normal values have been formulated for adults, and studies with body temperature gradients suggest that PFI can be a direct indicator of peripheral perfusion. The principle of pulse oximetry is based on two light sources with different wavelengths emitted through the cutaneous vascular bed of a finger or earlobe. Pulse oximetry is able to distinguish the pulsatile component of arterial oxygen saturation and overall haemoglobin concentration. The PFI is calculated as the ratio between the pulsatile component (arterial compartment) and the non-pulsatile component (other tissues).[126] It remains to be determined what the utility of this procedure is in young healthy individuals, particularly during exercise conditions.

Pulse oximetry is useful as a screening tool for the early detection of hypoxaemia and for continuous monitoring of oxygen saturation in clinical and exercise environments. In addition, it is quick, reliable, and non-invasive.[127] The limitations associated with pulse oximetry are as follows: (i) it does not detect the development of early hypoxaemia in individuals with a high partial pressure of O_2 as well;[127] (ii) other light-absorbing spectra, such as methaemoglobin, may interfere with the wavelength;[128] (iii) a significant source of error is motion artefact;[129] (iv) nail polishes may affect readings;[130] (v) severe hypotension, low cardiac output, vasoconstriction, and hypothermia reduce the pulsatile volume of blood in the tissue and may cause inaccurate readings;[131] (vi) the accuracy decreases with decreasing O_2 saturation and may be unreliable below 70%;[132] and (vii) although pulse oximeters are specified for use at particular frequencies, the values may be 15 nm above or below the actual intended signal.[133]

Near-infrared spectroscopy

Near-infrared spectroscopy (NIRS) is a non-invasive technique that operates in real time and is used for continuous monitoring of tissue oxygenation.[126,134] Similar to pulse oximetry, NIRS uses the principles of light transmission and absorption to measure the concentrations of haemoglobin and oxygen saturation. It has a greater tissue penetration than pulse oximetry and provides a global assessment of oxygenation in all vascular compartments.[126] NIRS has primarily been used to assess dynamic changes in the status of tissue oxyhaemoglobin, deoxyhaemoglobin, total blood volume, and the oxidation state of the copper moiety of mitochondrial cytochrome *c* oxidase in brain and muscle.[134] In healthy adults, NIRS produces reproducible measurements of tissue oxygenation during both arterial and venous occlusive events.[135]

NIRS has been used to examine muscle oxygenation trends during exercise, calculating the differences in the absorbency of haemoglobin and myogobin in the near-infrared range of the absorption spectrum. It has been used during incremental and steady-state exercise in various modes such as cycling,[136,137] rowing,[137] arm cranking,[138] and speed skating.[139] NIRS has also been used to study the acute changes in muscle oxygenation that occur with isotonic grip exercise,[140] upper extremity weight-lifting exercise,[141] and isometric contractions of the forearm,[142] and knee-extension exercises.[143] All of these investigations were carried out in adults. High correlations (r = 0.82–0.997) have been observed between the NIRS signal and oxyhaemoglobin saturation measured *in vitro* by co-oximetry, thereby validating this procedure.[136,144] When comparing NIRS to plethysmography and the Fick equation in the measurement of forearm blood flow, it was concluded that NIRS is a suitable tool to provide new insights into the heterogeneity of local muscle metabolism and that NIRS is able to discriminate between the resting and exercising states of the muscle and between the physically active and less active muscle.[145] Not all studies have found a good correlation between NIRS measurements and direct measurements of oxygen saturation. It has been documented that during exercise the NIRS signal initially desaturated and then resaturated. In the same studies, the direct measures of venous oxygen saturation initially decreased but did not increase as the NIRS signal did.[146,147]

Moalla *et al.*[148] examined the oxygenation responses of children during sustained isometric contractions. The NIRS probe was secured on the vastus lateralis (10–12 cm from the knee joint), parallel to the major axis of the thigh. The kinetics of muscle oxygenation and blood volume in the children were similar to the trends observed in adult studies for the same exercise mode.[149] Muscle oxygenation and blood volume decreased at the onset of exercise and reached the lowest point in the middle of the exercise duration. Immediately after exercise was terminated, a rapid increase in muscle oxygenation and blood volume which exceeded the resting values was noted.[148] Results in children have also demonstrated strong correlations between muscle oxygenation and blood volume.[148,150]

In children, a strong linear relationship has been found between ventilatory threshold determined by the V-slope method and NIRS, permitting the detection of ventilatory threshold in respiratory muscles.[151] While the participants exercised on a cycle ergometer, the NIRS probe was situated on the sixth intercostal space, at the anterior axillary line over the serratus anterior muscle. As demonstrated by NIRS, the respiratory muscles in children deoxygenate during incremental exercise.[151]

Blood flow can also be estimated using NIRS and indocyanine green dye as a tracer. Blood flow is quantified based on the ratio of tissue (indocyanine) to arterial (indocyanine); increases in tissue blood flow are defined by both a greater magnitude and rate of ICG accumulation in tissue for a given volume injected into the circulation.[152] This method has been used to measure blood flow during dynamic exercise in the calf and quadriceps muscles in adults.[134]

There is no gold standard to which NIRS data can be directly compared, and there is currently a variety of NIRS equipment available with different working systems.[126] There are also different methods of quantifying the NIRS signal; some studies present data in terms of absolute values whereas other studies present relative changes or physiological calibrations. Subcutaneous fat has a large impact on the NIRS signal whereby more fat results in less light absorption and a stronger signal.[124] Despite these limitations, NIRS allows for the accurate assessment of changes in regional tissue oxygenation and blood flow,[134] produces reliable measurements of tissue oxygenation during both arterial and venous occlusive events,[126] and is easily applied to investigate a variety of tissue regions in both healthy and diseased individuals,[152] including young people.[148]

Near-infrared technology has greatly advanced our understanding of regional tissue oxygenation and blood flow in adults. Data in young people are limited; however, NIRS may provide valuable insights into O_2 tissue transport and utilization at rest and during exercise as well as in health and diseased states.

Cardiovascular/vascular health

Blood pressure

Data from numerous studies provide convincing evidence of the direct relationship between resting blood pressure (systolic, diastolic, mean arterial, and pulse pressures) and CVD. Cardiovascular mortality increases progressively throughout the range of blood pressure, including the pre-hypertensive range (systolic blood pressure reading of 120–139 mmHg or diastolic blood pressure reading of 80–89 mmHg).[153] In addition, it has been suggested that blood pressure variability may also be an independent risk factor for cardiovascular morbidity.[153] Evidence shows that the antecedents of high blood pressure begin in childhood thus demonstrating the importance of monitoring at an early age.[154]

The traditional standard for clinical blood pressure measurement is readings taken by a trained health care provider, using a mercury sphygmomanometer and the Korotkoff sound technique (the auscultatory method). Compared to direct intra-arterial measurement, however, systolic blood pressure is underestimated and diastolic blood pressure is overestimated using this technique.[153] Due to tester error, the variability in blood pressure and the white-coat hypertension phenomenon, there has been increasing advocacy for the use of automated devices.[153]

There are numerous devices available for the assessment of blood pressure: (i) the mercury sphygmomanometer; (ii) the aneroid sphygmomanometer which is inherently less accurate than the mercury sphygmomanometer and requires frequent calibration; (iii) the hybrid sphygmomanometer, which combines some of the best features of both electronic and auscultatory devices and therefore has the potential to replace the mercury sphygmomanometer; (iv) the Finometer (formerly Finapres) which measures blood pressure at the finger, has been validated against intra-arterial pressures. This device is best suited for research investigations where short-term changes and variability in blood pressure are being measured, not clinical practice nor exercise conditions; (v) ultrasound techniques which are useful for detecting blood pressure in patients with very faint Korotkoff sounds; and (vi) tonometry-measured blood pressure at the wrist. This technique is not recommended for clinical use because comparisons with aortic pressure have shown considerable scatter between estimated and true values.[153,155]

Blood pressure and HR during submaximal exercise can be collected using a semi-automated blood pressure measurement device[155] or manual sphygmanometry in boys and girls.[156] At rest, no difference was found in blood pressure between genders.[156] During submaximal exercise, systolic blood pressure measured with a semi-automated blood pressure device increases linearly with progressive increases in workload in both genders with boys, demonstrating a higher blood pressure at each workload than girls. There was little to no change in diastolic blood pressure with incremental exercise protocols.[155]

A variety of blood pressure devices are available for the non-invasive assessment of vascular health. Automated machines are becoming increasingly popular, as they overcome limitations associated with the traditional method of assessment by a trained health professional. Blood pressure is a widely used technique that allows for early detection of CVD risk in children and provides important insight into children's cardiovascular response to stress (such as during exercise).

Endothelial function

The endothelium is a highly active tissue and plays an important role in the preservation of vascular tone and structure and in the regulation of cellular interactions contributing to the development of atherosclerosis.[157] Endothelial dysfunction can be broadly defined as an imbalance between factors contributing to vasodilatation and vasoconstriction.[158] In adults, endothelial dysfunction is associated with cardiovascular events, and the measurement techniques have contributed to the understanding of the atherosclerotic disease process. In children, endothelial dysfunction is associated with risk factors for CVD including obesity[159] and type I diabetes.[160] However, some have argued that the techniques to date are not adequately refined to use as screening tools or to make medical decisions.[157] Furthermore, there is still some debate as to the reproducibility[157] and normal ranges [161] of responses.

As reviewed by Deanfield *et al.*[157] and Anderson,[162] there are several methods used in the assessment of endothelial function. Cardiac catheterization and venous occlusion plethysmography (with pharmacological intervention) are invasive measures and therefore not advocated for use in children. Other common measures include ultrasound assessment of flow-mediated vasodilatation (FMD), laser Doppler flowmetry (LDF), and pulse-wave analysis. These techniques are all used in the assessment of vasomotion, that is, changes in vessel diameter and blood flow. Endothelial health can also be examined through the measurement of various blood factors (platelet aggregation and activation (flow cytometry), leukocyte adhesion (flow cytometry), circulating leukocyte adhesion molecules, cytokines, microparticles, progenitor endothelial cells, and C-reactive protein.[162] These techniques are also invasive in that they require blood samples and will not be covered here.

Flow-mediated vasodilatation

Flow-mediated vasodilation (FMD) measures the vasodilatory response of the arteries to increased blood flow (hyperaemia), typically after a period of occlusion.[158,163] It requires the use of a high resolution ultrasound, a HF linear array probe (5–13 MHz) and video-recording capabilities (for post-test analyses). Flow-mediated vasodilation is the most common and best validated technique[158] and is considered to be the gold standard in the assessment of endothelial biology,[157] but it is technically challenging and requires highly trained personnel and careful control of environmental and participant factors (such as room temperature, exercise, and diet) to ensure accuracy.[164]

Typically, the brachial artery is chosen for assessment because it is larger than the radial artery and more easily measured than the femoral artery.[161] The measurement of endothelial function in the brachial artery has been shown to be closely related to that of the carotid arteries,[165] which is important for research examining the relationship between endothelial function and CVD. There is also the potential for inaccurate determination of arterial diameter with small (<2.5 mm) arteries, such as those of young children.[166]

A complete description of the methods can be located elsewhere[158,163] but briefly, after at least 10 min of supine rest, baseline measurements are taken: 30 s to 1 min of pulsed-wave Doppler imaging at an angle of 70°.[163] Following this, a blood pressure cuff is inflated well above systolic blood pressure: 300 mmHg in adults, 200 mmHg in children, or 50 mmHg above the participant's systolic pressure. After 5 min, the cuff is rapidly deflated and the brachial artery diameter is assessed for 2–5 min. The results are calculated as percentage change in blood flow from baseline. In a simplified context, the influx of blood into the vessels produces a mechanical stress on the endothelium and the cells produce nitric oxide, a potent vasodilator, in response.[158] Normal values are not clearly defined but some researchers have previously defined endothelial dysfunction as FMD < 3%.[161] To distinguish endothelial dysfunction from smooth muscle dysfunction, a sublingual dose of nitric oxide (which acts independently of the endothelium to cause vasodilation) may be administered.[161,167]

Within-subject day-to-day variation in FMD responses is considerable but has been attributed to real variations in physiological function and not to measurement error; over the long-term FMD measures are considered reproducible[161] with one group reporting a between-visit coefficient of variation of 2.3%.[163] A comparison against pulse-wave analysis and pulse contour analysis[167] in healthy children and adults demonstrated that FMD was the most reproducible of the three. The authors noted that there was no correlation between the three methods and suggested that this may be due to differences in the regulation of vascular tone in each of the locations that the test was performed or that the tests were providing different information such as potential differences between conduit and resistance vessels.[168]

Overall, FMD appears to be an acceptable technique for evaluating endothelial function in children as it is non-invasive, well tolerated, and relatively affordable. More large-scale studies are needed to establish normal values for FMD as currently its use is limited to research purposes.

Cutaneous laser Doppler flowmetry

The endothelial function of the microvasculature (vessels with a lumen diameter 100–300 μm) can be evaluated continuously and non-invasively using laser Doppler flowmetry (LDF). In this technique, a probe is placed on the inner surface of the forearm and a laser is directed towards the skin surface. As the light hits moving blood cells, the wavelength changes (Doppler shift) and this, as well as the scatter, can be detected in the reflected beam.[169] Values obtained via LDF are in 'perfusion units' where 1 perfusion unit is equal to 10 mV. The values cannot be accurately converted to blood-flow values but should be expressed as conductance ($mV \cdot mmHg^{-1}$) or as a percentage of maximal flux, where maximal flux is induced by heating the laser Doppler probe to a temperature of 42–44°C.[170]

LDF has poor reproducibility if the measurement site is not standardized; but, otherwise, the coefficient of variation is similar to that of FMD (<10%).[169] Responses have been shown to be more reproducible when performed over a large area of skin as opposed to the single-point measures that are traditionally used.[171] Sex and percentage of body fat are associated with microvascular responses and may confound results if not controlled for statistically.[168]

Endothelium-dependent vasodilatation in the microvasculature can be induced in a manner similar to the FMD technique. That is, by occluding the vessels with a cuff inflated to greater than systolic blood pressure and measuring the hyperaemic response after restoration of flow.[169] Alternatively, vasoactive drugs, such as acetylcholine (an endothelial-dependent vasodilator), can be administered via iontophoresis.[172] In iontophoresis, a charged drug in solution is delivered transdermally by applying a low-intensity current.[173] Acetylcholine induced vasodilatation was shown to be larger and longer lasting than that induced by 4 min of arterial occlusion.[172] A final method of assessing vasodilatation in the microvasculature is the local application of heat,[169] in the same manner as obtaining maximal flux for the expression of blood flow as a percentage of maximal flow.

Blood flow through the microvasculature is not constant, but demonstrates periodic oscillations. This characteristic has been termed *flowmotion*, and a novel technique is to perform spectral analysis of the LDF signal using the wavelet transformation.[169] When the laser Doppler signal is examined in the frequency range of 0.0095–1.6 Hz, oscillations can be seen at 1, 0.3, 0.1, 0.04, and 0.01 Hz, and evidence suggests that these represent cardiac, respiratory, myogenic, neurogenic, and endothelium-independent influences, respectively. Should future studies confirm that oscillations in the 0.01 Hz range are endothelium dependent, this could be targeted to develop a test for endothelial function.[169] This technique has not yet been applied to children.

LDF shows promise as a non-invasive technique to evaluate microvascular function in children. However, strict attention to testing procedures (i.e. measurement site, subject position, room temperature) is required to ensure reproducible results.

Pulse-wave analysis

Pulse-wave analysis uses the technique of applanation tonometry to obtain a recording of the arterial pressure waveform non-invasively. The tonometer is placed over the artery (typically the radial artery) and once the anterior wall is flattened slightly, the pressure waveform is accurately recorded.[174] The peripheral waveform can be transformed to produce a central aortic waveform; however, this has only been validated in adults. The vascular response to glyceryl trinitrate and inhaled salbutamol (a β_2-agonist that elicits endothelial nitric oxide release) provides an estimate of global nitric oxide-dependent vascular reactivity.[174]

Pulse-wave analysis yields an 'augmentation index' which can be interpreted as a measure of arterial stiffness. The augmentation index is the ratio of the pulse pressures at the second and first systolic peaks.[174] Results can be expressed as the maximum change in augmentation index after drug administration.

This method is less reproducible in children than in adults,[167] and although it has the advantage of being relatively inexpensive and portable, it requires a skilled technician to ensure accurate and reliable results. There are virtually no data using pulse-wave analysis in children to assess endothelial function—the majority of current research using this technique in children is in the field of opthamology.

The use of tonometry to assess endothelial function is appealing for several reasons. The method is not as technically demanding as other methods and the equipment is portable and less expensive than that required for FMD. However, the analysis software is not set up to cope with sinus arrhythmia which is often observed in children and youth.[167] Moreover, tonometry is subject to motion artefacts which preclude use during exercise. Applanation tonometry also requires precise positioning and the external blood pressure measurement for calibration. As such, further research applying this technique to the evaluation of endothelial function in children is clearly warranted.

Arterial compliance

Arterial compliance is a measure of the buffering capacity of the arterial system and is calculated as the product of arterial size and distensibility of arterial walls.[175] Adults with major CVD risk factors[176] or CVD[177] have compromised arterial compliance. Small and large artery compliance are both significant predictors of morbid events.[176] Functional and structural changes occur within the arterial wall prior to the clinical evidence of chronic disease.[178] Thus, arterial compliance is an important early predictor of the risk for chronic vascular disease.[179]

The applanation tonometer is based on the modified Windkessel system.[177] The Windkessel theory treats the circulation as a central elastic reservoir into which the heart pumps and from which blood travels to the tissues through relatively non-elastic conduits.[180] The tonometer reports the capacitive or large compliance (C_1), oscillatory or small artery compliance (C_2), blood volume inertia and systemic vascular resistance, SV, capacitive compliance, proximal pressure, and distal pressure.[177] This device records radial arterial pulse waves with an arterial tonometer sensor array. The waveforms are calibrated by the oscillometric method with a cuff on the opposite arm and a calibration system internal to the machine. The tonometer sensor array adjusts itself automatically to obtain the optimal waveform and repeats the calibration until the waveform is stable. When the waveform is stable, a 30-s analog tracing of the radial artery waveform is digitized and stored. A beat-marking algorithm determines the beginning of systole, peak systole, onset of diastole, and end diastole for all beats in the 30-s measurement period, and an average beat is calculated and used in subsequent analyses.[177] The decay in the diastolic pressure waveform is calculated by an algorithm that consists of the sum of the exponential decay and the exponentially decaying sinusoidal term. From this algorithm, the compliance values are obtained.[181]

A comparison of radial tonometer waveforms and brachial intra-arterial waveforms (via invasive dye technique) yielded close correlations in 78 subjects with no signs or symptoms of heart failure. The waveforms displayed similar characteristics; however, the non-invasive waveform exhibited fewer HF components. There was a correlation of $r = 0.92$ between invasively and non-invasively measured ejection time and in 92% of the cases, estimated $\dot{Q}$ was within 25% of measured $\dot{Q}$. The correlations between C_1 and C_2 obtained from the two methods were significant ($r = 0.82$ and 0.62, respectively). The non-invasive technique tended to overestimate and underestimate $\dot{Q}$ if the measured $\dot{Q}$ was low or high, respectively. C_1 and C_2 were also overestimated; however, the investigators concluded that the technique could be widely applied as it appears to correctly identify vascular abnormalities, and its ability to correctly distinguish patients with and without vascular disease is more important than the absolute value.[177] Furthermore, arterial compliance assessed by applanation tonometry provides data that are both reproducible and have a good correlation with values obtained by magnetic resonance imaging.[182]

Both C_1 and C_2 are significantly and inversely correlated with age in adults[176,182] and in children arterial compliance increases approximately 2.5- fold from birth to 20 years of age.[183] The rate of change is non-linear in children with the most rapid increases occurring between the ages 3 and 7 years. Evidence that the ratio of arterial compliance to body surface area decreases with age suggests that this age-associated increase in arterial compliance is primarily due to increases in arterial size and decreases in arterial wall distensibility.[183]

Women have a greater age-related rise in arterial stiffness than men. Post menopause, women's large arteries are less compliant than those of age-matched men.[184] Sex steroids are relatively low in the post-menopausal years, suggesting that intrinsic gender differences exist in arterial compliance.[185] Similar evidence was found in pre- and post-pubertal youth. Central and peripheral large arteries are stiffer in prepubertal females compared with prepubertal males; however, post-puberty, females develop more compliant large arteries whereas large arteries in males become less compliant.[185] By contrast, the Minnesota Children's Blood Pressure Study found no sex differences in young adults (mean age 23.6 ± 0.1 years).[181]

In addition to the factors previously mentioned, arterial compliance in adults is associated with blood pressure, metabolic factors,[181] aerobic fitness,[186] race, and anthropometry.[187] In children, blood pressure,[181] anthropometry, and race[187] are associated with arterial compliance. A recent study documented that aerobic fitness, blood pressure, and height account for 37% of the variance in large artery compliance in children whereas weight, fitness, maturity, and blood pressure account for 44% of the variance in small artery compliance. Children with the highest fitness had 34% greater compliance than children with the lowest fitness.[179]

Despite the limitations associated with applanation tonometry (as discussed previously), the assessment of arterial compliance provides important information regarding the health of the vasculature. It also can be measured relatively easily in lab- and field-based settings with children.[179]

Conclusions

Various methods (both invasive and non-invasive) can be used to assess the cardiovascular function and health of young people. Many of these procedures were developed in clinical and/or adult populations and as such their utility with young healthy individuals is often limited. Fortunately, in recent years a series of non-invasive assessment tools have been developed, which allow for the comprehensive assessment of cardiovascular function and health in children at rest and during exercise conditions. As outlined throughout this chapter, there are strengths and weaknesses to each assessment tool. Ultimately, it is up to the individual researcher to determine the relative merits of each technology. This decision should be based on several factors including ease of administration with young people, versatility, non-invasiveness, reliability and validity, and the cost of usage of the procedure. We feel that a comprehensive assessment of cardiovascular function and health in young people would include measures of cardiac function (at rest and throughout incremental exercise), vascular health, and autonomic balance.

Summary

- Invasive measures of cardiac output are not recommended in healthy children given the accuracy, reliability, and relative ease of administration of various non-invasive procedures. The use of non-invasive measures, in particular, foreign gas rebreathing, is encouraged.
- Of the foreign gas rebreathing techniques, open- and closed-circuit acetylene rebreathing are recommended for assessing cardiac output in young people. These techniques permit spontaneous breathing, are reliable up to maximal exercise, and are easily tolerated by participants.
- Doppler echocardiography can be used to non-invasively determine cardiac output on a beat-by-beat basis and is not reliant on steady-state conditions. Questions, however, remain regarding the accuracy of the technique during strenuous and maximal exercise.
- Despite criticism regarding its theoretical construct, recent research has shown the ability of impedance cardiography to be used during exercise conditions. This technique is non-invasive, versatile, cost-effective, and suitable for beat-by-beat changes in cardiac function which makes it attractive for use with children.
- The arterial pulse contour analysis method appears to be capable of non-invasively measuring cardiac output at rest. Research examining its validity in the paediatric population and during exercise conditions is required.
- HRV and baroreflex sensitivity are non-invasive measures that can be used to predict cardiovascular risk.
- Two-dimensional and Doppler echocardiography can be used to non-invasively characterize changes in left ventricular function at rest and during exercise. This permits the assessment of left ventricular filling parameters, cardiac dimensions, wall thicknesses, wall motion velocities, and valve motion (to name a few).
- Indices of peripheral blood flow can be obtained by plethysmography (changes in limb volume), Doppler imaging (volume flow in a large artery), pulse oximetry (oxygen saturation), or NIRS (balance between local oxygen delivery and oxygen utilization).
- The measurement of blood pressure may allow for early detection of CVD risk in children and provides important insight into children's cardiovascular response to stress (such as during exercise).
- Endothelial dysfunction is associated with risk factors for CVD and can be measured non-invasively using FMD, LDF, or pulse-wave analysis.

References

1. Warburton DER, Haykowsky MJF, Quinney HA, Humen DP, Teo KK (1999). Reliability and validity of measures of cardiac output during incremental to maximal aerobic exercise. Part I: Conventional techniques. *Sports Med* **27**, 23–41.
2. Warburton DER, Haykowsky MJF, Quinney HA, Humen DP, Teo KK (1999). Reliability and validity of measures of cardiac output during incremental to maximal aerobic exercise. Part II: Novel techniques and new advances. *Sports Med* **27**, 241–60.
3. Gledhill N, Warburton D, Jamnik V (1999). Haemoglobin, blood volume, cardiac function, and aerobic power. *Can J Appl Physiol* **24**, 54–65.
4. Gledhill N, Warburton DER (2000). Hemoglobin, blood volume and endurance. In: Shephard RJ, Astrand PO (eds.), *Endurance in sport*, pp. 301–15. Blackwell Scientific Publications, Oxford.
5. Warburton DER, Gledhill N (2006). Comment on point-counterpoint: In health and in a normoxic environment, VO_2 max is limited primarily by cardiac output and locomotor muscle blood flow. *J Appl Physiol* **100,** 1415.

6. Ekblom B, Astrand PO, Saltin B, Stenberg J, Wallstrom B (1968). Effect of training on circulatory response to exercise. *J Appl Physiol* **24**, 518–28.
7. Baulig W, Bernhard EO, Bettex D, Schmidlin D, Schmid ER (2005). Cardiac output measurement by pulse dye densitometry in cardiac surgery. *Anaesthesia* **60**, 968–73.
8. Kusaka T, Okubo K, Nagano K, Isobe K, Itoh S (2005). Cerebral distribution of cardiac output in newborn infants. *Arch Dis Child Fetal Neonatal Ed* **90**, F77–8.
9. Aoyagi T (2003). Pulse oximetry: Its invention, theory, and future. *J Anesth* **17**, 259–66.
10. Bremer F, Schiele A, Tschaikowsky K (2002). Cardiac output measurement by pulse dye densitometry: A comparison with the Fick's principle and thermodilution method. *Intensive Care Med* **28**, 399–405.
11. Iijima T, Aoyagi T, Iwao Y, Masuda J, Fuse M, Kobayashi N, Sankawa H (1997). Cardiac output and circulating blood volume analysis by pulse dye-densitometry. *J Clin Monit* **13**, 81–9.
12. Imai T, Takahashi K, Fukura H, Morishita Y (1997). Measurement of cardiac output by pulse dye densitometry using indocyanine green: A comparison with the thermodilution method. *Anesthesiology* **87**, 816–22.
13. Imai T, Takahashi K, Goto F, Morishita Y (1998). Measurement of blood concentration of indocyanine green by pulse dye densitometry—comparison with the conventional spectrophotometric method. *J Clin Monit Comput* **14**, 477–84.
14. Nagano K, Kusaka T, Okubo K, Yasuda S, Okada H, Namba M, Kawada K, Imai T, Isobe K, Itoh S (2005). Estimation of circulating blood volume in infants using the pulse dye densitometry method. *Paediatr Anaesth* **15**, 125–30.
15. Taguchi N, Nakagawa S, Miyasaka K, Fuse M, Aoyagi T (2004). Cardiac output measurement by pulse dye densitometry using three wavelengths. *Pediatr Crit Care Med* **5**, 343–50.
16. Matsukawa K, Kobayashi T, Nakamoto T, Murata J, Komine H, Noso M (2004). Noninvasive evaluation of cardiac output during postural change and exercise in humans: Comparison between the Modelflow and pulse dye-densitometry. *Japanese J Physiol* **54**, 153–60.
17. Wyse SD, Pfitzner J, Rees A, Lincoln JCR, Branthwaite MA (1975). Measurement of cardiac output by thermal dilution in infants and children. *Thorax* **30**, 262–5.
18. McLuckie A, Murdoch IA, Marsh MJ, Anderson D (1996). A comparison of pulmonary and femoral artery thermodilution cardiac indices in paediatric intensive care patients. *Acta Paediatr* **85**, 336–8.
19. Pauli C, Fakler U, Genz T, Hennig M, Lorenz H-P, Hess J (2002). Cardiac output determination in children: Equivalence of the transpulmonary thermodilution method to the direct Fick principle. *Intensive Care Med* **28**, 947–52.
20. Tibby SM, Hatherill M, Marsh MJ, Morrison G, Anderson D, Murdoch IA (1997). Clinical validation of cardiac output measurements using femoral artery thermodilution with direct Fick in ventilated children and infants. *Intensive Care Med* **23**, 987–91.
21. Linton RA, Jonas MM, Tibby SM, Murdoch IA, O'Brien TK, Linton NWF, Band DM (2000). Cardiac output measured by lithium dilution and transpulmonary thermodilution in patients in a paedtric intensive care unit. *Intensive Care Med* **26,** 1507–11.
22. Jonas MM, Tanser SJ (2002). Lithium dilution measurement of cardiac output and arterial pulse waveform analysis: An indicator dilution calibrated beat-by-beat system for continuous estimation of cardiac output. *Curr Opin Crit Care* **8**, 257–61.
23. Warburton DER, Gledhill N, Jamnik VK (1998). Reproducibility of the acetylene rebreathe technique for determining cardiac output. *Med Sci Sports Exerc* **30**, 952–7.
24. Card N, Gledhill N, Thomas S (1996). A non-rebreathe technique for measuring cardiac output throughout progressive to max exercise. *Med Sci Sports Exerc* **28,** S120.
25. Zeidifard E, Godfrey S, Davies EE (1976). Estimation of cardiac output by an N_2O rebreathing method in adults and children. *J Appl Physiol* **41**, 433–8.
26. Johnson BD, Beck KC, Proctor DN, Miller J, Dietz NM, Joyner MJ (2000). Cardiac output during exercise by the open circuit acetylene washing method: comparison with direct Fick. *J Appl Physiol* **88**, 1650–8.
27. Bell C, Monahan KD, Donato AJ, Hunt BE, Seals DR, Beck KC (2003). Use of acetylene breathing to determine cardiac output in young and older adults. *Med Sci Sports Exerc* **35**, 58–64.
28. Dibski DW, Smith DJ, Jensen R, Norris SR, Ford GT (2005). Comparison and reliability of two non-invasive acetylene uptake techniques for the measurement of cardiac output. *Eur J Appl Physiol* **94**, 670–80.
29. Nassis GP, Sidossis LS (2006). Methods for assessing body composition, cardiovascular and metabolic function in children and adolescents: Implications for exercise studies. *Curr Opin Clin Nutr Metab Care* **9**, 560–7.
30. Zenger MR, Brenner M, Haruno M, Mahon D, Wilson AF (1993). Measurement of cardiac output by automated single-breath technique, and comparison with thermodilution and Fick methods in patients with cardiac disease. *Am J Cardiol* **71**, 105–9.
31. Thomas SG, Gledhill N, Jamnik V (1997). Single breath measurement of cardiac output: technique and reliability. *Can J Appl Physiol* **22**, 52.
32. Collier CR (1956). Determination of mixed venous CO_2 tensions by rebreathing. *J Appl Physiol* **9**, 25–9.
33. Defares JG (1958). Determination of $PvCO_2$ from the exponential CO_2 rise during rebreathing. *J Appl Physiol* **13**, 159–64.
34. Ferguson RJ, Faulkner JA, Julius S, Conway J (1968). Comparison of cardiac output determined by CO_2 rebreathing and dye-dilution methods. *J Appl Physiol* **25,** 450–4.
35. Beekman RH, Katch V, Marks C, Rocchini AP (1984). Validity of CO_2-rebreathing cardiac output during rest and exercise in young adults. *Med Sci Sports Exerc* **16**, 306–10.
36. Patterson DH, Cunningham DA (1976). Comparison of methods to calculate cardiac output using the CO_2 rebreathing method. *Eur J Appl Physiol* **35,** 223–30.
37. Sady SP, Freedson PS, Gilliam TB (1981). Calculation of submaximal and maximal cardiac output in children using the CO_2 rebreathing technique. *J Sports Med Phys Fitness* **21**, 245–52.
38. Patterson DH, Cunningham DA, Plyley MJ, Blimkie CJR, Donner AP (1982). The consistency of cardiac output measurement (CO_2 rebreathe) in children during exercise. *Eur J Appl Physiol* **49**, 37–44.
39. Pianosi P, Hochman J (1996). End-tidal estimates of arterial PCO_2 for cardiac output measurement by CO_2 rebreathing: A study in patients with cystic fibrosis and healthy controls. *Pediatr Pulmonol* **22**, 154–60.
40. Jacob SV, Hornby L, Lands LC (1997). Estimation of mixed venous PCO_2 for determination of cardiac output in children. *Chest* **111**, 474–80.
41. Rowland T, Obert P (2002). Doppler echocardiography for the estimation of cardiac output with exercise. *Sports Med* **32**, 973–86.
42. Welsman J, Bywater K, Farr C, Welford D, Armstrong N (2005). Reliability of peak VO_2 and maximal cardiac output assessed using thoracic bioimpedance in children. *Eur J Appl Physiol* **94**, 228–34.
43. Christie J, Sheldahl LM, Tristani FE, Sagar KB, Ptacin MJ, Wann S (1987). Determination of stroke volume and cardiac output during exercise: Comparison of two-dimensional and Doppler echocardiography, Fick oximetry, and thermodilution. *Circulation* **76**, 539–47.
44. Shaw JG, Johnson EC, Voyles WF, Greene ER (1985). Noninvasive Doppler determination of cardiac output during submaximal and peak exercise. *J Appl Physiol* **59**, 722–31.
45. Chew MS, Poelaert J (2003). Accuracy and repeatability of pediatric cardiac output measurement using Doppler: 20-year review of the literature. *Intensive Care Med* **29**, 1889–94.
46. Vinet A, Nottin S, Lecoq AM, Guenon P, Obert P (2001). Reproducibility of cardiac output measurements by Doppler echocardiography in prepubertal children and adults. *Int J Sports Med* **22**, 437–41.

47. Nottin S, Vinet A, Lecoq AM, Guenon P, Obert P (2000). Study of the reproducibility of cardiac output measurement during exercise in prepubertal children by doppler echocardiography and CO_2 inhalation [abstract only; article in French]. *Arch Mal Coeur Vaiss* **93**, 1297–303.
48. Rowland T, Whatley Blum J (2000). Cardiac dynamics during upright cycle exercise in boys. *Am J Hum Biol* **12,** 749–57.
49. Rowland TW, Melanson EL, Popowski BE, Ferrone LC (1998). Test-retest reproducibility of maximum cardiac output by Doppler echocardiography. *Am J Cardiol* **81,** 1228–30.
50. Ihlen H, Endresen K, Myreng Y, Myhre E (1987). Reproducibility of cardiac stroke volume estimated by Doppler echocardiography. *Am J Cardiol* **59**, 975–8.
51. Nicolosi GL, Pungercic E, Cervesato E, Pavan D, Modena L, Moro E, Dall'Aglio V, Zanuttini D (1988). Feasibility and variability of six methods for the echocardiographic and Doppler determination of cardiac output. *Brit Heart J* **59**, 299–303.
52. Lepretre PM, Koralsztein JP, Billat VL (2004). Effect of exercise intensity on relationship between VO_2 max and cardiac output. *Med Sci Sports Exerc* **36**, 1357–63.
53. Pianosi P (2004). Measurement of exercise cardiac output by thoracic impedance in healthy children. *Eur J Appl Physiol* **92**, 425–30.
54. Braden DS, Leatherbury L, Treiber FA, Strong WB (1990). Noninvasive assessment of cardiac output in children using impedance cardiography. *Am Heart J* **120**, 1166–72.
55. Edmunds AT, Godfrey S, Tooley M (1982). Cardiac output measured by transthoracic impedance cardiography at rest, during exercise and at various lung volumes. *Clin Sci (Lond)* **63**, 107–13.
56. Pianosi P, Garros D (1996). Comparison of impedance cardiography with indirect Fick (CO_2) method of measuring cardiac output in healthy children during exercise. *Am J Cardiol* **77**, 745–9.
57. Charloux A, Lonsdorfer-Wolf E, Richard R, Lampert E, Oswald-Mammosser M, Mettauer B, Geny B, Lonsdorfer J (2000). A new impedance cardiograph device for the non-invasive evaluation of cardiac output at rest and during exercise: Comparison with the "direct" Fick method. *Eur J Appl Physiol* **82**, 313–20.
58. Richard R, Lonsdorfer-Wolf E, Charloux A, Doutreleau S, Buchheit M, Oswald-Mammosser M, Lampert E, Mettauer B, Geny B, Lonsdorfer J (2001). Non-invasive cardiac output evaluation during a maximal progressive exercise test, using a new impedance cardiograph device. *Eur J Appl Physiol* **85**, 202–7.
59. Erlanger J, Hooker DR (1904). An experimental study of blood pressure and of pulse-pressure in man. *Johns Hopkins Hosp Rep* **12**, 145–378.
60. Kouchoukos NT, Sheppard LC, McDonald DA (1970). Estimation of stroke volume in the dog by a pulse contour method. *Circ Res* **26**, 611–23.
61. Antonutto G, Girardis M, Tuniz D, di Prampero PE (1995). Noninvasive assessment of cardiac output from arterial pressure profiles during exercise. *Eur J Appl Physiol* 72, 18–24.
62. Jellema WT, Imholz BP, Oosting H, Wesseling KH, van Lieshout JJ (1999). Estimation of beat-to-beat changes in stroke volume from arterial pressure: A comparison of two pressure wave analysis techniques during head-up tilt testing in young, healthy men. *Clin Auton Res* **9**, 185–92.
63. Linton NW, Linton RA (2001). Estimation of changes in cardiac output from the arterial blood pressure waveform in the upper limb. *Br J Anaesth* **86**, 486–96.
64. van Lieshout JJ, Wesseling KH (2001). Continuous cardiac output by pulse contour analysis? *Br J Anaesth* **86**, 467–9.
65. Rang S, de Pablo Lapiedra B, van Montfrans GA, Bouma BJ, Wesseling KH, Wolf H (2007). Modelflow: A new method for noninvasive assessment of cardiac output in pregnant women. *Am J Obstet Gynecol* **196**, 235 e1–8.
66. Wesseling KH, Purschke R, Smith NT, Wust HJ, de Wit B, Weber HA (1976). A computer module for the continuous monitoring of cardiac output in the operating theatre and the ICU. *Acta Anaesthesiol Belg* **27** Suppl, 327–41.
67. Stok WJ, Stringer RC, Karemaker JM (1999). Noninvasive cardiac output measurement in orthostasis: pulse contour analysis compared with acetylene rebreathing. *J Appl Physiol* **87**, 2266–73.
68. Bogert LWJ, van Lieshout JJ (2005). Non-invasive pulsatile arterial pressure and stroke volume changes from the human finger. *Exp Physiol* **90**, 437–46.
69. Kemmotsu O, Ohno M, Takita K, Sugimoto H, Otsuka H, Morimoto Y, Mayumi T (1994). Noninvasive, continuous blood pressure measurement by arterial tonometry during anesthesia in children. *Anesthesiology* **81**, 1162–8.
70. Bigger JT, Jr., Fleiss JL, Steinman RC, Rolnitzky LM, Kleiger RE, Rottman JN (1992). Frequency domain measures of heart period variability and mortality after myocardial infarction. *Circulation* **85**, 164–71.
71. Reed K, Warburton D, Whitney C, McKay H (2006). Differences in heart rate variability between Asian and Caucasian children living in the same Canadian community. *Appl Physiol Nutr Metab* **31**, 277–82.
72. Nagai N, Hamada T, Kimura T, Moritani T (2004). Moderate physical exercise increases cardiac autonomic nervous system activity in children with low heart rate variability. *Childs Nerv Syst* **20**, 209–14.
73. Gao YY, Lovejoy JC, Sparti A, Bray GA, Keys LK, Partington C (1996). Autonomic activity assessed by heart rate spectral analysis varies with fat distribution in obese women. *Obes Res* **4**, 55–63.
74. Aubert AE, Beckers F, Ramaekers D (2001). Short-term heart rate variability in young athletes. *J Cardiol* **37**, 85–8.
75. Gregoire J, Tuck S, Yamamoto Y, Hughson RL (1996). Heart rate variability at rest and exercise: Influence of age, gender, and physical training. *Can J Appl Physiol* **21**, 455–70.
76. Sinnreich R, Kark JD, Friedlander Y, Sapoznikov D, Luria MH (1998). Five minute recordings of heart rate variability for population studies: Repeatability and age-sex characteristics. *Heart* **80**, 156–62.
77. Umetani K, Singer DH, McCraty R, Atkinson M (1998). Twenty-four hour time domain heart rate variability and heart rate: Relations to age and gender over nine decades. *J Am Coll Cardiol* **31**, 593–601.
78. Huikuri HV, Valkama JO, Airaksinen KE, Seppanen T, Kessler KM, Takkunen JT, Myerburg RJ (1993). Frequency domain measures of heart rate variability before the onset of nonsustained and sustained ventricular tachycardia in patients with coronary artery disease. *Circulation* **87**, 1220–8.
79. Kienzle MG, Ferguson DW, Birkett CL, Myers GA, Berg WJ, Mariano DJ (1992). Clinical, hemodynamic and sympathetic neural correlates of heart rate variability in congestive heart failure. *Am J Cardiol* **69**, 761–7.
80. Petretta M, Marciano F, Bianchi V, Migaux ML, Valva G, De Luca N, Salemme L, Berardino S, Bonaduce D (1995). Power spectral analysis of heart period variability in hypertensive patients with left ventricular hypertrophy. *Am J Hypertens* **8**, 1206–13.
81. Martin GJ, Magid NM, Myers G, Barnett PS, Schaad JW, Weiss JS, Lesch M, Singer DH (1986). Heart rate variability and sudden death secondary to coronary artery disease during ambulatory ECG monitoring. *Am J Cardiol* **60**, 86–9.
82. Rollins MD, Jenkins JG, Carson DJ, McClure BG, Mitchell RH, Imam SZ (1992). Power spectral analysis of the electrocardiogram in diabetic children. *Diabetologia* **35**, 452–5.
83. Kazuma N, Otsuka K, Matsuoka I, Murata M (1997). Heart rate variability during 24 hours in asthmatic children. *Chronobiol Int* **14**, 597–606.
84. Finley JP, Nugent ST, Hellenbrand W, Craig M, Gillis DA (1989). Sinus arrhythmia in children with atrial septal defect: An analysis of heart rate variability before and after surgical repair. *Br Heart J* **61**, 280–4.
85. Massin M, von Bernuth G (1998). Clinical and haemodynamic correlates of heart rate variability in children with congenital heart disease. *Eur J Pediatr* **157**, 967–71.
86. van Ravenswaaij-Arts CMA, Kollee LAA, Hopman JCW, Stoelinga GBA, van Geijn HP (1993). Heart rate variability. *Ann Intern Med* **118**, 436–47.

87. Kleiger RE, Stein PK, Bigger JT (2005). Heart rate variability: Measurement and clinical utility. *Ann Noninvasive Electrocardiol* **10**, 88–101.
88. Task Force of the European Society of Cardiology and the North American Society of Pacing Electrophysiology (1996). Heart rate variability: standards of measurement, physiological interpretation, and clinical use. *Circulation* **93**, 1043–65.
89. Vinet A, Beck L, Nottin S, Obert P (2005). Effect of intensive training on heart rate variability in prepurbertal swimmers. *Eur J Clin Invest* **35**, 610–14.
90. Buchheit M, Simon F, Piquart F, Ehrhat J, Brandenberger G (2004). Effect of increased training load on vagal-related indices of heart rate variability: A novel sleep approach. *Am J Physiol Heart Circ Physiol* **287**, 2813–18.
91. Goto M, Nagashima M, Baba R, Nagano Y, Yokota M, Nishibata K, Tsuji A (1997). Analysis of heart rate variability demonstrates effects of development on vagal modulation of heart rate in healthy children. *J Pediatr* **130**, 725–9.
92. Mandigout S, Melin A, Fauchier L, N'Guyen LD, Courteix D, Obert P (2002). Physical training increases heart rate variability in healthy prepubertal children. *Eur J Clin Invest* **32**, 479–87.
93. Finley JP, Nugent ST, Hellenbrand W (1987). Heart rate variability in children. Spectral analysis of developmental changes between 5 and 24 years. *Can J Physiol Pharmacol* **65**, 2048–52.
94. Schwartz JB, Gibb WJ, Tran T (1991). Aging effects on heart rate variation. *J Gerontol* **46,** M99–106.
95. Rudiger H, Bald M (2001). Spontaneous baroreflex sensitivity in children and young adults calculated in time and frequency domain. *Auton Neurosci* **93**, 71–8.
96. Allen MT, Matthews KA, Kenyon K (2000). The relationships of resting baroreflex sensitivity, heart rate variability and measures of impulse control in children and adolescents. *Int J Psychophysiol* **37**, 185–94.
97. Farrell TG, Paul V, Cripps TR, Malik M, Polonіecki J, Bennett ED, Ward DE, Camm AJ (1991). Baroreflex sensitivity and electrophysiological correlates in patients after acute myocardial infarction. *Circulation* **83**, 945–52.
98. La Rovere M, Bigger J, Marcus F, Mortara A, Schwartz P (1998). Baroreflex sensitivity and heart-rate variability in prediction of total cardiac mortality after mycardial infarction. *Lancet* **351**, 478–84.
99. Frattola A, Parati G, Gamba P, Paleari F, Mauri G, Di Rienzo M, Castiglioni P, Mancia G (1997). Time and frequency domain estimates of spontaneous baroreflex sensitivity provides early detection of autonomic dysfunction in diabetes mellitus. *Diabetologia* **40**, 1470–5.
100. La Rovere MT (2000). Baroreflex sensitivity as a new marker for risk stratification. *Z Kardiol* **89**, 44–50.
101. Bertinieri G, DiRienzo M, Cavallazzi A, Ferrari AU, Pedotti A, Mancia G (1985). A new approach to analysis of the arterial baroreflex. *J Hypertens* **3**, S79–81.
102. Di Rienzo M, Castilioni P, Mancia G, Parati G, Pedotti A (1997). Critical appraisal of indices for the assessment of baroreflex sensitivity. *Methods Inf Med* **36**, 246–9.
103. Parati G, Di Rienzo M, Mancia G (2000). How to measure baroreflex sensitivity: From the cardiovascular laboratory to daily life. *J Hypertens* **18**, 7–19.
104. Watkins LL, Fainman C, Dimsdale J, Ziegler MG (1995). Assessment of baroreflex control from beat-to-beat blood pressure and heart rate changes: a validation study. *Psychophysiology* **32**, 411–4.
105. Pagani M, Somers V, Furlan R, Dell'Orto S, Conway J, Baselli G, Cerutti S, Sleight P, Malliani A (1988). Changes in autonomic regulation induced by physical training in mild hypertension. *Hypertension* **12**, 600–10.
106. Gerritsen J, Ten Voorde BJ, Dekker JM, Kostense PJ, Bouter LM, Heethaar RM (2000). Baroreflex sensitivity in the elderly: influence of age, breathing and spectral methods. *Clin Sci* **99**, 371–81.
107. Hayano J, Sakakibara Y, Yamada A, Mukai S, Fujinami T, Yokoyama K, Watanabe Y, Takata K (1991). Accuracy of assessment of cardiac vagal tone by heart rate variability in normal subjects. *Am J Cardiol* **67**, 199–204.
108. Di Rienzo M, Parati G, Castiglioni P, Tordi R, Mancia G, Pedotti A (2001). Baroreflex effectiveness index: An additional measure of baroreflex control of heart rate in daily life. *Am J Physiol* **280**, R744–51.
109. Rudiger H, Klinghammer L, Scheuch K (1999). The trigonometric regressive spectral analysis method for mapping of beat-to-beat recorded cardiovascular parameters on to frequency domain in comparison with Fourier transformation. *Comp Methods Prog Biomed* **58**, 1–15.
110. Hunt B, Farquhar W, Taylor J (2001). Does reduced vascular stiffening fully explain preserved cardio-vagal baroreflex function in older, physically active men? *Circulation* **103**, 2424–7.
111. Lenard Z, Studinger P, Mersich B, Kocsis L (2004). Maturation of cardiovagal autonomic function from childhood to young adult age. *Circulation* **110**, 2307–12.
112. Obert P, Mandigout S, Vinet A, N'Guyen LD, Stecken F, Courteix D (2001). Effect of aerobic training and detraining on left ventricular dimensions and diastolic function in prepubertal boys and girls. *Int J Sports Med* **22**, 90–6.
113. Sahn DJ, DeMaria A, Kisslo J, Weyman G (1978). Recommendations regarding quantitation in M-mode echocardiographic measurements. *Circulation* **58**, 1072–83.
114. Devereux R, Alonso D, Lutas E, Gottlieb G, Campo E, Sachs I, Reichek N (1986). Echocardiographic assessment of left ventricular hypertrophy: Comparison to necropsy. *Am J Cardiol* **57**, 450–8.
115. Dokainish H (2004). Tissue Doppler imaging in the evaluation of left ventricular diastolic function. *Curr Opin Cardiol* **19**, 437–41.
116. Rowland T, Heffernan K, Jae S, Echols G, Krull G, Fernhall B (2006). Cardiovascular responses to static exercise in boys: Insights from tissue Doppler imaging. *Eur J Appl Physiol* **97**, 637–42.
117. Rowland T, Heffernan K, Jae SY, Echols G, Fernhall B (2006). Tissue Doppler assessment of ventricular function during cycling in 7- to 12-yr-old boys. *Med Sci Sports Exerc* **38**, 1216–22.
118. Hayashi T (1987). Echocardiographic and electrocardiographic measures in obese children after an exercise program. *Int J Obes* **11**, 465–72.
119. Hollmann W, Rost R, Meirleir J, Liesen H, Heck H, Mader A (1986). Cardiovascular effects of extreme physical training. *Acta Med Scand* **711**, 193–203.
120. Greenan D, Gilliam T, Crowley D, Morehead-Steffiens C, Rosenthal A (1982). Echocardiographic measures in 6 to 7-year-old children after an 8 month exercise program. *Am J Cardiol* **49**, 1990–5.
121. Marshall SA, Weyman AE (1994). Doppler estimation of volumetric flow. In Weyman AE (ed.), *Principles and practice of echocardiography* (2nd ed.), pp. 955–78. Lea and Febiger, Philadelphia, PA.
122. Haugen BO, Berg S, Brecke KM, Torp H, Slordahl SA, Skaerpe T, Samstad SO (2002). Blood flow velocity profiles in the aortic annulus: A 3-dimensional freehand color flow Doppler imaging study. *J Am Soc Echocardiogr* **15**, 328–33.
123. Pemberton J, Xiaokui L, Kenny A, Davies CH, Minette MS, Sahn DJ (2005). Real-time 3-Dimensional Doppler Echocardiograph for the assessment of stroke volume: An in vivo human study compared with standard 2-Dimensional Echocardiography. *J Am Soc Echocardiogr* **18**, 1030–6.
124. McCully KK, Hamaoka T (2000). Near-infrared spectroscopy: What can it tell us about oxygen saturation in skeletal muscle? *Exerc Sport Sci Rev* **28**, 123–7.
125. Lima AP, Beelen P, Bakker J (2002). Use of a peripheral perfusion index derived from the pulse oximetry signal as a noninvasive indicator of perfusion. *Crit Care Med* **30**, 1210–13.
126. Lima AP, Bakker J (2005). Nonivasive monitoring of peripheral perfusion (review). *Intensive Care Med* **11**, 1316–26.

127. McMorrow R, Mythen M (2006). Pulse oximetry. *Curr Opin Crit Care* **12**, 269–71.
128. Barker S, Tremper K, Hyatt J (1989). Effects of methemoglobinemia on pulse oximetry and mixed-venous oximetry. *Anesthesiology* **70**, 112–17.
129. Reich D, Timcenko A, Bodian C, Kraidin J, Hofman J, Deperio M, Konstadt S, Kurki T, Eisenkraft J (1996). Predictors of pulse oximetry data failure. *Anesthesiology* **84**, 859–64.
130. Cole C, Goldstein E, Fuchsman W, Hoagin D (1989). The effect of nail polish on pulse oximetry. *Anesth Analg* **67**, 683–6.
131. Clayton D, Webb R, Ralston A, Duthie D, Runciman W (1991). A comparison of the performance of 20 pulse oximeters under conditions of poor perfusion. *Anaesthesia* **46**, 3–10.
132. Severnghaus J, Naifeh K, Koh S (1989). Errors in 14 pulse oximeters during profound hypoxemia. *J Clin Monit* **5**, 72–81.
133. Nickerson B, Sarkisian C, Tremper K (1988). Bias and precision of pulse oximeters and arterial oximeters. *Chest* **93**, 515–7.
134. Boushel R, Piantadosi CA (2000). Near-infrared spectroscopy for monitoring muscle oxygenation. *Acta Physiol Scand* **168**, 615–22.
135. Van Beekvelt MC, Colier WN, Wevers RA, Van Engelen BG (2001). Performance of near-infrared spectroscopy in measuring local O_2 consumption and blood flow in skeletal muscle. *J Appl Physiol* **90**, 511–19.
136. Belardinelli R, Barstow TJ, Porsasz J, Wasserman K (1995). Changes in skeletal muscle oxygenation during incremental exercise measured with near infrared spectroscopy. *Eur J Appl Physiol* **70**, 487–92.
137. Chance B, Dait M, Zhang C, Hamaoka T, Hagerman F (1992). Recovery from exercise-induced saturation in the quadriceps muscles of elite competitive rowers. *Am J Physiol* **262**, C766-75.
138. Jensen-Urstad M, Hallback I, Sahlin K (1995). Effect of hypoxia on muscle oxygenation and metabolism during arm exercise in humans. *Clin Physiol* **15**, 27–37.
139. Rundell K, Niola S, Chance B (1997). Hemoglobin/myoglobin desaturation during speed skating. *Med Sci Sports Exerc* **29**, 248–58.
140. Hamaoka T, Iwane H, Shimomitsu T, Katsumura T, Murase N, Nisho S, Osada T, Kurosawa Y, Chance B (1996). Noninvasive measures of oxidative metabolism on working human muscles by near-infrared spectroscopy. *J Appl Physiol* **81**, 1410 –17.
141. Tamaka T, Uchiyama S, Tamura T, Nakano S (1994). Changes in muscle oxygenation during weight lifting exercise. *Eur J Appl Physiol* **68**, 465–9.
142. Hampson N, Piantadosi C (1988). Near infrared monitoring of human skeletal muscle oxygenation during forearm ischemia. *J Appl Physiol* **62**, 2449–57.
143. Kennedy MD, Haykowsky MJF, Boliek CA, Esch BT, Scott JM, Warburton DE (2006). Regional muscle oxygenation differences in vastus lateralis during different modes of incremental exercise. *Dyn Med* **5**, 8.
144. Mancini DM, Bolinger L, Li L, Kendrick K, Chance B, Wilson JR (1994). Validation of near-infrared spectroscopy in humans. *J Appl Physiol* **77**, 2740–7.
145. Mireille CP, Van Beekvelt MC, Colier WN, Wevers RA, Van Engelen BG (2001). Performance of near-infrared spectroscopy in measuring local O_2 consumption and blood flow in skeletal muscle. *J Appl Physiol* **90**, 511–19.
146. Costes F, Barthelemy JC, Feasson L, Busso T, Geyssant A, Denis C (1996). Comparison of muscle near-infrared spectroscopy and femoral blood gases during steady-state exercise in humans. *J Appl Physiol* **80**, 1345–50.
147. MacDonald M, Tarnopolsky H, Green H, Hughson RL (1999). Comparison of femoral blood gases and muscle near-infrared spectroscopy at exercise onset in humans. *J Appl Physiol* **86**, 687–93.
148. Moalla W, Merzouk A, Costes F, Tabka Z, Ahmaidi S (2006). Muscle oxygenation and EMG activity during isometric exercise in children. *J Sports Sci* **24**, 1195–201.
149. Van Beekvelt M, Van Engelen B, Wevers R, Colier W (2002). In vivo quantitative near-infrared spectroscopy in skeletal muscle during incremental isometric handgrip exercise. *Clin Physiol Funct Imaging* **22**, 210–17.
150. Szmedra L, Nioka S, Chance B, Rundell K (2001). Hemoglobin/myoglobin oxygen desaturation during alpine skiing. *Med Sci Sports Exerc* **33**, 232–6.
151. Moalla W, Dupont G, Berthoin S, Ahmaidi S (2005). Respiratory muscle deoxygenation and ventilatory threshold assessments using near infrared spectroscopy in children. *Int J Sports Med* **26**, 576–82.
152. Boushel R, Langberg H, Olesen J, Gonzales-Alonzo J, Bulow J, Kjaer M (2001). Monitoring tissue oxygen availability with near infrared spectroscopy (NIRS) in health and disease. *Scand J Med Sci Sports* **11**, 213–22.
153. Pickering TG, Hall JE, Appel LJ, Falkner BE, Graves J, Hill MN, Jones DW, Kurtz T, Sheps SG, Roccella EJ (2005). Recommendations for blood pressure measurement in humans and experimental animals. Part 1: Blood pressure measurement in humans a statement for professionals from the subcommittee of professional and public education of the American Heart Association Council on High Blood Pressure Research. *Hypertension* **45**, 142–61.
154. National High Blood Pressure Education Program Working Group on Hypertension Control in Children and Adolescents (1996). Update on the 1987 Task Force Report on high blood pressure in children: A working group report from the national high blood pressure education program. *Pediatrics* **98**, 649–58.
155. Turley KR, Wilmore JH (1997). Cardiovascular responses to treadmill and cycle ergometer exercise in children and adults. *J Appl Physiol* **83**, 948–57.
156. Obert P, Mandigouts S, Nottin S, Vinet A, N'Guyen LD, Lecoq AM (2003). Cardiovascular responses to endurance training in children: effect of gender. *Eur J Clin Invest* **33**, 199–208.
157. Deanfield JE, Halcox JP, Rabelink TJ (2007). Endothelial function and dysfunction: Testing and clinical relevance. *Circulation* **115,** 1285–95.
158. Deanfield JE, Donald AE, Ferri C, Giannattasio C, Halcox JP, Halligan S, Lerman A, Mancia G, Oliver JJ, Pessina AC, Rizzoni D, Rossi GP, Salvetti A, Schiffrin EL, Taddei S, Webb DJ (2005). Endothelial function and dysfunction. Part 1: Methodological issues for assessment in the different vascular beds: A statement by the Working Group on Endothelin and Endothelial Factors of the European Society of Hypertension. *J Hypertension* **23,** 7–17.
159. Woo KS, Chook P, Yu CW, Sung RY, Qiao M, Leung SS, Lam CW, Metreweli C, Celermajer DS (2004). Effects of diet and exercise on obesity related vascular dysfunction in children. *Circulation* **109,** 1981–16.
160. Jarvisalo M, Raitakari M, Toikka JO, Putto-Laurila A, Rontu R, Laine S, Lehtimaki T, Ronnemaa T, Viikari J, Raitakari OT (2004). Endothelial dysfunction and increased arterial intima-media thickness in children with type 1 diabetes. *Circulation* **109**, 1750–5.
161. Jarvisalo M, Raitakari O (2005). Ultrasound assessment of endothelial function in children. *Vasc Health Risk Manag* **1**, 227–33.
162. Anderson TJ (2003). Nitric oxide, atherosclerosis and the clinical relevance of endothelial dysfunction. *Heart Fail Rev* **8**, 71–86.
163. Celermajer DS, Sorensen KE (1992). Non-invasive detection of endothelial dysfunction in children and adults at risk of atherosclerosis. *Lancet* **340**, 1111–15.
164. Corretti MC, Anderson TJ, Benjamin EJ, Celermajer D, Charbonneau F, Creager MA, Deanfield J, Drexler H, Gerhard-Herman M, Herrington D, Vallance P, Vita J, Vogel R (2002). International Brachial Artery Reactivity Task Force. Guidelines for the ultrasound assessment of endothelial-dependent flow-mediated vasodilation of the brachial artery: A report of the International Brachial Artery Reactivity Task Force. *J Am Coll Cardiol* **39**, 257–65.
165. Anderson TJ, Uehata A, Gerhard MD, Meredith IT, Knab S, Delagrange D, Lieberman EH, Ganz P, Creager MA, Yeung AC, Selwyn AP (1995). Close relation of endothelial function in the human coronary and peripheral circulation. *J Am Coll Cardiol* **26**, 1235–41.
166. Corretti MC, Plotnick GD, Vogel RA (1995). Technical aspects of evaluating brachial artery vasodilatation using high-frequency ultrasound. *Am J Physiol* **268**, 1397–404.

167. Donald AE, Charakida M, Cole TJ, Friberg P, Chowienczyk PJ, Millasseau SC, Deanfield JE, Halcox JP (2006). Non-invasive assessment of endothelial function. *J Am Coll Cardiol* **48**, 1846–50.
168. Khan F, Green FC, Forsyth JS, Greene SA, Morris AD, Belch JJ (2003). Impaired microvascular function in normal children: Effects of adiposity and poor glucose handling. *J Physiol* **551**, 705–11.
169. Cracowski J-L, Minson CT, Salvat-Melis M, Halliwill JR (2006). Methodological issues in the assessment of skin microvascular endothelial function in humans. *Trends Pharmacol Sci* **27**, 503–8.
170. Charkoudian N (2003). Skin blood flow in adult human thermoregulation: How it works, when it does not, and why. *Mayo Clin Proc* **78**, 603–12.
171. Newton DJ, Khan F, Belch JJ (2001). Assessment of microvascular endothelial function in human skin. *Clin Sci* **101**, 567–72.
172. Hansell J, Henareh L, Agewall S, Norman M (2004). Non-invasive assessment of endothelial function—relation between vasodilatory responses in skin microcirculation and brachial artery. *Clin Physiol Funct Imaging* **24**, 317–22.
173. Kaliea YN, Naik A, Garrison J, Guy RH (2004). Iontophoretic drug delivery. *Adv Drug Deliv Rev* **56**, 619–58.
174. Hayward CS, Kraidly M, Webb CM, Collins P (2002). Assessment of endothelial function using peripheral waveform analysis. *J Am Coll Cardiol* **40**, 521–8.
175. Cope FW (1960). An elastic reservoir theory of the human systemic arterial system using current data on aortic elasticity. *Bull Math Biophys* **22**, 19–40.
176. Grey E, Bratteli C, Glasser SP, Alinder C, Finkelstein S, Lindgren BR, Cohn JN. (2003) Reduced small artery but not large artery elasticity is an independent risk marker for cardiovascular events. *Am J Hypertens* **16**, 265 9.
177. Cohn JN, Finkelstein S, McVeigh G, Morgan D, LeMay L, Robinson J, Mock J (1995). Noninvasive pulse wave analysis for the early detection of vascular disease. *Hypertension* **26**, 503–8.
178. Ross R (1981). Atherosclerosis: A problem of the biology of arterial wall cells and their interactions with blood components. *Arteriosclerosis* **1**, 27–32.
179. Reed KE, Warburton DER, Lewanczuk RZ, Haykowsky MJF, Scott JM, C.L. W, McGavock JM, McKay HA (2005). Arterial compliance in young children: The role of aerobic fitness. *Eur J Cardiovasc Prev Rehabil* **12**, 492–7.
180. Oliver JJ, Webb DJ (2003). Noninvasive assessment of arterial stiffness and risk of atherosclerotic events. *Arterioscl Thromb Vasc Biol* **23**, 554–66.
181. Arnett DK, Glasser SP, McVeigh G, Prineas R, Finklestein S, Donahue R, Cohn JN, Sinaiko A (2001). Blood pressure and arterial compliance in young adults: The Minnesota Children's Blood Pressure Study. *Am J Hypertens* **14**, 200–5.
182. Resnick LM, Militianu D, Cunnings AJ, Pipe JG, Evelhoch JL, Soulen RL, Lester MA (2000). Pulse waveform analysis of arterial compliance: Relation to other techniques, age, and metabolic variables. *Am J Hypertens* **13**, 1243–9.
183. Senzaki H, Akagi M, Hishi T, Ishizawa A, Yanagisawa M, Masutani S, Kobayashi T, Awa S (2002). Age-associated changes in arterial elastic properties in children. *Eur J Pediatr* **161**, 547–51.
184. Waddell TK, Dart AM, Gatzka CD, Cameron JD, Kingwell BA (2001). Women exhibit a greater age-related increase in proximal aortic stiffness than men. *J Hypertens* **19**, 2205–12.
185. Ahimastos AA, Formosa M, Dart AM, Kingwell BA (2003). Gender differences in large artery stiffness pre- and post puberty. *J Clin Endocrinol Metab* **88**, 5375–80.
186. Boreham CA, Ferriera I, Twisk JW, Gallagher AM, Savage MJ, Murray LJ (2004). Cardiorespiratory fitness, physical activity, and arterial stiffness: The Northern Ireland Young Hearts Project. *Hypertension* **44,** 721–6.
187. Schutte AE, Huisman HW, van Rooyen JM, de Ridder JH, Malan NT (2003). Associations between arterial compliance and anthropometry of children from four ethnic groups in South Africa: The THUSA BANA study. *Blood Press* **12**, 97–103.

CHAPTER 8

Aerobic fitness

Neil Armstrong and Joanne R. Welsman

Introduction

At the onset of exercise, muscle contraction is supported by the energy released during the hydrolysis of adenosine triphosphate (ATP) but the intramuscular stores of ATP are limited and for exercise to be sustained, ATP must be rapidly re-synthesized. Anaerobic regeneration of ATP occurs almost instantaneously from phosphocreatine (PCr) and the rate of ATP re-synthesis from PCr reaches its peak within 2 s before declining. The anaerobic catabolism of glycogen/glucose to pyruvate is rapidly initiated and reaches maximal re-synthesis of ATP within 5 s. To sustain glycolysis, pyruvate is either converted to carbon dioxide (CO_2) and water by oxidative metabolism in the mitochondria or reduced to lactate. The rate of lactate formation during exercise is therefore dependent on the balance between anaerobic and aerobic metabolism of pyruvate. As exercise intensity increases, more pyruvate is reduced, lactate production in the muscle rises, and some of the muscle lactate diffuses into the blood where it can provide an indicator of aspects of aerobic fitness.

Aerobic re-synthesis of ATP, which is dependent upon oxygen (O_2) delivery to the muscles and the reactions of the tricarboxylic acid cycle, is sluggish to adapt to the demands of exercise and, in children, the time constant of the response to high intensity exercise is about 20 s. Although the rate at which ATP can be re-synthesized aerobically is much slower than through the anaerobic energy pathways, the aerobic pathway has a much greater capacity for energy generation. As a result, ATP regenerated from aerobic sources makes a relatively minor contribution to short-term high intensity exercise but the aerobic contribution to ATP re-synthesis increases with time and, in children, most of the energy during exercise longer than 1 min is derived from aerobic sources. Aerobic fitness supports the aerobic re-synthesis of ATP and may therefore be defined as the ability to deliver oxygen to the exercising muscles and to use it to generate energy during exercise.

Maximal oxygen uptake ($\dot{V}O_2$ max), the highest rate at which an individual can consume O_2 during exercise, is widely recognized as the best single measure of adults' aerobic fitness.[1,2] Maximal $\dot{V}O_2$ ultimately limits an individual's capacity to perform aerobic exercise but it does not describe fully all aspects of aerobic fitness. The transient kinetics of $\dot{V}O_2$ best reflect the integrated response of the O_2 delivery system and the metabolic requirements of the exercising muscle to rapid changes in exercise intensity. Furthermore, $\dot{V}O_2$ max is not the best index of an individual's ability to sustain submaximal aerobic exercise and despite its derivation from anaerobic metabolism, measures of blood lactate accumulation during submaximal exercise provide useful indicators of aerobic fitness.

As the assessment of $\dot{V}O_2$ kinetics is addressed in Chapter 22, in this chapter, we will focus on the assessment of $\dot{V}O_2$ max and blood lactate accumulation.

Maximal or peak oxygen uptake?

The first laboratory-based studies of boys' $\dot{V}O_2$ during treadmill running were carried out in the United States in the first half of the 20th century[3,4] and Åstrand's[5] classical investigation of physical working capacity in relation to sex and age, published in 1952, was the first major study to include girls as subjects. Since the publication of these pioneering papers, $\dot{V}O_2$ max has become the most researched variable in paediatric exercise science but its assessment has generated lively debate over many years.[6–8]

The traditional laboratory model used to determine $\dot{V}O_2$ max consists of a progressive exercise test to exhaustion in which the exercise intensity is incrementally increased. Oxygen uptake increases almost linearly with exercise intensity up to a point beyond which no further increase in $\dot{V}O_2$ takes place, even though a well-motivated subject is still able to increase his/her exercise intensity. Exercise beyond the point of levelling off of $\dot{V}O_2$ (a $\dot{V}O_2$ plateau) is assumed to be supported exclusively by anaerobic energy sources resulting in an intracellular accumulation of lactate, acidosis, and inevitably termination of the exercise.

In practice, an absolute levelling of $\dot{V}O_2$ with increasing exercise intensity seldom if ever occurs but even though both the methodological and theoretical bases of the plateau phenomenon have been challenged[9–12] it has retained primacy as the principal criterion for establishing $\dot{V}O_2$ max. A number of less rigorous criteria to define a $\dot{V}O_2$ plateau have been proposed,[13,14] and the most commonly applied criterion with young people is a body mass-related requirement for an increase in $\dot{V}O_2$ of not more than 2.0 $mL \cdot kg^{-1} \cdot min^{-1}$ for a 5–10% increase in exercise intensity.[15] However, as was first reported by Astrand,[5] regardless of the 'plateau criterion', only a minority of children and adolescents demonstrate a $\dot{V}O_2$ plateau during a progressive exercise test to exhaustion. Some authors have argued that the failure of children to elicit a $\dot{V}O_2$ plateau may be related to low levels of motivation or low anaerobic capacity[16,17] but recent data have demonstrated, with large samples of both children and adolescents, that those who plateau do not have higher $\dot{V}O_2$, heart rate (HR), or blood lactate accumulation than those not demonstrating a $\dot{V}O_2$ plateau.[18,19] Nevertheless, as the term $\dot{V}O_2$ max conventionally implies the existence of a $\dot{V}O_2$ plateau it has gradually become more common in paediatric exercise science to define the highest $\dot{V}O_2$ observed during a progressive exercise test to exhaustion as peak $\dot{V}O_2$.[6,20,21]

Two studies have addressed experimentally whether peak $\dot{V}O_2$ can be accepted as a maximal index of children's aerobic fitness. Armstrong *et al.*[22] determined the peak $\dot{V}O_2$ of 20 boys and 20 girls, mean age 9.9 years, on three occasions 1 week apart. On the first occasion, the children completed a discontinuous, incremental protocol on a treadmill with the belt speed held at 1.94 $m{\cdot}s^{-1}$ but the slope increasing every 3 min. The children exercised until voluntary exhaustion. Using a $\leq$2 $mL{\cdot}kg^{-1}{\cdot}min^{-1}$ increase in $\dot{V}O_2$ as the criterion, six boys and seven girls exhibited a $\dot{V}O_2$ plateau. No significant differences in either anthropometrical or peak physiological data were revealed between those who exhibited a $\dot{V}O_2$ plateau and those who did not. The second and third tests were performed at the same belt speed as test one (i.e. 1.94 $m{\cdot}s^{-1}$) but, following a 3 min warm-up running at 1.67 $m{\cdot}s^{-1}$, the children ran on slopes which were 2.5% and 5% greater, respectively, than the highest slope achieved on the first test. The children were strongly encouraged and the data were accepted if the child ran for at least 2 min on the higher slopes. Eighteen girls and 17 boys completed all tests and their data are presented in Table 8.1. Both boys and girls exhibited significantly higher blood lactate accumulation, minute ventilation, and respiratory exchange ratios (RER) in tests two and three than in test one but there were no significant differences in peak $\dot{V}O_2$ across the tests. Rowland[23] performed a similar study with nine children, aged 10–13 years, and reported the same outcomes.

These studies demonstrate that $\dot{V}O_2$ does not increase further in response to exercise intensities above the peak $\dot{V}O_2$ observed in a rigorously performed, progressive exercise test to voluntary exhaustion. Peak $\dot{V}O_2$ therefore reflects the limits of aerobic fitness in young people.

Peak oxygen uptake

The general principles underlying the determination of young people's peak $\dot{V}O_2$ are fundamentally the same as those which apply to adults, but with children and adolescents there are additional considerations which need to be addressed. These include ethics and pre-test preparation, respiratory gas analysis, appropriate ergometers and protocols, and defining a maximal effort. Subsequent sections will address these issues.

Ethics and pre-test preparation

The involvement of young people in non-therapeutic research raises complex issues which have been debated at length elsewhere[24–26] and a detailed discussion is presented in Chapter 1. In essence, researchers must consider carefully whether the procedures they wish to employ are ethical with young people, and whether the value of the knowledge gained clearly outweighs the risks, either physiological or psychological, to the child or adolescent. Young people should only participate in non-therapeutic research when the information required could not be gained by research with adults and when the risk to the child is negligible. Negligible risks have been defined as 'not greater than those ordinarily encountered in daily life or during the performance of routine physical or psychological examinations or tests' (see ref. 25, p. 14). Procedures suggested to represent negligible risk include observation of behaviour, non-invasive physiological monitoring, developmental assessments, physical examinations, changes in diet, and obtaining blood and urine samples.[25] The determination of healthy young people's peak $\dot{V}O_2$ and blood lactate accumulation clearly falls within these guidelines.

Children's and adolescents' participation in research involving the determination of peak $\dot{V}O_2$ should be through an informed willingness to cooperate rather than coercion. The legal age at

Table 8.1 Peak physiological data from 9-year-old children across three maximal treadmill exercise tests

	Test 1	Test 2	Test 3
Boys (n = 17)			
Oxygen uptake ($L{\cdot}min^{-1}$)	1.93 (0.23)	1.95 (0.24)	1.98 (0.17)
Oxygen uptake ($mL{\cdot}kg^{-1}{\cdot}min^{-1}$)	62 (6)	63 (8)	64 (7)
Minute ventilation ($L{\cdot}min^{-1}$)	63.6 (10.0)	68.7 (11.1)*	69.9 (11.1)*
Respiratory exchange ratio	0.99 (0.05)	1.15 (0.07)*	1.18 (0.09)*
Blood lactate ($mmol{\cdot}L^{-1}$)	5.7 (1.7)	8.4 (2.2)*	9.3 (1.9)*
Girls (n = 18)			
Oxygen uptake ($L{\cdot}min^{-1}$)	1.85 (0.28)	1.90 (0.26)	1.91 (0.35)
Oxygen uptake ($mL{\cdot}kg^{-1}{\cdot}min^{-1}$)	51 (6)	52 (7)	52 (7)
Minute ventilation ($L{\cdot}min^{-1}$)	60.7 (7.1)	66.2 (6.7)*	65.6 (11.2)*
Respiratory exchange ratio	1.00 (0.04)	1.13 (0.06)*	1.13 (0.06)*
Blood lactate ($mmol{\cdot}L^{-1}$)	6.4 (1.3)	8.3 (1.3)*	8.3 (2.1)*

Values are mean (standard deviation).

*Mean significantly different (p <0.05) from test 1 [from data in Armstrong *et al.*[22]].

which a minor can consent to participate in research projects varies from place to place but the young person's capacity to provide informed consent (assent) depends more upon his/her having sufficient understanding and intelligence to make that decision than chronological age. The responsibility to present the relevant information in a form that the child or adolescent can understand lies with the investigator. It is, however, prudent to ensure that parents or guardians are fully cognizant of all experimental procedures and give their informed consent before proceeding with the research programme.

It is advisable to invite parents and children to attend a pre-project meeting to discuss openly all aspects of the research. The preliminary meeting should be followed up by scheduling a visit to the laboratory by the young participants so that they can become familiar with the research team, the equipment, and the experimental procedures. At this meeting, a pre-test evaluation of each child may be performed according to recognized procedures.[2] If supporting materials such as purpose-written booklets with background information and space to fill in relevant data (e.g. stature, mass, etc.) are prepared in advance, the testing programme can be designed as an educational experience for the young child. The emphasis should, however, be on the young person enjoying the experience despite the need to exercise to exhaustion, which may be alien to many children and adolescents. The experience is enhanced if the laboratory is child-friendly, well-lit, appropriately decorated, spacious, with stable humidity (<60%) and temperature (20–22°C), and staffed with an experienced team who are able to maintain subject interest throughout the visit.

The involvement of local schools is often vital to the success of paediatric exercise science projects and this can be encouraged by giving schools the option of regular input into their curriculum by members of the research team. Although individual data must be held in confidence, descriptive data of samples of participants and interpretative project updates can be fed back to schools periodically both to enrich their curriculum and to promote long-term partnerships.

Calculation of oxygen uptake

The determination of $\dot{V}O_2$ is based on the ability to measure the volume of expired air per unit time ($\dot{V}_E$) and the fractions of oxygen (F_EO_2) and carbon dioxide (F_ECO_2) in the expired air. In addition, the barometric pressure, the gas temperature, and the water vapour pressure of the gases are required. Table 8.2 illustrates the calculations necessary to convert the measured variables into $\dot{V}O_2$ which is expressed under standard temperature and pressure, dry (STPD) conditions (i.e. temperature of 0°C, pressure of 760 mmHg, and completely dry). Measurement error in the determination of $\dot{V}O_2$ has been comprehensively discussed elsewhere[13] and this chapter will focus primarily on issues relevant to children and adolescents.

Respiratory gas analysis

Young people's $\dot{V}_E$, F_EO_2 and F_ECO_2 are often measured using systems which were designed for use with adults. Facemasks have a tendency to leak and mouthpieces and nose clips are usually preferred with young people although at least one study[27] has supported the use of facemasks and sealants with children as young as 8 years. However, regardless of whether a mouthpiece/noseclip system or a facemask is used, they must be matched to the size of the young subject's face/mouth. All breathing valves have a dead space and adult-sized valves may therefore cause children to inspire significant volumes of previously expired air during exercise. It has been suggested[28] that a valve dead space of 59 mL may be appropriate for children with body surface area >1.0 m^2 but that a dead space of 35 mL may be required for smaller subjects. The case to reduce valve dead space must, however, be balanced against the resulting increase in resistance to flow.

Table 8.2 Calculation of oxygen uptake from volume of expired air per minute and fraction of oxygen and carbon dioxide in expired air

1. Convert volume of expired air at ambient temperature and pressure, saturated (ATPS) to standard temperature and pressure, dry (STPD)

$$\dot{V}_E\,(\text{STPD}) = \dot{V}_E\,(\text{ATPS}) \times \frac{\text{Pb} - \text{Patm}(H_2O)}{760} \times \frac{273}{273 + \text{Ta}}$$

where $\dot{V}_E$ is volume of expired air in $L \cdot min^{-1}$, Pb is barometric pressure in mmHg, Patm(H_2O) is water vapour pressure in mmHg, and Ta is ambient temperature in °C.

2. Calculate volume of inspired air from volume of expired air

$$\dot{V}_I\,(\text{STPD}) = \frac{\dot{V}_E\,(\text{STPD}) \times (1 - F_EO_2 - F_ECO_2)}{0.7904}$$

where $\dot{V}_I$ is volume of inspired air in $L \cdot min^{-1}$, F_EO_2 is fraction of oxygen in expired air, F_ECO_2 is fraction of carbon dioxide in expired air, and 0.7904 is assumed to be the fraction of inert gases in the inspired air.

3. Calculate oxygen uptake

$$\dot{V}O_2\,(\text{STPD}) = [\dot{V}_I\,(\text{STPD}) \times F_IO_2 - \dot{V}_E\,(\text{STPD}) \times F_EO_2]$$

where $\dot{V}O_2$ is oxygen uptake in $L \cdot min^{-1}$, and F_IO_2 is fraction of oxygen in inspired air (often assumed to be 0.2093).

Many systems use a mixing chamber which stores gas over a given interval and with the help of baffles allows the fractions of O_2 and CO_2 to be mixed before being periodically sampled for measurement of FEO_2 and $FECO_2$. However, large mixing chambers may cause substantial errors in measurement of gas exchange variables as children have smaller exercise tidal volumes than adults. It has been recommended that mixing chambers should be tailored to the size of the subject[28] but appropriate dimensions in relation to tidal volume have not been established.

The development of rapidly responding flow meters, the ability to measure both inspired and expired ventilation, and the replacement of the traditional chemical analysis of gas fractions with fast response infrared CO_2 analysers and electrochemical O_2 analysers permit the measurement of gas exchange data on a breath-by-breath basis. These systems are becoming commonplace in paediatric exercise science laboratories but they are not without their problems. The phasic nature of breathing during exercise makes it difficult to measure ventilation in a rapidly breathing individual and flow meters need to be validated with flow rates ranging from what is observed for light through maximal exercise.[13,29] Similarly, gas analysers need to be calibrated carefully and a three-point calibration incorporating 0%, span and midrange values has been recommended for both gas analysers.[13]

Breath-by-breath data are providing new insights in paediatric exercise science (see Chapter 22) but they can also lead to confusion regarding data sampling. The variability in measuring $\dot{V}O_2$ is considerably greater as the sampling interval shortens[9,10] and this may be a particular problem with children with small peak $\dot{V}O_2$. Myers[29] recommended that if the determination of peak $\dot{V}O_2$ is the primary objective of a study, one should resist the temptation to use breath-by-breath data and configure the system to report test results using 30 s samples printed every 10 s. This smoothes the data but permits adequate resolution for analysis. However, regardless of the sample interval chosen, it should be reported as it will influence the $\dot{V}O_2$ observed.

Ergometers

Young people's peak $\dot{V}O_2$ has been determined using a wide range of ergometers.[7,30,31] But, although it is important to simulate competitive performance when testing young athletes,[30,32,33] the cycle ergometer and the treadmill remain the ergometers of choice in most paediatric exercise science laboratories.

Cycle ergometry provides a portable, relatively cheap, less noisy, and a more quantifiable mode of exercise than treadmill running and it may induce less anxiety in young subjects.[16,34,35] Limited upper body movement during cycle ergometry facilitates the measurement of ancillary variables such as HR, blood pressure, and blood lactate. Cycle ergometers may, however, need to be modified for young children[36] who often experience difficulty with the need to maintain a fixed pedal rate when cycling on mechanically braked ergometers.[5] Electronically braked ergometers which adjust resistance to pedalling frequency alleviate this difficulty to some extent but the increase in resistance required to maintain exercise intensity following a reduction in pedal rate may in itself cause problems with some youngsters.

Treadmill running engages a larger muscle mass than cycling and the peak $\dot{V}O_2$ obtained is therefore more likely to be limited by central rather than peripheral factors.[14,15] Peak $\dot{V}O_2$ is typically 8–10% higher during treadmill running than cycle ergometry[30,37,38] although some adolescents have been reported to achieve higher peak $\dot{V}O_2$ on a cycle ergometer.[30] Correlations between peak $\dot{V}O_2$ determined on a treadmill and a cycle are, normally about $r = 0.90$.[30,37,39]

The reported reliability of cycle and treadmill values for peak $\dot{V}O_2$ on repeated testing appears to be similar with correlation coefficients generally in the range 0.87–0.96.[7,40,41] However, the use of correlation coefficients to assess the variation in repeated measurements by the same method on the same subject has been criticized as they are a measure of the strength of the relationship between two measures, not of the repeatability in a test re-test model.[42–44] Welsman *et al.*[45] determined the peak $\dot{V}O_2$ of twenty 10-year-old children, on a cycle ergometer, across three tests each 1 week apart and reported the typical error expressed as a coefficient of variation as 4.1%, which compares favourably with the reliability of adults' $\dot{V}O_2$ max.

A major disadvantage of cycle ergometry with children is that a high portion of the total power output is developed by the quadriceps muscle,[46] and the effort required to push the pedals during the later stages of a progressive test is high in relation to muscle strength.[47] Blood flow through the quadriceps is restricted[48,49] resulting in increased anaerobic metabolism[37,50] and consequent termination of the test through peripheral muscle pain.[51]

At 10–12 years of age, sex differences in peak $\dot{V}O_2$ are generally less when determined on a cycle ergometer than when determined on a treadmill, whereas at 16 years of age, sex differences are consistent regardless of the ergometer used in the determination of peak $\dot{V}O_2$.[6] This might be a methodological artefact reflecting girls' earlier maturation and the tendency for cycle ergometer tests to be terminated by peripheral rather than central fatigue. The use of cycle ergometers to determine the true peak $\dot{V}O_2$ of children may therefore have clouded our understanding of the development of aerobic fitness and the treadmill appears to be the most appropriate mode of exercise in the laboratory determination of healthy young people's peak $\dot{V}O_2$.

Exercise protocols

Peak $\dot{V}O_2$ is a robust variable which has been shown, on a specific ergometer, to be generally independent of exercise protocol.[22,52,53] In clinical settings, standardized exercise protocols with published norms are popular[16,54,55] [see Chapter 31] but progressive exercise tests, with fixed incremental stages, which allow a series of submaximal parameters to be monitored are the most common with healthy children. However, research laboratories often use other protocols such as ramp tests[56] and maximal intensity tests[57] if they are best suited to the specific aims of the investigation and are appropriate for the age, size, and maturity of the subjects.

Progressive exercise tests to exhaustion may be continuous or discontinuous. Continuous tests reduce the total length of the test but the rest period during discontinuous stages facilitates ancillary measurements (e.g. blood sampling), allows the experimenters to encourage and motivate the subject, and compensates for children's shorter attention spans. The duration of each incremental stage may vary according to whether or not near steady-state measures of $\dot{V}O_2$ and blood lactate are required. A near steady-state in $\dot{V}O_2$ can be achieved within 2 min, but it may take up to 3 min for blood lactate to appropriately reflect the exercise intensity.[58]

General guidelines for the design of an appropriate exercise test for the determination of children's peak $\dot{V}O_2$ using a treadmill are outlined in Table 8.3.

Table 8.3 Guidelines for designing a treadmill exercise protocol to determine children's peak $\dot{V}O_2$

1. The time of day of the test does not appear to be critical (75) but the test should be conducted at least 2 hour after the consumption of solid food.
2. The subject should not have exercised vigorously on the day of testing and should be wearing physical education/sports kit and suitable footwear.
3. The subject should be habituated to the laboratory environment and familiar with treadmill running.
4. Throughout the test the child's safety and well-being are paramount. Contraindications to exercise must be ruled out before the test begins and experimenters should know what indications signal that the test should be terminated.
5. A low intensity exercise warm-up is advisable.
6. The child's age, maturity, and therefore attention span should be considered when designing the protocol. The optimal test duration is about 8 to 12 min of exercise following a warm-up and the exercise periods may be interspersed with standard rest periods (e.g. 1 min).
7. Ancillary measures such as blood sampling are facilitated by discontinuous tests although the length of each exercise stage should be at least 3 min for blood lactate to reflect the exercise intensity and at least 2 min for a near steady-state $\dot{V}O_2$
8. Changes in belt speed or slope should not be excessive and gradients and speeds should be appropriate to the size, age, and maturity of the subject.
9. Subjective and objective end-points should be decided prior to the test (e.g. facial flushing, sweating, hyperpnoea, steady gait, HR levelling off at about 200 beats min^{-1}, RER $\geq$ 1.0)
10. The subject should be allowed to gradually warm-down following the test.

Defining a maximal effort

Exercise tests with children and adolescents are normally terminated when the subject, despite strong verbal encouragement from the experimenters, is unable or unwilling to continue. The experimenters are then left, in the absence of a $\dot{V}O_2$ plateau, with the problem of deciding whether the young subject has delivered a maximal effort. Habituation to the laboratory environment, subjective criteria of intense effort (e.g. facial flushing, sweating, hyperpnoea, unsteady gait), and the paediatric exercise testing experience of the experimenters are vital ingredients in making this decision; however, supportive physiological indicators are also available.

Heart rate at peak oxygen uptake

During a progressive exercise, test HR rises in an almost linear manner with exercise intensity and $\dot{V}O_2$ and then from about 75% of peak $\dot{V}O_2$ it gradually levels off as peak $\dot{V}O_2$ approaches. HR therefore provides an indicator of effort but it is dependent on the exercise protocol[22,53,59] with HR at peak $\dot{V}O_2$ tending to be lower during cycle ergometry than treadmill running.[30,37,39] HR at peak $\dot{V}O_2$ is subject to wide individual variations but, during childhood and adolescence, it is independent of age,[19,60,61] maturation,[19,62,63] and sex.[18,64,65] Typical mean ± standard deviation HRs at peak $\dot{V}O_2$ for cycle and treadmill exercise respectively are 195 ± 7 and 200 ± 7 beats·min^{-1}.[19,66]

HR is used widely as an indicator of maximal performance with >85–90% of age predicted maximum HR often used as a criterion of maximal effort.[67,68] These criteria may not be rigorous enough to indicate a maximal effort with many young people and a recommendation of at least ≥95% of 195 or 200 beats·min^{-1} for cycling and treadmill running respectively, may be more appropriate, with the added proviso that HR should be levelling off over the final exercise stages.

Respiratory exchange ratio at peak oxygen uptake

RER rises during progressive exercise to reflect increased CO_2 production, through buffering lactate as well as substrate utilization, and can therefore indicate intense effort. An RER ≥ 1.00 has been advocated as the best criterion of maximal effort in both children and adults.[35] However, in a progressive exercise test, the standard deviation of RER at peak $\dot{V}O_2$ is about 0.06 with wide individual differences and some young subjects can provide an exhaustive effort with an RER at peak $\dot{V}O_2$ of <1.00.

The RER is ergometer dependent and, because of the greater anaerobic component, is often higher during cycling than running.[16,37] Furthermore, it is highly dependent on protocol regardless of the ergometer used.[22,23] This is clearly demonstrated in Table 8.1 where following a progressive treadmill protocol to exhaustion the mean RERs at peak $\dot{V}O_2$ of boys and girls were 0.99 and 1.00 respectively but, after a continuous 2 min treadmill run at the same speed but up a slope 5% higher than the previous test, the mean RERs were 1.18 and 1.13 respectively although the mean peak $\dot{V}O_2$ on the two tests was not significantly different. Nevertheless, an RER at peak $\dot{V}O_2$ ≥1.00 following a progressive exercise test is a valuable subsidiary indicator of near maximal effort in young people.

Blood lactate at peak oxygen uptake

High post-exercise blood lactate is routinely used to indicate maximal effort and some paediatric exercise testing laboratories recommend post-exercise blood lactates of 6–9 mmol·L^{-1} as a criterion of peak $\dot{V}O_2$ being accepted as a maximal index of aerobic fitness.[69,70] There is, however, considerable variability in the post-exercise blood lactates of children and adolescents with blood lactate at peak $\dot{V}O_2$ ranging from less than 4.0 mmol·L^{-1} to more than 13.0 mmol·L^{-1} using the same protocol, sampling, and assay techniques.[71] In the light of the methodological factors discussed later in this chapter and the dependence of blood lactate on mode of exercise,[37] protocols employed,[22] timing of post-exercise sampling relative to the cessation of the exercise,[72,73] and the low reliability of post peak $\dot{V}O_2$ blood lactates[74] the recommendation of minimum post-exercise blood lactates to validate children's peak $\dot{V}O_2$ as a maximal effort is untenable.

There is no easy solution to the problem of whether the child or adolescent has delivered a maximal effort. However, the view that if in a progressive exercise test to voluntary exhaustion, the subject demonstrates clear subjective symptoms of fatigue (e.g. hyperpnoea, sweating, facial flushing, unsteady gait), supported by a HR which is levelling off at about 200 beats min^{-1}, and an RER ≥ 1.00, a maximal effort can be assumed has received strong experimental support.[22,23,76]

Blood lactate

At rest and during exercise lactate is continuously produced in skeletal muscles and exercise driven increases in the glycolytic resynthesis of ATP result in a correspondingly greater production of lactate in the muscles. Lactate diffuses from the muscles into the blood where, both during and post-exercise, it can be sampled to provide information regarding, for example glycolytic stress[77] or changes in aerobic fitness.[78] For example, an 8 week training programme has been shown to elicit changes in blood lactate in young girls despite no changes in peak $\dot{V}O_2$.[78]

Although blood lactate is sampled with the aim of obtaining information about muscle lactate production, it is important to emphasize that lactate metabolism during exercise is a dynamic process in which lactate measured in blood cannot be assumed to have a consistent or direct relationship with either rates of muscle lactate production or muscle lactate concentration. In skeletal muscles, lactate may be produced in some muscle fibres while being simultaneously consumed by adjacent fibres within the same muscle; therefore, net lactate output from the muscles does not directly relate to the amount of lactate production.[79,80] For example, the high oxidative capacity of some type 1 muscle fibres allows some of the lactate produced in the initial stages of submaximal exercise to be reconverted to pyruvate and subsequently oxidized to CO_2 and water within the muscle. This explains why blood lactate accumulation often peaks in the early stages of submaximal exercise. Lactate which diffuses into the blood is removed by several processes, including oxidation in other skeletal muscles and the heart or used as a gluconeogenic precursor in the liver and kidneys.[81] The lactate accumulation measured in blood therefore reflects all those processes by which lactate is produced and eliminated. Consequently, blood lactate provides only a qualitative indication, and not a precise measure, of exercise-induced glycolytic activity.

During a progressive, incremental exercise test for the determination of peak $\dot{V}O_2$, blood lactate typically increases as illustrated in Fig. 8.1. The early stages of the test are associated with minimal change in blood lactate which does not significantly increase above resting values (1–2 mmol·L^{-1}). As the test progresses, a point is reached where blood lactate begins to increase rapidly with a subsequent steep rise until exhaustion. It cannot be inferred that the first increase in blood lactate reflects the onset of muscle lactate production; lactate production will have increased at low exercise intensities but where this is matched by increased removal and metabolism, the net result is no observable increase in blood lactate.[80]

As shown in Fig. 8.1, following appropriate training, the entire lactate curve is shifted to the right such that any given exercise intensity is achieved with lower blood lactate. This response forms the basis of the use of the blood lactate response to exercise as a sensitive and well-established measure of aerobic fitness in adults.[82] Children's blood lactate accumulation at the same relative exercise intensity is generally lower than that of adults[83,84] although definitive explanations for these differences remain elusive.[34,79] Some studies[85] have suggested that children have a faster elimination of lactate out of the blood compartment whereas others[86] have reported that although children may differ from adults in the production and accumulation of lactate, they do not differ in the rate of its elimination.

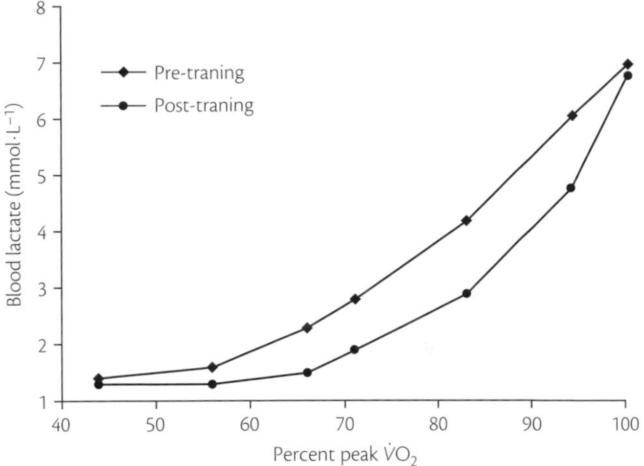

Fig. 8.1 Blood lactate response to exercise and training.

Blood lactate responses to exercise are highly influenced by methodological variations such as mode of exercise (e.g. cycle ergometer vs. treadmill), exercise protocol, site of blood sampling, blood treatment, and assay procedures. Evident in several comprehensive summaries of children's peak and submaximal lactate responses to exercise is a lack of inter-study standardization of methodology.[6,77,87] These differences must be considered when interpreting young people's blood lactate responses and are likely to have contributed to the controversy surrounding the interpretation of children's blood lactate responses to exercise in relation to age and maturation.[34]

Methodological considerations

Protocol effects

The concentration of lactate in blood and muscle is influenced by both a time-dependent and an intensity-dependent variation during exercise[88,89] therefore the duration of each exercise stage during an incremental protocol will influence the observed lactate level, particularly where the exercise intensity exceeds the maximal lactate steady state (MLSS). The exercise stage should be of sufficient duration to allow adequate diffusion of lactate from muscle to blood.[90,91] If sampled too soon, blood lactate measured will not accurately reflect the intensity of exercise and will influence the determination of fixed blood lactate reference values.[88,91] With adults, an incremental stage of at least 4 min is recommended,[92] but with young people a 3 min stage is considered sufficient.[82]

Safety issues

Strict procedures must be followed at all times in the sampling and handling of blood and the safety of both the child and the investigator is paramount. Detailed health and safety issues in haematology are beyond the scope of this chapter and readers can look up references 93 and 94 for further reading.

Site of sampling

Lactate generated in skeletal muscles during leg exercise diffuses into the femoral veins, and then rapidly appears in the arterial circulation. Thus blood sampled from the arteries of the arm provides the closest reflection of the extent of lactate diffusion into the systemic circulation.[95,96] The technical and medical hazards associated with arterial blood sampling preclude its use as a routine technique and the procedure is clearly not ethically defensible for research purposes with healthy young people [see Chapter 1].[97] However, it has been demonstrated that arterial lactate levels are closely reflected by capillary lactate levels during treadmill exercise[98] if a good blood flow is maintained at the sampling site. Capillary blood sampling from the fingertip[99] or earlobe[100] is the least invasive and traumatic sampling method, is suited to field situations, allows duplicate measurements, and has been extensively used with young people.[77,79] To induce vasodilation, the sampling site should be arterialized by immersion of the whole hand in hot water (42°C) in the case of the fingertip and by the use of a rubefacient in the case of the earlobe.[94] Squeezing the site to obtain an adequate blood sample must be avoided to prevent dilution of the sample by tissue fluid.[101] Similarly, the sampling site should remain clean and dry to prevent contamination by sweat.[102]

TO facilitate serial blood sampling, some investigators have drawn venous blood from a catheter inserted into an arm or hand vein. This is not recommended as several studies have shown that, in contrast to arterial blood, femoral lactate levels are not well reflected by venous blood.[103] Furthermore, during cycle ergometry, lactate in venous blood has been shown to be significantly lower than in simultaneously sampled arterial or capillary blood[104] with the discrepancy increasing at higher exercise intensities.[92,105] During steady-state submaximal treadmill exercise arterial-venous lactate differences appear less pronounced, but the trend towards an increasing discrepancy in values between sites remains.[98]

Assay methods

Despite its significant impact upon the value of blood lactate obtained, the nature and extent of differences between lactate assay methodologies remain poorly documented and infrequently acknowledged in the interpretation of young people's blood lactate responses during exercise.

Once sampled, blood may undergo a variety of treatments depending upon the analyser which may require preparation of serum, plasma, lysed blood, or a protein-free preparation (Table 8.4). The semi-automatic analysers used in many paediatric exercise laboratories are generally based on an enzymatic electrochemical assay which is usually used to analyse whole blood immediately following sampling. These analysers have many advantages; they are simple to use, do not require large amounts of blood (typically lactate is assayed in 25 mL of blood) and results are available rapidly (within 60–90 s). Portable versions of several models of analysers are available thus facilitating blood lactate measurement in field situations.

Before the availability of this methodology, lactate was often determined using an enzymatic-spectrophotometric assay which required the preparation of a protein-free filtrate. This is achieved by precipitating the blood proteins by the addition of ice-cold perchloric acid or trichloroacetic acid, centrifuging the sample and assaying lactate in the clear supernatant.

The variation in the results obtained from different assays may be considerable and depends on two main factors; first, whether or not the solids (cells, proteins, cellular debris, etc.) have been removed (as in plasma, serum, and protein-free preparations) or not (as in whole blood and lysed blood) and second whether the sample has been haemolysed to release erythrocyte lactate (as in lysed blood and protein-free preparations). The volume difference accounts for the largest variation in lactate levels observed. In whole blood assays, only the lactate in the plasma fraction is assayed but the sample still contains the solid fraction. Thus lactate levels in whole blood are substantially lower than in preparations from which the solids have been removed. Estimates quantifying the volume difference between protein-free and whole blood lactates have varied from 5 to 63% with the difference apparently reducing at high exercise intensities.[106] Lactate values in plasma are approximately 30% higher than in whole blood.[98,104]

The addition of a chemical lysing agent releases intracellular lactate, thus contributing an additional source of lactate to the sample. Therefore, in contrast to a whole blood assay where

Table 8.4 Blood preparations for lactate assay

Whole blood
Blood is collected into a capillary tube or cuvette coated with heparin to prevent clotting and is analysed, usually within minutes, without further treatment.
Plasma
Blood is collected as above and centrifuged to separate the liquid (plasma) and solid constituents of the blood. Lactate is then measured in the plasma.
Serum
Blood is allowed to clot and then centrifuged to separate the clear, straw-coloured serum which is assayed for lactate.
Lysed blood
Blood is treated with chemicals which break open (lyse) the red blood cells releasing the intracellular lactate. The blood is not separated before assay.
Protein-free preparation
The blood sample is chemically treated to break down blood proteins and then centrifuged to separate the solids and liquids. The liquid portion is then assayed for lactate

Reprinted from Armstrong and Welsman [34] with permission.

lactate is measured in the plasma compartment, protein-free and lysed blood assays measure total lactate (i.e. plasma plus erythrocyte lactate). Individual differences in haematocrit may, therefore, be a confounding factor in lactate levels observed.[104,105] Lactate in lysed blood tends to be higher than in whole blood, with the difference becoming more marked at higher lactate concentrations.[98]

The effect of different assay methodologies upon blood lactate values and the implications of these for performance evaluation can be clearly illustrated using the regression equations generated by Williams *et al.*[98] If a sample taken during exercise yields a whole blood lactate of 4 mmol^{-1}, simply lysing the blood would increase the lactate value to 4.4 mmol^{-1} and a value of 5.5 mmol^{-1} would be obtained if plasma was assayed.

Blood lactate measures of performance

Training-induced improvements in aerobic fitness result in a lower blood lactate response at all levels of submaximal exercise. Therefore, any point on the lactate curve (illustrated in Fig. 8.1) might be used to detect and monitor intra-individual improvements. However, in order to make comparisons among individuals or groups (e.g. by sex or maturity stage), blood lactate responses are often standardized to some measure of lactate threshold (T_{LAC}). Most often this term is used to describe the first observable increase in blood lactate above resting levels.[108] This can be determined from visual inspection of the inflection in blood lactate responses,[109] mathematical interpolation,[110–112] or by defining the point of inflection as a 1 mmol·L^{-1} increase over baseline level.[113] A clear inflection point may not be observable particularly during a discontinuous protocol where peak $\dot{V}O_2$ is attained within relatively few incremental stages (for example as in the data presented in Fig. 8.1 which are typical of a young person's blood lactate responses to incremental exercise). To avoid blood sampling, some authors have used non-invasive derivatives of the T_{LAC} such as the ventilatory threshold [see Chapters 6, 17 and 22].[114, 115] Others have recommended the use of a fixed blood lactate reference and in adults, a value of 4.0 mmol·L^{-1}, originally referred to as the 'onset of blood lactate accumulation',[116,117] has become an accepted assessment standard.[82] One justification for a 4 mmol·L^{-1} criterion was the suggestion that this corresponded to the MLSS[88] though subsequent evidence has demonstrated wide inter-individual variation, particularly in athletes.[118,119]

MLSS defines the highest exercise intensity which can be maintained without incurring a progressive increase in blood lactate. As processes of lactate accumulation and elimination are in equilibrium, although elevated above resting levels, exercise can continue for prolonged periods at or below the MLSS and it represents a sensitive and informative measure of aerobic fitness.

It is important to re-emphasize that the exercise intensity at which a given threshold or reference occurs is highly specific to both the exercise protocol and the methods used to assess blood lactate accumulation. Much of the original work into blood lactate responses which resulted in the general acceptance of a 4 mmol·L^{-1} reference criterion determined lactate in a protein-free preparation. Given that young people respond to any given exercise intensity with lower blood lactate accumulation than adults and that the majority of paediatric laboratories assay lactate in whole blood,[77] the validity of a 4 mmol·L^{-1} reference level to assess aerobic fitness in children and adolescents may be questioned. In both trained[109,120] and untrained[71,121,122] young people, a whole blood lactate level of 4 mmol·L^{-1} might not be attained until 90% of peak $\dot{V}O_2$.

In response to this, Williams *et al.*[71] proposed the use of a 2.5 mmol^{-1} whole blood criterion and demonstrated that physiological responses to exercise eliciting this value of blood lactate closely represent those at the MLSS in 13 year old boys and girls.[99] In this study, the MLSS, defined as a change in blood lactate of $\leq$0.5 mmol^{-1} between minutes 5 and 10 of a 10 min continuous exercise bout, occurred at 2.1 and 2.3 mmol^{-1} in boys and girls, respectively. The MLSS in young people has not been documented extensively but studies with boys have reported lactate levels at the MLSS ranging from 3.1 to 5.0 mmol^{-1}.[100,123–125] These studies used a protein-free assay, and hence the higher values reported are not unexpected. Further sources of inter-study variation in results may include the use of cycle ergometry[124,125] versus treadmill running[99,123] and continuous[97,124] versus discontinuous[100, 123] exercise stages. The value of blood lactate obtained has also been shown to vary according to the duration of each exercise stage and the specific criterion used to define the MLSS.[125] In the light of the methodological problems described, the application of fixed reference blood lactates as putative indicators of young people's MLSS needs to be carried out with extreme caution.

Several studies have investigated children's and adolescents' blood lactate responses to exercise but a precise description of changes with age and maturation remains elusive largely as a result of inconsistent exercise protocols, threshold definitions, blood sampling and assay techniques, and small and/or single sex samples.[34,87]

Blood lactate responses to exercise and age

Apparent age-related differences have been noted in several small studies of boys. Tanaka and Shindo[126] observed a significant inverse relationship between HR at the T_{LAC}, expressed as a percentage of HR max, and chronological age in 8–15-year olds. Similarly, Izumi and Ishiko[127] noted that during cycle ergometry, the T_{LAC} occurred much closer to peak $\dot{V}O_2$ in teenage boys than in adults. Atomi *et al.*[128] found T_{LAC} as a % of peak $\dot{V}O_2$ to decrease in seven boys from age 10.5 to 11.8 years. A comparison of teenage boys with adults reported higher HRs at the exercise intensity corresponding to a 4.0 mmol^{-1} blood lactate in the younger subjects, although differences became negligible when expressed in relative terms.[129]

Williams and Armstrong[121] studied 149 11- to 16-year-old boys and girls and found no significant relationship between age and % peak $\dot{V}O_2$ at a blood lactate of 4.0 mmol^{-1} ; however this criterion occurred so close to peak $\dot{V}O_2$ to be of questionable value as a marker of submaximal performance. Interestingly, a significant, although very low, correlation was obtained between age and % peak $\dot{V}O_2$ at a lower reference of 2.5 mmol^{-1} in the same boys ($r = -0.226$) and girls ($r = -0.272$). An absence of an age effect has also been noted with respect to the MLSS. Beneke *et al.*,[122] observed no significant relationship between either blood lactate or % peak $\dot{V}O_2$ at the MLSS determined during cycle ergometry and age in 34 males aged 11–20 years. Data are sparse, but there is no evidence of significant sex differences in performance at fixed submaximal blood lactates during childhood and adolescence.[121]

Blood lactate responses to exercise and maturation

Despite early indications that muscle and blood lactate responses are related to indices of maturational age[130] and animal studies suggesting androgenic dependency of muscle glycolytic capacity and consequent lactate production,[131,132] the role of maturation in determining young people's blood lactate responses to exercise remains inconclusive. Studies examining specific relationships between maturation and blood lactate indices of aerobic performance are sparse but consistent in failing to identify an independent maturational effect. For example, Welsman *et al.*[133] used a regression approach to examine the effects of body size and salivary testosterone on blood lactate indices including % peak $\dot{V}O_2$ at a 2.5 mmol^{-1} reference in 12- to 16-year-old boys whose maturation ranged from 1 to 5 in the stages described by Tanner.[134] No significant independent effect of testosterone on submaximal blood lactate levels was observed. Similarly, no significant differences in the % peak $\dot{V}O_2$ at blood lactates of 2.5 and 4.0 mmol^{-1} were observed in a sample of 119 boys and girls compared by maturity group.[121] Thus it would appear that factors other than hormonal changes with sexual maturation regulate developmental changes in blood lactate responses during exercise.

Summary

- Maximal $\dot{V}O_2$ is widely recognized as the best single indicator of aerobic fitness but only a minority of children and adolescents demonstrate the $\dot{V}O_2$ plateau conventionally associated with $\dot{V}O_2$ max. There is therefore a growing conviction that peak $\dot{V}O_2$ is the appropriate term to use with young people.
- Peak $\dot{V}O_2$ may be accepted as a maximal measure of young people's aerobic fitness provided appropriate subjective criteria of exhaustion are fulfilled and supported by the achievement of specific HR and/or RER values
- Prior to a determination of peak $\dot{V}O_2$ ethical issues, pre-test preparation, and technical and methodological aspects of respiratory gas analysis need to be addressed.
- The treadmill is the ergometer of choice for the determination of peak $\dot{V}O_2$, but the specific exercise protocol should be designed with reference to the aims of the study and the age, size, and maturity of the participants. The precise methodology, apparatus, and criteria of maximal effort used in the determination of peak $\dot{V}O_2$ should be carefully reported.
- Lactate measured in the blood cannot be assumed to have a consistent or direct relationship with rates of either muscle lactate production or muscle lactate concentration. However, blood lactate accumulation during submaximal exercise does provide a measure which may be more sensitive to training-induced improvements in aerobic fitness than peak $\dot{V}O_2$.
- Strict safety procedures must be followed at all times in the sampling and handling of blood. Much of the variability in the interpretation of blood lactate accumulation during exercise is attributable to differences in the site of blood sampling and assay methodology.
- Blood lactate responses to exercise can be interpreted using the T_{LAC} and MLSS but direct comparisons of these parameters across studies are not always possible through lack of standardization of appropriate methodology. Lactate threshold and MLSS are extensively used as the lower and upper criterion respectively of the heavy exercise domain in the interpretation of $\dot{V}O_2$ kinetics. (see Chapter 22).
- Children's blood lactate accumulation is generally lower than that of adults during comparable exercise but the evidence relating blood lactate to age, maturation, and sex during childhood and adolescence is equivocal and further research is required.

References

1. Astrand PO, Rodahl K (1986). *Textbook of work physiology*. McGraw-Hill, New York.
2. American College of Sports Medicine (1995). *ACSM's guidelines for exercise testing and prescription*. Williams and Wilkins, Baltimore.
3. Robinson S (1938). Experimental studies of physical fitness in relation to age. *Arbeitsphysiol* **10**, 251–323.
4. Morse M, Schlutz FW, Cassels DE (1949). Relation of age to physiological responses of the older boy to exercise. *J Appl Physiol* **1**, 683–709.
5. Åstrand PO (1952). *Experimental studies of physical working capacity in relation to sex and age*. Munksgaard, Copenhagen.
6. Armstrong N, Welsman J (1994). Assessment and interpretation of aerobic fitness in children and adolescents. *Exerc Sport Sci Rev* **22**, 435–76.
7. Rivera-Brown AM, Frontera WR (1998). Achievement of plateau and reliability of $\dot{V}_{O2}$ max in trained adolescents tested with different ergometers. *Pediatr Exerc Sci* **10**, 164–75.
8. Rowland TW (2005). *Children's exercise physiology*, pp. 92–94. Human Kinetics, Champaign, IL.
9. Myers J, Walsh D, Buchanan N, Froelicher VF (1989). Can maximal cardiopulmonary capacity be recognised by a plateau in oxygen uptake. *Chest* **96**, 1312–6.
10. Myers J, Walsh D, Sullivan M, Froelicher V (1990). Effect of sampling on variability and plateau in oxygen uptake. *J Appl Physiol* **68**, 404–10.
11. Byung-kon Y, Kravitz L, Robergs R (2007). $\dot{V}_{O2}$ max, protocol duration, and the $\dot{V}_{O2}$ plateau. *Med Sci Sports Exerc* **39**, 1186–92.
12. Noakes TD (1997). Challenging beliefs: ex Africa semper aliquid novi. *Med Sci Sports Exerc* **29**, 571–90.
13. Howley ET, Bassett DR, Welch HG (1995). Criteria for maximal oxygen uptake: Review and commentary. *Med Sci Sports Exerc* **27**, 1292–301.
14. Shephard RJ (1984). Tests of maximum oxygen intake. A critical review. *Sports Med* **1**, 99–124.
15. Shephard RJ (1971). The working capacity of schoolchildren. In: Shephard RJ (ed.), *Frontiers of fitness* (pp. 319–45). Thomas, Springfield, IL.
16. Rowland TW (1993). Aerobic exercise testing protocols. In: Rowland TW (ed.), *Pediatric laboratory exercise testing in children*, pp. 19–42. Human Kinetics, Champaign, IL.
17. Krahenbuhl GS, Skinner JS, Kohrt WM (1985). Developmental aspects of maximal aerobic power in children. *Exerc Sport Sci Rev* **13**, 503–38.
18. Armstrong N, Kirby BJ, McManus AM, Welsman JR (1995). Aerobic fitness of pre-pubescent children. *Ann Hum Biol* **22**, 427–41.
19. Armstrong N, Williams J, Balding J, Gentle P, Kirby B (1991). The peak oxygen uptake of British children with reference to age, sex and sexual maturity. *Eur J Appl Physiol* **62**, 369–75.
20. Armstrong N, Davies B (1984). The metabolic and physiological responses of children to exercise and training. *Phys Educ Rev* **7**, 90–105.
21. Armstrong N, Welsman JR (1997). The assessment and interpretation of aerobic fitness in children and adolescents: An update. In: Froberg K, Lammert O, St. Hansen H, Blimkie CJR (eds.), *Exercise and fitness—benefits and limitations*, pp. 173–80. University Press, Odense, Denmark.

22. Armstrong N, Welsman J, Winsley R (1996). Is peak $\dot{V}O_2$ a maximal index of children's aerobic fitness? *Int J Sports Med* **17**, 356–9.
23. Rowland TW (1993). Does peak $\dot{V}O_2$ reflect $\dot{V}O_2$ max in children? Evidence from supramaximal testing. *Med Sci Sports Exer* **25**, 689–93.
24. Nicholson RH (1986). *Medical research with children*. Oxford University Press, Oxford.
25. Working Party on Ethics of Research in Children (1980). Guidelines to aid ethical committees considering research involving children. *BMJ* **280**, 229–31.
26. Working Party on Research in Children (1991). *The ethical conduct of research in children*. Medical Research Council, London.
27. Mahon AD, Stolen KQ, Gay JA (1998). Using a facemask and sealant to measure respiratory gas exchange in children during exercise. *Pediatr Exerc Sci* **10**, 347–55.
28. Staats BA, Grinton SF, Mottram CD, Driscoll DJ, Beck KC (1993). Quality control in exercising testing. *Prog Pediatr Cardiol* **2**, 11–7.
29. Myers JN (1996). *Essentials of cardiopulmonary exercise testing*. Human Kinetics, Champaign, IL.
30. Armstrong N, Davies B (1981). An ergometric analysis of age group swimmers. *Brit J Sports Med* **15**, 20–6.
31. Chan OL, Duncan MT, Sundsten JW, Thinakaran T, Noh MNBC, Klissouras V (1976). The maximum aerobic power of the Temiars. *Med Sci Sports Exerc* **8**, 235–8.
32. Al-Hazza HM, Al-Refaee SA, Sulaiman MA, Dafterdar MY, Al-Herbish AS, Chukwuemeka AC (1998). Cardiorespiratory responses of trained boys to treadmill and arm ergometry: Effects of training specificity. *Pediatr Exerc Sci* **10**, 264–76.
33. Armstrong N, Welsman JR (1995). Laboratory testing of young athletes. In: Maffulli N (ed.), *Color atlas and textbook of sports medicine in childhood and adolescence*, pp. 109–22. Mosby-Wolfe, London.
34. Armstrong N, Welsman JR (1997). *Young people and physical activity*. Oxford University Press, Oxford.
35. Léger L (1996). Aerobic performance. In: Docherty D. (ed.), *Measurement in pediatric exercise science*, pp. 183–223. Human Kinetics, Champaign, IL.
36. Howell ML, MacNab RBJ (1968). *The physical work capacity of Canadian children aged 7 to 17*. Canadian Association for Health, Physical Education and Recreation, Toronto, Ontario.
37. Boileau RA, Bonen A, Heyward VH, Massey BH (1977). Maximal aerobic capacity on the treadmill and bicycle ergometer of boys 11–14 years of age. *J Sports Med Phys Fitness* **17**, 153–62.
38. Turley KR, Rogers DM, Wilmore JH (1995). Maximal treadmill versus cycle ergometry testing in children: Differences, reliabilities and variability of responses. *Pediatr Exerc Sci* 7, 49–60.
39. Bloxham SR, Welsman JR, Armstrong N (2005). Ergometer-specific relationships between peak oxygen uptake and short-term power output in children. *Pediatr Exerc Sci* **17**, 136–48.
40. Golden JC, Janz KR, Clarke WR, Mahoney LT (1991). New protocol for submaximal and peak exercise values for children and adolescents: The Muscatine Study. *Pediatr Exerc Sci* **3**, 129–40.
41. Baggley G, Cumming GR (1972). Serial measurement of working and aerobic capacity of Winnipeg schoolchildren during a school year. In: Cumming GR, Taylor AW, Snidal D. (eds.), *Environmental effects of work performance*, pp. 173–86. Canadian Association of Sport Sciences, Toronto, Ontario.
42. Hopkins WG (2000). Measures of reliability in sports medicine and science. *Sports Med* **30**, 1–15.
43. Atkinson G, Nevill AM (1998). Statistical methods for assessing measurement error (reliability) in variables relevant to sports medicine. *Sports Med* **26**, 217–38.
44. Atkinson G, Nevill AM (2000). Typical error versus limits of agreement. *Sports Med* **30**, 375–81.
45. Welsman JR, Bywater K, Farr C, Welford D, Armstrong N (2005). Reliability of peak $\dot{V}O_2$ and maximal cardiac output assessed using thoracic bioimpedance in children. *Eur J Appl Physiol* **94**, 228–34.
46. Kay C, Shephard RJ (1969). On muscle strength and the threshold of anaerobic work. *Arbeitsphysiol* **27**, 311–28.
47. Hoes M, Binkhorst RA, Smeekes-Kuyl A, Vissurs AC (1968). Measurement of forces exerted on a pedal crank during work on the bicycle ergometer at different loads. *Arbeitsphysiol* **26**, 33–42.
48. Katch FI, Girandola FN, Katch VL (1971). The relationship of body weight to maximum oxygen uptake and heavy work endurance capacity on the bicycle ergometer. *Med Sci Sports Exerc* **3**, 101–6.
49. Glassford RC, Bayford GHY, Sedgwick AW, McNab RBJ (1965). Comparison of maximal oxygen uptake values determined by predicted and actual methods. *J Appl Physiol* **20**, 509–13.
50. Skinner JS, McLellan TH (1980). The transition from aerobic to anaerobic metabolism. *Res Q* **51**, 234–48.
51. Wirth A, Trager E, Scheele K, Mayer D, Diehm K, Reisch K (1978). Cardiopulmonary adjustment and metabolic response to maximal and submaximal physical exercise of boys and girls at different stages of maturity. *Eur J Appl Physiol* **39**, 229–40.
52. Skinner JS, Bar-Or O, Bergsteinova V, Bell CW, Royer D, Buskirk ER (1971). Comparison of continuous and intermittent tests for determining maximal oxygen intake in children. *Acta Paediatr Scand* **217**, 24–8.
53. Sheehan JM, Rowland TW, Burke EJ (1987). A comparison of four treadmill protocols for determination of maximal oxygen uptake in 10 to 12 year old boys. *Int J Sports Med* **8**, 31–4.
54. Freedson PS, Goodman TL (1993). Measurement of oxygen consumption. In: Rowland TW (ed.), *Pediatric laboratory exercise testing*, pp. 91–113. Human Kinetics, Champaign, IL.
55. Herbestreit H (2004). Exercise testing in children—What works, what doesn't, and where to go? *Pediatr Resp Rev* **5**, S11–4.
56. 56. Fawkner SG, Armstrong N (2004). Longitudinal changes in the kinetic response to heavy intensity exercise in children. *J Appl Physiol* **97**, 460–6.
57. Williams CA, Ratel S, Armstrong N (2005). Achievement of peak $\dot{V}O_2$ during a 90-s maximal intensity cycle sprint in adolescents. *Can J Appl Physiol* **30**, 157–71.
58. Williams J, Armstrong N (1991). The maximal lactate steady state and its relationship to performance at fixed blood lactate reference values in children. *Pediatr Exerc Sci* **3**, 333–41.
59. Cumming GR, Langford S (1985). Comparison of nine exercise tests used in pediatric cardiology. In Binkhorst RA, Kemper HCG, Saris WHM (eds.), *Children and exercise XI*. pp. 58–68. Human Kinetics, Champaign, IL.
60. Bailey DA, Ross WD (1978). Size dissociation of maximal aerobic power during growth in boys. *Med Sport* **11**, 140–51.
61. Bale P (1981). Pre- and post-adolescents' physiological response to exercise. *Br J Sports Med* **15**, 246–9.
62. Armstrong N, Welsman JR, Kirby BJ (1998). Peak oxygen uptake and maturation in 12-year-olds. *Med Sci Sports Exerc* **30**, 165–9.
63. Armstrong N, Welsman JR (2001). Peak oxygen uptake in relation to growth and maturation. *Eur J Appl Physiol* **28**, 259–65.
64. Andersen KL, Seliger V, Rutenfranz J, Skrobak-Kaczynski J (1976). Physical performance capacity of children in Norway. Part IV—The rate of growth in maximal aerobic power and the influence of improved physical education of children in a rural community. *Eur J Appl Physiol* **35**, 49–58.
65. Vinet A, Mandigout S, Nottin S, Nguyen L-D, Lecoq A-M, Courteix D, Obert P (2003). Influence of body composition, hemoglobin concentration, and cardiac size and function on gender differences in maximal oxygen uptake in prepubertal children. *Chest* **124**, 1494–9.
66. Armstrong N, Balding J, Gentle P, Williams J, Kirby B (1990). Peak oxygen uptake and physical activity in 11 to 16 year olds. *Pediatr Exerc Sci* **2**, 349–58
67. Dencker M, Thorsson O, Karlsson MK, Linden C, Eiberg S, Wollmer P, Andersen LB (2007). Gender differences and determinants of aerobic fitness in children aged 8–11 years. *Eur J Appl Physiol* **99**, 19–26.

68. Froberg K, Andersen LB, Lammert O (1991). Maximal oxygen uptake and respiratory functions during puberty in boy groups of different physical activity. In: Frenkl R, Szmodis I (eds.), *Children and exercise pediatric work physiology XV*, pp. 265–80. National Institute for Health Promotion, Budapest, Hungary.
69. Cumming GR, Hastman L, McCort J, McCullough S (1980). High serum lactates do occur in children after maximal work. *Int J Sports Med* **1**, 66–9.
70. Docherty D, Gaul CA (1990). *Critical analysis of available laboratory tests used in evaluating the fitness of children and youth*. Fitness Canada, Ottawa.
71. Williams J, Armstrong N, Kirby B (1990). The 4 mM blood lactate level as an index of exercise performance in 11–13 year old children. *J Sports Sci* **8**, 139–47.
72. Chia M, Armstrong N, Childs D (1997). The assessment of children's anaerobic performance using modifications of the Wingate anaerobic test. *Pediatr Exerc Sci* **9**, 80–9.
73. Shephard RJ, Allen C, Bar-Or O, Davies CTM, Degre S, Hedman R, Ishii K, Kaneko M, LaCour JR, di Prampero PE, Seliger V (1969). The working capacity of Toronto schoolchildren, I. *Can Med Assoc J* **100**, 560–6, 705–14.
74. Rowland TW, Cunningham LN (1992). Oxygen uptake plateau during maximal treadmill exercise in children. *Chest* **101**, 485–9.
75. Cunnigham DA, Van Waterschoot B, Paterson DH, Lefcoe M, Sangal SP (1977). Reliability and reproducibility of maximal oxygen uptake measurements in children. *Med Sci Sports Exerc* **9**, 104–7.
76. Cumming GR (1967). Current levels of fitness. *Can Med Assoc J* **88**, 351–5.
77. Welsman J, Armstrong N (1998). Assessing postexercise blood lactates in children and adolescents. In: Van Praagh E (ed.) *Pediatric anaerobic performance*, pp. 137–53. Human Kinetics, Champaign, IL.
78. Welsman JR, Armstrong N, Withers S (1997). Responses of young girls to two modes of aerobic training. *Br J Sports Med* **31**, 139–42.
79. Pfitzinger P, Freedson P (1997). Blood lactate responses to exercise in children: Part 2. Lactate threshold. *Pediatr Exerc Sci* **9**, 299–307.
80. Brooks GA (1991). Current concepts in lactate exchange. *Med Sci Sports Exerc* **23**, 895–906.
81. Stainsby WN, Brooks GA (1990). Control of lactic acid metabolism in contracting muscles and during exercise. *Exerc Sports Sci Rev* **18**, 29–63.
82. Bird S, Davison R (eds.). (1997) *Guidelines for the physiological testing of athletes* (3rd ed.) BASES, Leeds.
83. Eriksson BO, Saltin B (1974). Muscle metabolism during exercise in boys aged 11–16 years compared to adults. *Acta Paediatr Belg* **28** (Suppl.), 257–65.
84. Martinez LR, Haymes EM (1992). Substrate utilization during treadmill running in prepubertal girls and women. *Med Sci Sports Exerc* **24**, 975–83.
85. Beneke R, Hutler M, Jung M, Leithauser RM (2005). Modeling the blood lactate kinetics at maximal short-term exercise conditions in children, adolescents and adults. *J Appl Physiol* **99**, 499–504.
86. Dotan R, Ohana S, Bediz C, Falk B (2003). Blood lactate disappearance dynamics in boys and men following exercise of similar and dissimilar peak lactate concentrations. *J Pediatr Endocrinol Metab* **16**, 419–29.
87. Pfitzinger P, Freedson P (1997). Blood lactate responses to exercise in children: Part 1. Peak lactate concentration. *Pediatr Exerc Sci* **9**, 210–22.
88. 88. Heck H. Mader A, Hess G, Mucke S, Muller R, Hollman W (1985). Justification of the 4 $mmol^{-1}$ lactate threshold. *Int J Sports Med* **6**, 117–30.
89. Campbell ME, Hughson RL, Green HJ (1989). Continuous increase in blood lactate concentration during different ramp exercise protocols. *J Appl Physiol* **66**, 1104–7.
90. Karlsson J, Jacobs, I (1982). Onset of blood lactate accumulation during muscular exercise as threshold concept. I. Theoretical consideration. *Int J Sports Med* **3**, 190–201.
91. MacDougall JD, Wenger, HA, Green HJ (eds.). (1991). *Physiological testing of the high-performance athlete*. Human Kinetics, Champaign, IL.
92. Yoshida T (1984). Effect of exercise duration during incremental exercise on the determination of anaerobic threshold and the onset of blood lactate accumulation. *Euro J Appl Physiol* **53**, 196–9.
93. Maughan RJ, Leiper JB, Greaves M (2001). Haematology. In: Eston RG, Reilly TP (eds.), *Kinanthropometry and exercise physiology laboratory manual* (pp. 99–115). E & FN Spon, London.
94. Maughan RJ, Shirreffs SM, Leiper JB (2007). Blood sampling. In: Winter EM, Jones AM, Daison RCR, Bromley PD, Mercer TH (eds.), *Sport and physiology testing guidelines. Volume 1: Sport testing*, pp. 25–9. Routledge, London.
95. Newton JL, Robinson S (1965). The distribution of blood lactate and pyruvate during work and recovery. *Fed Proc* **24**, 590.
96. Saltin B, Blomqvist G, Mitchell JH, Johnson RL Jr, Wildenthal K, Chapman C (1968). Response to exercise after bed rest and after training. *Circulation* **38 (Suppl 5)**, 1–78.
97. Bar-Or O (1984). The growth and development of children's physiologic and perceptional responses to exercise. In: Ilmarinen J, Valimaki I (eds.), *Children and sport*, pp. 3–17. Springer-Verlag, Berlin.
98. Williams JR, Armstrong N, Kirby BJ (1992). The influence of the site of sampling and assay medium upon the measurement and interpretation of blood lactate responses to exercise. *J Sports Sci* **10**, 95–107.
99. Williams JR, Armstrong N (1991). Relationship of maximal lactate steady state to performance at fixed blood lactate reference values in children. *Pediatr Exerc Sci* **3**, 333–41.
100. Mocellin R, Heusgen M, Gildein HP (1991). Anaerobic threshold and maximal steady-state blood lactate in prepubertal boys. *Eur J Appl Physiol* **62**, 56–60.
101. Tietz NW (1986). *Textbook of clinical chemistry.* WB Saunders, Philadelphia.
102. Thoden JS (1982). Testing aerobic power. In: MacDougall JD, Wenger HA, Green HJ. (eds.), *Physiological testing of the high-performance athlete*, pp. 107–74 Human Kinetics, Champaign, IL.
103. Gisolfi C, Robinson, S (1970). Venous blood distribution in the legs during intermittent treadmill work. *J Appl Physiol* **29**, 368–73.
104. Foxdal P, Sjödin B, Rudstam H, Östman C, Östman B, Hedenstierna GC (1990). Lactate concentration differences in plasma, whole blood, capillary finger blood and erythrocytes during submaximal graded exercise in humans. *Eur J Appl Physiol* **61**, 218–22.
105. Yoshida T, Suda Y, Takeuchi N (1982). Endurance training regimen based upon arterial blood lactate: Effects on anaerobic threshold. *Eur J Appl Physiol* **49**, 223–30.
106. Weil MH, Leavy JA, Rackow EC, Halfman CJ (1986). Validation of a semi-automated technique for measuring lactate in whole blood. *Clin Chem* **32**, 2175–7.
107. Soutter WP, Sharp F, Clark DM (1978). Bedside estimation of whole blood lactate. *Br J Anaesthesia* **50**, 445–50.
108. Wasserman K, Whipp BJ, Koyal SN, Beaver WL (1973). Anaerobic threshold and respiratory gas exchange during exercise. *J Appl Physiol* **35**, 236–43.
109. Maffulli N, Testa V, Lancia A, Capasso G, Lombardi S (1991). Indices of sustained aerobic power in young middle distance runners. *Med Sci Sports Exerc* **23**, 1090–6.
110. Davis JA, Caiozzo VJ, Moore JL, Hawksworth CA Prietto CA, McMaster WC (1983). Accuracy of the subjective determination of the anaerobic threshold discerned from gas exchange measurements. *Int J Sports Med* **4**, 137.
111. Gladden LB, Yates, JW, Stremel RW, Stamford BA (1985). Gas exchange and lactate anaerobic threshold: Inter and intra evaluator agreement. *J Appl Physiol* **58**, 2082–9.
112. Beaver WL, Wasserman K, Whipp BJ (1985). Improved detection of lactate threshold during exercise using a log-log transformation. *J Appl Physiol* **59**, 1936–40.

113. Coyle EF, Martin WH, Ehsani AA, Hagberg JM, Bloomfield SA, Sinacore DR, Holloszy JO (1983). Blood lactate threshold in some well-trained ischemic heart disease patients. *J Appl Physiol* **54**, 18–23.
114. Hebestreit H, Staachen B, Hebestreit A (2000). Ventilatory threshold: A useful method to determine aerobic fitness in children. *Med Sci Sports Exerc* **32**, 164–9.
115. Fawkner SG, Armstrong N, Childs DJ, Welsman JR (2002). Reliability of the visually assessed ventilatory threshold and V-slope in children. *Pediatr Exerc Sci* **14**, 181–2.
116. Sjodin B, Jacobs I, Karlsson J (1981). Onset of blood lactate accumulation and enzyme activities in m. vastus lateralis in man. *Int J Sports Med* **2**, 166–70.
117. Sjodin B, Schele R, Karlsson J, Linnarsson D, Wallensten R (1982). The physiological background of onset of blood lactate accumulation. In: Komi P (ed.), *Exercise and sport biology*, pp. 43–55. Human Kinetics, Champaign, IL.
118. Stegmann H, Kindermann W (1982). Comparison of prolonged exercise tests at the individual anaerobic threshold and the fixed anaerobic threshold of 4 $mmol^{-1}$. *Int J Sports Med* **3**, 105–10.
119. Haverty M, Kenny WL, Hodgson JL (1988). Lactate and gas exchange responses to incremental and steady state running. *Br J Sports Med* **2**, 51–4.
120. Yoshizawa S, Honda H, Urushibara M, Nakamura N (1989). Aerobic-anaerobic energy supply and daily physical activity level in young children. In: Oseid S, Carlsen K-H (eds.), *Children and exercise XIII*, pp. 47–56. Human Kinetics, Champaign, IL.
121. Williams JR, Armstrong N (1991). The influence of age and sexual maturation on children's blood lactate responses to exercise. *Pediatr Exerc Sci* **3**, 111–20.
122. Fernhall B, Kohrt W, Burkett LN, Walters S (1996). Relationship between the lactate threshold and cross-country run performance in high school male and female runners. *Pediatr Exerc Sci* **8**, 37–47.
123. Mocellin R, Heusgen M, Korsten-Reck U (1990). Maximal steady state blood lactate levels in 11-year-old boys. *Eur J Pediatr* **149**, 771–3.
124. Beneke R, Heck H, Schwarz V, Leithäuser, R (1996). Maximal lactate steady state during the second decade of age. *Med Sci Sports Exerc* **28**, 1474–8.
125. Beneke R, Schwarz V, Leithäuser R, Hütler M, von Duvillard SP (1996). Maximal lactate steady state in children. *Pediatr Exer Sci* **8**, 328–36.
126. Tanaka H, Shindo M. Running velocity at blood lactate threshold of boys aged 6–15 years compared with untrained and trained young males (1985). *Int J Sports Med* **6**, 90–4.
127. Izumi I, Ishiko T (1984). Lactate threshold in pubescent boys. *Japanese J Phys Educ* **28**, 309–14.
128. Atomi Y, Iwaoka K, Hatta H, Miyashita M, Yamamoto Y (1986). Daily physical activity levels in preadolescent boys related to $\dot{V}O_2$ max and lactate threshold. *Eur J Appl Physiol* **55**, 156–61.
129. Simon G, Berg A, Dickhuth HH, Simon-Alt A, Keul J (1981). Bestimmung der anaeroben schwelle in abhangigkeit von alter und von der leistungsfahigkeit. (Determination of the anaerobic threshold depending on age and performance potential). *Deutsche Zeitschrift Sportsmed* **32**, 7–14.
130. Eriksson BO, Karlsson J, Saltin B (1971). Muscle metabolites during exercise in pubertal boys. *Acta Paediatr Scand* **217(Suppl)**, 154–7.
131. Dux L, Dux E, Guba F (1982). Further data on the androgenic dependency of the skeletal musculature: The effect of prepubertal castration of the structural development of the skeletal muscles. *Hormone Metabol Res* **14**, 191–4.
132. Krotkiewski M, Kral JG, Karlsson J (1980). Effects of castration and testosterone substitution on body composition and muscle metabolism in rats. *Acta Physiol Scand* **109**, 233–7.
133. Welsman JR, Armstrong N, Kirby BJ (1994). Serum testosterone is not related to peak $\dot{V}O_2$ and submaximal blood lactate responses in 12–16 year old males. *Pediatr Exerc Sci* **6**, 120–7.
134. Tanner JM (1962). *Growth at adolescence* (2nd ed.). Blackwell Scientific Publications, Oxford.

CHAPTER 9

Field tests of fitness

Grant R. Tomkinson and Timothy S. Olds

Introduction

At one time, short-duration exercise requiring maximal effort was thought to be solely fuelled by anaerobic metabolism, and longer-duration exercise requiring maximal (or near- maximal) effort solely by aerobic metabolism. Anaerobic metabolism—the resynthesis of adenosine triphosphate (ATP) in the absence of oxygen—responds more quickly to the energy demands of exercise but results in a relatively small energy yield. Aerobic metabolism—the resynthesis of ATP in the presence of oxygen—yields by far more ATP, but produces energy more slowly than anaerobic metabolism. However, irrespective of the intensity or duration of the exercise, energy for muscular work is produced by both anaerobic and aerobic metabolism (see Fig. 9.1).

While sophisticated laboratory equipment and appropriate testing protocols are required for the most valid assessment of aerobic and anaerobic fitness, properly conducted field tests offer a simple, feasible, practical, reasonably valid, and reliable alternative. Despite possessing numerous advantages over laboratory-based tests, field tests are not without their disadvantages. There are various factors which influence field test performances, including practice, environmental conditions, motivation, pacing (in the case of many aerobic tests), clothing and field surfaces, pre-test instructions, and the purpose and context of testing. Even so, aerobic and anaerobic field tests have been administered to children and adolescents for over 100 years, with interest in fitness testing accelerating since the Second World War.[2,3] This chapter will focus on field tests which are commonly used to estimate aerobic and anaerobic fitness in children and adolescents. The discussion will be limited to field tests requiring maximal effort, such as distance running tests of aerobic fitness and jumping and sprint running tests of anaerobic fitness (see Chapters 5 and 8 for an analysis of laboratory assessment of these variables). There will also be a discussion of secular changes in aerobic and anaerobic performance.

Aerobic field tests

Aerobic fitness relates to an individual's ability to perform large muscle group exercise of moderate to high intensity for long periods. Performance on tests of aerobic fitness depends on pulmonary, cardiovascular, and haematological components to deliver oxygen to the working muscles and to use the delivered oxygen to generate energy for exercise. There are three major components:

i) Maximum oxygen uptake ($\dot{V}O_2$ max), which is the highest rate at which an individual can consume oxygen during exercise.

ii) Mechanical efficiency or economy, which is the metabolic cost (measured as the oxygen cost) of any given intensity of exercise.

iii) Fractional utilization, which is the percentage of $\dot{V}O_2$ max which can be sustained for any given length of time.

These variables describe the physiological limits of exercise intensity for an individual.[4] The vast majority of paediatric fitness research has concentrated on aerobic fitness. This canalized focus is the result of convincing adult evidence relating aerobic fitness to health outcomes,[5,6] and evidence showing that aerobic fitness and other cardiovascular disease risk factors track (though only moderately well) from childhood and adolescence into adulthood.[7,8] However, because disease risk factors do not generally manifest in childhood or adolescence, it is difficult to relate aerobic fitness to health outcomes directly in children and adolescents. Consequently, paediatric research has focussed on the association between aerobic fitness and cardiovascular disease risk. Several, but not all, studies of children and adolescents have found that low aerobic fitness is related to cardiovascular disease risk.[9,10]

In adults, directly measured $\dot{V}O_2$ max is generally accepted as the gold standard measure of aerobic fitness. In children and adolescents, directly measured peak oxygen uptake (peak $\dot{V}O_2$) is commonly used as the criterion because only a minority of children and adolescents exhibit a plateau in $\dot{V}O_2$ during graded exercise[see Chapter 8]. [11]Directly measured peak $\dot{V}O_2$ testing is time consuming and complicated, requiring sophisticated laboratory procedures and is, therefore, not a practical tool for mass testing. In response to the need for mass testing, as well as the need for simple, feasible, easy, and practical alternatives, numerous field tests of aerobic fitness have been developed. The three main types of aerobic fitness tests commonly administered to children and adolescents are:

i) the *distance run*, where performance is measured as the time taken to cover a fixed distance (e.g. the 1600-m run test);

ii) the *timed run*, where performance is measured as the distance covered in a fixed time (e.g. the 9-min run test); and

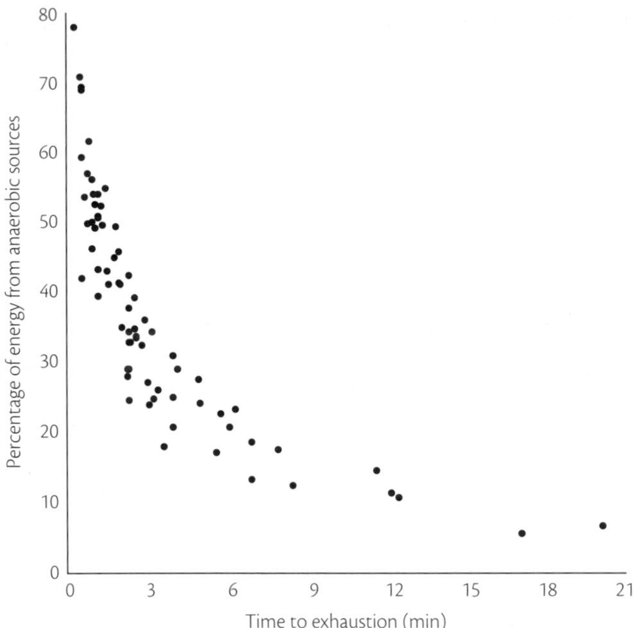

Fig. 9.1 A summary of 20 studies which have quantified the anaerobic contribution to exercise using the oxygen-deficit method. Data were available on adults (active, sprint-trained or endurance-trained) tested using different ergometers (arm–leg, cycle, and treadmill). The references can be found in Olds.[1]

iii) the *endurance shuttle run*, where performance is measured as the number of completed laps of a fixed distance with progressively increasing running speed (e.g. the 20-m shuttle run test).

Though it is acknowledged that other field tests (e.g. step tests) are used to assess aerobic fitness, only running tests requiring maximal effort (i.e. distance, timed, and endurance shuttle runs) will be reviewed in this section.

Distance and timed running tests

Performances on distance and timed running tests have long been used to indicate aerobic fitness in children and adolescents, with published data dating back at least 90 years.[12] Depending on the length or duration of the test, paediatric running performances requiring maximal effort can last from a few to as many as 20 min. Using adult data, in 3 min of maximal-intensity exercise, about 70% of the energy comes from aerobic sources. In 20 min, this rises to above 90% (Fig. 9.1). (Note, although children are typically more aerobic than are adults,[13] these data can be used as a rough guide because comparable paediatric data are sparse) Distance and timed running tests are very easy to administer, requiring only a hand-held stopwatch and a flat marked field (usually a grass oval or running track).

The popularity of distance and timed running tests has evolved over time. In the United States, for example, the 549-m run (600 yards) was the aerobic fitness test described in the first American Alliance for Health, Physical Education and Recreation (AAHPER) Youth Fitness Test Manual.[14] However, construct validation and factor analytic research in the 1970s revealed that the 549-m run was not a good measure of aerobic fitness, and consequently, optional distance (e.g. 1600 and 2400 m) and timed (e.g. 9 and 12 min) runs were included in subsequent AAHPER fitness test batteries. Similarly, in Australia, the most popular distance running test for children and adolescents in the 1960s and the 1970s was the 549-m run. However, since the early 1980s, the 1600-m run test has been the most popular.[15] While this evolving popularity is characteristic of many countries, it is not common to all, with some aerobic tests standing the test of time. In New Zealand for example, the 549-m run test has been the test of choice for numerous national, regional, and local health and fitness surveys of children and adolescents since the early 1960s.[3]

Distance running tests require participants to run (or walk) as fast as possible on a flat marked outdoor course (typically circular) of fixed distance. Performances are recorded as the time to the nearest second. For children and adolescents, distance running tests typically vary in length from several hundred metres to several kilometres. The protocol for the timed running tests is identical to that for distance running tests, except that distance, rather than time, is used as the criterion variable. In a timed running test, participants are instructed to run (or walk) as far as possible in a fixed period of time on a flat marked outdoor course, with distance to the nearest metre recorded. Timed running tests typically range from about 6 to 12 min. From a logistical standpoint, distance runs are preferred over timed runs because the time taken to complete a known distance can be measured more easily than the distance covered in a fixed time period. Furthermore, being able to visualize the distance to be covered offers participants a more precise end point.[16] Performances on distance and timed run tests are often used to estimate $\dot{V}O_2$ max (see ref. 17,18) for prediction equations).

While distance run performances are often expressed in time, and timed run performances in distance, given that speed equals distance divided by time, running performances can also be expressed as average running speed ($m \cdot s^{-1}$). Since mass-specific $\dot{V}O_2$ and $\dot{V}O_2$ max vary linearly with speed and maximal speed, average running speed should better reflect $\dot{V}O_2$, that is, the oxygen cost of the performance. There is certainly some evidence of this, with average running speed over 1600 m reported to be a significantly better predictor of $\dot{V}O_2$ max than running time.[19] In addition, running speed is typically more normally distributed than time or distance, and hence, it is more amenable to parametric statistical analysis.

Numerous studies have reported on the validity of distance and timed running tests in children and adolescents. Fig. 9.2 summarizes 22 studies which have reported the correlation between running performance (nine different distance and timed running tests) and directly measured mass-specific peak $\dot{V}O_2$ ($mL \cdot kg^{-1} \cdot min^{-1}$) in children and adolescents [see 3 for references). The *y* axis shows the coefficient of determination (i.e. the percentage of variance in distance run performance explained by variance in measured peak $\dot{V}O_2$ and the *x* axis the average run distance (for timed runs, the average distance covered was estimated from the reported descriptive summary statistics). The best-fit curve shows tests which require running over longer distances (or running for longer periods of time) are the most valid estimators of peak $\dot{V}O_2$. The strongest relationships occur when the average run distance is about 1600–2400 m, or for timed runs, when the average test duration is about 9–15 min. Performance on longer distance running tests incur an additional time cost for both tester and child. Tests of longer distance or duration may be less feasible and may detract from motivation, especially in younger children. At best, only about 50–60% of the variance in distance run performance is explained by peak

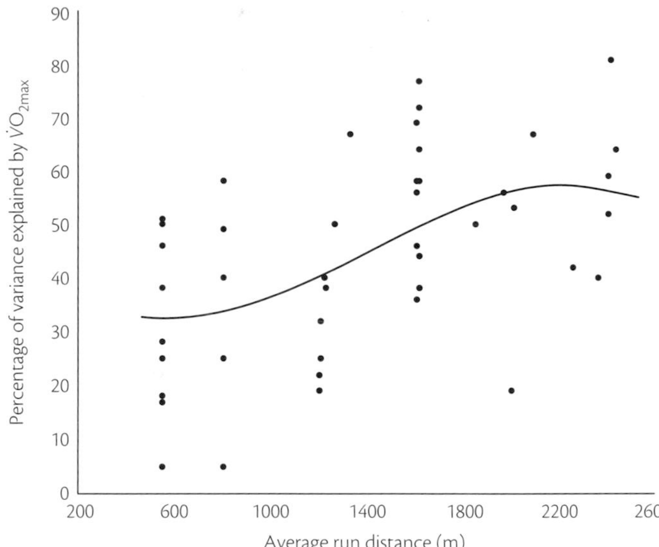

Fig. 9.2 A summary of 22 studies which have reported the correlation between distance run performance (nine different distance and timed runs tests) and directly measured peak $\dot{V}O_2$ (mL·kg^{-1}·min^{-1}) in children and adolescents (see 3). The *y* axis shows the coefficient of determination (%) and the x axis the average run distance(s). (Note, in timed run tests, the average distance covered was estimated from the reported descriptive summary statistics). The line of best fit is shown as a third-order polynomial.

$\dot{V}O_2$ These data confirm that factors other than peak $\dot{V}O_2$ contribute to distance running performance. Running economy,[20] fractional utilization,[21] $\dot{V}O_2$ kinetics,[22] lactate threshold,[23] anaerobic capacity,[24] maximal running speed,[21,25] fat mass,[25] and psychosocial factors such as pacing, self-efficacy, and motivation,[26] have all been associated with distance running performance in children and adolescents. Moreover, different distance run tests impose different physiological and psychosocial demands. For example, factors such as $\dot{V}O_2$ kinetics and anaerobic capacity will be relatively more important for shorter distance runs (see Fig. 9.1)—though the effect will be very small over distances of more than several hundred metres[22]—and peak $\dot{V}O_2$ relatively more important for longer distance runs.

Distance and timed running tests are highly reliable. In a review of 10 reliability studies of distance and timed running tests, Safrit *et al.* [27] reported a sample weighted average coefficient of determination (r^2) of +0.80. These data compare favourably to reliability data on criterion measures of aerobic fitness (e.g. peak $\dot{V}O_2$) [see ref. 27 and Chapter 8].

Methodologically, there are many similarities and differences among the various distance and timed running tests extant today. In a meta-analysis of paediatric aerobic performance, Tomkinson[3] reported that all reviewed test protocols recommend scoring performances based on a single run, standardized to a standing start, and in the case of distance run performances, recorded using a handheld stopwatch. However, the running course is not always standardized. Take the 1600-m run for example. Some test protocols recommend that the 1600-m distance be run as four laps of a 400-m course, others as eight laps of a 200-m course, a difference which could conceivably affect performance. Practice can significantly affect distance running performance. Watkins and Moore[28,29] reported that Scottish school boys and girls (aged 12–15 years) improved their 1609-m (1 mile) run times by 7–8% over three trials in the space of 2 weeks, presumably due to improved tactical awareness. It is also conceivable that differences in the actual test name (e.g. run test vs. run/walk test) could result in different types of performance. Environmental factors such as temperature, humidity, and ground conditions are rarely controlled or reported by testers and are, therefore, likely to increase performance variability.

Distance run performance improves as children grow. Analysis of Australian data cumulated across 10 studies (N = 39,239) shows that between the ages of 7 and 16 years, there is an age-related improvement of 35% and 21% in 1600-m run performance of boys and girls, respectively. Boys' performance continues to improve until about the age of 15 years whereas girls' performance stabilizes around the age of 13 years. But what is causing this age-related performance improvement? At present, the picture is unclear. Examination of age-related changes in factors which underscore distance run performance may provide some clues. While peak $\dot{V}O_2$ explains a moderate to large proportion of distance running performance cross-sectionally, it provides little insight longitudinally. The reviews of Armstrong and Welsman[30] and Krahenbuhl *et al.*[31] indicated that as children grow, mass-specific peak $\dot{V}O_2$ remains relatively stable in boys and declines (by about 30%) in girls. On the other hand, cross-sectional and longitudinal studies examining running economy in children indicate that older children are more economical than younger children.[32–34] This means that older children can perform longer at the same speed, or faster over the same distance. Another answer may lie with fractional utilization. Krahenbuhl *et al.*[34] reported that the superior 9-min running performances of older boys was partly explained by their better ability to sustain a higher fraction of peak $\dot{V}O_2$. While a number of alternative models have been proposed, few have been extensively tested experimentally.[35]

Endurance shuttle running tests

Since its description in 1984 by Léger *et al.*,[36] the 20-m shuttle run test (20mSRT) with 1-min stages [note, the test was originally described with 2-min stages—see ref. 37] has been widely used to assess the aerobic fitness of children, adolescents, and adults. The test consists of a number of stages (also called levels), each lasting about 1 min and comprising a number of 20-m laps (also called shuttles), paced by beeps on a cassette or CD. At each stage, the required running speed increases, until the participant can no longer reach the 20-m distance on cue. Each stage includes seven or more laps, depending on the required running speed and exact protocol used. The test has been shown to be a reliable and valid method of estimating peak $\dot{V}O_2$ in children and adolescents. A recent review of 15 reliability and validity studies reported a sample weighted average coefficient of determination (r^2) of 0.51 for validity (relative to directly measured peak $\dot{V}O_2$), and 0.73 for reliability.[38] Today, the 20mSRT is probably the most widely used aerobic field test with children and adolescents.

Relative to distance and timed running tests, the 20mSRT offers several advantages. First, the running course for the 20mSRT is shorter; therefore, less space is required. Second, the 20mSRT can be conducted indoors, where the environmental conditions (e.g. temperature) can be more easily controlled. Third, because the 20mSRT is externally paced, cognitive aspects of maximal performance are less likely to be important. And fourth, participants can be more closely monitored by testing personnel. On the down side, and as a function of the shorter course, the 20mSRT requires participants to run back and forth along a 20-m course, by pivoting at the end of each lap to change direction. This intermittent style of running may lead to exhaustion through localized leg fatigue rather than central fatigue. Also, for some children, especially younger children, the initial stages may be set at too fast a pace, leading to premature onset of fatigue.

Although the 20mSRT is widely used, there are numerous methodological issues associated with it, including the existence of a number of variant forms of the test, small differences in the conduct of the test, and the use of different metrics for expressing performances. Some of these issues are briefly described below. However, for a thorough review of these methodological issues, the reader is referred to the extensive review of Tomkinson *et al.*.[39]

Tomkinson *et al.*[39] described the three major variants of the 1-min stage test extant today as follows:

i) Léger's original 1-min protocol[36] which starts at a speed of 8.5 km·h^{-1}, and increases in speed by 0.5 km·h^{-1} each minute.

ii) The protocol used by the Eurofit,[40] the Australian Coaching Council,[41] the British National Coaching Foundation,[42] and the American Progressive Aerobic Cardiovascular Endurance Run (PACER)[43] system, among others. In this protocol, participants start at a speed of 8.0 km·h^{-1}, the second stage is at 9.0 km·h^{-1}, and thereafter increases in speed by 0.5 km·h^{-1} each min.

iii) The Queen's University of Belfast protocol (QUB)[44] which starts at 8.0 km·h^{-1}, and increases in speed by 0.5 km·h^{-1} each minute.

In addition, there are often several different cassettes or CDs (often produced in-house) used for the same protocol. Methodological variations on these cassettes (e.g. calling the stage number at the start versus the finish of each stage; using only full minutes versus both full minutes and half minutes to indicate completed stages) means that identical performances are reported in different ways. In addition to variation in protocols, there has been variation in how results have been reported. Individual results have been reported as the number of completed stages, the running speed at the last completed stage, the number of completed laps (or stages plus laps), the number of minutes the test lasted, or as an estimated $\dot{V}O_2$ max based on regression equations.[42,45,46] In order to minimize methodological variability, Tomkinson *et al.* 39 recommend the use of single-test protocol (e.g. Léger's original protocol), or at least that the protocol used should be accurately reported, and that 20mSRT performances should ideally be expressed as running speed at the last completed 1-min stage.

World percentile ranks for the 20mSRT [speed (km·h^{-1}) at the last completed 1-min stage] among healthy 7- to 18-year-old boys and girls are shown in Tables 9.1 and 9.2, respectively. 20mSRT data were collected using the 1-min stage protocol [standardized to Léger's protocol—see ref. 39 for details] on 417,991 children and adolescents from 37 countries (across six continents) between 1981 and 2003 (see ref. 47–49). Higher percentile values represent superior 20mSRT performance. Over the 1981–2003 period, paediatric 20mSRT performances declined globally at –0.43% per annum (p.a.).[39] It is, therefore, likely that these data, with a median measurement year of 1999, would overestimate 20mSRT performances in 2007 by approximately 3.4%. As with distance run peformances, 20mSRT performances improve as children grow (Fig. 9.3), although the improvement is somewhat less for 20mSRT performance than for distance run performance. Between the ages of 7 and 18 years, boys' 20mSRT performances improved by about 30%, increasing every year of age until 18 years. In girls, the age-related improvement is less than half as great (13%), with performance stabilizing from about the age of 15 years.

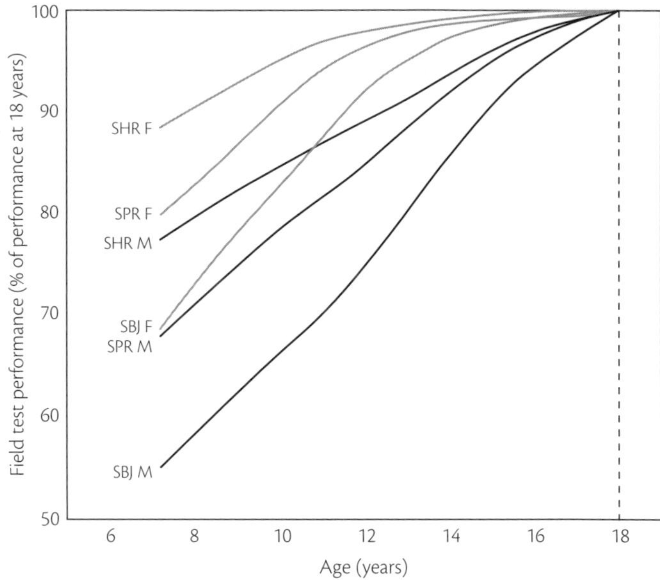

Fig. 9.3 The age-related changes in standing broad jump, 50-m sprint running and 20-m shuttle running performance in 7- to 18-year-olds. Performances are represented as a percentage of the performances at the age of 18 years. Smoothed (fitted) lines are shown for each sex × test group. Data are cross-sectional and were taken from Jürimäe *et al.*,[47] Olds *et al.*,[48] Tomkinson[74] and Tomkinson *et al.*.[49] Note, SHR F = 20-m shuttle run (females); SHR M = 20-m shuttle run (males); SBJ F = standing broad jump (females); SBJ M = standing broad jump (males); SPR F = 50-m sprint (females); and SPR M = 50-m sprint (males).

Anaerobic field tests

The vast majority of research into paediatric fitness has focused on aerobic fitness rather than anaerobic fitness. This is not surprising given that aerobic fitness is better defined, easier to study, and has been linked to health outcomes.[5] However, this lop-sided focus leaves many with the misguided belief that anaerobic fitness is not important. Anaerobic fitness may be just as important as aerobic fitness in maintaining overall health and function,[50] especially in children and adolescents. Short-duration activities make up the bulk of the daily physical activities of children and adolescents. Bailey *et al.*,[51] in an observational study of 6- to 10-year-old children in natural conditions, found that children more often engaged in very intense, short-duration activities than in less intense activities of longer duration. The average duration of activities of all intensities was 6 s, with 95% of all intense activities lasting < 15 s. These results are similar to those reported by Baranowski *et al.*[52] and Gilliam *et al.*.[53] The importance of anaerobic fitness to success in a range of sports, particularly intermittent sports such as basketball, hockey, football, and soccer, is well established.[54,55] Since the majority of paediatric physical activities involve high-intensity

Table 9.1 Percentile ranks for 20-m shuttle run [speed ($km \cdot h^{-1}$) at the last completed 1-min stage] for 7–18-year-old boys

Percentile	7 years	8 years	9 years	10 years	11 years	12 years	13 years	14 years	15 years	16 years	17 years	18 years
99	11.5	12.0	12.5	13.0	13.5	14.0	14.5	14.5	15.0	15.5	15.5	15.5
95	11.0	11.5	12.0	12.5	12.5	13.0	13.5	13.5	14.0	14.5	14.5	14.5
90	10.5	11.0	11.5	12.0	12.0	12.5	13.0	13.0	13.5	14.0	14.0	14.0
80	10.0	10.5	11.0	11.5	11.5	12.0	12.5	12.5	13.0	13.0	13.5	13.5
75	10.0	10.5	11.0	11.0	11.5	12.0	12.0	12.5	12.5	13.0	13.0	13.0
70	10.0	10.5	10.5	11.0	11.5	11.5	12.0	12.0	12.5	13.0	13.0	13.0
60	9.5	10.0	10.5	10.5	11.0	11.5	11.5	12.0	12.0	12.5	12.5	12.5
50	9.5	10.0	10.0	10.5	11.0	11.0	11.0	11.5	12.0	12.0	12.0	12.0
40	9.0	9.5	10.0	10.0	10.5	10.5	11.0	11.0	11.5	11.5	12.0	12.0
30	9.0	9.5	9.5	10.0	10.0	10.5	10.5	11.0	11.0	11.5	11.5	11.5
25	9.0	9.0	9.5	9.5	10.0	10.0	10.5	10.5	11.0	11.0	11.5	11.5
20	8.5	9.0	9.0	9.5	9.5	10.0	10.0	10.5	11.0	11.0	11.0	11.0
10	8.5	8.5	9.0	9.0	9.0	9.5	9.5	10.0	10.0	10.5	10.5	10.5
5	8.0	8.0	8.5	8.5	9.0	9.0	9.0	9.5	9.5	10.0	10.0	10.0
1	8.0	8.0	8.0	8.0	8.0	8.0	8.0	8.0	8.5	8.5	9.0	9.0
Mean	9.5	9.9	10.1	10.5	10.7	10.9	11.2	11.5	11.8	12.1	12.2	12.3
SD	0.9	1.0	1.1	1.1	1.2	1.2	1.3	1.3	1.3	1.4	1.4	1.4
n	10,138	9562	12,935	18,886	16,050	26,369	28,085	27,702	23,028	13,757	15,430	8,580

Note: Data were available for boys from 37 countries (across six continents) tested between 1981 and 2003. Higher percentile values indicate superior performances.

Source: Based on data from Jürimäe *et al.*,[47] Olds *et al.*,[48] and Tomkinson *et al.*[49]

Table 9.2 Percentile ranks for 20-m shuttle run [speed ($km \cdot h^{-1}$) at the last completed 1 min stage] for 7–18-year-old girls.

Percentile	7 years	8 years	9 years	10 years	11 years	12 years	13 years	14 years	15 years	16 years	17 years	18 years
99	11.0	11.5	12.0	12.0	12.5	12.5	13.0	13.0	13.0	13.0	13.0	13.0
95	10.5	11.0	11.0	11.5	12.0	12.0	12.0	12.0	12.0	12.0	12.0	12.0
90	10.0	10.5	11.0	11.0	11.5	11.5	11.5	12.0	12.0	12.0	12.0	12.0
80	10.0	10.0	10.5	10.5	11.0	11.0	11.0	11.5	11.5	11.5	11.5	11.5
75	9.5	10.0	10.5	10.5	11.0	11.0	11.0	11.0	11.0	11.0	11.0	11.0
70	9.5	10.0	10.0	10.5	10.5	11.0	11.0	11.0	11.0	11.0	11.0	11.0
60	9.5	9.5	10.0	10.0	10.5	10.5	10.5	10.5	10.5	10.5	10.5	10.5
50	9.0	9.5	9.5	10.0	10.0	10.0	10.0	10.5	10.5	10.5	10.5	10.5
40	9.0	9.5	9.5	9.5	10.0	10.0	10.0	10.0	10.0	10.0	10.0	10.0
30	9.0	9.0	9.0	9.5	9.5	9.5	9.5	10.0	10.0	10.0	10.0	10.0
25	8.5	9.0	9.0	9.5	9.5	9.5	9.5	9.5	9.5	9.5	9.5	9.5
20	8.5	9.0	9.0	9.0	9.5	9.5	9.5	9.5	9.5	9.5	9.5	9.5
10	8.5	8.5	8.5	9.0	9.0	9.0	9.0	9.0	9.0	9.0	9.0	9.0
5	8.0	8.0	8.0	8.5	8.5	8.5	8.5	8.5	8.5	8.5	8.5	8.5
1	8.0	8.0	8.0	8.0	8.0	8.0	8.0	8.0	8.0	8.0	8.0	8.0
Mean	9.2	9.5	9.7	9.9	10.1	10.2	10.3	10.3	10.4	10.4	10.5	10.4
SD	0.7	0.8	0.9	0.9	1.0	1.0	1.1	1.1	1.0	1.0	1.2	1.1
n	10,168	10,868	12,700	18,409	16,016	27,105	27,697	25,565	20,747	13,988	15,293	8,913

Note: Data were available for girls from 34 countries (across six continents) tested between 1981 and 2003. Higher percentile values indicate superior performances.

Source: Based on data from Jürimäe *et al.*,[47] Olds *et al.*,[48] and Tomkinson *et al.*.[49]

bursts requiring the production of anaerobic energy, monitoring and tracking of anaerobic performance may provide meaningful information about the status of, and changes in, these natural daily physical activities. As Rowland[35] argued, anaerobic activities should be the focus of efforts to improve paediatric physical activity.

Anaerobic performance tests can be divided into tests which measure anaerobic power (the maximum rate at which anaerobic energy can be supplied during short-duration, maximal-intensity exercise) and anaerobic capacity (the maximum amount of anaerobic energy which can be supplied during short-duration, maximal-intensity exercise). Tests which measure efforts lasting up to about 10 s are typically thought of as anaerobic power tests, while tests measuring efforts lasting longer than 10 s (and up to about 60 s) are typically thought of as anaerobic capacity tests (ref. 26 and see Chapter 5).

A plethora of tests have been developed to assess anaerobic power and capacity. The vast majority of these tests have been developed to assess lower body/leg power and capacity, with few developed for upper body/arm power and capacity.[56] While a number of laboratory tests are available (e.g. monarticular force–velocity tests, staircase-running tests, and friction-loaded and isokinetic cycle ergometer tests), field testing alternatives have been limited principally to the assessment of anaerobic power (e.g. jumping and sprint running tests). (For a thorough review of laboratory-based tests of anaerobic performance see ref. 57,58 and Chapter 5) As Van Praagh[57] suggested, it is maximal-intensity performance which should be the focus of anaerobic assessment. Though it is acknowledged that jumping and sprint running tests are not exclusively field tests (e.g. vertical jump performance can be measured in the field or in the laboratory using a force platform), this section will focus only on the field test variants. The discussion will be limited to field tests requiring maximal effort, such as jumping (e.g. jumping for maximal vertical height and horizontal distance) and sprint running (e.g. short-distance sprint running) tests.

Jumping tests

Since its original description in 1921,[59] the vertical jump test has been widely used to indicate explosive muscular power. This is based on the assumption that the energy needs of a single, maximal jump are met by anaerobic energy sources (i.e. the ATP-phosphocreatine system). The test requires participants to use a double-leg take-off to jump, using a countermovement (i.e. a rapid knee bending preparatory to the jump), as high as possible vertically (with fingers extended). Jump height is taken to be the vertical distance between the height of the jump and the height reached by the participant when standing erect with arms and fingers extended vertically. Performances are recorded to the nearest centimetre and typically scored as the better of two, or best of three, jumps. While many variants to Sargent's vertical jump protocol exist today, most mimic it closely. Vertical jump performance can be measured with minimal equipment, using a piece of chalk with which to strike a wall-mounted board and a measuring tape, or more precisely with the use of electronic pressure sensors placed over a wall-mounted board. In addition, because vertical jump performance has the dimension of work (i.e. the distance through which a force—the weight of the body—is moved), not power, it has been strongly criticized as test of explosive muscular power. (Note, the Lewis formula[60] can be used to convert vertical jump performance to power output, although the validity of this procedure is questionable see ref. 61). Nevertheless, the vertical jump test is considered a criterion of explosive muscular power.[35]

Numerous jump tests other than the vertical jump have been proposed to assess explosive muscular power. These include single- and multiple-jump tests for maximum vertical and horizontal distance, using a single- or double-leg take-off.[56] Of these, the standing broad jump is most often used in lieu of the vertical jump. It has long been used as a test of explosive power in many performance-test batteries (e.g. the Eurofit, AAHPER Youth Fitness Test) and is frequently used as part of fitness surveys of children and adolescents. Using a double-leg take-off, the standing broad jump test requires participants to use a countermovement to jump as far as possible horizontally. Jump distance is measured using a measuring tape from the front edge of the starting line to the point where the back of the heel nearest to the starting line lands. As with the vertical jump, performances are recorded to the nearest centimetre and depending on the protocol, scored as the better of two, or best of three, jumps.

Few studies have reported on the validity and reliability of jump tests, in part due to the problem of identifying appropriate criterion measures. Safrit [62] reported a very high correlation ($r = 0.78$) between vertical jump performance and four power events in track and field, although it is not clear which athletic events were used. A high correlation ($r = 0.92$) has also been reported between field- and laboratory-based (measured by force platform) vertical jump tests.[63] Bar-Or [64] reported that the correlation between vertical jump performance and peak power measured on the Wingate anaerobic test in 48 adolescent boys was very high ($r = 0.77$). A strong link between the standing broad jump test and an unspecified 'pure' power test ($r = 0.61$) has also been reported.[65] Using one test as a criterion for the other, Larson[66] reported that the standing broad and vertical jumps were very highly correlated ($r = 0.79$). Considering reliability, a review of seven reliability studies of the standing broad and vertical jumps reported a sample weighted average coefficient of determination (r^2) of +0.83.[67]

A considerable amount of intersubject variability in jump performance can be linked to differences in test methodologies. For example, significant differences in jump heights have been reported for different vertical jump tests[68] and between jump heights recorded in the laboratory and the field.[69,70] Jump test performances are also affected by differences in countermovements and scoring methods. Bosco and Komi[69,70] reported that countermovement jumps (e.g. with rapid preparatory knee bending) are typically superior (by about 10%) to crouch jumps where countermovements are minimized likely because of the reuse of elastic energy and the stretch-reflex potentiation. The magnitude and rate of the countermovement is also important.[71] There is also some evidence that jumps which allow rapid arm swinging are superior (again by about 10%) to jumps which minimize arm swinging.[72] It is also possible that differences in the magnitude of trunk extension will affect vertical jump performance.[73] Furthermore, jump test performances are highly dependant on the scoring method used (e.g. the number of trials allowed). While jump performances are typically scored as either the better of two jumps or the best of three (and rarely scored as a single jump), systematic differences have been reported between different scoring methods.[3] It is likely that these differences are a function of learning and recovery. For example, if enough time were allowed between jumps to maximize a learning effect and minimize fatigue, then performance would

Table 9.3 Percentile ranks for standing broad jump performances (cm) for 7–18-year-old European boys

Percentile	7 years	8 years	9 years	10 years	11 years	12 years	13 years	14 years	15 years	16 years	17 years	18 years
99	169	176	184	195	208	221	235	248	258	266	272	277
95	157	162	170	180	191	204	217	230	240	249	255	260
90	149	155	162	171	183	195	208	220	231	239	246	250
80	140	145	153	162	173	185	197	209	220	228	235	240
75	137	142	149	158	169	181	193	205	215	224	231	236
70	134	139	146	155	165	177	189	201	211	220	227	232
60	128	134	141	149	159	171	182	194	204	213	220	225
50	123	128	135	144	154	165	176	187	197	206	213	219
40	118	123	130	139	148	159	170	181	191	200	207	213
30	112	118	125	133	142	153	163	174	183	192	200	206
25	109	115	121	130	139	149	159	170	179	188	196	202
20	105	111	118	126	135	145	155	165	175	184	191	198
10	96	102	109	117	126	135	144	154	163	171	179	187
5	88	95	102	110	118	127	135	144	153	161	170	178
1	74	81	88	95	103	119	118	126	134	142	150	158
Mean	123	128	139	144	154	165	176	187	197	206	213	219
SD	21	21	21	22	23	23	24	25	26	26	27	27
n	5448	6735	7472	13,439	10,045	15,313	12,052	12,415	12,137	8067	7656	4246

Note: Data were available for boys from 22 European countries tested between 1982 and 2003. Higher percentile values indicate superior performances.

Source: Based on Eurofit data from Tomkinson *et al.*.[49]

Table 9.4 Percentile ranks for standing broad jump performances (cm) for 7–18-year-old European girls

Percentile	7 years	8 years	9 years	10 years	11 years	12 years	13 years	14 years	15 years	16 years	17 years	18 years
99	159	166	176	187	199	207	213	216	218	219	219	219
95	147	153	162	173	183	190	196	199	200	201	202	202
90	139	146	155	165	174	182	187	190	191	192	193	193
80	130	137	146	155	164	171	176	179	181	182	183	183
75	127	134	142	152	161	167	172	175	177	179	179	180
70	124	131	139	149	157	164	169	172	174	175	176	176
60	119	125	134	143	151	158	163	166	168	169	170	170
50	114	120	128	137	145	152	157	160	162	164	164	165
40	109	115	123	132	140	146	151	154	157	158	159	159
30	103	110	118	126	134	140	145	148	150	152	153	153
25	100	107	115	123	130	136	141	145	147	148	149	150
20	97	104	111	119	126	133	137	141	143	145	146	146
10	88	95	103	111	117	123	127	130	133	134	136	136
5	80	88	96	103	109	114	119	122	124	126	127	128
1	65	74	82	89	95	99	103	105	108	109	110	111
Mean	114	120	129	137	145	152	157	160	162	164	164	165
SD	19	20	21	22	22	23	23	23	23	23	23	22
n	5408	6583	7033	12,912	9933	16,198	12,143	12,139	11,755	8046	7557	4097

Note: Data were available for girls from 23 European countries tested between 1981 and 2003. Higher percentile values indicate superior performances.

Source: Based on Eurofit data from Tomkinson *et al.*,[49]

likely improve with successive jumps. However, if successive jumps were not spaced far enough apart to facilitate recovery, then the effect of fatigue may outweigh the learning effect and result in poorer successive jump performance. It is also possible that differences in testing equipment (e.g. wall-mounted boards vs. portable devices) could affect jump height, although no supporting data are available.

European percentile ranks for the standing broad jump (cm) among healthy 7- to 18-year-old boys and girls are shown in Tables 9.3 and 9.4, respectively. Standing broad jump data were collected using the Eurofit protocol[40] on 228,829 young Europeans from 23 countries between 1981 and 2003 (see ref. 49) for references but note that because of differences in test methodologies, only Eurofit data were used]. Higher percentile values represent superior jumping performance. It should be noted that over the 1981–2003 period, jumping performances declined in young Europeans at −0.20% p.a..[74] It is, therefore, likely that these data, with a median measurement year of 1997, would overestimate standing broad jump performances in 2007 by approximately 2%.

Using cumulated cross-sectional Eurofit data, Fig. 9.3 graphically illustrates the age-related changes in standing broad jump performances of boys and girls. Standing broad jump performances improved by 81% and 46% in boys and girls between the ages of 7 and 18 years, respectively. The age-related improvement for boys was linear, with performances increasing for each year of age through to age of 18 years. For girls, jump performances increased until about the age of 14 years and plateaued thereafter. Klausen *et al.*[75] reported similar longitudinal changes. Analysis of cross-sectional data on vertical jump performance shows a parallel age-related pattern of change.[76] These age-related improvements in jump test performance appear to match age-related changes in body mass.[75] For example, Klausen *et al.*[75] reported no significant age-related change in mass-corrected vertical jump performances of 10- to 12-year-old boys and girls, and 13- to 15-year-old boys. However, there was a significant age-related decline in 13- to 15-year-old girls.

Sprint running tests

Sprint running tests have traditionally been used as a measure of maximal running speed, and thus they are thought to reflect short-duration, maximal-intensity anaerobic power. Intuitively, this makes sense, because the duration of the most commonly used sprints running tests (e.g. 30–50 m) is typically less than about 12 s, leaving performances highly dependant on anaerobic energy sources (see Fig. 9.1). Sprint running tests are very easy to administer and can be performed with minimal equipment, indoors or outdoors, and in little time. Sprint running, like jumping, is a natural activity for children and adolescents and is typical of many athletic endeavours. However, given that power is the product of force and velocity, sprint running tests cannot be considered a true power test because the force component is not measured.[77]

Sprint running tests require participants to run as fast as possible over a flat marked course of short distance. Tests ranging from 20 to 100 m have been described, with 30–50-m sprints the most commonly used. Generally, sprint running tests can not only be performed outdoors on a grass field or a running track but can also be performed indoors, provided there is sufficient room for the sprint run and post-run braking. It is common for the sprint run to be performed only once, using a standing start, with the time taken recorded to the nearest 0.01 s.[3] While few studies have reported on the validity and reliability of sprint running tests, general face validity has been accepted.[65] Van Praagh *et al.* [78] reported a very high correlation ($r = 0.80$) between peak power measured on a cycle force–velocity test and 30-m sprint performance in 7- to 12-year-old boys and girls, although the correlation was significantly lower when only the girls' data were analysed. In a review of four reliability studies of the 46-m (50 yards) sprint, Docherty[67] reported a sample weighted average coefficient of determination (r^2) of +0.71.

Sprint performance, like any other field test performance, is highly dependant on the test methodology used. While methodological issues common to all field tests have been outlined above, sprint performances are specifically affected by differences in recording methods, the scoring methods, and sprint starting position. Consider first differences in recording methods. Traditionally, handheld stopwatches have been used to record sprint times, but in recent years, electronic timers have increased in popularity. Harman *et al.*[79] reported that the correlation between electronic and stopwatch times in 37-m (40 yards) sprint performance of 70 male American football players was nearly perfect ($r = 0.98$). On average, stopwatch times are 0.23 s faster than electronic times—the likely function of human reaction time. The effect of this will be quantitatively larger for shorter sprint runs. This difference might account for as much as 10 percentile points (see Tables 9.5 and 9.6). Second, despite that most test protocols recommend scoring sprint performances based on a single sprint, some protocols recommend the use of multiple trials (e.g. better of two or best of three). It is, therefore, conceivable that differences in scoring methods could lead to systematic differences between performances. However, data from several reliability studies of the 46-m (50 yards) sprint show no practice effect.[80–82] Third, while it is conceivable that differences in starting positions (e.g. crouch start vs. standing start) could systematically affect sprint performances, no quantifiable data are available.

World percentile ranks for the 50-m sprint (s) among healthy 7- to 18-year-old boys and girls are shown in Tables 9.5 and 9.6, respectively. Sprint running data were collected using the same protocol (stopwatch-timed sprints from a standing start) on 1,982,731 children and adolescents from nine countries (across four continents) between 1980 and 2003 (see ref. 74 for references). Higher percentile values represent superior sprint running performance. Note, over the 1980–2003 period, paediatric sprint running performances declined globally at −0.05% p.a..[74] It is, therefore, likely that these data, with a median measurement year of 1990, would overestimate 50-m sprint running performances in 2007 by approximately 0.9%.

Numerous studies have described age-related improvements in sprint performance. While some studies have shown the age-related improvements to be similar for boys and girls, most show greater age-related improvements in boys. Summarizing the data from Tables 9.5 and 9.6, Fig. 9.3 shows the age-related changes in 50-m sprint performance for boys and girls. In boys, average 50-m sprint performance improved by 47% between the ages of 7 and 18 years, while for girls, average sprint performance improved by 26%. Analysis of longitudinal data shows similar age-related changes.

The mechanistic factors underlying these age-related improvements in sprint performance are not altogether clear. This is

Table 9.5 Percentile ranks for 50-m sprint run performances (s) for 7–18-year-old boys

Percentile	7 years	8 years	9 years	10 years	11 years	12 years	13 years	14 years	15 years	16 years	17 years	18 years
99	8.5	8.3	8.1	7.8	7.6	7.3	7.0	6.8	6.7	6.6	6.5	6.4
95	9.1	8.8	8.5	8.2	7.9	7.6	7.3	7.1	7.0	6.8	6.7	6.6
90	9.4	9.1	8.8	8.4	8.1	7.8	7.5	7.3	7.1	7.0	6.9	6.8
80	9.8	9.5	9.1	8.7	8.4	8.1	7.8	7.5	7.3	7.2	7.0	6.9
75	10.0	9.6	9.2	8.8	8.5	8.2	7.9	7.6	7.4	7.3	7.1	7.0
70	10.1	9.8	9.4	9.0	8.6	8.3	8.0	7.7	7.5	7.3	7.2	7.1
60	10.4	10.0	9.6	9.2	8.8	8.4	8.1	7.9	7.6	7.5	7.3	7.2
50	10.7	10.3	9.8	9.4	9.0	8.6	8.3	8.0	7.8	7.6	7.4	7.3
40	11.0	10.6	10.1	9.6	9.2	8.8	8.5	8.2	7.9	7.7	7.6	7.4
30	11.3	10.9	10.4	9.9	9.4	9.0	8.7	8.4	8.1	7.9	7.7	7.5
25	11.6	11.0	10.5	10.0	9.6	9.2	8.8	8.5	8.2	8.0	7.8	7.6
20	11.8	11.2	10.7	10.2	9.7	9.3	8.9	8.6	8.3	8.1	7.9	7.7
10	12.5	11.8	11.2	10.6	10.1	9.7	9.3	8.9	8.6	8.3	8.1	7.9
5	13.0	12.3	11.6	11.0	10.5	10.0	9.6	9.2	8.9	8.6	8.3	8.1
1	14.2	13.3	12.5	11.8	11.2	10.7	10.2	9.7	9.4	9.0	8.7	8.5
Mean	10.8	10.4	9.9	9.5	9.1	8.7	8.4	8.1	7.8	7.6	7.5	7.3
SD	1.2	1.1	1.0	0.9	0.8	0.7	0.7	0.6	0.6	0.5	0.5	0.5
n	57,659	69,795	69,084	89,652	97,304	90,687	87,278	95,292	88,564	88,544	90,710	72,142

Note: Data were available for boys from nine countries (across four continents) tested between 1980 and 2003. Higher percentile values indicate superior performances.

Source: Based on data from Tomkinson.[74]

Table 9.6 Percentile ranks for 50-m sprint run performances(s) for 7–18-year-old girls

Percentile	7 years	8 years	9 years	10 years	11 years	12 years	13 years	14 years	15 years	16 years	17 years	18 years
99	9.0	8.7	8.4	8.1	7.9	7.8	7.7	7.7	7.7	7.7	7.6	7.6
95	9.5	9.2	8.8	8.5	8.2	8.1	8.0	8.0	8.0	8.0	8.0	8.0
90	9.8	9.5	9.1	8.7	8.5	8.3	8.2	8.2	8.2	8.2	8.2	8.2
80	10.2	9.9	9.5	9.0	8.7	8.6	8.5	8.4	8.4	8.4	8.4	8.4
75	10.4	10.0	9.6	9.2	8.9	8.7	8.6	8.6	8.5	8.5	8.5	8.5
70	10.6	10.2	9.7	9.3	9.0	8.8	8.7	8.6	8.6	8.6	8.6	8.6
60	10.9	10.5	10.0	9.5	9.2	9.0	8.9	8.8	8.8	8.8	8.8	8.8
50	11.2	10.8	10.2	9.7	9.4	9.2	9.1	9.0	9.0	9.0	9.0	9.0
40	11.6	11.1	10.5	10.0	9.6	9.4	9.3	9.2	9.2	9.2	9.2	9.2
30	12.0	11.4	10.8	10.3	9.9	9.7	9.6	9.5	9.4	9.4	9.4	9.4
25	12.2	11.6	11.0	10.4	10.1	9.8	9.7	9.6	9.6	9.6	9.5	9.5
20	12.5	11.8	11.2	10.6	10.2	10.0	9.8	9.8	9.7	9.7	9.7	9.7
10	13.2	12.5	11.8	11.2	10.7	10.5	10.3	10.2	10.1	10.1	10.1	10.1
5	13.9	13.2	12.4	11.7	11.2	10.9	10.7	10.6	10.5	10.5	10.5	10.5
1	15.3	14.6	13.7	12.9	12.2	11.8	11.5	11.4	11.3	11.2	11.2	11.2
Mean	11.4	10.9	10.4	9.9	9.5	9.3	9.2	9.1	9.1	9.1	9.1	9.1
SD	1.3	1.2	1.1	1.0	0.9	0.9	0.8	0.8	0.8	0.8	0.7	0.7
n	57,206	68,228	67,626	87,851	95,724	89,301	86,605	94,115	88,228	88,834	90,748	71,554

Note: Data were available for girls from nine countries (across four continents) tested between 1980 and 2003. Higher percentile values indicate superior performances.

Source: Based on data from Tomkinson.[74]

primarily because there are few experimental studies which have examined the development of paediatric sprint running performance. The consensus is that the vast majority of the age-related improvement in sprint performance is explained by increases in body size (e.g. height). Numerous other factors, such as stride length[83] (itself a function of increases in body size), force production,[84] muscle strength,[85] muscle fibre typing,[86] and neural factors,[87] have also been implicated. Furthermore, while sprint running is highly dependent on anaerobic energy supply, adult data suggest that anaerobic capacity is not rate limiting.[88] Therefore, it appears that physical factors, rather than metabolic factors, are primarily responsible for the age-related performance improvements. [Note, this explanation may not hold true for other short-duration activities (e.g. swimming) and cross-sectional comparisons of paediatric sprint performance.] The reader is referred to Rowland[35] for a thorough review of the mechanistic factors summarized here.

Recommendations

- Whatever field test is used, children and adolescents should be given the opportunity to practise the test to minimize the potential influence of cognitive and affective factors, such as pacing and motivation.
- Aerobic tests should ideally cover at least 1600 m to minimize the influence of anaerobic contributions.
- It is preferable, other things being equal, to select tests for which substantial reference data are available. The Eurofit test battery[40] offers a widely used collection of tests with a wide range of reference data across ages and countries.
- Reference to norms should take into account secular changes in fitness test performance. Using norms established several years ago may underestimate the relative performance of children today.
- Results of running tests, both short and long duration should be expressed as speeds for analysis. In particular, the results of the 20mSRT should be expressed as the running speed at the last completed 1-min stage.

Secular changes in aerobic and anaerobic performance

There has been considerable interest in both the popular and scientific literature regarding whether today's children and adolescents are fitter than yesterday's children and adolescents. On the back of considerable anecdotal and lay speculation, it is widely believed that the fitness of children and adolescents has declined in recent decades. Sedentary technologies, the easy availability of energy-rich food, and declines in community-based physical activity have been implicated.[89] While there is certainly some scientific evidence which argues that paediatric fitness has declined,[90,91] not all available evidence is supportive, with some authors arguing that it has not changed at all[92,93] or that we cannot be confident either way (see ref. 94 and see Chapter 20).

The fact that most of the available scientific evidence has made only informal secular comparisons, with occasional rigorous statistical treatment, means that very little is known about secular changes in paediatric fitness. Many studies provide only local, temporally limited snapshots, which are restricted to narrow age bands and a single fitness component (typically aerobic fitness). Furthermore, only a handful of studies have actually reported on secular changes in criterion measures of fitness (e.g. directly measured peak $\dot{V}O_2$). Unfortunately, these studies have had to rely on comparisons across relatively small samples of volunteers for maximal exercise who are athletically inclined.[95] The paucity of representative criterion data has hindered our understanding of secular changes in construct fitness.

While it is acknowledged that all of these factors make it difficult to draw any confident conclusions regarding secular changes in paediatric fitness, some clues can be gleaned by examining secular changes in fitness test performance. Hitherto, the reviews of Tomkinson[74] and Tomkinson and Olds[38] provide the most complete commentary on secular changes in paediatric aerobic and anaerobic fitness test performances requiring maximal effort. These studies are reviewed below. Using a meta-analytical strategy, Tomkinson[74] and Tomkinson and Olds[38] reviewed 42 studies which examined the secular changes in power (single-jump tests), speed (sprint running and sprint-agility running tests) and aerobic (distance running, timed running, and endurance shuttle running tests) test performance. The reviews included only studies which explicitly commented on secular changes across at least two time points, spanning a minimum range of 3 years, on comparable populations. Secular changes were calculated at the country × age × sex × test level using least squares regression weighted by the square root of sample size and were expressed as a percentage of the weighted mean value for all data points in the regression. (Note, it is acknowledged that not all secular changes are linear, and the use of linear regression analysis to estimate secular changes may not have always been the most appropriate) Negative values were used to indicate performance declines, and positive values performance improvements.

Secular changes in power (n = 20, 802, 925), speed (n = 28, 320, 308) and aerobic (n = 25, 455, 527) performance were calculated for 6- to 19-year-olds from 32 countries (representing five geographical regions) between 1958 and 2003. Over the 45-year period, power and speed test performances improved at +0.03% and +0.04% p.a., respectively, while aerobic performances declined at –0.36% p.a..[38,74] Performance changes were strikingly similar for boys and girls, and children (<13 years) and adolescents (≥13 years), and reasonably similar for different geographical regions, and developed and developing countries. The secular changes, however, have not always been consistent over time (Fig. 9.4a). Changes for both power and speed were initially positive (i.e. improvements); however, at about 1985 there was a crossover from positive to negative (i.e. declines) for power, and a drop from positive to zero (i.e. no change) for speed. Aerobic changes were also initially positive, from the late 1950s through to about 1970, where changes crossed from positive to negative, increasing in magnitude every decade thereafter. Fig. 9.4b describes the time-related patterns of performance, standardized to 1958 = 100. Power test performances consistently improved from the late 1950s until the early 1980s, stabilizing until the late 1980s, followed by a 15-year decline. Speed test performances on the other hand have steadily risen over the 1958–1985 period, and plateaued thereafter. Aerobic performances improved sharply from the late 1950s until the mid-1960s, where there was a performance shoulder until the mid-1970s, followed by a 25–30-year decline.

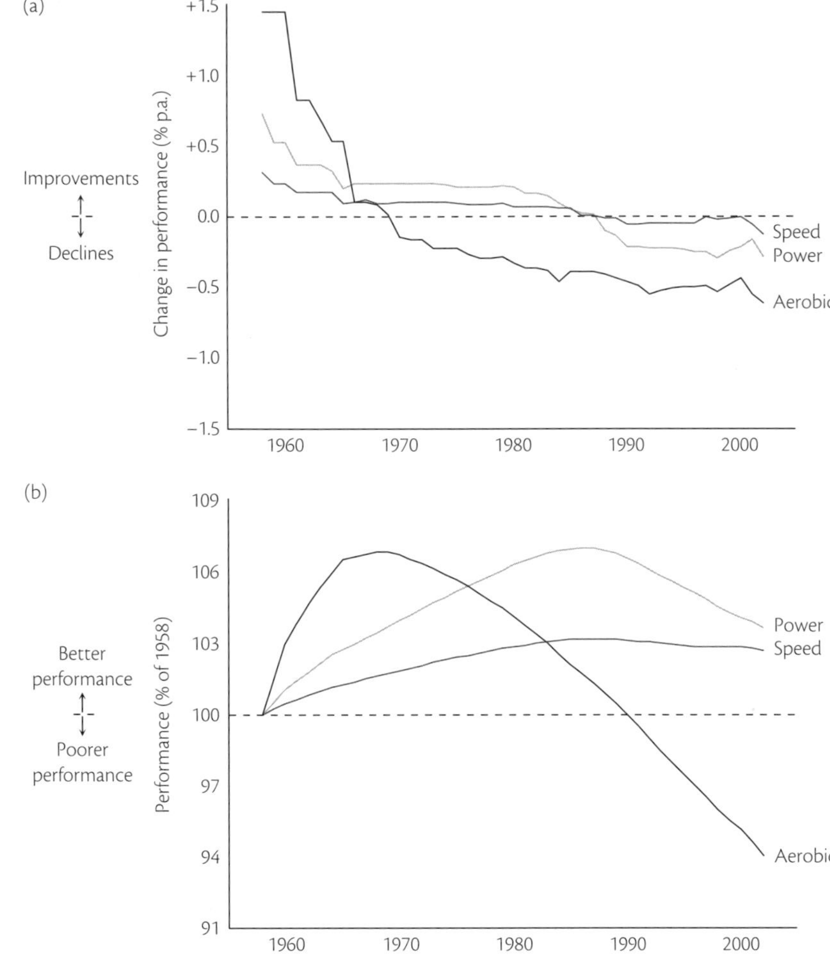

Fig. 9.4 Global time-related patterns of (**a**) change and (**b**) performance for aerobic fitness tests (black lines) and anaerobic fitness tests of power (light grey lines) and speed (dark grey lines) for the period 1958–2002. The power and speed test data are from Tomkinson [74] and the aerobic test data from Tomkinson and Olds.[38] In (a) higher values (i.e. those greater than zero) indicate improvements in performance; in (b) higher values (i.e. those greater than 100) indicate better performance. Adapted by permission from Tomkinson[74] and Tomkinson and Olds.[38]

While the results of Tomkinson[74] and Tomkinson and Olds[38] described secular changes in average fitness test performance, secular changes in the distribution of fitness test performances are less clear. Knowledge of this issue is potentially important in understanding both how the decline in aerobic performance came about and how best to address it.[96] There is evidence that the variability (operationalized as the coefficient of variation) of fitness test performance is increasing.[3,97] Unfortunately, secular changes in performance variability do not describe what has been happening at the tails of the distribution, nor do they describe changes in skewness. Several studies have commented on distributional changes in fitness test performances,[96,98–100] particularly distributional changes in aerobic performances. Collectively, they suggest that secular changes have not always been consistent across the entire distribution, particularly in aerobic fitness tests, where it appears that it is the poorly performing tail of the distribution which is dragging the average performances down.

It should be noted that secular analysis of fitness test performance data is not without its limitations. Various factors (e.g. practice, environmental conditions, effort, motivation, tests instructions etc.) influence fitness test performance and could lead to spurious conclusions regarding secular changes. Further contaminating secular changes are differences in sampling methods, errors of measurement (e.g. calibration and type of equipment, methodological drift, allowances for diurnal variation), differences in the reporting of age, the number of performance trials allowed, and the scoring of performances (e.g. one trial, the better of two, or the best of three). Without any evidence of systematic time-related changes in such factors, estimates of mean changes should not be biased, although our confidence in these estimates will be reduced. Nevertheless, evidence presented above shows that there is good reason to believe that field tests are reliable and reasonably valid estimators of underlying fitness components.

Causes, correlates, and mechanisms of change

The comprehensive reviews of Tomkinson[74] and Tomkinson and Olds[38] suggest that, particularly over the past three decades, there has been a sharp decline in aerobic performance and relative stability in anaerobic performance. So what is causing this recent decline in aerobic performance? It has been suggested that secular declines in aerobic performance requiring maximal effort are caused by a network of social, behavioural, physical, psychosocial, and physiological factors (see ref. 38 and Fig. 9.5). Though this section will review a possible causal model, it is important to note that it is the secular changes in paediatric fitness test performance which are important, rather than the mechanistic factors underlying those

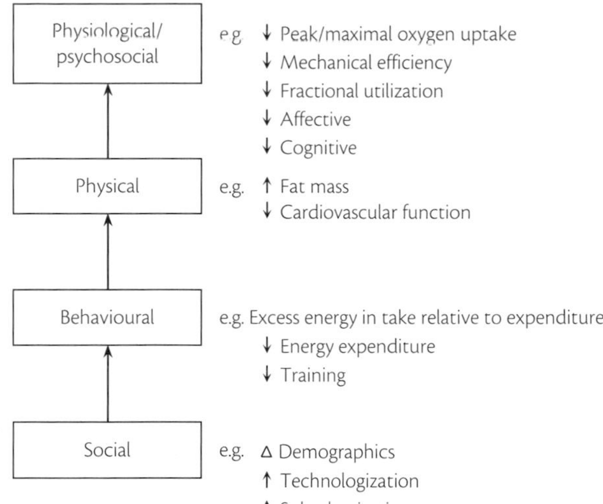

Fig. 9.5 Flowchart showing potential factors causing the decline in aerobic performance. Reprinted by permission from Tomkinson and Olds.[38]

performances. It is the ability to run fast, play harder, and keep moving longer which is important for children's physical activity levels, irrespective of the underlying mechanisms responsible for the changes.

Consider first the likely physiological causes. Proximate causes of declines in maximal aerobic performance are essentially changes in peak $\dot{V}O_2$, mechanical efficiency and fractional utilization.[20,21,101] For example, a decrease in mass-specific peak $\dot{V}O_2$ (mL·kg^{-1}·min^{-1}) will impair running performance. Second, a reduction in mechanical efficiency (or running economy) will change the running speed-$\dot{V}O_2$ relationship, increasing the oxygen cost at any given running speed. Third, a reduction in fractional utilization will mean that only reduced exercise intensity can be maintained for any given length of time. Furthermore, a reduction in affective (e.g. lack of motivation) and/or cognitive (e.g. inability to judge pace) aspects of maximal aerobic performance may also be important.[102]

Given this plausible physiological argument, is there any evidence for declines in these physiological factors (i.e. aerobic fitness)? Though secular data on directly measured criterion measures of aerobic fitness in children and adolescents are few, some secular data are available for peak $\dot{V}O_2$. Armstrong *et al.*[92] found little secular change in directly measured peak $\dot{V}O_2$ (both absolute and mass specific) of 433 11–16-year-olds from the United Kingdom between 1975 and 1991. Similarly, Eisenmann and Malina,[103] who extended the study of Freedson and Goodman,[104] reported that both absolute and mass-specific peak $\dot{V}O_2$ has remained relatively stable over the period 1938–1995 in 2878 US children aged 6–19 years. However, further examination of Eisenmann and Malina's [103] data suggests that both absolute and mass-specific peak $\dot{V}O_2$ has declined in recent decades in girls.[105] Fredriksen *et al.* [106] compared the mass-specific peak $\dot{V}O_2$ values of 617 young Norwegians (8–16 years) between 1952 and 1997. Over the 45 year period, peak $\dot{V}O_2$ declined at −0.12% p.a. Miyashita and Sadamoto [107] reported that the mass-specific peak $\dot{V}O_2$ of 10- to12-year-old Japanese children declined at −1.24% p.a. between 1969 and 1979.

Despite analysing directly measured peak $\dot{V}O_2$ data, these studies have been criticized for making secular comparisons among small samples (typically comprising only volunteers who are willing to exercise to exhaustion) and undifferentiated age ranges, and for mixing data from different ergometers (e.g. cycle and treadmill).[95,105] Regardless, these studies suggest that there has been little secular change in absolute and mass-specific peak $\dot{V}O_2$ in children and adolescents, with small declines in some groups more recently. It should be noted that secular changes in mass-specific peak $\dot{V}O_2$ might reflect changes in the denominator (i.e. body mass) rather than changes in the numerator (i.e. absolute peak $\dot{V}O_2$).[95]

Further insight into secular changes in paediatric peak $\dot{V}O_2$ may be gleaned by examining secular data on maximal-intensity laboratory-based aerobic fitness tests which are very highly correlated with peak $\dot{V}O_2$. The watt–max test, for example, an incremental maximal cycle ergometer test which has been validated against peak $\dot{V}O_2$ (r^2 = 0.89; 108), has been used to examine secular changes in the aerobic fitness of Danish children and adolescents.[100,109,110] Using a stratified, proportional sample of 1020 Danish children (aged 8–10 years) and adolescents (aged 14–16 years) tested in 1997–1998, Wedderkopp *et al.* [100] and Wedderkopp[110] compared the watt–max test results to 1369 children in 1985–1986 and 1260 adolescents in 1983–1984, respectively. Estimated mass-specific peak $\dot{V}O_2$ reportedly declined at −0.27% p.a. in children and improved at +0.13% p.a. in adolescents. Møller *et al.* [109] reported increases of +0.25% p.a. in maximal power output (W·kg^{-1}) in 968 8–10-year-old Danish children tested between 1997 and 2004. These data also suggest that mass-specific peak $\dot{V}O_2$ has been relatively stable in recent decades. It is acknowledged, however, that although this discussion on secular changes in aerobic fitness has concentrated solely on changes in peak $\dot{V}O_2$, aerobic fitness is not exclusively related to peak $\dot{V}O_2$.[4] Unfortunately, there are no available secular trend data on paediatric mechanical efficiency or fractional utilization.

But do the recent secular declines in aerobic performance reflect secular declines in aerobic fitness? Using the validity coefficients from 22 studies comparing distance run performance (both distance and timed runs) and directly measured peak $\dot{V}O_2$ (mL·kg^{-1}·min^{-1}) in children and adolescents, Fig. 9.2 shows that peak $\dot{V}O_2$ can explain a moderate to large (35–60%) part of the variability in distance run performance. Peak $\dot{V}O_2$ is relatively more important in tests requiring children to run over longer distances, or to run for longer periods of time, whereas anaerobic capacity and $\dot{V}O_2$ kinetics are relatively more important for tests over shorter distances or tests requiring running for less time. A similar proportion of 20mSRT can be explained by peak $\dot{V}O_2$.[38] Given that aerobic fitness tests are reasonably valid estimators of peak $\dot{V}O_2$, secular declines in aerobic performance are at least suggestive of secular declines in peak $\dot{V}O_2$. Nevertheless, it is important to remember that other physiological factors (e.g. mechanical efficiency, fractional utilization, anaerobic capacity, and $\dot{V}O_2$ kinetics) and psychosocial factors (e.g. pacing skills, motivation, and self-efficacy) also contribute to aerobic performance. While it is conceivable that there have been secular changes in these factors, no data are available.

Tomkinson and Olds[38] suggested that changes in the physiological mechanisms underlying aerobic performance are caused by physical changes, such as increased fat mass and reduced cardiovascular function. There is now overwhelming evidence that paediatric fatness has increased in recent decades.[111–113] A number of authors have indicated increases in fatness as a cause of declines in weight-bearing aerobic performance.[98,114–117] There are good reasons for making this causal connection: plausible mechanistic links, significant cross-sectional correlations, and parallel secular changes in weight-bearing aerobic performance and fatness (see ref. 102 for a review). Recently, however, two studies[102,118] have addressed the causal connection between changes in fatness and changes in aerobic performance directly. Using a matching analysis, where children and adolescents tested for aerobic fitness at one time period are matched for sex, age, and fatness with their peers tested years later, Olds and Dollman [102] and Tomkinson *et al.*[118] attempted to quantify the contribution of changes in fatness (operationalized as the triceps skinfold and body mass index [BMI]) to changes in aerobic performance (1600-m run and 20mSRT performance). Collectively, these studies concluded that increases in fatness explained 29–61% of the observed declines in aerobic performance. Therefore, while changes in fatness account for a moderate to large proportion of the variance in aerobic performance, other factors (e.g. lower levels of physical activity or less experience with maximal sustained efforts) must also be at work.

Secular comparisons of aerobic and anaerobic performance

A consistent finding in the literature dealing with secular changes in paediatric fitness test performance is that, in recent decades, there has been (i) little change in anaerobic performance and more marked change in aerobic performance and (ii) inconsistencies in the direction of change in anaerobic performance and consistent declines in aerobic performance.[38,74,114,116,119–129] These secular differences are best illustrated by examining the time-related patterns of change for power, speed, and aerobic test performance over the period 1958–2002 (Fig. 9.4 a and b). So why have aerobic performances declined, and power and speed performances remained relatively stable? It is not obvious why these secular differences are observed, but the answers may lie with the differential effects on fitness test performances of (i) fat mass and fat-free mass, (ii) maturational advances, and (iii) motor skills.

Consider first the differential effects of fat mass and fat-free mass on anaerobic and aerobic performances.[38] With overwhelming evidence of a global increase in paediatric BMI,[113] it is likely that increases in BMI reflect increases in both fat mass and fat-free mass. There is certainly some evidence of this, with increases in BMI, fat mass and fat-free mass found in 10–11-year-old Australians between 1985 and 1997.[74] From a mechanistic point of view, increases in fat mass should impair performance to a greater extent in distance running than in sprint running or jumping, while increases in fat-free mass should assist performances requiring strength and power, such as sprint running and jumping, as opposed to distance running. Using data from several large health and fitness surveys of Australian youth (n = 28,804), Tomkinson *et al.* [130] reported that (i) there is a strong negative relationship between fat mass and distance running, and only a moderate negative relationship between fat mass and sprint running and jumping; and (ii) there is a strong positive relationship between fat-free mass and sprint running and jumping, and only a weak positive relationship between fat-free mass and distance running. These data suggest that for distance running, the positive effect of increasing fat-free mass may not be enough to match the negative effect of increasing fat mass, hence the declines over time. While for sprint running and explosive jumping, the positive effect of increasing fat-free mass may counteract the negative effect of increasing fat mass, hence the relative stability over time.

Second, advances in the rate of maturation may also help explain the secular differences. Since the end of the nineteenth century, the age of sexual maturity (indicated by menarche and voices breaking in boys) has been advancing by about 0.2–0.4 years every decade,[131,132] although in some countries the trend appears to have slowed or stopped in the last few decades.[76] Assuming the trend towards earlier maturation is continuing, and since older children typically perform better than younger children on anaerobic and aerobic fitness tests (see Fig. 9.3), today's children would be expected to perform better than their peers of 30–40 years ago based on maturational advances alone. Analysis of several large health and fitness surveys of Australian youth shows that the age-related improvements in jumping (3.4–8.5% for each year of age between 9 and 15 years) and sprint running (1.1–3.8%) are larger than the age-related improvements in distance running and endurance shuttle running (0.6%–2.9%).[130] Examination of Fig. 9.3 confirms this. Therefore, the effect of maturational change will be quantitatively larger for secular changes in anaerobic performances (especially power test performance) than for changes in aerobic performances. In addition, without correction for maturational change, the reported declines in aerobic performance may be somewhat underestimated, and the apparent stability in anaerobic performance might mask an 'underlying' decline (for more details, see Ref 38, 130).

Third, it is also possible that skill contributes more to paediatric anaerobic performance than to paediatric aerobic performance. Without evidence of a secular change in motor skills, anaerobic performances could be less susceptible to secular change. Though not complete, these are at least three reasons why there are secular differences in anaerobic and aerobic performances.

Summary

- Field tests of aerobic and anaerobic power show high reliability and moderate validity with reference to laboratory-based tests of putative underlying physiological concepts.
- When interpreting the results of field tests, the tendency to simplistically map the results of tests onto physiological constructs such as energy systems should be avoided. While aerobic field tests are a reasonable proxy for $\dot{V}O_2$ max, many other factors contribute to performance. Similarly, sprint and jump tests are not pure measures of anaerobic power.
- The two main types of maximal effort aerobic field test are the run with either distance or time as an end point, and the endurance shuttle run tests.
- Maximal effort run tests should ideally last at least 10 min (or about 1600 m) to minimize the contribution of anaerobic energy supply.
- It is important to standardize methodologies when conducting maximal effort aerobic and anaerobic field tests. This includes the amount of practice, the number of trials, ground and weather conditions, and procedural variants such as the use of a countermovement in jump tests. In particular, testers should be alert to methodological variants of the 20mSRT, and be careful to express their results in metrics which are comparable with other data.

- There are substantial reference databases for the 1600-m run test, 20mSRT, vertical jump, standing broad jump and 40- and 50-m sprints.
- Performance in both aerobic and anaerobic tests improves with age, but at different rates in boys and girls, and in different kinds of tests. Age-related improvements in sprint and jumping performances are more rapid than in aerobic running tests.
- There have been distinct secular changes in the performance of children and adolescents on field tests over the last 50 years. Aerobic performance improved until 1970 and has since been falling rapidly at the rate of about 4–5% per decade. Performance on power (mainly jumping) tests peaked close to 1985 and has since been falling. Performance on sprint tests plateaued towards 1985.
- These secular changes are driven in part by increasing paediatric fatness, but it is likely that other factors such as lack of familiarity with maximal efforts are also involved.

References

1. Olds TS (1996). *Mathematical modeling of cycling performance*. Unpublished PhD dissertation. University of New South Wales, Sydney.
2. Morrow JR (2005). Are American children and youth fit? It's time we learned. *Res Q Exerc Sport* **76**, 377–88.
3. Tomkinson G (2004). *Secular trends in fitness performance of Australasian children and adolescents*. Unpublished PhD dissertation. University of South Australia, Adelaide.
4. Léger L (1996). Aerobic performance. In: Docherty D (ed.), *Measurement in pediatric exercise science*, pp. 183–223. Human Kinetics, Champaign, IL.
5. United States Department of Health and Human Services (1996). *Physical activity and health: A report of the Surgeon General*. United States Department of Health and Human Services, Centers for Disease Control and Prevention, National Center for Chronic Disease Prevention and Health Promotion, Atlanta, GA.
6. Williams PT (2001). Physical fitness and activity as separate heart disease risk factors: A meta-analysis. *Med Sci Sports Exerc* **33**, 754–61.
7. Andersen LB, Haraldsdottir J (1993). Tracking of cardiovascular disease risk factors including maximal oxygen uptake and physical activity from late teenage to adulthood: An 8-year follow-up study. *J Intern Med* **234**, 309–15.
8. Malina RM (2001). Physical activity and fitness: Pathways from childhood to adulthood. *Am J Hum Biol* **13**, 162–72.
9. Eiberg S, Hasselstrom H, Gronfeldt V, Froberg K, Cooper A, Andersen LB (2005). Physical fitness as a predictor of cardiovascular disease risk factors in 6- to 7-year old Danish children: The Copenhagen school child intervention study. *Pediatr Exerc Sci* **17**, 55–64.
10. Eisenmann JC, Katzmarzyk PT, Perusse L, Tremblay A, Despres JP, Bouchard C (2005). Aerobic fitness, body mass index, and CVD risk factors among adolescents: The Quebec family study. *Int J Obes* **29**, 1077–83.
11. Åstrand PO (1952). *Experimental studies of physical fitness in relation to age and sex*. Munksgaard, Copenhagen.
12. Ikai M, Fukunaga T (1975). Imbalance between growth and physical fitness. In: Asahina K, Shigiya R (eds.), *Physiological adaptability and nutritional status of the Japanese: B; growth, work capacity and nutrition of Japanese*, pp. 26–30. University of Tokyo Press, Tokyo.
13. Hebestreit H, Mimura K, Bar-Or O (1983). Recovery from anaerobic muscle power following 30-s supramaximal exercise: Comparison between boys and men. *J Appl Physiol* **74**, 2875–80.
14. Hunsicker PA (1958). *AAHPER youth fitness test manual*. American Association for Health, Physical Education, and Recreation, Washington, DC.
15. Olds TS, Tomkinson GR (2003). The aerobic fitness of 9–15 year old South Australian children: Norms, trends and international comparisons. *ACHPER Healthy Lifestyles J* **50**, 25–30.
16. Cooper CB, Storer TW (2001). *Exercise testing and interpretation: A practical approach*. Cambridge University Press, Cambridge.
17. Cooper KH (1968). A means of assessing maximal oxygen intake. *JAMA* **203**, 201–4.
18. Massicotte DR, Markon P, Gauthier R (1985). Prediction du $\dot{V}O_2$ max a partir des courses de 800, 1600 et 2400 metres chez les jeunes ages de 6 a 17 ans [$\dot{V}O_2$ max prediction in 800, 1600 and 2400 metre racing performance of 6 to 17 year old youth]. *CAHPER J* **51**, 25–9.
19. Krahenbuhl GS, Pangrazi RP, Petersen GW, Burkett LN, Schneider MJ (1978). Field testing of cardiorespiratory fitness in primary school children. *Med Sci Sports* **10**, 208–13.
20. Lussier L, Buskirk ER (1977). Effects of an endurance training regimen of assessment of work capacity in prepubertal children. *Ann NY Acad Sci* **301**, 734–47.
21. Krahenbuhl GS, Pangrazi RP, Chomokos EA (1979). Aerobic responses of young boys to submaximal running. *Res Q* **50**, 413–21.
22. Péronnet F, Thibault G (1989). Mathematical analysis of running performance and world records. *J Appl Physiol* **67**, 453–65.
23. Sjödin B (1982). The relationship among running economy, aerobic power, and onset of blood lactate accumulation in young boys (11–15 years). In: Komi PV (ed.), *Exercise and sport biology*, pp. 57–60. Human Kinetics, Champaign, IL.
24. Mayers N, Gutin B (1979). Physiological characteristics of elite prepubertal cross-country runners. *Med Sci Sports* **11**, 172–6.
25. Cureton KJ, Boileau RA, Lohman TG, Misner JE (1977). Determinants of distance running performances in children: Analysis of a path model. *Res Q* **42**, 270–9.
26. Powers SK, Howley ET (2007). *Exercise physiology: Theory and application to fitness and performance* (6th ed.). McGraw-Hill, New York.
27. Safrit MJ, Hooper LM, Ehlert SA, Glaucia Costa M, Patterson L (1988). The validity of generalization of distance run tests. *Can J Sports Sci* **13**, 188–96.
28. Watkins J, Moore B (1983). The performance of Scottish boys in the one mile run test. *Scottish J Phys Educ* **11**, 4–10.
29. Watkins J, Moore B (1996). The effects of practice on performance in the one mile run test of cardiorespiratory fitness in 12–15 year old girls. *ACHPER Healthy Lifestyles J* **43**, 11–4.
30. Armstrong N, Welsman JR (1994). Assessment and interpretation of aerobic fitness in children and adolescents. *Exerc Sports Sci Rev* **22**, 435–76.
31. Krahenbuhl GS, Skinner JS, Kohrt WM (1985). Developmental aspects of maximal aerobic power in children. *Exerc Sports Sci Rev* **13**, 503–38.
32. Daniels J, Oldridge N (1971). Changes in oxygen consumption of young boys during growth and running training. *Med Sci Sports Exerc* **3**, 161–5.
33. Daniels J, Oldridge N, Nagle F, White B (1978). Differences and changes in $\dot{V}O_2$ among young runners 10 to 18 years of age. *Med Sci Sports Exerc* **10**, 200–3.
34. Krahenbuhl GS, Morgan DW, Pangrazi RP (1989). Longitudinal changes in distance-running performance of young males. *Int J Sports Med* **10**, 92–6.
35. Rowland TW (2005). *Children's exercise physiology* (2nd ed.). Human Kinetics, Champaign, IL.
36. Léger L, Lambert J, Goulet A, Rowan C, Dinelle Y (1984). Capacité aérobic des Québécois de 6 à 17 ans—test navette de 20 mètres avec paliers de 1 minute. *Can J Appl Sport Sci* **9**, 64–9.
37. Léger LA, Lambert J. (1982). A maximal multistage 20m shuttle run test to predict $\dot{V}O_2$ max. *Eur J Appl Physiol* **49**, 1–12.
38. Tomkinson GR, Olds TS (2007). Secular changes in pediatric aerobic fitness test performance: The global picture. *Med Sport Sci* **50,** 46–66.

39. Tomkinson GR, Léger LA, Olds TS, Cazorla G. (2003). Secular trends in the performance of children and adolescents (1980–2000): An analysis of 55 studies of the 20 m shuttle run in 11 countries. *Sports Med* **33**, 285–300.
40. Council of Europe (1988). *Eurofit: Handbook for the Eurofit tests of physical fitness*. Council of Europe, Rome.
41. Australian Sports Commission (1999). *20 m shuttle run test: A progressive shuttle run test for measuring aerobic fitness*. Australian Coaching Council, Belconnen, ACT.
42. Brewer J, Ramsbottom R, Williams C (1988). *Multistage fitness test: A progressive shuttle-run test for the prediction of maximum oxygen uptake*. National Coaching Foundation, Leeds.
43. Cooper Institute for Aerobics Research (1992). *The Prudential FITNESSGRAM test administration manual*. Cooper Institute for Aerobics Research, Dallas, TX.
44. Riddoch CJ (1990). *The Northern Ireland health and fitness survey—1989: The fitness, physical activity, attitudes and lifestyles of Northern Ireland post-primary schoolchildren*. The Queen's University of Belfast, Belfast.
45. Barnett A, Chan LYS, Bruce IC (1993). A preliminary study of the 20-m multistage shuttle run as a predictor of peak $\dot{V}O_2$ in Hong Kong Chinese students. *Pediatr Exerc Sci* **5**, 42–50.
46. Léger LA, Mercier D, Gadoury C, Lambert J (1988). The multistage 20 metre shuttle run test for aerobic fitness. *J Sports Sci* **6**, 93–101
47. Jürimäe T, Volbekiene V, Jürimäe J, Tomkinson GR (2007). Changes in Eurofit test performance of Estonian and Lithuanian children and adolescents (1992–2002). *Med Sport Sci* **50,** 129–42.
48. Olds TS, Tomkinson GR, Léger LA, Cazorla G (2006). Worldwide variation in the performance of children and adolescents: An analysis of 109 studies of the 20 m shuttle run test in 37 countries. *J Sports Sci* **24**, 1025–38.
49. Tomkinson GR, Olds TS, Borms J (2007). Who are the Eurofittest? *Med Sport Sci* **50**, 104–28.
50. Armstrong N, Welsman JR (1997). *Young people and physical activity*. Oxford University Press, Oxford.
51. Bailey RC, Olson J, Pepper SL, Porszasz J, Bartsow TJ, Cooper DM (1995). The level and tempo of children's physical activities: An observational study. *Med Sci Sports Exerc* **27**, 1033–41.
52. Baranowski T, Hooks P, Tsong Y, Cieslik C, Nader PR (1987). Aerobic physical activity among third- to sixth-grade children. *J Dev Behav Pediatr* **8**, 203–6.
53. Gilliam TB, Freedson PS, Geenan DL, Shahraray B (1981). Physical activity patterns determined by heart rate monitoring in 6- to 7-year-old children. *Med Sci Sports Exerc* **13**, 65–7.
54. Kirkendall DT (2000). Physiology of soccer. In: Garrett WE, Kirkendall DT (eds.). *Exercise and sport science*, pp. 875–84. Williams and Wilkins, Philadelphia, PA.
55. Kraemer WJ, Gotshalk LA (2000). Physiology of American football. In: Garrett WE, Kirkendall DT (eds.). *Exercise and sport science*, pp. 795–813. Williams and Wilkins, Philadelphia.
56. Kirby RF (1991). *Kirby's guide to fitness and motor performance tests*. BenOak, Cape Girardeau, MO.
57. Van Praagh E (2007). Anaerobic fitness tests: What are we measuring? *Med Sport Sci* **50,** 26–45.
58. Van Praagh E, França NM (1995). Measuring maximal short-term power output during growth. In: Van Praagh E (ed.), *Pediatric anaerobic performance*, pp. 155–89. Human Kinetics, Champaign, IL.
59. Sargent DA (1921). The physical test of a man. *Am Phys Ed Rev* **26**, 188–94.
60. Fox EL, Mathews DK (1981). *The physiological basis of physical education and athletics*. Saunders College, Toronto, ON.
61. Harman EA, Rosenstein MT, Frykman PN, Rosenstein RM, Kraemer WJ (1991). Estimation of human power output from vertical jump. *J App Sport Sci Res* 5, 116–20.
62. Safrit MJ (1990). The validity and reliability of fitness tests for children. *Pediatr Exerc Sci* **2**, 9–28.
63. Davies CTM, Young K (1984). Effects of external loading on short-term power output in children and young male adults. *Eur J Appl Physiol* **52**, 351–4.
64. Bar-Or O (1996). Anaerobic performance. In: Docherty D (ed.), *Measurement in pediatric exercise science*, pp. 161–82. Human Kinetics, Champaign, IL.
65. Johnson BL, Nelson JK (1986). *Practical measurement for evaluation in physical education* (4th ed.). Burgess International, Edina, MN.
66. Larson LA (1974). *Fitness, health and work capacity: International standards for assessment*. MacMillan, New York.
67. Docherty D (1996). Field tests and test batteries. In: Docherty D (ed.). *Measurement in pediatric exercise science*, pp. 285–334. Human Kinetics, Champaign, IL.
68. Vandewalle H, Pérès G, Monod H (1987). Standard anaerobic exercise tests. *Sports Med* **4**, 268–89.
69. Bosco C, Komi PV (1979). Mechanical characteristics and fiber composition of human leg extensor muscles. *Eur J Appl Physiol* **41**, 275–84.
70. Bosco C, Komi PV (1980). Influence of aging on the mechanical behavior of leg extensor muscles. *Eur J Appl Physiol* **45**, 209–19.
71. Bosco C, Komi PV (1981). Influence of countermovement amplitude in potentiation of muscular performance. In: Morecki AA, Fidelus K, Kedzior K, Wit A (eds.). *Biomechanics VII*, pp. 129–35. University Park Press, Baltimore, MD.
72. Harman EA, Rosenstein MT, Frykman PN, Rosenstein RM (1990). The effects of arms and countermovement on vertical jumping. *Med Sci Sports Exerc* **22**, 825–33.
73. Luhtanen P, Komi PV (1978). Segmental contribution to forces in vertical jump. *Eur J Appl Physiol* **38**, 181–8.
74. Tomkinson GR (2007). Global changes in anaerobic fitness test performance of children and adolescents (1958–2003). *Scand J Med Sci Sports* 17, 497–507.
75. Klausen K, Schibye B, Rasmussen B (1989). A longitudinal study of changes in physical performance of 10- to 15-year-old girls and boys. In: Oseid S, Carlsen KH (eds.), *Children and exercise XIII*, pp. 113–22. Human Kinetics, Champaign, IL.
76. Malina RM, Bouchard C, Bar-Or O (2004). *Growth, maturation and physical activity* (2nd ed.). Human Kinetics, Champaign, IL.
77. Wilkie DR (1950). The relation between force and velocity in human muscle. *J Physiol* **110**, 249–80.
78. Van Praagh E, Fellmann N, Bedu M, Falgairette G, Coudert J (1990). Gender difference in the relationship of anaerobic power output to body composition in children. *Pediatr Exerc Sci* **2**, 336–48.
79. Harman E, Garhammer J, Pandorf C (2000). Principles of test selection and administration. In: Baeche T, Earle R (eds.). *Essentials of strength and conditioning*, pp. 275–86. Human Kinetics, Champaign, IL.
80. Klesius SG (1968). Reliability of the AAHPER youth fitness test items and relative efficiency of the performance measures. *Res Q* **39**, 809–11.
81. Marmis C, Montoye H, Cunningham D, Kozar A (1969). Reliability of the multi-trial items of the AAHPER youth fitness test. *Res Q* **40**, 240–5.
82. Safrit MJ (1986). *Introduction to measurement in physical education and exercise science*. Mosby, St Louis, MO.
83. Mero A (1998). Power and speed training in childhood. In: Van Praagh E (ed.), *Pediatric anaerobic performance*, pp. 241–67. Human Kinetics, Champaign, IL.
84. Shephard RJ, Lavallee H, LaBarre R (1980). On the basis of data standardization in prepubescent children. In: Ostyn M (ed.), *Kinanthropometry II*, pp. 306–16. Karger, Basel.
85. Thorland WG, Johnson GO, Cisar CJ, Housh TJ, Tharp GD (1987). Strength and anaerobic responses of elite young female sprint and distance runners. *Med Sci Sports Exerc* **19**, 56–61.
86. Mero A, Jaakola L, Komi PV (1991). Relationships between muscle fibre characteristics and physical performance capacity in trained athletic boys. *J Sports Sci* **9**, 161–71.

87. Blimke CJR (1989). Age- and sex- associated variation in strength during childhood: Anthropometric, morphological, neurological, biomechanical, endochronologic, genetic, and physical activity correlates. In: Gisolfi CV, Lamb DR (eds.), *Perspectives in exercise science and sports medicine. Vol. 2 (Youth, exercise and sport)*, pp. 99–164. Benchmark Press, Indianapolis, IN.
88. Weynard PG, Lee CS, Martinez-Ruiz R, Bundle MW, Bellizzi MJ, Wright S (1999). High speed running performance is largely unaffected by hypoxic reductions in aerobic power. *J Appl Physiol* **86**, 2059–64.
89. French SA, Story M, Jeffery RW (2001). Environmental influences on eating and physical activity. *Annu Rev Public Health* **22**, 309–35.
90. DiNubile NA (1993).Youth fitness—problems and solutions. *Prev Med* **22**, 589–94.
91. Strong WB (1990). Physical activity and children. *Circulation* **81**, 1697–701.
92. Armstrong N, Williams J, Balding J, Gentle P, Kirby B (1991). The peak oxygen uptake of British children with reference to age, sex, and sexual maturity. *Eur J Appl Physiol* **62**, 369–75.
93. Corbin CB, Pangrazi RP (1992). Are American children and youth fit? *Res Q Exerc Sport* **63**, 96–106.
94. Rowland T (2002). Declining cardiorespiratory fitness in youth: Fact or supposition? *Pediatr Exerc Sci* **14**, 1–8.
95. Rowland TW (2007). Evolution of maximal oxygen uptake in children. *Med Sport Sci* **50**, 200–9.
96. Dollman J, Olds TS (2007). Distributional changes in the performance of Australian children on tests of cardiorespiratory endurance. *Med Sport Sci* **50**, 210–25.
97. Noi S, Masaki T (2002). The educational experiments of school health promotion for the youth in Japan: Analysis of the 'sport test' over the past 34 years. *Health Promot Int* **17**, 147–60.
98. Dollman J, Olds T, Norton K, Stuart D (1999). The evolution of fitness and fatness in 10–11-year-old Australian schoolchildren: Changes in distributional characteristics between 1985 and 1997. *Pediatr Exerc Sci* **11**, 108–21.
99. McNaughton L, Morgan R, Smith P, Hannan G (1996). An investigation into the fitness levels of Tasmanian primary schoolchildren. *ACHPER Healthy Lifestyles J* **43**, 4–10.
100. Wedderkopp N, Froberg K, Hansen HS, Andersen LB (2004). Secular trends in physical fitness and obesity in Danish 9-year-old girls and boys: Odense School Child Study and Danish substudy of the European Youth Heart Study. *Scand J Med Sci Sports* **14**, 150–5.
101. Sjödin B, Svedenhag J (1985). Applied physiology of marathon running. *Sports Med* **2**, 83–99.
102. Olds TS, Dollman J (2004). Are changes in distance-run performance of Australian children between 1985 and 1997 explained by changes in fatness? *Pediatr Exerc Sci* **16**, 201–9.
103. Eisenmann JC, Malina RM (2002). Secular trends in peak oxygen consumption among United States youth in the 20th century. *Am J Hum Biol* **14**, 699–706.
104. Freedson PS, Goodman TL (1993). Measurement of oxygen consumption. In: Rowland TW (ed.). *Pediatric laboratory exercise testing*, pp. 91–114. Human Kinetics, Champaign, IL.
105. Malina RM (2007). Physical fitness of children and adolescents in the United States: Status and secular change. *Med Sport Sci* **50**, 67–90.
106. Fredriksen PM, Thaulow E, Nystad W, Ingjer F (1998). Aerob kapasitet hos barn og unge—Nordiske resultater gjennom 45 år [Aerobic capacity among children and adolescents – Nordic results over the past 45 years]. *Tidsskr Nor Loegeforen* **118**, 3106–10.
107. Miyashita M, Sadamoto T (1987). The current problems of physical fitness in Japanese children: In comparison with European and North American children. *J Sports Med* **27**, 217–22.
108. Riddoch C, Edwards D, Page A, Froberg K, Anderssen SA, Wedderkopp N, Brage S, Cooper AR, Sardinha LB, Haro M, Klasson-Heggebø L, Van Mechelen W, Boreham C, Ekelund U, Andersen LB (2005). The European Youth Heart Study—cardiovascular disease risk factors in children: Rationale, aims, study design and validation of methods. *J Phys Activity Health* **2**, 115–29.
109. Møller NC, Wedderkopp N, Kristensen PL, Andersen LB, Froberg K (2008). Secular trends in cardiorespiratory fitness and body mass index in Danish children: The European Youth Heart Study. *Scand J Med Sci Sports, 17, 331–9.*
110. Wedderkopp N (2001). *Atherosclerotic cardiovascular risk factors in Danish children and adolescents: A community based approach with a special reference to physical fitness and obesity*. Unpublished PhD dissertation. University of Southern Denmark, Denmark.
111. Olds TS, Ridley K, Tomkinson GR (2007). Declines in aerobic fitness: Are they only due to increasing fatness? *Med Sport Sci* **50**, 226–40.
112. Olds T, Tomkinson G, Dollman J (2007). Secular trends in the skinfold thicknesses of young people in developed countries. *J Hum Ecol* **15**, 41–9.
113. World Health Organisation (1998). *Obesity: Preventing and managing the global epidemic*. Geneva, World Health Organisation.
114. Bunc V, Jansa P, Kluka D (1997). Prognosis of boys' physical fitness development in the Czech Republic to 2001. *ICHPER-SD J* **33**, 51–4.
115. Rode A, Shephard RJ (1984). Growth, development and acculturation—A ten year comparison of Canadian Inuit children. *Hum Biol* **56**, 217–30.
116. Watanabe T, Yamamoto Y, Miyashita M, Mutoh Y (1998). Secular change in running performance of Japanese adolescents: A longitudinal developmental study. *Am J Hum Biol* **10**, 765–79.
117. Westerstahl M, Barnekow-Bergkvist M, Hedberg G, Jansson E (2003). Secular trends in body dimensions and physical fitness among adolescents in Sweden from 1974 to 1995. *Scand J Med Sci Sports* **13**, 128–37.
118. Tomkinson GR, Olds TS, Gulbin J (2003), Secular trends in physical performance of Australian children: Evidence from the Talent Search program. *J Sports Med Phys Fitness* **43**, 90–8.
119. Cilia G, Bellucci M, Riva M, Venerucci I (1996). *Eurofit 1995*. Istituto Superiore Statale di Educazione Fisica, Roma.
120. Dawson K, Hamlin M, Ross J, Duffy D (2001). Trends in the health-related physical fitness of 10–14 year old New Zealand children. *J Phys Educ NZ* **34**, 26–39.
121. Hamlin MJ, Ross JJ, Hong S-W (2002). Health-related fitness changes and gender differences in 6–12 year old New Zealand children. *NZ J Sports Med* **30**, 4–11.
122. Lefèvre J, Bouckaert J, Duquet W (1998). De barometer van de fysieke fitheid van de Vlaamse jeugd 1997: De resultaten [The barometer of the physical fitness of Flemish youth 1997: Results]. *Sport (Bloso Brussel)* **4**, 16–22.
123. Mészáros J, Mahmoud O, Szabó T (1999). Secular trend and motor performance scores in Hungarian school-boys. *Facta Universitatis Phys Educ* **1**, 43–9.
124. Ministry of Culture and Tourism (1998). *National survey of physical fitness*. Korean Sport Science Institute, Seoul.
125. Przeweda R (2000). Generation changes of physical fitness in Polish children and youth during the last two decades. *Scripta Periodica* **3**, 99–108.
126. Quek JJ, Menon J, Tan S, Wang B (1993). Review of National Physical Fitness Award (NAPFA) norms. In: *Optimising performance: Proceedings of the International Sports Science Conference 1993*, pp. 161–212. Singapore Sports Council, Singapore.
127. Saranga S, Prista A, Maia J (2002). Mudança nos níveis de aptidão física em função de alterações políticas e sócio-económicas de 1992–1999 [Changes in physical fitness levels as a function of political and socio-economic alterations between 1992 and 1999]. In: Prista A, Maia J, Saranga S, Marques A (eds.), *Saúde, crescimento e desenvolvimento: um estudo epidemiológico em crianças e jovens de Moçambique [Health, growth and development: An epidemiological study in boys and girls from Mozambique]*, pp. 71–87. FCDEF—Universidade do Porto/FCEFD—Universidade Pedagógica, Porto.

128. Tomkinson GR, Olds TS (2007). Secular changes in aerobic fitness test performance of Australasian children and adolescents. *Med Sport Sci* **50**, 168–82.
129. Updyke WF, Willett MS (1989). *Physical fitness trends in American youth 1980–1989: Report summary*. Chrysler Fund-AAU Physical Fitness Program, Bloomington, IL.
130. Tomkinson GR, Hamlin MJ, Olds TS (2006). Secular trends in anaerobic test performance in Australasian children and adolescents. *Pediatr Exerc Sci* **18**, 314–28.
131. Himes JH (1979). Secular changes in body proportions and composition. In: Roche AF, ed. *Secular trends in human growth, maturation and development*, pp. 28–58. Society for Research in Child Development, Chicago, IL.
132. Norton K, Olds T, Olive S, Craig N (1995). Anthropometry and sports performance. In: Norton K, Olds T (eds.), *Anthropometrica*, pp. 287–364. University of New South Wales Press, Sydney.

CHAPTER 10

Physical activity

Kirsten Corder and Ulf Ekelund

Introduction

In this chapter, we discuss the assessment and interpretation of physical activity in young people in three main sections. The first section is an introduction to why we need to measure physical activity more accurately with definitions of various terminologies commonly used in the field of physical activity research. Then we move on to describe methods used to measure habitual physical activity in children and adolescents, summarizing advantages and limitations of each. In the last section we discuss the issues surrounding the interpretation of physical activity data in young people.

The strength of the relationship between physical activity and health varies considerably; this is at least partly due to challenges surrounding the accurate measurement of physical activity. The relationship between physical activity and health is weaker in children than in adults and is therefore harder to determine.[1] This difference may be due to higher activity levels in children and a longer lifetime of exposure for an adult, with more time for disease to develop. Inaccurate measurement with non-differential error leads to an underestimation of the true association between the exposure and outcome in observational studies.[2] Figure 10.1, adapted from Wong *et al.*,[2] illustrates how accuracy of measurement, of both the exposure and outcome, impacts the sample size required to find an association with 95% power at a significance level of $p < 0.0001$. These calculations were done in reference to gene–environment interactions, but the principle that more accurate measurement requires a smaller sample size to find an association is applicable to all forms of epidemiological measurement.

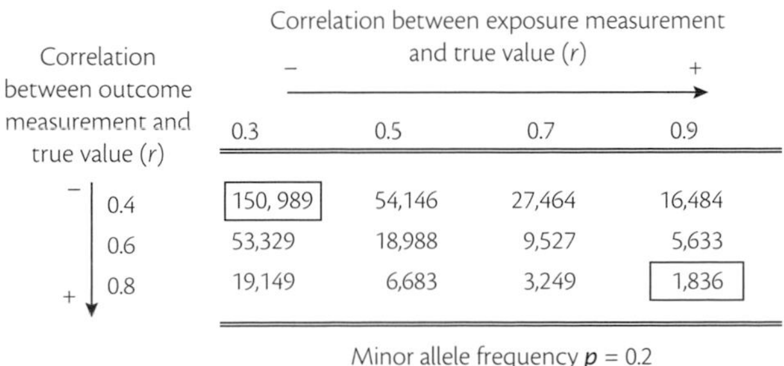

Correlation between outcome measurement and true value (r) (– to +)	Correlation between exposure measurement and true value (r) (– to +): 0.3	0.5	0.7	0.9
0.4	150, 989	54,146	27,464	16,484
0.6	53,329	18,988	9,527	5,633
0.8	19,149	6,683	3,249	1,836

Minor allele frequency **p** = 0.2
Gene misclassification, 0.025

Fig. 10.1 How the accuracy of measurement, of both the exposure and outcome, impacts the sample size required to find an association.

A concise summary of why we need to assess physical activity more accurately is given below as defined by Wareham and Rennie:[3]

- To specify which aspect of physical activity is important for a particular health outcome.
- To estimate more accurately the effect size.
- To make cross-cultural comparisons.
- To monitor temporal trends in physical activity.
- To monitor the effect of interventions.

Despite much progress with physical activity assessment in young people in recent years, substantial limitations still exist for the accurate and feasible assessment of habitual physical activity in children, especially in large populations. These limitations are amplified in young people and some are unique to this age group as children's physical activity is different from that in adults due to considerable differences in physiology and the nature of their physical activity. Children's physical activity tends to be sporadic and of more variable intensity than that of adults, also generally consisting of less planned, time-bound and organized activity. Subsequently, the assessment of physical activity in young people is not synonymous with that in adults and should be considered as a separate entity.

Physical activity definitions

Physical activity is a complex behaviour [4] and the term is often used interchangeably with energy expenditure, exercise, and physical fitness. For clarity and consistency, we refer to these terms as defined by Casperson *et al.*,[4] summarized below:

- *Physical activity* is 'any bodily movement produced by skeletal muscles that results in energy expenditure'.
- *Exercise* is 'a subset of physical activity that is planned, structured, and repetitive and has as a final or an intermediate objective the improvement or maintenance of physical fitness'.
- *Physical fitness* is 'a set of attributes either health- or skill related' and this is not synonymous with physical activity.

As defined above, physical activity is the bodily movement that produces associated energy expenditure; physiological energy expenditure is numerically presented in joules or calories whereas body movement can be numerically summarized in various ways. Physical activity is a complex behaviour, comprising various dimensions. Different research questions will require assessments of different dimensions of physical activity, and different methods of assessment will only be able to assess certain dimensions. Consequently, the dimension of activity required for a particular study will heavily influence the type of measurement method chosen. It is not possible to assess every aspect of physical activity at once and definitely not with only one method. The term physical activity is often subdivided and some of these commonly used terms are defined below for consistency:

- *Frequency* is the number of physical activity bouts during a specific period of time.
- *Duration* is the time of participation in a single bout of physical activity.
- *Intensity* is the physiological effort involved in carrying out physical activity. The intensity of physical activity can be defined in absolute and relative terms and can be normalized for differences in body size. A commonly used absolute intensity categorization is that of multiples of resting metabolic rate (1 MET or 3.5 $mLO_2 \cdot kg^{-1} \cdot min^{-1}$). Moderate intensity activity refers to a level of 3–6 METS in adults [5] and 5–8 METS for youth.[6] These levels broadly correspond to 40–55% of maximal oxygen uptake or 60–70% of maximal heart rate (HR) in adolescents,[7] which are examples of intensity expressed in relative terms.
- *Type* or *mode* of physical activity is what physical activity is being carried out; it is usually assessed with self-report methods, such as questionnaires, diaries, and interviews, or by direct observation.

Energy expenditure measured in joules (or calories) can also be a misleading term and is often subdivided into categories. These categories are described as follows:

- *Total energy expenditure* (TEE) is the total amount of energy required by an individual measured in joules or calories usually expressed per day.
- *Basal metabolic rate* (BMR) is the amount of energy required by an individual when completely at rest, usually measured immediately after waking in the morning and at least 12 h after the last meal, measured in joules or calories and expressed per day.[8]
- *Resting energy expenditure* (REE) is often used interchangeably with BMR, but it is the amount of energy required at rest, not subject to such a stringent measurement protocol as BMR. REE may include the thermic effect of feeding (TEF); however, BMR and REE usually differ by less than 10% and are measured in joules or calories.[8]
- *TEF* or diet-induced thermogenesis (DIT) is the increment in energy expenditure above BMR due to the cost of processing food for storage and use.[9]
- *Physical activity energy expenditure* (PAEE) is the amount of energy required to carry out physical activity, this is usually calculated as PAEE = TEE–BMR or PAEE = (0.9×TEE)–BMR to account for the TEF (commonly assumed to be approximately 10% of the TEE).[10]
- *Physical activity level* (PAL) calculated as PAL = TEE / RMR.
- *Physical activity intensity*, PAI = PAEE per unit time.

Physical activity domains

Physical activity can also be subdivided into different domains (i.e. where the activity takes place). These include home-time, school-time, school-break-time, sports- or leisure-time, and habitual physical activity. Despite the importance of studies carried out in controlled and short-term environments for the improvement and optimization of data collection and analysis techniques, these studies are not often directly applicable to the assessment of habitual physical activity. The accuracy of measurement tends to be greater in controlled environments but small samples are often used to allow for the use of more expensive methods of assessment and this can limit generalizability. It is generally easier to assess physical activity in domains with a shorter time frame as they are easier to remember or are done by choice, or for a predetermined period of time. For example, physical activity during school-break-time is a defined and bounded period of time lending itself to direct observation studies and potentially easily controlled intervention opportunities.

Habitual physical activity is logically the most important dimension for health outcomes and the primary focus here is the assessment and subsequent interpretation of habitual physical activity in young people. Here we refer to habitual physical activity as the assessment of the usual physical activity carried out in normal daily life in every domain and any dimension, either assessed as a frequency, intensity, and duration or mode of activity or as PAEE assessed during free-living. It is not possible to directly measure habitual or usual physical activity so it must be estimated by the measurement of free-living physical activity for a defined period of time.

How active are young people?

The current physical activity recommendation for young people is 60 min of at least moderate intensity activity every day;[11,12] various studies have sought to determine whether this recommendation is correct and whether they are actually reaching these recommendations.[13] The answers to these questions at least partly depend on the assessment method and subsequent interpretation of the physical activity data.

Most results indicate that young people are not sufficiently active when compared to these recommendations, but there is some disparity. However, it is generally agreed that the overweight are less active than the lean,[14–16] boys are more active than girls, and physical activity decreases with age.[13,17,18] Different methods of measurement and analysis mean that estimates of physical activity from different sources are not always comparable, making comparisons about PALs across studies and populations challenging.

Table 10.1 summarizes some studies which have assessed habitual physical activity levels in young people. All studies used the same objective method (accelerometry) when estimating the levels of activity undertaken. Summary values are used as average counts per minute (cpm), which is an integrated measure of the overall daily intensity level, and also as time spent in moderate to vigorous physical activity (MVPA), a measure of duration and intensity

Table 10.1 Free-living actigraph-assessed PALs

Citation	Population	Gender	*N*	Age (years)	Counts per minute (cpm)	Minutes at MVPA	MVPA cut-point used (cpm)
Metallinos-Katsaras *et al.*[88]	Massachusetts, USA	Boys and Girls	51	2–5	744.0 (165.7)	272.2 (60.1)	615
Reilly *et al.*[45]	Glasgow, UK	Boys	128	4.2 (0.3)	773 (151)	44.6[a]	3200
Reilly *et al.*[45]	Glasgow, UK	Girls	140	4.2 (0.3)	694 (165)	33.1[a]	3200
Janz *et al.*[15]	Iowa, USA	Boys	176	5.6 (0.5)	782 (164)	304	Freedson equation
Janz *et al.*[15]	Iowa, USA	Girls	202	5.7 (0.5)	719 (159)	291	Freedson equation
Janz *et al.*[15]	Iowa, USA	Boys	176	8.5 (0.5)	734 (194)	203	Freedson equation
Janz *et al.*[15]	Iowa, USA	Girls	202	8.6 (0.5)	628 (163)	176	Freedson equation
Riddoch *et al.*[13]	Denmark, Portugal, Estonia and Norway	Girls	2185 (Boys and girls aged 9 and 15)	9.6 (0.4)	649 (204)	160 (54)	1000
Riddoch *et al.*[13]	Denmark, Portugal, Estonia and Norway	Boys	2185 (Boys and girls aged 9 and 15)	9.7 (0.4)	784 (282)	192 (66)	1000
Ness *et al.*[16]	Bristol, UK	Boys and Girls	5500	11.7	604.7	19.7	3600
Riddoch *et al.*[13]	Denmark, Portugal, Estonia and Norway	Girls	2185 (Boys and girls aged 9 and 15)	15.4 (0.6)	491 (163)	73 (32)	1500
Riddoch *et al.*[13]	Denmark, Portugal, Estonia and Norway	Boys	2185 (Boys and girls aged 9 and 15)	15.5 (0.5)	615 (228)	99 (45)	1500

[a] Original paper states % of time (*t*) in MVPA, values above calculated as (1440/10).

of activity. The total cpm values should be relatively comparable between studies, depending whether any 'not-worn' time has been discounted. Minutes spent in MVPA are not necessarily comparable between studies as the thresholds for identifying the intensity corresponding to MVPA vary across studies.[19] The major caveats of using PAI cut-points and of discounting 'not-worn' time will be discussed later. In Table 10.1, the average number of minutes spent in MVPA varies from 20.8 to 272.2 min per day, theoretically ranging from very inactive to very active children. Part of this difference in activity levels between studies is real but it is impossible to make firm conclusions about the differences in activity levels since the thresholds used to define this MVPA are ranging between 615 and 3600 cpm.

Little is known about the strength of any temporal trends in children's physical activity levels, due to the lack of historical objective data on physical activity. Existing longitudinal physical activity data are limited and consist of self-reported or proxy measures.[20–22] Self-reported methods are useful to assess some aspects of physical activity, but have limited accuracy for use in children, especially in those under the age of 10 years.[23]

Validity and reliability of physical activity assessment methods

Validity and reliability are different concepts and are sometimes wrongly used interchangeably. Validity is the extent to which a measurement instrument assesses the true exposure of interest.[24] Criterion validity is the extent of the association between the method tested and a more accurate method.[25] Absolute validity is when the absolute outcome [i.e. energy expenditure (EE) or time spent in activity] is compared to data from an objective instrument which provides the same outcome measure. The association is usually reported as the degree of agreement.[26]

Reliability is the extent to which an instrument gives the same result on different occasions.[24] Test–retest reliability is mainly used for self-report instruments such as questionnaires; this is the comparison of repeated administrations of the same instrument to the same population. Test–retest reliability is presented in various ways, using intra-class correlation coefficients, the actual units of measurement, or as a proportion of the measured values.[27] Inter-investigator reliability is the degree to which different investigators agree on measurements, this is relevant to methods with investigator-determined subjective components such as direct observation and interviews.

With objective methods, there is often variation between the outputs of different monitors of the same brand, model, or make, and this can be tested using a standard mechanical calibration procedure. All monitors should be mechanically and uniformly calibrated before use in the field, and a monitor-specific calibration factor can be used to 'correct' the output if necessary. This could especially be a problem if the inter-monitor error is intensity specific; consequently, it would be ideal to use the same monitor for each individual at all stages of a longitudinal study. Inter-instrument reliability should be established by multiple routinely scheduled mechanical calibrations.

An important issue with all objective measurement methods is the number of days of assessment required to obtain a reliable estimate of habitual physical activity. There is some evidence that 4–9 full days of monitoring, including 2 weekend days is probably the minimum number required for a reliable estimate.[28] Seven days of continuous monitoring seems logical but as protocol adherence decreases with days of wear, it may be more feasible to opt for 4 full days, as is often the case in large studies; unfortunately, this is again a trade-off between feasibility and accuracy. Seasonality, due to school terms, school holidays, and possibly also climate are an important consideration for a habitual estimate of physical activity; a single measurement occasion may not adequately reflect children's habitual physical activity as there may be considerable annual intra-individual variation.[29]

Validation of physical activity instruments

The exposure of interest for a validation study, and any assessment of physical activity should be explicitly defined *a priori*.[3] Also, the criterion and test instruments must measure the same exposure for a validation study to be worthwhile; however, the methods should not be too similar, specifically without correlated error. A validation of a questionnaire against an activity diary or an accelerometer against another accelerometer may therefore not be the preferred option. Validation studies of physical activity assessment methods in children tend to broadly occur in four situations: in a controlled environment on a treadmill, during various 'lifestyle' activities, in a semi-controlled environment such as a school, or in a free-living environment. It will be free-living validations and their application to assessment of habitual physical activity that will be discussed here.

Large differences in activity behaviour are likely to be present between age groups, populations, and ethnic groups meaning that the population chosen for a validation study should be as representative as possible to where the technique is to be applied. It is not feasible to have a validation study for every population, and some free-living validation studies have no choice but to use limited populations due to the expensive nature of criterion methods and time constraints. Similarly, healthy populations are often used for validation studies, again often due to convenience or the voluntary nature of the recruitment process but limiting to generalizability. These factors should all be considered when choosing a measurement method as, for example, a method valid for use in lean children may not be suitable for assessing the same exposure in the obese.[10]

Correlation coefficients are the traditional outcome variable used in validation studies; however, they do not allow for investigation of direction of error, systematic bias, or any heteroscedasticity. The limitations of using correlations are widely accepted and more appropriate statistics for use in physical activity measurement are discussed in detail elsewhere.[30] Bland–Altman plots with limits of agreement are increasingly used to determine the direction of error and to estimate heteroscedasticity in comparative studies.[26] The main types of error experienced in validation studies are displayed graphically in Bland–Altman plots (Fig. 10.2). The concept of validity itself is subjective and fluid, and each study and method should be considered carefully before use, irrespective of a positive validation outcome.

Methods of physical activity assessment

Physical activity assessment methods can be split clearly into two groups: subjective or self-report methods and objective monitoring.

Subjective methods such as questionnaires, interviews, and activity diaries may be influenced by opinion and perception, from the participant, investigator, or both.

Objective methods record a physiological or biomechanical parameter and use this to estimate physical activity; these methods are not influenced by opinion or perception but are susceptible to measurement error.

Not only the validity but also the cost, feasibility, investigator, and participant burden need to be considered when choosing a measurement method. Unfortunately, in reality, this is always a compromise between feasibility and accuracy.[3] All methods have limitations but it is generally accepted that objective methods are the more accurate way to assess physical activity, but the expense and expertise required limits feasibility. Various objective methods are used to assess PAEE and the intensity, frequency, and duration of activity but are not able to assess mode or type of activity. Unfortunately, there is a negative relationship between the accuracy and the feasibility and ease of use of a method. This relationship is demonstrated in Fig. 10.3, however, this is just an illustration of the relationship, which is not necessarily linear.

Criterion methods

The criterion methods, namely, doubly labelled water (DLW) and indirect calorimetry both derive their estimates of physiological energy expenditure from oxygen consumption and/or carbon

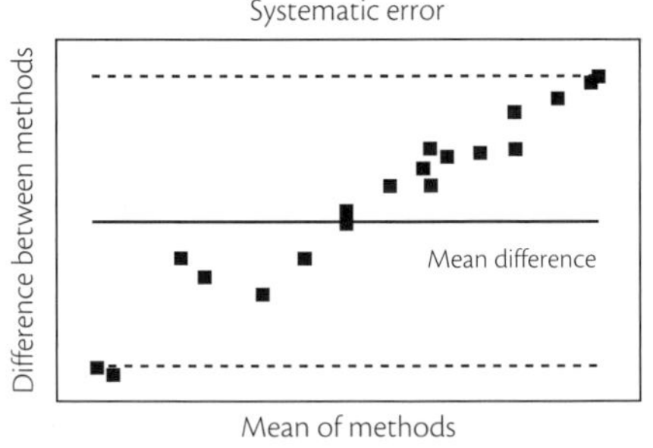

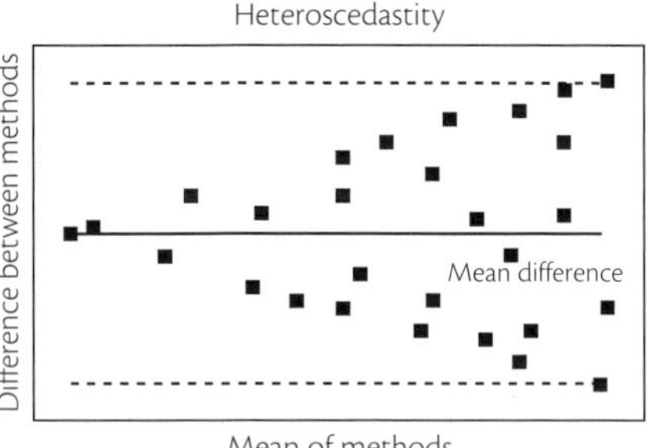

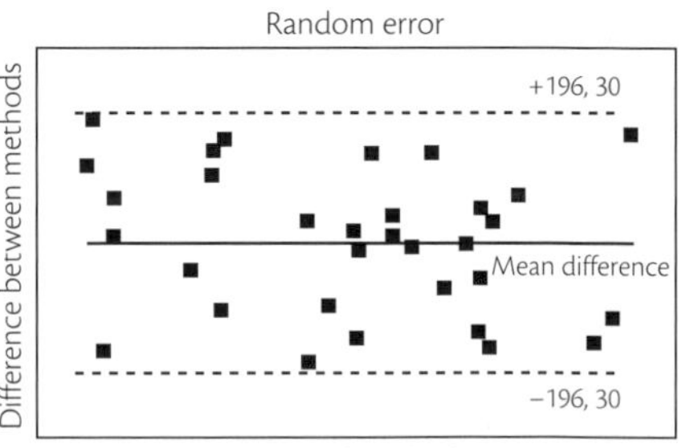

Fig. 10.2 Graphical representation of error. Systematic error—error that is not due to chance but is introduced by biases in the measurement method or by human factors; the error may have a directional bias dependent on *x* values. Heteroscedasticity––when the error at each *x*-value is not the same and is therefore greater at some *x*-values than others. Random or non-differential error—the distribution of measurement errors is randomly distributed and usually results in a dilution of association.

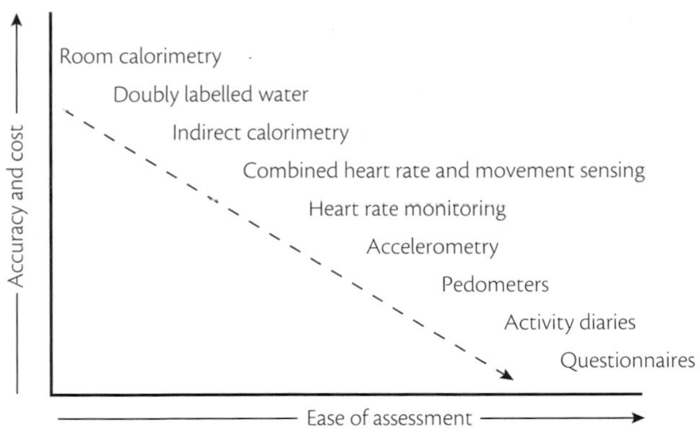

Fig. 10.3 The accuracy of an assessment method is inversely associated with the cost and ease of assessment.

dioxide production, but they are estimated from different sources. Indirect calorimetry relies on the measurement of oxygen consumption and expired carbon dioxide, usually in the laboratory. The DLW method requires urine or saliva samples, usually provided daily, from which carbon dioxide production is calculated. The DLW method is valid and suitable for assessing free-living energy expenditure over 1–3 weeks.

Doubly labelled water

The DLW method was developed in the late 1940s and early 1950s by Lifson *et al.*,[31] but it was not until relatively recently that it was used to assess energy metabolism and to act as the criterion for the assessment of daily energy expenditure.[32] The DLW method made it possible to prove that obese people do not have lower energy requirements than lean people [33] and that physical activity is the most variable component of TEE, compared to BMR and the TEF.[32] However, measurement error can usually account for 5–10% of the estimate of TEE from DLW, and the accuracy of these estimates are to some extent dependent on protocol adherence regarding sample collection. This error is still substantially less than other methods and this method is now undoubtedly the gold standard for the assessment of free-living energy expenditure in humans.[32]

The use of the DLW method to estimate human energy expenditure is described in detail elsewhere.[32,34] In summary, energy expenditure is calculated from estimations of carbon dioxide production determined after dosing with water labelled with known amounts of the stable isotopes deuterium (^{2}H) and ^{18}O. In simple terms, the deuterium is eliminated from the body as water and the ^{18}O as both water and carbon dioxide; consequently, the difference in elimination rates is the amount of carbon dioxide production. This method requires collection of urine or saliva samples, usually daily over 7–14 days, thus, barely disrupting daily life. The levels of isotopes in the samples are measured using a mass spectrometer; the need for this machine and the specific training and skills required further restrict the use of the DLW method. Energy expenditure is then calculated from this estimate using equations from indirect calorimetry.[35] As TEE is assessed using DLW, the amount of that energy used for activity (PAEE) is calculated by subtracting the measured or predicted REE or BMR from TEE. Despite the high accuracy of this method, it is restricted to relatively small samples due to the high costs of isotopes and analyses.

Calorimetry

Direct and indirect room calorimetry are not suitable for assessing habitual physical activity in children as they require confinement to a metabolic chamber.[36] Detailed descriptions of these methods are available elsewhere.[36] The former method uses the heat transfer from the body to the environment and the latter uses the measurement of all expired gases to calculate energy expenditure. Both methods are able to provide very accurate estimates of energy expenditure but unfortunately in unnatural environments and at high cost. For validating energy expenditure prediction equations and maybe also deriving equations from accelerometry or HR, a metabolic chamber would be suitable, possibly even for young children. A metabolic chamber has been used successfully to determine sleeping metabolic rate during a 1–2 h afternoon nap in young children under 2 years old, and the measurement was successful in 86% of tests.[37]

Indirect calorimetry uses standard equations[35] to predict energy expenditure from oxygen consumption and carbon dioxide production. Expired air is collected via a face mask, mouthpiece, or hood covering the head. Mobile and laboratory methods of indirect calorimetry are more feasible for use in children but are still unable to provide free-living estimates of physical activity. Validation studies of methods in a controlled environment, such as on a treadmill or using structured activities, often use these methods, either with the analyser stationed next to the exercise apparatus or mounted on the volunteer's back. Despite the size of the equipment, this latter method has been used successfully in comparison to an accelerometer during structured laboratory activities in 3- to 5-year-old children.[38]

Objective methods

Movement sensing

Movement sensing is certainly the most common objective method used to assess physical activity, especially in population studies. Here we have used the term 'movement sensing' broadly to mean any method assessing body movement. There are many brands of movement sensor and it would be impractical to discuss every one that has been used in physical activity research, we will mainly focus on general principles and issues associated with accelerometry and pedometry.

Accelerometry

Acceleration is a change in velocity over time ($m{\cdot}s^{-2}$) and therefore quantifies the volume and intensity of movement.[39] Broadly, accelerometry uses the measurement of the amplitude and frequency of the vertical acceleration by a piezometer;[40] this is usually enclosed in a solid casing and attached to the body with a strap at the hip, lower back, ankle, wrist, or thigh.

Accelerometer type

The way in which accelerometers are classified varies according to the direction in which the accelerometer measures. The terms uniaxial, biaxial, triaxial, and omni-directional describe the direction in which acceleration is assessed. Uniaxial accelerometry measures in one direction, usually in the vertical plane, biaxial in two directions, generally transverse and longitudinal, triaxial in three directions, and so on. An omni-directional accelerometer is fundamentally uniaxial as it is most sensitive to movement in the vertical plane, despite being sensitive to movement in all directions.[41] There is limited evidence that the extra measurement ability of triaxial over uniaxial accelerometers warrants the extra cost and size.[42]

Monitor placement and multiple accelerometers

Monitor placement is very relevant to uniaxial accelerometry as movement is only assessed in one axis and the dominant direction of movement varies according to activity type. Most commonly, accelerometers are placed around the waist, usually at the hip or the lower back and there appears to be no difference in monitor output from the two locations in free-living adults.[43] Accelerometers can be placed on the ankle and/or wrist to capture different activities, but the hip is the position of choice for a solo accelerometer. In adults, multiple accelerometers explain slightly more variance in activity than one alone, but the extra burden is unlikely to be worth the increase in accuracy.[28] This has not been investigated fully in children, which is unfortunate considering that their activity style is more varied than most adult's predominantly ambulatory activity.[28]

Epoch length

Most investigations regarding the best epoch length to use have occurred with respect to uniaxial accelerometry but they are also relevant to other methods. Generally the shortest epoch possible should be used,[44] at least 15 s but preferably shorter, to capture as much variation in activity levels as possible. New technology enables accelerometers to have memory capacity allowing data storage for over a week of continuous data collection at 5-s epochs and this short epoch captures significantly more time spent at MVPA than when using 60-s epochs.[44]

Accelerometry can accurately determine time spent in ambulatory activities, time in different activity intensities, and time spent sedentary.[45] Uniaxial accelerometry cannot accurately record the limited vertical movement of some activities, such as cycling, and also that of different running speeds.[46,47] Limitations when using accelerometry to assess energy expenditure, suggest that it may be most useful to use uniaxial accelerometry to derive physical activity rather than energy expenditure outcomes. The large majority of validation studies for predicting PAEE using uniaxial accelerometry have either used treadmill locomotion or activities all with mainly vertical movements and sedentary activities to derive the equations.[41,48–50] This serves to perhaps falsely enhance the apparent validity of these monitors to assess PAEE accurately in varied situations such as free-living. The issues regarding the interpretation and analysis of accelerometry data will be discussed below.

Pedometers

The use and validity of pedometers in physical activity research has been systematically reviewed.[25] Electronic pedometers usually consist of a horizontal spring-suspended lever arm that moves with the vertical acceleration of the hips during ambulation.[25] The two main advantages of pedometers are that they are objective and of low cost; however, they are only able to accurately assess ambulatory activity. Pedometer data have been used to estimate energy expenditure against DLW in adults,[51] but the fundamental differences between these two outputs limit the validity of this. To our knowledge, pedometers have not been validated to assess physical activity during free-living in children. Pedometers also are susceptible to noise during activities such as cycling or driving on uneven surfaces. Unlike accelerometers, which record and store data by epoch, pedometers usually give an overall estimate of 'steps taken' per day, limiting the output to overall daily summary scores of physical activity.

Correlations between pedometer step counts and oxygen uptake ($\dot{V}O_2$) are generally good; the median correlation between EE and pedometer counts in a recent review was $r = 0.62$.[52] However, in 9-year-old children during treadmill activity and unregulated play, correlations were as high as $r = 0.78$ and 0.92.[42] Comparative studies of different pedometer brands show that accuracy is good at faster speeds, generally above about 80 m·min^{-1}, but below this speed error is generally quite substantial.[53,54] Pedometer data will not necessarily be comparable across different age groups due to different heights and therefore stride lengths; a child with a stride length of 50 cm would walk approximately 2.5 km less in 10,000 steps than one with a stride length of 75 cm, which may correspond to about 30 min of moderate intensity activity.

Pedometers cannot assess intensity, duration, or frequency of activity and have errors when assessing EE. However, they do give an overall indication of ambulatory activity, are cheap, and have also been used successfully as a motivational tool in children.[55]

Heart rate monitoring

Traditional HR monitors generally use watches to display and record HR from a chest-band transmitter with participants able to see their HR during the assessment. HR monitors are becoming smaller and more discrete and now have the ability to internally store minute-by-minute data for over a week while not displaying HR, reducing the chance of altered behaviour due to measurement effect.

The relationship between HR and energy expenditure is fundamentally linear during activity, but not at low intensity activity and while sedentary. Consequently, HR is often used to predict energy expenditure or to determine time spent when physically active, with heart beats per minute above a certain level. HR data theoretically require more processing than movement data if they are to be used for the assessment of physical activity. Some sort of individual calibration is generally necessary due to individual variation in resting HRs and fitness levels which influence the slope and intercept of the regression line between HR and energy expenditure.[56] This may be impractical in free-living studies as simple calibration procedures explain a substantial proportion of the between-individual variance in the PAEE–HR relationship.[57] Despite validation studies of HR monitoring for assessing physical activity in children, both in controlled and free-living environments,[42,58] research using HR data has not been anywhere near as prolific as that with movement sensing. This is probably due to the higher proportion of missing and erroneous data and the need for individual calibration. The question of what to do with missing data and issues with individual calibration are discussed in more detail.

New technology and combined methods

There is an emerging generation of methods to assess physical activity and energy expenditure using new technologies, which are often able to measure and combine accelerometry with a physiological parameter using one device. These include combined HR and movement sensors, combined movement and temperature sensors, and multi-sensor devices to determine body position. It is logical that combined parameters would capture more variance in activity than one alone, if the increase in accuracy is worth the often substantial extra cost of these new technologies. Currently, the high cost of some of these methods inhibits their use for large-scale epidemiological studies, but they can nevertheless provide very interesting information on body positioning and are useful in clinical populations.

Novel methods are now also being used for the enhancement of physical activity assessment, including the use of global positioning systems to map movement, environmental characteristics, and even determinants of physical activity.[59] This has great potential in the field of physical activity research with its use sure to increase as the technology develops.

Combined heart rate and movement sensing

Movement sensing is able to relatively accurately assess physical activity at lower activity intensities, as it has the ability to easily determine whether someone is moving or not. However, movement sensing has significant limitations during certain activities where the majority of movement is not vertical. HR monitoring is accurate during active periods but has limitations at lower intensity levels; therefore it is logical that a combination of these two methods would provide a more accurate assessment of physical activity than either method used alone.[24,60]

The simultaneous use of HR monitoring and movement sensing using two separate devices has been done in adults[61–66] in children[42,67] and using combined methods in adults[68–70] and children.[50] Consequently, compared to either method used alone, this is a relatively unexplored area of physical activity research. HR monitors can be relatively bulky, so the development of new technology is essential for the progress of this area of research as combined monitors reduce participant and investigator burden.

The combination of HR and movement sensing has been shown to be more accurate than either method used alone in controlled environments in children.[50,71] Free-living studies using combined and separate HR and movement sensing are necessary to determine whether the accuracy of the prediction is increased enough relative to the increased cost and complexity of analysis of the combined method.

Subjective methods

Questionnaires

Self-report methods of physical activity assessment, specifically questionnaires and activity diaries are the cheapest and arguably the simplest method of assessing physical activity, but they have some unavoidable limitations. Self-report methods are subject to recall bias. This can either be intentional or accidental false recall, missed recall, or differential reporting accuracy of different intensities, dimensions, and domains of activity. The subjective classification of intensity is also a problem with all subjective methods, and it contributes to the large variation in error in individual estimates of energy expenditure.

Age is a significant factor in determining the method of administration, for example, children under the age of 10 years are known not to provide accurate self-report data.[23] Therefore, parental and teacher-reported questionnaires or proxy-reports are often used. However, recall of children's physical activity is difficult for adults [72] and unique limitations and errors are associated with this method as neither a parent nor a teacher will be able to constantly monitor any one child for elongated periods, and they may also be in charge of other children.

Many questionnaires only measure one aspect of physical activity such as sport participation or MVPA. Participation in discrete activities are generally more accurately recalled by self-report methods as the individual has made a conscious decision to carry out that activity in a defined period of time. However, the outcome of interest here, habitual or usual activity, is much more difficult to capture accurately with self-report methods.

Correlations between criterion and subjective methods indicate that questionnaires have severely limited ability to accurately assess and quantify physical activity and PAEE. However, for certain types of activity, such as MVPA, the correlations between methods can be quite respectable (i.e. $r > 0.5$).[73,74] Some questionnaires may be appropriate to rank the EE of children, but the absolute validity is likely to be very poor.[73]

Activity diaries

Activity diaries are inexpensive and have been shown to be valid to assess PAEE on a group level in 15-year-old adolescents[75,76] and to record bouts of MVPA[76,77] and also physical activity type. However, there is a relatively high participant burden associated with the completion of an activity diary, which could possibly affect habitual behaviour. The nature of a diary, writing what activity was carried out for the majority of a bound time segment, will inevitably lead to minor or short-term activities being omitted. However, recall periods shorter than 15 min have been found to be too intensive and to not get fully completed.[75] Activity diaries have only been successfully used in adolescents probably as younger children are unlikely to cope as well with the task of accurately completing a diary.

Direct observation

Direct observation is often used as a criterion method for the assessment of physical activity but not energy expenditure in children.[78] An observer will watch the children using one of many observational systems available to record physical activity, these systems have been reviewed elsewhere.[72,78] Direct observation has much utility for the assessment of physical activity in controlled environments, such as during school break-times, and for short-term validation studies. However, substantial investigator burden associated with this method makes it unsuitable for the assessment of habitual or free-living activity. The position, mode, duration, and location of physical activity can be assessed relatively well using this method but the assessment of activity intensity is fraught with problems due to the subjective nature of classification, especially at the mid-ranges of intensity levels. Also, the addition of an observer to the habitual environment can easily lead to reactivity of the subject and consequently altered behaviour. Many observational systems are available,[72,78] but like questionnaires, it seems to make good sense to use already existing observational systems, implementing alterations and improvements if necessary, rather than producing new methods to add to the ever-increasing number available.

No one method will be suitable for all situations, and all methods have limitations, often these are limitations that seriously affect the feasibility and validity of the methods. The measurement of physical activity in both children and adults is always a trade-off between feasibility and accuracy. The most accurate method possible should be used when considering the resources available and after careful consideration of the physical activity outcome required. A summary of key points for each method are summarized in Table 10.2.

Data analysis and interpretation

It is not just the correct choice and use of a measurement method but also choosing the most suitable method of interpretation that is of importance in physical activity research. Physical activity out-

Table 10.2 Summary of key points for physical activity assessment methods

	DLW	Calorimetry	Accelerometry	Pedometers	Heart rate monitoring	Combined heart rate and movement	Questionnaires	Activity diaries	Direct observation
Can it assess free-living physical activity?	Yes	No, laboratory based	Yes	Yes	Yes	Yes	Yes	Yes	No, used in controlled environments
Invasiveness and burden	Not invasive	Bulky equipment and invasive with use of mask	Not invasive	Not invasive	Can be bulky	Not invasive	Not invasive	Very time consuming	High burden for investigators
Cost	Very expensive	Very expensive	Moderate	Inexpensive	Moderate	Moderate to expensive	Inexpensive	Inexpensive	Expensive
Dimensions assessed	Total energy expenditure	Total energy expenditure, intensity, frequency, duration	Activity counts: intensity, frequency, duration, EE can be predicted	Total steps, total daily PA	Intensity, frequency, duration, EE can be predicted	Intensity, frequency, duration, EE can be predicted	Type, possibly frequency and duration of sports and leisure activities and to rank EE	Total EE, type, duration, frequency	Type, duration, frequency
Length of measurement	Usually between 7 and 14 days	Short term. Up to 24 h in a metabolic chamber	1 to 14 days Usually up to seven days	Up to 14 days (usually less)	1 to 14 days Usually 4 days	1 to 14 days	From 1 day to habitual	4 to 7 days	Short term in controlled environments, less than 24 h
Accuracy	Very accurate	Very accurate	Accurate during flat locomotion and for sedentary activities	Accurate during most walking speeds	Good at higher activity intensities but poor at low activity intensities	Should be accurate across all intensity levels	Only suitable in those over 10 years old	Only in older adolescents	Accurate in short term

puts can be broadly grouped into two main categories: the estimation of energy expenditure or another physical activity outcome. Energy expenditure outcomes generally use TEE and predicted or measured BMR or REE to derive PAEE and related outcomes. Conversely, the physical activity outcomes are variable and the ability to assess these strongly depends on the method of measurement used. Some of the most common outcome measures of EE and physical activity (PA) are listed, but it is not necessarily an exhaustive list.

Energy expenditure outcomes

- PAEE = TEE − BMR or = 0.9·TEE–BMR (e.g. kJ, kcal).
- PAL = TEE / BMR.
- PAI = EE per unit of time (e.g. kJ·min,$^{-1}$ kcal·min,$^{-1}$ or min·d^{-1}).

Physical activity outcomes

- Time spent physically active (e.g. min·d^{-1}).
- Intensity of physical activity (e.g. sedentary, light, moderate, vigorous).
- Total counts (per unit time) or average cpm.
- Total steps (per unit time).
- Duration of bouts of physical activity.
- Frequency of physical activity.
- Mode or type of physical activity.

Accelerometry

Owing to the volume of publications using uniaxial accelerometry to derive PAEE and other physical activity outcomes, the task of interpreting output from uniaxial accelerometers is something constantly under discussion.[79] Choosing the most accurate and appropriate method for the interpretation of accelerometry data is possibly one of the biggest challenges facing researchers, due to the multitude and variety of published methods.

Substantial error can be introduced by choosing unwise and poorly considered methods of analysis and interpretation. For example, it is easy, with the same dataset, to label a population very inactive or sufficiently active, as demonstrated in Fig. 10.4. Using three commonly used cut-points for defining MVPA using accelerometry data, this sample of 28 children aged 12–13 years old are shown to have very different activity levels. Using one set of cut points [80] indicates that both boys and girls are doing 60 min of MVPA a day on average. However, using other thresholds for different intensity levels neither boys nor girls are carrying out 30 min of MVPA a day,[81] with a third set of cut-points showing that boys but not girls are carrying out 30 min of MVPA a day.[82] The difference between these activity thresholds varies depending on the activities performed when establishing the relationship between counts and energy expenditure.

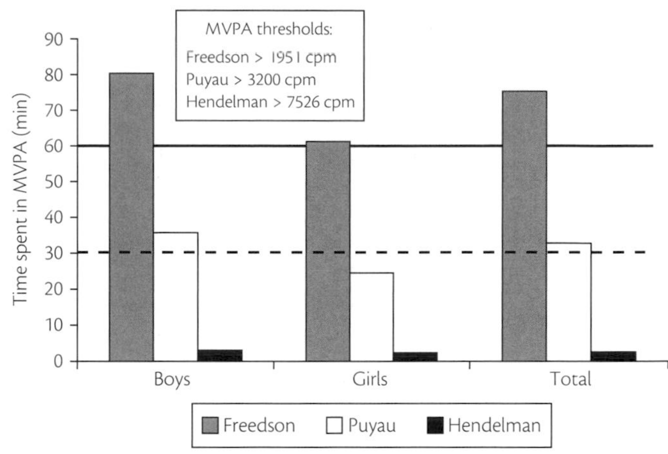

Fig. 10.4 The effect of different physical activity thresholds on time spent at moderate and vigorous intensity physical activity intensity in 12- to 13-year-old children.

Defining worn time

The standard instruction to those wearing an accelerometer is usually to wear it only during waking hours, removing it for sleeping, bathing, showering, and swimming if the monitor is not water proof. Consequently, the definition of worn time and time when the monitor was potentially removed, including during sleep, is an important consideration. As sleep usually accounts for approximately 8 h every day, it can make a big difference whether these data are included or not. Twenty-four hours of data can be included in analyses for each valid day, even if it is suspected that the monitor was not worn, or data can be excluded when it is suspected that the monitor was removed. Various methods are used to exclude data:

- Data consisting of continuous zeros can be deleted.
- Data can be removed after comparison with a diary of wear time.
- Data can be removed from assumed standard sleep times.

If excluding data based on numbers of continuous zeros, the number of zeros chosen may increase with age, due to the sporadic and frequent nature of young children's physical activity. The minimum number of continuous zeros to confidently discount time as 'not-worn' is likely to be about 10 min in young children, probably increasing to about 20 min in adolescents and even higher in adults. All methods have limitations, as one is either making assumptions or putting trust in a diary. Whatever method is chosen, it should be taken into consideration when making cross-study comparisons. For example, when an accelerometry equation was used to estimate PAEE from free-living data, it overestimated by 83% using 24 h of accelerometry data with none excluded, and the same equation underestimated PAEE by no more than 3% when using only awake time, with sleep time discounted. However, in the latter case a systematic error was introduced.[83]

Defining valid days

If any data are being discounted, the amount of 'worn time' constituting a valid day of wear has to be decided. A threshold is defined for the minimum number of minutes when the monitor is thought to have been worn, and below this threshold the day is discounted. Again, there is not a widely used value for this but around 600 min or 10 h of worn time is often used.[13,84] A recent study in 5-year-old children examined the reliability of uniaxial accelerometry data finding that reliability increased up to 80% when including 10 h of data per day over 7 days, but reliability was very similar (79%) when only including data for 3 h per day.[85] If including data for 4 days, reliability was 69% when including either 3 or 10 h of monitoring per day. Consequently, it may be possible to obtain reliable data for even very young children with relatively short measurement periods.[85]

Intensity thresholds

Cut-points are levels of movement (counts·min^{-1}) that are equivalent to different activity intensities. The wide variety in these cut-points unfortunately affects the comparability between studies. Upper limits for sedentary behaviour range from 100 to 1100 counts·min^{-1} [80,86,87] and the lower cut-points for moderate intensity activity range from 615 to 7526 counts·min^{-1}.[81,88] Table 10.3 gives some examples of published cut-points used when assessing physical activity by the Actigraph accelerometer; some adult-derived cut-points are included as they lie within the range of the child-derived cut-points, except for the moderate cut-point derived by Hendelman *et al.*[81] which is substantially higher. The cut-points available vary widely, and when used in the same population, they can give substantially different results regarding activity level,[19] as indicated in Fig. 10.4.

Probably the most important decision that could be made by the physical activity research community would be to agree on a universal standard cut-point. It seems sensible not to keep deriving more but to compare and utilize existing ones and it is quite possible that cut-points are population and age-group specific. However, the large inter-individual variation in accelerometer output for a given exercise task[89] may be greater than the between group variation.

Activity counts have been used successfully to define sedentary behaviour in comparison to direct observation;[87] this is a relatively novel use of movement data and cut-points. This has great potential as it does not introduce error and assumptions; sedentary behaviour should have less inter-individual variation than MVPA and is an exposure likely to be very important for health.

Fig. 10.5 shows that when using equations derived from different activities to predict EE, the same cut-point corresponds to very different energy expenditures and the predicted energy expenditures vary by approximately 700 J·min·kg^{-1} at high intensity activity.

Summary scores from accelerometry data

Movement data are also commonly used as a summary score of average cpm, or total count 5 per minute, removing the need for cut-points; however, this gives no information about patterns of activity and how activity is distributed over a specific time period. The estimates of average cpm will be substantially lower if the entire measurement time is used with no 'not-worn' time discounted, and this will obviously affect comparability between studies. Regardless, this summary score of average intensity is significantly associated with individual metabolic risk factors and clustered metabolic risk independent of adiposity in children.[90,91]

Activity bouts

Bouts of activity maintained above a certain intensity level (usually moderate intensity) and maintained for a period of time (often 5 or 10 min) are also used to display accelerometry data. There are both commercially and researcher developed software programs available which will automatically summarize data into user-defined variables including bouts of activity dependent on various conditions.

A consideration is whether every minute or epoch of data within the bout has to remain above the defined threshold or whether 1 or 2 min of data can drop below, without the bout being discounted. This is especially important with young children when sporadic activity could influence the stability of activity bouts. The summation of accelerometry data as bouts of activity maybe particularly useful in certain situations, such as when examining the associations between physical activity and specific health outcomes if it is shown that physical activity needs to be accumulated in bouts of a certain intensity. Future studies should address this issue in children.

Prediction of energy expenditure

Accelerometry

The prediction of PAEE from biomechanical and physiological variables such as accelerometry and HR requires significant assumptions to be made. An EE prediction model will always have error so the aim should be to minimize the error and produce uniformly accurate estimates over the whole spectrum of activity levels. Predictions of PAEE are often subject to systematic error and heteroscedasticity which can limit their ability to predict PAEE in anything but a controlled environment and homogenous population. Energy expenditure prediction equations vary considerably and the situation where a prediction equation is applied and subsequently derived will affect accuracy, as shown in Fig. 10.5.

The accuracy of equations derived in a laboratory environment and then applied in a different situation is dependent on the activities carried out and the similarity of the two situations.[92] This is likely to be more of a problem with accelerometry than HR or combined HR and movement sensor (HR+M) equations.[71] Even

Table 10.3 Physical activity MVPA thresholds for uniaxial accelerometry

Citation	Sedentary threshold (counts·min^{-1})	Moderate threshold (counts·min^{-1})	Derivation age group (years)	Derivation activities
Freedson *et al.*,[79]	<100	>1951	Adults	Treadmill walking and jogging
Hendelman *et al.*,[80]	<191	>7526	Adults	Walking and household activities
Metallinos-Katsaras *et al.*,[20]	–	>615	6	Equivalent to 3 METS, from laboratory study
Puyau *et al.*,[81]	<800	>3200	6–16	Structured activities
Reilly *et al.*,[86]	<1100	>3200	4	Sedentary from nursery activity, moderate from Puyau *et al.*[81]
Treuth *et al.*,[85]	<100	>3000	13–14	Structured activities

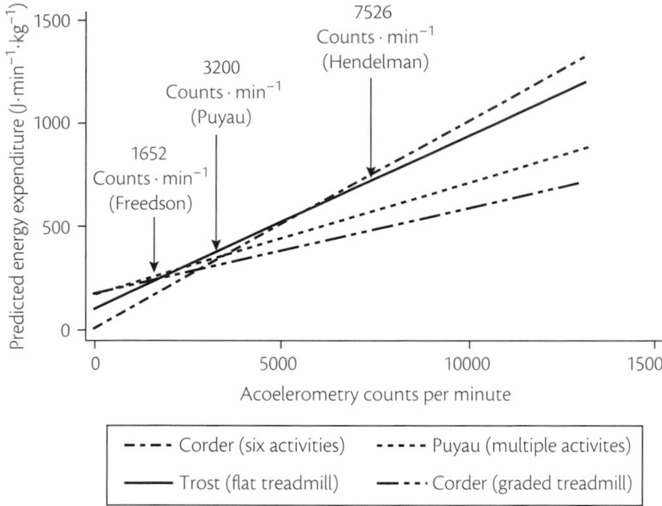

Fig. 10.5 Mean physical activity energy expenditure predicted by four different equations in relation to accelerometry counts per minute.

when equations are derived and applied in a similar situation, other factors such as the activity levels of both groups and data treatment processes will affect the accuracy. Energy expenditure prediction equations based on laboratory assessments of the relationship between energy expenditure and activity significantly differ from equations derived from the relationship between activity counts and DLW measured PAEE when applied to the same group of children.[83] Equations derived in the laboratory, both during ambulatory and 'lifestyle' calibration activities, should be used with caution for the prediction of free-living PAEE. When used in the field, equations derived during flat treadmill activity tend to underestimate PAEE and those based on lifestyle activities tend to overestimate PAEE.[93] This is due to the gradient of the regression line; an equation derived during lifestyle activities tends to have a flatter slope, such as the Puyau equation in Fig. 10.5,[82] unless the regression line is anchored at zero such as the Corder, six activity equation also included in Fig. 10.5.[71,94] A PAEE–activity count relationship with a flatter slope will overestimate PAEE during low intensity activities, and this is the majority of activity for most people during free-living.

Novel methods are now being used to predict energy expenditure with greater precision including the progression from the 'traditional' linear equations to a two regression method for accelerometry [94] or branched modelling for combined HR+M.[95] Although these methods have been developed on adult data, they would also be applicable for use with children. The first of these methods uses the coefficient of variation of accelerometer counts to determine whether activity recorded is ambulatory or not. Two different prediction equations are subsequently used depending on the classification of activity.[94] If the activity produced low number of counts, the non-ambulatory equation was used to anchor the regression line at zero [94] and avoid biologically implausible results for activities producing low count values. This method provides a more accurate prediction of EE than previously published linear equations.[94] Others have also used a prediction equation with linear and quadratic terms to account for the decrease in the movement count–EE relationship with increasing activity intensity.[96]

Despite all of this work on PAEE prediction equations using movement counts, although relatively accurate predictions are possible at a group level, predicting EE accurately on an individual level from solely movement counts is only likely to work moderately well at best.[39] Furthermore, newly derived approaches needs to be validated against free-living PAEE measured by the DLW method.

Heart rate monitoring

The relationship between HR and EE is relatively linear during activity, but unfortunately not when sedentary. A 'flex point' is often used to define the point at which the relationship of HR and energy expenditure becomes linear. The relationship between HR and energy expenditure below the flex point is variable as HR can be increased by environmental conditions such as anxiety, stress, or increased temperature without an increase in energy expenditure.[95] Unfortunately, this is where the majority of free-living and habitual energy expenditure lies, especially in sedentary populations. The flex HR method is valid for estimating group TEE averages but generally not on an individual level in children.[58]

Traditionally a HR–PAEE (HR–$\dot{V}O_2$) relationship is derived in a laboratory environment and then applied to predict PAEE in a free-living situation. This individual calibration is time consuming and still may not be valid to assess free-living PAEE, as the choice of activities in the calibration protocol will again affect the accuracy of the prediction.[92] As the HR–PAEE relationship will be affected by fitness,[97] some form of individual calibration is necessary if individual estimates of PAEE are required. In situations where indirect calorimetry is not feasible as a calibration procedure, simple step tests with a standard workload can be used for a simple individual calibration.[57] An even easier way of calibration is the sleeping HR. This is assessed by default if HR monitors are worn overnight and may explain substantial variation in the HR–PAEE relationship, negating the need for long laboratory individual calibration procedures.[57] During free-living, HR monitoring is probably the most likely method of physical activity measurement to record spurious data, with some monitors affected by electrical interference from household devices or a bad connection with the skin. The 'cleaning' of HR data, including the identification of erroneous data points and their subsequent deletion or interpolation can introduce error. However, a reduction in the need for complicated and expensive individual calibration substantially increases the feasibility of HR monitoring or combined HR and movement sensing in large free-living populations.

Combined heart rate and movement data

New methods have been used to improve the accuracy of PAEE prediction, including combining HR and movement data. Branched modelling has been used to account for the limitations in accuracy of the two methods at different activity intensities. A detailed account of this method is available elsewhere[95] but briefly, PAEE from separate accelerometry and HR equations are weighted in four different weightings for HR and acceleration, depending on the level of HR and activity counts. Branched modelling has shown a reduction in the error of energy expenditure prediction in adults[95,98] and 12- and 13-year-old children in controlled environments.[50]

Correction for body size

PAEE is influenced by body weight and movement efficiency, so PAEE is not necessarily reflective of the intensity of the activity.

Consequently, it is necessary to correct for body size when making PAEE comparisons.[33] PAEE can be corrected by dividing or scaling body weight, this is especially important if comparing between those of different body size.[99] This is important in children as physical activity measured as body movement by accelerometry decreases with age [100] while absolute PAEE increases.[101] PAEE is also greater in the obese than the normal-weight but they have a lower physical activity.[14] Fat-free mass may be the most appropriate variable by which to scale PAEE as it may account for sex differences in body composition.[102]

Subjective methods

The physical activity output from a questionnaire is subject to substantial interpolation and assumption; consequently, it may be best to not impute too much and to use the data as raw as possible. It is not recommended to estimate PAEE or activity intensity using a questionnaire, especially in young children as far too many assumptions need to be made, on top of the already subjective data. For adults, MET levels for various questionnaires have been summarized[103] but no such resource is available for use with children and young people. Owing to a lack of a comprehensive alternative for youth, these standard MET levels are still commonly used in young people despite the differences between METs for the same activities in adults and children.[104,105] However, when expressed as multiples of REE, not using 1 MET as an oxygen uptake of 3.5 $\text{mL}\cdot\text{kg}^{-1}\cdot\text{min}^{-1}$, the ratio of EE to REE is comparable in children and adults.[104]

Questionnaires can accurately determine the type or mode of activity and can be used to adequately rank, group, or categorize physical activity levels,[73,106] and possibly even assess some aspects of MVPA[74,107] if no objective assessment is available. The use of questionnaires is vital in the collection of behavioural and determinant physical activity data but should not be used if possible when quantification of PAEE is required.

Activity diaries are able to predict PAEE and MVPA bouts on a group, but not individual level, and to define subgroups based on TEE.[75] However, subjective methods of measurement should not be used in preference to an objective method if quantification of PAEE is the primary purpose of the study.

Summary

- Energy expenditure and physical activity are different constructs and are not synonymous.
- It is important to define the dimension of physical activity to be assessed *a priori*.
- Carefully consider the validity of available measurement methods, with regard to the exact exposure that you require and the specific population.
- The aim in physical activity research, regarding self-report methods, direct observation, and accelerometry should be to optimize existing methods, rather than to create new ones.
- Uniaxial accelerometry and combined HR+M, are currently the methods with the most potential to accurately assess physical activity and PAEE, respectively, in epidemiological physical activity research.
- Non-linear modelling of energy expenditure, using accelerometry and HR+M, is a growing area of research and does hold great potential for the increased accuracy of energy expenditure prediction in the future.
- Questionnaires are able to assess type or mode of activity and possibly sports and vigorous activities to rank activity levels but are not able to give accurate estimates of PAEE or physical activity intensity.
- Subjective methods should not be used in preference to an objective method if quantification of intensity, frequency, duration, and PAEE is the primary purpose of the study.

References

1. Harro M, Riddoch C (2000). Physical activity. In: Armstrong N, van Mechelen W (eds.), *Paediatric exercise science and medicine* (1st ed.), pp. 77–84. Oxford University Press, Oxford.
2. Wong M, Day N, Luan J, Chan K, Wareham N (2003). The detection of gene–environment interaction for continuous traits: Should we deal with measurement error by bigger studies or better measurement? *Int J Epidemiol* **32**, 51–7.
3. Wareham N, Rennie K (1998). The assessment of physical activity in individuals and populations: Why try to be more precise about how physical activity is assessed? *Int J Obes* **22(Suppl 2)**, S30–S8.
4. Caspersen C, Powell K, Christensen G (1985). Physical activity, exercise, and physical fitness: Definitions and distinctions for health-related research. *Pub Health Rep* **100**, 126–31.
5. Pate R, Pratt M, Blair S, Haskell W, Macera C, Bouchard C, Buchner D, Ettinger W, Heath G, King A. (1995). Physical activity and public health. A recommendation from the Centers for Disease Control and Prevention and the American College of Sports Medicine. *JAMA* **273**, 402–7.
6. Pate R (1998). Physical activity for young people. *President's Council on Physical Fitness and Sports Research Digest* **3**, 1–8.
7. Ekelund U, Poortvliet E, Yngve A, Hurtig-Wennlov A, Nilsson A, Sjostrom M (2001). Heart rate as an indicator of the intensity of physical activity in human adolescents. *Eur J Appl Physiol* **85**, 244–9.
8. NRC (1989). *Recommended dietary allowances (dietary reference intakes)* (10th ed.). National Research Council, The National Academies Press, Washington, DC.
9. Denzer C (2003). The effect of resistance exercise on the thermic effect of food. *Int J Sport Nutr Exerc* **13**, 396–402.
10. Maffeis C, Schutz Y, Schena F, Zaffanello M, Pinelli L (1993). Energy expenditure during walking and running in obese and nonobese prepubertal children. *J Pediatr* **123**, 193–9.
11. Biddle S, Gorely T, Stensel D (2004). Health-enhancing physical activity and sedentary behaviour in children and adolescents. *J Sports Sci* **22**, 679–701.
12. Strong W, Malina R, Blimkie C, Daniels S, Dishman R, Gutin B, Hergenroeder A, Must A, Nixon P, Pivarnik J, Rowland T, Trust S, Trudeau F. (2005). Evidence based physical activity for school-age youth. *J Pediatr* **146**, 732–7.
13. Riddoch CJ, Bo Andersen L, Wedderkopp N, Harro M, Klasson-Heggebo L, Sardinha LB, Cooper AR, Ekelund U. (2004). Physical activity levels and patterns of 9- and 15-yr-old European children. *Med Sci Sport Exerc*, **36**, 86–92.
14. Ekelund U, Aman J, Yngve A, Renman C, Westerterp K, Sjostrom M (2002). Physical activity but not energy expenditure is reduced in obese adolescents: A case-control study. *Am J Clin Nutr* **76**, 935–41.
15. Janz K, Burns T, Levy S (2005). Tracking of activity and sedentary behaviors in childhood. The Iowa Bone Development Study. *Am J Prev Med* **29**, 171–8.
16. Ness A, Leary S, Mattocks C, Blair S, Reilly J, Wells J, Ingle S, Tilling K, Davey-Smith G, Riddoch C. (2007). Objectively measured physical activity and fat mass in a large cohort of children. *PLOS Med* **4**, 476–84.

17. Armstrong N, Welsman JR (2006). The physical activity patterns of European youth with reference to methods of assessment. *Sports Med* **36**, 1067–86.
18. McMurray R, Harrell J, Bangdiwala S, Jianhua H (2003). Tracking of physical activity and aerobic power from childhood through adolescence. *Med Sci Sport Exerc* **35**, 1914–22.
19. Guinhouya C, Hubert H, Soubrier S, Vilhelm C, Lemdani M, Durocher A (2006). Moderate-to-vigorous physical activity among children: Discrepancies in accelerometry-based cut-off points. *Obesity* **14**, 774–7.
20. Nelson M, Neumark-Stzainer D, Hannan P, Sirard J, Story M (2006). Longitudinal and secular trends in physical activity and sedentary behavior during adolescence. *Pediatrics* **118**, e1627–e34.
21. Gordon-Larsen P, Nelson M, Popkin B (2004). Longitudinal physical activity and sedentary behavior trends adolescence to adulthood. *Am J Prev Med* **27**, 277–83.
22. Twisk J, Kemper H, van Mechelen W (2000). Tracking of activity and fitness and the relationship with cardiovascular disease risk factors. *Med Sci Sport Exerc* **32**, 1455–61.
23. Sallis JF (1991). Self-report measures of children's physical activity. *J School Health* **61**, 215–9.
24. Rennie KL, Wareham NJ (1998). The validation of physical activity instruments for measuring energy expenditure: Problems and pitfalls. *Pub Health Nutr* **1**, 265–71.
25. Tudor-Locke C, Williams J, Reis J, Pluto D (2002). Utility of pedometers for assessing physical activity. Convergent validity. *Sports Med* **32**, 795–808.
26. Bland JM, Altman DG (1986). Statistical methods for assessing agreement between two methods of clinical measurement. *Lancet* **8**, 307–10.
27. Baumgarter T (1989). Norm-referenced measurement: Reliability. In: Safrit M, Wood T, (eds.), *Measurement concepts in physical education and exercise science*, pp. 45–72. Human Kinetics, Champaign, IL.
28. Trost S, McIver K, Pate R (2005). Conducting accelerometer-based activity assessments in field-based research. *Med Sci Sport Exerc* **37**, 531–43.
29. Mattocks C, Leary S, Ness A, Deere K, Saunders J, Kirkby J, Blair S, Tilling K, Riddoch C. (2007). Intraindividual variation of objectively measured physical activity in children. *Med Sci Sport Exerc* **39**, 622–9.
30. Atkinson G, Nevill A (1998). Statistical methods for assessing measurement error (reliability) in variables relevant to sports medicine. *Sports Med* **26**, 217–38.
31. Lifson N, Gordon C, Visscher M, Nier A (1955). Measurement of total carbon dioxide production by means of D_2O.[18] *J Appl Physiol* **7**, 704–10.
32. Schoeller D (1999). Recent advances from application of doubly labeled water to measurement of human energy expenditure. *J Nutr* **129**, 1765–8.
33. Prentice A, Black A, Coward W, Cole T (1996). Energy expenditure in overweight and obese adults in affluence societies: An analysis of 319 doubly-labelled water measurements. *Eur J Appl Physiol* **50**, 72–92.
34. Schoeller D, van Santen E (1982). Measurement of energy expenditure in humans by doubly labeled water method. *J Appl Physiol* **53**, 955–9.
35. de Weir JB (1949). New methods for calculating metabolic rate with special reference to protein metabolism. *J Physiol* **109**, 1–9.
36. Murgatroyd P, Shetty P, Prentice A (1993). Techniques for the measurement of human energy expenditure: A practical guide. *Int J Obes* **17**, 549–68.
37. Butte N, Wong M, Hopkinson J, Heinz C, Mehta N, Smith E (2000). Energy requirements derived from total energy expenditure and energy deposition during the first 2 y of life. *Am J Clin Nutr* **72**, 1558–69.
38. Pate R, Almeida M, McIver K, Pfeiffer K, Dowda M (2006). Validation and calibration of an accelerometer in preschool children. *Obesity* **14**, 2000–6.
39. Freedson P, Pober D, Janz K (2005). Calibration of accelerometer output for children. *Med Sci Sport Exerc* **37**, S523–S30.
40. Melanson E, Freedson P (1995). Validity of the computer science and applications, Inc. (CSA) activity monitor. *Med Sci Sport Exerc* **27**, 934–40.
41. Puyau M, Adolph AL, Vohra F, Zakeri I, Butte NF (2004). Prediction of activity energy expenditure using accelerometers in children. *Med Sci Sport Exerc* **36**, 1625–31.
42. Eston RG, Rowlands AV, Ingledew DK (1998). Validity of heart rate, pedometry, and accelerometry for predicting the energy cost of children's activities. *J Appl Physiol* **84**, 362–71.
43. Yngve A, Nilsson A, Sjostrom M, Ekelund U (2003). Effect of monitor placement and of actvity setting on the MTI accelerometer output. *Med Sci Sport Exerc* **35**, 320–6.
44. Nilsson A, Ekelund U, Yngve A, Sjostrom M (2002). Assessing physical activity among children with accelerometers using different time sampling intervals and placements. *Pediatr Exerc Sci* **14**, 75–84.
45. Reilly J, Kelly L, Montgomery C, Williamson A, Fisher A, McColl J, (2006). Physical activity to prevent obesity in young children: Cluster randomised controlled trial. *BMJ* **333**, 1041–3.
46. Brage S, Wedderkopp N, Andersen L, Froberg K (2003). Influence of step frequency on movement intensity predictions with the CSA accelerometer: A field validation study in children. *Pediatr Exerc Sci* **15**, 277–87.
47. Rowlands A, Stone M, Eston R (2007). Influence of speed and step frequency during walking and running on motion sensor output. *Med Sci Sport Exerc* **39**, 716–27.
48. Trost S, Ward D, Moorehead S, Watson P, Riner W, Burke J (1998). Validity of the computer and science and applications (CSA) activity monitor in children. *Med Sci Sport Exerc* **30**, 629–33.
49. Mattocks C, Leary S, Ness A, Deere K, Saunders J, Tilling K, Kirkby J, Blair S, Riddoch C (2007). Calibration of an accelerometer during free-living activities in children. *IJPO*, 214, 218–26.
50. Corder K, Brage S, Wareham NJ, Ekelund U (2005). Comparison of PAEE from combined and separate heart rate and movement models in children. *Med Sci Sport Exerc* **37**, 1761–7.
51. Leenders N, Sherman W, Nagaraja H, Kien C (2001). Evaluation of methods to assess physical activity in free-living conditions. *Med Sci Sport Exerc* **33**, 1233–40.
52. Tudor-Locke C, Ainsworth BE, Thompson R, Matthews C (2002). Comparison of pedometer and accelerometer measures of free-living physical activity. *Med Sci Sport Exerc* **34**, 2045–51.
53. Crouter S, Schneider P, Karabulut M, Bassett DJ (2003). Validity of 10 electronic pedometers for measuring steps, distance and energy cost. *Med Sci Sport Exerc* **35**, 1455–60.
54. Beets M, Patton M, Edwards S (2005). The accuracy of pedometer steps and time during walking in children. *Med Sci Sport Exerc* **37**, 513–20.
55. Oliver M, Schofield G, MvEvoy E (2006). An integrated curriculum approach to increasing habitual physical activity in children: A feasibility study. *J School Health* **76**, 74–9.
56. Rowland T (1996). *Developmental exercise physiology*. Human Kinetics, Champaign, IL.
57. Brage S, Ekelund U, Brage N, Hennings M, Froberg K, Franks P, Wareham NJ (2007). Hierarchy of individual calibration levels for heart rate and accelerometry to measure physical activity. *J Appl Physiol* 103, 682–92.
58. Livingstone MB, Coward WA, Prentice AM, Davies AM, Strain JJ, McKenna PG, Mahoney CA, White JA, Stewart CM, Kerr MJ (1992). Daily energy expenditure in free-living children: Comparison of heart-rate monitoring with the doubly labelled water (2H2(18)O) method. *Am J Clin Nutr* **56**, 343–52.
59. Rodriguez D, Brown A, Troped P (2005). Portable global positioning units to complement accelerometry-based physical activity monitors. *Med Sci Sport Exerc* **37**, S572–S81.
60. Brage S, Brage N, Franks P, Ekelund U, Wareham NJ (2005). Reliability and validity of the combined heart rate and movement sensor Actiheart. *Eur J Clin Nutr* **59**, 561–70.

61. Avons P, Garthwaite P, Davies HL, Murgatroyd PR, James WP (1988). Approaches to estimating physical activity in the community: Calorimetric validation of actometers and heart rate monitoring. *Eur J Clin Nutr* **42**, 185–96.
62. Meijer G, Westerterp K, Koper H, Ten Hoor F (1989). Assessment of energy expenditure by recording heart rate and body acceleration. *Med Sci Sport Exerc* **21**, 343–7.
63. Moon J, Butte N (1996). Combined heart rate and activity improve estimates of oxygen consumption and carbon dioxide production. *J Appl Physiol* **81**, 1754–61.
64. Strath S, Bassett D, Swartz A, Thompson D (2001). Simultaneous heart rate-motion sensor technique to estimate energy expenditure. *Med Sci Sport Exerc* **33**, 2118–23.
65. Strath S, Bassett D, Thompson D, Swartz A (2002). Validity of the simultaneous heart rate-motion sensor technique for measuring energy expenditure. *Med Sci Sport Exerc* **34**, 888–94.
66. Brage S, Brage N, Wedderkopp N, Froberg K (2003). Reliability and validity of the computer science and applications accelerometer in a mechanical setting. *Meas Phys Educ Exerc Sci* **7**, 101–19.
67. Treuth MS, Adolph AL, Butte NF (1998). Energy expenditure in children predicted from heart rate and activity calibrated against respiration calorimetry. *Am J Physiol* **275**, E12–E8.
68. Haskell WL, Yee MC, Evans A, Irby PJ (1993). Simultaneous measurement of heart rate and body motion to quantitate physical activity. *Med Sci Sport Exerc* **25**, 109–15.
69. Luke A, Maki KC, Barkey N, Cooper R, McGee D (1997). Simultaneous monitoring of heart rate and motion to assess energy expenditure. *Med Sci Sport Exerc* **29**, 144–8.
70. Rennie KL, Rowsell T, Jebb SA, Holburn D, Wareham NJ (2000). A combined heart rate and movement sensor: Proof of concept and preliminary testing study. *Eur J Clin Nutr* **54**, 409–14.
71. Corder K, Brage S, Mattocks C, Ness A, Riddoch C, Wareham N, Ekelund U. (2007). Comparison of two methods to assess PAEE during six activities in children. *Med Sci Sport Exerc* **39**, 2180–8.
72. Pate R (1993). Physical activity assessment in children and adolescents. *Crit Rev Food Sci* **33**, 321–6.
73. Slinde F, Arvidsson D, Sjoberg A, Rossander-Hulthen L (2003). Minnesota leisure time activity questionnare and doubly labeled water in adolescents. *Med Sci Sport Exerc* **35**, 1923–8.
74. Philippaerts R, Matton L, Wijndaele K, Balduck A, De Bourdeaudhuij I, Lefevre J. (2006). Validity of a physical activity computer questionnaire in 12- to 18-year-old boys and girls. *Int J Sports Med* **27**, 131–6.
75. Bratteby L, Sandhagen B, Fan H, Samuelson G (1997). A 7-day activity diary for assessment of daily energy expenditure validated by the doubly labelled water method in adolescents. *Eur J Clin Nutr* **51**, 585–91.
76. Ekelund U, Yngve A, Sjostrom M (1999). Total daily energy expenditure and patterns of physical activity in adolescents assessed by two different methods. *Scand J Med Sci Sport* **9**, 257–64.
77. Weston A, Petosa R, Pate R (1997). Validation of an instrument for measurement of physical activity in youth. *Med Sci Sport Exerc* **29**, 138–43.
78. Sirard J, Pate R (2001). Physical activity assessment in children and adolescents. *Sports Med* **31**, 439–54.
79. Troiano R (2005). A timely meeting: Objective measurement of physical activity. *Med Sci Sport Exerc* **37**, S487–S9.
80. Freedson P, Melanson E, Sirard J (1998). Calibration of the computer science and applications, Inc. accelerometer. *Med Sci Sport Exerc* **30**, 777–81.
81. Hendelman D, Miller K, Baggett C, Debold E, Freedson P (2000). Validity of accelerometry for the assessment of moderate intensity physical activity in the field. *Med Sci Sport Exerc* **32**, S442–S9.
82. Puyau M, Adolph A, Vohra F, Butte N (2002). Validation and calibration of physical activity monitors in children. *Obes Res* **10**, 150–7.
83. Nilsson A, Brage S, Riddoch C, Anderssen S, Sardinha L, Wedderkopp N, Anderson L, Ekelund U (2008). Comparison of equations for predicting energy expenditure from accelerometer counts in children. *Scand J Med Sci Sport*. Jan 14 (Epub ahead of print) PMID: 18248534 [PubMed as supplied by publisher]
84. Ekelund U, Sardinha LB, Anderssen SA, Harro M, Franks PW, Brage S, Cooper AR, Anderson LB, Riddoch C, Froberg K. (2004). Associations between objectively assessed physical activity and indicators of body fatness in 9- to 10-y-old European children: A population-based study from 4 distinct regions in Europe (the European Youth Heart Study). *Am J Clin Nutr* **80**, 584–90.
85. Penpraze V, Reilly J, MacLean C, Montgomery C, Kelly L, Paton J, Aitchinson T, Grant S (2006). Monitoring of physical activity in young children: How much is enough? *Pediatr Exerc Sci* **18**, 483–91.
86. Treuth M, Schmitz K, Catellier D, McMurray R, Murray D, Almeida M, Going S, Normal J, Pate R (2004). Defining thresholds for activity intensities in adolescent girls. *Med Sci Sport Exerc* **36**, 1259–66.
87. Reilly J, Coyle J, Kelly L, Burke G, Grant S, Paton J (2003). An objective method for measurement of sedentary behaviour in 3- to 4-year olds. *Obes Res* **11**, 1155–8.
88. Metallinos-Katsaras E, Freedson P, Fulton J, Sherry B (2007). The association between an objective measure of physical activity and weight status in preschoolers. *Obesity* **15**, 686–94.
89. Ekelund U, Aman J, Westerterp K (2003). Is the ArteACC index a valid indicator of free-living physical activity in adolescents? *Obes Res* **11**, 793–801.
90. Andersen L, Harro M, Sardinha L, Froberg K, Ekelund U, Brage S, Anderssen S (2006) Physical activity and clustered cardiovascular risk in children: A cross-sectional study (The European Youth Heart Study). *Lancet* **368**, 299–304.
91. Ekelund U, Brage S, Froberg K, Harro M, Anderssen S, Sardinha L, Riddoch C, Anderson L (2006). TV viewing and physical activity are independently associated with metabolic risk in children: The European Youth Heart Study. *PLoS Medicine* **3**, e488.
92. Livingstone MB, Robson PJ, Totton M (2000). Energy expenditure by heart rate in children: An evaluation of calibration techniques. *Med Sci Sport Exerc* **32**, 1513–9.
93. Welk G, McClain J, Eisenmann J, Wickel E (2007). Field validation of the MTI Actigraph and BodyMedia armband monitor using the IDEEA monitor. *Obesity* **15**, 918–28.
94. Crouter S, Clowers K, Bassett D (2006). A novel method for using accelerometer data to predict energy expenditure. *J Appl Physiol* **100**, 1324–31.
95. Brage S, Brage N, Franks PW, Ekelund U, Wong MY, Andersen LB, Froberg K, Wareham NJ (2004). Branched equation modeling of simultaneous accelerometry and heart rate monitoring improves estimate of directly measured physical activity energy expenditure. *J Appl Physiol* **96**, 343–51.
96. Schmitz K, Treuth MS, Hannan P, McMurray R, Ring K, Catellier D, Pate R (2005). Predicting energy expenditure from accelerometry counts in adolescent girls. *Med Sci Sport Exerc* **37**, 155–61.
97. Ekelund U, Poortvliet E, Nilsson A, Yngve A, Holmberg A, Sjostrom M (2001). Physical activity in relation to aerobic fitness and body fat in 14- to 15-year-old boys and girls. *Eur J Appl Physiol* **85**, 195–201.
98. Thompson D, Batterham A, Bock S, Robson C, Stokes K (2006). Assessment of low-to-moderate intensity physical activity thermogenesis in young adults using synchronized heart rate and accelerometry with branched-equation modeling. *J Nutr* **136**, 1037–42.
99. Schoeller D, Jefford G (2002). Determinants of the energy costs of light activities: Inferences for interpreting doubly labeled water data. *Int J Obes* **26**, 97–101.

100. Trost S, Pate R, Sallis J, Freedson P, Taylor W, Dowda M, Sirard J (2002) Age and gender differences in objectively measured physical activity in youth. *Med Sci Sport Exerc* **25**, 350–5.
101. Hoos M, WJM G, Kester A, Westerterp K (2003). Physical activity levels in children and adolescents. *Int J Obes* **27**, 605–9.
102. Ekelund U, Yngve A, Brage S, Westerterp K, Sjostrom M (2004). Body movement and physical activity energy expenditure in children and adolescents: How to adjust for differences in body size and age. *Am J Clin Nutr* **79**, 851–6.
103. Ainsworth B, Haskell W, Whitt M, Irwin M, Swartz A, Strath S, O'Brien W, Bassett DJ, Schmitz K, Emplaincourt P, Jacobs DJ, Leon A (2000) Compendium of physical activities: An update of activity codes and MET intensities. *Med Sci Sport Exerc* **32**, S498–504.
104. Harrell J, McMurray R, Baggett C, Pennell M, Pearce P, Bangdiwala S (2005). Energy costs of physical activities in children and adolescents. *Med Sci Sport Exerc* **37**, 329–36.
105. Spadano J, Must A, Bandini L, Dallal G, Dietz W (2003). Energy cost of physical activities in 12-y-old girls: MET values and the influence of body weight. *Int J Obes* **27**, 1528–33.
106. Arvidsson D, Slinde F, Hulthen L (2004). Physical activity questionnaire for adolescents validated against doubly labelled water. *Eur J Clin Nutr* **59**, 376–83
107. Telford A, Salmon J, Jolley D, Crawford D (2004). Reliability of physical activity questionnaires for children: The children's leisure activities study survey (CLASS). *Pediatr Exerc Sci* **16**, 64–78.

CHAPTER 11

Effort perception

Kevin L. Lamb, Gaynor Parfitt, and Roger G. Eston

Introduction

Individuals possess a well-developed system for sensing the strain involved in physical effort. Effort perception and perceived exertion are synonymous terms which can be defined as the act of detecting and interpreting the sensations arising from the body during physical exertion.[1] The ability to detect and interpret these sensations has been studied in a wide range of populations in a variety of activities and exercise tasks. The plethora of research activity on perceived exertion in adults in the last 30 years has been the subject of several comprehensive reviews.[2–6] However, research on the efficacy of using perceived exertion in children is still relatively new. This has been the subject of critical review papers by the authors[7–9] and others,[10] and some of the information presented here will utilize material from these reviews.

Although there have been over 40 studies of children's perceptions of physical effort, our understanding remains underdeveloped. It was only just over a decade ago that researchers realized that adult-derived methods and applications of the rating of perceived exertion (RPE) notion are not appropriate for use with children. When writing for the first edition of this text, we observed that prior to 2000, most investigators had conducted their research in the same vein as that performed in greater volume on adults, and we appealed for progress in this regard. While we can report that significant progress has been made in the intervening years, there remains, regrettably, a lack of consensus in terms of how data should be gathered (which tools and protocols are appropriate) and analysed statistically, making interpretations of validity and reliability quite difficult. In the past 10 years existing scales have been refined and 'new' ones have been constructed and promoted across a range of exercise modalities. The following sections describe these advances and controversies and present the current status of the application of effort perception research in the paediatric exercise domain.

Application and description of traditional RPE scales

A description of the most common methods of assessing perceived exertion and how this information is used to assess and regulate the intensity of exercise follows. A variety of scales have been developed in an attempt to assess perceived exertion. The ubiquitous 15-point alpha–numeric RPE category scale, developed by Borg in 1970,[11] later revised in 1986,[12] and Borg's lesser-used 12-point Category Ratio 10 (CR 10) scale,[13] are the most commonly used RPE scales. These scales can be used to assess *overall* feelings of exertion or they can be used to *differentiate* between respiratory–metabolic (central) and peripheral (local) signals of exertion. For example, *differentiated* ratings of perceived exertion may be used to segregate the sensations arising from the upper body and the lower body during cycle ergometry exercise or during rowing, running, or stepping.

In the traditional 15-point and CR 10 scales, numbers are anchored to verbal expressions. However, in the CR 10 scale, the numbers have a fixed relationship to one another. For example, an intensity judgement of three would be gauged to be one-third that of nine. On this scale, there is a point above 10 (extremely strong, almost maximal) which may be assigned any number in proportion to 10 which describes the proportionate increase in perceived exertion. For example, if the exercise intensity feels 30% harder than 10 on the CR 10 scale, the RPE would be 13. This type of scale has been suggested to reflect the incremental pattern of effort perception in relation to ventilatory drive during exercise, which is discussed later.

Estimation and production of effort

It is generally observed that RPE measured during an exercise bout increases as exercise intensity increases. Reviews of studies have confirmed the existence of a strong positive association between RPE and indices of metabolic demand in adults[1–6,14] and children,[7–10] particularly when the exercise stimulus is presented in an incremental fashion. Such relationships have been most frequently observed using the so-called passive *estimation* paradigm. In this way, a RPE is given in response to a request from the exercise scientist or clinician to indicate how 'hard' the exercise feels. The information is frequently used to compare responses between exercise conditions or after some form of intervention. It may also be used to assist the clinician or coach to prescribe exercise intensities. For example, an exercise intensity [e.g. heart rate (HR), work rate or oxygen uptake ($\dot{V}O_2$)], which coincides with a given RPE, may be prescribed by the clinician. Alternatively, an active *production* paradigm can be employed whereby the individual is requested to regulate his/her exercise intensity to match specified RPE values.

Measures of metabolic demand can then be compared at each RPE-derived exercise intensity. Several studies on adults[15–21] and children[22–33] show support for the use of RPE in this way.

Evidence suggests that the accuracy of RPE in estimation and production procedures is improved with practice, although there are surprisingly few studies which have explored this fundamental concept in adults,[16] and only two[31,33] which have attempted to adequately address this issue in children. As this is deemed to be an important area of research by the authors, it is appropriate here to consider some of the issues relating to the process of learning. Consideration of the validity and reliability of an RPE scale for children should not ignore age, reading ability, experience, and conceptual understanding. The latter is a developmental issue, which has been the subject of a recently published review by Groslambert and Mahon.[10] In addition, a confounding factor recognized by two of the leading proponents of RPE, Borg,[34] and Bar-Or,[35] 30 years ago is the extent to which children's direct experiences of exercise (their exposure to different exercise intensities) influence their perceptions of exertion.

Surprisingly, however, few investigations of perceived exertion in children have incorporated all of these issues into their design. For a child to perceive effort accurately, and then reliably produce a given intensity at a given RPE, it is logical to assume that learning must occur. Implicit in the process of learning is practice (of the skill) and the cognitive ability of the child. According to Piaget's stages of development, children around the age of 7–10 years can understand categorization but find it easier to understand and interpret pictures and symbols rather than words and numbers. Recently, investigators have incorporated various symbols to emulate categories of effort and acute fatigue into paediatric versions of an RPE scale. These developments have also recognized the need for verbal descriptors and terminology which are more pertinent to a child's cognitive development, age, and reading ability.

The study of perceived exertion in children: A historical perspective

Oded Bar-Or[35] is credited with being the pioneer of research on perceived exertion in children. In 1975, he presented RPE data on 589 children (aged 7–17 years) at the First International Symposium on Physical Work and Effort, recorded during continuous, incremental cycle ergometry. All six age-groups (7–9, 8–10, 10–11, 11–12, 13–14, and 16–17 years) reported higher RPEs with increases in power output. However, compared with adults, the children tended to report a lower RPE for a given relative exercise intensity.

This research acquired a near-definitive status for the next 10 years. With a few exceptions, notably an abstract by Kahle *et al.*[36] which reported an increase in the reproducibility of RPE in healthy girls as they got older, a study by Davies *et al.*[37] which observed that anorexic girls could use RPE to discriminate between differences in exercise intensity, and Eston's[38] somewhat prescient discussion paper on the potential for using RPE in the secondary-school physical education curriculum, there were no further reports in the academic literature until 1986. In that year, there were at least five simultaneous published reports from Canada, England, Japan, and the United States.[39–43] With the exception of the paper by Eston,[38] researchers focused on the RPE-objective effort (HR, work rate) relationship in the laboratory setting and in the passive 'estimation' mode, described above. From 1990, however, pre-specified RPEs were used to compare objective effort measures in children.[22]

The development of child-specific rating scales

Important advances in the study of effort perception in children have occurred in the last 20 years. Despite recognition that experience of exercise was an important determinant for accurate perception of exercise intensity,[34,35,44] little regard was given to the creation of a more developmentally appropriate scale using meaningful terminology and symbols until 1989. In that year, Nystad *et al.*[45] published an illustrated RPE scale with all the written descriptors removed. Six stick figures depicted various stages of effort for use with a group of 10–12-year-old asthmatic children. Despite these attempts to improve the relatively incomprehensible nature of the 6–20 scale, children were still confused by the scale. The investigators concluded that the children lacked physical experience and awareness of different exercise intensities, and therefore, could not understand the concept of perceived exertion. A similar idea was adopted by Mutrie and colleagues (unpublished) using caricatures at various stages of animation (Fig. 11.1). In both versions of the scale, the original wording used by Borg[11] has been retained, although the scale used by Mutrie and colleagues adopted vernacular terms, indigenous to the Glasgow area. At present, there

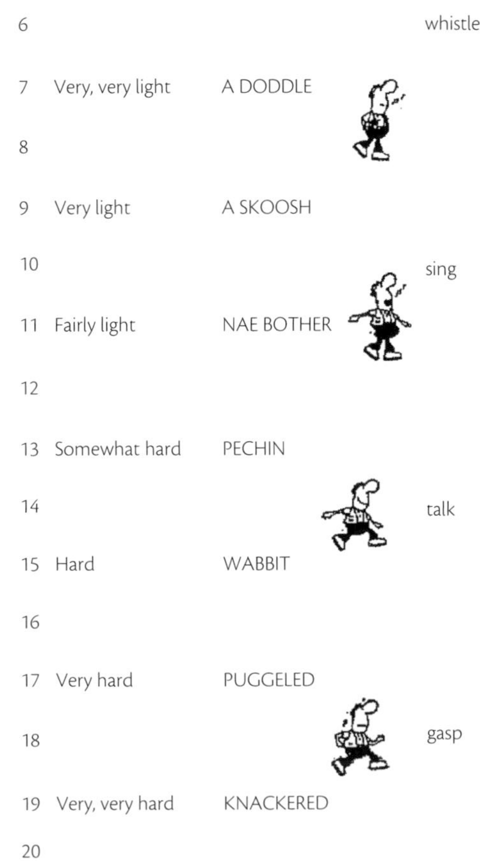

Fig. 11.1 The Glasgow adapted Borg RPE scale

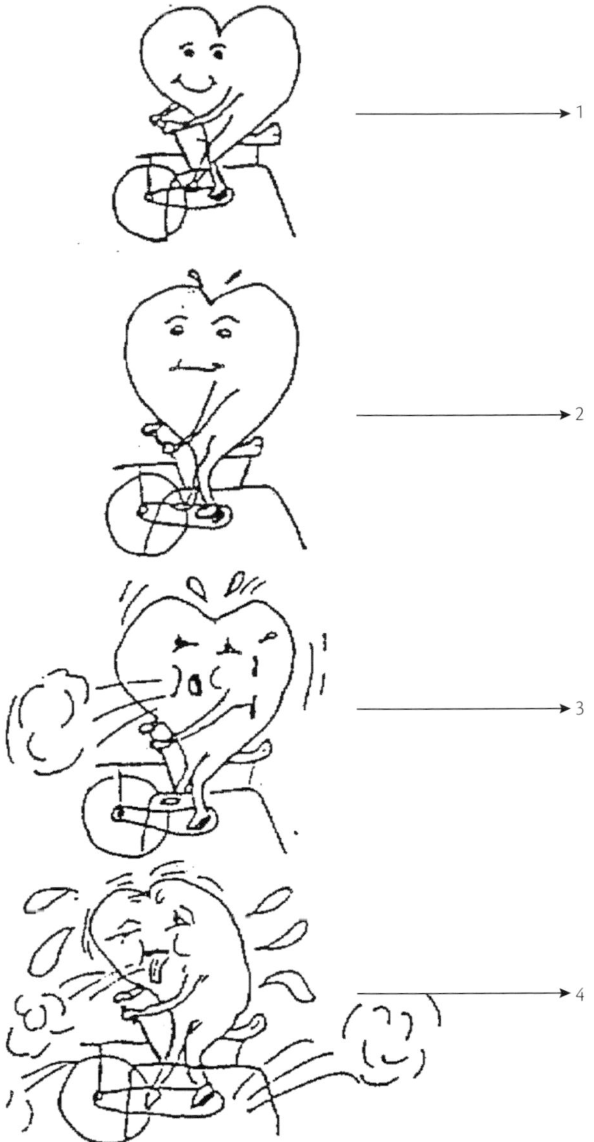

Fig.11.2 Exercising heart RPE scale

are no validity or reliability data on this particular version of the scale.

Other illustrated RPE scales have been applied, including a four-point exercising heart scale developed in a pilot study of 20 boys and girls (aged 9–11 years) during discontinuous cycling (Fig. 11.2). This scale utilizes images of a heart exercising on a cycle in progressively increasing states of exertion. Although not shown here, the scale also uses the colour red to reinforce the notion of exertion. The relationship between effort ratings and HRs (0.62; $p < 0.01$) and power output (0.67; $p < 0.01$) suggests that this scale, with its limited selection of exertion categories, may be worthy of further investigation (Lowry A., The development of a pictorial scale to assess perceived exertion in school children. Unpublished BSc thesis, University College Chester).

Following earlier recommendations by Williams *et al.*[25] in 1991 for a more simple 1–10 perceived exertion scale, a significant development in the measurement of children's effort perception occurred in 1994 with the publication of two papers which proposed and validated an alternative child-specific rating[26,27] (Fig. 11.3). Compared to the Borg scale, the children's effort rating table (CERT) has five fewer possible responses, a range of numbers [1–10] more familiar to children [than 6–20] and verbal expressions chosen by children as descriptors of exercise effort. The CERT soon became recognized as a notable advancement in the study of paediatric effort perception.[46] Studies comparing the 6–20 RPE and CERT in children aged 5–9 years[47] during stepping and 8–11 years[27,28,48,49] during cycling exercise provided support for the CERT. The latter study on 69 Chinese children utilized Chinese-translated (Cantonese) versions of both the Borg 6–20 RPE and the CERT and observed that the validity correlations for CERT, power output, HR, and $\dot{V}O_2$ were consistently higher than those for the 6–20 RPE scale. Leung *et al.*[49] also reported CERT ratings that were more reliable than RPE across two identical continuous, incremental cycling tests.

1	Very, very easy
2	Very easy
3	Easy
4	Just feeling a strain
5	Starting to get hard
6	Getting quite hard
7	Hard
8	Very hard
9	Very, very hard
10	So hard I'm going to stop

Fig. 11.3 Children's effort rating table [from Williams *et al.* [26]]

Pictorial versions of the CERT

The CERT initiative for a simplified scale containing more 'developmentally appropriate' numerical and verbal expressions led to the development of scales which combined numerical and pictorial ratings of perceived exertion. All of these scales depict four to five animated figures, portraying increased states of physical exertion. Like the CERT, the scales have embraced a similar, condensed numerical range and words or expressions which are either identical to [Pictorial-CERT[30], Fig. 11.4], abridged from [Cart and Load Effort Rating (CALER),[33] Bug and Bag Effort (BABE) Rating,[50,51] Eston-Parfitt Curvilinear[8]], or similar in context to the CERT [OMNI[46,52]]. The rationale for the development of these scales and their application is described below.

The principle of presenting a scale that is readily assimilated by children on the basis of their own experiences and stages of development is very important. Using this principle as a basis for the conceptual framework of an alternative illustrated scale, Fig. 11.5 presents a child pulling a cart that is loaded progressively with bricks [CALER scale]. The number of bricks in the cart is commensurate with numbers on the scale. The wording was selected from the CERT to accompany some of the categories of effort. In the study by Eston *et al.*,[33] 20 children aged 7–10 years performed

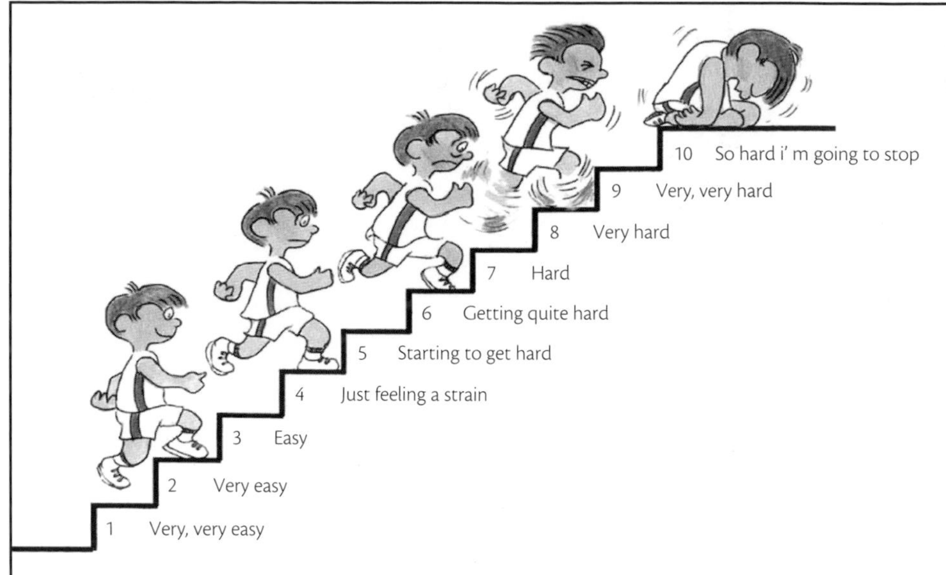

Fig. 11.4 Pictorial children's effort rating table (PCERT) [from Yelling *et al.* [30]]

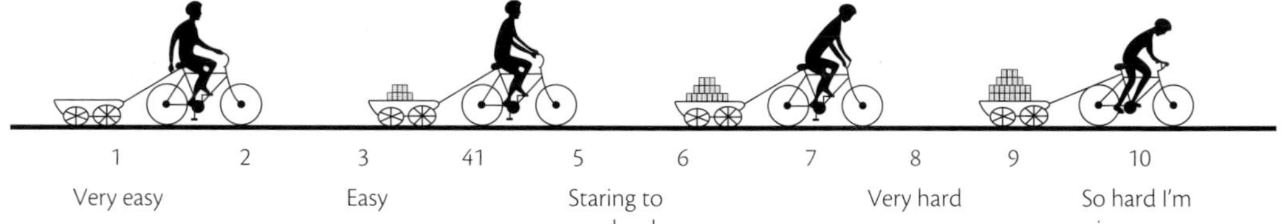

Fig. 11.5 Cart and load effort rating table (CALER) scale [from Eston *et al.* [33]]

four intermittent, incremental active production tests at CALER 2, 5, and 8 over a 4 week period. To reach the specific CALER level, the child instructed the experimenter, in the first 2–3 min, to adjust the cycling resistance by adding or taking away weights (not visible to the child). Each bout was 3 min, separated by 2.5-min rest intervals. An increase in power output across trials (44, 65, and 79 W at CALER 2, 5, and 8, respectively), confirmed that the children understood the scale. Analysis (via limits of agreement and intraclass correlation) between trials indicated that the reliability of the efforts produced improved with practice. This study was the first to apply more than two repeated effort production trials in young children and provides strong evidence that practice improves the reliability of effort perception in children of this age.

The BABE scale (Fig. 11.6), developed by Eston and colleagues,[50,51] depicts a cartoon bug-like character at various stages of exertion stepping up and down on a bench. The character carries a backpack that is progressively loaded with rocks. Like the CALER, the number of coloured rocks in the backpack is commensurate with numbers on the linear scale. The limited verbal descriptors are also the same as those used for the CALER scale. Preliminary validity data for the BABE scale were collected from children (7–10 years) over three repeated trials.[50] The children performed three separate intermittent effort production protocols, 1–2 weeks apart, which involved stepping up and down on a bench (0.30-m high) for 2–3 min at a cadence of 25 steps.min^{-1}. Bouts were separated by 5-min rest periods. Exercise intensities were adjusted by loading a backpack fitted to the subject with loads equivalent to 0, 5, 10, 15, 20, and 25% of body mass. While stepping, randomly ordered target-effort ratings equating to levels 3, 5, and 8 were requested of the children, who asked the investigator to add or remove weights to the backpack until their targets were reached. At this point (within 2–3 min), stepping was continued for a further minute during which time HR and power outputs were recorded. Analysis revealed that power outputs and HRs increased across the three BABE ratings, confirming that the children understood how to use the scale in this mode. Moreover, and in accordance with earlier findings with the CALER scale, the reliability of the efforts produced was good and improved with practice.

More recently, the validity and reliability of the CALER and BABE scales for intra and intermodal regulation of effort production has been investigated.[51] This study utilized a triple repeated, randomized, intermittent, production paradigm using cycling and stepping protocols among 30 boys and girls (aged 7–11 years) randomly allocated into a CALER or BABE group. Each group performed an effort production protocol on six occasions (1 week apart); the first three trials involved cycling and the second three stepping (in the manner described above). As in the initial validation study, the children were required to regulate their exercise intensity to levels 3, 5, and 8. Increases in power outputs and HRs across the three effort levels reaffirmed the validity of each scale in both modes of exercise. In addition, mean HR responses during each type of exercise did not differ between the BABE and CALER groups, suggesting the children could use the scales interchangeably. Reliability

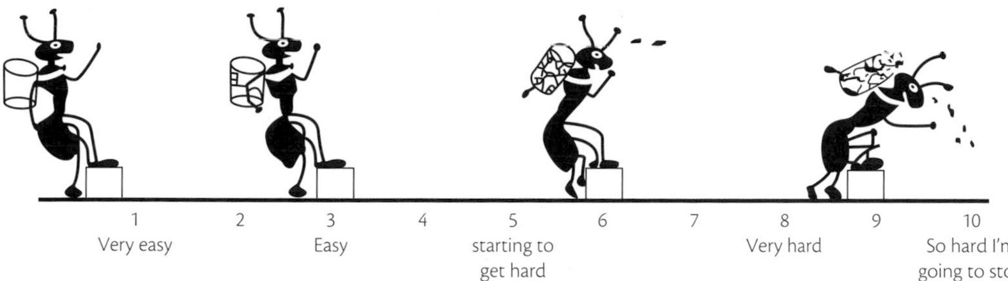

Fig. 11.6 Bug and bag effort rating (BABE) scale [from Parfitt *et al.* [51]]

statistics offered a favourable interpretation for both scales, and in the cycling exercise, the aforementioned practice effect was again noticed, with efforts produced being more consistent between the second and third trials.

A further pictorial version of the CERT (PCERT), initially described by Eston and Lamb,[53] has been validated for both estimation and production tasks during stepping exercise in adolescents.[30] The scale depicts a child running up a 45-degree stepped gradient at five stages of exertion, corresponding to CERT ratings of 2, 4, 6, 8, and 10. Yelling first proposed the PCERT at a perceived exertion symposium hosted by the authors and Gunnar Borg at the University of Wales in 1999. The scale had immediate appeal and was considered to be a significant improvement on the CERT. To facilitate the development of the PCERT, Yelling *et al.*[30] engaged 48 boys and girls (aged 12–15 years) in a series of play and running activities. Throughout the lessons, the children were asked to focus on the exercise sensations of breathlessness, body temperature, and muscle aches. Immediately afterwards, the children were presented with a copy of the CERT in the form of a stepped gradient and five pictorial descriptors and asked to locate the positions which best reflected their own perceptions of effort. The frequency with which the children positioned the visual character at given points along the scale was recorded and the most commonly chosen format was selected, resulting in the pictorial scale.

The validity of the PCERT was determined in a separate group of 48 similarly aged boys and girls in two exercise trials separated by 7–10 days.[30] In trial 1, the children completed 5 × 3 min incremental stepping exercise bouts interspersed with 2-min recovery periods. HR and RPE were recorded in the final 15 s of each bout. They observed that perceived exertion increased as exercise intensity increased. This was also reflected by simultaneous significant increases in HR. In trial two, the children were asked to regulate their exercise intensity during four intermittent 4-min bouts of stepping to match randomly assigned ratings of perceived exertion at 3, 5, 7, and 9. Bouts were separated by a 2-min recovery period. The desired step heights and frequency were determined in the first 2 min of the 4-min exercise bout by verbal feedback from the child. HR and power output were recorded in the last 15 s of each bout. The HR and power output produced at each of the four prescribed effort levels were also significantly different. Yelling *et al.*[30] concluded that the children could discriminate between the four different exercise intensities and regulate their exercise intensity according to the four prescribed ratings from the PCERT.

The utility of the PCERT has been augmented by the findings of two rather different studies, one involving an innovative application of the scale in a U.K. physical education setting,[32] and the other, a comparison with the Borg CR 10 scale among Bulgarian children.[54] The latter study examined the concurrent validity of the PCERT and CR 10 scales during incremental (estimation) laboratory treadmill running in 50 boys and girls in the age group of 10–17 years. The children completed identical trials separated by 1 month, reporting their effort perceptions with one scale in the first trial and the other scale in the second trial. The analysis of the associations between effort ratings and physiologic measures ($\dot{V}O_2$, HR, and minute ventilation) revealed significantly higher correlations overall (r = 0.62–0.82) for the PCERT than the Borg CR 10 scale (r = 0.51–0.71). In the way that the original CERT scale had been shown to be more valid than the 6–20 Borg scale over 10 years ago,[48] these findings lead to the conclusion that the PCERT is more appropriate for estimating exercise effort among such children than the Borg scale.

In the field-based study of Preston and Lamb,[32] 21 boys (aged 13 years) were requested to regulate their exercise outputs during structured (intermittent) physical education activities to match PCERT levels 3, 9, 5, and 7 (in that order). The activity corresponding to PCERT 9 was repeated a week later to assess the children's ability to reproduce their exercise efforts. Analysis of HRs recorded during the exercise bouts revealed that the children could distinguish between level 3 ('easy') and level 9 ('very, very hard'), but not so between the other levels. In addition, while the reliability of effort at PCERT 9 was at best modest overall, some of the children were able to reproduce efforts that were within a relatively narrow range of HRs. These data were encouraging and represent one of the very few attempts there have been to apply effort perception in circumstances of practical value.

OMNI scale

In recognition of the advantages of using a comparatively narrow numerical range to assess perceived exertion, such as that used in the CERT, Robertson[46] proposed the idea of using pictorial descriptors along the scale for assessing perceived exertion in children. As part of a special symposium on effort perception at the European Pediatric Work Physiology Conference in 1997, he presented the idea for a 1–10 pictorial scale (now 0–10) which would be applicable to variations in race, gender, and health status, hence the term OMNI scale. His original idea was to employ, 'pictorially interfaced cognitive anchoring procedures, eliminating the need for mode-specific maximal exercise tests to establish congruence between stimulus and response ranges' (p. 35). However, since then, a number of different pictorial scales have been validated for various modes of exercise in children—for example, cycling,[52] walking/running,[55] and stepping.[56]

In the original OMNI scale validation study,[52] four equal groups of 20 healthy African American and White boys and girls aged 8–12 years, performed a continuous, incremental exercise test on a cycle ergometer. Exercise intensities were increased by 25 W every 3 min. Differentiated (chest and legs) and undifferentiated (whole body) RPE, HR, and $\dot{V}O_2$ were monitored in the final minute of each test stage. The authors reported similarly high positive linear associations between HR, $\dot{V}O_2$, and RPE for each gender/race cohort of children. Their values for the entire cohort ranged from 0.85 to 0.94 for the relationships between RPE, HR, and $\dot{V}O_2$. The RPE for the legs was significantly higher than the chest RPE and overall RPE values. Consequently, this study formed the basis for a number of subsequent validation studies (see above) with various forms of the OMNI scale being employed in estimation protocols. To date, only one study has focused on the validity of the children's OMNI scale in production mode.[29]

Although they were developed independently, there are marked similarities between the PCERT and the OMNI scale. With the exception of the '0' starting point on the OMNI scale, there is the same limited range of numbers, a linear gradient and culturally familiar verbal cues derived from common verbal expressions used by the children in the two respective countries (United Kingdom and United States) to describe their feelings of exertion. With regard to the specificity of the verbal anchors, it is important to note that the original derivation and validation of the CERT was based on children aged 5–9 years of age in the United Kingdom, whereas the OMNI was based on children aged 8–12 years of age in the United States. This difference in maturational status and cognitive development, in addition to cultural semantics and socio-economic status, should be taken into account regarding the differences in terminology that were originally derived for the two scales.

The common cue throughout the OMNI scale is 'tired', the degree of which is indicated by various adverbs: *0—not tired at all, 2—a little tired, 4—getting more tired, 6—tired, 8—really tired, 10—very, very tired.* In the initial validation of the scale, this trunk word appeared 475 times out of a total of 1582 verbal expressions.[52] Conversely, the verbal cues derived for use in the CERT describe degrees of exertion according to various levels of being 'easy' or 'hard' to the extent that the exercise becomes so hard that the child will stop ('so hard I am going to stop'). The appropriateness of the latter term is supported by frequent observations by the authors that young children will often stop exercising when it becomes too uncomfortable. Sometimes, there is little pre-warning of this occurrence.

The connotations of the wording in the two scales are quite distinct. In this regard, the OMNI scale assumes a baseline level of 'tiredness' from the starting point of 0. From a purely semantic and literal perspective, feeling *tired* is a term used to describe a general condition or state of fatigue, weariness, or sleepiness rather than effort. It is not an indication of exertion. Anchoring the scale around the central condition of varying states of 'feeling tired' could be perceived as portraying a negative perspective on the feelings experienced during physical activity, such as that experienced in children's play. Indeed, feeling tired is a common psychological barrier to engaging in physical activity. We, therefore, feel that the use of this term to describe states of physical exertion is somewhat inapt. It is notable that the more recent adult versions of the OMNI scale developed initially for resistance exercise and later to be re-illustrated for cycling, utilize the terms 'easy' and 'hard'. The authors did not divulge the rationale for changing the terminology in the adult scales, although we are of the opinion that these terms are much better suited for purpose. These are the terms used in the CERT.

Independent validation of scales

In recognition of the dearth of data for the OMNI walking/running scale[55] and the PCERT scale in young children,[30] Roemmich *et al.*[57] have recently examined the two scales during sub-maximal exercise. In their study, 51 boys and girls aged 11–12 years performed a perceptual estimation paradigm, comprising a five-stage incremental treadmill test to elicit about 85% of the HR max. Increases in the PCERT and OMNI scales were correlated with increases in $\dot{V}O_2$ ($r = 0.90$ and $r = 0.92$) and HR ($r = 0.89$ and $r = 0.92$), respectively. There was no difference in the slopes of the PCERT and OMNI scores when regressed against HR or $\dot{V}O_2$. There was also no difference in the percentage of maximal PCERT and OMNI at each exercise stage. In effect, the results showed that the two scales could be used with equal validity.

In a further study by Barkley and Roemmich[58] on 16 boys aged 9–10 years, the validity of the CALER and OMNI scales was confirmed against HR and $\dot{V}O_2$ during an incremental exercise test on a cycle ergometer to exhaustion. Increases in scores on both scales were associated with increases in $\dot{V}O_2$ ($r = .92$ and .93) and HR ($r = 0.88$ and $r = 0.89$). These results are not that surprising since the scales utilize basically the same number range. This observation raises the question as to where the child's focus of attention is based. Is it mainly based on the number scale, the figures, or equally combined between the two? If attention is focused primarily on the limited number range, it perhaps questions the need for pictorial scales of perceived exertion for children of this age range.

All the pictorial scales considered above have used either a horizontal line or one that has a linear slope. Following earlier suggestions by the authors in the previous edition of this text, a curvilinear scale has been presented by Eston and Parfitt[8] for consideration and evaluation. Our rationale for exploring the use of such a scale was originally founded on its inherently obvious face validity. It is readily conceivable that a child will recognize from previous learning and experience that the steeper the hill, the harder it is to ascend. This may also be helpful in the process of 'anchoring' effort perceptions (see below). Further, as ventilation is a physiological mediator for respiratory–metabolic signals of exertion during endurance exercise, and given that this variable rises in a curvilinear fashion with equal increments in work rate, a curvilinear gradient may be appropriate. The study of Barkley and Roemmich[58] provides data to support the development of a curvilinear scale. Their data showed that the proportions of maximal CALER (75%) and maximal OMNI (74%) were substantially less ($p < 0.001$) than the proportion of HR max (94.5%). In other words, the children in their study did not indicate a proportion of the RPE scales (CALER, OMNI) which was equivalent to the proportion of physiological effort. They concurred with the suggestion that linear scales may benefit from modification to their upper range either by changing the verbal descriptors, or changing the linearity of the scales so the final stages of the scale increase at a greater rate. Readers are referred to the chapter by Eston and Parfitt[8] for further description and initial pilot work on a curvilinear scale for children.

Anchoring effort perceptions

Whatever scale is used, it is important to provide the child with an understanding of the range of sensations that correspond to categories of effort within the scale. This is known as 'anchoring'. There are three ways by which perceptual anchoring may be accomplished—from memory, by definition or from actual physical experience. The memory method requires the child to remember the easiest and hardest experiences of exercise and use these as the anchor values on the scale. The 'definition' method involves the experimenter defining the anchors with terms such as 'the lowest effort imaginable' for the low anchor or the 'greatest effort imaginable' as the high anchor. The third method (experience) allows the child to physically experience a range of perceptual anchors. In 2000, Eston and Lamb[53] stated that the experiential method is the preferred of the three methods. They recommended that the child should be exposed to a range of intensities that can be used to set the perceptual anchor points at 'low' and 'high' levels. This can be achieved during habituation to the test or exercise procedures. In particular, it was suggested that, following a warm-up, the child should be allowed to experience exercise that is perceived as being 'hard' or 'very hard'. To avoid fatigue, a period of time should be allowed to regain full recovery. However, a recent study by Lamb *et al.*[31] has questioned this assertion. In their study, 41 boys and girls aged 11–13 years, randomly assigned to either an experiential anchor group or a non-anchor group, undertook two identical production-only trials (three 3-min cycle ergometer bouts at randomized CERT levels 3, 6, and 8). Before each trial, the anchor group received an experiential exercise trial to provide a frame of reference for their perceived exertions, at levels 2, 1, and 9, in that order. The authors reported slightly better test–retest reproducibility for HR and power output in the non-anchor group, with intraclass correlation (ICC) values ranging from .86–.93 and .81–.95, respectively. Importantly, limits of agreement analysis indicated no marked differences between the two groups in the amount of bias and within-subject error. The implementation of an experiential anchoring protocol therefore, had no positive effect on the reproducibility of the children's ability to self-regulate exercise using prescribed CERT levels. Further research on this theme would seem to be merited.

Validity of effort perception: Problems with comparing values from estimation and production paradigms during continuous and intermittent procedures

The majority of investigations have typically studied children's perceptions of effort during a passive estimation process (perceptual estimation paradigm). The effort perceptions have then been compared against objective measures of physiological strain, such as HR, power output, or $\dot{V}O_2$, using either intermittent or continuous protocols. Most studies on RPE have used a continuous testing protocol in preference to an intermittent testing protocol. The CERT, for example, was developed and validated using a continuous protocol,[26] as was the OMNI scale.[52]

Few studies have applied effort production procedures in which children are requested to regulate their exercise output to match experimenter-prescribed effort ratings. These studies have included continuous exercise protocols [6–20 RPE scale,[25] CERT[26,27,59]] and intermittent protocols [6–20 RPE scale,[22–24] CERT,[28,59] CALER,[33] and PCERT[30,32]]. It has been fairly common to compare the objective indicators of effort with expected values derived from a previous estimation trial.[22–24,27] In this so-called estimation-production paradigm, the ability of children to use perceptions of effort to actively self-regulate exercise-intensity levels using predetermined RPEs has, in our opinion, been inappropriately compared to their ability to passively appraise exercise intensity from a previous test.

It is, therefore, difficult to appraise children's ability to reliably and accurately produce a given objective effort from these studies. For example, in the first full paper published on this theme,[22] it was concluded that 9–15-year-old overweight children could discriminate between four work rates based on predetermined RPE values of 7, 10, 13, and 16. However, it was reported that the children produced work rates that were significantly different to expected (or 'criterion') values. It is necessary to point out that these criterion values were derived from a different perceptual process. Similar findings were reported in later studies.[23,24] These observations lead us to recommend that validity studies should focus on either production data only, or estimation data only, and not confound the issue by comparing data derived from a passive perceptual process on one occasion to an active perceptual process on a subsequent occasion.[8] Noble's[60] argument that this involves two dissimilar psychophysical processes is highly pertinent. Furthermore, the disparity between the two psychophysical processes is most likely attenuated by the extent of children's limited perceptual experience. This mismatch has since been recognized as a lack of 'prescription congruence'.[29]

The assessment of perceived exertion using a repeat-production paradigm examines a child's ability to discern between different target RPEs while self-regulating exercise intensity on more than one occasion.[28,31–33,50,51,59] Studies by Eston and colleagues[33,50,51] are the only ones to apply three or more repeated-effort production trials in young children (7–11 years). The increase in the size of ICCs between paired comparisons of the successive production trials in both studies support the importance of practice. For example, in the 2000 study,[33] the ICCs improved from 0.76 to 0.97 and the overall bias and limits of agreement narrowed from -12 ± 19 W to 0 ± 10 W. These data provide the strongest evidence available to date to demonstrate that practice improves the reliability of effort perception in children of this age.

Lamb *et al.*[59] used a production-only paradigm to assess the influence of a continuous and intermittent exercise protocol on the relationship between perceived exertion (CERT) and objective effort in children aged 9–10 years. Common to both groups was the requirement to regulate exercise intensity to match a range of four randomly presented effort-rating levels [3, 5, 7, and 9]. The children were allowed 2 min to settle on the appropriate resistance before cycling for a further 1 min at the prescribed RPE. For subjects allocated to the discontinuous group, each bout was separated by a 3-min rest period. The provision of 3-min recovery periods between exercise bouts produced higher relationships between CERT and HR ($r = 0.66$ vs. $r = 0.46$, for the intermittent and continuous protocol, respectively). HRs tended to be lower in the discontinuous protocol. These results indicate that children may be more able to use effort ratings to control exercise intensity when the exercise is intermittent rather than continuous in nature. Surprisingly, a study to compare the effects of an intermittent versus a continuous incremental exercise protocol on perceived exertion using a passive estimation paradigm (on the same group of children) has yet to be conducted. However, we have limited (unpublished) data to suggest that an intermittent protocol may be preferred.

Much of our understanding of children's effort perceptions has evolved from measuring responses to a situation in which they realize that the exercise is getting progressively harder. Studies which have allowed rest periods between exercise bouts,[33,36,42,61–63] and thereby reduced the influence of fatigue on effort perceptions, have all been incremental in nature. Few studies have randomized the order of presentation of work loads.[22,30,40,59] Logically, the 'accuracy' and reliability of effort perceptions and objective markers of effort produced at specified effort ratings will be influenced by test protocol (continuous or intermittent), the order of the load presentation (incremental or random) and the timing of the data collection. Furthermore, future investigations into children's effort perception should not disregard the manner in which the exercise is applied, the duration of the exercise bout, nor the number of practice periods, as these factors seem to have a bearing on the outcome measures.

Concluding comments

As the importance of encouraging physical activity in children is recognized, it makes sense to study the accuracy and reliability of effort perception in this population. While the breadth of research into children's effort perception has expanded over the past 5 years in particular, studies have still to extend beyond the laboratory and consistently use appropriate methods of assessing the relationships between effort perception and objective markers of effort. Moreover, attention needs to be paid to issues involving the type of perceptual paradigm, the temporal nature of the exercise protocol, and the influences of learning and practice on scale comprehension. Future studies should focus on the extent to which children of various ages and health status can learn to use effort perceptions in a variety of tasks.

Summary

- While effort perception research amongst paediatric populations has been in existence for 30 years, it has been only since 1994 that exercise scientists have endeavoured to develop rating scales that are suited to children's cognitive abilities.
- It is now generally regarded that the universally recognized Borg 6–20 RPE scale is unsuitable for use with children of most ages.
- RPE scales constructed with children in mind have followed the example set by the 1–10 CERT and typically include words and/or pictures to reflect varying degrees of exercise effort.
- A conceptual inconsistency has emerged with the recent appearance of the OMNI scale and its focus on ratings of tiredness rather than the established notion of effort.
- Strong evidence now exists to support the validity of paediatric scales against objective indicators of effort (HR, $\dot{V}O_2$ and power output) when applied via a perceptual estimation paradigm, often involving continuous incremental protocols, and to a lesser extent intermittent protocols.
- Studies employing child-specific RPE scales via a production paradigm have been relatively scarce, though the evidence thus far has offered encouragement that children can use their understanding of perceived exertion to help them regulate their exercise outputs.
- Attention to the important measurement issue of the reliability of scale application has been limited, and until very recently confounded by the use of inappropriate statistical techniques. Importantly, research has emerged showing that practice of using the RPE scale has a beneficial effect on the consistency of its application in both estimation and production paradigms.
- The effects of adopting recognized preparatory anchoring techniques on scale application have been virtually overlooked, though one study has reported no positive consequences.
- Despite the growth of research activity in this field, few studies have explored the efficacy of using a child scale in a practical (e.g. physical education) setting. It is time to consider the external validity of such scales.

References

1. Noble BJ, Robertson RJ (1996). *Perceived exertion*. Human Kinetics, Champaign, IL.
2. Carton RL, Rhodes EC (1985). A critical review of the literature on rating scales for perceived exertion. *Sports Med* **2**, 198–222.
3. Watt B, Grove R (1993). Perceived exertion: Antecedents and applications. *Sports Med* **15**, 225–41.
4. Williams JG, Eston RG (1989). Determination of the intensity dimension in vigorous exercise programmes with particular reference to the use of the rating of perceived exertion. *Sports Med* **8**, 177–89.
5. Eston RG, Connolly DA (1996). Use of ratings of perceived exertion for exercise prescription in patients receiving beta-blocker therapy. *Sports Med* **21**, 176–90.
6. Chen MJ, Fan X, Moe ST (2002). Criterion-related validity of the Borg rating of perceived exertion scale in healthy individuals: a meta-analysis. *J Sports Sci* **20**, 873–899
7. Lamb KL, Eston RG (1997). Effort perception in children. *Sports Med* **23**, 139–48.
8. Eston RG, Parfitt G (2006). Effort perception. In: Armstrong N (ed.), *Paediatric exercise physiology*, pp. 275–97. Elsevier, London.
9. Lamb KL, Eston RG (1997). Measurement of effort perception: Time for a new approach. In: Welsman N, Armstrong N, Kirby B (eds.), *Children and exercise XIX Volume II*, pp. 1–23. Washington Singer Press, Exeter.
10. Groslambert A, Mahon A D (2006). Perceived exertion: Influence of age and cognitive development. *Sports Med* **36**, 911–28.
11. Borg G (1970). Perceived exertion as an indicator of somatic stress. *J Rehab Med* **2**, 92–8.
12. Borg G (1986). Psychophysical studies of effort and exertion: Some historical, theoretical, and empirical aspects. In: Borg G, Ottoson D (eds.), *The perception of exertion in physical work*, pp. 3–14. Macmillan, London.
13. Borg G (1982). Psychophysical basis of perceived exertion. *Med Sci Sport Exerc* **14**, 371–81.
14. Pandolf KB (1983). Advances in the study and application of perceived exertion. *Exerc Sport Sci Rev* **11**, 118–58.

15. Eston RG, Davies BL, Williams JG (1987). Use of perceived effort ratings to control exercise intensity in young healthy adults. *Eur J Appl Physiol* **56**, 222–4.
16. Eston RG, Williams JG (1988). Reliability of ratings of perceived effort for regulation of exercise intensity. *Br J Sports Med* **22**, 153–4.
17. Dunbar CC, Robertson RJ, Baun R, Blandin MF, Metz K, Burdett R, Goss FL (1992). The validity of regulating exercise intensity by ratings of perceived exertion. *Med Sci Sport Exerc* **24**, 94–9.
18. Glass S, Knowlton R, Becque MD (1992). Accuracy of RPE from graded exercise to establish exercise training intensity. *Med Sci Sport Exerc* **24**, 1303–7.
19. Parfitt G, Eston RG, Connolly DA (1996). Psychological affect at different ratings of perceived exertion in high- and low-active women: A study using a production protocol. *Percept Motor Skills* **82**, 1035–42.
20. Williams JG, Eston RG (1996). Exercise intensity regulation. In: Eston RG, Reilly T (eds.), *Kinanthropometry and exercise physiology laboratory manual: Tests, procedures and data,* pp. 221–35. E and FN Spon, London.
21. Eston RG, Thompson M (1997). Use of ratings of perceived exertion for predicting maximal work rate and prescribing exercise intensity in patients receiving atenolol. *Br J Sports Med* **31**, 114–9.
22. Ward DS, Bar-Or O (1990). Use of the Borg Scale in exercise prescription for overweight youth. *Can J Sports Sci* **15**, 120–5.
23. Ward DS, Jackman JD, Galiano FJ (1991). Exercise intensity reproduction: Children versus adults. *Pediatr Exerc Sci* **3**, 209–18.
24. Ward DS, Bar-Or O, Longmuir P, Smith K (1995). Use of ratings of perceived exertion (RPE) to prescribe exercise intensity for wheelchair-bound children and adults. *Pediatr Exerc Sci* **7**, 94–102.
25. Williams JG, Eston RG, Stretch C (1991). Use of rating of perceived exertion to control exercise intensity in children. *Pediatr Exerc Sci* **3**, 21–7.
26. Williams JG, Eston RG, Furlong B (1994). CERT: A perceived exertion scale for young children. *Percept Motor Skills* **79**, 1451–8.
27. Eston RG, Lamb KL, Bain A, Williams M, Williams JG (1994). Validity of a perceived exertion scale for children: A pilot study. *Percept Motor Skills* **78**, 691–7.
28. Lamb KL (1996). Exercise regulation during cycle ergometry using the CERT and RPE scales. *Pediatr Exerc Sci* **8**, 337–50.
29. Robertson RJ, Goss JL, Bell FA, Dixon CB, Gallagher KI, Lagally KM, Timmer JM, Abt KL, Gallagher JD, Thompkins T (2002). Self-regulated cycling using the children's OMNI scale of perceived exertion. *Med Sci Sport Exerc* **34**, 1168–75.
30. Yelling M, Lamb K, Swaine IL (2002). Validity of a pictorial perceived exertion scale for effort estimation and effort production during stepping exercise in adolescent children. *Eur Phys Educ Rev* **8**, 157–75.
31. Lamb KL, Eaves SJ, Hartshorn JE (2004). The effect of experiential anchoring on the reproducibility of exercise regulation in adolescent children. *J Sports Sci* **22**, 159–65.
32. Preston S, Lamb KL (2005). Perceptually-regulated exercise responses during physical education lessons. *J Sports Sci* **23**, 1214–5.
33. Eston RG, Campbell L, Lamb KL, Parfitt G (2000). Reliability of effort perception for regulating exercise intensity: A study using the Cart and Load Effort Rating (CALER) scale. *Pediatr Exerc Sci* **12**, 388–97.
34. Borg G (1977). *Physical work and effort.* Pergamon Press, Oxford.
35. Bar-Or O (1977). Age-related changes in exercise perception. In: Borg G, ed. *Physical work and effort*, pp. 255–66. Pergamon Press, Oxford.
36. Kahle C, Ulmer HV, Rummel L (1977). The reproducibility of Borg's RPE scale with female pupils from 7 to 11 years of age. *Pflugers Archiv Eur J Physiol* **368**, R26.
37. Davies CTM, Fohlin L, Thoren C (1980). Perception of exertion in anorexia nervosa patients. In: Berg K, Eriksson BO (eds.), *Children and exercise IX,* pp. 327–32. University Park Press, Baltimore.
38. Eston RG (1984). A discussion of the concepts: Exercise intensity and perceived exertion with reference to the secondary school. *Phys Educ Rev* **7**, 19–25.
39. Bar-Or O, Reed S (1986). Rating of perceived exertion in adolescents with neuromuscular disease. In: Borg G, Ottoson D (eds.), *The perception of exertion in physical work*, pp. 137–48. Macmillan Press, Basingstoke.
40. Eston RG, Williams JG (1986). Exercise intensity and perceived exertion in adolescent boys. *Br J Sports Med* **20**, 27–30.
41. Miyashita M, Onedera K, Tabata I (1986). How Borg's RPE scale has been applied to Japanese. In: Borg G, Ottoson D (eds.), *The perception of exertion in physical work*, pp. 27–34. Macmillan Press, Basingstoke.
42. Van Huss WD, Stephens KE, Vogel P, Anderson D, Kurowski T, Jones JA, Fitzgerald C. (1986). Physiological and perceptual responses of elite age group distance runners during progressive intermittent work to exhaustion. In: Weiss M, Gould D (eds.), *Sport for children and youth,* pp. 239–46. Human Kinetics Publishers, Champaign, IL.
43. Ward DS, Blimkie CJR, Bar-Or O (1986). Rating of perceived exertion in obese adolescents. *Med Sci Sport Exerc* **18**, S72.
44. Bar-Or O, Ward DS (1989). Rating of perceived exertion in children. In: Bar-Or O (ed.), *Advances in pediatric sports sciences,* pp. 151–68. Human Kinetics, Champaign, IL.
45. Nystad W, Oseid S, Mellbye EB (1989). Physical education for asthmatic children: The relationship between changes in heart rate, perceived exertion, and motivation for participation. In: Oseid S, Carlsen K (eds.), *Children and exercise XIII,* pp. 369–77. Human Kinetics, Champaign, IL.
46. Robertson RJ (1997). Perceived exertion in young people: Future directions of enquiry. In: Welsman J, Armstrong N, Kirby B (eds.), *Children and exercise XIX,* Vol. II, pp. 33–9. Washington Singer Press, Exeter.
47. Williams JG, Furlong B, MacKintosh C, Hockley TJ (1993). Rating and regulation of exercise intensity in young children. *Med Sci Sport Exerc* **25**, S8 .
48. Lamb KL (1995). Children's ratings of effort during cycle ergometry: An examination of the validity of two effort rating scales. *Pediatr Exerc Sci* **7**, 407–21.
49. Leung ML, Cheung PK, Leung RW (2002). An assessment of the validity and reliability of two perceived exertion rating scales among Hong Kong children. *Percept Motor Skills* **95**, 1047–62.
50. Eston RG, Parfitt G, Shepherd P (2001). Effort perception in children: Implications for validity and reliability. In: Papaionnou A, Goudas M, Theodorakis Y (eds.), *Proceedings of 10th World Congress of Sport Psychology*, pp. 104–6. Skiathos, Greece.
51. Parfitt G, Shepherd P, Eston RG (2007). Control of exercise intensity using the children's CALER and BABE perceived exertion scales. *J Exerc Sci Fitness* **5**, 49–55.
52. Robertson RJ, Goss FL, Boer NF, Peoples JA, Foreman AJ, Dabayebeh IM, Millich NB, Balasekaran G, Riechman SE, Gallagher JD, Thompkins T (2000). Children's OMNI Scale of perceived exertion: Mixed gender and race validation. *Med Sci Sport Exerc* **32**, 452–8.
53. Eston RG, Lamb KL (2000). Effort perception. In: Armstrong N, Van-Mechelen W (eds.), *Paediatric exercise science and medicine,* pp. 85–91. Oxford University Press, Oxford.
54. Marinov B, Mandadjieva S, Kostianev S (2008). Pictorial and verbal category ratio scales for effort estimation in children. *Child Care Health Dev* **34**, 35–43.
55. Utter AC, Robertson RJ, Nieman DC, Kang J (2002). Children's OMNI scale of perceived exertion: walking/running evaluation. *Med Sci Sport Exerc* **34**, 139–44.
56. Robertson RJ, Goss JL, Andreacci JL, Dubé JJ, Rutkowksi JJ, Snee BM, Kowallis RA, Crawford K, Aaron DJ, Metz KF (2005). Validation of the

children's OMNI RPE Scale for stepping exercise. *Med Sci Sport Exerc* **37**, 290–8.

57. Roemmich JN, Barkley JE, Epstein LH (2006). Validity of the PCERT and OMNI-walk/run ratings of perceived exertion scales. *Med Sci Sport Exerc* **38**, 1014–19.
58. Barkley JE, Roemmich JN (2008). Validity of the CALER and OMNI bike ratings of perceived exertion. *Med Sci Sports Exerc* **40**, 760–9.
59. Lamb KL, Eston RG, Trask S (1997). The effect of discontinuous and continuous testing protocols on effort perception in children. In: Armstrong N, Kirby B, Welsman J (eds.), *Children and exercise XIX*, pp. 258–64. E and FN Spon, London.
60. Noble BJ (1982). Clinical applications of perceived exertion. *Med Sci Sport Exerc* **14**, 406–11.
61. Tolfrey K, Mitchell J (1996). Ratings of perceived exertion at standard and relative exercise intensities in prepubertal, teenage and young adult males. *J Sports Sci* **14**, 101–2.
62. Ueda T, Kurokawa T (1991). Validity of heart rate and ratings of perceived exertion as indices of exercise intensity in a group of children while swimming. *Eur J Appl Physiol* **63**, 200–4.
63. Meyer F, Bar-Or O, Wilk B (1995). Children's perceptual responses to ingesting drinks of different compositions during and following exercise in the heat. *Int J Sport Nutr* **5**, 13–24.

PART II

Developmental Aspects of Paediatric Exercise Science

CHAPTER 12

Growth and maturation

Adam D.G. Baxter-Jones

Introduction

The concepts of a child's growth and maturation are central to all studies related to paediatric exercise science. It is, therefore, imperative that any study recording the acute and chronic responses of the child and adolescent to exercise and/or physical activity takes into consideration the growth and maturity status of the participant. Morphological parameters and physiological functions, such as heart volume, lung function, aerobic power, and muscular strength, develop with increasing age and body size. Furthermore, physical fitness parameters (e.g. muscular, motor, and cardio respiratory) also change with growth and maturation. Thus, the effects of growth and maturation may mask or be greater than the exercise and/or physical activity effects under investigation.

Interest in the effects that physical activity and/or exercise has on a child's growth and maturation has a long history. At the beginning of the twentieth century, D'Arcy Thompson wrote his classic treatise *On Growth and Form*, suggesting that exercise was a direct stimulus to growth.[1] In 1964, James Tanner published *The Physique of the Olympic Athlete*, in which he concluded that 'the basic body structure must be present for the possibility of being an athlete to arise'.[2] Other authors who have subsequently measured the growth and maturation of young athletes have agreed with this statement, and concluded that body size is most probably genotypic and reflects selection at a relatively young age for the size demands of the sport.[3] However, a number of studies, especially with aesthetic sports such as gymnastics, have suggested that when heavy training regimens are started at a young age the growth and maturation of the child may be affected adversely.[4] Thus, the nature versus nurture debate continues.

It should be emphasized that regular exercise is only one of many factors that may influence a child's growth and maturation. Growth and maturation are maintained primarily by genes, hormones, energy, and nutrients, which interact among themselves and also with the environment in which the individual lives. Since the process of gene–environmental interactions developing through time is non-linear, it is important to realize that the same genes will be expressed differently when exposed to different environmental conditions.[5] To fully understand the potential of exercise or physical activity on a child's growth, a sound understanding of the general principles of childhood growth and maturation, otherwise termed auxology, is required.

Growth refers to changes in the size of an individual, as a whole or in parts. As children grow, they become taller and heavier, they increase their lean and fat tissues, and their organs increase in size. Changes in size are a result of three cellular processes: (i) an increase in cell number, or hyperplasia; (ii) an increase in cell size, or hypertrophy; and (iii) an increase in intercellular substances, or accretion. All the three processes occur during growth but the predominance of one process over another varies with chronological age and the tissue involved.[6]

Maturation is the progressive achievement of adult status and comprises a subset of developmental changes that include morphology, function, and complexity. The acquisition of secondary sexual characteristics, such as breast development in girls and facial hair in boys, are common examples of maturation during adolescence. Size and morphological changes can also be scaled relative to the achievement of adult status and can be used as a continuous scale of maturation; for example, percentage of adult height attained.[7] The major distinction between size *per se* and maturation is that all children eventually achieve the same adult maturity, whereas adult size and body dimensions vary considerably. It is therefore important to remember that growth and maturation occur simultaneously and interact; however, they may not follow the same time line. A young person could appear to be tall for their age but also be delayed in biological maturation, or vice versa.

The process of maturing has two components: timing and tempo. The former refers to when specific maturational events occur [e.g. age when menarche is attained, age at the beginning of breast development, age at the appearance of pubic hair, or age at maximum growth in height during the adolescent growth spurt (peak height velocity, PHV)]. Tempo refers to the rate at which maturation progresses (i.e. how quickly or slowly an individual passes from the initial stages of sexual maturation to the mature state). Maturation occurs in all biological systems in the body but at different rates. Furthermore, the timing and tempo of maturity vary considerably among individuals, with children of the same chronological age differing dramatically in their degree of biological maturity.

The terms 'growth' and 'maturation' are used broadly to include all developmental processes, for example, cognitive growth and social maturation;[8] however, this chapter uses a stricter definition and limits its focus to physical aspects, primarily the growth at the organism level, that is, the level of the whole child. In the growth and maturity literature, life leading up to maturity is split into three stages: the prenatal period, childhood, and adolescence. The period of prenatal life is vitally important to the child's well-being;[9] however, it will not be covered in this chapter, as discussion will focus on the first two decades of post-natal life. The terms adolescence and puberty are used frequently in the paediatric literature to explain the later period of growth and maturity, often with no clear distinction in their definitions. Some authors refer to adolescence when talking about psychosocial changes and puberty when talking about the physical changes. However, as most of the literature use these terms interchangeably, this chapter will use adolescence synonymously with puberty.

The curve of growth

One of the most famous records of human growth is that of a boy known simply as De Montbeillard's son. Between 1759 and 1770, the Count Philibert Gueneau De Montbeillard successively measured his son at approximately 6-month intervals. Although initially published in 1778 in the French units of that time, it was not until 1927 that the measurements were translated into centimetres and plotted in the form of a chart by R.E. Scammon (Fig. 12.1).[10] This is known as a height distance or height for age curve.

If you think of growth in terms of a journey, then the curve describes the distance travelled from birth to 18 years of age; you can therefore see that a child's height at any particular age is a reflection of how far that child has progressed towards the mature adult state. The pattern of the growth curve to a large extent is related to the frequency of data collection. If only two data points have been collected, say at birth and 18 years of age, then the line between them would be linear. However, in this case data were collected approximately every 6 months, and this clearly illustrates that growth is not a linear process, that is, we do not gain the same amount of height during each calendar year. Figure 12.1 also illustrates the fact that between birth and 18 years of age, the distance curve is made up of a number of different shaped curves with different slopes. Relatively rapid growth is observed in infancy, which gradually declines by 5 years of age, that is, the slope of the line decreases. This is followed by steady growth in childhood (between 5 and 10 years of age) and then rapid growth during adolescence (between 10 and 16 years of age). During adolescence an S-shaped, or sigmoid, curve is observed. Finally, very slow growth is observed as the individual approaches an asymptote at 19 years of age. Although this distance curve shows the continuous rate of magnitude of change with age, in terms of our journey it only tells us where we are at any particular point in time. No information is provided as to how we reached this point; thus, the distance point is largely dependent on how much the child has grown in all proceeding years.

What is therefore required is a measure of growth that describes the speed of our journey at any one point in time. To get an idea of speed, the data have to be expressed in terms of a rate of growth (cm per year) (Fig. 12.2).[10] Velocity of growth is a better reflection of the child's state at any particular time than the distance achieved. This is important to the paediatric exercise scientist because substances whose amounts change with age, such as the concentrations of metabolites in blood or tissue physiology, will most probably show similar patterns of growth to the velocity rather than the distance curve.

From the curve you can see that following birth two distinct increases in growth rates occur. The first of these is the juvenile or mid-growth spurt occurring between 6 and 8 years of age. The

Fig. 12.1 The growth in height of de Montbeillard's son 1759–1777: distance curve. Redrawn from data reported by Scammon.[10]

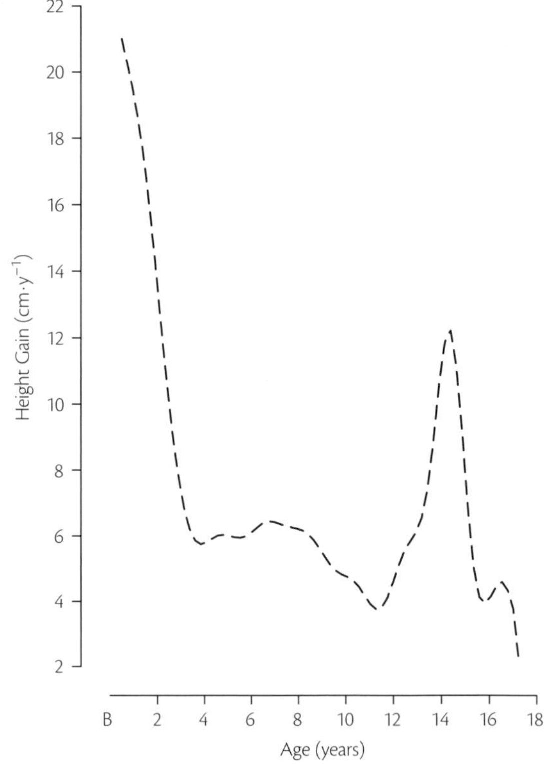

Fig. 12.2 The growth in height of de Montbeillard's son 1759–1777: velocity curve. Redrawn from data reported by Scammon.[10]

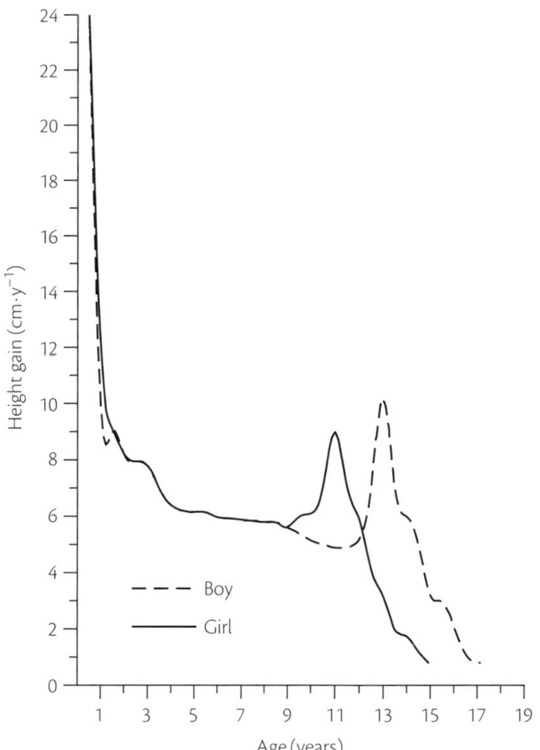

Fig. 12.3 Typical individual height velocity curves for boys and girls, representing the velocity of the typical boys and girls at any given instance. Redrawn from data reported by Malina *et al.*[6]

second, more dramatic, increase occurs between 11 and 18 years and is called the adolescent growth spurt. Whilst the juvenile growth spurt varies in magnitude between individuals, it occurs at roughly the same age both within and between sexes. The adolescent growth spurt, however, varies in both magnitude and timing within and between the sexes. Males enter their adolescent growth spurt almost 2 years later than females and have a slightly greater magnitude of height gain (Fig. 12.3).[6] This extra 2 years of growth before adolescence, in combination with a greater magnitude of growth during adolescence, explains in part the increased final adult height observed in males. At the same time, other skeletal changes occur that result in gender difference in adulthood, such as wider shoulders in males and wider hips in females. Males also demonstrate rapid increases in muscle mass whilst females accumulate greater amounts of fat, thus as a result of natural biological development by the end of adolescence males are stronger. The increase in size also gives males other physiological advantages over females such as increased lung capacity.

Types of growth data

When describing a growth curve, it is important to distinguish between a curve fitted to a single individual's data (longitudinal data) and curves of yearly averages derived from different children measured only once (cross-sectional data), as each of these curves will have a different shape.[11] Cross-sectional studies are attractive as they can be carried out quickly and include larger numbers of children. Unfortunately, although cross-sectional studies provide information about a static picture of the population variation in growth variables (the distance curve), they provide little information about individual growth rates or the timing of particular phases of growth. This is important because the individual differences, timing and tempo, in growth velocity are important to throw light on the genetical control of growth and the correlation of growth with physical development. Most of the seminal growth research has been longitudinal in design. Longitudinally measuring the same participants over time, allows one to ascertain part or the entire growth pattern of an individual. A pure longitudinal design is where a cohort of children born within the same year is followed continuously and assessed on at least three separate occasions. In practice, it is virtually impossible to measure exactly the same group of children every year for a prolonged period; inevitably some children leave the study, some can join, and others come and go. This type of study is called a mixed longitudinal study and is a compromise between cross-sectional and longitudinal design. The mixed longitudinal design consists of a number of relatively short longitudinal studies that interlock and cover a whole age range (e.g. 8–10 years, 9–11 years, 10–13 years, and so on). Mixed longitudinal studies provide information on status and rate of growth; however, sophisticated statistical techniques are required to interpret the data accurately. The advantage of longitudinal over cross-sectional designs is that within individual variance can be obtained and thus the timing and tempo of an individual's pattern of growth identified. When conducting longitudinal research, it is important to remember that two measures separated by a time period do not constitute longitudinal data; true longitudinal data have at least three measures and thus two velocities. Unfortunately, longitudinal research is often impractical for paediatric exercise research as the process is laborious, expensive, and time consuming for both the participants and the investigators. This means that most knowledge in paediatric exercise science is based on cross-sectional research. Therefore, although valuable in itself for describing distance curves, it can be in some respects misleading. Because of the large variation observed in the timing and tempo of growth average, velocity data inevitably produce growth curves that are smoothed or flattened and distance curves that are distorted because they do not rise sufficiently in periods of rapid growth, such as adolescence.[11]

Growth in stature

Stature is made up of sitting height (distance from the sitting surface to the top of the head) and leg length, or subischial length (distance between the hip joint to the floor). The exact landmark of the hip joint is sometimes hard to locate; therefore, leg length is most often calculated by subtracting sitting height from standing height. Stature varies during the course of the day, with greater readings in the morning that decrease throughout the day. Shrinkage during the day occurs because the intervertebral discs become compressed as a result of weight bearing, thus the diurnal variation may be as much as 1 cm or more.[6]

During the first year of life, infants grow at a fast rate, approximately 25 ($cm \cdot y^{-1}$), in fact during the first 6 months of life the velocity may be even faster, around 30 $cm \cdot y^{-1}$. During the second year of life, there is growth of another 12–13 cm in stature. This accelerated growth means that by 2 years of age boys have attained approximately 50% of their adult stature. Girls are always closer to their mature status, even at birth, than boys and reach 50% of their final adult stature by 18 months of age (Fig. 12.3).[6] From then on there is a steady deceleration in growth, dropping to a rate of about 5–6 cm·y^{-1} before the initiation of the adolescent growth spurt. Between 6.5 and 8.5 years, there is a small but distinct increase in growth rate, known as the juvenile or mid-growth spurt. During adolescence the maximum velocity of growth is known as PHV. Girls, on average, attain PHV approximately 2 years earlier than boys with their onset of PHV occurring between 8.2 and 10.3 years (Fig. 12.4).[6] On average PHV is reached between 11.3 and 12.2 years. Corresponding ages for boys are 10.0–12.1 years and 13.3–14.4 years.[11] By PHV individuals have attained 92% of their adult height.

Upon reaching final adult height males are on average 13 cm taller than females; however, up until the initiation of PHV the sex differences in height are small (Fig. 12.4).[6] Therefore, boys achieve their height advantage during the adolescent period. Specifically, boys on average, experience about 2 years more preadolescent growth, approximately 5 cm·y^{-1}, than girls. This is approximately 10 cm of growth that girls do not experience. Boys also achieve a slightly greater (on average 2 cm) magnitude of height at PHV. Both of these growth differences cause males, on average, to have a greater adult stature. Girls stop growing in stature by about 16 years of age and boys by about 18 or 19 years of age. However, these ages may be spuriously young as many growth studies stop measuring youth at 17 or 18 years of age, and it is known that many youth continue to grow into their early- to mid-20s.

These curves of growth in height reflect the growth patterns found in all healthy children who live in a normal environment. As mentioned, individuals will differ in absolute height of growth velocity (i.e. adult heights) and in the timing of the adolescent growth spurt; however, to reach their destined final height each individual will go through a similar pattern of human growth.

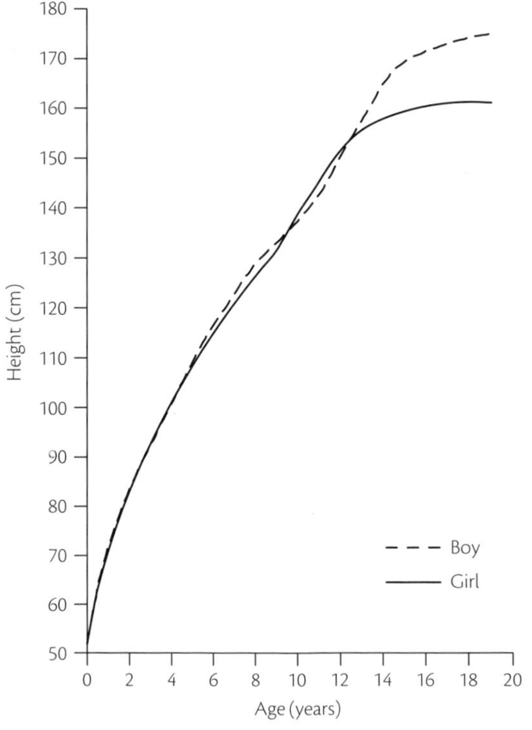

Fig. 12.4 Typical individual distance curves for boys and girls. Redrawn from data reported by Malina *et al.*[6]

Patterns of growth

Statural growth, as demonstrated in Fig. 12.4, shows only one of several patterns of growth found within the human body.[6] Different parts of the body grow at different rates and at different times.[12] It has been proposed that all tissues and systems follow four patterns of growth: (i) neurological (e.g. brain and head), (ii) reproductive (e.g. reproductive organs), (iii) lymphoid (e.g. lymph glands, tonsils, and appendix), and (iv) general (e.g. stature and heart size).[12] Brain and head growth (neural tissue) exhibits the most rapid early growth. At birth a child's head is roughly half its adult size. From birth there is steady growth up until 7 years of age, by 8 years of age neural tissue growth is almost complete. In contrast, reproductive tissue does not really start to increase in size until 12–14 years of age. The reproductive curve includes primary sex characteristics (e.g. uterus, vagina, and fallopian tubes in females; prostate and seminal vesicles in males) and secondary sex characteristics (e.g. breasts in females, facial hair in males, and axillary and pubic hair in both sexes). The reproductive curve shows some growth during infancy followed by reduced growth during childhood; by 10–12 years of age reproductive organs are only 10% of their adult size. During adolescence (puberty) there is a rapid growth in genital tissues. The lymphoid tissues, which act as a circulatory system for tissue fluid, are involved with the immunological capacities of the child and show a different growth curve from the rest of the body. There is a remarkable increase in size of the lymphoid tissue until the early adolescent years (~11–13 years). The relative size of the tissue then steeply declines during puberty, probably a result of the up-regulation of sex hormones during this period. The general curve of growth includes many tissues and systems in the body, such as skeletal tissue, the respiratory system, and the digestive system. As illustrated by the shape of stature shown in Fig. 12.4, the general curve follows a sigmoid curve of growth and reflects a rapid growth during infancy and early childhood, steady growth during mid-childhood, rapid growth during early adolescence, and asymtoping in late adolescence.[12]

Growth in body mass

Body mass is made up of a composite of tissues, including fat, lean, and bone tissue, that accrue at different rates and times. Significant changes in body composition occur during growth and maturation, especially during infancy and puberty. This is an important point and indicates why body composition assessment in children is far more challenging than in adults.[13] Changes in body mass are a result of changes in fat or fat-free mass and also changes in body water concentrations (dehydration or overhydration). The relative proportions and distributions of fat and fat-free components depend on age, sex, and other environmental and genetic factors. Body mass is a very sensitive and thus fluctuating measurement, in the sense that it can change from one day to another due to minor alterations in body composition. Furthermore, body mass, similar to stature, also shows diurnal variation. An individual is lightest in the morning, upon voiding the bladder.[14] Throughout the day body mass increases and is affected by diet and physical activity. In menstruating adolescent girls, the phase of the menstrual cycle can also affect body mass.[6]

As seen with the development of height, body mass follows a four-phase growth pattern: rapid growth in infancy and early childhood, rather steady gain during mid-childhood, rapid gain during adolescence, and usually a slower increase into adulthood. The water content of the foetus is high and represents about 75% of body weight at birth, much of this is lost during the first few days of life declining to 45% and by puberty water represents approximately 19% of total body weight. At birth the brain represents 13% of body weight compared to 2% in adulthood. Thus, the brain along with other organ tissue makes a greater contribution to body weight and lean body mass during infancy. During the first year of life body mass doubles and by the end of the second year it has quadrupled. Most children show the lowest annual increment in body mass around 2–3 years of age; from this point to the onset of adolescence body mass increases, but at a slower rate. At the onset of adolescence there is a rapid gain in the velocity of body mass development. The precise timing of the adolescent growth spurt in body mass is generally less clear than it is for height. It has been estimated that peak velocity in body mass normally occurs 0.2–0.4 years after PHV in boys and 0.3–0.9 years after PHV in girls.[15]

Boys and girls follow the same pattern in body mass development. Before the adolescent growth spurt, boys are slightly heavier than girls. Girls then experience an earlier growth spurt and thus for a short time are heavier. As soon as boys go through their adolescent growth spurt they catch up and thus become and remain heavier than girls. It is important to remember that there is a normal range of individual variation in body mass resulting in some girls being heavier than most boys at virtually all ages.

In boys, the growth spurt in body mass is primarily due to gains in muscle mass and skeletal tissue with fat mass remaining fairly stable. Girls, however, experience a less dramatic rise in muscle mass and skeletal tissue but experience a continuous rise in fat mass during adolescence. Specifically, before adolescence boys have a slightly larger lean body mass than girls; however, during the adolescent growth spurt the magnitude of the velocity of change is greater and more prolonged. One of the consequences of this pattern of growth is that by young adulthood males have 50% more lean body mass than females. Although sex differences in skeletal tissue may be present during infancy and childhood,[16] they become far more pronounced during adolescence.[17] Approximately 40% of peak bone mass (the maximum amount of bone in the body) is attained during adolescence. This is due to the growth and expansion of the skeleton; the density of bones also changes. When aligned by chronological age no sex differences are observed until 14 years of age, after which boys have approximately 10% more bone mineralization. When the confounders of body size and lean mass are controlled, boys have significantly great bone mineralization at all ages during adolescence, suggesting that much of this difference between the sexes is due to boys' greater stature and lean mass.[18]

With regard to fat mass development, in mid-foetal life body fat is 1% of total body weight. Subcutaneous fat begins to be laid down in the foetus at about 34 weeks and increases continuously thereafter, so that by birth fat represents 15% of total body weight, 25% at 6 months, and 30% at 1 year of age. Skinfold thickness, an index of subcutaneous fat, peaks about 9 months after birth. After 9 months, the skinfolds decrease until age 6–8 years when they begin to rise again. This pattern showing a flow, ebb, and a flow is termed the adiposity rebound.[19] The rebound occurs earlier in children at higher percentiles for fatness and there is a tendency for children with an early rebound to have higher fatness at the end of growth. In general, girls have higher skinfold thickness than boys, even at birth, but the divergence becomes marked by 8 years of age. Both boys and girls experience a prepubescent adipose tissue gain but more so in girls than in boys. Girls' skinfolds continue to increase through adolescence. In contrast, during mid-pubescence, boys' skinfolds decrease, particularly at the triceps and to a lesser extent at the subscapular. During childhood, the ratio of trunk and extremities skinfolds is relatively stable but at adolescence both sexes gain proportionally more on the trunk. The gain is less in girls and boys experience a decrease at the extremity sites. The result of this is that by the end of adolescence boys have relatively more subcutaneous adipose tissue on the trunk.[20]

Although the timing and magnitude of peak velocity of the different tissues differ between the sexes, the pattern of growth of the different tissues is consistent between sexes. Peak lean velocity is attained first, approximately 0.3 years after PHV, followed by peak fat and peak bone mineralization. Because total body mass represents the composite of lean, fat, and bone, peak body mass occurs after lean and fat mass peaks but before the peak in bone mass.[15]

Development of shape

In contrast to changes in size, which just shows a child's progression in terms of a percentage of adult status, the concept of change in shape reflects the changes in proportionality of body segments from infancy to adulthood. From these growth gradients can be identified. As already indicated, there is a two-fold increase in head size from birth to maturity; however, other segments show different patterns. The trunk increases three-fold, the arms four-fold, and the legs at maturity are five times their length at birth. These changes illustrate that there is a head–trunk–legs gradient. In early foetal growth, the head growth is fastest, in infancy trunk growth accelerates, and in childhood leg growth accelerates. However within the trunk itself no cephalocaudal gradients are found, as it has been found that abdominal growth proceeds growth in the thorax and the last vertebral epiphyses to fuse are the second to seventh thoracic. Since change in shape is difficult to measure ratios are often used to characterize physiological age, for example, volume of trunk/volume of head and volume of trunk/length of limbs. Since the increase in these physical parameters occurs at different times and tempos, these ratios thus increase with increasing age and can be used to measure shape maturity. Other gradients of growth are also observed; within the limbs, during childhood and adolescence, growth occurs distal to proximal. For example, the hand and feet experience accelerated growth first, followed by the calf and the forearm, the hips, and the chest, and finally the shoulders. Thus, during childhood there may be a period where children appear to have large hands and feet in relation to the rest of their body. However, once the adolescent growth spurt has ended, hands and feet are a little smaller in proportion to arms, legs, and stature. Most body dimensions, with the exception of subcutaneous adipose tissue and the dimensions of the head and face, follow a growth pattern similar to that of stature; however, there are wide variations in the timing of growth spurts. From childhood to adolescence, the lower extremities (legs) grow faster than the upper body (trunk). This results in sitting height contributing less to stature as age progresses. During the adolescent growth spurt the legs experience a growth spurt earlier than the trunk. Thus, for a period during early adolescence a youth will have relatively long legs, but the appearance of long-leggedness disappears with the later increase in trunk length. Sex differences in leg length and sitting height are small during childhood. For a short time during the early part of adolescence, girls, on average, have a slightly longer leg length than boys, due to girls experiencing adolescence on average 2 years earlier. By about 12 years of age boys' leg length exceeds girls, but boys do not catch up in sitting height until about 14 years of age. The longer period of preadolescent growth in boys is largely responsible for the fact that men's legs are longer than women's in relation to trunk length.[11]

Other shape differences also occur during adolescence between girls and boys. Boys experience a broadening of the shoulders relative to the hips and girls experience a broadening of the hips relative to the shoulders. These sex differences are evident during childhood but become accentuated during adolescence. During the adolescent growth spurt boys gain more in shoulder (biacromial) breadth (~2.3 cm), whereas girls gain slightly more in hip (bicristal) breadth (~1.2 cm).[6] Boys catch up to girls in their bicristal breadth in late adolescence. The timing and speed of these changes in body dimensions may have a dramatic effect on several aspects of physical performance. An increase in shoulder width can result in increased muscle mass in the upper body in boys. This is one reason why sex differences in strength are much greater in the upper body compared with the lower body. Furthermore, this greater upper body muscle combined with longer arms could explain why older boys are better at throwing, racquet sports, and rowing than girls. Girls tend to have a lower centre of gravity, due to the relative broadening of the hips, which may contribute to their better sense of balance.[21]

Adolescence and puberty

As described previously, maturation is the progressive achievement of adult status. Adolescence or puberty refers to the time period that sees the onset of adult reproductive capacity. This is a dramatic period involving rapid transformation of anatomy, physiology, and behaviour.[22] The progressive acquisition of secondary sexual characteristics, such as breast development in girls and facial hair in boys, are common examples of maturation during adolescence. In these examples, the progress of sexual maturation is determined by the attainment of stages, a qualitative term[23,24] in contrast size and morphological variables can be scaled continuously, for example, percentage of adult height attained or age of attainment of PHV. Growth at adolescence is characterized by the presence of the adolescent, or pubertal, growth spurt and is a time of greatest sex differentiation since the early intrauterine months. There is wide variation among populations, individuals, and the two sexes as to the timing of the adolescent growth spurt, its magnitude and the age at which mature size is reached. When large numbers of individual velocity curves are compared, it soon become apparent that some children reach PHV earlier than others. In 1930, Boas[25] coined the expression tempo of growth drawing the analogy with classical music: some children are marked *allegro* (fast), others *lento* (slow). The empirical finding from this study was that adult height, in general, did not differ, indicating that there are two independent patterns of growth: size and maturation.

Often within exercise physiology there is an interest in examining the trainability of the child, or the association between physical activity and health outcomes. However, interpretation of these outcomes must consider the process of normal growth and maturation, particularly during adolescence, before any definitive conclusion can be reached. Unless body size and biological maturity indicators are considered, one cannot definitively identify the independent effects of physical activity or training on the outcome (see Chapters 39 and 40).

Regulation of growth and maturation

The regulation of growth and maturation involves the complex and continuous interaction of genes, hormones, nutrients, and the physical environment. A genotype is the group of genes making up an individual. Simply, an individual's genotype can be thought of as a potential for growth and maturation.[5] Whether a child achieves that potential, however, depends on the conditions (i.e. environment) in which the child is born into and subsequently raised. An individual's phenotype is the observed physical or physiological characteristics/traits that are produced by the genotype in conjunction with the environment.[5] General health and well-being of the child is paramount to normal growth, in turn normal growth is a strong indicator of the overall good health of the child. Essential to normal growth and development are adequate levels of several hormones. Hormones are therefore essential for a child to reach his/her full genetic potential.

There are a large number of hormones which are of particular importance in the initiation and regulation of pubertal events (i.e. maturation of secondary sex characteristics, attainment of reproduction function, and PHV). Recent scientific advances in endocrinology have shed light on the mechanisms, actions, and interactions among hormones and highlight the complexity of these processes. Some of the most prominent hormones involved in the regulation of growth and maturation include testosterone (primarily from the Leydig cells of the testes and also the adrenal cortex), oestrogen (primarily from the ovarian follicle and also the adrenal cortex), thyroxine (from the thyroid gland), cortisol and adrenal androgens (from the adrenal cortex), insulin (from the β-cells of the Islets of Langerhans of the pancreas), and a series of hormones from the pituitary glands. The pituitary hormones include adrenocorticotrophin (ACTH), follicle-stimulating hormone (FSH), growth hormone (GH) (or somatotrophin), luteinizing hormone (LH), and thyrotrophin [thyroid stimulating hormone (TSH)]. This list is by no means exhaustive. There are many other hormones, growth factors, and cytokines that are also actively involved in the regulation of growth and maturation, which are beyond the scope of this chapter.

Post-natal growth is a result of GH secretion and the final component of post-natal growth, puberty, when GH interacts with gonadal steroids.[26] GH and thyroid hormones are the primary hormones for growth prepubertally. GH is secreted in a pulsatile fashion from the somatotrophins in the anterior pituitary gland. GH is regulated by GH-releasing hormone, which causes release and synthesis of GH and somatostatin, which inhibits GH release. In humans, there is a dose-dependent relationship between the amount of GH secreted over a 24-hour period and the growth rate of an individual. Although GH has direct effects on some cells, many of its effects are mediated by the local generation of insulin-like growth factor 1 (IGF-1).[26] Prepubertal growth is, therefore, largely dependent on the thyroid hormones and the GH/IGF-1 axis. IGF-1 plays an important role in muscle tissue growth through the stimulation of glycogen accumulation and the transfer of amino acids into cells for protein synthesis. IGF-1 also promotes connective tissue, cartilage, and bone growth through the stimulation of cartilage growth and the formation of collagen.[27]

During the final component of post-natal growth, namely pubertal growth, sex steroids modulate growth. Since puberty is not an instantaneous event but rather a process integrating the antecedent and development of immaturity and adulthood, it is quite difficult to clearly identify either its beginning or its end.[21] What is observed is a rapid and profound trajectory of change from the immature to mature state. The central feature of puberty is the maturation of the primary reproductive endocrine axis. This is composed of hypothalamus, pituitary gland, and gonad. This three part system is known as the HPG (hypothalamic–pituitary–gonadal) axis. The secondary features of puberty include the development of secondary sexual characteristics, the development of sexual dimorphic anatomical features, and the acceleration and cessation of linear growth. Virtually, all these secondary changes of puberty are downstream consequences of the maturation of the HPG axis.

The central features of the HPG axis are shown diagrammatically in Fig. 12.5,[22] although it should be noted that the details are far more complex than is shown. Hormone signals flow between the components of the HPG axis. The hypothalamus serves as the main enabling centre, its primary signal is a hormone known as gonadotrophin-releasing hormone (GnRH) or LH-releasing hormone (LHRH) that is released in a pulsatile fashion.[28] Conceptually, the hypothalamus is seen as the primary on–off switch controlling reproductive function and is thought to be influenced by a vast range of stimuli. The effect of GnRH release is to simulate production and release two gonadotrophins from the pituitary, FSH and LH.[29,30] In the ovary, LH stimulates testosterone production and FSH stimulates the conversion of testosterone to oestradiol. At the same time, inhibin is secreted which has a suppressive effect on FSH. After ovulation progesterone is secreted. The combined effect of these steroids and inhibin is to inhibit the pituitary.[31] In the testis, LH stimulates testosterone production and FSH stimulates inhibin secretion, which act as feedback controls on the pituitary. Gonadal function is also regulated by a number of metabolites including insulin, cortisol, GH, and IGF-1.[32]

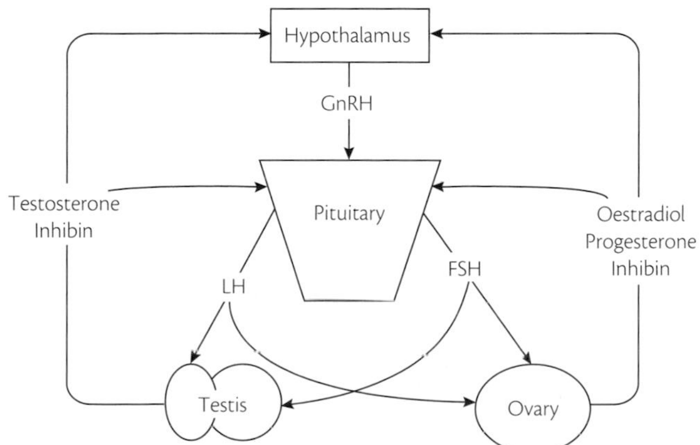

Fig. 12.5 The hypothalamic–pituitary–gonadal axis and its principal hormones. Redrawn from data reported by Ellison.[22]

Circulating levels of FSH are much higher in girls, compared to boys during infancy, whereas no sex differences are noted in LH. During childhood the levels of FSH and LH remain stable, with girls maintaining slightly higher levels of FSH than boys. In late childhood, the hypothalamus stimulates the anterior pituitary gland to release FSH and LH, causing the blood concentrations to increase substantially. Thus, one of the first detectable signs of biological maturity, related to a change in HPG axis activity, is the appearance of sleep-associated increased LH pulse amplitude. On average LH concentrations will rise first in girls at about 8–9 years of age, reflecting their earlier onset of puberty, and then in boys 1–2 years later.[33]

Elevations of gonadotrophin are associated with gonadal maturation, as evidenced in boys by increasing testicular volume. The resultant rise in testosterone levels stimulates a host of other pubertal changes, including the appearance of pubic, axillary, and facial hair, voice changes, accelerated linear growth, and increase in muscle mass. In girls, increased LH stimulation leads to increase in ovarian steroid production with oestradiol levels approaching those characteristic of women in the follicular phase. As a result of an increase in steroid production, pubic and axillary hair develop, breasts enlarge, linear growth accelerates, the pelvic remodels, an increase in adiposity occurs, and menarche is attained.

In late puberty, the secretion of FSH and LH becomes cyclic in females. In boys, LH stimulates testosterone production and FSH stimulates growth of tubules and sperm production. In contrast to the cyclic secretion of FSH and LH in females with the attainment of sexual maturity, in males FSH and LH secretion remains constant. Blood levels of gonadotrophins increase with puberty in both males and females. On average, girls experience a three-fold increase in the secretion of FSH and LH by stage 4 of breast and pubic hair development. Boys, on average, experience a six-fold increase by stage 5 of genital and pubic hair development (i.e. attainment of sexual maturity).[6]

Oestradiol, produced in the ovaries, is the most potent oestrogen in females. Testosterone is also present in females, but in small amounts compared to boys. In males testosterone is synthesized in the testes. Although testosterone is the most abundant androgen in males, the most potent androgen is dihydrotestosterone which is derived from testosterone. Circulating androgens are also converted to oestrogens in the peripheral tissues of males.

Levels of testosterone and oestradiol differ considerably during infancy, childhood, and puberty. During infancy, boys demonstrate higher levels of testosterone than girls. Compared to infancy, levels of testosterone and oestradiol are reduced during childhood, with no marked sex differences. During the prepubertal years oestradiol increases gradually, demonstrating a rapid spurt at the onset of sexual maturation (puberty). In addition to oestrogen, other less potent oestrogenic hormones are produced, which also contribute to sexual maturation. Similar to the production of gonadotrophic hormones in females, oestrogen production becomes cyclic during late puberty. In boys, circulating testosterone increases steadily during puberty. The sex differences in hormones are accentuated during puberty (i.e. increased oestradiol levels in girls and increased testosterone levels in boys).

Both oestradiol and testosterone affect GH production by augmenting GH pulse amplitude. Increases in IGF-1, the major mediator of GH action on skeletal growth, are correlated with secondary sex stages of pubertal development and gonadal steroid levels. GH and IGF-1 also have stimulatory effects on gonadal steroid production, and gonadal steroids have independent effects on skeletal growth not mediated by the somatotrophic axis.[34,35] Thus, the somatotrophic axis and the HPG axis function synergistically in promoting the adolescent growth spurt. However, it must be remembered that the initial stimulation comes from the maturation of the HPG axis.[22]

Oestrogens and androgens increase anabolism through nitrogen retention. Androgens, however, are much more potent anabolic hormones than oestrogen and most probably contribute to the sex differences in body size that occurs during puberty. During puberty, males experience a dramatic growth spurt in muscle and fat-free mass, which is primarily due to the rise in circulating levels of testosterone. Females' more modest gain in muscle mass during puberty is primarily caused by the lower levels of adrenal androgens produced. The increased fat disposition in females during puberty is due to the rising levels of oestrogens at this time.

As indicated previously, androgens and oestrogens also promote bone growth and skeletal maturation. Androgens stimulate longitudinal growth and increased thickness of bones. Greater growth is experienced during puberty in boys and is primarily due to the actions of testosterone. Oestrogen has little effect on linear growth but has an important role to play in bone formation and maturation. Oestrogens stimulate the production of bone matrix and act to maintain a positive calcium balance. Most importantly, oestrogens are responsible for the final stage of skeletal maturation (i.e. epiphyseal closure).

The causes and correlates of HPG axis maturation are still debatable. However, what is known is that changes in hypothalamic function are responsible for pubertal activation of the HPG axis and that puberty is not limited by the maturational status of either the pituitary or the gonad. What is uncertain is the process that leads to the establishment of the mature pattern of GnRH release. Although it has been suggested that at puberty, the hypothalamus becomes less sensitive to the negative feedback effects of gonadotrophins and steroids,[36] this hypothesis has been questioned.[37] The alternative hypothesis is that there is a positive stimulation of gonadotrophin production. However, neither of these hypotheses resolves the question as to what causes the maturational changes of the hypothalamus. However what is important is that when considering this question, the researcher adequately distinguishes potential causes of HPG axis maturation, such as training, from correlated and consequent events, such as menarche.

Biological maturity

As indicated previously, there is wide variation amongst children both within and between genders as to the exact timing and tempo of maturation. Therefore to adequately distinguish the effects of physical activity or exercise on a group of children, biological maturity needs to be controlled. When considering how to assess biological maturation it is first important to understand that 1 year of chronological time does not equal 1 year of maturational time. Whilst every individual passes through the same stages of maturity they do so at differing rates, resulting in children of the same chronological age differing in their degree of maturity, this is reflected in Fig. 12.6.[38] The top photographs show two girls both 11 years of age; however, what is not apparent is the fact that they differ considerably in their degree of maturity. At 11 years of age they are similar in height (girl on the left 1.56 m; girl on the right 1.58 m); however, the second set of photos of the same individuals at 35 years of age indicate that adult heights are significantly different (girl on the left 1.81 m; girl on the right 1.65 m). It is, therefore, apparent that at 11 years of age the girl on the right was very close to her final adult height, 7 cm of growth remaining, and thus close to full maturity. In contrast, at 11 years of age the girl on the left still had 25 cm of growth to go and thus was less mature at 11 years of age. This illustrates the point that the size of an individual is not an accurate indicator of maturity. Certainly, in very general terms, size is associated with maturity, in that a bigger individual is likely to be chronologically older and thus be more mature than a smaller individual. However, it is well recognized that size does not play a part in the assessment of maturity.

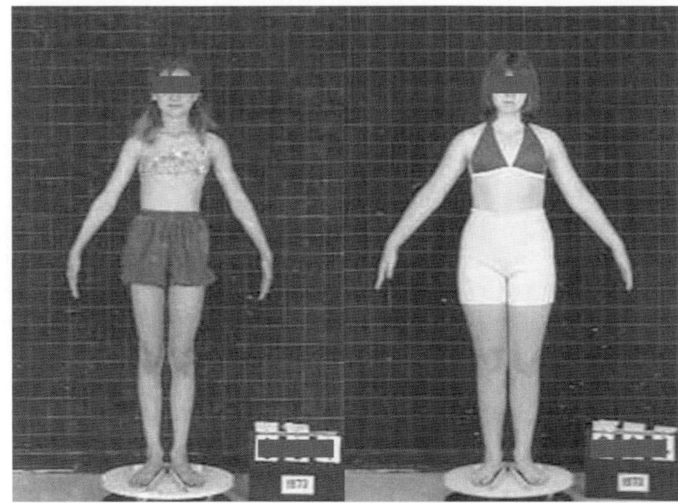

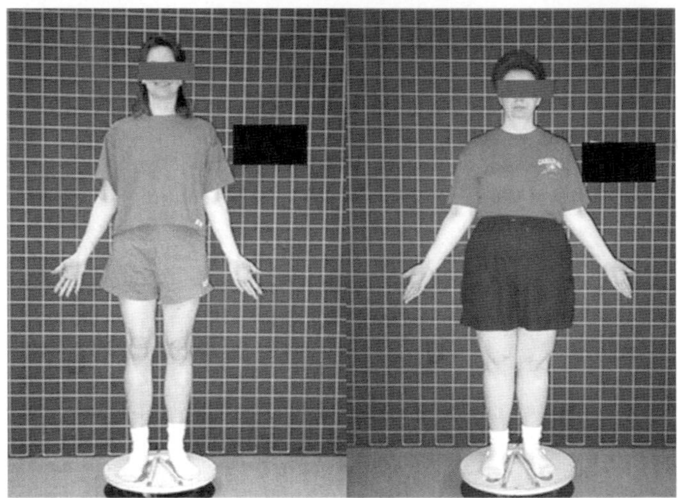

Fig. 12.6 Two girls photographed at the same chronological ages (11 and 35 years). At 11 years of age the girl on the left has 25.2 cm of growth in stature remaining and the girl on the right 6.5 cm of statural growth remaining. Data taken from two individuals who participated in the Saskatchewan Growth and Development Study (1964–1998).[37]

To adequately control for maturity, an indicator of maturity needs to be incorporated into the research methodology. The maturity indicator chosen should be any definable and sequential change in any part of the body that is characteristic of the progression of the body from immaturity to maturity.[39] The most commonly used methods to assess maturity are skeletal maturity, sexual maturity, biochemical and hormonal maturity, somatic or morphological maturity, and dental maturity. The technique of choice varies with the study design. Each method, with its associated limitations, is described in Chapter 3.

The interrelationships among the various indicators of biological maturation are complex, because only skeletal maturity and percentage of adult stature span the entire maturation period from birth to adulthood. During puberty, a number of other indicators become apparent, such as somatic and sexual maturity both of which are related to skeletal maturity. The various ages of the timing and tempo of a number of pubertal events are illustrated in Fig. 12.7.[40,41] The upper portion of Fig. 12.7 shows the average age in girls when the various biological events take place[40] and the range of variation in the ages when these events occur. In girls, the first event to be noticed is the start of breast development; the time when prepubertal girls in breast stage 1 enter breast stage 2, the advent of the breast bud. This occurs on average around 11.0 years of age (range 8.0–13.0 years). The onset of pubic hair development is a little later; although in about one third of girls pubic hair appears before the breast bud.[11] Menarche, the first menstrual period, occurs relatively late in puberty, between 12.8 and 13.2 years; although in normal healthy girls it can occur as early as 10.5 years and as late as 15.5 years. When menarche occurs most girls are in breast stage 4 and pubic hair stages 3 or 4; however, some girls can be in pubic hair stage 1 and others in pubic hair stage 5. The relationship between menarche and PHV is much stronger, occurring at the time of maximum deceleration of height velocity.

Beginning testicular enlargement is usually the first sign of puberty in boys, accompanied by changes in the texture and colour of the skin of the scrotum, this occurs on average around 11.5 years of age (range 9.5–15.5 years). A little later, the penis starts to enlarge and pubic hair starts to appear. Acceleration of penis growth begins on average at about 12.5 years (range 10.5–14.5 years) with the completion of growth by 14.4 years (range 12.5–16.5 years). It is, therefore, possible for a late maturing boy to start penis growth after the earliest maturer has completed it. On average, pubic hair development starts around 12 years of age (stage 2) and is completed by 15 years of age (stage 5). The adolescent growth spurt starts on

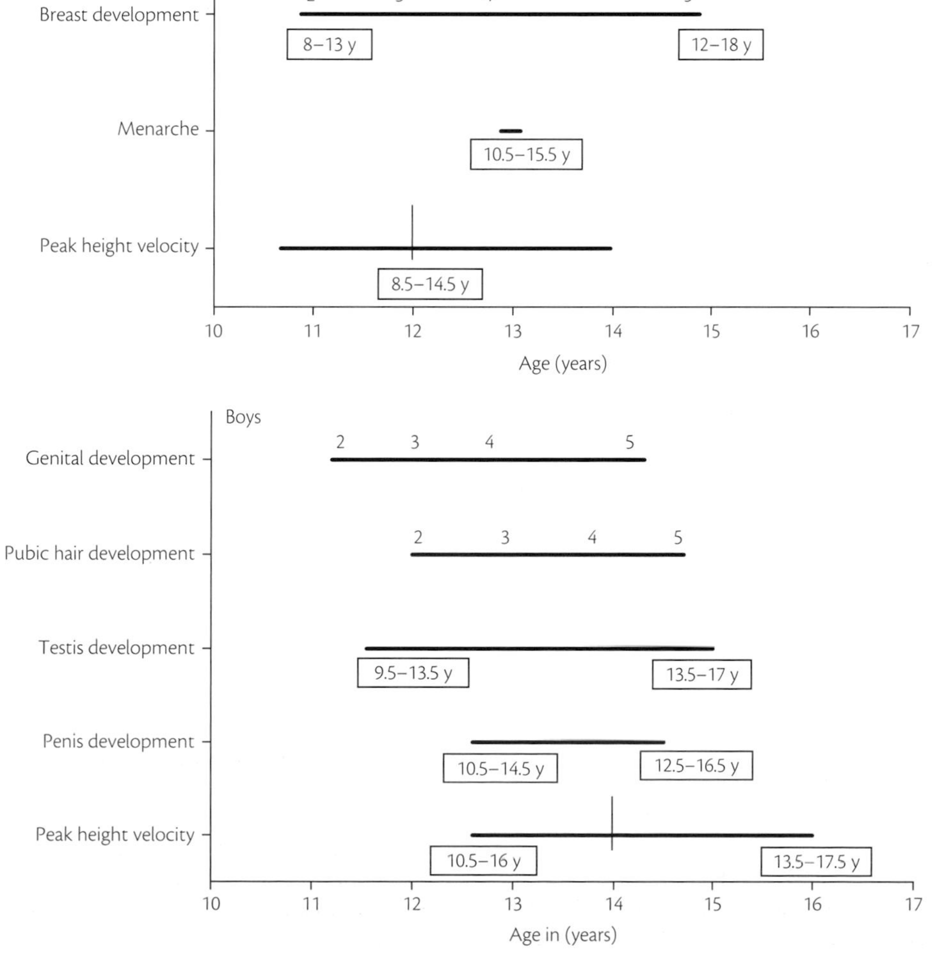

Fig. 12.7 Diagram of sequence of events at puberty in girls and boys. Redrawn from data reported by Marshall and Tanner.[40,41]

average at around 12.5 years, a year after the first signs of testicular enlargement and reaches its peak (PHV) at around 14 years of age when genitalia development is between stages 4 and 5, and pubic hair between stages 3 and 4. Facial hair appears somewhat later as does the breaking of the voice, a relatively late pubertal event.[11]

Figure 12.7 illustrates the fact that a number of pubertal events are occurring at the same time, all under the control of various endocrine systems and ultimately controlled by genetic expression. However, the timing of pubertal events varies between individuals of the same sex. Apart from individual variation, there is also a marked sex difference in the timing of somatic and sexual maturation. Girls enter and end puberty approximately 2 years before boys. It is also important to be aware that pubertal events do not occur in the same sequence between the sexes. For example, when comparing pubic hair growth to statural growth PHV is a relatively early event in girls and a relatively late event in boys.[42] As indicated, boys' PHV occurs, on average, during pubic hair stages 4 and 5, whereas girls' PHV usually occur during pubic hair stages 3 and 4. This suggests that the timing of sexual and somatic maturation is not the same between girls and boys.

Aligning individuals by secondary sex characteristics is used frequently in the paediatric exercise science literature because it does not require longitudinal observations, is easy to administer, cost effective, and non-invasive (with the replacement of physician assessment with self-assessment). However, a common misuse of secondary sex characteristics when controlling for maturity is to analyse categories as if they were continuous variables. For example, an individual in the early phase of stage 3 of pubic hair development is rated the same as an individual in the late phase of this stage. It is rare that the point in time at which the change from one stage to another stage is ever measured; what is actually being reported is the interval between two stages. This provides even less information when you consider that the length of time it takes to move through a stage varies considerably among individuals.[42] In addition, there is no relationship between the age at which a secondary sex characteristic begins and the length of time that it takes to pass through the stage. Another concern with the use of secondary sex staging relates to possible misuse in alignment of individuals. Many paediatric studies align boys and girls on (i) the same secondary sex characteristic, (ii) on different secondary sex characteristics, or (iii) more than one secondary sex characteristics to develop a composite score of sexual development. The assumption behind these strategies is that the order and timing of the appearance of the same secondary sex characteristic and/or different sex characteristics are identical in both sexes. It further presumes that the sequence of the appearance of secondary sex characteristics between sexes with other maturity indicators is also identical. However, as described previously, there is a considerable difference in timing and tempo of somatic and sexual development between sexes during adolescence. This means that all three of these alignment strategies are inappropriate when making comparisons between boys and girls. Furthermore, different maturity events occur at different times during adolescence. For example, genitalia development and breast development occur early in adolescence; whereas menarche in girls and axillary and facial hair in boys occur late in adolescence. An individual who is at stage 3 for breast development will not necessarily be at stage 3 for pubic hair development. Likewise, a boy at stage 3 for genital development is not necessarily of the same biological age as a girl who is at stage 3 for breast development. Hence, it is unfounded to make comparisons between individuals using different secondary sex characteristics; thus, it is important for researchers to detail which secondary sex characteristic is being used as the maturity indicator.

When controlling for the confounding effects of biological maturity between genders, boys and girls are most often aligned on pubic hair stages, as this is the only sex characteristic that is present in both boys and girls (apart from axillary hair growth, which proves to be problematic if girls remove underarm hair). In addition to other cautions outlined previously, one should be aware that pubic hair development represents the onset of adrenarche (an increased secretion of sex hormones by the adrenal cortex) and not necessarily the onset of true pubertal development. As stated previously, onset of breast development in girls and testicular volume in boys are the first true signs of centrally mediated puberty. Thus if individuals are aligned only on pubic hair development, caution should be taken when interpreting individuals classified into the early stages. Therefore, although any of the maturity indicators can be used when making comparisons within sexes, for gender comparisons studies should either use skeletal age or some form of somatic maturity.[7]

Correlations between the timing of maturity indicators are generally moderate to high, suggesting that there is a general maturity factor underlying the tempo of growth and maturation during adolescence in both boys and girls (Fig. 12.7). However, there is sufficient variation to suggest that no single system (i.e. sexual, skeletal, or somatic) provides a complete description of the tempo of maturation during adolescence. Furthermore, although sexual maturation and skeletal development are associated, an individual in one stage of secondary sexual development cannot be assumed to be in a set stage of skeletal development. The apparent discord among the aforementioned indicators reflects individual variation in the timing and tempo of sexual and somatic maturity, and the methodological concerns in the assessment of maturity.

Relationship of maturity to body size and function

From what has been described previously, it should now be obvious that a child's maturity status will influence measures of growth and performance. Early maturing individuals of both sexes are taller and heavier than average maturing and late maturing individuals of the same chronological age. If a youth's height was expressed as a percentage of their adult height, early maturing individuals would be closest to their adult height at all ages during adolescence. Early maturing individuals also have a greater weight for height at each age. The height advantage of the early maturing individual is primarily due to an earlier attainment of PHV and also a greater magnitude of peak height gain. Studies have repeatedly shown little or no correlation between the timing of the adolescent growth spurt (i.e. maturity status) and adult stature, suggesting that early, average, and late maturing children reach, on average, the same adult height. This is not the same for weight. Early maturing individuals have, on average, greater body weights as young adults. Early maturing individuals and late maturing individuals also vary in body shape. Late maturers tend to have relatively longer legs (i.e. legs account for a greater percentage of adult stature) than early maturers. Furthermore, early maturing girls and boys tend to have relatively wider hips and relatively narrower shoulders. In contrast, late maturing individuals tend to have relatively narrower hips and relatively wider shoulders.

The average age at which the velocity in growth of lean mass and fat mass peak occurs is earliest in early maturers, late in average maturers, and latest in late maturers.[14] In both sexes early maturing youngsters have, on average, larger measurements of muscle and fat. The differences between children of contrasting maturity groups are primarily due to size differences, because early maturers are taller and heavier than late maturers of the same chronological age. When muscle widths are expressed relative to height the differences between maturity groups are often eliminated. However, there is some evidence that during the later adolescent years early maturing boys have larger muscle widths even after taking into account height differences. On the other hand, early maturing individuals of both sexes appear to have greater fat widths at all ages through adolescence, even when height differences are controlled.[6] In summary, at any given chronological age during adolescence, early maturing boys and girls are on average taller, heavier, have greater fat-free mass (especially in boys), total body fat, and % body fat (especially in girls) than their less mature peers. The maturity-associated differences in body size and body composition are especially marked during adolescence and influence strength and aerobic power.

Strength increases during adolescence are associated with the natural development in lean mass, and generally reach a peak at the same time as PHV in girls and a year after PHV in boys. Studies have shown that early maturing boys are stronger than late maturing boys during adolescence. Early maturing girls tend to be slightly stronger than late maturing girls early in adolescence (11 through 13 years of age), but as adolescence continues the difference between maturity groups disappears. When strength is expressed relative to height, the difference among maturity groups persists in boys, probably due to the early maturers rapid growth in muscle mass. On the other hand, when strength is expressed relative to height in girls, the differences between maturity groups disappear.

It has been shown that early maturing individuals, when compared to late maturing individuals of the same chronological age, have a higher absolute peak oxygen uptake (peak $\dot{V}O_2$). Although the size advantage of the early maturing individual is reflected in a greater peak $\dot{V}O_2$, a maturity effect, independent of body size, has been demonstrated. This difference in peak $\dot{V}O_2$ between contrasting maturity groups is more pronounced in males than in females which may be due to males developing greater muscle mass, red blood cells, haemoglobin, lung capacity, pulmonary ventilation, and $\dot{V}O_2$ than females during adolescence.[43] When both early and late maturers are fully grown, and have achieved the same stature, the differences in peak $\dot{V}O_2$ disappears (see Chapter 20).

General conclusion

Paediatric exercise science examines the acute and chronic responses of the child and adolescent to exercise and/or physical activity. Of primary interest are the physiological changes, physical activity, and health-related outcomes during childhood and adolescence, and the differences of the aforementioned between sexes, and between children and adults. Because children of the same age do not all follow the same tempo and timing of biological maturity (i.e. there are early, average, and late maturers), it is essential to consider growth and maturity confounders when studying paediatric exercise physiology. For example, many studies have found that participation in physical activity decreases during adolescence and that the decline in physical activity is more pronounced in girls than in boys.[44,45] However, when aligned by biological age (years from PHV) physical activity measured either subjectively[46] or objectively[47] is not significantly different at any biological age between the sexes.

Summary

- The process of growth and maturation is continuous throughout childhood and adolescence, with girls, on average, experiencing the onset of puberty about 2 years in advance of boys.
- Although all young people follow the same pattern of growth from infancy to full maturity, there is considerable variation both between and within sexes in the timing and magnitude of these changes.
- During adolescence boys become considerably larger and acquire broader shoulders, whereas girls enlarge their pelvic diameter and have increased deposits of fat in various places such as the breast.
- Adolescent males lay down a considerably greater amount of lean tissue compared to girls, this increase in skeletal size and muscle mass leads to increased strength in males.
- Within an age group, early maturers are, on average, taller and heavier and have a larger fat-free mass (especially boys) and fat mass (especially girls) than late maturers.
- The effects of a child's maturation, in a biological context, may mask or be greater than the effects associated with the exposure to physical activity or exercise, the paediatric exercise scientist must therefore include an assessment of biological age in their study design.
- Indicators of skeletal, sexual, and somatic maturation are moderately to highly correlated during adolescence, however, no one indicator gives a complete description of the tempo of growth and maturation.
- It is recommended that for gender-specific comparisons any of the discussed methods are appropriate, however, for studies that make gender comparisons either skeletal age or one of the somatic indices should be used.

References

1. Thompson D'AW (1942). *On growth and form*. Cambridge University Press, Cambridge.
2. Tanner JM (1964). *The physique of the Olympic athlete*. George Allen and Unwin Ltd., London.
3. Malina RM (1994). Physical growth and biological maturation of young athletes. *Exerc Sport Sci Rev* **22**, 389–434.
4. Caine D, Bass SL, Daly R (2003). Does elite competition inhibit growth and delay maturation in some gymnasts? Quite possibly. *Pediatr Exerc Sci* **15**, 360–72.
5. Thomis MA, Towne B (2006). Genetic determinants of prepubertal and pubertal growth and development. *Food Nutr Bull* **27**(Suppl. 4), S257–79.
6. Malina RM, Bouchard C, Bar-Or O (2004). *Growth, maturation, and physical activity* (2nd ed.). Human Kinetics, Champaign, IL.

7. Baxter-Jones ADG, Eisenmann JC, Sherar LB (2005). Controlling for maturation in pediatric exercise science. *Pediatr Exerc Sci* **17**, 18–30.
8. Salkind NJ (2002). *Child development*. Macmillan, New York.
9. Cameron N, Demerath EW (2002). Critical periods in human growth and their relationship to disease of aging. *Yearbook Phys Anthrop* **45**, 159–84.
10. Scammon RE (1927). The first seriatim study of human growth. *Am J Phys Anthrop* **10**, 329–36.
11. Tanner JM (1989). *Foetus into man*. Castlemead Publications, London.
12. Scammon RE (1930). The measurement of the body in childhood. In: Harris JA, Jackson CM, Paterson DG, Scammon RE (eds.), *The measurement of man*, pp. 173–215. University of Minnesota Press, Minneapolis, MN.
13. Zemel B, Barden E (2004). Measuring body composition. In: Hauspie RC, Cameron N, Molinari L (eds.), *Methods in human growth research*, pp. 141–78. Cambridge University Press, Cambridge.
14. Jones PRM, Norgan NG (1994). Anthropometry and the assessment of body composition. In: Harries M, Williams C, Stanish WD, Micheli LJ (eds.), *Oxford textbook of sports medicine*, pp. 149–60. Oxford University Press, Oxford.
15. Iuliano-Burnes S, Mirwald RL, Bailey DA (2001). Timing and magnitude of peak height velocity and peak tissue velocities for early, average, and late maturing boys and girls. *Am J Hum Biol* **13**, 1–8.
16. Rupich RC, Specker BL, Lieuw AF, Ho M (1996). Gender and race differences in bone mass during infancy. *Calcif Tissue Int* **58**, 395–7.
17. Maynard LM, Guo SS, Chumlea WC, Roche AF, Wisemandle WA, Zeller CM, Towne B, Siervogel RM (1998). Total-body and regional bone mineral content and areal bone mineral density in children aged 8–18 y: The Fels Longitudinal Study. *Am J Clin Nutr* **68**, 1111–17.
18. Baxter-Jones ADG, Mirwald RL, McKay HA, Bailey DA (2003). A longitudinal analysis of sex differences in bone mineral accrual in healthy 8 to 19 year old boys and girls. *Ann Hum Biol* **30**, 160–75.
19. Rolland-Cachera M-F (1998). Adiposity rebound and prediction of adult fatness. In: Ulijaszek SJ, Johnston FE, Preece MA (eds.), *The Cambridge encyclopedia of human growth and development*, pp. 51–3. Cambridge University Press, Cambridge.
20. Norgan NG (1998). Body composition. In: Ulijaszek SJ, Johnston FE, Preece MA (eds.), *The Cambridge encyclopedia of human growth and development*, pp. 212–15. Cambridge University Press, Cambridge.
21. Armstrong N, Welsman JR (1997). *Young people and physical activity*. Oxford University Press, Oxford.
22. Ellison PT (2002). Puberty. In: Cameron (ed.), *Human growth and development*, pp. 65–84. Academic Press, San Diego, CA.
23. Reynolds EL, Wines JV (1951). Physical changes associated with adolescence in boys. *Am J Dis Child* **82**, 529–47.
24. Tanner JM (1962). *Growth at adolescence* (2nd ed.). Blackwell Scientific Publications, Oxford.
25. Boas F (1930). Observations on the growth of children. *Science* **72**, 44–8.
26. Hindmarsh P (1998). Endocrinological regulation of post-natal growth. In: Ulijaszek SJ, Johnston FE, Preece MA (eds.), *The Cambridge encyclopedia of human growth and development*, pp. 212–15. Cambridge University Press, Cambridge.
27. Rogol AD, Roemmich JN, Clark PA (2002). Growth at puberty. *J Adolesc Health* **31**, 192–200.
28. Matsuo H, Babba Y, Nair RMG, Arimura A, Schaly AV (1971). Structure of the porcine LH- and FSH-releasing hormone. *Biochem Biophy Res Commun* **43**, 1334–9.
29. Carmel PW, Araki S, Ferin M (1976). Pituitary stalk portal blood collection in rhesus monkeys: Evidence for pulsatile release of GnRH. *Endocrinology* **99**, 243–8.
30. Beil JD, Patton JM, Dailey RA, Tsou RC, Tindall GT (1977). Luteinizing hormone releasing hormone (LHRH) in pituitary portal blood of rhesus monkeys: Relationship to level of LH release. *Endocrinology* **101**, 430–4.
31. Yen SSC (1991). The human menstrual cycle: Neuroendocrine regulation. In: Yen SSC, Jaffe RB (eds.), *Reproductive endocrinology* (3rd ed.), pp. 273–308. Saunders, Philadelphia, PA.
32. Hall PF (1988). Testicular steroid synthesis: Organization and regulation. In: Knobil E, Neill JD (eds.), *The physiology of reproduction*, pp. 975–98. Raven Press, New York.
33. Boyar RM (1978). Control of the onset of puberty. *Ann Rev Med* **29**, 509–20.
34. Libanti C, Baylink DJ, Lois-Wenzel E, Srinvasan N, Mohan S (1999). Studies on the potential mediators of skeletal changes occurring during puberty in girls. *J Clin Endocrinol Metab* **84**, 2807–14.
35. Lackey BR, Gray SL, Henricks DM (1999). The insulin-like growth factor (IGF) system and gonadotropin regulation: Actions and interactions. *Cytokine Growth Factor Rev* **10**, 201–17.
36. Kulin HE, Grumbach MM, Kaplan SL (1969). Changing sensitivity of the pubertal gonadal hypothalamic feedback mechanism in man. *Science* **166**, 1012–13.
37. Plant TM (1988). Puberty in primates. In: Knobil E, Neill JD (eds.), *The physiology of reproduction*, pp. 1763–88. Raven Press, New York.
38. Mirwald RL (1978). Saskatchewan growth and development study. In Ostyn M, Beunen G, Simons J (eds.), *Kinanthropometry II*, pp. 289–305. University Park Press, Baltimore, MD.
39. Cameron N (2002). Assessment of maturation. In: Cameron (ed.), *Human growth and development*, pp. 65–84. Academic Press, San Diego, CA.
40. Marshall WA, Tanner JM (1969). Variations in the pattern of pubertal changes in girls. *Arch Dis Child* **44**, 291–303.
41. Marshall WA, Tanner JM (1970). Variations in the pattern of pubertal changes in boys. *Arch Dis Child* **45**, 13–23.
42. Sherar LB, Baxter-Jones AD, Mirwald RL (2004). Limitations to the use of secondary sex characteristics for gender comparisons. *Ann Hum Biol* **31**, 586–93.
43. Kemper HC, Verschuur R (1981). Maximal aerobic power in 13- and 14-year-old teenagers in relation to biologic age. *Int J Sports Med* **2**, 97–100.
44. Riddoch CJ, Andersen LB, Wedderkopp N, Harro L, Klasson-Heggebo L, Sardinha LB, Cooper AR, Ekelund U (2004). Physical activity levels and patterns of 9- and 15-yr-old European children. *Med Sci Sports Exerc* **36**, 86–92.
45. Trost SG, Pate RR, Sallis JF, Freedson PS, Taylor WC, Dowda M, Sirard J (2002). Age and gender differences in objectively measured physical activity in youth. *Med Sci Sports Exerc* **34**, 350–5.
46. Thompson AM, Baxter-Jones AD, Mirwald RL, Bailey DA (2003). Comparison of physical activity in male and female children: Does maturation matter? *Med Sci Sports Exerc* **35**, 1684–90.
47. Sherar LB, Esliger DW, Baxter-Jones ADG**,** Tremblay MS (2007). Age and gender related differences in childhood physical activity: Does physical maturity matter? *Med Sci Sports Exerc* **39**, 830–5.

CHAPTER 13

Developmental biodynamics: the development of coordination in children

James Watkins

Introduction

Human movement is brought about by the musculoskeletal system under the control of the nervous system. By coordinated activity between the various muscle groups, forces generated by the muscles are transmitted by the bones and joints to enable the individual to maintain an upright or partially upright posture and bring about voluntary controlled movements.[1] Biomechanics of human movement is the study of the relationship between the external forces (due to body weight and physical contact with the external environment) and internal forces (active forces generated by muscles and passive forces exerted on other structures) that act on the body and the effect of these forces on the movement of the body.[2]

The brain coordinates and controls movement via muscular activity.[3] Coordination refers to the timing of relative motion between body segments and control refers to the optimization of relative motion between body segments, that is, the extent to which the kinematics of segmental motion and, consequently, the motion of the whole-body centre of gravity (CG), matches the demands of the task.[4] For example, the mature form of coordination of the leg action in a countermovement vertical jump, as shown in Fig. 13.1, is characterized by simultaneous flexion of the hips, knees, and ankles in the countermovement phase [Fig. 13.1(a–c)] followed by simultaneous extension of the hips, knees, and ankles in the propulsion phase [Fig. 13.1(c–e)]. This pattern of coordination normally occurs between 3 and 4 years of age.[4] However, whereas all normal mature individuals exhibit similar coordination in the standing vertical jump (and other whole-body movements) there are considerable differences in the extent to which individuals can control the movement, that is, optimize the relative motion of the body segments in order to match the task demands.

If the objective in performing a countermovement vertical jump is to maximize height jumped (upward vertical displacement of the whole-body CG measured from the floor), then control of the movement is concerned with maximizing the height of the CG at take-off (h_1) and maximizing the upward vertical displacement of the CG after take-off (h_2) [Fig. 13.1(e) and (f)]. h_1 is determined by body position which, in turn, is determined by the range of motion in the joints and the extent to which the available range of motion is used. h_2 is determined by the vertical velocity of the CG at take-off, the greater the take-off velocity, the greater h_2. Take-off velocity is determined by the impulse of the ground reaction force (the force exerted between the feet and the floor) prior to take-off, the larger the impulse the greater the velocity. The impulse Ft of the ground reaction force F is determined by the magnitude of F and its duration t; the larger the force and the longer its duration the larger the impulse. The magnitude of F will depend on the strength of the muscles, especially the extensor muscles of the hips, knees, and ankles. The duration of F will depend on the range of motion in the hips, knees, and ankles, and the extent to which the available range of motion is used. Clearly, restricted ranges of motion in any of the joints, especially hips, knees, and ankles, and lack of strength in any of the muscles, especially the extensor muscles of the hips, knees, and ankles, will adversely affect an individual's ability to control the movement and, consequently, result in less than optimal performance.

There are numerous studies of jumping performance in adults, especially elite athletes.[5,6] However, there are relatively few studies on the development of coordination and control of jumping in young children. Jensen *et al.*[4] investigated coordination and control in the countermovement vertical jump in two groups of young children (mean ± SD age = 3.4 ± 0.5 years) and a group of skilled adults. The two groups of children ($n_1 = n_2 = 9$) were selected from a larger group ($n = 32$) on the basis of their take-off angle (angle of velocity vector of the whole-body CG at take-off) into a high take-off group (HT0) and low take-off group (LT0). Take-off angle is a key control variable, since to maximize vertical displacement after take-off the take-off angle should be 90° (with respect to the horizontal). The criterion for inclusion in the HT0 and LT0 groups was a take-off angle at least 1 SD greater or less than the total group mean, respectively. All jumps were performed on a force platform to measure the ground reaction force. To encourage maximum effort, a suspended ball, just out of reach, was used as a visual target. Coordination was examined in terms of the timing of reversals

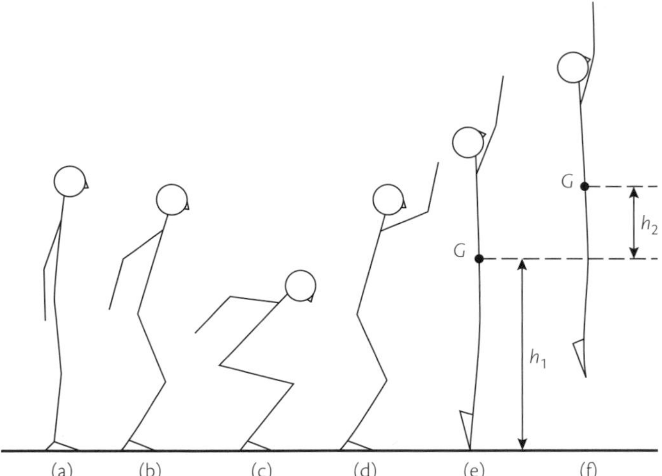

Fig. 13.1 Stick figure sequence of a countermovement vertical jump from a standing position: (a) to (c) = countermovement or dip phase; (c) to (e) = propulsion phase. G = whole-body centre of gravity; h_1 = height of G above the floor at take-off; h_2 = upward vertical displacement of G after take-off.

(between the countermovement and propulsion phases of the jump) of the hip, knee, and ankle joints and the timing of the peak extension velocities of the hip, knee, and ankle joints. Control was examined in terms of the body position at three significant events in the propulsion phase; the time of maximum acceleration downwards (minimum ground reaction force), the time of maximum acceleration upwards (maximum ground reaction force), and take-off.

No significant differences were found between the three groups with regard to the coordination variables. This finding is consistent with the results of a study by Clark *et al.*[7] for 3-, 5-, 7-, and 9-year-old children involving the same task and methodology. The mean take-off angles for the adults, HT0 and LT0 groups, 91.8° ± 3.8°, 82.0° ± 3.5°, and 61.2° ± 5.6°, respectively, were significantly different from each other and the mean of the adult group was close to the theoretically desired angle of 90°. There were also significant differences between the groups in some of the other control variables (hip, knee, and ankle angles) at one or more of the three events, in particular, ankle angle between adults and both child groups at take-off and knee angle between all three groups at take-off. The small angle of take-off of the LT0 group was found to be associated with a large (relative to the adults and HT0 groups) forward displacement of the CG during the countermovement and propulsion phases, that is, the trajectory of the CG was V-shaped, downward and forward then upward and forward. In contrast, the trajectory of the CG of the adults was U-shaped, downward and very slightly forward then upward and very slightly forward. The trajectory of the CG of the HT0 group was in between those of the adult and LT0 groups. In general, the smaller the forward displacement of the CG the greater the take-off angle and vice versa. Whereas the HT0 and LT0 groups had smaller take-off angles than the adult group the HT0 and LT0 groups still accomplished a clearly recognizable vertical jump, the jumps were simply not optimized for maximum vertical displacement of the CG. Jensen *et al.*[4] concluded that the performances of the children were coordinated but poorly controlled, perhaps due to inadequate strength of the leg extensor muscles, especially during the braking period of the countermovement phase (the period when the downward velocity of the CG is reduced to zero).

Development of coordination and control

The human neuromusculoskeletal system consists of approximately 10^{11} neurons, 10^3 muscles, and 10^2 moveable joints.[3,8] The way that the nervous system organizes movement in the face of such complexity has been viewed historically from two viewpoints: the neuromaturational perspective and the information-processing perspective.[8]

The neuromaturational perspective has been used primarily to explain motor development in infants and children. The neuromaturational perspective arose from the work of Gesell and Thompson[9] and McGraw,[10] who observed and described the gradual and sequential development of motor skills in infants from apparently unintentional reflex movements through the development of intentional movements such as crawling, sitting, standing, and walking. Gesell and McGraw came to the view that the gradual development of motor skills reflected the gradual maturation of the nervous system. This view became widely held and the age norms for the emergence of motor skills in infants and children produced by Gesell and McGraw became, and still are, widely used.[11] Whereas neuromaturation is undeniably a major determinant of motor development in infants and children, it does not explain skill acquisition in adults where the nervous system is considered to be fully mature.[12]

Traditionally, the information-processing perspective has dominated theories of skill acquisition in adults.[13] From the information-processing perspective, the brain is regarded rather like a computer with a very large number of motor programmes which can be executed at will to match the specific demands of each movement task as defined by the available sensory information. However, similar to the neuromaturational perspective, the information-processing perspective does not account for the great flexibility demonstrated by individuals in accommodating rapidly changing task demands, especially in the context of sports.

The deficiencies of the neuromaturational and information-processing perspectives were pointed out by Bernstein.[14] He argued that the complexity of the neuromusculoskeletal system was such that there could not be a one-to-one relationship between activity in the nervous system and actual movements. He also pointed out that a particular set of muscular contractions is not always associated with the same movement pattern, and that not all movements are controlled by the nervous system. For example, if you raise your arm to the side by activity in the shoulder abductor muscles and then relax the muscles, the arm will fall down under its own weight without any involvement of the nervous system. Similarly, if you hold your arm with the upper arm horizontal, the lower arm vertical, and the wrist relaxed, and then alternately slightly flex and extend the elbow fairly rapidly, the hand will flail about the wrist due to its own inertia and the force exerted on the hand at the wrist by the movement of the lower arm, without any involvement of the nervous system. At any particular point in time, each body segment may be acted on by four kinds of forces which can be classified in two ways: internal (muscle, articular) and external (weight, contact) forces, and active (muscle) and passive (articular, weight, contact) forces. Articular forces are passive forces exerted between articular surfaces and by joint support structures due to movement of adjacent segments. Contact forces are forces resulting from contact with surfaces external to the body, such as the floor.

Reference axes and degrees of freedom

In describing the movement of a joint it is useful to refer to three mutually perpendicular axes: anteroposterior, transverse, and vertical (Fig. 13.2). With respect to the three reference axes there are six possible directions, called degrees of freedom, in which, a joint, depending on its structure, may be able to move. There are three possible linear directions (along the axes) and three possible angular directions (about the axes). Most of the joints in the body have between one and three degrees of freedom. Most movements of the body involve simultaneous movement in a number of joints and the degrees of freedom of the whole segmental chain is the sum of the degrees of freedom of the individual joints in the chain. For example, if the wrist (which is composed of eight small irregular shaped bones) is regarded as a single joint with two degrees of freedom (flexion–extension and abduction–adduction), then the arm has approximately 25 joints (joints of the shoulder, elbow, wrist, and fingers) and approximately 35 degrees of freedom.

Coordination and degrees of freedom

Bernstein[14] described the development of coordination as a progressive increase in mastery of the very many degrees of freedom in a particular movement. He suggested that the development of skill in any particular task-oriented movement could be divided into two stages. The first stage involves the development of functional synergies between the muscle groups in the segmental chain, which is characterized by joint couplings between the joints in the segmental chain; the joint couplings result in reciprocal movement between the joints, that is, coordinated movement of the linked segments, which effectively considerably reduces the number of degrees of freedom. In addition, coordination is further simplified, at least initially, by restricting the range of motion in the joints. The second stage involves the development of control, that is, the functional synergies and ranges of motion in the joints gradually become optimized to maximize effectiveness in terms of task demands and maximize movement efficiency in terms of energy expenditure. This process involves neural integration of the active and passive forces in a manner which minimizes energy expenditure (the work done by muscles) and maximizes energy conservation (by facilitating energy transformation, potential to kinetic and vice versa, and energy transfer between segments).

Most of the muscles (muscle–tendon units) of the body cross over more than one joint. These muscles, such as the rectus femoris and hamstrings, are usually referred to as biarticular muscles, since muscles that cross over more than two joints function in the same way as muscles that cross over just two joints.[15] Biarticular muscles are too short to fully flex or fully extend all the joints that they cross over simultaneously. For example, the hamstrings are too short to fully extend the hip and fully flex the knee at the same time; indeed, hip extension is usually associated with knee extension and hip flexion is usually associated with knee flexion, as in a countermovement vertical jump (Fig. 13.1). Ingen Schenau[16] has suggested that correct use of biarticular muscles is of prime importance in the development of functional synergies (Fig. 13.3).

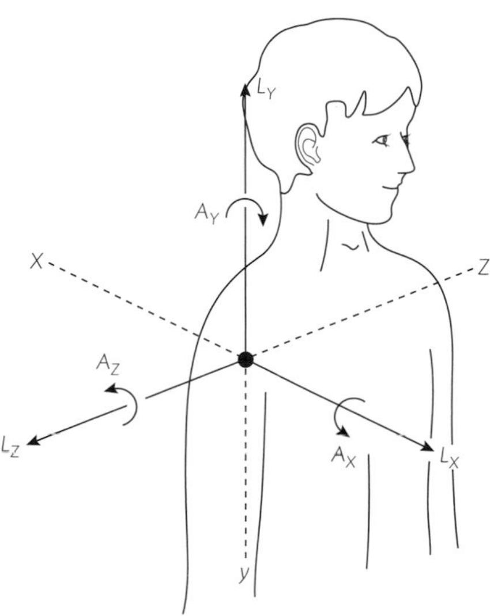

Fig. 13.2 Linear and angular degrees of freedom with respect to the shoulder joint. X = anteroposterior axis; Y = vertical axis; Z = transverse axis; L_X = linear motion along X axis; L_Y = linear motion along Y axis; L_Z = linear motion along Z axis; A_X = angular motion about X axis; A_Y = angular motion about Y axis; A_Z = angular motion about Z axis.

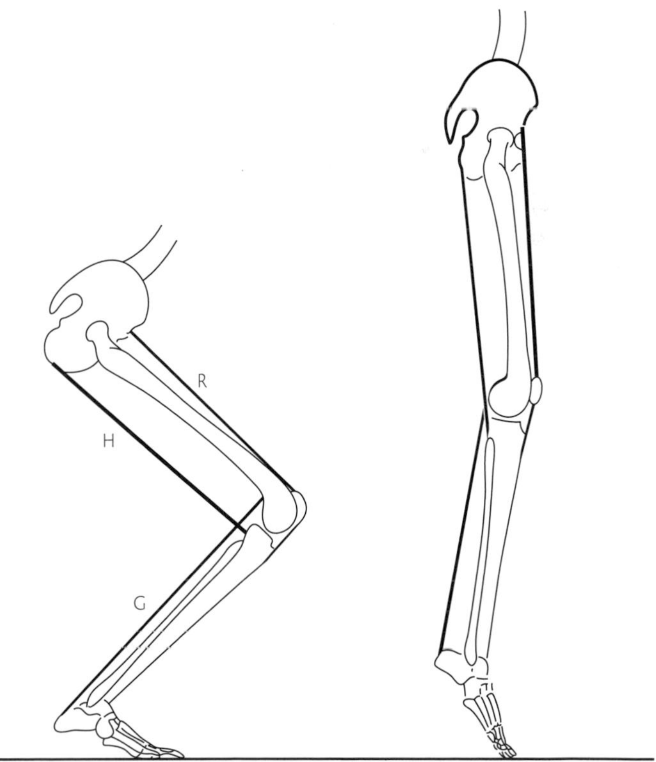

Fig. 13.3 Coupling of the trunk, upper leg, and lower leg by the rectus femoris, hamstrings, and gastrocnemius. The trunk is linked to the lower leg by the hamstrings (H) and the rectus femoris (R), and the upper leg is linked to the foot by the gastrocnemius (G). If the lengths of H, R and G are appropriately set, hip extension will result in simultaneous knee extension and ankle plantar flexion (adapted from Ingen Schenau[16]).

Research on Bernstein's ideas was quite limited until fairly recently (past 15 years) due, it would appear, to a combination of factors including the hypothetical nature of some biomechanical concepts, such as resultant joint moment,[16] and difficulties associated with modelling the human body for the purpose of biomechanical analysis[17,18] Recent advances in modelling capability and increased use of biomechanical analysis techniques by motor development researchers has resulted in more research on the biomechanics of coordination.[19,20] However, there would appear to be few studies which have related kinematics to kinetics, investigated the effects of practice, or involved children.

Kinematics of coordination

Whereas control of movement is essential to maximize performance, the development of coordination is a necessary precursor to the development of control. This was demonstrated by Anderson and Sidaway[21] in a study of the effects of practice on performance in kicking. A novice group of right foot dominant subjects, five males and one female (mean age 20.3 years, age range 18–22 years), was selected on the basis of no previous experience of organized soccer or soccer training. An expert group of three males (mean age 25.2 years, age range 22–30 years), each with more than 10 years experience of organized soccer, was included in the study in order to determine whether the coordination of the three experts was similar and to compare the pre- and post-practice coordination of the novices with the experts. The task to be learned (only the novice group took part in the practice sessions) was a right-footed instep drive at a 2 m^2 target placed 5 m from the ball following a two-step approach. The primary goal was to maximize the velocity of the ball while trying to hit the target. The subjects practised twice a week for 10 weeks and had between 15 and 20 trials during each session. Prior to and after the practice period, three trials of each subject were videotaped with a single camera placed perpendicular to the plane of motion on the right side of the subject. By using markers on the right shoulder, right hip, right knee, and right small toe (Fig. 13.4), the angular displacement and angular velocity of the hip and knee and linear velocity of the foot (toe) was found for each subject at 60 Hz throughout each trial. From the linear and angular velocity data and angular displacement data, three velocity measures, three timing measures, and two ranges of motion were derived for each subject in each trial (as defined in Table 13.1). Since each subject exhibited a high degree of consistency with regard to the eight variables, the data were averaged across the three trials.

Table 13.1 shows the group means and standard deviations for the eight variables for the novices, pre- and post-practice, and the experts, together with percentage changes pre- and post-practice for the novices, and percentage comparison of the novices, pre- and post-practice, with the experts. It is clear that the performance of the novices, in terms of maximum foot linear velocity (which reflects ball velocity), improved considerably with practice (47%) but was still well below that of the experts (85%) post-practice. However, the 47% increase in maximum foot linear velocity was associated with much smaller increases in maximum hip angular velocity (2.1%), maximum knee angular velocity (12.3%), hip range of motion (19.8%), and knee range of motion (14.5%). These changes, especially the angular velocity changes, suggest that improvement in performance resulted largely from a change in coordination

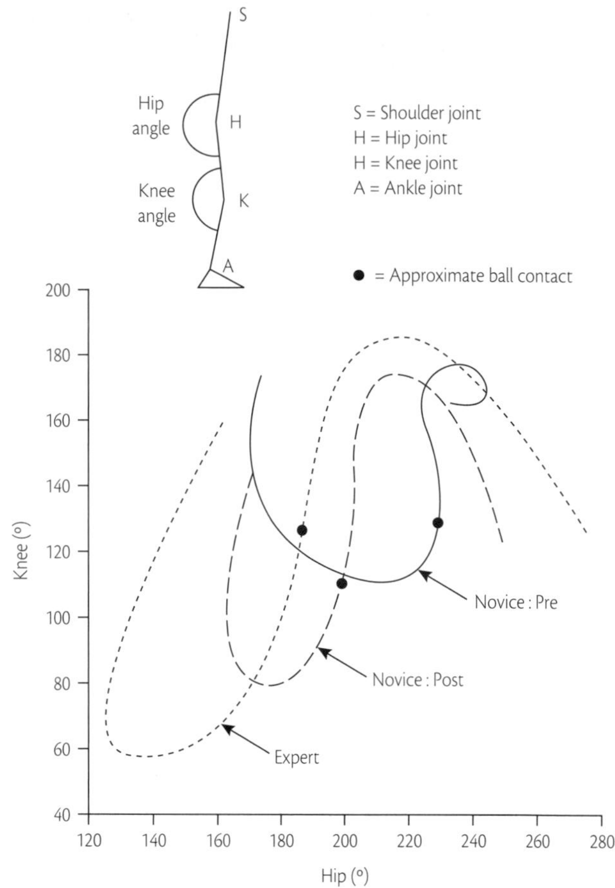

Fig. 13.4 Kicking a soccer ball: hip angle–knee angle diagrams for one representative novice's performance, pre- and post-practice, and one representative expert's performance (adapted from Anderson and Sidaway,[21] with permission).

rather than an increase in the speed of execution of the pre-practice movement pattern. This interpretation is supported by the change in the timing variables which were much closer to those of the experts post-practice than pre-practice (see Table 13.1). It is also supported by the change in relative motion of the thigh and lower leg as reflected in the representative knee angle–hip angle diagrams shown in Fig. 13.4. The post-practice pattern was similar to that of the experts which suggests that the novices had developed coordination. However, comparison of the novice post-practice and expert linear and angular velocities and ranges of motion in Table 13.1 indicates that control was less than optimal. The results of the study provide support for Bernstein's two-stage theory of skill acquisition, that is, development of coordination followed by development of control.

Kinetics of coordination

A kinematic analysis describes the way an object moves. In order to understand why an object moves the way that it does, it is necessary to carry out a kinetic analysis, that is, an analysis of the impulses and timing of the impulses of the forces acting on the object during the movement. With regard to human movement this involves analysis of the active and passive forces acting on each segment.

Table 13.1 Kicking a soccer ball: means, standard deviations, and comparative data for velocity, timing, and range of motion variables for novice and expert subjects

	Novice							Expert	
	Pre-practice			Post-practice					
	Mean	SD	%E	Mean	SD	%E	%pp	Mean	SD
MFLV ($m{\cdot}s^{-1}$)	14.9	1.7	58	21.9	1.5	85	47	25.6	1.1
MHAV ($deg{\cdot}s^{-1}$)	671	77	78	685	168	79	2.1	864	49
MKAV ($deg{\cdot}s^{-1}$)	1146	213	77	1287	251	86	12.3	1494	115
SKE/IMHAV	1.02	0.06	117	0.89	0.05	102	−13	0.87	0.03
IMHAV/IMFLV	0.61	0.1	77	0.69	0.03	87	13	0.79	0.01
IMKAV/IMFLV	1.14	0.06	109	1.04	0.05	100	−8.7	1.04	0.03
HIP ROM (deg)	86	14	64	103	21	77	19.8	135	9.5
KNEE ROM (deg)	90	16	75	104	13	86	14.5	121	5.7

MFLV: maximum foot linear velocity; MHAV: maximum hip angular velocity; MKAV: maximum knee angular velocity; SKE: start of knee extension; I: instant of; %E: per cent of expert value; %pp: per cent difference between pre and post.

Adapted from Anderson and Sidaway.[21]

Modelling

Each body segment is composed of hard and soft tissues. Whereas the segment may deform to a certain extent during movement, the amount of deformation is usually very small and, as such, for the purpose of biomechanical analysis the body segments may be regarded as rigid.[22] Consequently, the human body may be regarded as a system of rigid segments with the main segments (head, trunk, upper arms, forearms, hands, thighs, lower legs, feet) linked by freely moveable joints.

Free body diagram

Jensen *et al.*[23] carried out kinetic analyses of spontaneous leg movements in infants while reclined at 45°, as shown in Fig. 13.5(a). Figure 13.5(b) and (c) shows free body diagrams of the thigh and the combined lower leg and foot of the right leg, that is, sketches of the segments showing all of the forces acting on them. It is assumed that the movement of the legs takes place in the sagittal plane (X–Y plane with respect to Fig. 13.5). There are no contact forces acting on the segments and, as such, the only forces shown are the weights of the segments acting at the segmental CGs, and the force distributions around the hip and knee joints. It can be shown that any force distribution is equivalent to the resultant force R acting at an arbitrary point P together with a couple C equal to the resultant moment of the force distribution about P. The combination of R (acting at P) and C is referred to as the equipollent of the force distribution. In a kinetic analysis of human movement, it is usual to show the force distribution around a joint as the equipollent with respect to the joint centre. In Fig. 13.5(b) and (c), the equipollent of the force distribution around the hip joint is shown as F_H and M_H, and the equipollent of the force distribution around the knee joint is shown as F_K and M_K. In Fig. 13.5(d) and (e), the resultant forces through the hip and knee joint centres are replaced by their horizontal (F_{HX}, F_{KX}) and vertical (F_{HY}, F_{KY}) components.

Components of net joint moment

Each segment will move in accordance with Newton's laws of motion. Consequently, with respect to the lower leg and foot segment,

$$F_X = ma_x \quad (13.1)$$

$$F_Y = ma_y \quad (13.2)$$

$$M_Z = I\alpha \quad (13.3)$$

where F_X = resultant of horizontal forces acting on the segment; F_Y = resultant of vertical forces acting on the segment; a_x = horizontal component of the linear acceleration of the CG of the segment; a_y = vertical component of the linear acceleration of the CG of the segment; M_Z = resultant moment about the Z axis through the CG of the segment; I = moment of inertia of the segment about the Z axis through the CG of the segment; and α = angular acceleration of the segment about the Z axis through the CG of the segment.

From Eqns (13.1), (13.2), and (13.3), it follows that

$$F_{KX} = ma_x \quad (13.4)$$

$$F_{KY} - W_S = ma_y \quad (13.5)$$

$$M_K - F_{KX}d_1 - F_{KY}d_2 = I\alpha \quad (13.6)$$

From Eqn (13.5),

$$F_{KY} = ma_y + W_S \quad (13.7)$$

By substitution of F_{KX} from Eqn (13.4) and F_{KY} from Eqn (13.7) into Eqn (13.6),

$$M_K - ma_xd_1 - (ma_y + W_S)d_2 = I\alpha$$

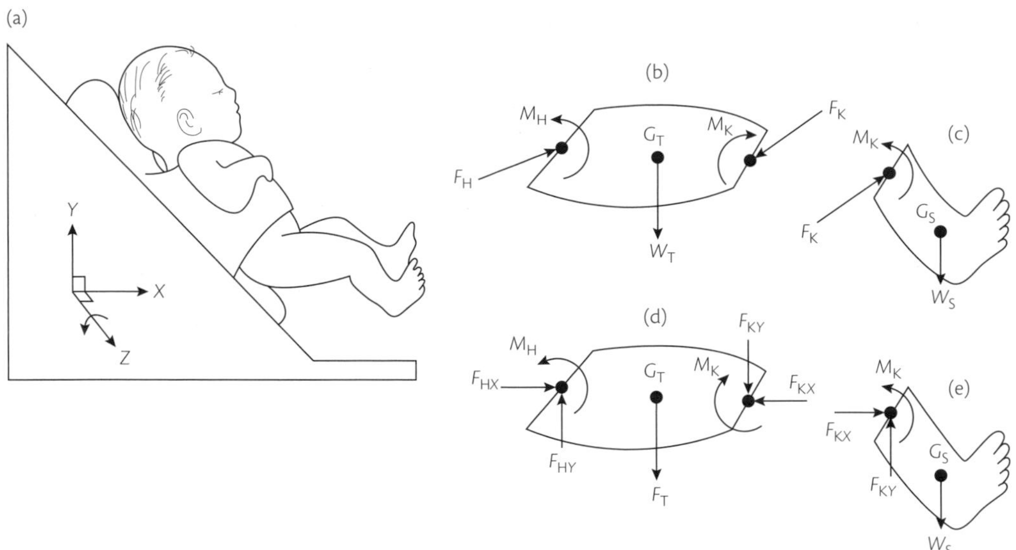

Fig. 13.5 Free body diagrams of the thigh and combined lower leg and foot of the right leg of a 3-month-old infant inclined at 45°: (a) infant inclined at 45°; (b) free body diagram of right upper leg; (c) free body diagram of combined right lower leg and foot; (d) free body diagram of right upper leg with resultant joint forces replaced by horizontal and vertical components; (e) free body diagram of combined right lower leg and foot with resultant joint forces replaced by horizontal and vertical components. IF_H = force distribution (muscle and articular) about the hip joint; IF_K = force distribution (muscle and articular) about the knee joint; M_H = moment of IF_H about the Z axis through the hip joint centre; M_K = moment of IF_K about the Z axis through the knee joint centre; F_H = resultant of IF_H acting through the hip joint centre; F_{HX} = horizontal component of F_H; F_{HY} = vertical component of F_H; F_K = resultant of IF_K acting through the knee joint centre; F_{KX} = horizontal component of F_K; F_{KY} = horizontal component of F_K; G_T = centre of gravity of the upper leg; G_S = centre of gravity of the combined lower leg and foot; W_T = weight of upper leg; W_S = weight of combined lower leg and foot; d_1 = moment arm of F_{KX} about the Z axis through G_S; d_2 = moment arm of F_{KY} about the Z axis through G_S.

$$M_K - ma_xd_1 - ma_yd_2 - W_Sd_2 = I\alpha$$

$$M_K - (ma_xd_1 + ma_yd_2) - \mathrm{W}sd_2 = I\alpha$$

M_K = Generalized Muscle Moment (*MUS*): the resultant moment of the force distribution about the Z axis through the knee joint centre, that is, the moment exerted by the muscle and articular forces about the joint. $(ma_xd_1 + ma_yd_2)$ = Motion Dependent Moment (*MDM*): the moment acting on the segment as a result of the motion of adjacent segments, that is, the thigh. W_Sd_2 = Gravitational Moment (*GRAV*): the moment acting on the segment due to its weight. $I\alpha$ = Net Joint Moment (*NET*): the resultant of *MUS*, *MDM*, and *GRAV* moments acting on the segment.

In the above example, there is no external contact force, such as the ground reaction force in walking or running, acting on the lower leg and foot segment. However, when there are contact forces, these must be included in the analysis of the components of joint moment. Consequently, the general equation relating the components of joint moment may be expressed as

$$NET = MUS + GRAV + MDM + EXT \qquad (13.8)$$

EXT represents the moments about the joint exerted by one or more external contact forces. The *NET* is the resultant of the active (*MUS*) and passive (*GRAV*, *MDM*, *EXT*) components and can be thought of as the joint moment required to accomplish the task. The actual signs of the components in Eqn (13.8) would depend on the directions of the components. The relationship between *MUS*, *GRAV*, *MDM*, and *EXT* is usually referred to as the biodynamics of joint movement.[14] It is clear from Eqn (13.8) that the inertial (*MDM*) and environmental (*GRAV*, *EXT*) components may significantly influence the movement of a joint.

With current technology it is not possible to directly measure the forces that contribute to *MUS* or, therefore, to measure the separate contributions of muscle and articular forces to the *MUS*. However, since the *MUS* comprises the only active (muscle) component of the *NET*, the *MUS* is particularly important for understanding coordination. Whereas *MUS* cannot be measured directly it can be determined indirectly, that is, *MUS* = *NET* – *MDM* – *GRAV* – *EXT*.

EXT can usually be measured. For example, ground reaction force can be measured by a force platform. *NET*, *MDM*, and *GRAV* can be calculated directly by kinematic analysis of the movement involving the following stages:

(i) Digitization of film or videotape of the movement with respect to a suitable X–Y frame of reference to obtain joint centre displacement–time data.

(ii) Calculation of segmental angular displacement–time data and CG displacement–time data (by use of published data concerning location of segmental CG in relation to joint centres, e.g. Dempster[24] and Hatze[25]).

(iii) Calculation of a_x and a_y from CG displacement–time data.

(iv) Calculation of α from angular displacement–time data.

(v) Calculation of moment arms of forces from the joint centre and CG displacement–time data.

(vi) Estimation of m and I values from published data.[17,18]

This indirect method of determining MUS is referred to as indirect dynamics or inverse dynamics.[26] The converse of indirect dynamics, that is, the determination of kinematics from directly measured kinetic (forces and moments of force) data is referred to as direct dynamics.

In the study by Jensen *et al.*[23] of spontaneous leg movements in children reclined at 45°, it was found that the infants naturally produced kicks of varying degrees of vigour and range of motion. In general, the infants exhibited a consistent pattern of relative

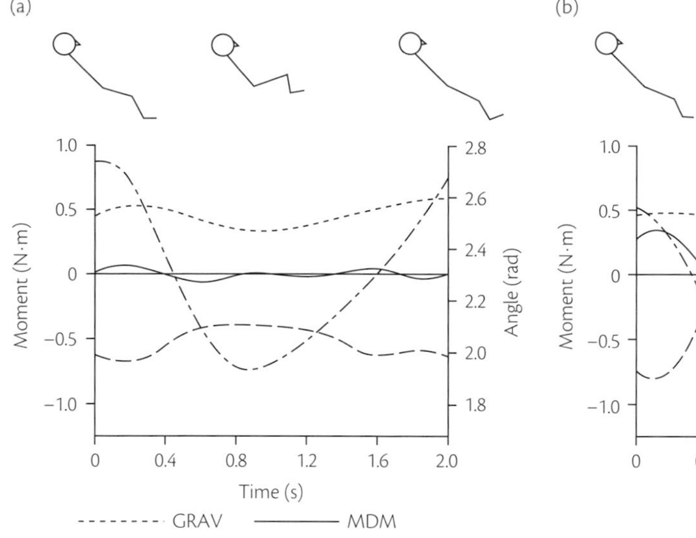

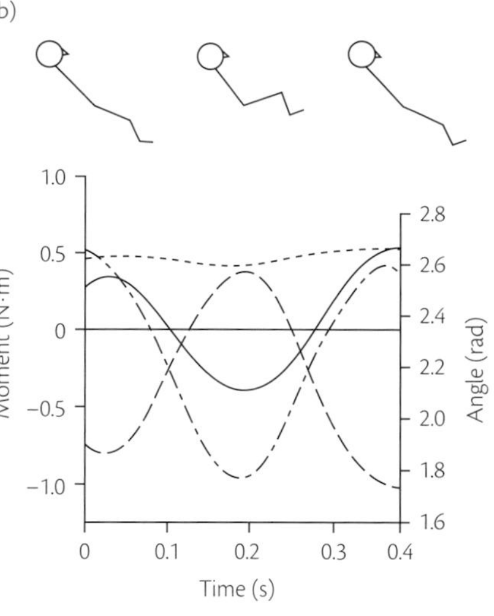

Fig. 13.6 Profiles of generalized muscle moments (*MUS*), motion dependent moments (*MDM*), and gravitational moments (*GRAV*) about the hip joint in relation to hip joint angle for an infant performing (a) a spontaneous nonvigorous kick and (b) a vigorous kick (adapted from Kamm *et al.*,[12] with permission).

motion between trunk, thigh, and lower leg segments suggesting a high level of coordination. With regard to kinetics, the relationship between the *MUS*, *MDM*, and *GRAV* profiles was similar at the hip and knee joints. At slow speeds of movement, the *MDM* were very small and the *MUS* served mainly to counteract the *GRAV* [Fig. 13.6(a)]. The *GRAV* profile, as expected, was similar at all kicking speeds. However, at fast speeds the *MUS* and *MDM* profiles were sinusoidal and out of phase by approximately 180° suggesting that as speed of movement increased the main function of the MUS was to counteract the *MDM* [Fig. 13.6(b)]. The *MUS* profile was also found to be approximately 180° out of phase with the change in joint angle, that is, the peaks of the *MUS* profile corresponded to changes in direction of movement of the segment. Since change in direction of movement is associated with eccentric muscle activity during the deceleration phase, the correspondence between the profiles of joint angle, *MUS* and *MDM*, suggest that coordinated movement tends to exploit the capacity of muscle–tendon units to store energy (in the elastic components during eccentric contractions) which, in turn, is likely to enhance energy conservation and reduce the energy expenditure of the muscles. Schneider *et al.*[27] found similar correspondence between the profiles of joint angle (shoulder, elbow, and wrist), *MUS* and *MDM* in adults performing a rapid reciprocal precision hand-placement task. The studies by Jensen *et al.*[23] and Schneider *et al.*[27] support the now generally held view that the development of coordination and control involves a process of optimization of the passive and active components of joint moment around each joint in order to maximize the use of passive moments which, in turn, decreases the contribution of active moments and, therefore, decreases energy expenditure. This process was expressed by Bernstein[14] as follows:

> The secret of coordination lies not in wasting superfluous force in extinguishing reactive phenomena but, on the contrary, in employing the latter in such a way as to employ active muscle forces only in the capacity of complementary forces. In this case, the same movement (in the final analysis) demands less expenditure of active force. (p. 109)

Lockman and Thelen[19] introduced the term developmental biodynamics to describe the development of coordination and control in infants, that is, how infants learn to coordinate joint biodynamics.

Energy generation and absorption by muscles

Just as it is not possible to directly measure the forces which contribute to *MUS* it is not possible to directly measure the work done by and on the individual muscles which contribute to *MUS*. However, the net work done by and on the muscles within *MUS* can be determined indirectly by integration of the power–time curve associated with the *MUS* around each particular joint. The power *P* at a joint is the product of the *MUS* and angular velocity ω, that is, $P = MUS\omega$. Power is positive (power output) if *MUS* and ω are of the same polarity, that is, net concentric activity; for example, hip flexion coinciding with a hip flexor moment. Power is negative (power absorption) if *MUS* and ω are of opposite polarity, that is, net eccentric activity; for example, hip flexion coinciding with a hip extensor moment. Winter[28] investigated the energy generated and absorbed by the muscles around the hip, knee, and ankle in adult subjects while walking at fast (n =10, mean cadence 125.4 steps·min^{-1}), natural (n = 9, mean cadence 104.4 steps·min^{-1}), and slow (n = 9, mean cadence 85.9 steps·min^{-1}) speeds of walking. Figure 13.7 shows typical power–time curves at the hip, knee, and ankle for one stride (heel contact to heel contact of the same foot) for one subject walking at a fast cadence. The net energy generated and absorbed by the muscles around each joint is represented by the positive and negative areas of the curves, respectively. The actual amounts of energy generated and absorbed in the various phases, as shown in the figure, indicate that over the complete stride the hip muscles (+20 J, −35 J) and knee muscles (+20 J, −70 J) were net energy absorbers and the ankle muscles (+35 J, −7 J) were net energy generators. Patterns of energy generation and absorption at the hip were not consistent, but the patterns at the knee (net energy absorbers) and ankle (net energy generators) were consistent across all subjects and all cadences. It is not possible to determine how much of the absorbed energy was subsequently released in energy generation. However, it is likely that greater utilization of stored energy, that is, recycling of absorbed energy, is made at a preferred (natural) cadence since energy

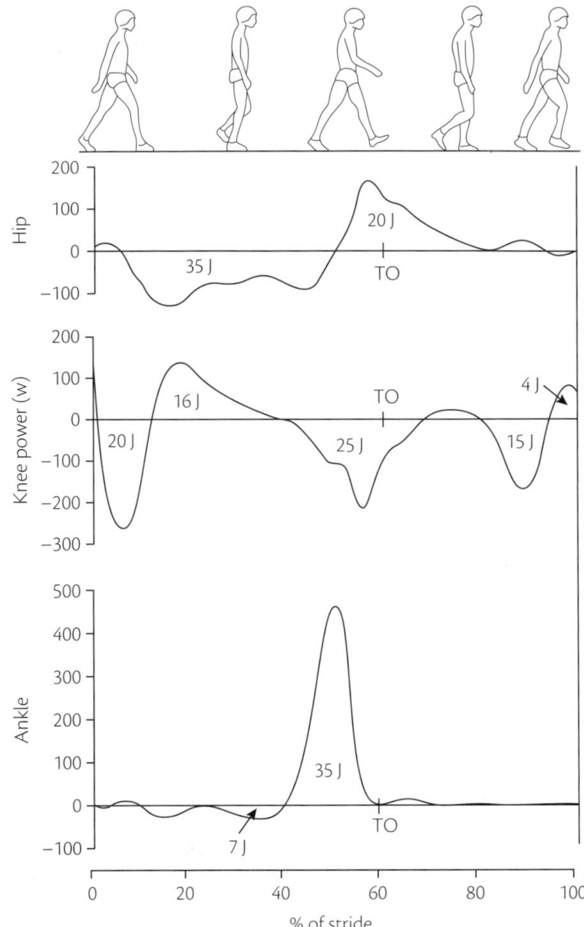

Fig. 13.7 Power generation and absorption at the hip, knee, and ankle joints during one stride (heel-strike to heel-strike of the right leg, TO = toe-off) while walking (adapted from Winter,[28] with permission).

expenditure (oxygen consumption) has been shown to be lowest at preferred cadence for the same speed of walking in adults and children.[29,30]

Dynamical systems approach to development of coordination

Studies of spontaneous kicking[23] and reaching[31] clearly indicate that infants have a high level of coordination in spontaneous (non-task oriented, non-intentional) multijoint limb movements, which suggests an intrinsic ability of the body segments to self-organize their relative motion.[32] Self-organization is a key feature of complex dynamical systems which, similar to the human body, have many degrees of freedom and are subject to a range of constraints.[33] Dynamical systems theory was developed nearly 100 years ago to try to explain how physical systems including, for example, weather patterns, change over time.[8] The dynamical systems approach was first applied to coordination of human movement by Kugler *et al.*,[34] since then concepts from dynamical systems have been increasingly used to explain the development of coordination.[13,35]

Self-organization and constraints

From a neuromaturational perspective of motor development, a child's movement is considered to result from gradually maturing predetermined patterns in the nervous system and that the level of skill displayed is reflected in the maturational status of the nervous system, that is, the more mature the nervous system, the greater the level of skill. Similarly, from an information-processing perspective of motor learning in adults, movement is assumed to result from the triggering of established motor programmes. In contrast, the dynamical systems perspective views human movement (and the movement of all other animals) as emerging from the intrinsic self-organizing properties of the dynamical system consisting of the person, the person's environment, and the desired movement.[7,36,37]

Self-organization refers to the spontaneous integration of the dynamical properties of the subsystems that comprise a system and results in the spontaneous establishment of a pattern of activity.[38] The actual pattern that emerges is dependent on the constraints on the system. With regard to human movement, a constraint is any influence that serves to decrease the number of degrees of freedom that need to be controlled, that is, the constraints acting on the system limit the types of movement that can emerge.[39] Constraints can be broadly classified into three groups: task, environmental, and organismic.[40]

There are essentially two types of task constraints, extrinsic and intrinsic.[39] Extrinsic task constraints refer to the mechanical requirements of the tasks, that is, the speed (e.g. running for a bus) and/or precision (e.g. threading a needle) needed to successfully complete the task. Intrinsic task constraints refer to the individual's perception of the potential costs (e.g. energy expenditure and risk of injury) of particular types of movement that could be used to complete the task. There is clear evidence that individuals normally move in ways that tend to minimize energy expenditure (e.g. walk rather than run) and risk of injury (e.g. walk slowly rather than quickly on a slippery surface). Environmental constraints arise from the physical and sociocultural environment.[8] Physical environmental constraints include weather conditions, conditions of light and heat, surface conditions, and the availability of protective clothing (e.g. in industry and sport). Sociocultural environmental constraints include peer pressure and the pressure to behave in culturally acceptable ways.

Organismic constraints, also referred to as individual constraints, refer to the limitations imposed by the current status of the individual in terms of all aspects of physical, cognitive, and affective functions.

All organisms within a species, such as humans, share a common gene pool (the sum total of all the genes in a species).[41] However, the genome of each individual organism (the genes and assembly of genes) is slightly different from all other organisms within the species. The genome determines ontogenesis, that is, the innate process of development of the individual towards maturity.[42] Ontogenesis is similar for all organisms within a species, but not exactly the same due to differences in genomes, that is, ontogenesis imposes organismic constraints on development. Development is simultaneously influenced by environmental constraints; different environments tend to result in different rates of development.[43] Consequently, the actual development of an organism, referred to as epigenesis,[42] is the result of the interaction of organismic and environmental constraints.

In terms of human movement, a propensity to develop those behaviours that enable the infant to explore and interact with the environment (locomotion and manipulation skills) would appear to be central to ontogenesis. Most normally developing infants experience similar motor development outcomes in terms of the timing and types of motor skills that emerge. From a dynamical systems perspective, these predictable early milestones are viewed as the result of species-similar constraints.[7] From this perspective, the maturational status of the nervous system is regarded as a major organismic constraint, but only one of many organismic constraints that together with task and environmental constraints determine the form of movement that emerges. For example, infants normally learn to crawl and then stand before walking. However, there is no predetermined programme for crawling. Crawling emerges as the best available solution to a particular motor problem (to travel in a particular direction), to be replaced by a more effective and efficient solution, that is, walking, as a result of changes in individual constraints.[43] Furthermore, as the constraints are continually changing, the system as a whole is in a constant state of flux so that no two movements are exactly the same.

The appropriateness of the dynamical systems approach to understanding motor development was clearly shown by Thelen and her colleagues[44–48] (see Chapter 14) in a series of studies on infant locomotion. Thelen monitored the spontaneous behaviours of infants and found that certain behaviours appeared, disappeared, and then reappeared after some time.[49] For example, she found that infants exhibit kicking movements when lying on their backs and stepping movements when they are held upright, more-or-less from birth. She also observed that stepping disappeared within the first 3 months, only to reappear a few weeks later, while kicking continued and increased in frequency over the same period. She also observed that infants who gained weight fastest were the first to stop stepping. Thelen reasoned that if the appearance and disappearance of stepping was due solely to nervous system maturation, then changing the prevailing environmental constraints, such as the effect of gravity, should not affect the behaviour. She tested the hypothesis by artificially increasing and decreasing the weight of the legs of the infants. She found that stepping behaviour can be made to disappear by artificially increasing the weight of the legs of infants by attaching small weights to the ankles and that removing the weights restores the stepping behaviour. Furthermore, she found that the stepping behaviour could be restored in infants who had stopped stepping by submerging the infants' legs in water. The buoyancy provided by the water artificially reduces the weight of the infants' legs which, in turn, increases the leg strength:leg weight ratio to a level that restores the stepping behaviour. These observations clearly indicate that strength:weight ratio is an important organismic constraint that influences the motor behaviour of infants.

Most researchers agree that the development of strength and postural control are major influences on the rate of development of walking in infants and that body growth, neural maturation, and practice of walking determine strength and postural control.[50] However, there is less agreement and little empirical research on the relative importance of body growth, neural maturation, and walking practice on the development of strength and postural control. The lack of empirical research would appear to be due, at least in part, to methodological difficulties associated with assessing neural development and practice and in separating out the effects of body growth, neural maturation, and walking practice which are all constantly changing. Adolph *et al.*[51] investigated the relative contribution to improvements in walking of body growth (height, weight, leg length, head circumference, crown–rump length, ponderal index), neural maturation (assumed to be reflected in chronological age), and practice in walking (assumed to be reflected in the number of days since the onset of walking defined as the first day that the infant could walk at least 3 m independently) in a part-longitudinal and part cross-sectional study. The subjects were 210 infants (101 girls, 109 boys) aged 9–17 months and, for comparison, 15 children (8 girls, 7 boys) aged 5–6 years and 13 adults (10 women, 3 men). Using robust statistical methods based on hierarchical regression analyses, the results showed that body growth did not explain improvements in walking skill independent of neural maturation and walking practice. Similarly, neural maturation did not explain improvements in walking skill independent of body growth and walking practice. In contrast, walking practice played the single most important role in the improvements in walking skill. It was concluded that the magnitude, distributed nature, and variability of infants' walking experience facilitate the exploration of passive forces and differentiation of perceptual information which, in turn, promote the development of postural control.

In accordance with the dynamical systems approach, Clark[8] pointed out that motor skill acquisition takes place throughout the whole of the life of the individual and that the process underlying the emergence of new skills is basically the same at any age. Consequently, to describe the process of children learning to walk as motor development and that of adults learning a new sports technique as motor learning is to make an unnecessary artificial distinction between the way that children and adults learn new motor skills.

Coordinative structures, control parameters, and order parameters

According to the principles of dynamical systems, the movement pattern of the human body that emerges in response to the need to solve a particular movement task, such as reaching, pointing, walking, running, hopping, skipping, jumping, and landing, is the result of self-organization of the task, environmental and organismic constraints on the system. For a particular movement task, self-organization assembles the muscles/joints of the body into functional groups (referred to by Bernstein[14] as functional synergies) that together form a coordinate structure for the whole body[34] (see Fig. 13.8). The muscles/joints in each functional group move together (e.g. extend simultaneously or flex simultaneously), which dramatically reduces the number of degrees of freedom within the functional group and, as such, dramatically reduces the number of degrees of freedom in the coordinate structure. The smaller the number of degrees of freedom in the coordinate structure, the lower the demand on the nervous system. The coordinate structure sets the timing (relative phasing) of the movements of the body segments.

Different task constraints give rise to different coordinative structures. For example, for speeds of locomotion up to about 2.0 $m \cdot s^{-1}$ most humans naturally adopt a walking pattern (bipedal alternate right–left–right–left stepping) rather than another form of locomotion such as running or hopping. The coordinate structure for walking is characterized by two double support phases

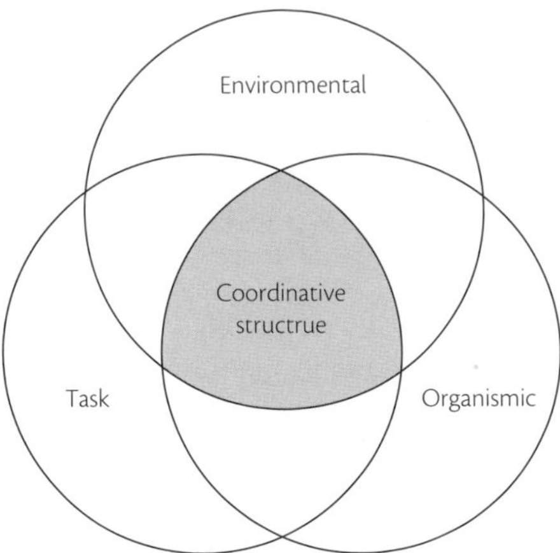

Fig. 13.8 The formation of a coordinate structure resulting from self-organization of the task, environmental, and organismic constraints on the system.

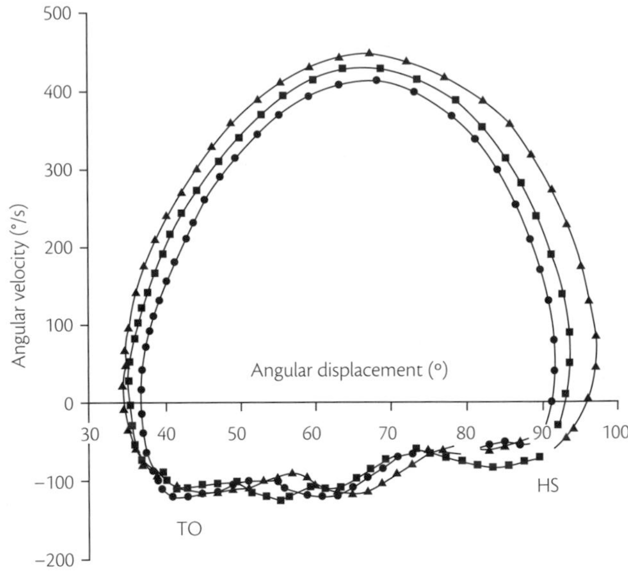

Fig. 13.9 Phase plane of the sagittal plane movement of the shank in three successive stride cycles of an infant four weeks after starting to walk (adapted from Clark and Phillips,[55] with permission). HS: heel-strike; TO: toe-off.

(both feet in contact with the ground at the same time) and separate single support and swing phases of each leg during each stride. Different forms of locomotion, such as walking, running, hopping, skipping, and jumping, have different coordinative structures. A coordinative structure is stable over particular ranges (or scaling) of certain constraints (referred to as control parameters) so that the observed movement pattern may change qualitatively (reflected in changes in order parameters) while the coordinate structure remains the same.[52] For example, as walking speed (control parameter) increases up to about 2.0 $m{\cdot}s^{-1}$, the movement pattern changes qualitatively (change in the order parameters of stride length and stride frequency), but the coordinative structure (walking) remains the same. However, as the speed of walking increases above 2 $m{\cdot}s^{-1}$, the walking pattern becomes increasingly unstable, reflected in increasing variability of the relative phasing of the body segments and increasing asymmetry between the movements of the left and right sides of the body. At about 2.3 $m{\cdot}s^{-1}$, there is an abrupt change from walking to running, that is, a change to a new coordinative structure that is characterized by two flight phases (instead of two double support phases as in walking) and separate single support and swing phases of each leg during each stride. This coordinate structure remains stable over most of the 2.3 $m{\cdot}s^{-1}$ to maximum speed range.

The abrupt change from walking to running illustrates a major characteristic of dynamical systems, that is, changes in coordinative structure are triggered by instability resulting from a change in the scaling of one or more control parameters. In the case of bipedal locomotion, speed is a control parameter that determines the most appropriate coordinative structure, that is, walking or running, for a given speed.

Patterns, attractors, and stability

Coordinate structures result in stable patterns of activity, which are likely to be reflected in the activity of the system as a whole and/or in the activity of the subsystems. In human movement, the pattern of activity resulting from a particular coordinative structure is likely to be manifest in a very wide range of kinematic (e.g. the movement of each body segment), kinetic (e.g. peak force at heel-strike, rate of loading during the passive phase of ground contact), physiological (e.g. tidal volume, breathing rate, stoke volume, heart rate, rate of oxygen consumption), and neuromusculoskeletal (e.g. intensity and duration of contractions of individual muscles) indicators. Kinematic indicators are likely to show highly repeatable whole-body movement patterns (CG), highly repeatable movement patterns of individual body segments, and low variability in the relative phasing (coordination) of the movement of body segments.

The stability of a movement pattern can be illustrated and quantified in a number of ways.[53] One of the most frequently used dynamical systems techniques for illustrating the movement pattern of a body segment is the phase plane (also referred to as phase portrait, phase plane trajectory, and parametric phase plot). A phase plane captures the space–time pattern of the movement of the segment by plotting the velocity (linear or angular) of the segment as a function of the displacement of the segment.[54] For example, Fig. 13.9 shows a phase plane of the movement of the shank of an infant in the sagittal plane, 4 weeks after the infant started to walk.[55] The phase plane shows the angular velocity–angular displacement trajectory of the shank in three successive stride cycles. It is clear that there is some overlap between the trajectories, but no direct mapping of one trajectory on to the next. In dynamical systems terminology, the pattern of movement exhibited by the shank occupies a region in the state space.[56] The state space encompasses all possible patterns, that is, all possible trajectories of the shank in the state space. The state space is defined by the relevant state variables. In this example, the state variables are the angular velocity and angular displacement of the shank which define a two-dimensional state space.

The trajectories of the shank define a region in the state space referred to as the attractor, that is, the region of the state space in which the movement of the shank is most stable. The stability of the attractor, that is, the stability of the movement pattern of the shank from cycle to cycle is reflected in the bandwidth of the attractor. The narrower the bandwidth, the more stable the attractor. The standard deviation of the length of the angular velocity–angular displacement vectors (determined at the same frequency as the data used to plot the phase plane) over a number of cycles provides an estimate of the bandwidth; the lower the standard deviation, the more stable the attractor.

Another frequently used dynamical systems technique for estimating the stability of a movement pattern is the variability of the relative phase between two events in the movement pattern over a number of trials or cycles. For example, in running, the relative phasing of the movement of the knee and ankle joints of each leg could be determined by the time difference between peak knee flexion and peak ankle dorsiflexion during the ground contact phase expressed as a proportion of ground contact time (Fig. 13.10). A similar measure of relative phase could be obtained for any pair of joints in the same leg during each ground contact phase (hip–knee, knee–ankle, hip–ankle) or for corresponding joints in the left and right legs during each stride (left hip–right hip, left knee–right knee, left ankle–right ankle). The stability of each measure of relative phase is reflected in the standard deviation of the relative phase over a number of cycles; the smaller the standard deviation, the more closely coupled is the movement of the two joints and, therefore, the more stable is the movement pattern.

Cyclicity in biological systems

The dynamical systems approach emphasizes the thermodynamic nature of biological systems and how thermodynamic laws guide behaviour.[54] Biological systems obey the second law of thermodynamics, that is, all systems tend towards instability and disorder which, in the case of a living organism, culminates in death. However, during life a biological system can maintain an ordered state by a cyclical process of generation, transformation, and dissipation of energy which occurs at all levels of the system including circadian rhythms, cardiac rhythms, respiratory rhythms, and locomotion.[57] It is believed that the oscillatory nature of biological systems is analogous to inanimate self-organizing oscillatory systems.[58] This viewpoint has led to the application of the physics of pendulums to such systems.

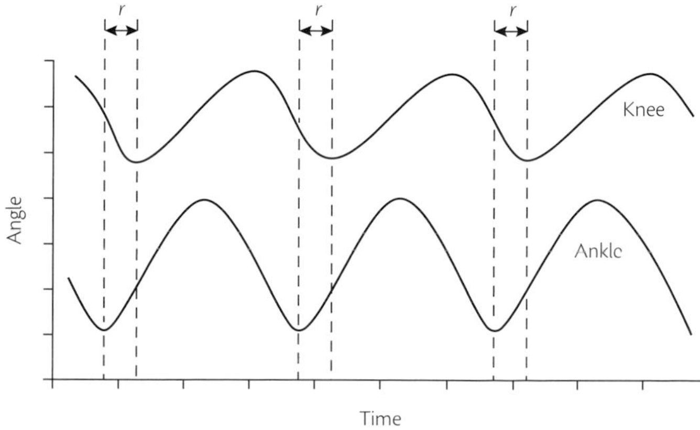

Fig. 13.10 Determination of the relative phase (r) between peak knee flexion and peak ankle dorsiflexion during the ground contact phase in running (adapted from Holt and Jeng[54]).

Any object that is free to oscillate about a horizontal axis is a pendulum. For example, a pendulum in a clock usually consists of a long light bar or rod that supports a small dense mass. The idealized form of this type of pendulum, referred to as a simple pendulum, consists of a mass-less rod of length L that supports a point mass m. As the rod has no mass, the centre of mass of a simple pendulum is at the centre of mass of the point mass. Consequently, the distance D from the axis of rotation to the centre of mass of the pendulum is equal to L. The moment of inertia I of the pendulum about the axis of rotation through its point of support is given by $I = mL^2$, where L is the radius of gyration of the pendulum about the axis of rotation. A real pendulum is usually referred to as a compound pendulum. In a compound pendulum, L is always longer than D.

If a pendulum (simple or compound) is displaced from its vertical resting position and then released, it will oscillate about the vertical rest position with a constant period, that is, the duration of each cycle of movement will be constant even though the amplitude of movement will gradually decrease (due to friction around its axis of rotation and, to a lesser extent, air resistance). The period τ of a simple pendulum is given by $\tau = 2\pi(L/g)^{1/2}$. An oscillator that has a constant period, similar to a swinging pendulum, is referred to as a harmonic oscillator.

The period (seconds per cycle) of a pendulum is entirely determined by its physical properties, in particular, the distribution of the mass of the pendulum. For a given mass, a change in the distribution of mass will result in a change in the moment of inertia of the pendulum with respect to its axis of rotation, that is, a change in L, which, in turn, will result in a change in the period. The reciprocal of the period is the frequency of oscillation (cycles per second). As the period of a pendulum is constant, its frequency of oscillation is referred to as natural frequency or resonant frequency.

If there was no friction around the axis of rotation of a pendulum and no air resistance, the pendulum would oscillate with constant amplitude and the energy of the system would be entirely conserved at the level it had at the point of release. In practice, there would be some friction around the axis of rotation and some air resistance such that a certain amount of energy would be dissipated (lost to the pendulum in the form of heat and movement of the air) during each oscillation. Consequently, the amplitude of oscillation would gradually decrease and the pendulum would eventually come to rest and hang vertically. A pendulum is a very simple example of a dynamical system, that is, the movement of the system after release is self-organized (amplitude and frequency of oscillation), entirely predictable, and energy is conserved (to a level determined by friction and air resistance). Similarly, if a metal spring is stretched or compressed and then released, then the spring will oscillate in a predictable manner and come to rest at its equilibrium position; there is no brain controlling its movement which is determined completely by its physical properties of stiffness and damping. Just as the physical properties of a pendulum and a spring determine their movement when allowed to oscillate freely, it is reasonable to assume that the movement of the arms and legs might be determined in a similar manner in certain movements. For example, in walking, if the stiffness and damping levels of the legs are set by the muscles that control the hips, knees, and ankles, then the oscillation of the legs will be determined to a certain extent by their physical properties, which is likely to simplify neural control of the movement.[33]

Force driven harmonic oscillators

If a child's swing is set in motion, its swing amplitude will gradually decrease due to friction around its axis of rotation and to air resistance. In order to maintain a constant swing amplitude, the swing must receive a brief push at the start of each swing to replace the energy lost due to friction and air resistance in the preceding swing. A harmonic oscillator, similar to a child's swing, that requires energy input at the start of each oscillation in order to maintain a constant amplitude of oscillation is referred to as a force driven harmonic oscillator (FDHO).

The motion of the legs in constant speed walking is quasi-periodic (alternate oscillation of the legs with similar swing time and similar swing amplitude). However, the body as a whole loses energy in each step due to damping, that is, kinetic energy transformed into strain energy during the period of double support as a result of eccentric muscle contraction is partially dissipated as heat. Unless replenished, the loss of energy during each step would quickly bring the body to rest. The continued oscillation of the legs is maintained by a burst of muscular activity at the start of each leg swing (to replace the energy lost in the previous step). Consequently, the motion of the legs in constant speed walking is similar to that of a FDHO.

In a FDHO, there is a particular frequency, referred to as the resonant frequency, which requires minimal force to maintain oscillations. In human movement, muscle forces (intensity, duration, and frequency of muscular activity) determine energy expenditure. There is considerable evidence that adults and children naturally adopt a stride frequency and stride length in walking that minimizes energy expenditure and maximizes stability.[29,30,59–61] Furthermore, the preferred stride frequency can be predicted from the resonant frequency of an FDHO model of the leg swing[30,60], where the period $\tau = 2\pi(L/2g)^{1/2}$.[33] Similarly, Ledebt and Breniere[62] found that in 4- to 8-year-old children, gait initiation (from the start of movement to maximum horizontal velocity in the first step) can be closely predicted from the resonant frequency of an FDHO model of the movement over the grounded foot. Even very young children appear to adopt movement patterns at resonant frequency in certain situations. For example, Goldfield *et al.*[63] showed that infants bouncing up and down in a jumper device tend to adopt resonant frequency as modelled by an FDHO mass-spring system.

Self-optimization of coordinative structures

The observation that cyclic human movement such as walking tends to be performed at resonant frequency has led to the suggestion that coordination is self-optimized in relation to so-called optimality criteria to which the individual is sensitive in adopting a particular movement pattern.[29,60] The optimality criteria reflect the prevailing intrinsic task constraints and result in movement patterns that minimize the 'costs' to the system.[39] The main optimality criterion would appear to be energy expenditure, but others have been suggested including stability, bilateral symmetry, and shock absorption at foot-strike.[30,64] For example, at a particular walking speed, minimal expenditure usually occurs at preferred stride frequency in children and adults and is usually associated with high stability and high bilateral symmetry.[29,30]

With regard to symmetry, Clark *et al.*[59] investigated coordination in walking in a cross-sectional study involving seven groups of subjects: new walkers (capable of three independent steps) with support and new walkers without support, children who had been walking for 2 weeks, 1 month, 3 months, and 6 months, and a group of adults. There were five subjects in each group. The average age of onset of walking in the infant subjects was 11.2 months. Interlimb coordination, at preferred speed of walking, was assessed by measuring the step time:stride time ratio (temporal phase) and the step length:stride length ratio (distance phase). It was expected that in a mature walking gait, the temporal phase and the distance phase would be close to 50% and that a low variability (measured as the standard deviation of each phase) would indicate a stable coordinative structure. The results showed that there was no significant difference in mean temporal phase or mean distance phase (all close to 50%) across all age groups and that variability decreased with age with no significant difference in variability between the 3 months, 6 months, and adult groups. The variability of the supported new walkers (two-handed support by a parent) was not significantly different from the 2 weeks, 1 month, and 3 months groups in temporal phase and not significantly different from the 3 months and 6 months groups in distance phase. Clark *et al.*[59] concluded that (i) the coordinative structure for interlimb coordination used by new walkers is similar to, but not as tightly coupled as that used by adults and (ii) practice of walking increases postural stability which, in turn, increases the stability of the coordinative structure. The results of the study suggested that bilateral symmetry is a feature of coordination in walking.

Jeng *et al.*[30] investigated energy expenditure, stability, and symmetry in walking in 3- to 12-year-old children and adults. There were six groups of subjects with nine subjects in each group: 3–4 years, 5–6 years, 7–8 years, 9–10 years, 11–12 years, and 20–21 years. The subjects were carefully selected to represent the full range of body sizes in each age group. After familiarization, each subject was required to walk for 8 min on a treadmill at preferred walking speed (established in overground walking) at three stride frequencies in time with a metronome: preferred stride frequency (PSF), PSF – 25%, and PSF + 25%. The physiological cost of steady-state walking at each stride frequency was assessed by the physiological cost index (the ratio of the difference between resting heart rate and steady-state heart rate during walking and walking speed).

Coordination was assessed at each stride frequency via symmetry and relative phase. Bilateral symmetry was assessed by the ratio of the durations of the stance phases of each leg in each stride, the ratio of the durations of the swing phases of each leg in each stride, and the ratio of the duration of the right step to the stride duration in each stride. The mean of each ratio was calculated over 10 consecutive stride cycles during steady-state walking. The relative phase (time difference between the occurrences of the maximum angles of each pair of joints in each stride as a percentage of stride time) was determined for the hip–knee, knee–ankle, and hip–ankle joint couplings. The mean of each relative phase was calculated over 10 consecutive stride cycles during steady-state walking. Stability was assessed as the standard deviation of each of the symmetry and relative phase measures.

The results clearly indicated that physiological cost, symmetry, and stability were all optimal at preferred stride frequency for all age groups and that preferred stride frequency was consistent with resonant frequency as predicted by an FDHO model of the leg swing.[33] Seven of the 3–4 year olds and four of the 5–6 year

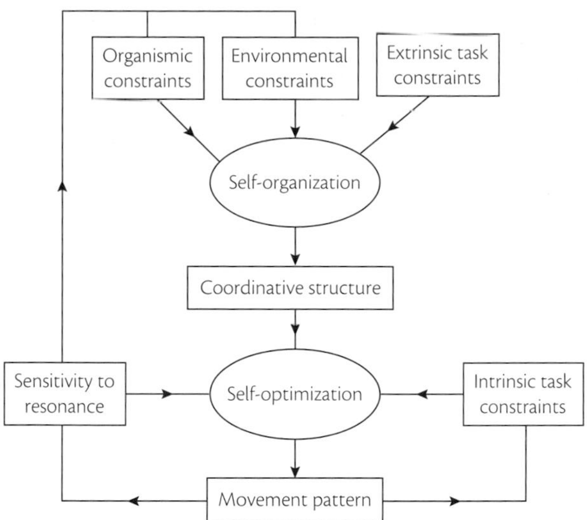

Fig. 13.11 A model of the emergence of motor behaviour based on the dynamical systems approach to motor development.

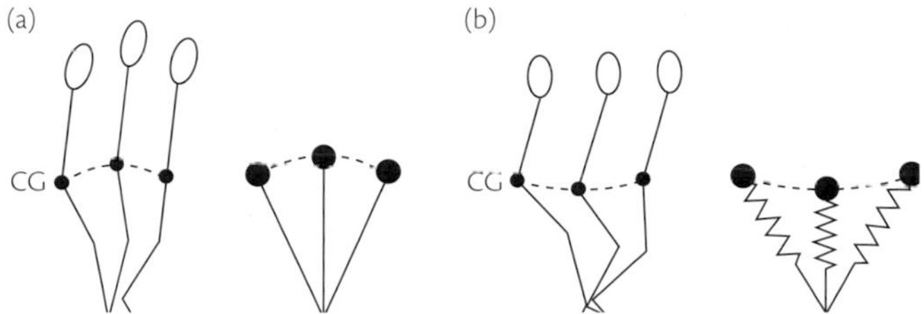

Fig. 13.12 (a) Pendulum dynamics is the predominant form of energy conservation in walking. (b) Spring dynamics is the predominant form of energy conservation in running (adapted from Farley and Ferris[70]). CG: whole-body centre of gravity.

olds had difficulty in modulating their stride frequency at the non-preferred stride frequencies. All of the other subjects were able to modulate their stride frequency at the non-preferred stride frequencies. Jeng *et al.* concluded that the ability to self-optimize walking appears to be established by 7 years of age and seems to involve three stages. Stage 1 (1–4 years of age) is characterized by early sensitivity to resonance and difficulty in modulating stride frequency to non-preferred frequencies. Stage 2 (4–6 years of age) is characterized by a progressive increase in the ability to modulate stride frequency and a decrease in stability, which may be due to the need to adapt to marked changes in body composition that are characteristic of this period. Stage 3 (6–7 years of age) is characterized by the ability to consistently modulate stride frequency.

Jeng *et al.*[65] suggested that sensitivity to resonance (an awareness of how to minimize energy expenditure by maximizing energy conservation in energy exchanges between and within body segments) may be a mechanism underlying the development of self-optimization in walking. They also suggested that sensitivity to resonance is a function of the individual's sensitivity to the physical properties of her/his body and to the environment. Sensitivity to personal physical properties would suggest awareness of the anthropometric (size and shape), inertial (mass and distribution of mass), viscoelastic (stiffness and damping), and gravitational (weight) properties of body segments and combinations of body segments. Sensitivity to the environment would suggest awareness of what movements are possible in a given environment such as, for example, negotiating an obstacle or moving through a confined space. Awareness of the possibilities afforded by a particular environment has been referred to by Gibson[66] as affordance. Figure 13.11 presents a model of the emergence of motor behaviour based on the dynamical systems approach.

Dynamic resources

As shown by Adolph *et al.*,[51] the rapid improvement in walking ability in the first month following the onset of walking would appear to be largely due to the effects of practice. According to Fonseca *et al.*[67] and Holt *et al.*,[68] practice of walking enables toddlers to explore their dynamic resources, that is, the sources of energy available to them to maintain upright posture and forward progression. The dynamic resources available may be categorized as (i) energy generation by concentric muscular contractions; (ii) conservation of energy in soft tissues, that is, the potential to store and then release strain energy in muscle–tendon units (spring dynamics); and (iii) conservation of energy by interchange of kinetic energy and gravitational potential energy within and between body segments (pendulum dynamics). The gait (walking movement pattern) that emerges will reflect the relative contribution of the three sources of energy.

There are potentially a number of ways of using these resources to maintain upright posture and forward progression. For example, pendulum dynamics is more evident in walking than in running and spring dynamics is more evident in running than in walking[69,70] (Fig. 13.12).

Figure 13.13 shows a picture sequence of a young boy walking at preferred speed from just after heel-strike of the right foot to just after heel-strike of the left foot. From toe-off of the left foot (TO_L) to heel-strike of the left foot (HS_L) (single support phase of the right leg, approximately 40% of the stride cycle) the body rotates forward over the right foot similar to an inverted pendulum [Fig. 13.12(a) and Fig. 13.13(a–e)]. During the period TO_L to mid-stance [Fig. 13.13(a–c)], kinetic energy is converted to gravitational potential energy and during the period from mid-stance to HS_L [Fig. 13.13(c–e)], gravitational potential energy is converted to kinetic energy. There will be some loss of energy during these phases due to damping in soft tissues (dissipated as heat inside the body and then to the surrounding air), but energy will largely be conserved due to pendulum dynamics.

During the period HS_R to TO_L [Fig. 13.13(a) and (b)] (double support phase prior to left swing phase, approximately 10% of the stride cycle), kinetic energy is converted to strain energy in the right leg (the leg is compressed like a spring). Most of the strain energy will be immediately returned as kinetic energy and gravitational potential energy, but some of the strain energy will be lost due to damping in the soft tissues. Simultaneous to the storage and release of strain energy in the right leg, active plantar flexion of the left ankle (the push-off of the left foot) generates new energy (kinetic and gravitational). To maintain forward progression, the new energy generated by the push-off must be sufficient to replace the energy that was lost due to damping in soft

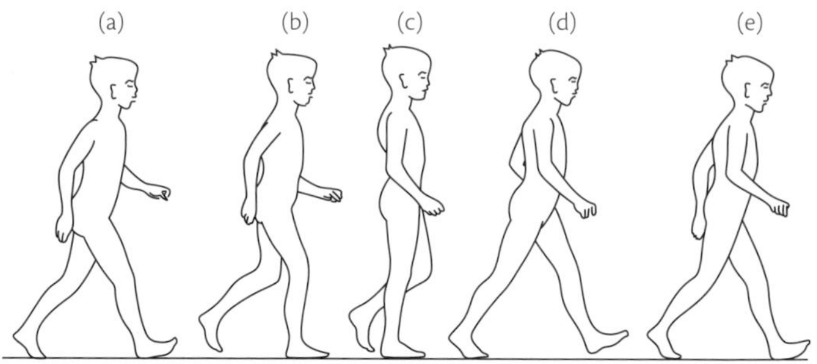

Fig. 13.13 A young boy walking at preferred speed from just after heel-strike of the right foot to just after heel-strike of the left foot.

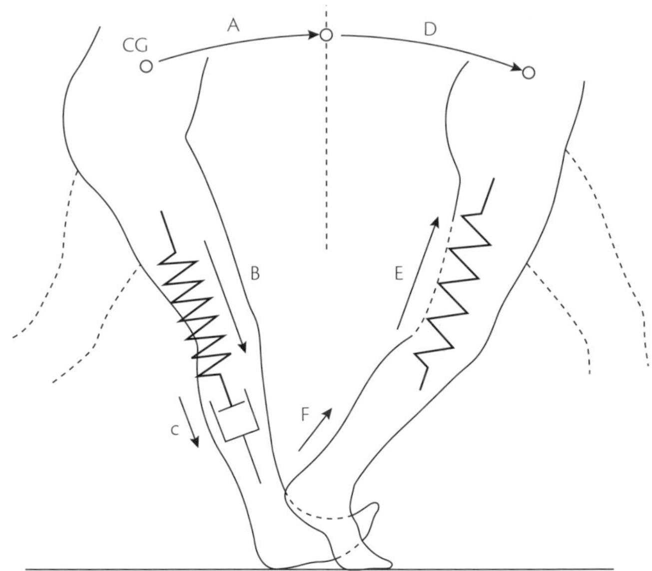

Fig. 13.14 The energy changes between heel-strike and toe-off of each foot during walking (adapted from Holt *et al.*[36]). A: conversion of kinetic energy to gravitational potential energy; B: storage of strain energy in the muscle–tendon units and other soft tissues; C: loss of some strain energy as heat; D: conversion of gravitational potential energy to kinetic energy; E: release of remaining strain energy; F: push-off; CG: whole-body centre of gravity.

tissues. The energy changes between HS and TO of each foot are illustrated in Fig. 13.14.

Walking at resonant frequency will result in minimal loss of energy and therefore minimal energy expenditure. As in any FDHO, correct timing of the push-off (referred to by Holt *et al.*[68] as the escapement force) is necessary to produce resonant frequency in walking. To produce resonance, the push-off should begin as the landing foot strikes the ground at the start of the double support phase, that is, the period of generation of new energy should correspond to the period when energy is lost due to compression of the lead leg.

Holt *et al.*[68] investigated the use of pendulum dynamics and spring dynamics in new walkers. The subjects were seven infants who were encouraged to walk on a walkway in a laboratory while being videotaped from the side. The infants were videotaped on seven visits to the laboratory at 1-month interval. The first videotaping of each infant occurred as soon as possible after the infant could perform 3–6 independent steps. The mean age of the infants was 11 months at the first visit and 17 months at the last visit. The timing of the push-off (referred to as escapement timing) was assessed in terms of the time difference ($t_c - t_a$) between foot-strike (t_c) and peak forward acceleration of the whole-body CG (t_a). A negative escapement time indicates that t_a occurs after t_c, that is, during double support when the push-off would be most effective (correspondence between the new energy generation phase of the rear leg and the energy loss phase of the lead leg). However, a positive escapement time indicates that t_a occurs before t_c, indicating lack of correspondence between the energy generation phase and the energy loss phase of the lead leg. At visit 1, mean escapement time was positive with high variability. At visit 2, mean escapement time was negative with high variability. In visits 3–7, the mean escapement time was consistently negative with much lower variability than in visits 1 and 2. Consequently, in contrast to visit 1, escapement time in visits 2–7 was consistent with effective forward propulsion.

The changes in the effectiveness of escapement over visits 1–7 were reflected in changes in walking speed, stride length, and stride frequency. There were significant increases in speed of walking (0.18–0.59 $m \cdot s^{-1}$), stride length (0.21–0.42 m), and stride frequency (0.85–1.4 Hz) between visits 1 and 2, but no significant changes in any of the three variables over visits 2–7. There were no significant differences in weight, standing height, and sitting height of the subjects between visits 1 and 2, but there were significant increases in all three variables over visits 2–7. The results suggested that in the early stages of walking (within the first month after the onset of walking) infants rapidly learn to provide active force (via appropriate escapement timing) in a way that is consistent with the utilization of pendulum and spring dynamics to optimize energy expenditure.

A dynamical systems perspective of walking in children with cerebral palsy

The major task constraints in walking are the maintenance of an upright posture and continued oscillation of the legs despite energy loss. As a result of weakness in the calf muscles (ankle plantar flexors), children with spastic diplegia, a condition of cerebral palsy, are unable to generate the same amount of new energy during push-off in walking as normally developing children. The reduced new energy available from the push-off makes the use of a pendulum gait pattern almost impossible.[67] As energy generation (concentric muscle contractions), pendulum dynamics, and spring dynamics are the only dynamic resources that are potentially available, and energy generation and pendulum dynamics are severely restricted, it follows that forward progression can only be maintained by increasing the amount of energy available from spring dynamics. Consequently, it should be no surprise that children with spastic diplegia tend to adopt a gait that is more similar to running (a bouncing pattern) than walking as spring dynamics is predominant in running whereas pendulum dynamics is predominant in walking.

The increase in energy available via spring dynamics is the result of increased stiffness of the legs due to co-contraction of the flexors and extensors of the hips, knees, and ankles and an equinus foot position (plantar-flexed ankles). The increase in energy available via spring dynamics is the result of the body being projected upwards following each bounce which increases the amount of gravitational potential energy available at mid-stance (relative to walking) and, even allowing for loss of strain energy as heat during the subsequent compression phase of the lead leg, results in sufficient energy being returned to maintain forward progression. The bouncing gait requires a higher level of energy expenditure than normal walking, but it is reasonable to assume that such a gait is optimal in relation to the dynamic resources available. There is evidence that the efficiency of the bouncing gait is increased over time by adaptive morphological changes that increase the tendon length:muscle length ratio in the leg extensor muscles which, in turn, increases the resilience of the muscle–tendon units and, therefore, reduces the amount of energy that is lost.[71]

Traditional therapy for such gait abnormalities has been directed at normalizing the abnormal kinematics. For example, attempts have been made to reduce the equinus foot position in children with spastic diplegia by electrical stimulation of the tibialis anterior (to dorsiflex the ankle). However, such intervention has largely been unsuccessful.[36] From a dynamical systems perspective, the lack of success of traditional therapy is not surprising; all of the abnormal joint movements in an abnormal gait will be the result of a particular coordinative structure and, consequently, all of the abnormal joint movements will be symptoms of the underlying cause, that is, abnormal organismic constraints in the form of abnormal dynamic resources. The corollary is that therapy directed at normalizing the abnormal dynamic resources is likely to be more effective than therapy directed at normalizing the abnormal kinematics. There is evidence in support of this view. For example, electrical stimulation of the gastrocnemius–soleus group to improve the push-off in children with spastic diplegia (which might have been expected to worsen the equinus gait) has been shown to result in a more normal gait that included a normal heel-strike.[72,73] The implication of these findings is that normalizing the dynamic resources results in a more normal coordinative structure which, in turn, produces a more normal gait.

Summary

- The brain coordinates and controls movement via muscular activity. Coordination refers to the timing of relative motion between body segments and control refers to the optimization of relative motion between body segments.
- The development of coordination has been viewed historically from two viewpoints, the neuromaturational perspective (in relation to motor development in children) and the information-processing perspective (in relation to motor learning in adults). However, these approaches fail to account for the great flexibility demonstrated by individuals in accommodating rapidly changing task demands.
- The deficiencies of the neuromaturational and information-processing perspectives were pointed out by Bernstein.[14] He showed that all joint movements are the result of active (muscle) and passive (motion dependent, gravitational, and external) components of joint moments (referred to as joint biodynamics) and that coordination results in utilization of the passive components to minimize energy expenditure.
- Bernstein's biodynamical approach was a major influence on the currently widely held dynamical systems view of the development of coordination. The dynamical systems perspective views human movement as emerging from the intrinsic self-organizing properties of the dynamical system consisting of the person, the person's environment, and the desired movement.
- Self-organization refers to the spontaneous integration of the dynamical properties of the subsystems that comprise a system and results in the spontaneous establishment of a coordinative structure or functional synergy within and between the subsystems which, in turn, results in a pattern of activity. The actual pattern that emerges is dependent on the constraints on the system. In human movement, constraints can be broadly classified into three groups: task, environmental, and organismic.
- There is considerable evidence that coordination is self-optimized in relation to optimality criteria to which the individual is sensitive in adopting a particular movement pattern. The main optimality criterion would appear to be energy expenditure, but there is clear evidence of others, including, for example, stability, bilateral symmetry, and shock absorption at foot-strike in walking.
- Traditional therapy for gait abnormalities has been directed at normalizing the abnormal kinematics. However, such intervention has been largely unsuccessful. From a dynamical systems perspective, the lack of success of traditional therapy is not surprising; all of the abnormal joint movements in an abnormal gait will be the result of a particular coordinative structure and, consequently, all of the abnormal joint movements will be symptoms of the underlying cause, that is, abnormal organismic constraints in the form of abnormal dynamic resources. The corollary is that therapy directed at normalizing the abnormal dynamic resources is likely to be more effective than therapy directed at normalizing the abnormal kinematics. There is increasing evidence in support of this view.

References

1. Watkins J (1999). *Structure and function of the musculoskeletal system.* Human Kinetics, Champaign, IL.
2. Watkins J (2007). *An introduction to biomechanics of sport and exercise.* Churchill Livingstone, Edinburgh.
3. Turvey MT (1990). Coordination. *Am Psychol* **45**, 938–53.
4. Jensen JL, Phillips SJ, Clark JE (1994). For young jumpers, differences are in movement's control, not in coordination. *Res Q Exerc Sport* **65**, 258–68.
5. Bobbert MF, van Ingen Schenau GJ (1988). Coordination in vertical jump. *J Biomech* **21**, 249–62.
6. Hay JG (1993). Citius, altius, longius (faster, higher, longer): The biomechanics of jumping for distance. *J Biomech* **26** (Suppl 1), 7–21.
7. Clark JE, Phillips SJ, Petersen R (1989). Developmental stability in jumping. *Dev Psychol* **25**, 929–35.
8. Clark JE (1995). On becoming skillful: Patterns and constraints. *Res Q Exerc Sport* **66**, 173–83.
9. Gesell A, Thompson H (1938). *The psychology of early growth including norms of infant behavior and a method of genetic analysis.* Macmillan, New York.
10. McGraw MB (1943). *The neuromaturation of the human infant.* Columbia University Press, New York.
11. Thelen E (1995). Motor development: A new synthesis. *Am Psychol* **50**, 79–85.
12. Kamm K, Thelen E, Jensen JL (1990). A dynamical systems approach to motor development. *Phys Ther* **70**, 763–75.

13. Handford C, Davids K, Bennett S, Button C (1997). Skill acquisition in sport: Some implications of an evolving practice ecology. *J Sports Sci* **15**, 621–40.
14. Bernstein N (1967). *The coordination and regulation of movements.* Pergamon, London.
15. Lieber RL (1992). *Skeletal muscle structure and function.* Williams and Wilkins, Baltimore, MD.
16. Ingen Schenau GJV (1989). From translation to rotation: Constraints on multijoint movements and the unique action of biarticular muscles. *Hum Mov Sci* **8**, 301–37.
17. Schneider K, Zernicke RF (1992). Mass, centre of mass, and moment of inertia estimates for infant limb segments. *J Biomech* **25**, 145–8.
18. Sun H, Jensen RK (1994). Body segment growth during infancy. *J Biomech* **27**, 265–75.
19. Lockman JJ, Thelen E (1993). Developmental biodynamics: Brain, body and behavior connections. *Child Dev* **64**, 953–9.
20. Zernicke RF, Schneider K (1993). Biomechanics and developmental neuromotor control. *Child Dev* **64**, 982–1004.
21. Anderson DI, Sidaway B (1994). Coordination changes associated with practice of a soccer kick. *Res Q Exerc Sport* **65**, 93–9.
22. Andrews JG (1974). Biomechanical analysis of human motion. In: Hay JG (ed.), *Kinesiology IV*, pp. 32–42. American Alliance for Health, Physical Education and Recreation, Reston, VA.
23. Kamm K, Thelen E, Jensen JL (1990). A dynamical systems approach to motor development. *Phys Ther* **70**, 763–75.
24. Dempster WT (1955). *Space requirements of the seated operator: Geometrical, kinematic and mechanical aspects of the body with special reference to the limbs. WADT Technical Report No. 55–159.* Wright Patterson Air Force Base, OH.
25. Hatze H (1980). A mathematical model for the computational determination of parameter values of anthropometric segments. *J Biomech* **13**, 833–43.
26. Winter DA (1990). *Biomechanics and motor control of human movement.* John Wiley, New York.
27. Schneider K, Zernicke RF, Schmidt RA, Hart TJ (1989). Changes in limb dynamics during the practice of rapid arm movements. *J Biomech* **22**, 805–17.
28. Winter DA (1983). Energy generation and absorption at the ankle and knee during fast, natural, and slow cadences. *Clin Orthop* **175**, 147–54.
29. Holt KG, Hamill J, Andres RO (1991). Predicting the minimal energy costs of human walking. *Med Sci Sport Exerc* **23**, 491–8.
30. Jeng S-F, Liao H-F, Lai J-S, Hou J-W (1997). Optimization of walking in children. *Med Sci Sport Exerc* **29**, 370–6.
31. Thelen E, Corbetta D, Kamm K, Spencer J, Schneider K, Zernicke RF (1993). The transition to reaching: Mapping intention and intrinsic dynamics. *Child Dev* **64**, 1058–98.
32. Jensen JL, Thelen E, Ulrich BD (1989). Constraints on multijoint movements: From spontaneity of infancy to the skill of adults. *Hum Mov Sci* **8**, 393–402.
33. Kugler PN, Turvey MT (1987). *Natural law, and the self assembly of rhythmic movement.* Erlbaum, Hillside, NJ.
34. Kugler PN, Kelso JAS, Turvey MT (1980). On the concept of coordinative structures as dissipative structures: I. Theoretical lines of convergence. In: Stelmach GE, Requin J (ed.), *Tutorials on motor behavior*, pp. 3–47. North Holland, New York.
35. Davids K, Glazier P, Araujo D, Bartlett R (2003). Movement systems as dynamical systems: The functional role of variability and its implications for sports medicine. *Sports Med* **33**, 245–60.
36. Holt KG, Obusek JP, Fonseca ST (1996). Constraints on disordered locomotion: A dynamical systems perspective on spastic cerebral palsy. *Hum Mov Sci* **15**, 177–202.
37. Dickinson MH, Farley CT, Full RJ, Koehl MAR, Kram R, Lehman S (2000). How animals move: An integrative view. *Science* **288**, 100–6.
38. Madore BF, Freedman WL (1987). Self-organizing structures. *Am Sci* **75**, 252–59.
39. Holt KG (1998). Constraints in the emergence of preferred locomotory patterns. In: Rosenbaum DA, Collyer CE (ed.), *Timing of behavior: Neural, psychological, and computational perspectives*, pp. 261–91. MIT Press, Cambridge, MA.
40. Newell KM (1986). Constraints on the development of coordination. In: Wade MG, Whiting HTA (ed.), *Motor development in children: Aspects of coordination and control*, pp. 341–60. Martinus Nijhoff, Dordrecht.
41. Clugston MJ (1998). *The new penguin dictionary of science.* Penguin, London.
42. Sipper M, Sanchez E, Mange D, Tomassini M, Perez-Uribe A, Stauffer A (1997). A phylogenetic, ontogenetic, and epigenetic view of bio-inspired hardware systems. *IEEE Trans Evol Comput* **1**, 83–97.
43. Smith LB, Thelen E (2003). Development as a dynamic system. *Trends Cogn Sci* **7**, 343–8.
44. Thelen E (1981). Kicking, rocking and waving: Contextual analysis of stereotyped behaviour in normal infants. *Anim Behav* **29**, 3–11.
45. Thelen E (1985). Developmental origins of motor coordination: Leg movements in human infants. *Dev Psychobiol* **18**, 1–22.
46. Thelen E (1986). Treadmill-elicited stepping in seven-month-old infants. *Child Dev* **57**, 1498–506.
47. Thelen E, Fisher DM (1982). Newborn stepping: An explanation for a "disappearing reflex." *Dev Psychobiol* **18**, 760–75.
48. Thelen E, Fisher DM, Ridley-Johnson R (1984). The relationship between physical growth and a newborn reflex. *Infant Behav Dev* **7**, 479–93.
49. Spencer JP, Corbetta D, Buchanan P, Clearfield M, Ulrich B, Schoner G (2006). Moving toward a grand theory of development: In memory of Esther Thelen. *Child Dev* **77**, 1521–38.
50. Adolph KE (2002). Learning to keep balance. In: Kail R (ed.), *Advances in child development and behavior*, Vol. 30, pp. 1–40. Elsevier Science, Amsterdam.
51. Adolph KE, Vereijken B, Shrout PE (2003). What changes in infant walking and why. *Child Dev* **74**, 475–97.
52. Kelso JAS, Holt KG, Kugler PN, Turvey MT (1980). On the concept of coordinative structures as dissipative structures: II. Empirical lines of convergence. In: Stelmach GE, Requin J (ed.), *Tutorials on motor behavior*, pp. 49–70. North Holland, New York.
53. Hamill J, Haddad JM, McDermott WJ (2000). Issues in quantifying variability from a dynamical systems perspective. *J Appl Biomech* **16**, 407–18.
54. Holt KG, Jeng S-F (1992). Advances in biomechanical analysis of the physically challenged child: Cerebral palsy. *Pediatr Exerc Sci* **4**, 213–35.
55. Clark JE, Phillips SJ (1993). A longitudinal study of intralimb coordination in the first year of independent walking: A dynamical systems analysis. *Child Dev* **64**, 1143–57.
56. van Emmerik REA, van Wegen EEH (2000). On variability and stability in human movement. *J Appl Biomech* **16**, 394–406.
57. Morowitz HJ (1978). *Foundations of bioenergetics.* Academic, New York.
58. Beek PJ, Wieringen PCWV (1994). Perspectives on the relation between information and dynamics: An epilogue. *Hum Movement Sci* **13**, 519–33.
59. Clark JE, Whitall J, Phillips SJ (1988). Human interlimb coordination: The first 6 months of independent walking. *Dev Psychobiol* **21**, 445–56.
60. Holt KG, Hamill J, Andres RO (1990). The force driven harmonic oscillator as a model for human walking. *Hum Mov Sci* **9**, 55–68.
61. Holt KG, Jeng S-F, Ratcliffe RJ, Hamill J (1995). Energetic cost and stability during human walking at the preferred stride frequency. *J Motor Behav* **27**, 164–78.
62. Ledebt A, Breniere Y (1994). Dynamical implication of anatomical and mechanical parameters in gait initiation process in children. *Hum Mov Sci* **13**, 801–15.
63. Goldfield EC, Kay BA, Warren WH (1993). Infant bouncing: The assembly and tuning of action systems. *Child Dev* **64**, 1128–42.

64. Ratcliffe RJ, Holt KG (1997). Low frequency shock absorption in human walking. *Gait Posture* **5**, 93–100.
65. Jeng S-F, Holt KG, Fetters L, Certo C (1996). Self-optimization of walking in nondisabled children and children with spastic hemiplegic cerebral palsy. *J Motor Behav* **28**, 15–27.
66. Gibson EJ (1982). The concept of affordances in perceptual development: The renascence of functionalism. In: Collins WA (ed.), *Minnesota symposia on child psychology*, Vol. 15, pp. 55–80. Erlbaum, Hillsdale, NJ.
67. Fonseca ST, Holt KG, Fetters L, Saltzman E (2004). Dynamic resources used in ambulation by children with spastic hemiplegic cerebral palsy: Relationship to kinematics, energetics, and asymmetries. *Phys Ther* **84**, 344–54.
68. Holt KG, Saltzman E, Ho C-L, Kubo M, Ulrich BD (2006). Discovery of the pendulum and spring dynamics in the early stages of walking. *J Motor Behav* **38**, 206–18.
69. Alexander R McN (1991). Energy-saving mechanisms in walking and running. *J Exp Biol* **160**, 55–69.
70. Farley CT, Ferris DP (1998). Biomechanics of walking and running: Center of mass movements to muscle action. *Exerc Sport Sci Rev* **26**, 253–85.
71. Holt KG, Fonseca ST, LaFiandra ME (2000). The dynamics of gait in children with spastic hemiplegic cerebral palsy: Theoretical and clinical implications. *Hum Mov Sci* **19**, 375–405.
72. Carmick J (1995). Managing equinus in children with cerebral palsy: Electrical stimulation to strengthen the triceps surae muscle. *Dev Med Child Neurol* **37**, 965–75.
73. Comeaux P, Patterson N, Rubin M, Meiner R (1998). Effect of neuromuscular electrical stimulation during gait in children with cerebral palsy. *Pediatr Phys Ther* **9**, 103–9.

CHAPTER 14

Motor development

David A. Sugden and Helen C. Soucie

Introduction

The development, performance, and learning of motor skills are lifelong processes that show both obvious and more subtle changes in the individual. One has only to informally view a young child from infancy through to 4 or 5 years of age to recognize the huge changes that take place in the area of motor competence, with these changes being clear and obvious in the growing child, but both adolescents and adults continue to adapt and refine their motor skills as they strive for the most proficient route to effective movement.[1] According to Keogh and Sugden,[2] development involves the adaptive change towards competence, and these adaptations and alterations to our movements are constantly in flux even though the adaptations are not always apparent to the human eye. Changes occur in biological, physical, and social environments to enable individuals and their surroundings to become congruous, with a constant transaction taking place between the resources the child brings to any given movement problem, the context in which the problem is based and the problem or the task that is being solved. Thus behaviour, in this case motor behaviour, is the cumulation of many intrinsic influences, including psychological, sociological, biological, physiological, cognitive, and mechanical changes, all transacting with the extrinsic constraints of the task to be performed set in an environmental context.[2,3]

This chapter examines motor development from a number of perspectives. The first two sections overview a description followed by possible explanations of motor development. These sections are predicated on the assumption that two major questions permeate motor development: the first question asks what happens during development, describing and analysing the changes that occur; the second, a more difficult question, examines the possible explanations as to what are the mechanisms that are driving these changes. A third section provides an overview of recent work in the area of infant and early childhood development utilizing concepts from dynamic systems theory and ecological psychology. A fourth part examines two relatively recent ideas from early childhood and motor development. The first one promotes the idea of embodied cognition where a child's physical, social, and linguistic interaction with the environment may be the root of flexible intelligent behaviour. The second one looks at the way in which some development is atypical, through an examination of precursors in early infancy being possible predictors for later problems. Finally, an example of atypical development is illustrated through a description of the condition known as developmental coordination disorder.

Description of change

Motor development begins with conception and continues through to adulthood. It is often considered age-related, but as individuals and environments differ so extensively, development is best viewed as a continuous process of change, with age being simply one indicator of development. Dramatic changes in individuals are seen as the newborn baby develops into the young child with self-help skills and into adult life as our movements adapt to meet the demands of our environment. These descriptions of change are well documented and detailed summaries are available from a number of sources.[1,2]

Examples from early development are present in the areas of locomotion and manual skills. *Locomotion* is not present in the newborn but develops though gaining postural control with the result that by the time the child is around 1 year of age he/she is walking and using other forms of locomotion to explore the environment. By 2 years of age, the child is performing rudimentary jumps and moving towards running. These fundamental skills continue to develop and by the time the child is 6 or 7 years of age, one could state that by this age all of the fundamental motor skills are in place in a rudimentary fashion. These skills include running, jumping, hopping, skipping, galloping, climbing, throwing, and catching. The argument continues that after this age the child does not develop new fundamental locomotor skills, but refines, plays with, modifies, and generally improves the ones that are already present. A related assertion here notes that if this is the case, there is a very strong argument for skilled teaching of physical activity between the ages of 3 and 7. After the age of 7 these fundamental skills are honed and refined, made use of in game, recreational, and leisure activities and utilized in contexts where maximum performance is required. Again, descriptions of these changes are well documented.[1,2]

In the area of *manual skills* a similar pattern is seen. The newborn has crude but goal-directed manual skills that involve both manipulation and reaching and grasping. Classic studies by Connolly and Elliott[4] have described how finger and thumb opposition occurs early in life. The very young infant will grasp an object with the palm and the ulnar side of the hand and during the first year of life this changes to the more radial and distal location with eventually the grasp being a combination of the thumb and index finger in true opposition. A similar trajectory of change to locomotion occurs in the early years; by the age of 6 or 7 the child can perform often in a rudimentary fashion, most of the basic and fundamental manual skills. They have a range of grips that will vary according to environmental demands; they can form letters, often words, can draw and paint, cut with scissors, and manipulate a range of objects. Not all of these skills are performed with dexterity but they are present by these ages and continue to improve throughout childhood, being used flexibly, becoming more accurate, increasing in speed, and being used adaptively in numerous and different environmental contexts.[1,2]

If we take drawing as a further example of how a child develops, we note that the first attempts begin around 18 months of age. These are usually 'scribble' type often appearing to be random in nature. By 3 years of age, lines and circles begin to appear and by 4 years of age a simple cross can be drawn. It is interesting to note here that around this time a child who has difficulty in drawing/copying a square will be able to copy one using four matchsticks; it is as though the ongoing simultaneous acts of copying and drawing take the full capacity of the child, whereas simply copying through the positioning of the matchsticks is much less complex. This type of task shows that the difficulty the child is having with drawing not being a straightforward perceptual one. By 5 years of age, the child can draw a square and very often a triangle. As the child progresses, the drawings also start to include faces and other more complex pictures.[5]

Another manual skill that is acquired early in life and continues, especially, in western cultures, is feeding with a spoon. The act of using a spoon is more complicated than we typically realize. It involves ensuring that the concave side of the spoon faces upwards, and this position is kept throughout the act; it involves loading the spoon, transporting it to the mouth, inserting the spoon and emptying it in the mouth, removing it from the mouth, and transporting it back to the bowl where the food is. This cycle is then repeated. In the first year of life most of the feeding responsibility is taken by the parent but gradually this is taken over by the infant. There are many reports of the infant 'playing' with the spoon, putting it in the mouth empty, banging it on the table, and dropping on the ground and these may be exploratory activities for the most appropriate actions. This is an area of infant behaviour that would benefit from more detailed examination.[6]

Another upper limb action that appears to be universal is throwing, an activity that is also common in the primate population. Throwing develops in terms of form, distance, and accuracy. Studies have shown a consistent linear increase in maximum velocity from 5 to 12 years of age for both boys and girls with boys having an increasing advantage with age.[7] In the same age range, the maximum distance attained also has a linear increase with boys at six throwing approximately 9 m rising to 30 m by 12; the comparable figures for girls are 6 and 18 m.[7,8] The two variables of maximum velocity and maximum distance are highly correlated[9] although accuracy is another variable that is also relevant. An interesting finding in examining accuracy is that for most ages up to adulthood, individuals when asked to throw for accuracy would adjust their velocity to about 75% of maximum for the throw,[7] but again with a similar trend of increasing accuracy with age and boys performing better than girls. This difference between genders before puberty in throwing is more pronounced than other attributes and has been attributed to evolutionary adaptation.[10–12] Changes in form in throwing behaviour have been analysed by researchers using various methodologies from early film studies to later biomechanical techniques.[7,13] Changes in form in throwing behaviour do change with age and at different rates for boys and girls with detailed descriptions available.[7,14,15] In all of the studies noted above, although the emphasis has been on the changes in the resources of the child, that is by age, there is also evidence to show that other variables are at work that produce the changes such as the environmental context and task constraints, topics that we will address in the section on explanation of development.

Explanation of change

Maturational explanations

For many years, a child's motor development has involved accounts of their physical growth patterns. Early researchers concluded that the regularity of the emerging motor skills seen in children reflected the genetically driven process common to all normally developing children, namely, that of brain maturation.[16,17] This process of maturation was responsible for coordinated movements to emerge in an orderly fashion, and this was usually cephalo-to-caudal and central-to-distal as cortical control increasingly took over from lower reflexes with the movements taking on a more coordinated form. This view inferred, and offered findings to support such a claim, that it was autonomous changes in the nervous system that supported motor skill development. Dennis and Dennis[16] demonstrated that even when children had their movements restricted, as did the Hopi children on cradleboards, the genetically driven timetable for motor skill development, in this case walking, would continue unabated. In another early study Peiper[18] reports on a 6-month-old girl who had a bilateral congenital hip dislocation and was put in a cast until she was 18 months old. One day after the cast was removed the girl started to walk.

The scientific study of motor development can be traced back to the 1930s and 1940s when pioneer developmental scientists such as Shirley,[17] Gesell and Amatruda,[5] and McGraw[19,20] spent many years observing and reporting how infants gain control of their movements. Shirley[17] compiled individual movement biographies cataloguing the movements of 25 babies from birth to 2 years of age through regular home visits of at least once per week. The child's movements were recorded graphically and by long hand. The detail amounted to an intensive, longitudinal study of early walking development. Gesell and Amatruda[5] also collected observations of child development, so much so, that their data were used to produce developmental scales on which a diagnosis of development could be based. McGraw[19,20] and the other early developmentalists were not the only observers of children, they were also theorists. They noted that children universally pass through a series of motor milestones and that these movements occur in sequence. For example, McGraw felt that the consistencies seen in the emerging motor skills of young children were due to a genetically driven process, that of the brain maturing.

This all led to the conclusion that development was attributed to the maturation of the nervous system, that movement coordination was a gradual unfolding of predetermined patterns, and cortical control was taking over from lower brain stem and spinal reflexes.

However, as we explain below, these conclusions and interpretations are now being re-evaluated.

Ulrich[21] notes that there are sound reasons to cast doubt upon maturation and simple neural development being the sole cause of changes in motor development. She comments that some maturationists maintain that because people pass through similar sequences, a 'programme' for this is prepared in advance and is genetically determined. The assumption is that this information for development is encoded genetically. She argues that logically this would be such a cumbersome system for humans to deal with; assigning sets of neurons for the development of movement patterns is not a parsimonious way of dealing with the complex issue of evolving development. In addition, as will be explained later, an end movement product is not just the result of the firing of neurons. A final note on the maturational view concerns the contribution this line of research did engender. It established motor milestones and expectancies for the developing child giving us great insight into the changes that take place through their meticulous observation; however, the stability of these milestones and the reasons for them has been questioned.

Cognitive explanations

Explanations from cognitive perspectives have long been favourites in many quarters of psychology and related fields. Early and influential work by Piaget[22] looked at ages and stages of development noting that there is an order to them and that they are rarely skipped. Of great influence, and a topic that will be revisited later in the chapter is the influence that movement and motor development have on other developing aspects of the child. Possibly of greater influence than Piaget in the specific field of motor development and motor behaviour in general is the body of knowledge that comes under the general heading of *information processing systems* (IPS). These approaches have had major influences on the manner by which we examine motor behaviour and continue to do so with influential texts such as Schmidt and Lee[23] providing comprehensive coverage and explanations of the processes involved in motor performance and learning. The essence of IPS is that information flows through a system that eventually puts out a movement product. There are many variations of IPS but they have a number of characteristics in common. First, they are all component based, that is, information is taken in through the senses and is gradually transformed through a series of operations before a movement outcome is achieved. These components will differ according to who is proposing the model but many will contain the following.

The mechanisms for how information in the environment is brought into the system are usually through vision and kinaesthesis but also touch and auditory senses are used to influence movement. Information is attended to and selected out as being of relevance to the task on hand. This information is held in a working memory as it is compared to previous experiences in order to be used to prepare a plan of action. This plan is often labelled as a programme and is often purported to contain such parameters as force, timing, spatial characteristics, and other variables that may influence the movement outcome. The motor programme is 'run off' to produce the movement which in turn produces various types of feedback that are used to evaluate the movement and prepare for any subsequent action. Other characteristics of IPS include the principle of being time determined, that is, some of the components require performance at speed for optimum effect. Activities involving fast ball games are good examples of this where detection, selection, reaction, preparation of a programme, and movement speed are all crucial to effectiveness. Many models propose the concept of limited processing space whereby a person can become overloaded with information which in turn can lead to a detriment in performance. Early models of IPS were linear in nature with simple sequential processing, but recent ones are much more sophisticated and complex models are commonplace with multiple simultaneous channels of processing.

The major assumption from IPS models surrounding the explanation of motor development and the improvement in performance as the child gets older is that children become better and more accomplished in the various components of the IPS models. For example, as the child improves memory through the use of various cognitive strategies, this improvement in memory will aid in the transformation of information through the processing system and thus has a beneficial effect on the movement outcome. Another example is reaction time; as the child develops, reaction times decrease from around 600 ms at the age of 5 or 6 to half that by the time the child reaches 12 years of age. This has obvious implications for a child performing fast activities.[2]

IPS approaches have given a tremendous boost to the study of motor behaviour and thus have been massively influential in the field of motor development. They have allowed researchers to take a much more scientific approach to the study of movement and actions by allowing more controlled experiments, the isolation of variables for study, resulting in a massive accumulation of knowledge.

However, they have not been without their critics. Ulrich[21] notes that IPS approaches are essentially prescriptive in nature and rely on pre-existing structures such as motor programmes but do not explain how they originate. In a sense, they are simply descriptions at a deeper level. The lack of explanation of the motor components of motor behaviour has come in for specific criticism. Much of the work on IPS systems has mirrored work in cognition without paying particular attention to the most distinctive feature of motor behaviour, that is, the control of movement itself.

Dynamic systems and ecological explanations

Views of motor development in the 1980s and 1990s stress the roles of exploration, and the selection of solutions to the demands of novel tasks. These new views in contrast with the traditional maturational accounts of motor development by proposing that the so-called phylogenetic skills, such as reaching, crawling, and walking, are in fact learnt by adapting current dynamics through exploration and selection of possible movements to fit the new task.[24] Changes in behaviour are not brought about by prescribed genetic instructions as earlier thought, but rather are motivated by a task, such as moving across a room to join other people, and recruiting the available resources to do this. It is the matching of the internal resources of the child together with the challenging contextual demands and requirements which promote development.

These approaches have been generated from sources such as dynamic systems theory and ecological perspectives on motor behaviour. There is a move away from looking at performance variables, such as crawling, and relating those behaviours to age or stage of development, to moving towards investigating the processes by which a child develops and learns new skills.

Through the imposition and presentation of novel tasks, there is an emphasis on how an infant explores, discovers, adapts, and remembers transitions from one behaviour to the next. The nervous system, in this new approach, is seen as dynamic and self-organizing, using repeated cycles of perception and action to facilitate new forms of behaviour. The approach represents a move away from explanations which rely alone upon internal mechanisms such as genes, programmes, and cognitive structures suggesting a blueprint for behavioural change.

As Thelen[24] notes

> The study of the acquisition of motor skills, long moribund in developmental psychology, has seen a renaissance in the last decade. Inspired by contemporary work in movement science, perceptual psychology, neuroscience, and dynamics systems theory, multidisciplinary approaches are affording new insights into the processes by which infants and children learn to control their bodies ... Studies are concerned less with how children perform and more with how the components cooperate to produce stability or engender change. Such process approaches make moot the traditional nature-nurture; debates. (p. 79)

Ideas and theories proposed by Adolph *et al.*,[25] Goldfield *et al.*,[26] Jensen *et al.*,[27] Sporns and Edelman,[28] Stoffregen *et al.*,[29] Thelen,[24] and Turvey and Fitzpatrick,[30] for example, bring together a new synthesis of information attempting to explain motor skill development from a multicausal perspective emphasizing the contextual and self-organizing nature of development through the roles of exploration–action–perception cycles, degrees of freedom equations, and brain plasticity, working together with environmental constraints. A greater emphasis is placed upon the role of the child, and the link of perception to the development of skills from the learner's explorations, in other words, there is a unity of perception, action, and cognition through the process of exploration.[24]

The thrust of this view of motor development is that through repeated cycles of perception and action, new behaviours emerge that are not explained by a pre-existing genetic plan. Given normal development, we all discover walking rather than jumping as a more efficient means of locomotion most of the time, but the style with which we walk is quite idiosyncratic. Walking as a solution to moving from point A to point B is not just the result of pre-programming, but rather walking develops because of the constraints we as humans find anatomically, biomechanically, and environmentally. These constraints can include those in the environment, those personal to the performer, the present state of the nervous and musculoskeletal system, the masses and lengths of limbs, the material properties of environmental objects, and the ever present gravitational field.[26] Walking is viewed then as an inevitable solution to the demands of the task. One of the principles of dynamic systems is the multiple components that contribute to the final movement solution.

Perception–action links

The perception–action relationship, proposed by Gibson,[31,32] appears to play a major role in the control of movements through the repeated cycle of exploration–perception–action, with the child being an active participant in the process that affords change. As we perceive the environment, the activity of seeing, for example, creates an optical flow field providing both space and time information. The rate of image expansion given by the light hitting the retina offers us direct information about oncoming objects for instance. Gibson[31] believes that the information from the rate of image expansion offers direct perception of objects colliding or the timing of interceptions without the need for higher-order cortical calculations. In visual cliff experiments, Gibson and Walk[33] demonstrated the use of direct perception and the relationship between affordances in the environment and personal affordances in the control of movements, even from this early age. The perception–action link is one of the integrated branches of an ecological perspective on motor development.

Synergies, coordinative structures, and self-organization

Another branch of the new synthesis considers the question asked by Bernstein[34] about how humans, or indeed animals, control the many degrees of freedom possible in our movements. Degrees of freedom, in this sense, refer to the very many possibilities a person may have in their movements by the fixing or releasing the limb joints. This grouping of degrees of freedom is referred to as synergies or coordinated structures. The development of synergies to accomplish a task does not demand the use of higher cortically processed instructions to carry out a movement, rather the process relies to an extent on the physical properties of our dynamic system as we self-organize, such as the spring-like properties of our muscles, the nature of the performer's environment, and the demands of the task. The more degrees of freedom used in a movement, in most cases, the finer the movement can be, provided that the person has control of these multiple joint movements. The fewer degrees of freedom used, the more fixed the movement is. A person reaching for an object with fixed elbow and wrist joints uses fewer degrees of freedom, so possibly making the reaching easier to control but allowing fewer options in the manner in which they reach. As the infant explores its environment, the movements they use change from simply exploratory to more refined and purposeful movements which result in an efficiency not seen earlier. The movements that developing children use are seen to adapt to the degrees of freedom equation, altering and adapting these synergies to suit the task in hand and their changing resources. The self-assembly of the synergies required to meet the demands of the task in the case of the developing child is dependent on the child's own resources, such as postural control, muscular strength, and attractiveness of the task. This particular approach to the explanation of motor control and change examines development from a multicausal perspective, always looking for information on how our complex, dynamic, and evolving system supports the environmental task.

The notion of exploration and selection as processes involved in development includes a view of the brain as a changing, developing organ that is itself moulded through experience. This is referred to as 'plasticity' of the brain, where individual perception and action act as fodder for brain change, which in turn opens new opportunities for experience. As Sporns and Edelman[28] write,

> There is overwhelming evidence that the emergence of coordinated movements is intimately tied both to the growth of the musculoskeletal system and to the development of the brain. Thus, neural development and learning cannot be considered outside of their biomechanical context. (p. 967)

Sporns and Edelman[28] refute the idea that development evolves from genetic instructions, and instead propose that through periods of instability (where many options to solve a motor problem are experienced) and stability (where far fewer options are used to solve a motor problem) humans select solutions which strengthen certain connections or groups of neurones through use. Selection is experience dependent, with diversity providing the raw material. Sporns and Edelman[28] also believe that there are reciprocal and recursive signals from many areas of the brain that integrate messages from multiple senses to give a coordinated response. Thelen[24] has referred to this as a kind of mapping of maps. Basically, this neural diversity and cross entries of sensory information allows the nervous system to recognize and categorize signals through a dynamic and self-organizing system. The brain develops through experiences, rather than through genetic maturation. Adopting this theory of development, individual differences can be accounted for. The reason for some children not crawling before they walk can be explained, for under these terms not every child is timetabled to go through certain inevitable motor milestones.

Studies from the ecological perspective or new synthesis are worthy of elaboration as they emphasize the notion of active learning from a multidisciplinary, multicausal position. In addition, these studies, whilst concentrating upon changes seen in infants and young children, offer a model for change throughout the lifespan not simply related to childhood. If experience and resources afford adaptation, if exploration leads to selection and further exploration develops into retention of preferred actions, the same model can be applied to the acquisition of new or adapted skills learnt by adults. If young children alter and adapt the degrees of freedom used to accomplish a task as they experiment with the nature of the task and their own constraints, then it may be possible for this process to be applied to the learning adult or older child too. Our resources and our ideas on solutions to the motor skill questions asked of us are continually evolving and self-organizing through our dynamic system.

Infant development and early childhood

At birth, a baby is reliant on adults for moving position but there are significant movement patterns that serve a number of functions. First, reflex mechanisms seen in the early months stabilize joints and can, for instance, prevent possible damage by fast movements. Second, Thelen[35] noted the seemingly random leg kicks, arm waves, and body rolling of young babies. These movements, known as spontaneous movements, are not reflexes or involuntary movements, yet for a long time were viewed by researchers as apparently serving no purpose or use in the goal-directed sense. Both reflexive movements and spontaneous movements have been viewed as possible precursors to later voluntary movements. For example, Thelen *et al.*[36] measured the spontaneous movements seen in young babies and noted that the kinematics of the spontaneous kicking movements resemble the spatial and temporal components of mature walking patterns.

Reflexes and spontaneous movements

The early or primitive reflexes found in babies are related to infant survival and are nourishment-seeking as well as protective actions. These subcortically controlled reflex movements are present in newborn babies, and the rate and strength at which they appear and disappear are considered as indicators of healthy development or early indicators of central nervous system disorders. Some researchers also believe that there is a link between these subcortical reflex behaviours, such as the crawling, primary stepping, and swimming reflexes, and later cortically processed voluntary movements, such as actual walking, swimming, and climbing.[37] This is despite there being a gap between the disappearance of the reflexive behaviours and the appearance of the voluntary movements. However, in the case of spontaneous leg movements there is no disappearance of the movements before the onset of locomotion. The reflexive movements seen in the stepping reflex disappear with time, but the spontaneous kicking of a child laid on his/her back remains.[24]

Thelen[24] proposes a different explanation for the disappearance of the so-called newborn stepping reflex. This stepping action occurs when a newborn infant is held upright with their feet on a support surface and they perform alternating step-like movements. Thelen[24] believes this appearance and subsequent disappearance of the stepping behaviour can be explained by looking at the multicausality of action rather than depending on the maturation hypothesis.

Traditionally, the disappearance of this so-called stepping reflex was attributed to maturation of the voluntary cortical centres which inhibited reflexive movements and then later facilitated the movements under a different and higher level of control[20] This was a long-held view to explain the onset of this stepping 'reflex', its disappearance, and its reappearance towards the end of the child's first year. Taking a multicausal view of the disappearance of the so-called stepping reflex Thelen and Fisher[38,39] noted that first the random, spontaneous kicking actions that infants perform when laid on their backs had very similar movement patterns to the stepping 'reflex', but unlike the stepping 'reflex' these spontaneous kicks continued and did not disappear after a few months. The comment Thelen[24] makes is that these two movements, the so-called reflexive stepping and the spontaneous kicking, were the same movements performed in two different postures. So why would the cortex supposedly inhibit one movement, the stepping reflex, but not the other, the spontaneous kicking? The explanation according to Thelen and Fisher[38,39] lies not in a maturational timetable taking hold of the infant, but because of the dynamics of the situation for the infant at that moment in their lives. Considering the dynamics, such as the task demands, the resources of the infant at that particular age, and the development of the musculoskeletal system, another explanation for the disappearing reflex was proposed.

At the same time as the stepping reflex disappears infants experience a rapid gain in mass, most of which is subcutaneous fat rather than muscle tissue. It was suggested, therefore, that in order for the infant to move their legs in a step-like movement they required the postural support from a prone or supine position, as quite simply, the legs had become too heavy for the infants to move them while upright. Thelen and Fisher[39] experimented with the infant's mass against gravity by either submerging the infant in warm water to 'restore' the stepping, or by adding weights to 'inhibit' stepping, thereby simulating the developmental changes by simple physical means. The relationship between gravity and weight gain was therefore seen to combine to afford or not afford the stepping actions from different support positions.

Other studies support Thelen's proposals demonstrating that the child's resources are brought to bear on the task in hand as they respond adaptively to the constraints within and before them. Goldfield *et al.*[26] monitored the development of infants learning to use a 'baby bouncer' as they adjusted their kicking to gain optimal bounce. The results of the kinematic analysis provided evidence that:

> infants assemble and tune a periodic kicking system akin to a forced mass-spring, homing in on its resonant frequency. (p. 1137)

Basically, the infants in this study moved to an optimized attractor state where they got the maximal bounce for minimal energy input. It appears that through vision and perception, the infants sensed the timing and force necessary to get what Thelen[24] describes as 'the most bounce for the ounce'.

Environmental affordances

In an examination of the environmental context, Adolph *et al.*[25] investigated the perceived affordances of toddlers aged 14 months when presented with ascending or descending sloping walkways of differing angles. We have all seen how young children, and even adults, adapt their methods of locomotion to suit the terrain or explore the unknown. Developing children relatively new to locomotion have many new challenges presented to them, with the question of high balance on their agenda. The toddlers in this study were able to walk unaided for 3 m, and initially they were required to walk towards one of their parents on a flat walkway. This walkway was then angled to form an ascending or descending slope in the middle of two flat pathways. The children were then beckoned by one of their parents again. The results of the study indicate that toddlers perceive affordances for walking over slopes. The children overestimated their ability to ascend slopes, falling often but picking themselves up, altering their style of locomotion to include climbing but continuing with the task to completion. On the descents the children chose alternative methods to get down the slope other than walking, they altered their locomotion to include sliding positions and it was noted that in contrast to their ascents the toddlers asked for help when descending. The toddlers had few falls and actively explored alternative means to achieve the task, so demonstrating their perception of affordance.

A similar experiment with infant crawlers reported that younger children did not explore alternative means to descend the slopes before plunging down! Even though they had the ability to alter their method of locomotion to backward scooting, they did not make use of that option. This is in direct contrast to the toddlers who rarely fell because of their appropriately adapted movements. Adolph *et al.*[25] suggest that infant crawlers are less attentive to their own postural ability than toddlers who are possibly more focused because of the demand for balancing on two legs. In addition, it is suggested that the infant crawlers seeing the supportive nature of the flat walkway below the slope felt the descent would be safe and that at this moment in their development they were unable to relate the steepness of the descending slope to their own locomotor abilities.

Stoffregen *et al.*[29] examined whether young children, with only a few weeks of standing experience, were able to maintain and adapt their standing posture to the constraints placed upon them by different support surfaces. The children used complex movements to maintain postural control including movements of the hips (not previously thought possible until 3–4 years of age) and the ankles, and use of the arms and hands. The children used a wide variety of coordination modes in the maintenance of their stance.

In a study of 3-month-old infants, Thelen[40] found that babies were in fact able to direct movements towards a novel task; in this case, moving an overhead mobile. Her study suggests that, even at this early stage in life, learning processes are in place, once again supporting the view that new movements seen in infants are not simply the result of autonomous brain maturation. This study by Thelen[40] represents an excellent example of the evolving resources of the infant and the developing dynamic system used to find a solution to the presented motor problem. The babies were placed lying on their backs under an attractive overhead mobile. When the infants were allowed to control the movement of the mobile by their left ankles being tethered by soft elastic to the mobile, it was found that all the babies kicked more and faster as their kicks were reinforced by the mobile movement. This was not the only finding from the study. Thelen[40] decided to join the tethered left ankle to the right ankle so making it possible for the infant to alter their previous style of independent leg kicks to an in-phase pattern that would recruit the strength from both legs to move the mobile. Not only did Thelen[40] find that the babies kicked more when their movements made the mobile move but she also found that those babies with the right ankle yoked to the left increasingly kicked in a simultaneous or in-phase fashion. Thelen[40] states in her discussion:

> In everyday learning of new motor skills, tasks and constraints also appear and disappear. Opportunities for action depend on the presence of desired objects, suitable support surfaces, postures available to the infant, helping social support, and so on. Thus, in Gibsonian terms, a certain class of objects affords reaching or mouthing, or certain surfaces afford crawling upon. What is important for understanding development is how infants discover and learn new patterns in a specific situation, as demonstrated in this experiment: how those patterns are remembered: and then how classes of solutions are generalized to novel, but similar situations. (p. 284)

The children in these studies demonstrated an awareness of their environment, its constraints, and an ability to link their perceptions with their actions and develop solutions. The children's motor activities provided the means to explore their environment and the opportunity to learn about its properties. As each new solution was gained, it opened up opportunities for further perceptual motor exploration, and so the children built on their knowledge from the demands of the tasks. Therefore, once again this perspective of motor development disputes the notion of inevitable stages in motor development and emphasizes the dynamic and ecological nature of development.

Fundamental skills

From a dynamical perspective, the fundamental skills that children develop from birth to around their second birthday, and onwards, have arisen because of the relationship that exists between the child's physical development and the ever changing action–perception cycles. These relationships have engendered stability and instability to produce change as the child has sought out solutions to the motor problems presented to them.

Fundamental skills do not follow a predetermined plan of occurrence, rather they develop from the child finding new solutions to new tasks as their human resources afford them. Using the example of throwing, a baby soon learns how to get rid of an implement held in their hands. This develops into transporting hand-held objects to destinations further away than simply dropping them, often it seems, simply for the pleasure of seeing an adult retrieve it! As these developments take place, the child is learning categories of movements which can be applied to a constrained task. These constraints require the young child to freeze the degrees of freedom used in the act of throwing, and over time the synergies developed reveal how those degrees of freedom are freed as their experiences and resources.

The younger child tends to limit the throwing action to one mainly from the elbow with little rotary movement. The child's body mass is not really transferred into the throw and the feet tend to remain stationary. If the same child without the adult resources attempted to use a more mature technique to throw, they would probably end up in a heap on the floor, so the child freezes the degrees of freedom in order to keep control of the movement. This self-organizing system is demonstrating the resource the child has at this moment in time and how they are adapting to the internal and external constraints placed upon them. The coordinative structures or synergies seen in the developing child of fixed or locked joints later include greater flexibility enabling more adaptive movements. As the child learns that moving more of the arm is beneficial to the throw, and that the non-throwing arm can be used to stabilize the increased movement, so more rotation comes into play and a definite shift of body mass supports the additional movements. The child is freeing some degrees of freedom as their resources now enable them to and a new category of movements make a higher level association. Therefore, the story continues, as the throwing action becomes more dynamic, the arm movements become more extensive and there is a greater awareness of how these additional degrees of freedom can be controlled and used to produce a more efficient throw, in a variety of contexts. The child's movements are being tuned to their ever evolving resources. (Exactly the same argument can be made to explain how an ageing adult with arthritis, for example, redefines their actions to within their resources and the demands of the task.)

The 6-year-old child normally uses many more degrees of freedom when throwing than the 2-year-old would, but this is not always the case. The 6-year-old child can return to the status of the 2-year-old when the constraints of the environment are such that the many degrees of freedom developed would lead to an inaccurate or inefficient movement. For example, if a child was running fast to throw a ball in an atmosphere of much excitement and tripped *en route*, he/she would be very likely to revert to the pattern of throwing seen in the 2-year-old. Therefore, although the child learns to free their many degrees of freedom in order to produce more efficient movements, they also become aware of what conditions demand the freezing of them. Vereijken *et al.*[41] have demonstrated exactly this process of freeing and freezing degrees of freedom as a task is learnt, in this case a simulated ski task, where the novice first freezes at the knee and ankle joints and latter frees the joints for a more efficient movement once previous constraints have been overcome. One would hypothesize that should the skier meet with a very steep slope, next to a vertical drop, scattered with moguls and bumps, that the actions from the easier ski runs would be seriously adapted to meet the demands of the task, demonstrating that actions alter not only as we acquire a skill but also upon the conditions in which the acquired task is performed.

Early childhood motor development

Research into the general capabilities of young infants and children has expanded greatly in recent years, and this has been mirrored by developments in the motor domain and related fields. The research, rather than concentrating simply on developments and progressions in the motor area, has started to take on a wider brief by an examination of not only how motor links with other areas of human development but also how much early signs of difficulties in the motor domain are predictive of later problems. Two areas are briefly explored: the first, embedded cognition, involves the view that cognitive processes are initiated by the body's interactions with the world. The second, General Movements (GMs), are explored as early indicators of difficulties that emerge in both early and later childhood.

Embodied cognition

The term 'embodied cognition' is one that is used to describe the idea that intelligence or cognition emerges in the early years as an interaction between the sensorimotor actions of a baby with his/her environmental context.[42,43] This is not a new idea as Piaget[22] made similar notes, but researchers have taken this further with the rationale for this claim lying in a number of areas. They note and would encourage children to make contact with the physical world through multiple senses creating redundancy such that the loss of one sensory component does not affect overall function. Multiple sensory inputs, such as through handling and sight, also reinforces the whole experience of an event such as picking up a toy. The two or even multiple systems start to map on to each other thus reinforcing and enabling higher processes to continually evolve such that when a object is visually perceived it automatically evokes physical connections with that object and vice versa. These multimodal interactions change over time with a 4-month-old having different sensory and motor experiences than a 1-year-old which in turn will affect the developmental outcome. For example, self locomotion changes the nature of the type of visual, tactile, and auditory inputs of the infant which in turn has a profound effect on cognition.[42,43] To illustrate this, babies when they are able to self-locomote do not make the same errors of conservation of place of object that occurs when they cannot self-locomote.[42]

Random exploration is a second example, where babies learn about their world and reciprocally develop actions. For example, in reaching and grasping there is a continuous process of arousal to an object, exploration by the hand and arms leading to different solutions. This in turn leads to new tasks and challenges being attempted and consequently new solutions being derived. Smith and Gasser[42] noted that young mammals move in a variety of ways often for no apparent reason; these movements often called play are exploring new avenues that are essential to the building of intelligence and cognitive operations.

Third, infant and mother interactive gaze, imitation, and the progressive action transaction between mother and child from this are other areas whereby the dynamics of context affect development. Parents and children look at each other, parents introduce a toy to a child, it is moved and waved and named, and this range of modality input in a social setting help to establish the concept of the object in the world. Finally, action and language are linked in the manners similar to action and sensory and social areas. Young infants possess multiple sensory and action systems that develop as the infant explores the environmental context and interacts with others. Intelligence and cognition emerge from these interactions or more accurately transactions; this intelligence is embedded in these multiple systems and develops in a dynamic manner where all of the components change and interact.

Wilson[43] has proposed the notion of off-line embodied cognition as a powerful force in the development of cognition. Off-line embodied cognition involves those activities where the sensorimotor activity is simulated in the cognitive action. For example, all forms of imagery provide good examples of simulating external events with recent work with children showing coordination difficulties showing interesting ways forward for intervention. In off-line embodied cognition, episodic memory involving the visual, kinaesthetic, and motor impressions is linked to our bodies' experiences with the world; other examples are available in the area of problem solving and reasoning.

General movements as early indicators of later difficulties

Conditions such as cerebral palsy, minor neurological dysfunction, and attention deficit hyperactivity disorder (ADHD) are very difficult to diagnose early and this difficulty is reflected in the diversity of methods used to assess the brain at an early age. These methods include bedside examination involving neurological examinations with little equipment, to technical assessments using a variety of technological aids such as various forms of brain imaging. The task of predicting is made more difficult by the fact that the developing brain is constantly changing and does not reach full maturity till way past childhood. The clinical consequences of the changing neural attributes require age-specific neurological assessment and the way in which any neural dysfunction changes with age make predictions difficult although this does not underestimate the need for such predictions.

In the light of the above any predictions that have high validity would have high value for a number of reasons not the least would be early identification leading to appropriate early intervention. Work on GMs has provided promising results in this area.[44–46] GMs are a series of gross movements involving all parts of the body but do not have the usual sequences seen in coordinated movements. They emerge *in utero* from about 28 weeks, before isolated limb movements and at this time they have great variation in speed and amplitude. From 36 to 38 weeks, the initial GMs are replaced by ones that are forceful writhing movements. A second change takes place around 6–8 weeks post-term when the writhing movements become more 'fidgety' in character.

Four different types of GMs have been defined: two forms of normal GMs, normal optimal and normal suboptimal; and two forms of abnormal GMs, mildly abnormal and definitely abnormal. In a series of papers, researchers at the University of Groningen, for example, Hadders-Algra and Groothuis,[45] have made some interesting links between GMs and a range of subsequent behaviours and difficulties later in childhood. They found that definitely abnormal GMs at the fidgety stage, that is, 2–4 months post-term were associated with a high risk of the children developing cerebral palsy and those with mildly abnormal GMs had an association with the development of minor neurological dysfunction and ADHD and aggressive behaviour between the ages of 4 and 9 years. Further research confirmed that these predictions held true for older children aged 9–12 years with the quality of the GMs being related to the types and severity of neurological outcome.[44]

Research on embedded cognition and GMs is indicative of the different approaches to analysing motor development. It is using the knowledge we have about motor behaviour in the developing child and applying it to related and relevant fields. By doing this two advances in the field are promoted. First, it is becoming apparent that the motoric development of the child has implications beyond the motor domain. Second, by closely scrutinizing these implications and relationships there is a more in depth analysis of motor development itself.

Developmental coordination disorder

Most children on entry into school have developed a range of movement competencies that equip them for the requirements of the school environment. They have been exposed to the normal demands at home and in play situations and they have developed locomotor and manual skills that will carry over into the school contexts where they will be used in novel situations much of the time involving other children. There are some children, however, who do not develop fully in this way; they have no outward signs of physical disability and rarely show movements that are pathological such as the jerkiness or continuous motion often seen in cerebral palsy, yet their motor skills are poor and appear to lag behind those of their peers.[47]

Over the years these children have been associated with numerous labels such as the clumsy child, perceptual motor dysfunction, movement difficulties, dyspraxia with the current term—developmental coordination disorder (DCD)—being the one that is most widely used world wide. Although all labels bring with them various negative connotations and simplistic descriptions, the term DCD is logical in that the condition is developmental and it is concerned with coordination.[48,49]

The core characteristic of DCD is that the children show poor motor performance in comparison to their peers. Indeed the first criterion of the DSM IV-TR diagnosis[50] is that the children have significant motor difficulties that are over and above that what would be expected for their age and intelligence. The second criterion states that the impairment detailed above significantly and negatively affects activities of daily living and/or academic achievement. The third and fourth criteria are ones of exclusion noting that any impairment cannot be explained and is over and above that of any learning difficulty, and is not better explained by a known medical condition such as cerebral palsy or another pervasive developmental disorder.

Descriptions of children with DCD change as the children develop. In the younger years, there are parent reports of the children having great problems dressing in the morning, being disorganized, and having difficulties with their clothes and bathroom activities. At school they are often poor and slow at handwriting and in the playground are reluctant to engage in normal playground activities even if they are invited, which they are often not. As they enter middle childhood, such social activities as bicycle riding present difficulties while very often the writing problem continues. This latter trait is a particular hindrance to the pupil as they enter secondary school where the ability to write legibly and fast is usually a requirement. We have recent evidence to show that difficulties continue into emerging adulthood with the social consequences of motor problems being at the forefront, with the specific case of driving being a challenging issue.[51]

We know little about the underlying aetiology of DCD but it is anticipated that functional magnetic resonance imaging, genetic studies, and improved kinematic analysis may bring about a greater understanding. The current situation is that the prevalence figure is approximately 4–5% in primary schools although this varies depending on the criteria that is being used. The DSMIV-TR[50] figure is 6% for children between the ages of 6 and 11. Whatever criteria are used the prevalence of boys is usually at least twice that of girls and often three to four times.[50]

Although the database is not as strong as in other conditions, the evidence suggests that without adequate intervention, children do not grow out of the condition. They very often compensate by not engaging in activities where they know failure awaits them, or by participating in alternative activities. However, there have been numerous intervention studies with varying degrees of success. Many have used specialists trained in the area such as occupational therapists while others have employed teachers and parents to work with the children. An example of the latter showed that a 16-week intervention of three to four times a week of 20–30 min duration produced gains in the majority of the 31 children. Moreover, after a 2-year period, half of the children had remained out of the category of DCD following intervention, while another quarter remained out during the intervention period but *a priori* it was not possible to predict which group the children would fit into. A final quarter was variable in their performance over time with two children seemingly not improving at all. It may be that these children required different intervention from specialists such as occupational therapists. The conclusion from this set of studies was that most children can be helped by non-specialists and that gains stayed with most of them, but that intervention should become a way of life, built into the routines of the family and should be low key over a long period of time. Comparisons with diet and losing weight and keeping it off are quite appropriate rather than a quick fix that will soon dissipate once the programme has stopped.[52,53]

The condition of DCD is not as yet identified as a constitutional disorder with an organic base and fixed abnormal symptoms. Children do acquire many of the skills that are necessary for activities of daily living, but they often acquire them slowly, do not reach high levels of competence and fail to acquire the ability to adapt them to new and novel situations. Future work examining the causality of the condition involving ideas from complex and dynamic systems is a possible way forward.

The children who are diagnosed as DCD do not form an homogeneous group, with some being severe and others having only mild symptoms; in addition, the nature of the disorder is not constant, some have problems in all motor activities while others are of a more specific variety such as poor balance and agility skills, or have problems with manual activities such as handwriting. There have been a few studies examining the intragroup characteristics of children with DCD by analysing the subgroups that emerge from factor and cluster analytic studies. These have generally found that children with DCD do have different profiles but currently there are not enough strong data to precisely determine the subtypes.[54–56]

Many studies have been carried out to determine differences in such areas as information processing between groups of children with DCD and those who have typical development. Some studies have found deficits in visual and kinaesthetic abilities while others have shown the central decision making capacity of children with DCD not to be as efficient as those in children with typical development. Most of our studies examining intergroup differences have concentrated on information processing paradigms, but suggestions from some researchers have led to investigations that have been more from a dynamic perspective.[57]

Although the core characteristic of children with DCD is that of movement difficulties, there is overlap with other conditions with many of the children identified as having DCD also possessing co-occurring characteristics. Over the past 15 years children with DCD have also been identified as having co-occurring conditions of reading and attention difficulties, social and emotional problems, and speech and language impairment. For example, Sweden Gillberg and his colleagues[58] have used the term DAMP (deficits in attention, motor, and perception) to describe some developmental disorders and within this category there was a 40% overlap between DCD and ADHD.

Summary

- The study of motor development has been seen to move away from phylogenetic and ontogenetic explanations and into a process-orientated approach, where self-organizing dynamic systems are tuned to the constraints of the environment and the resources of the mover, through individual action and perception. The growing child is regarded far more as an intricate part of the evolution and development of the relationship between affordance and developing motor skills, and definitely not simply a product of a predetermined genetic map.
- Motor development is starting to be seen as an integral part of overall development. It has been customary to view development as a series of changes in specific areas such as perception, cognition, social, language, and motor. Detailed descriptions are available in all of these areas.
- Using frameworks from ecological psychology and dynamical systems, it is now possible to take a holistic view. We have described how cognition is linked to motor actions through multiple inputs and how this in turn influences the next interaction the child has with the environment. Thus, one sense is changed and the child's reference point for their next action, thought or sense is also modified. It is a complex system.
- Recent work examining predictions of difficulties from early movements has implications not only for the early identification and hence early intervention of children with difficulties, but also for the understanding of typical development and how early signs are related to later behaviours.
- The utility of looking at holistic development is shown when we look at a specific motor difficulty such as children with developmental coordination disorder. This is a difficulty with motor problems at the core but in many of the cases there are co-occurring characteristics such as language difficulties, problems in attention, social and behavioural concerns, and academic difficulties. Thus, we are noting the importance of motor behaviour as an area in its own right but in addition the crucial contribution it makes along with other attributes to the total developing child.

References

1. Haywood KM, Getchell N (2001). *Life span motor development* (3rd ed.). Human Kinetics, Champaign, IL.
2. Keogh JF, Sugden DA (1985). *Movement skill development*. Macmillan, New York.

3. Newell KM (1986). Constraints on the development of coordination. In: Wade MG, Whiting HTA (eds.), *Motor development in children: Aspects of coordination and control*, pp. 341–60. Martinus Nijhoff, Dordrecht.
4. Connolly KJ, Elliott JM (1972). The evolution and ontogeny of hand function. In: Burton-Jones N (ed.), *Ethological studies of child behaviour*, pp. 329–83. Cambridge University Press, Cambridge.
5. Knobloch H, Pasamanick, B (1974). Gesell and Amatruda's developmental diagnosis: The evaluation and management of normal and abnormal neuropsychologic development in infancy and early childhood (3rd edition). Harper Row, New York.
6. van Roon D, van der Kamp J, Steenbergen B (2003). Constraints in children's learning to use spoons. In: Savelsbergh G, Davids K, van der Kamp J, Bennett S (eds.), *Development of movement co-ordination in children*, pp. 79–93. Routledge, London.
7. Burton AW, Rodgerson RW (2003). The development of throwing behaviour in children. In: Savelsbergh G, Davids K, van der Kamp J, Bennett S (eds.), *Development of movement co-ordination in children*, pp. 225–40. Routledge, London.
8. Keogh JF (1969). *Change in motor performance during early school years*. Technical Report No. 2–69, United States Public Health Service Grant HD 01059. Department of Physical Education, UCLA.
9. Rippee NE, Pangrazi RP, Corbin CB, Borsdorf L, Peterson G, Pangrazi D (1991). Throwing profiles of first and fourth grade boys and girls. *Phys Educ* **47**, 180–5.
10. Thomas JR (2000). Children's control, learning, and performance of motor skills. *Res Q Exerc Sport* **71**, 1–9.
11. Geary DC (1998). *Male, female: The evolution of human sex differences*. American Psychological Association, Washington, D.C.
12. Wilson FR (1998). *The hand: How its use shapes the brain, language and human culture*. Pantheon, New York.
13. Wild MR (1931). The behavior pattern of throwing and some observations concerning its development in children. *Res Quart* **9**, 2–24.
14. Langerdorfer SJ, Roberton MA (2000). Does the backswing limit development of differentiated trunk rotation in throwing? *J Sport Exerc Psychol* **22**, S67.
15. Sakurai S, Miyashita M (1983). Developmental aspects of overarm throwing related to age and sex. *Hum Mov Sci* **2**, 67–76.
16. Dennis W, Dennis M (1940). The effect of cradling practices upon the onset of walking in Hopi children. *J Genet Psychol* **56**, 77–86.
17. Shirley MM (1931). *The first two years: A study of twenty-five babies, Vol. 1: Postural and locomotor development*. University of Minnesota Press, Minneapolis, MN.
18. Peiper A (1963). *Cerebral function in infancy and childhood*. Consultants Bureau, New York.
19. McGraw MB (1935). *Growth: A study of Johnny and Jimmy*. Appleton-Century, New York.
20. McGraw MB (1943). *The neuromuscular maturation of the human infant*. Colombia University Press, New York.
21. Ulrich BD (1997). Dynamic systems theory and skill development in infants and children. In: Connolly KJ, Forssberg H (eds.), *Neurophysiology and neuropsychology of motor development*, pp. 319–45. Mackeith Press, London.
22. Piaget J (1952). *The origins of intelligence in children*. International Universities Press, New York.
23. Schmidt RA, Lee TD (2005). *Motor control and learning: A behavioral emphasis*. Human Kinetics, Champaign, IL.
24. Thelen E (1995). Motor development a new synthesis. *Am Psychol* **50**, 79–95.
25. Adolph KE, Eppler MA, Gibson EJ (1993). Crawling versus walking infants' perception of affordances for locomotion over sloping surfaces. *Child Dev* **64**, 1158–74.
26. Goldfield EC, Kay BA, Warren WH Jr (1993). Infant bouncing: The assembly and tuning of action systems. *Child Dev* **64**, 1128–42.
27. Jensen JI, Thelen E, Ulrich BD, Schneider K, Zernicke RF (1995). Adaptive dynamics of the leg movement patterns of human infants: III. Age-related differences in limb control. *J Motor Behav* **27**, 366–74.
28. Sporns O, Edelman GM (1993). Solving Bernstein's problem: A proposal for the development of coordinated movement by selection. *Child Dev* **64**, 960–81.
29. Stoffregen TA, Adolph K, Thelen E, Gorday KM, Sheng YY (1997). Toddlers' postural adaptations to different support surfaces. *J Motor Control* **1**, 119–37.
30. Turvey MT, Fitzpatrick P (1993). Commentary: Development of perception-action systems and general principles of pattern formation. *Child Dev* **64**, 1175–90.
31. Gibson JJ (1979). *The ecological approach to visual perception*. Houghton Mifflin, Boston, MA.
32. Gibson EJ (1982). The concept of affordances in development: The renaissance of functionalism. In: Collins WA (ed.), *The concept of development. Minnesota symposium on child psychology*, Vol. 15, pp. 55–81. Erlbaum, Hillsdale, NJ.
33. Gibson EJ, Walk RD (1960). The 'visual cliff'. *Sci Am* **202**, 64–71.
34. Bernstein N (1967). *The coordination and regulation of movements*. Pergamon, London.
35. Thelen E (1979). Rhythmical stereotypes in normal human infants. *Anim Behav* **27**, 699–715.
36. Thelen E, Bradshaw G, Ward JA (1981). Spontaneous kicking in month old infants: Manifestation of a human central locomotor program. *Behav Neural Biol* **32**, 45–53.
37. Zelazo P (1976). From reflexive to instrumental behavior. In: Lipsitt PL (ed.), *Developmental psychobiology: The significance of infancy*, pp. 87–106. Erlbaum, Hillsdale, NJ.
38. Thelen E, Fisher DM (1982). New-born stepping: An explanation for a 'disappearing reflex'. *Dev Psychol* **18**, 760–75.
39. Thelen E, Fisher DM (1983). The organization of spontaneous leg movements in new-born infants. *J Motor Behav* **15**, 353–77.
40. Thelen E (1994). Three-month-old infants can learn task-specific patterns of interlimb coordination. *Psychol Sci* **5**, 280–5.
41. Vereijken B, van Emmerik REA, Whiting HTA, Newell KM (1992). Free(z)ing degrees of freedom in skill acquisition. *J Motor Behav* **24**, 133–42.
42. Smith L, Gasser M (2005). The development of embedded cognition: Six lessons from babies. *Artif Life* **11**, 13–30.
43. Wilson M (2002). Six views of embodied cognition. *Psychon B Rev* **9**, 625–36.
44. Groen SE, de Blecourt ACE, Postema K, Hadders-Algra M (2005). General movements in early infancy predict neuromotor development at 9 to 12 years of age. *Dev Med Child Neurol* **47**, 731–8.
45. Hadders-Algra M, Groothuis AMC (1999). Quality of general movements in infancy is related to neurological dysfunction, ADHD, and aggressive behaviour. *Dev Med Child Neurol* **41**, 381–91.
46. Hadders-Algra M (2004). General movements: A window for early identification of children at high risk of developmental disorders. *J Pediatr* **145**, 12–18.
47. Sugden DA, Wright HC (1998). *Motor coordination disorders in children*. Sage, Thousand Oaks, CA.
48. Polatajko HJ, Fox AM, Missiuna C (1995). An international consensus on children with developmental coordination disorder. *Can J Occup Ther* **62**, 3–6.
49. Sugden DA (ed.) (2006). *Leeds consensus statement: Developmental coordination disorder as a specific learning difficulty*. DCD-UK/ Dyscovery Centre, Leeds.
50. American Psychiatric Association (2000). *DSM-IV-TR diagnostic and statistical manual of mental disorders*. American Psychiatric Association, Washington, D.C.

51. Cousins M, Smyth MM (2005). Progression and development in developmental coordination disorder. In: Sugden DA, Chambers ME (eds.), *Children with developmental coordination disorders*, pp. 119–33. Whurr, London.
52. Sugden D, Chambers ME (2003). Intervention in children with developmental coordination disorder: The role of parents and teachers. *Br J Educ Psychol* **73**, 545–61.
53. Sugden DA, Henderson SE. (2007). *Ecological intervention*. Harcourt Brace, London.
54. Wright HC, Sugden DA (1996). The nature of developmental coordination disorder: Inter and intra group differences. *Adapt Phys Act Quart* **13**, 358–74.
55. Dewey D, Kaplan BJ (1994). Subtyping of developmental motor deficits. *Dev Neuropsychol* **10**, 265–84.
56. Hoare D (1994). Subtypes of developmental coordination disorder. *Adapt Phys Act Quart* **11**, 158–69.
57. Geuze RH (2005). Cognitive explanations of the planning and organization of movement. In: Sugden DA, Chambers ME (eds.), *Children with developmental coordination disorders*, pp. 47–71. Whurr, London.
58. Gillberg K, Gillberg C, Groth J (1989). Children with preschool minor neurodevelopmental disorders. V: Neurodevelopmental profiles of age 13. *Dev Med Child & Neurol*, 31, 14–24.

CHAPTER 15

Muscle strength

Mark B. A. De Ste Croix

Introduction

Muscle strength is a multifaceted, performance-related fitness component, which is underpinned by muscular, neural, and mechanical factors. The complex interaction of these components makes the study of the increase in muscle strength during growth and maturation challenging. As strength is an essential component of most aspects of performance, it is surprising that we know little about the factors associated with strength development during childhood in comparison to other physiological variables. This may be attributed to the difficulty in measuring internal forces and the inherent methodological problems associated with determining external force. As there are no physiological markers to confirm that a maximal effort has been given, the methodology and assessment tool are critical in paediatric studies of muscle strength, as reviewed in Chapter 4.

Despite a relatively limited understanding of the factors associated with strength development, advances in equipment, and increased understanding of growth and maturation issues, have provided new insights into paediatric muscle strength development. Strength testing of children is performed routinely by researchers to monitor the determinants and development of strength throughout childhood, and also by physiotherapists to assess the degree of muscle disability and to diagnose the rate of recovery. It is important for strength test administrators to be equipped with knowledge of the normal age- and sex-associated variations in strength and the factors attributable to that variation. As described in Chapter 2, it is important that a size-free strength variable is used for interpretive purposes for comparisons to be made between individuals of different sizes. From a strength perspective, the key issue to be addressed when scaling for body size differences is the body size variable with which the performance variable is scaled [e.g. body mass, fat-free mass (FFM), or muscle cross-sectional area (mCSA)] and the method to be employed (e.g. ratio standard or allometric scaling). For a detailed review of adjusting for body size on strength variables, the reader is directed to the paper by Jaric.[1] Over time, the use of differing techniques to adjust for body size has changed our perspective of the historical concept of the age- and sex-associated differences in muscle strength. Likewise, the development of more sophisticated techniques to determine muscle size and body composition has allowed researchers to explore the factors associated with the development of strength during growth with a greater degree of validity.

Muscle growth

Jones and Round[2] suggested that childhood is a time when young people progressively become less physically dependent on their parents, until puberty when the young person equals or challenges the physical abilities of their parents. The growth of muscle mass and strength is central to this process. There are three main reasons for studying the growth of human muscle. First, as a matter of complementing previous work on the normal patterns of growth and increasing strength in children; second, to provide normative data with which the progress or potential of children whether they need to be trained, recover from an injury, or disabled can be judged; and third, because childhood offers the opportunity to observe muscle as it undergoes the unique process of rapid growth, development, and maturation.[2]

The maximum force producing capacity of a muscle is determined by the number of sarcomeres in parallel, that is, mCSA and not the number of sarcomeres in series, that is, length. Therefore, in the following discussion on muscle size measurement, it is the CSA aspect of muscle size rather than muscle volume that is of interest. Strictly speaking, maximal muscle force is proportional to the physiological CSA (pCSA), which is a function of the number of sarcomeres in parallel and the angle of pennation. Since the angle of pennation and therefore pCSA cannot easily be determined *in situ*, estimates of anatomical CSA (aCSA) have been most commonly used. A close relationship has been shown between the two areas as determined by ultrasound scanning[3] and computed tomography (CT)[4] of arm muscles. It should be recognized, however, that aCSA and pCSA will be more similar when the muscle in question is parallel fibred such as the biceps brachii and less similar in pennate muscles such as quadriceps femoris. Some authors have begun to determine the pCSA of muscle in adults using magnetic resonance imaging (MRI) and ultrasonography.[5] However, to date there appear to be no studies that have utilized these techniques to calculate pCSA in paediatric subjects. Therefore, when mCSA is referred to in this chapter we will be drawing upon studies examining aCSA rather than pCSA.

The origins of the diversity in muscularity in adults occur early in foetal development, approximately at the fifth week of gestation when some mesodermal cells differentiate into myoblasts. Most of the myoblasts fuse to form myotubes containing multiple nuclei that attach to the developing skeleton to form primordial muscles.

The primordia of most muscle groups are well defined by the end of the ninth week of gestation. The others stay as mononucleate cells that become the satellite cells of more mature muscle, responsible for muscle cell repair. Within the myotubes of primordial muscles, a chain of central nuclei forms and soon after the contractile proteins, actin and myosin, with their characteristic striations, are synthesized. From 11 to 18 weeks, hypertrophy of the muscles occurs due to both the multiplication of myofibrils and the addition of sarcomeres on to the ends of the muscle. By 23 weeks, the nuclei of mature myotubes have moved to the edges of the muscle cell.

At about 10 weeks of gestation, outgrowths from the spinal motor neurones begin to innervate the developing muscle fibres. What initially begins with multiple synapses ends up with only one neuromuscular junction, usually in the centre of the fibre. The fibre type or the contractile and metabolic characteristics are determined at this early stage since muscle is a slave to its innervation or electrical frequency of stimulation. Generally, about half of the developing fibres express slow myosin isoforms and the other half express fast isoforms. Muscle fibre differentiation usually occurs after about 32 weeks of gestation but is not fully complete until a few months after birth. The muscularity of an individual is reliant on the size and number of muscle fibres. The number of muscle fibres is due to the number of foetal myoblasts, with a significant genetic component. The question of whether increases in muscle size during growth are due to hypertrophy or hyperplasia has been difficult to answer *in situ* because of the ethics of muscle biopsy and also limitations of non-invasive imaging techniques. It is clear from cross-sectional studies of whole autopsied vastus lateralis muscle that despite wide interindividual variation, the average total number of fibres remains stable across age groups.[6] Therefore in normal growth and development, increases in mCSA are generally agreed to be due to increased fibre size or hypertrophy rather than cellular hyperplasia.

The quantification of mCSA has not only been used to investigate the role that muscle size may play in the age- and sex-associated development of strength but also to clinically evaluate growth and maturational states of children,[7] muscle wastage,[8] and the effect of interventions on muscle hypertrophy and atrophy.[9]

Determining muscle size—Measurement techniques

When measuring mCSA in children for research purposes, the technique used should be non-invasive with no potential side effects. Many studies with children have used anthropometric techniques to estimate mCSA because they are low cost, equipment is easily accessible and often easily portable, and measurement protocols take little time and manpower which is important if the number of subjects is large.[10,11] Every effort should be made to ensure accuracy and standardization of techniques and measurements should always be made by the same trained observers, especially if measurements are to be taken over time, in order to safeguard the validity and usefulness of the data.

At the simplest level coaches have been known to take circumference measurements alone to estimate mCSA but circumference measurements ignore the obvious fact that limb circumference is influenced by fat and bone cross-sections as well as muscle, such that a large circumference need not mean a large muscle. Efforts have been made to take into account the contribution of fatness to the circumference measurement by incorporating skinfold thickness into the equation.[12–14]

The technique described by Jones and Pearson[12] is the most widely used anthropometric technique for estimating thigh muscle volume plus bone in children although more recent equations by Housh *et al.*[10] for determining total mCSA plus bone have also become popular. The main problem with both of these techniques is that the regression equations have been derived from adult data and therefore cannot be confidently applied to children. Work exploring the reliability of the Jones and Pearson[12] technique in children, comparing the anthropometric technique to muscle volumes determined using MRI, found that the anthropometric technique underestimates lean thigh volume by 31% (range 14–46%).[15] Limits of agreement further support this conclusion by identifying a consistent bias towards an underestimation in total thigh volume.[15] Therefore, while anthropometric estimates may be valid for a 'snapshot' of mCSA plus bone or for characterizing various populations, they are not acceptable for monitoring changes over time[10] particularly in studies examining changes during growth and maturation.

Radiography is a technique which can potentially provide estimates of mCSA but due to the radiation exposure required to produce well-defined radiographs, ethical considerations mean this technique is generally unsuitable for use with healthy children. In any case, conventional radiographs depict a three-dimensional object as a two-dimensional image so that overlying and underlying tissues are superimposed on the image which makes determination of mCSA difficult.

Computerized tomography (CT) overcomes this problem by scanning thin slices of the body with a narrow x-ray beam which rotates around the body, producing an image of each slice as a cross-section of the body and showing each of the tissues in a thin slice. Unlike conventional radiography, CT can distinguish well between muscle, bone, and fat. However, children are particularly sensitive to radiation; therefore, this technique is contraindicated in paediatric populations (see Chapter 1).

Ikai and Fukunaga[3] made the first measurement of strength per mCSA using ultrasonography with children. The technique has also been applied in studies concerned with fibre pennation of the quadriceps muscle after training,[16] mCSA of the calf of the dominant leg of junior soccer players,[17] and the effect of strength training on upper arm mCSA of children.[18] Some of the major issues of ultrasonography include the difficulty in distinguishing tissue boundaries, the difficulty in determining individual muscles/muscle groups, and that images in obese subjects are not clear.

MRI is a technique that in recent years has offered exciting opportunities for the study of gross structure and metabolism of healthy and diseased muscle. With MRI, ethical constraints are avoided unlike CT and radiography. aCSA can be accurately measured by MRI, distinct muscle groups can be differentiated and it appears to be more suitable than other imaging techniques used for the examination of mCSA. With unparalleled picture clarity (Fig. 15.1), it is possible to differentiate individual muscle/muscle groups and identify both intramuscular fat and blood vessels.

By using an infrared mouse on a gridded mouse mat, it is possible to trace around relevant areas of interest to determine the CSA of different tissues. Despite the high cost numerous studies have recently used MRI with children and adolescents to determine muscle volume and mCSA.[19–24]

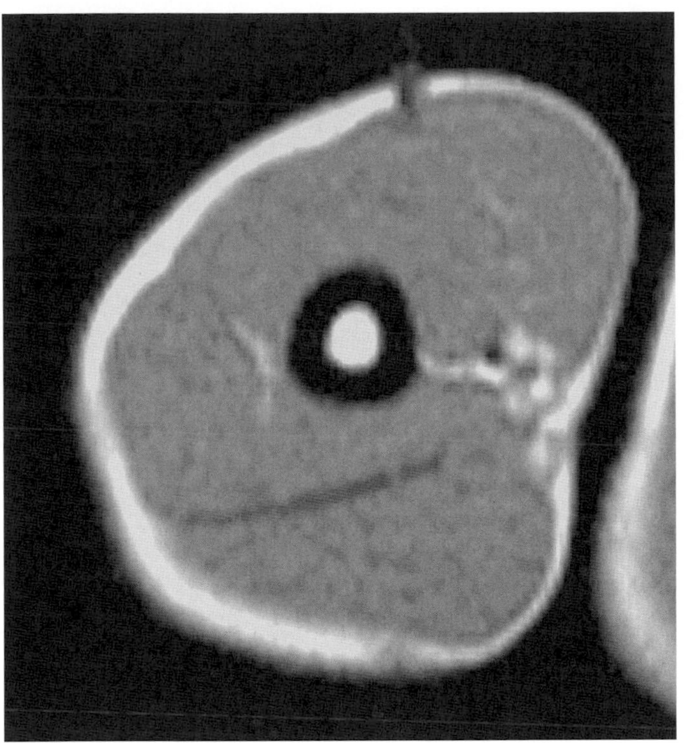

Fig. 15.1 MRI scan of the mid-upper arm of a 16-year-old male.

Site of mCSA measurement

A methodological problem with many previous studies of force or torque per mCSA with growth and maturation is that the optimal site for the measurement of maximum mCSA within and between subjects has not been clearly identified. Instead, an arbitrary location on the limb has been used for mCSA determination of mid femur in the case of thigh muscles and mid humerus in the elbow flexors and extensors.[11,24] Adult data suggest that for the knee extensors (KE), two thirds upper femur height and one third lower femur height for the knee flexors (KF) should be used as the site of maximal mCSA. However, whether this site is suitable for the growing child, when anatomical structures develop at differing rates, has been largely ignored until recently. De Ste Croix *et al.*[19] measured the maximal mCSA of each individual subject using MRI and found maximal thigh mCSA to occur between 51% and 69% of ascending femur length in 10–14 year olds. The same research group demonstrated that there are age differences in the MRI-determined location of maximal mCSA of the elbow extensors in 9 year olds, 16 year olds, and adults.[21] In order for age, sex, and muscle group comparisons to be made, an optimal site of mCSA needs to be individually determined for the paediatric population. Therefore, the site chosen to determine mCSA should be taken into account when interpreting the age- and sex-associated development in mCSA.

Age- and sex-associated development in mCSA

The CSAs of muscle fibres reach their maximal adult size by age 10 years in girls and 14 years in boys. Although muscle fibres appear to reach their maximal CSA early in childhood, this does not mean that muscle has reached its maximal length as muscle will continue to grow in length simultaneously with growth in limb length (LL) segments. For example, Round *et al.*[25] have proposed that testosterone may play an indirect role in the size of the muscle during growth by promoting development in the length of the humerus as part of the general development of the male upper limb girdle. They suggested that the increase of tension on the muscle from bone growth will in turn provide a stimulus for the muscle fibre to increase in size.

The Harpenden Growth study examined age and sex differences in radiographically determined upper arm and calf widths of British children from infancy to 18 years of age.[26] Boys' muscle widths appeared greater than those of girls during childhood but the difference was small. MRI studies have also found no significant sex difference in knee and elbow mCSA up until 13–14 years.[19,21] The Harpenden study observed that girls exhibited their adolescent spurt before the boys at age 11 years, at that time they had a temporary advantage in size in calf muscle width. Arm muscle width demonstrated less of a growth spurt in the girls so that the sex difference was only temporarily reduced. The sex difference was magnified when the boys underwent their adolescent spurt at the age of approximately 13 years. Boys' calf width eventually overtook that of the girls at about 15 years of age and both arm and calf width were still rising but at a slower rate at 18 years of age. In girls, both muscle widths peaked at 17 years and began to show a slight decrease by 18 years. The sex differences in muscle widths persisted into adulthood and were more apparent for musculature of the upper extremity. This has been supported in a large cross-sectional study using MRI which demonstrated a significant age effect in elbow mCSA up until 24 years.[21] These data indicate that from 9 to 24 years elbow extensor and flexor mCSA increase by 207% and 210% in males and 65% and 78% in females, respectively. Likewise, one of the few longitudinal studies examining sex differences in upper body mCSA showed non-significant differences in elbow extensor and flexor mCSA at 13 years but significant difference was observed 2 years later.[22] By adulthood, CT-determined muscle size showed that the mCSA of the arm and thigh of adult females was about 57% and 73%, respectively, that of adult males.[27] Changes in mCSA with age and sex, determined using MRI, are illustrated in Fig. 15.2.

Defining muscle strength

There are various definitions of muscle strength probably attributable to the numerous factors that interact to form the expression of strength. However, during dynamic movements we know that both concentric and eccentric muscle actions occur. Given the significance of these muscle actions in everyday life, investigations of age- and sex-associated strength development should consider concurrently the ability of the individual to perform both types of action. Underpinning the choice of muscle action to examine should be the activity or sport-specific component under investigation. For example, in sports where maximal strength is an important component it may be wise to assess children's strength at very slow velocities, on the basis of the force–velocity relationship. However, during activities where fast velocity movements are common it may be prudent to assess functional strength at faster velocities rather than maximal strength.

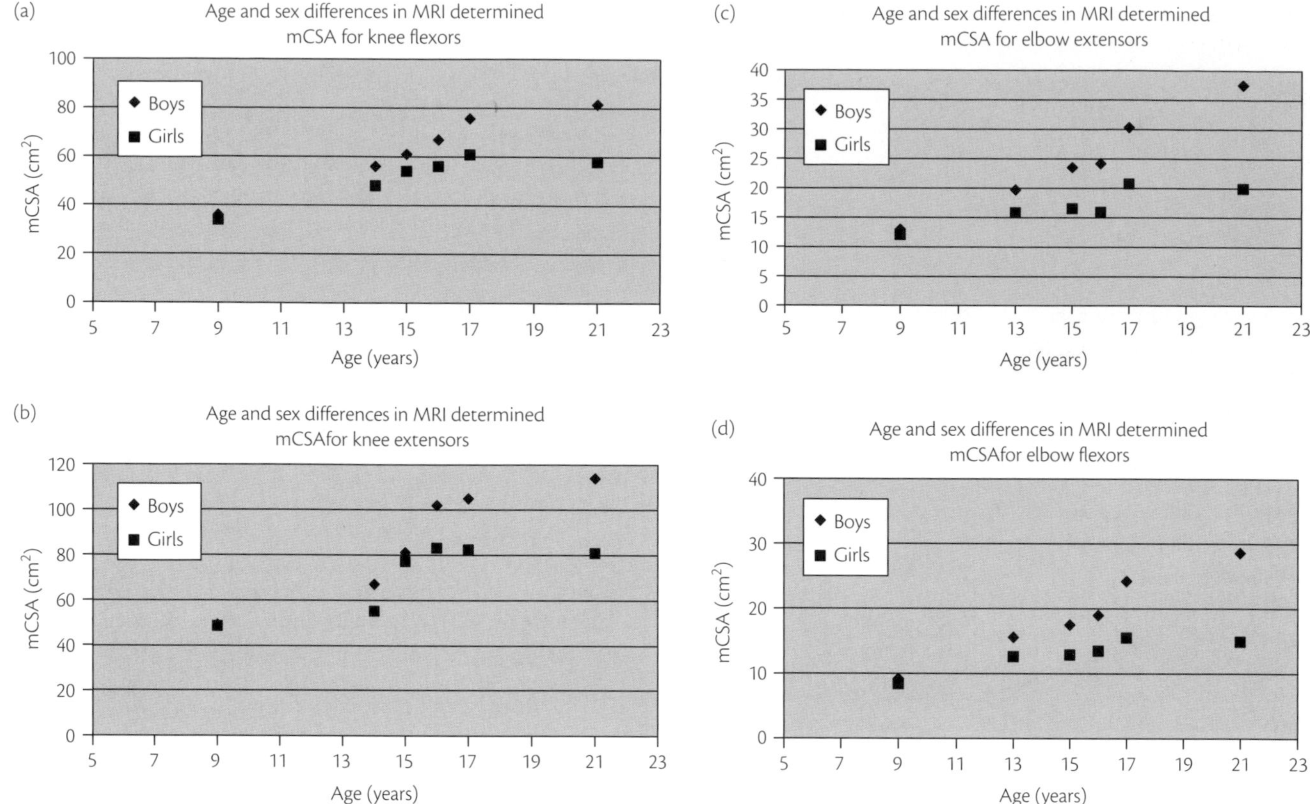

Fig. 15.2 Age- and sex-associated changes in MRI-determined muscle cross-section for the knee and elbow muscles. Data from De Ste Croix *et al.*,[19] Deighan *et al.*,[21] and Wood *et al.*[22]

Eccentric testing

As highlighted in Chapter 4, eccentric actions occur in everyday life as often as concentric actions. As such, the KE play a significant role in shock absorption during walking, running, and jumping and the KF play the role of a 'brake' as the knee extends during walking, kicking, and running. The range of commercial isokinetic dynamometers currently available has allowed the researcher to isolate eccentric muscle actions during a range of joint movements. Even though eccentric data on children are relatively sparse, the technological advances in isokinetic dynamometry have opened up avenues to explore the age- and sex-associated changes in eccentric muscle actions, as well as to examine the eccentric/concentric ratio to examine joint stability.[28,29]

Eccentric/concentric ratio and knee stability

The knee is a complex, multiaxial joint and the muscles around this joint play an important role in absorbing and transmitting large forces.[30] Adult studies have shown that the co-activation of the hamstrings work synergistically with the knee ligaments to assist joint stability and reduce the magnitude of net anterior shear.[31,32] Despite the important role that the knee muscles play in dynamic joint stability, very few studies have examined this role in the growing child.[28,29,33,34] Conventionally, the hamstring/quadriceps ratio is calculated by dividing the torque of KE and KF at identical angular velocity and contraction mode. However, previous authors have suggested that to evaluate muscular balance of the knee the eccentric/concentric actions of the KF and KE should be examined (ECC_{KF}/CON_{KE} or CON_{KF}/ECC_{KE} ratio) and referred to as a functional ratio rather than the conventional ratios often used (ECC_{KF}/CON_{KF} or ECC_{KE}/CON_{KE} ratio).[28,35] The examination of reciprocal muscle group ratios provides information on knee function, injury risk and, most importantly, knee joint stability.[28] One previous study that used conventional ratios of the knee demonstrated that an ECC/CON ratio of less than 60% at 1.04 rad·s^{-1} represents a 77.5% probability of knee injury in elite adult soccer players.[36] There appear to be no available data from functional ratios on relative risk of injury in children and non-elite performers.

As dictated by the force–velocity relationship, the ECC/CON ratio will increase as angular velocity increases[37,38] but if measured at one velocity it is possible to make comparisons of peak torque ratios between age groups and sexes. Meaningful interpretation of the ECC/CON ratio in relation to age and sex have been problematic due to the order of action cycling in an isokinetic protocol. For example, during ECC/CON cycles the ECC action may theoretically potentiate the following CON action.[39,40] Despite this concern, some authors have described the functional ECC/CON ratio using appropriate methods. It cannot be assumed that the relationship between CON and ECC actions is the same across ages during childhood and puberty because children may have immature neuromuscular systems due to the incomplete myelination of nerve fibres during childhood.[41] However, probably due to ethical issues surrounding invasive testing procedures, the neuromuscular system of children is poorly understood and requires further investigation.

Dvir[42] proposed that ECC_{KF}/CON_{KE} ratios derived from low/medium test velocities are typically within the range of 0.95–2.05 for healthy adults. The few studies that have measured the ECC/CON ratio in children have all found significantly higher ECC compared to CON strength[39,43–45] with ratios ranging from 1.17 at the slowest velocity to 1.47 at the highest velocity. However, in these studies, the ECC/CON ratio has been determined using ECC and CON KE strength rather than functional ratios. One study that used the functional ratio reported a non-significant age effect on functional ratios between 12- and 17-year-old trained male basketball players.[28]

Some studies have indicated that sex differences in adults in the conventional ECC/CON ratio of the knee joint are due to differences in percentage motor unit activation (%MUA) during maximal voluntary actions, with women having a lower %MUA than men during CON actions,[38,46] but not ECC actions, possibly because the actions have separate neural control mechanisms.[47] Others have suggested that the sex difference is due to a lower capacity for CON rather than a higher capacity for ECC force production in females.[48] There is contrary evidence, however, in the form of a superior ability of females compared to males in utilizing stored elastic energy in the muscle–tendon unit.[49] Hirohawa *et al.*[32] examined the age- and sex-associated changes in the functional ratio in prepubertal children, teenagers, and adults. In this study, females' functional ratio was significantly lower than males' at both slow and fast velocities and was a product of lower concentric torque as opposed to high eccentric torque producing capability. This is in conflict with previous data that suggested females have higher eccentric force producing capability compared to males. Adults demonstrated significantly lower CON_{KF}/ECC_{KE} than teenagers at 0.52 $rad{\cdot}s^{-1}$ and lower than the prepubertal and teenager groups at 3.14 $rad{\cdot}s^{-1}$. However, for ECC_{KF}/CON_{KE} at 3.14 $rad{\cdot}s^{-1}$ prepubertal ratios were significantly lower than teenagers and adults.[32] These data showed for the first time that during fast velocity movements, prepubertal children have a lower capacity for generating eccentric compared to concentric torque. The lower CON_{KF}/ECC_{KE} ratio in adults appears to be due to a greater ability to generate large eccentric torques during slow and fast movement velocities. Longitudinal data are needed to examine how the functional ratio changes through the pubertal years.

Interpretation of strength data

It has become common in the literature to express strength in absolute terms, with isometric data expressed in Newtons (N) and isokinetic data expressed in Newton metres (N·m). In the study of muscle strength in relation to growth and maturation, comparisons are made between individuals of different sizes. It is therefore important that a size-free strength variable is used for interpretive purposes. Current methods used for scaling for differences in body size are discussed in detail in Chapter 2.

The most commonly used technique in the strength literature to partition out differences in size is the ratio standard with body mass as the most widely used denominator. However, stature and FFM have also featured as covariates.[25,50] Others have used allometric scaling techniques to examine the theory that mCSA and strength are a function of the second power of stature.[51] The *b* exponents identified in the study of Kanehisa *et al.*[51] ranged from 2.4 to 3.6, which were significantly higher than the predicted 2.0 and the authors concluded that strength should be scaled to stature^3, or body mass.

Three longitudinal studies have used multilevel modelling to examine a number of known covariates to determine their influence on the age- and sex-associated changes in muscle strength.[19,22,25] Most authors currently support the view that suitable scaling factors should be derived from careful modelling of individual data sets, and therefore be sample specific rather than adopting assumed scaling indices.

Development of muscle strength: age- and sex-associated changes

Much of our early understanding of the age- and sex-associated development in strength was restricted to physical performance tests. Historically, field tests have been advocated as a measure of muscle strength, however, they must be viewed with caution as they frequently measure endurance rather than strength. Field tests tend to lack measurement sensitivity and often result in a high percentage of zero scores. As strength testing is dependent on motivation, field tests may not be sensitive enough to detect the more generalized gains in strength. A good example of this is the data presented in the National Child and Youth Fitness Study[52] in which 60% of girls aged 10–18 years failed to do one pull-up. As field tests require the resistance or movement of the individual's body mass it follows that children with a larger mass will be disadvantaged. Studies that have used pull-ups as the criterion measure for determining sex differences in muscle strength have therefore clouded our understanding of strength development during growth and maturation.

It is important to bear in mind that our understanding of the development of strength with age will be influenced by the nuances of the testing procedures used, such as subject positioning, degree of practice, level of motivation, lateral dominance, and level of understanding about the purpose and nature of the test.

When examining data relating to changes in strength due to growth and maturation, it is important to remember that the majority of data have been derived from isometric testing.[11,25,53–55] Children may not produce maximal force during isometric actions, and this has been attributed to inhibitory mechanisms that preclude children from giving a maximal effort due to a feeling of discomfort caused by the rapid development of force during isometric actions. Therefore, the whole motor pool may not be activated due to a reduction in the neural drive under high tension loading conditions.[56]

The literature on strength during childhood has been derived largely from cross-sectional studies as there are few longitudinal studies available. However, recent years have seen an increase in the number of longitudinal studies, which have focused predominantly on knee function,[19,24,25,57,58] but there are also studies on elbow strength[22,25] and back strength.[59,60] Others have used cross-sectional studies with large sample sizes, over a wide age range, to develop normative age-related data for strength development.[54,61]

Data from isometric actions indicate that in both boys and girls, strength increases in a fairly linear fashion from early childhood until the onset of puberty in boys and until about the end of the pubertal period in girls. The marked difference seen between boys and girls is a strength spurt in boys throughout the pubertal period, which is not evident in girls. Girls' strength appears to increase during puberty at a rate similar to that seen during the prepubertal phase and then appears to plateau postpuberty. There is some disagreement about the age at which sex differences become evident and this will be discussed in more detail later; however, although conflicting evidence is available it is generally agreed that before the male adolescent growth spurt there are considerable overlaps in strength values between boys and girls. By the age of 16–17 years few girls outperform boys in strength tests with boys demonstrating 54% more strength on average than girls (see Figs. 15.3 and 15.4).

Throughout childhood and puberty, particularly in males, isometric elbow flexor and KE strength are highly correlated with chronological age.[62] Although there are some data on the age-related changes in the KE and KF of children, the trends affecting these muscle groups are limited. In line with isometric data, most cross-sectional and longitudinal studies of changes in dynamic strength have demonstrated a significant increase with age.[19–22,24,57,58,61,63] For example, increases in males' and females' absolute KE (314% and 143%) and KF (285% and 131%) strength have been noted from 9 to 21 years of age.[63] A recent 11-year longitudinal study in healthy male soccer players, from 10 to 21 years, also showed large increases in absolute isokinetic knee extension (257%) and knee flexion (264%).[57]

Some studies have suggested that age exerts an independent effect on strength development over and above maturation and stature.[64] Others have indicated that even when mCSA is accounted for using a multilevel modelling procedure, age explains a significant amount of the additional variance for isometric elbow extensors.[22] It was suggested that this positive age term may be explained by the shared variance with maturation as maturation was not included in the model. However, another longitudinal data set, using multilevel modelling, suggested that age is a non-significant explanatory variable of isokinetic knee torque once stature and mass are accounted for.[19] This is probably attributable to differing rates of anatomical growth and maturation which vary independently and thus their effects on strength do not correlate simply with chronological age. It would appear that although there is a strong correlation between strength and age, a large portion of this association is probably attributable to the shared factors of biological and morphological growth rather than chronological age itself.[65]

There is little consensus about when sex differences in muscle strength become apparent. Some authors have suggested that sex differences in muscle strength are evident from as early as 3 years, or at least by 9–10 years.[24,66] Other studies have shown clear sex differences by 13–14 years.[11,62,67] A recent large cross-sectional study of 1140 boys and girls aged 9–17 years demonstrated that sex differences in absolute dynamic knee strength occur at 14 years.[61] This is further supported by a well-controlled longitudinal study, which used multilevel modelling to control for known covariates, and indicated that there are no sex differences in dynamic strength up until the age of 14 years.[19] After 14 years boys outperform girls in muscle strength irrespective of the muscle action examined even with body size accounted for. It is important at this point to remind ourselves that factors relating to biological growth and maturation probably play a key role in the factors behind the timing of sex differences in strength development. For example, some authors have attributed the non-significant sex difference observed at 13–14 years to earlier biological maturation in girls, and the associated neural maturation that accompanies biological maturation.[19,25] However, as little is known about neural maturation it is probably more likely that the well-recognized relationship between

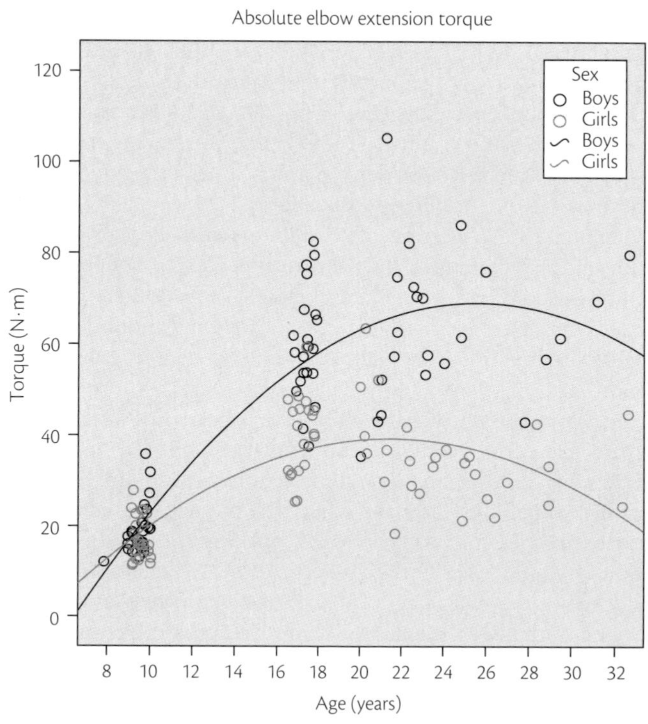

Fig. 15.3 Absolute peak elbow extension torque by age and sex. Data from Deighan *et al.*[77]

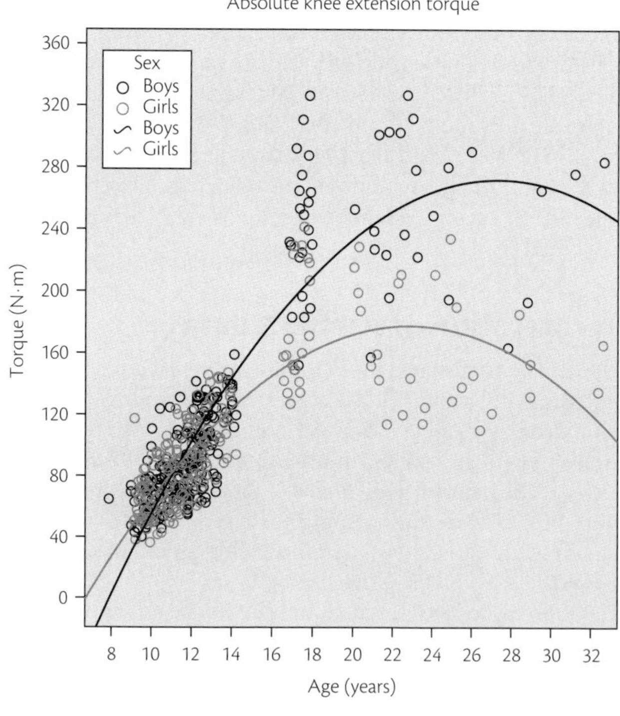

Fig. 15.4 Absolute knee extension torque by age and sex. Data from De Ste Croix *et al.*[19] and Deighan *et al.*[20,77]

peak strength velocity (PSV) and peak height velocity (PHV) play a key role in sex differences. As can be seen in Fig. 15.5, PSV occurs about a year after PHV at about 11.4–12.2 years in girls and 13.4–14.4 years in boys.

Therefore, 13- to 14-year-old girls are more likely to have benefited from peak strength gains while boys are still in the PHV phase and will have not experienced a strength spurt. In addition, there is evidence that PSV, in boys at least, lags behind peak gains in muscle mass velocity by 0.4 year and thus boys do not gain an advantage in strength, based on the growth in muscle size, until about 15 years of age.[68]

Isometric data indicate that sex differences in strength are relatively greater in muscles of the upper body compared to the lower body in children. Gilliam *et al.*[66] reported no significant sex difference in 15–17 year olds' knee extension peak torque but sex differences were apparent for the elbow extensors. This has been attributed to the weight-bearing role of the leg muscle. It has also been suggested that during growth and maturation boys use their upper body more than girls through habitual physical activities (such as climbing). This sociocultural explanation has recently been brought into doubt as there is no overlap in strength between sexes as would be expected with physically active girls and sedentary boys if this contention was true.[25] A recent longitudinal study also demonstrated that sex differences are apparent in elbow flexion and extension from 13 to 15 years, even when stature and arm length are accounted for. However, when mCSA was accounted for, sex differences disappeared, leading the authors to conclude that the use of linear dimensions to account for sex differences in upper body strength has clouded our understanding. Thus, caution must be exercised when describing sex-associated differences in upper and lower body strength during childhood.

Determinants of strength development

Many factors have been associated with the age- and sex-associated development in muscle strength but the complex interaction of these factors remains challenging to identify. There are few longitudinal studies of strength development that have spanned early childhood to adulthood and examined these variables concurrently using appropriate scaling methods.

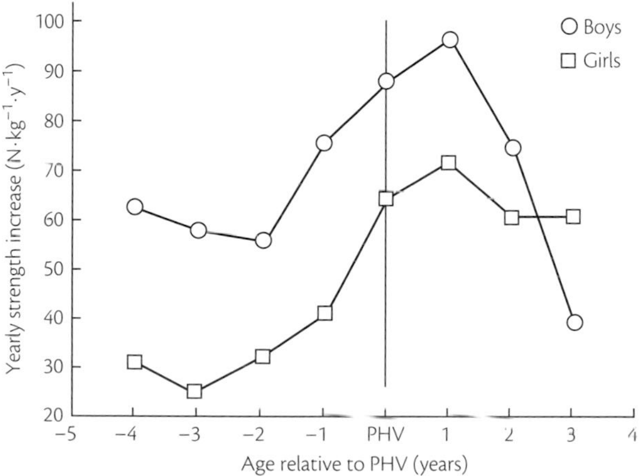

Fig. 15.5 Peak strength velocity in relation to peak height velocity by sex. Adapted from Froberg and Lammert,[87] with permission.

Stature, mass, and strength development

The influence of gross body size on strength development has been examined in several studies. Stature and mass are traditionally the size variables of choice because they can be quickly and easily measured. Early longitudinal studies reported that isometric strength per body mass varied only slightly during childhood and through puberty in girls.[52,69] Whereas from the time of boys' PHV (i.e. about age 14 years), an increase in strength per body mass in boys which was still increasing by age 18 years was demonstrated.[69]

Body mass has been found to be highly correlated with maximal voluntary isometric strength of elbow flexors and KE in males aged 9–18 years.[62] Figure 15.6 demonstrates the strong positive correlation between isokinetic knee and elbow extension torque and body mass in 7- to 32-year-old males and females.

However, age-specific correlation coefficients between strength and body mass for males are generally low to moderate during the mid-childhood years, then increase and peak during puberty, and abate in the late teens.[70] Data on this relationship are sparse for females but moderate positive coefficients between strength and body mass for females during the prepubertal years and at the onset of puberty and low correlations at the end of puberty and during puberty have been reported.[69,70] Others have found the relationship between female strength and body mass to be high during the teen years and to decline during young adulthood.[63] When related to shorter periods of growth (in which the range of anthropometric variables is small), correlations become weaker. This reliance of the correlation coefficient on the characteristics of the sample shows that comparison of correlation coefficients between studies should be undertaken cautiously. It is worth noting here that when isokinetic knee extension and flexion torque were adjusted for body mass using the ratio standard the rate of change in strength between 9

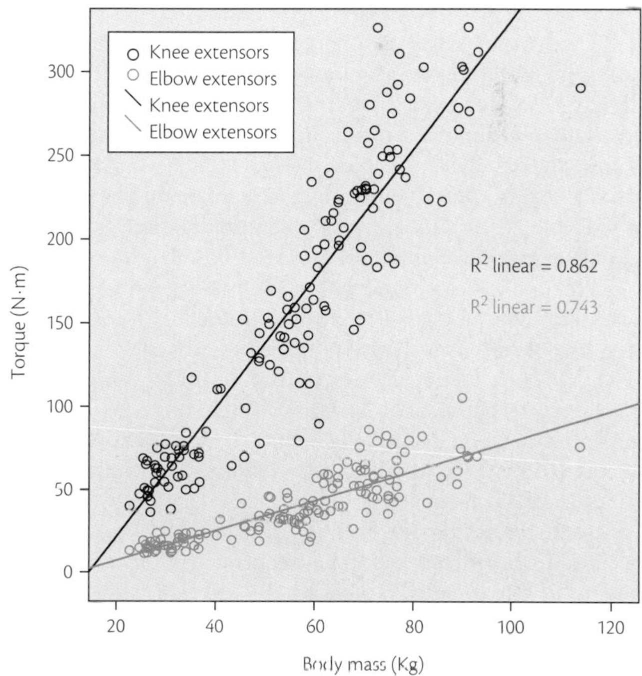

Fig. 15.6 Relationship between knee and elbow extension torque and body mass. Data from Deighan *et al.*[20,77]

and 21 years was underestimated compared to mass-adjusted data using allometric techniques.[63]

Three recent longitudinal studies, one examining isometric strength and two examining isokinetic strength, have used multilevel modelling to examine the influence of stature and body mass on strength development. Round *et al.*[25] reported that isometric KE strength in girls increased in proportion to the increase in stature and mass in 8–13 year olds. De Ste Croix *et al.*[19] also demonstrated that stature and mass are significant explanatory variables of isokinetic knee extension and flexion torque in 10–14 year olds. This was further reinforced by Wood *et al.*[22] who demonstrated a significant influence of stature on the development of isometric and isokinetic elbow flexion and extension on 13–15 year olds. Conflicting data are available and the study of Round *et al.*[25] suggested that in boys the strength of the KE was disproportionate to the increase in body size. This difference was explained once testosterone was added to the multilevel model.

Although both stature and mass appear to be important explanatory variables of the age- and sex-associated development in strength, it may be the simultaneous development of other biological factors that are contributing to this increase. For example, it has been postulated that the linear increase in bone with age produces a stimulus for muscle growth and therefore increases in stature with age are associated with increases in muscle size. Similarly, the changes in proportions of body fat and lean tissue, as a percentage of total body mass, are important factors in the expression of strength with age. Therefore, although simple body dimensions appear to be important in the development of strength with age only between 40% and 70% of the variance in strength of 5- to 17-year-old children could be accounted for by age, sex, stature, and body mass, which leaves a large portion of the variance unexplained.[62]

Maturation and hormonal influences on strength development

De Ste Croix *et al.*'s[19] longitudinal study of 10–14 year olds indicated that maturation was a non-significant explanatory variable in the development of isokinetic knee extension and flexion, once stature and mass were accounted for. However, the authors acknowledged that their sample consisted of a narrow range of maturational stages. Nevertheless, supporting data on young athletes are available, with studies reporting that maturation did not exert an independent effect upon isometric strength development in 10- to 18-year-old athletes[64] and 12- to 14-year-old football players[71] once age and body size had been controlled for.

An important consideration regarding the development of muscle function is the effect of endocrine adaptations typical of sexual maturation such as increased levels of testosterone and growth hormone (GH). There is both direct and indirect evidence to demonstrate the association between testosterone and strength development during puberty.

Testosterone has been shown to stimulate anabolic processes in skeletal muscle and appears to be the principal hormone responsible for the development of strength. Round *et al.*[25] proposed that testosterone accounts for the sex difference existing in isometric strength even after making allowances for body size. They observed that there was an increase of 0.7% in isometric knee extension strength for every unit of circulating testosterone ($nmol \cdot L^{-1}$). The analysis showed that the young men in the sample were 15–20% stronger as a result of the testosterone than might be expected from their overall body stature. In contrast, the same analysis for biceps showed that sex differences could not be fully accounted for by the effects of testosterone in teenage boys. These authors speculated that the linear measure inserted into the model for biceps should be humerus length as opposed to stature. Their plausible suggestion was based on the well-known increase in the upper limb girdle dimensions in boys during puberty that provides an additional stimulus for muscle growth with the direct action of testosterone in the muscle. Jones and Round[2] indicated that increasing levels of oestrogen in girls causes inhibition of muscle growth as a result of a speedier skeletal maturation, which removes the lengthening stimulus for muscle growth.

Ramos *et al.*[72] also reported that body mass did not eliminate the age effect in isokinetic peak torque in boys. Testosterone increased with age in boys but not in girls and this increase in testosterone preceded the gains in muscle strength but perhaps more importantly there was a moderate positive correlation ($r = 0.64$) between serum testosterone and isokinetic angle specific torque. Although conflicting data are available it may be the role that testosterone plays in increasing muscle size that is important in examining the relationship between circulating hormones and muscle strength in the growing child. Well-controlled longitudinal studies that concurrently examine testosterone and maturation, alongside other known variables, are still needed before firm conclusions about the independent influence of maturation on strength development can be established.

Fat free mass and strength development

Typically, during childhood and adolescence, strength increases coinciding with changes in FFM.[62] Moderate to strong correlations have been found between knee extension and flexion torque and FFM in 8- to 13-year-old wrestlers.[73] However, some studies have reported age-related increases in torque per FFM for KE and elbow extensors and flexors that could not be accounted for by changes in FFM.[74,75] The age effect for increases in strength, independent of FFM, may be attributable to an increase in muscle mass per unit of FFM or neural maturation which allows for a greater expression of strength. The proportion of FFM, which is skeletal muscle, has been suggested to increase with age. In addition, the proportion of muscle mass that is distributed at various sites is thought to vary and at birth approximately 40% of total muscle mass is located in the lower extremities, increasing to approximately 55% at sexual maturity in both boys and girls.

Studies that have used anthropometric estimations of total body muscle mass have reported that estimated total body muscle mass cannot account for the age-related increase in strength and that non-significant correlations exist between age and estimated muscle mass co-varied for FFM.[73] This suggests that there are nearly proportional increases in total body muscle mass and FFM across age and that age-related increases in strength are not due to an increase in muscle mass per unit of FFM. It is possible that the anthropometric equations in these studies were not sensitive enough to detect a change across age in the contribution of muscle mass to FFM.

If conclusions are made about the factors affecting strength development based on age- or sex-related differences in strength per FFM, then the assumption must be that a muscle or muscle group mCSA is always the same proportion of FFM across ages and between sexes. It may be that regional mCSA increases from prepuberty to postpuberty at the same rate as FFM and not that total muscle mass increases at the same rate as FFM. This has led most researchers to bypass FFM and investigate changes in mCSA as the key variable in the age- and sex-associated development in strength.

Strength development and muscle cross-sectional area

There are considerable data that support the contention that differences in muscle size account for differences in muscle strength during growth. One of the earliest studies examined the relationship between isometric elbow flexion strength and mCSA determined by ultrasonography in 12–29 year olds.[3] Although correlation coefficients were not reported, the authors indicated that strength 'is fairly proportional' to elbow flexor mCSA regardless of age or training status. The relationship appeared weaker for girls than boys. Others have reported a strong positive correlation between muscle size, and isometric knee strength ($r = 0.87$), isokinetic knee strength ($r = 0.73$), isokinetic elbow strength ($r = 0.82$), and isokinetic triceps surae strength ($r = 0.91$).[10,11,51,76] In addition, based on children's grip strength data, the sex-related growth curve patterns for body muscle are virtually identical to those for strength, suggesting a strong association between muscle growth and gains in strength. Numerous longitudinal studies have shown that as an independent covariate mCSA is a significant explanatory variable in the age-associated development in strength.[19,22] However, as we will go on to discuss, it would appear that when additional variables are examined concurrently alongside mCSA its influence lessens or disappears.

Age differences in strength per muscle cross-sectional area

There is still some debate about whether strength per mCSA increases with age. Early studies demonstrated increasing strength per mCSA from age 7 to 13 years. Also, Kanehisa *et al.*[51] suggested that isokinetic strength per mCSA, measured using ultrasonography, was greater in older age groups (18 years) than in younger age groups (7 years) in every muscle group measured. It was hypothesized that children in the early stages of puberty may not develop strength in proportion to their muscle aCSA. It is likely that the deficiency of strength per mCSA in the younger age groups is related to a lack of ability to mobilize the muscle voluntarily. The same authors found that the isometric strength of the ankle dorsi flexors and plantar flexors per mCSA measured by ultrasonography in boys and girls aged 7–18 years was significantly greater only for plantar flexion in 16- to 18-year-old boys compared to the other groups. In a cross-sectional study, Deighan *et al.*[20,77] have reported a significant increase in isokinetic knee and elbow torque per MRI-determined mCSA from 9 to 16 years but no significant difference from 16 to 24 years. Further investigation is required to establish whether these differences in torque per mCSA are due to biomechanical or neuromuscular factors. What these data do suggest is that torque per mCSA of the elbow and KE and KF are at adult levels by 16 years. Conflicting data are available indicating that, despite smaller MRI-determined triceps surae mCSA, early pubertal boys torque scaled to muscle size is not different from adult males.[78] These conflicting data emphasize the need to measure the strength per mCSA ratio in a variety of muscles as the strength development characteristics of one muscle or group of muscles may not be the same as another, even within the same joint.

Sex differences in strength per muscle cross-sectional area

Whether sex differences exist in strength per mCSA is debatable. Early work reported that absolute isometric strength differences between sexes disappeared when data were normalized to anthropometric muscle (plus bone) CSA in 9–12 year olds. Sunnegardh *et al.*[11] showed that boys had significantly greater torque per CSA than girls at age 13 years. Deighan *et al.*[77] recently reported significant sex differences in isokinetic elbow flexion per mCSA in 9–10 year olds and 16–17 year olds. These studies are in contrast to others that have demonstrated similar strength to mCSA ratios between sexes.[3,22] Deighan *et al.*[20,77] reported no significant sex differences in isokinetic torque per mCSA of the KE and KF and elbow flexors in 9–10 year olds, 16–17 year olds, and adults. Using multilevel modelling procedures on longitudinal data, Wood *et al.*[22] also reported that sex effects for isokinetic elbow extensors and flexors became non-significant once mCSA was controlled for. The majority of recent studies would lead us therefore to the conclusion that there is no significant sex difference in strength per mCSA irrespective of the muscle joint or action examined. It would appear that factors in addition to mCSA may account for the age- and sex-associated development in strength.

For example, the peak gain in muscle strength in boys occurs more often after peak stature and mCSA velocity but there is no such trend for girls. Therefore, particularly in boys there may be factors other than mCSA that affect strength expression during puberty. It has been shown that the sex differences that occur in the strength of boys and girls of the same stature cannot be accounted for by muscle size alone. A longitudinal study of upper arm area and elbow flexor strength has shown that boys have muscles approximately 5% greater in area but which produce approximately 12% more strength.[22] Others have indicated that mCSA is a non-significant explanatory variable once stature and mass are accounted for.[19]

Consequently, this would seem to suggest either a biomechanical effect or a qualitative change in muscle tissue as puberty progresses and perhaps a neuromuscular maturation affecting the volitional demonstration of strength.

Biomechanical factors and strength development

The mechanical advantage of the musculoskeletal system is variable across different muscle groups and is considered unfavourable because the measured force or torque is somewhat smaller than the corresponding tension developed in the muscle tendon. Another unfavourable biomechanical influence on the measured force lies in the internal muscle architecture, that is, the greater the angle of pennation to the long axis of the muscle the smaller proportion of force in the muscle fibres that is transmitted to the muscle tendon. The age-associated relationships between these factors have not yet been extensively investigated in children.

It is probable that small differences between subjects in the location of the centre of rotation of the joint or in the length of the lower limb could contribute to the observed variability in the ratio of muscle strength to mCSA. It is difficult to account for biomechanical factors but some authors have divided strength values by the product of mCSA and stature (Nm·cm^{-3}), that is, the product of mCSA and possible differences in moment arm length or mechanical advantage which they assumed to be proportional to stature.[20,76,77] There are few published data on the relationship between strength per mCSA and mechanical advantage covering different age groups, both sexes and different muscle groups but it seems sensible to correct strength for possible differences in mechanical advantage, especially if comparing children of different sizes by normalizing to mCSA*LL.[79] One of the major assumptions with using this method is that muscle moment arm and LL are proportional to one another.

Kanehisa *et al.*[76] found that isokinetic torque was significantly correlated to mCSA*thigh length ($r = 0.72–0.83$). These data suggest that at least part of the age-associated variability in voluntary strength may be attributed to differences in mechanical advantage that occur with growth.

Blimkie[62] reported that age effects were the same whether dividing torque by the product of mCSA and stature or just mCSA. Young adults have been found to have significantly higher ratios of isokinetic knee extension torque per unit of mCSA*thigh length than children with the difference becoming greater with increasing velocity of movement. Deighan *et al.*[20,77] proposed that the influence of mechanical advantage on the development of isokinetic strength may be muscle group specific. Data showed a non-significant age effect for the elbow extensors and flexors but a significant difference between 9–10 year olds and 16–17 year olds in knee extension and flexion torque per mCSA*LL. The knee data suggested that mCSA*LL alone cannot account for the age differences in strength. It is difficult to attribute physiological reasons to the muscle group differences but it is possible that part of the explanation may lie in the differing function of the arms and legs. For example, there is some evidence to suggest that the extent of MUA of the arm muscles remains essentially unchanged with growth but increases in the muscles of the thigh.[80]

Early work indicated that sex differences in absolute torque remained statistically significant, although diminished, when expressed per unit mCSA*thigh length. Kanehisa *et al.*[76] reported no significant sex differences in young children but that sex differences became apparent in adulthood when expressing torque per mCSA*LL. Deighan *et al.*[20,77] reported non-significant sex differences for the knee and elbow extensors and flexors in torque per mCSA*LL in 9–10 year olds, 16–17 year olds, and adults. Recent data therefore suggest that sex differences, at least for dynamic strength, can be accounted for by the product of mCSA and LL. Further investigation is needed to examine whether this pattern remains in relation to isometric strength.

There has been speculation that the angle of muscle pennation plays a role in the group differences in strength per mCSA.[62] Conventional scanning techniques all measure mCSA at right angles to the limb, that is, anatomical mCSA. However, the maximum force a whole muscle or muscle group can produce is a function of the tension generated by each individual fibre in the direction of the muscle's line of pull. Therefore, physiological mCSA is thought to be a better predictor of force producing capacity than anatomical mCSA. However, true physiological mCSA cannot easily be determined *in vivo* and to date there are no paediatric studies that have examined physiological mCSA.

Neuromuscular factors and strength development

Some authors who have not fully accounted for the age- and sex-associated changes in muscle strength by controlling for muscle size have suggested that possible changes in neural maturation may account for the difference. However, it is generally unclear about what these authors mean by 'neural maturation', which is supposed to accompany sexual maturation. Asmussen[81] has suggested that maturation of the central nervous system (CNS) with age can improve static and dynamic motor skill performance; however, the mechanisms by which CNS maturation may influence strength development remains unclear.

We know that measured voluntary strength depends highly on the degree of %MUA. The ideal way to measure the contractile capacity of a muscle is to record the force developed during supramaximal electrical stimulation of the nerve innervating the muscle. When an electrical stimulus is applied to a motor nerve near the muscle, the resultant muscle force is free of any inhibitory influence from above the point of stimulation. On the other hand, force or torque measured during a voluntary action is the result of neuromuscular influences from the brain and inhibitory reflex influences from the spinal cord in addition to the maximum force producing capacity of the muscle. The results of tetanic electrical stimulation may not be comparable to voluntary muscle actions, since in the former method synergistic muscles may not be excited and the procedure is very painful leading to reduced compliance and, with child as subjects, ethical concerns.

Owing to these problems with tetanic stimuli of children's muscles, most studies that have investigated maximum force producing capacity in children have used twitch stimuli because various properties of an electrically evoked twitch reveal information about intrinsic muscle properties and %MUA. Assuming that %MUA stays constant with age, then the ratio of evoked twitch force to voluntary force should stay constant with age. On the basis of this assumption, Davies[82] measured both evoked twitch force and maximum voluntary force in groups of 9-, 11-, 14-, and 21-year-old males and females. The twitch torque/voluntary torque ratio of the triceps surae was similar in boys and girls aged 9 years but it gradually decreased with age in the males. However, no conclusion of a greater %MUA with increasing age in boys could be made because there was also a change in the twitch to evoked tetanus ratio with increasing age. On examination of the tetanic/voluntary ratio it appeared that %MUA may vary with age but not sex. The possibility that an inability to fully recruit the available motor unit pool may be reflected in smaller strength per mCSA scores in children than in adults has not been extensively investigated.

Blimkie[62] used the interpolated twitch technique (ITT) on maximum voluntary isometric actions of the elbow extensors and KF and reported that %MUA of the KE increased with age in boys from 77.7% to 95.3% over the age range 10–16 years, an increase in %MUA of 17.6%. A different pattern was found for the elbow flexors whose respective values at 10 and 16 years were 89.4% and 89.9%, indicating no change in the %MUA of elbow flexors. No studies appear to have investigated this phenomenon in females and thus explanations for sex differences in %MUA in children remain to be identified.

In adults, a sex difference has been demonstrated in the rate of force development which is an important factor for dynamic muscle actions in which there is limited time to generate force. Recent data examining isokinetic time to reach peak torque suggest that there are non-significant sex differences in the knee and elbow extensor and flexor muscles.[83] In the same study, age-related changes in time to peak torque were muscle group and muscle action specific leading the authors to the conclusion that care must be taken when making assumptions on differing muscle groups and muscle actions.

Time to peak twitch torque and twitch relaxation indices can be used as a measure of rate of energy turnover and fibre type composition. Twitch relaxation times have been shown to be similar in boys and girls and are not influenced by age. Also, it has been found that time to peak twitch force and relaxation times were the same regardless of age during childhood.[84] Likewise, similar time to peak twitch tension was demonstrated in 3 year olds as in 25 year olds. These data suggest that muscle fibre composition and muscle activation speed are similar between these age groups and that there is no difference in the fibre type distribution from the age of about 7 years. Previous authors have suggested that the neuromuscular system is still maturing with respect to the myelination of the nerves in younger children.[85] Also muscle fibre conduction velocity has been seen to increase with age in children. The influence that neuromuscular factors have on the development of muscle strength, concurrently with other known variables, remains to be established.

Conclusions

There is a clear need for further longitudinal investigation into the static and dynamic development of muscle strength through childhood and adolescence into adulthood. The major difficulty in describing the age- and sex-associated development in strength is that much of the current data reveal muscle group and muscle action specific differences in the relationships described. For example, the factors responsible for the development of isokinetic eccentric elbow flexion may be different from isometric knee extension. Despite this, the age-associated development of strength is reasonably consistent, irrespective of the muscle group or action examined. There is slight disagreement about when sex differences occur. Importantly, many of the factors discussed in this chapter play a role in strength development when examined as independent variables.

It would appear that for dynamic muscle actions in particular that mechanical factors may play a large role in the development of muscle torque and accurate investigation of the muscle moment arm, employing MRI techniques, would provide us with a clearer picture of the age- and sex-associated development. The greatest challenge is to elucidate the factors that contribute to the age- and sex-associated development in strength concurrently with other known explanatory variables.

Future directions

There are still unexplained factors that may contribute to the age- and sex associated development in strength. We know relatively little about muscle fibre types in children, probably due to the invasive nature of muscle biopsies (see Chapter 16) and the associated ethics that preclude the use of such techniques with paediatric subjects (see Chapter 1). There has been some tentative exploration into the use of MRI to determine fibre type in adults[85] but this technique has not been validated for use with children and requires further investigation. Researchers are turning to new technologies to advance our understanding of the mechanisms that contribute to the development of force. For example, studies with adults have used ultrasonography and muscle pennation angle[5] to calculate pCSA. Other studies of adults have begun assessing muscle–tendon stiffness using ultrasonography[86] but as yet there appear to be no longitudinal studies that have examined the age- and sex-associated changes in muscle–tendon stiffness in children.

There is no doubt that development in techniques to measure muscle forces (e.g. isokinetic dynamometers), muscle size (MRI), and newer techniques for controlling for differences in body size (allometric scaling and multilevel modelling) have contributed to greater understanding of the age- and sex-associated development in strength. However, there is still much we do not know and continuing advances and access to sophisticated technologies, for example, Dual energy X-ray absorptiometry (DEXA), MRI, and ultrasonography, may elucidate new thoughts in this area over the coming decade.

Summary

- Measurement of muscle size in children using anthropometric techniques underestimates muscle volume by 31%.
- There are overlaps in muscle size in boys and girls up until the ages of 13–14 years when boys demonstrate a spurt in muscle size. Girls' muscle size increases at a slower rate up until about 17 years when it plateaus. Boys' muscle growth continues into the mid-20s.
- There are distinct differences in static and dynamic strength characteristics in children which must be acknowledged when examining age- and sex-associated changes in strength.
- Functional ECC/CON ratio is important for knee stability and should be investigated longitudinally through the pubertal years.
- The age-associated development in strength is attributable to the shared variance in growth and maturation. Sex differences appear at around 14 years and very few girls outperform boys in strength tests at 18 years.
- The age- and sex-associated development in muscle strength, combined with the factors that contribute to this development appear to be muscle group and muscle action specific.
- Stature and mass appear to be important explanatory variables in the development of muscle strength. Peak height velocity is a particularly important time for maximal gains in strength during childhood.
- Sexual maturation has not been shown to exert an influence on strength development once body size is controlled for but circulating hormones, such as testosterone stimulate development in muscle size.
- Muscle CSA exerts an independent effect on strength development but is a non-significant explanatory variable once body size is accounted for.
- The muscle moment arm is possibly the most important factor in the development of muscle strength with age but further longitudinal studies using MRI are needed.
- Neuromuscular maturation is poorly understood but may contribute to the improvement in motor unit activation with age.
- The influence of physiological CSA and tendon stiffness need to be investigated as explanatory factors in the age- and sex-associated development of strength.

References

1. Jaric S (2002). Muscle strength testing: Use of normalisation for body size. *Sports Med* **32**, 615–31.
2. Jones DA, Round JM (2000). Strength and muscle growth. In: Armstrong N, Van Mechelen W (eds.), *Paediatric exercise science and medicine*, pp. 133–42. Oxford University Press, Oxford.
3. Ikai M, Fukunaga T (1968). Calculation of muscle strength per unit cross-sectional area of human muscle by means of ultrasonic measurement. *Int Z Angew Physiol Einschl Arbeitsphysiol* **26**, 26–32.
4. Schantz P, Randal-Fox E, Hutchinson W, Tyden A, Astrand PO (1983). Muscle fibre distribution, muscle cross-sectional area and maximal voluntary strength in humans. *Acta Physiol Scand* **117**, 219–26.
5. Maganaris CN, Baltzopoulos V, Ball D, Sargeant AJ (2001). *In vivo* specific tension of human skeletal muscle. *J Appl Physiol* **90**, 865–72.
6. Lexell J, Sjostrum M, Nordlund A, Taylor CC (1992). Growth and development of human muscle: Morphological study of whole vastus lateralis from childhood to adult age. *Muscle Nerve* **15**, 404–9.
7. Gurney JM, Jeliffe DB (1973). Arm anthropometry in nutritional assessment; nomogram for rapid calculation of muscle circumference and cross-sectional muscle and fat areas. *Am J Clin Nutr* **26**, 912–15.
8. Young A, Stokes M, Round JM, Edwards RHT (1983). The effect of high-resistance training on the strength and muscle cross-sectional area of human quadriceps. *Eur J Clin Invest* **13**, 411–17.
9. Narici MV, Roi GS, Landoni L (1989). Changes in force, cross-sectional area and neural activation during strength training and detraining of the human quadriceps. *Eur J Appl Physiol* **59**, 310–19.
10. Housh DJ, Housh TJ, Weir JP, Weir LL, Stout JR, Johnson GO (1995). Anthropometric estimation of thigh muscle cross-section. *Med Sci Sports Exerc* **27**, 784–91.
11. Sunnegardh J, Bratteby LE, Nordesjo LO, Nordgren B (1988). Isometric and isokinetic muscle strength, anthropometry and physical activity in 8 and 13 year old Swedish children. *Eur J Appl Physiol* **58**, 291–7.
12. Jones PRM, Pearson J (1969). Anthropometric determination of leg fat and muscle plus bone volumes in young male and female adults. *J Physiol* **240**, 63–6.
13. Heymsfield SB, McManus C, Smith C, Stevens J, Nixon DW (1982). Anthropometric measurement of muscle mass: Revisited equations for calculating bone free arm muscle area. *Am J Clin Nutr* **36**, 680–90.
14. Koning FL, Binkhorst RA, Kauer JMG, Thijssen HOM (1986). Accuracy of an anthropometric estimate of the muscle and bone area in a transversal cross-section of the arm. *Int J Sports Med* **7**, 246–9.
15. Winsley RJ, Armstrong N, Welsman JR (2003). The validity of the Jones and Pearson anthropometric method to determine thigh volumes in young boys: A comparison with magnetic resonance imaging. *Revista Portuguesa de Ciencias do Desporto* **3**, 74–5.
16. Rutherford OM, Jones DA (1992). Measurement of fibre pennation using ultrasound in the human quadriceps *in vivo*. *Eur J Appl Physiol* **65**, 433–7.
17. Kearns CF, Isokawa M, Abe T (2001). Architectural characteristics of dominant leg muscles in junior soccer players. *Eur J Appl Physiol* **85**, 240–3.
18. Kawakami Y, Abe T, Kuno S, Fukunaga T (1995). Training induced changes in muscle architecture and specific tension. *Eur J Appl Physiol* **7**, 37–43.
19. De Ste Croix MBA, Armstrong N, Welsman JR, Sharpe P (2002). Longitudinal changes in isokinetic leg strength in 10–14 year olds. *Ann Hum Biol* **29**, 50–62.
20. Deighan MA, Armstrong N, De Ste Croix MBA (2003). Peak torque per MRI-determined cross-sectional area of knee extensors and flexors in children, teenagers and adults. *J Sports Sci* **21**, 236.
21. Deighan, MA, De Ste Croix MBA, Armstrong N (2006). Measurement of maximal muscle cross-sectional area of knee and elbow extensors and flexors in children, teenagers and adults. *J Sports Sci* **24**, 543–6.
22. Wood LE, Dixon S, Grant C, Armstrong N (2004). Elbow flexion and extension strength relative to body size or muscle size in children. *Med Sci Sports Exerc* **36**, 1977–84.
23. Wood LE, Dixon S, Grant C, Armstrong N (personal communication). Elbow strength, muscle size and leverage in adolescence.
24. Kanehisa H, Kuno S, Katsuta S, Fukunaga T (2006). A 2-year follow-up study on muscle size and dynamic strength in teenage tennis players. *Scand J Med Sci Sports* **16**, 93–9.
25. Round JM, Jones DA, Honour JW, Nevill AM (1999). Hormonal factors in the development of differences in strength between boys and girls during adolescence: A longitudinal study. *Ann Hum Biol* **26**, 49–62.
26. Tanner JM, Hughes PCR, Whitehouse RH (1981). Radiographically determined widths of bone, muscle and fat in the upper arm and calf from age 3–18 years. *Ann Hum Biol* **8**, 495–517.
27. Miller AEJ, MacDougall JD, Tarnopolsky MA, Sale DG (1993). Gender differences in strength and muscle fibre characteristics. *Eur J Appl Physiol* **66**, 254–62.
28. Gerodimos V, Mandou V, Zafeiridis A, Ioakimidis P, Stavropoulos N, Kellis S (2003). Isokinetic peak torque and hamstring/quadriceps ratio in young basketball players. *J Sports Med Phys Fitness* **43**, 444–52.
29. De Ste Croix MBA, Deighan MA, Armstrong N (2007). Functional eccentric-concentric ratio of knee extensors and flexors in pre-pubertal children, teenagers and adults. *Int J Sports Med* **28**, 768–72.
30. Osternig L (2000). The role of coactivation and eccentric activity in the ACL-injured knee. In: Lephart SM, Fu FH (eds.), *Proprioception and neuromuscular control in the joint stability*, pp. 385–92. Human Kinetics, Champaign, IL.
31. Baratta RM, Solomonow BH, Zhou ED, Letson R, Chuinard R, D'Ambrosia R (1988). Muscular coactivation: The role of the antagonist musculature in maintaining knee stability. *Am J Sports Med* **16**, 113–22.
32. Hirohawa S, Solomonow M, Lou Z, Lu Y, D'Ambrosia R (1991). Muscular co-contraction and control of knee stability. *J Electronyog Kinesiol* **1**, 199–208.
33. Noyes FR, Barber-Westin SD (2005). Isokinetic profile and differences in tibial rotation strength between male and female athletes 11 to 17 years of age. *Iso Exerc Sci* **13**, 251–9.
34. Kellis E, Unnithan VB (1999). Co-activation of vastus lateralis and biceps femoris muscles in pubertal children and adults. *Eur J Appl Physiol* **79**, 504–11.
35. Aagaard P, Simonsen EB, Magnusson SP, Larsson B, Dyhre-Poulsen P (1998). A new concept for isokinetic hamstring: Quadriceps muscle strength ratio. *Am J Sports Med* **26**, 231–7.
36. Dauty M, Potiron-Josse M, Rochcongar P (2003). Identification of previous hamstring injury by isokinetic concentric and eccentric torque measurement in elite soccer players. *Iso Exerc Sci* **11**, 134–44.
37. Colliander EB, Tesch PA (1989). Bilateral eccentric and concentric torque of quadriceps and hamstring muscles in females and males. *Eur J Appl Physiol* **59**, 227–32.
38. Griffin JW, Tooms RE, Zwaag RV, Bertorini TE, O'Toole ML (1993). Eccentric muscle performance of elbow and knee muscle groups in untrained men and women. *Med Sci Sports Exerc* **25**, 936–44.
39. Hildebrand KA, Mohtadi NG, Kiefer GN, Tedford K, Massey A, Brant R (1994). Thigh muscle strength in preadolescent girls. *Clin J Sport Med* **4**, 108–12.
40. Mohtadi NGH, Kiefer GN, Tedford K, Watters S (1990). Concentric and eccentric quadriceps torque in pre-adolescent males. *Can J Sport Sci* **15**, 240–3.
41. Brooks GA, Fahey TD (1985). *Exercise physiology: Human bioenergetics and its application.* MacMillan, New York.
42. Dvir Z (1995). *Isokinetics: Muscle testing, interpretation and clinical applications.* Churchill Livingstone, New York.
43. Seger JY, Thorstensson A (1994). Muscle strength and myoelectric activity in prepubertal and adult males and females. *Eur J Appl Physiol* **69**, 81–7.

44. Calmels P, VanDenBorne I, Nellen M, Domenach M, Minaire P, Drost M (1995). A pilot study of knee isokinetic strength in young, highly trained, female gymnasts. *Iso Exerc Sci* **5**, 69–74.
45. Kellis E, Kellis S, Gerodimos V, Manou V (1999). Reliability of isokinetic concentric and eccentric strength in circumpubertal soccer players. *Pediatr Exerc Sci* **11**, 218–28.
46. Westing S, Seger J (1989). Eccentric and concentric torque-velocity characteristics, torque output comparisons and gravity effect corrections for the quadriceps and hamstring muscles in females. *Int J Sports Med* **10**, 175–80.
47. Enoka RM (1996). Eccentric contractions require unique activation strategies by the nervous system. *J Appl Physiol* **81**, 2339–46.
48. Seger JY, Thorstensson A (2000). Muscle strength and electromyogram in boys and girls followed through puberty. *Eur J Appl Physiol* **81**, 54–61.
49. Komi PV, Bosco C (1978). Utilization of stored elastic energy in leg extensor muscles by men and women. *Med Sci Sports* **10**, 261–5.
50. Weir JP, Housh TJ, Johnson GO, Housh DJ, Ebersole KT (1999). Allometric scaling of isokinetic peak torque: The Nebraska wrestling study. *Eur J Appl Physiol* **80**, 240–8.
51. Kanehisa H, Ikegawa S, Tsunoda N, Fukunaga T (1995). Strength and cross-sectional areas of reciprocal muscle groups in the upper arm and thigh during adolescence. *Int J Sports Med* **16**, 54–60.
52. Ross JG, Gilbert CG (1985). The National Children and Youth Fitness Study: A summary of findings. *J Phys Educat Recreat Dance* **56**, 45–50.
53. Carron AV, Bailey DA (1974). Strength development in boys from 10 through 16 years. *Monogr Soc Res Child Dev* **39**, 1–37.
54. Eek MN, Kroksmark AK, Beckung E (2006). Isometric muscle torque in children 5 to 15 years of age: Normative data. *Arc Phys Med Rehab* **87**, 1091–9.
55. Parker DF, Round JM, Sacco P, Jones DA (1990). A cross-sectional survey of upper and lower limb strength in boys and girls during childhood and adolescence. *Ann Hum Biol* **17**, 199–211.
56. Backman E, Henriksson KG (1988). Skeletal muscle characteristics in children 9–15 years old: Force, relaxation rate and contraction time. *Clin Physiol* **8**, 521–7.
57. Holm I, Steen H, Olstad M (2005). Isokinetic *muscle* performance in growing boys from pre-teen to maturity. An eleven-year longitudinal study. *Iso Exerc Sci* **13**, 153–6.
58. Kanehisa H, Abe T, Fukunaga T (2003). Growth trends of dynamic strength in adolescent boys. A 2-year follow-up survey. *J Sports Med Phys Fitness* **43**, 459–64.
59. Peltonen JE, Taimela S, Erkintalo M, Salminen JJ, Oksanen A, Kujala UM (1998). Back extensor and psoas muscle cross-sectional area, prior physical training, and trunk muscle strength—A longitudinal study in adolescent girls. *Eur J Appl Physiol* **77**, 66–71.
60. Newcomer K, Sinaki M, Wollan P (1997). Physical activity and four year development of back strength in children. *Am J Phys Med Rehab* **76**, 52–8.
61. Barber-Westin SD, Noyes FR, Galloway M (2006). Jump-land characteristics and muscle strength development in young athletes a gender comparison of 1140 athletes 9 to 17 years of age. *Am J Sports Med* **34**, 375–84.
62. Blimkie CJR (1989). Age and sex-associated variation in strength during childhood: Anthropometric, morphologic, neurologic, biomechanical, endocrinologic, genetic and physical activity correlates. In: Gisolf CV, Lamb DR (eds.), *Perspectives in exercise science and sports medicine: Youth, exercise and sport*, Vol. 2, pp. 99–163. Benchmark Press, Indianapolis, IN.
63. De Ste Croix MBA, Armstrong N, Welsman JR (1999). Concentric isokinetic leg strength in pre-teen, teenage and adult males and females. *Biol Sport* **16**, 75–86.
64. Maffulli N, King JB, Helms P (1994). Training in elite youth athletes: Injuries, flexibility and isometric strength. *Brit J Sports Med* **28**, 123–36.
65. Davies CTM (1985). Strength and mechanical properties of muscle in children and young adults. *Scand J Sport Sci* **7**, 11–15.
66. Gilliam TB, Villanacci JF, Freedson PS, Sady SP (1979). Isokinetic torque in boys and girls ages 7 to 13: Effect of age, height and weight. *Res Q* **50**, 599–609.
67. Falk B, Tenenbaum G (1996). The effectiveness of resistance training in children: A meta-analysis. *Sports Med* **22**, 176–86.
68. Rasmussen B, Kalusen K, Jespersen B, Jensen K (1990). A longitudinal study of development in growth and maturation of 10- to 15-year old girls and boys. In Oseid S, Carlsen HK (eds.), *Children and exercise XIII*, pp. 103–11. Human Kinetics, Champaign, IL.
69. Faust MS (1977). Somatic development of adolescent girls. *Soc Res Child Dev* **42**, 1–90.
70. Parker DF, Round JM, Sacco P, Jones DA (1990). A cross-sectional survey of upper and lower limb strength in boys and girls during childhood and adolescence. *Ann Hum Biol* **17**, 199–211.
71. Hansen L, Klausen K, Muller J (1997). Assessment of maturity status and its relation to strength measurements. In: Armstrong N, Kirby BJ, Welsman J (eds.), *Children and exercise XIX: Promoting health and well-being*, pp. 325–30. E&FN Spon, London.
72. Ramos E, Frontera WR, Llopart A, Feliciano D (1998). Muscle strength and hormonal levels in adolescents: Gender related differences. *Int J Sports Med* **19**, 526–31.
73. Housh TJ, Johnson GO, Housh DJ, Stout JR, Weir JP, Weir LL (1996). Isokinetic peak torque in young wrestlers. *Pediatr Exerc Sci* **8**, 143–55.
74. Housh TJ, Stout JR, Housh DJ, Johnston GO (1995). The covariate influence of muscle mass on isokinetic peak torque in high school wrestlers. *Pediatr Exerc Sci* **7**, 176–82.
75. Housh TJ, Stout JR, Weir JP, Weir LL, Housh DJ, Johnson GO (1995). Relationships of age and muscle mass to peak torque in high school wrestlers. *Res Q Exerc Sport* **66**, 256–61.
76. Kanehisa H, Ikegawa S, Tsunoda N, Fukanaga T (1994). Strength and cross-sectional area of knee extensor muscles in children. *Eur J Appl Physiol* **68**, 402–5.
77. Deighan MA, Armstrong N, De Ste Croix MBA (2002). Peak torque per arm muscle cross-sectional area during growth. In: Koskolou M, Geladas N, Klissouras V (eds.), *7th Annual Congress of the European College of Sport Science*, p. 47. Pashalidis Medical Publisher, Athens.
78. Tolfrey K, Morse C, Thom J, Vassilopoulos W, Narici M (2003). Plantar flexion torque per unit muscle cross-sectional area is similar in boys and young men. *Revista Portuguesa de Ciencias do Desporto* **3**, 78–9.
79. Blimkie CJR, Macauley D (2000). Muscle strength. In: Armstrong N, Van Mechelen W (eds.), *Pediatric exercise science and medicine*, pp. 23–36. Oxford University Press, Oxford.
80. Blimkie CJR, Ebbesen B, MacDougall D, Bar-Or O, Sale D (1989). Voluntary and electrically evoked strength characteristics of obese and non-obese preadolescent boys. *Hum Biol* **61**, 515–32.
81. Asmussen E (1973). Growth in muscular strength and power. In: Rarick GL (eds.), *Physical activity: Human growth and development*, pp. 60–79. Academic Press, New York.
82. Davies CTM (1985). Strength and mechanical properties of muscle in children and young adults. *Scand J Sport Sci* **7**, 11–15.
83. De Ste Croix MBA, Deighan MA, Armstrong N (2004). Time to peak torque for knee and elbow extensors and flexors in children, teenagers and adults. *Iso Exerc Sci* **12**, 143–8.
84. Davies CTM, White MJ, Young K (1983). Muscle function in children. *J Appl Physiol* **52**, 111–4.
85. Houmard JA, Smith R, Jendrasiak GL (1995). Relationship between MRI relaxation time and muscle fibre composition. *J Appl Physiol* **78**, 807–9.
86. Kubo K, Ohgo K, Takeishi R, Yoshinaga K, Tsunoda N, Kanehisa H, Fukunaga T (2006). Effects of series elasticity on the human torque-angle relationship *in vivo*. *Res Q Exerc Sport* **77**, 408–16.
87. Froberg K, Lammert O (1996). Development of muscle strength during childhood. In: Bar-Or O (ed.), *The child and adolescent athlete*, pp. 25–41. Blackwell Scientific, London.

CHAPTER 16

Exercise metabolism

Neil Armstrong and Samantha G. Fawkner

Introduction

Paediatric exercise physiologists working with healthy children are normally limited to examining blood and respiratory gas markers of exercise metabolism and, although these studies have enhanced knowledge, ethical considerations have restricted potentially more informative studies at the level of the muscle cell. Much of what we know of exercise metabolism during growth and maturation has therefore been derived from measures of maximal (or peak) anaerobic and aerobic performance. However, although metabolic profiles founded on maximal intensity ('anaerobic') exercise and peak oxygen uptake ($\dot{V}O_2$) tests are useful indicators of exercise metabolism, they require confirmation at the muscle level and do not provide the quality or specificity of data required to tease out growth- and maturation-related changes in metabolism during exercise of various intensities and durations.

In this chapter, to better understand the interplay of anaerobic and aerobic exercise metabolism during growth and maturation, we will

(i) compare and contrast the development of maximal measures of anaerobic and aerobic performance,

(ii) analyse relevant data from muscle biopsy investigations,

(iii) review studies of substrate utilization during exercise, and

(iv) explore recent insights into muscle metabolism provided by rigorous analyses of breath-by-breath respiratory gases and ^{31}P-magnetic resonance spectroscopy (^{31}P-MRS) spectra.

Maximal (or peak) anaerobic and aerobic performance

Measures of anaerobic and aerobic fitness and performance during growth and maturation are comprehensively discussed and referenced in Chapters 5, 8, 9, 17, and 20 and will, therefore, only be summarized briefly here with a focus on their comparative development.

The physiological and methodological problems associated with the estimation of maximal anaerobic performance (or more appropriately maximal intensity exercise) are reviewed in Chapter 5 and it is apparent that direct measures of young people's maximal anaerobic performance are not available. Research has primarily focused on the assessment of what has been called short-term power output and the Wingate anaerobic test (WAnT), which enables the determination of cycling peak power (PP), usually over a 1- or 5-s period, and mean power (MP), over the 30-s test period, is the most popular means of assessment. Cross-sectional data are equivocal and longitudinal data sparse but a consistent finding in both girls and boys is an increase in PP and MP with age. Sex differences appear to be minimal until about 12 years of age, but this finding might be clouded by the fact that few studies have simultaneously considered the stage of maturation of the participants. The PP and MP are correlated with body size, body composition, and thigh volume, age exerts an additional positive effect but an additional, independent effect of maturation remains to be demonstrated. However, both sexes benefit from an enhanced increase in PP and MP during adolescence with the effect being more marked in boys (ref. 1 and see Chapter 17).

Boys' ability to recover faster than men following high-intensity running[2,3] and cycling exercise[3,4] is well-documented, and research with females, although less comprehensive, has reported a lower decrement in power output in 13-year-old girls than in adult women over a series of maximal cycling bouts interspersed with short rest periods.[5] Some authors have suggested that factors such as faster phosphocreatine (PCr) resynthesis, greater oxidative capacity, better acid–base regulation, faster readjustment of initial cardiorespiratory parameters, and lower production and/or higher removal of metabolic by-products may explain children's faster recovery following high-intensity exercise.[6,7] Other researchers have focused on methodological limitations of the maximal intensity exercise models used to compare children and adults and concluded that children's faster recovery is likely a direct consequence of their limited capacity to generate power[8] (see Chapter 17).

In contrast to maximal anaerobic performance, the assessment and interpretation of aerobic fitness during childhood and adolescence is comprehensively documented with extensive cross-sectional and longitudinal peak $\dot{V}O_2$ data in relation to age readily available. Data are consistent and, with body size appropriately controlled for (ref. 9 and see Chapter 2), boys' peak $\dot{V}O_2$ increases with age from childhood into young adulthood whereas girls' peak $\dot{V}O_2$ tends to level off at about 14 years of age. Maturation induces increases in peak $\dot{V}O_2$ in both sexes independent of those explained by body size, body composition, and age. Boys' peak $\dot{V}O_2$ is higher than girls', at least from age 8 years, and sex differences progressively increase with age (ref. 10 and see Chapters 8 and 20).

Although measures reflecting both peak anaerobic and aerobic metabolism increase with age, the data indicate age- and sex-related changes that are not synchronous and both boys and girls experience a more marked increase in maximal anaerobic metabolism than aerobic metabolism as they move from childhood, through adolescence, and into young adulthood. Comparative anaerobic and aerobic data are available in a single mixed longitudinal study where the PP, MP, and peak $\dot{V}O_2$ of the same participants were determined at 12, 13, and 17 years.[1,11] The PP and MP increased, respectively, by 121% and 113% in boys and 66% and 60% in girls, whereas the corresponding increases in peak $\dot{V}O_2$ were somewhat less at 70% and 50% for the boys and girls, respectively.

Muscle biopsy studies

The muscle biopsy technique was first introduced in the early 1900s to study muscular dystrophy but it was Bergstrom's reintroduction of the biopsy needle to exercise science in 1962 which stimulated research into muscle biochemistry during exercise.[12–14] The technique involves local anaesthesia followed by a small incision through the skin, subcutaneous tissue, and fascia. A hollow needle is inserted into the belly of the muscle and, via a plunger in the centre of the needle, a small piece of muscle is excised and the needle containing the muscle withdrawn. The muscle sample is cleaned and quickly frozen for subsequent microscopy or biochemical analysis. Despite problems related to the size of the muscle sample,[15] the depth of the incision in relation to muscle size[16] and the variability of fibre type distributions within and between human muscles[17,18] muscle biopsies have greatly enhanced our understanding of muscle biochemistry. In many laboratories, muscle biopsies are used almost routinely in adult investigations but ethical considerations have limited the number of healthy children subjected to the technique (see Chapter 1).

Muscle fibre types

Muscle fibres consist of a continuum of biochemical and contractile features but they are conventionally classified into type I (slow twitch), type IIa (fast twitch–fatigue resistant), and type IIX (fast twitch–fatiguable) fibres. It is sometimes possible to detect type IIc fibres but they normally account for less than 1% of the total muscle fibre pool. Type I fibres have a high oxidative capacity and are characterized by a rich capillary blood supply, numerous mitochondria, and high activity of oxidative enzymes. The high triglyceride content of type I fibres supports lipid oxidation during submaximal exercise with a glycogen sparing effect. Type II fibres are better equipped for high-intensity exercise with higher glycolytic enzyme activity and greater glycogen and PCr stores than type I fibres. In type II fibres, the rate of pyruvate production by glycolysis is greater than the rate at which it can be oxidized and the excess pyruvate is reduced to lactate to allow regeneration of nicotinamide adenine dinucleotide and the continuation of glycolysis. Type I fibres have a low threshold of activity and preferentially respond to low-intensity exercise but type IIa and type IIX fibres are better equipped to support more severe exercise and they are sequentially recruited as exercise intensity increases.

It has been suggested that maturation of skeletal muscle fibre patterns might account for growth-related changes in the metabolic response to high-intensity exercise[19] but published studies of muscle biopsies with children are sparse, generally involve few participants and the interpretation of data has been confounded by large interindividual variations in fibre profiles.[20,21] Nevertheless, some patterns have emerged from the extant literature.

Muscle fibre size appears to increase linearly with age from birth to adolescence[22] and, in males, into young adulthood.[15] Some studies have indicated that during adolescence muscle fibre areas for all fibre types are larger in boys than in girls but girls' values are similar to those of young adult females.[21,23]

In an early study, which is often cited, Bell *et al.*[24] obtained biopsies from the vastus lateralis of thirteen 6-year-old Swiss children and reported that the fibre type distribution pattern was not different from normal adult tissue. However, it should be noted that the 'normal adult tissue' data referred to was extracted from previous studies performed by others elsewhere. Eight years later, Oertel[25] reported data from an autopsy study of 113 subjects, aged from 1 week to 20 years, and revealed that the % of type I fibres in the vastus lateralis muscle of some 15–20 year olds tended to be lower than in younger subjects. This trend was strongly supported by Lexell *et al.*[15] in a similar autopsy study of 22 previously healthy males, aged 5–37 years. They observed a highly significant negative relationship between the % of type I fibres in the vastus lateralis and age. The % of type I fibres decreased from about 65% at age 5 years to about 50% at age 20 years. Glenmark *et al.*[23] provided further support for an age-related decline in the % of type I fibres, at least in males, in what appears to be the only published study involving young people in which data have been collected longitudinally. Biopsies taken from the vastus lateralis of 55 males and 28 females at age 16 years and again at 27 years were analysed for fibre type. The % of type I fibres significantly decreased with age in males but no significant change in females was observed.

Jansson[16] critically reviewed the extant literature to examine the hypothesis that the % of type I fibres in the vastus lateralis is a function of age. She concluded that the % of type I fibres decreases in sedentary to moderately active males without any known diseases between the ages of 10 and 35 years. No clear age-related fibre type changes were observed in females but she commented that this might be a methodological artefact as so few data on girls and young women are available.

Studies comparing the muscle fibre distribution of boys and girls are particularly sparse. Small participant samples, including fewer girls than boys, and large interindividual differences cloud statistical analyses. Significant sex differences in the % of type I fibres have not been recorded but there is a consistent trend with adolescent boys and young male adults exhibiting, on average, 8–15% more type I fibres in the vastus lateralis than similarly aged girls in the same study[20,24,26] (Table 16.1). No published study has indicated that girls have a higher % of type I fibres than boys.

Methodological concerns suggest that paediatric muscle biopsy data should be treated cautiously but the extant data are consistent in showing an age-related decline in the % of type I fibres from childhood to young adulthood and published work indicates a trend in which adolescent boys present a higher % of type I fibres than girls. Further research is clearly warranted and the introduction of magnetic resonance imaging (MRI) as a means of estimating muscle fibre types might provide an ethical means of resolving key issues concerning age- and sex-related differences in muscle fibre type.[27,28]

Table 16.1 Percentage of type I fibres in the vastus lateralis by age

Citation	Age (years)	Males		Females		Sex difference (%)
		n	% Type I fibres (mean ± SD)	*n*	% Type I fibres (mean ± SD)	
Komi and Karlsson[20]	15–24	20	55.9 ± 11.9	11	49.1 ± 7.7	13.8
du Plessis *et al.*[26]	14–16	28	52.9 ± 15.6	6	46.2 ± 13.5	14.5
Glenmark *et al.*[23]	16	55	55 ± 12	28	51 ± 9	7.8

Muscle metabolism

In a series of innovative muscle biopsy studies of 11- to 16-year-old boys, Eriksson and co-workers[29–34] made a significant contribution to understanding young people's muscle metabolism. They focused on energy stores and enzyme activity in the muscle at rest, following exercise of different intensities, and post-training. Their data, which have often been interpreted uncritically, have influenced paediatric exercise science for almost 40 years.

Energy stores

Eriksson and Saltin[33] took muscle biopsies from the lateral part of the quadriceps femoris muscle of boys aged 11.6 years ($n = 8$), 12.6 years ($n = 9$), 13.5 years ($n = 8$), and 15.5 years ($n = 8$), and analysed the samples for concentrations of adenosine triphosphate (ATP), PCr, glycogen, and lactate at rest and immediately after both submaximal exercise and exercise to peak $\dot{V}O_2$ ('maximal exercise') on a cycle ergometer. They reported resting ATP stores of about 5 mmol·kg^{-1} wet weight of muscle which did not change with age and were similar to values others had recorded in adults. The concentration of ATP remained essentially unchanged following 6-min bouts of submaximal exercise but minor reductions were observed following maximal exercise.

The authors concluded that boys' PCr concentration at rest was similar to that of adults but closer scrutiny of the data suggests an age-related change in PCr stores. The PCr concentration of the 11 year olds was 14.5 mmol·kg^{-1} wet weight of muscle but that of the 15 year olds was 63% higher at 23.6 mmol·kg^{-1} wet weight of muscle and comparable with values recorded in men in earlier studies. The PCr concentration gradually declined following exercise sessions of increasing intensity with values of less than 5 mmol·kg^{-1} wet weight of muscle observed following maximal exercise. In an earlier study, Eriksson *et al.*[31] trained eight boys, aged 11.5 years at onset, for 4 months and noted that following the training programme stores of ATP and PCr increased significantly (see Chapter 40 for further details of this study).

In the 11 year olds, muscle glycogen concentration at rest averaged 54 mmol·kg^{-1} wet weight of muscle and progressively increased with age reaching 87 mmol·kg^{-1} wet weight of muscle in the 15 year olds which is comparable to muscle glycogen concentrations, but not absolute values, previously observed in men. With exercise a gradual decrease in glycogen was observed in all groups but the decrease was three times greater in the oldest compared to the youngest boys thus suggesting enhanced glycolysis with age.[33] Following 4 months of training, resting glycogen stores significantly increased in eight 11-year-old boys but it is not apparent whether any attempt was made to control diet.[31]

Lactate production and concentration

Lactate is continuously produced in skeletal muscles, even at rest, but the onset of exercise stimulates glycolysis and lactate production increases as a function of the imbalance between the anaerobic and aerobic metabolism of pyruvate. Lactate metabolism is a dynamic process and while some fibres produce lactate adjacent fibres consume it as an energy source. The net muscle lactate concentration derived from a muscle biopsy is therefore not a direct measure of lactate production but it reflects the glycolytic contribution to the resynthesis of ATP during exercise. There are very few data on young people's muscle lactate concentration either at rest or after exercise.

In the initial report of their muscle biopsy studies, Eriksson *et al.*[29] observed, in 13-year-old boys, a mean resting muscle lactate concentration of 1.3 mmol·kg^{-1} wet weight of muscle. At low exercise intensities lactate concentration increased very little but at exercise intensities above 60% of peak $\dot{V}O_2$ (presumably above the boys' anaerobic threshold) a more rapid increase was observed. When the research was extended to 11- to 15-year-old boys,[33] it was noted that muscle lactate concentration increased with increasing relative exercise and that the lactate concentration immediately following submaximal exercise was higher in older boys. The age-related increase in the glycolytic contribution to metabolism after maximal exercise described earlier was reflected by observations of muscle lactate concentrations of 8.8, 10.7, 11.3, and 15.5 mmol·kg^{-1} wet weight of muscle for boys aged 11.6, 12.6, 13.5, and 15.5 years, respectively.[33]

Eriksson *et al.*[30] commented that boys' blood lactate accumulation reflected their muscle lactate concentration and they suggested a possible maturation effect on muscle lactate as, at age 13.6 years, those with the higher muscle lactate concentrations had the greater testicular volume, although this relationship was only 'almost significant'. In subsequent paediatric studies, blood lactate accumulation has conventionally been used to provide a window into muscle lactate concentration but the limits of this assumption are examined in Chapter 8. There is some recent evidence which suggests that age-related differences in the kinetics of blood lactate concentration reflect a faster elimination of lactate out of the blood compartment in children rather than differences in muscle lactate[35] but this interpretation has been criticized on methodological grounds[8] and conflicting data are available.[36] The interpretation of blood lactate accumulation, as a surrogate of muscle lactate concentration, in relation to sex, age, and maturation is also clouded by methodological issues (see Chapter 8) and whereas there appears to be a positive relationship between age and blood lactate accumulation during both submaximal and maximal exercise a direct relationship with maturation has proved elusive to establish. Some studies have indicated that girls exhibit a greater accumulation of blood lactate during both submaximal and maximal exercise but data are equivocal and sex differences remain to be proven[37–39] (see Chapter 8).

In the present context, the work of Pianosi *et al.*[40] who monitored the blood lactate and pyruvate concentrations of 28 young people following 6 min of cycling at two thirds of maximal exercise is worthy of note. Pianosi *et al.*[40] analysed their data in relation to three age groups: 7–10 year olds ($n = 6$), 11–14 year olds ($n = 12$), and 15–17 year olds ($n = 10$). They reported that following exercise, blood lactate accumulation increased out of proportion to that of blood pyruvate such that the lactate/pyruvate ratio rose in an age-related manner. These data suggest an age-related enhanced glycolytic function rather than a compromised oxidative capacity with increasing age. On the other hand using the WAnT as an exercise model, Beneke *et al.*[41] concluded that lower post-exercise blood lactate concentrations in children reflect a lower muscle mass combined with a facilitated aerobic metabolism.

Enzyme activity

Pioneering research by Eriksson and his associates[32] described the levels of succinic dehydrogenase (SDH) and phosphofructokinase (PFK) activity in the vastus lateralis of five boys, mean age 11.2 years before and after a 6-week training programme. They demonstrated a 29% increase in SDH and an 83% increase in PFK activity after training (see Chapter 40 for further details). However, it was the pre-training activities of SDH and PFK, which were observed to be 20% higher and 50% lower, respectively, than adult values reported by the same research group,[42] which generated the most interest among paediatric exercise physiologists. Despite the small sample size, the fact that the muscle biopsies were carried out at rest, and Eriksson's[31] comment in his thesis that his results must be interpreted with caution, numerous authors (particularly of textbooks) have uncritically cited these data to unequivocally support the view that children have a low glycolytic and enhanced oxidative capacity during exercise. Subsequent studies of enzyme activity in the vastus lateralis have provided more comprehensive analyses of young people's enzyme activity.

In a series of well-designed studies Haralambie[43,44] determined the activities of a number of enzymes from biopsies of the vastus lateralis taken at rest. He acknowledged the limitations of extrapolating *in vitro* data to *in vivo* conditions and focused on measuring enzyme activity as near as possible to optimal conditions including physiological temperature. To maximize insights into the mechanisms controlling the functional characteristics and capacity of muscle, he emphasized the importance of investigating as many enzyme activities of a specific metabolic pathway as possible.

Haralambie[43] compared enzyme activity in twelve 11- to 14-year-old girls with ten 36-year-old women. He reported significantly higher activity of two tricarboxylic acid cycle enzymes, namely, fumarase and isocitrate dehydrogenase (ICDH), in the girls and he concluded that this may reflect a trend to enhanced oxidation of substrate in the younger participants. He also observed higher lactate dehydrogenase (LDH) activity in the girls but commented somewhat glibly that this, 'simply suggests a daily physical activity directed towards more intensity than endurance in this group' (p. 265).

In a more comprehensive investigation, Haralambie[44] determined the activity of 22 enzymes involved in energy metabolism in seven boys and seven girls, aged 13–15 years; and seven women and seven men, aged 22–42 years. The activity of glycolytic enzymes was not significantly different between adults and adolescents. In contrast with his earlier report, Haralambie observed no significant age difference in LDH activity and his observation of no age-related change in PFK activity was in direct conflict with Eriksson *et al.*'s findings.[32] The activity of enolase was lower in females in both age groups, but no difference due to age was noted and this was the only sex difference in enzyme activity recorded. Of the oxidative enzymes studied by Haramblie,[44] only citrate synthase (CS) showed no difference between adults and adolescents with all other oxidative enzymes more active in adolescents. The relationship of the activities of CS, ICDH, and fumarase were markedly different in adolescents compared to adults with adolescents exhibiting significantly higher fumarase and ICDH activity relative to CS activity. No significant adult–adolescent differences were noted in activities of three enzymes involved in fatty acid metabolism but enzymes involved in amino acid metabolism showed a tendency to higher activity in adolescents. Haralambie hypothesized that as activities of adults' and adolescents' glycolytic enzymes did not differ but several tricarboxylic acid (TCA) cycle enzymes had higher activity in adolescents than adults (e.g. ICDH activity was 44% higher in adolescents), the ratio 'pyruvate to lactate'/'pyruvate oxidized' is lower than in adults (in accordance with Pianosi *et al.*'s observations[40] of an age-related blood lactate/blood pyruvate ratio). He suggested that this is one of the factors contributing to lower blood lactate accumulation in adolescents than in adults during exercise and to adolescents' faster $\dot{V}O_2$ kinetics at the onset of exercise.

Berg and his associates[45,46] biopsied resting samples from the vastus lateralis and determined the activity of creatine kinase (CK), hexose phosphate isomerase, aldolase, pyruvate kinase (PK), LDH, CS, and fumarase in 33 participants categorized into three groups by age, that is, children (four males, four females), age 6.4 ± 2.1 years; juveniles (five males, seven females), age 13.5 ± 1.3 years; and young adults (five males, eight females), age 17.1 ± 0.8 years. The activity of the glycolytic enzymes was positively correlated with age and the activity of the TCA cycle enzymes was negatively correlated with age, although all correlations were not statistically significant. Mean activity increases of 32%, 85%, 48%, 143%, and 25% were observed in CK, aldolase, PK, LDH, and hexose phosphate isomerase, respectively, from 6 to 13 years, although with wide intragroup standard deviations changes were only significant for aldolase, PK, and LDH. With the exception of LDH, which decreased in activity from 13 to 17 years but remained significantly higher than at age 6 years, there were no significant changes from 13 to 17 years. The activity of TCA cycle enzymes, CS, and fumarase declined by 28% and 40%, respectively, from 6 to 17 years with the decrease in fumarase activity being statistically significant.

The work of Haralambie[43,44] and Berg *et al.*[45,46] provides the opportunity for further insights into muscle metabolism through the exploration of ratios of specific glycolytic/oxidative enzyme activities. A recalculation of Berg's data indicates PK/fumarase ratios of 3.585, 3.201, and 2.257 for adults, juveniles (adolescents), and children, respectively. In other words, the glycolytic/oxidative enzyme activity ratio was 59% higher in young adults than in children. Haralambie's data allow a comparison of the activity of potential rate-limiting enzymes of glycolysis and the TCA cycle, namely, PFK and ICDH. Unfortunately data are only available on eight adolescents and eight adults but the ratio PFK/ICDH was reported to be 93% (and significantly) higher in adults than in adolescents at 1.633 and 0.844, respectively.

Jansson and Hedberg[21] observed significantly higher SDH activity in 16-year-old boys than in similarly aged girls but no significant sex differences in PFK or 3-hydroxyacyl-CoA-dehydrogenase activity, although the boys' values tended to be higher. Kaczor *et al.*[47] collected samples of the obliquus abdominis muscle from twenty 3- to 11-year-old and twelve 29- to 54-year-old hernia patients and determined the enzyme activity of adenylate kinase (AK), CK, carnitine palmitoyltransferase (CPT), LDH, and 2-oxoglutarate dehydrogenase (OGDH), a rate-limiting enzyme in the TCA cycle. They reported lower activity of the 'anaerobic' enzymes (AK, CK, and LDH) in children and suggested that this difference, particularly in LDH, is likely to be a major factor in children's lower anaerobic performance (and muscle/blood lactate concentration) compared to adults. They observed OGDH activity to be slightly lower in children and CPT activity to be similar for children and adults but when the data were expressed in relation to protein content, there were no significant differences. The ratio of CPT/LDH was much greater in children and the ratio of CPT/OGDH tended to be higher in children. The authors commented that their results indicate that children have a greater ability than adults to oxidize lipids during exercise.

In summary, despite methodological limitations and some equivocal data, muscle biopsy studies have provided valuable insights into muscle metabolism, and the ratios of various glycolytic and oxidative enzyme activities are of particular interest. The weight of evidence suggests that young children have lower glycolytic enzyme activity than adolescents but, although the data are less clear, on balance, glycolytic enzyme activity in adolescents does not appear to be significantly less than in adults. However, the reported activity of oxidative enzymes indicates that children are able to oxidize pyruvate and free fatty acids (FFAs) at a higher rate than adolescents and that adolescents have an enhanced oxidative capacity compared to adults. A consistent finding is that the ratio of glycolytic/oxidative enzyme activity is higher in adults than in adolescents and children.

Substrate utilization

The relative contribution to total energy derived from carbohydrate and lipid during submaximal, steady-state exercise can be computed from the respiratory exchange ratio (RER) measured at the mouth and non-protein respiratory quotient values.[48] Studies have consistently reported significantly lower RER values (and therefore a higher lipid contribution to energy) in boys than in men during exercise at the same relative[49,50] and absolute intensity.[51,52] Two studies of females, however, have observed no significant difference in the RER of 9- to 13-year-old girls during cycling[53] or treadmill[54] exercise at the same relative exercise intensity compared with young women whereas a third study[55] reported significantly lower RER values in 9-year-old girls compared to young women running at the same relative exercise intensity. The conflicting female data on lipid utilization during exercise might be related to the menstrual cycle as oestrogen and progesterone have been shown to influence substrate utilization.[56,57]

Stephens *et al.*[58] investigated the effect of maturation on substrate utilization by observing the RER responses of males, between the ages of 9 and 27 years, at four different stages of maturation, during cycling exercise at 30–70% peak $\dot{V}O_2$. They reported higher lipid and lower carbohydrate utilization in a mid-pubertal (mean age 12 years and pubic hair stage 2 or 3)[59] group compared to late-pubertal (mean age 15 years and pubic hair stage 4 or 5) and young adult (mean age 22 years and assumed to have reached pubertal maturity) groups. However, no significant differences in fuel utilization between the early (mean age 10 years and pubic hair stage 1) and mid-pubertal groups at most of the submaximal exercise intensities were observed. Stephens *et al.*[58] concluded that the development of an adult fuel-utilization profile occurs sometime in the transition between mid-puberty and late-puberty and is complete on reaching full maturity. The authors acknowledged, however, that other uncontrolled factors (e.g. chronological age) in addition to maturation may also play a role in substrate utilization during exercise.

In a series of innovative studies, Timmons *et al.*[60–62] used both RER and ^{13}C stable isotope methodology to investigate substrate utilization during exercise. In their initial study, they examined the responses of ten 22-year-old men and twelve 9-year-old boys during 60 min of cycling at 70% peak $\dot{V}O_2$. They observed that the boys utilized about 70% more lipid and 23% less carbohydrate than the men during the final 30 min of the exercise. As part of the experimental design they also examined the pattern of substrate utilization when exercise was performed with external carbohydrate feeding (a ^{13}C-enriched 6% carbohydrate beverage). The boys were shown to oxidize relatively more exogenous carbohydrate than the men but to maintain higher relative rates of total lipid oxidation compared with men, even when fed with external carbohydrate.

In subsequent studies,[61,62] they compared the responses of 12-year-old girls with 14-year-old girls[61] and 12-year-old boys with 14-year-old boys[62] during 60-min cycling at 70% peak $\dot{V}O_2$ with and without carbohydrate supplementation (^{13}C-enriched 6% carbohydrate beverage). In the non-enriched carbohydrate trials, they observed higher lipid and lower carbohydrate oxidation rates during exercise in the younger compared to the older children. However, in contrast to the boys the girls' reliance on exogenous carbohydrate was not found to be age-dependent. Timmons *et al.*[60–62] synthesized their findings and, although they stressed the need for further studies, concluded that in childhood sex differences exist in substrate utilization during exercise. Furthermore, they argued that their data did not support the idea of an underdeveloped glycolytic flux in children but rather an underdeveloped depot of intramuscular fuels.

The responses of hormones to exercise will influence substrate utilization but it is difficult to assess the precise effect of a hormone upon a metabolic pathway during exercise. As reviewed by Boisseau and Delamarche,[19] an increase in plasma concentration of a hormone or substrate does not necessarily reflect an increase in secretion, but may be caused by a decrease in metabolic clearance rate or a decrease in plasma volume. Hormone activity also depends on receptor availability and sensitivity.

During exercise the plasma concentration of catecholamines rises and the balance of evidence suggests a lower sympathetic response in children than in adults[63,64] although there are contrasting data.[65] Lower sympathetic activity during childhood may reduce glycolytic activation but data are sparse and they are both inconsistent and confounded by the wide intraindividual variability of circulating catecholamines and should be treated with caution.[19,45] Circulating testosterone concentration increases with maturation and may promote glycolytic activity but the extant literature is equivocal.[66,67]

In a study of young swimmers, Wirth *et al.*[68] determined the plasma insulin, FFA, and glucose concentrations of prepubertal, pubertal, and post-pubertal boys and girls at rest and during exercise at 70% of peak $\dot{V}O_2$. They reported that insulin levels decreased during exercise in the prepubertal children, remained constant in pubertal children and increased in the post-pubertal groups. Higher insulin concentration during exercise may increase plasma glucose uptake by the muscles and inhibit FFA mobilization and could contribute to maturation-related differences in substrate utilization. However, Wirth *et al.*[68] observed that, despite differences in insulin concentration, neither plasma glucose nor plasma FFA concentrations changed during exercise and differences between sexes or stages of maturation were not present. Wirth *et al.*'s findings[68] on plasma glucose concentrations are consistent with the extant literature which notes that, although children might experience difficulty in maintaining a constant plasma glucose concentration at the onset of submaximal exercise,[63,69] no clear age- or maturation-dependent plasma glucose differences are apparent during more prolonged submaximal exercise.[70,71]

Data on plasma FFAs and glycerol are less clear with some studies reporting similar exercise-induced responses in plasma FFA and glycerol concentrations.[55,70] Martinez and Haymes[55] showed similar FFA:glycerol ratios in girls and women but they concluded on the basis of their RER data that during submaximal exercise girls rely more on lipid utilization and less on carbohydrate utilization than women. Others have measured plasma FFA and glycerol and demonstrated greater FFA utilization in children than in adults.[63,69] Berg and Keul[45] reported reduced FFA:glycerol ratios during exercise in boys, which implies improved FFA utilization relative to men. On balance, the data suggest that children rely more on FFAs for energy provision during submaximal exercise than adults and in their comprehensive review of the topic, Boisseau and Delamarche[19] concluded that, 'this greater fat utilization may compensate for reduced glycolytic capacity and may allow children to maintain appropriate plasma glucose levels during exercise' (p. 415).

In summary, RER, ^{13}C stable isotope methodology, and studies of plasma concentration of glucose and FFAs during submaximal, steady-state exercise indicate an age- and maturation-related effect with children demonstrating a greater reliance than adults on lipids as an energy source. Boys' data are more consistent than those from girls and there may be sex-related differences in the balance between lipid and carbohydrate utilization during childhood and adolescence, as has been demonstrated in adults.[72] Enhanced use of lipids as an energy source during childhood may be a carbohydrate-sparing response to low muscle glycogen content. There are few data on hormonal responses to exercise during childhood (but see Chapter 38) and the impact of hormones on substrate utilization during childhood and adolescence is difficult to interpret.

Oxygen uptake kinetics

Pulmonary $\dot{V}O_2$ kinetic responses to step changes in exercise intensity have been shown to provide a non-invasive window into metabolic activity at the muscular level.[73] A high degree of rigour is required to assess and interpret $\dot{V}O_2$ kinetics in children and in Chapter 22 and elsewhere[74–78] we have addressed these methodological issues and critically analysed the extant literature of $\dot{V}O_2$ kinetics during childhood and adolescence. Here, we will briefly outline the characteristics of $\dot{V}O_2$ kinetic responses and focus on the insights into exercise metabolism which have been provided by rigorous studies.

Characteristics of the oxygen uptake kinetic response to exercise

Oxygen uptake kinetics are studied in the laboratory by the use of a step transition where a period of low-intensity exercise (e.g. unloaded pedalling on a cycle ergometer) is followed by a sudden increase in exercise intensity to a pre-determined level. The $\dot{V}O_2$ kinetic response to the step increase in exercise intensity is then interpreted in relation to four exercise domains which are called moderate, heavy, very heavy, and severe and set in relation to clear demarcation thresholds (see Fig. 22.1). The upper threshold of moderate exercise is the anaerobic threshold or a suitable derivative such as the lactate threshold or, more often with children, the non-invasive ventilatory threshold, (T_{VENT}) (see Figs. 6.3 and 6.4).[79] The T_{VENT} acts as the lower threshold of the heavy exercise domain with the maximal lactate steady state (MLSS)[10] (see Chapter 8) or the critical power (CP)[80] as the upper marker. As determination of the MLSS requires multiple blood sampling and determination of the CP is very demanding and time consuming, the upper threshold of the heavy exercise domain is normally defined as 40% of the difference between T_{VENT} and peak $\dot{V}O_2$, which has been shown to be appropriate for heavy intensity exercise studies with most children.[81] Exercise above CP but below peak $\dot{V}O_2$ falls into the very heavy exercise domain and $\dot{V}O_2$ rises until peak $\dot{V}O_2$ is achieved. In the severe exercise domain, the projected $\dot{V}O_2$ is greater than peak $\dot{V}O_2$ and the $\dot{V}O_2$ kinetic response is terminated with the rapid achievement of peak $\dot{V}O_2$. As rigorously determined data from children are only available for moderate and heavy exercise we will focus on these domains.

At the onset of a step transition in exercise there is an almost immediate increase in cardiac output which occurs prior to the arrival at the lungs of venous blood from the exercising muscles. This cardiodynamic phase (phase 1) which, in children, lasts about 15 s is independent of $\dot{V}O_2$ at the muscle ($\dot{Q}O_2$) and reflects an increase in pulmonary blood flow with exercise. Phase 2, the primary component, is a rapid exponential increase in $\dot{V}O_2$ that arises with hypoxic and hypercapnic blood from the exercising muscles arriving at the lungs. Phase 2 kinetics are described by the time constant (τ) which is the time taken to achieve 63% of the change in $\dot{V}O_2$. In phases 1 and 2, ATP resynthesis cannot be fully supported by oxidative phosphorylation and the additional energy requirements of the exercise are met from O_2 stores, PCr and glycolysis. The O_2 equivalent of these energy sources is the O_2 deficit and the faster the τ the smaller is the O_2 deficit. Phase 2 $\dot{V}O_2$ kinetics have been shown to closely reflect $\dot{Q}O_2$ despite some disassociation due to muscle utilization of O_2 stores and differences in blood flow at the muscles and lungs.[73]

During moderate intensity exercise, pulmonary $\dot{V}O_2$ reaches a steady state (phase 3) within about 2 min with an O_2 cost (gain) of about 10 $mL{\cdot}min^{-1}{\cdot}W^{-1}$ above that found during unloaded pedalling. During heavy intensity exercise, the primary phase 2 gain is similar to that observed during moderate exercise but the O_2 cost of exercise increases over time as a slow component of $\dot{V}O_2$ is superimposed upon the primary component and the achievement of a steady state might be delayed by 10–15 min (see Fig. 22.1). Data on the slow component in children are sparse and confounded by inappropriate methodology[81–86] (see Chapter 22) but the phenomenon has been clearly demonstrated during heavy intensity exercise with prepubertal children.[82,83] The mechanisms underlying the slow component remain speculative but appear to be a function of muscle fibre distribution, motor unit recruitment and the matching of O_2 delivery to active muscle fibres[87] (see Chapter 22).

Oxygen uptake kinetics during moderate intensity exercise

The effect of age on the phase 2 $\dot{V}O_2$ response to moderate exercise has been investigated in several studies. Methodological inadequacies limit other than cautious interpretation of the outcomes and the data are equivocal but two recent reviews of the extant literature have demonstrated a clear trend towards a faster τ in children than adults.[78,88]

To date, only one study[89] of children's $\dot{V}O_2$ kinetic response to moderate intensity exercise has used breath-by-breath analysis, reduced the 'noise' by averaging multiple transitions, used appropriate modelling techniques, exhibited strict adherence to well-defined exercise domains, and reported the 95% confidence intervals of their data. After excluding from the study those in whom the 95% confidence interval exceeded 5 s, the authors compared the $\dot{V}O_2$ kinetic responses to a step increment to exercise at 80% of T_{VENT} of 12 boys and 11 girls (aged 11–12 years) with 13 men and 12 women (aged 19–25 years). They demonstrated that the primary τ was significantly faster in boys (19.0 ± 2.0 s) than men (27.9 ± 8.6 s) and in girls (21.0 ± 5.5 s) than women (26.0 ± 4.5 s) with no sex differences observed in either children or adults. The $\dot{V}O_2$ amplitude, O_2 deficit, and O_2 deficit relative to $\dot{V}O_2$ amplitude were all significantly higher in men than boys and in women than girls. The authors suggested that children's faster τ and therefore higher aerobic contribution to ATP resynthesis during phase 2 might be due to a greater relative capacity for O_2 utilization at the muscle, a more efficient O_2 delivery system or both. Although in studies using dye dilution (see Chapter 7), Koch[90,91] indicated that muscle blood flow during exercise may decrease in boys from the age of 12 to 14 years, there is no strong evidence to indicate that the delivery of O_2 to the mitochondria is enhanced in children compared to adults or that increased availability of O_2 to the muscles increases the rate of $\dot{V}O_2$ kinetics during moderate intensity exercise. It is, therefore, likely that the children's faster τ and lower O_2 deficit reflect an enhanced capacity for oxidative phosphorylation.

In their comprehensive review of published studies, Barstow and Scheuermann[88] concluded that despite concerns about the rigour of the methodology of several investigations, the literature supports a pattern for a higher O_2 cost (gain) in prepubertal children than in adults. An age-dependent effect on the O_2 gain of the primary component during moderate intensity exercise would also indicate an enhanced capacity for oxidative phosphorylation in children but further evidence is required for confirmation of this hypothesis.

Oxygen uptake kinetics during heavy intensity exercise

Two studies[85,86] have compared the $\dot{V}O_2$ kinetic responses to exercise above T_{VENT} of children to adults and, although the experimental designs and methodology used have been criticized,[79,88] both studies observed significantly faster primary τs and greater O_2 gains in children than in adults.

Fawkner and Armstrong[82] carefully investigated prepubertal children's responses to a step change from unloaded pedalling to exercise at 40% of the difference between T_{VENT} and peak $\dot{V}O_2$. Only participants with 95% confidence intervals not exceeding 5 s following multiple transitions were included in the analysis. They monitored changes in 13 boys' and 9 girls' $\dot{V}O_2$ kinetic responses over a 2-year period. On the first test occasion, when all the children were at stage 1 for pubic hair,[59] a significantly greater O_2 gain during phase 2 and a significantly faster τ were observed in both the boys (17.1 ± 6.2 vs. 22.5 ± 4.8 s) and girls (21.9 ± 8.3 vs. 25.9 ± 8.3 s) than on a subsequent test 2 years later. A slow component of $\dot{V}O_2$ was observed on both test occasions, contributing about 10% of the final $\dot{V}O_2$ after 9 min on the first occasion and increases to about 15% 2 years later. The O_2 gain at the end of the exercise was equal on both test occasions suggesting that the phosphate turnover required to maintain the exercise was independent of age and that the older children achieved a lower proportion of the required O_2 in phase 2.

Using exactly the same methodology as in their earlier study Fawkner and Armstrong[83] demonstrated sex differences in the $\dot{V}O_2$ kinetic responses to heavy intensity exercise of prepubertal children (25 boys and 23 girls). The primary τ was significantly faster in boys (17.6 ± 5.8 s) than girls (21.9 ± 8.2 s) and the $\dot{V}O_2$ slow component was significantly greater in girls than boys (11.8% vs. 8.9%).

Changes in the size of the O_2 gain of the primary component, the magnitude of the $\dot{V}O_2$ slow component, and the speed of the τ with age are consistent with the presence of a developmental influence on the muscles' potential for O_2 utilization and therefore support an enhanced oxidative function during childhood. These responses are also characteristic of subjects with a high ratio of type I to type II muscle fibres (see Fig. 22.4 which shows a remarkable similarity between $\dot{V}O_2$ gain in relation to age and fibre type). Why sex differences in $\dot{V}O_2$ kinetic responses to heavy but not moderate intensity exercise have been observed is not readily apparent but they may be related to sex differences in muscle fibre types (see Table 16.1). In adults, the % of type I fibres has been shown to be negatively related to τ during exercise above but not below T_{VENT}.[92] The $\dot{V}O_2$ kinetic findings are therefore consistent with the trend for boys to have a greater % of type I fibres than similarly aged girls but more research is required to substantiate the relationship if it exists.

In summary, there are few rigorously designed and executed studies of children's $\dot{V}O_2$ kinetics but the technique has the potential to provide new insights into exercise metabolism during growth and maturation. Children's faster τ during both moderate and heavy intensity exercise, greater O_2 cost of heavy (and possibly moderate) exercise and smaller $\dot{V}O_2$ slow component are consistent with an enhanced oxidative function during childhood. The independent effects of maturation on $\dot{V}O_2$ kinetic responses to moderate and heavy exercise remain to be explored.

Magnetic resonance spectroscopy

Magnetic resonance spectroscopy (MRS) is a non-invasive technique that provides in real time and *in vivo* a window through which muscle can be interrogated during exercise. The safety of MRS for research with human participants is well-documented[93] and as no ionizing radiation or injected labelling agents are involved rigorous application of the technique using the naturally occurring phosphorus nucleus (^{31}P) has the potential to provide unique insights into exercise metabolism during growth and maturation.

Methodological issues

MRS studies are constrained by exercising within a small bore tube and the need to synchronize the acquisition of data with the rate of muscle contraction and this can be challenging with young participants. To illustrate some of the methodological issues, we will describe techniques used in our laboratory with children during exercise studies.

We have constructed a to-scale replica of our MR scanner which both allows young participants to overcome any fears of exercising within a tube and to habituate to the required exercise regimen without using expensive magnet time.[94] While lying in the replica scanner, the child's foot is fastened securely with Velcro to a padded foot brace which is connected to a non-magnetic ergometer incorporating a load basket which provides via a pulley system a variable resistance against which unilateral knee extensions can be performed while lying prone. To standardize the exercise protocol the children practise following an image of a vertical metronomic cursor, projected on to a visual display in front of them, using a second vertical cursor under their control. To ensure interrogation of the quadriceps muscles for metabolic changes always occurs in the same volume of interest (VOI), the frequency of the cursor is set to 40 pulses per minute to ensure that the children practise knee extensions over the prescribed range at a cadence in unison with the magnetic pulse sequence typically used in the MR scanner. It is only when the children are comfortable in the enclosed space of the replica scanner, fully habituated to the exercise regimen, and capable of maintaining the required knee cadence that they are transferred to the MR scanner.

In the MR scanner, the child's foot is again securely attached to a non-magnetic ergometer with Velcro and to prevent displacement of the quadriceps VOI relative to the MRS coil and to minimize adjacent muscles contributing to the exercise task, the child's legs, hips, and lower back are secured in position using Velcro straps. The magnetic field is activated and following a period of rest, single leg quadriceps muscle exercise is initiated and carefully monitored. Once the magnet is activated the nuclei of atoms align with the magnetic field, a second oscillating magnetic field is applied and the subsequent nuclear transitions allow spectral analysis of the interrogated muscles. Molecules produce their own individual spectra and once the molecules have been identified changes in the spectral lines can be interpreted. The principal nucleus used in metabolic studies is the naturally occurring phosphorus nucleus, ^{31}P which enables the monitoring of the molecules that play a central role in exercise metabolism, namely, ATP, PCr, and inorganic phosphate (Pi). Typical ^{31}P-MRS spectra obtained during rest, incremental exercise, and recovery are shown in Fig. 16.1, where, from left to right, the spectral peaks represent Pi, the single phosphorus nucleus of PCr, and the three phosphate nuclei of ATP. During incremental exercise, Pi increases with a corresponding decline in PCr. Spectral areas are quantified and exercise-induced changes in PCr and Pi are expressed as the percentage change from baseline using the PCr and Pi spectral areas obtained during the preceding rest period.

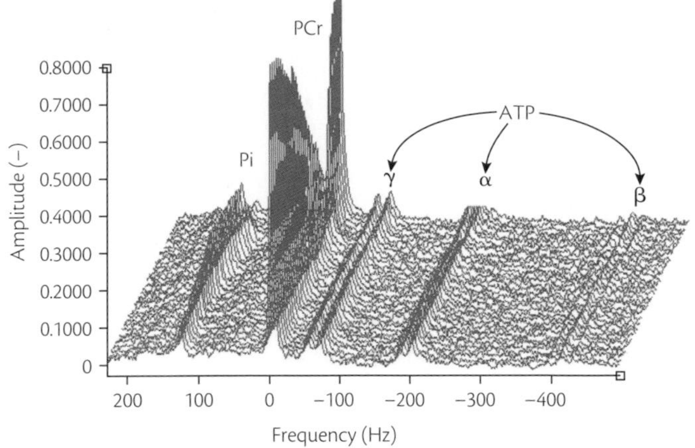

Fig. 16.1 ^{31}P-magnetic resonance spectra obtained from a 9-year-old child during rest, exercise, and recovery. From left to right the peaks represent free organic phosphate (Pi), phosphocreatine (PCr), and the three phosphorus nuclei of adenosine triphosphate (ATP). Reprinted from Armstrong and Welsman,[96] with permission.

The chemical shift of the Pi spectral peak relative to the PCr peak reflects the acidification of the muscle and intracellular pH can be determined using the relationship:

$$\text{pH} = 6.75 + \log (\sigma—3.27)/(5.96—\sigma)$$

where σ represents the chemical shift in parts per million between the Pi and the PCr resonance peaks.[95] The change in pH during exercise provides an indication of muscle glycolytic activity but it is not a direct measure of glycolysis.

A typical progressive, incremental exercise test to exhaustion in our MR scanner follows a 2 min resting baseline measurement period and starts with an initial basket load of 0.5 kg. The basket load is increased in steps of 0.5 kg each minute using brass weights until the child can no longer comply with the required knee extensor rate. Increments of 0.5 kg used as pilot work has demonstrated that this protocol ensures, with children, exhaustion within 7–12 min. Following time alignment of data to the start of the exercise test, work done is interpolated second by second and averaged every 30 s to coincide with the resolution used for metabolite acquisition. Power output is derived from each data bin by dividing the work done by time. Spectra are obtained every 1.5 s and 20 measurements are performed leading to a spectra being acquired every 30 s. Using resting values as a baseline the changes in spectral areas in Pi/PCr and pH during exercise are quantified and each variable is plotted as a function of power output as shown in Fig. 16.2.

An incremental exercise test to exhaustion results in non-linear changes in the ratio Pi/PCr plotted against power output and in pH plotted against power output. As power output increases, an initial shallow slope is followed by a second steeper slope and the transition point is known as the intracellular threshold (IT). ITs are valuable indicators of children's metabolism during incremental exercise and they occur at a relative exercise intensity similar to the T_{VENT} during incremental cycle ergometer exercise. For example, Barker *et al.*[97] observed the ^{31}P-MRS determined Pi/PCr IT to occur at 59% of maximal power output and the cycle ergometer T_{VENT} to occur at 58% of peak $\dot{V}O_2$ in the same 9–11 year olds. Using this

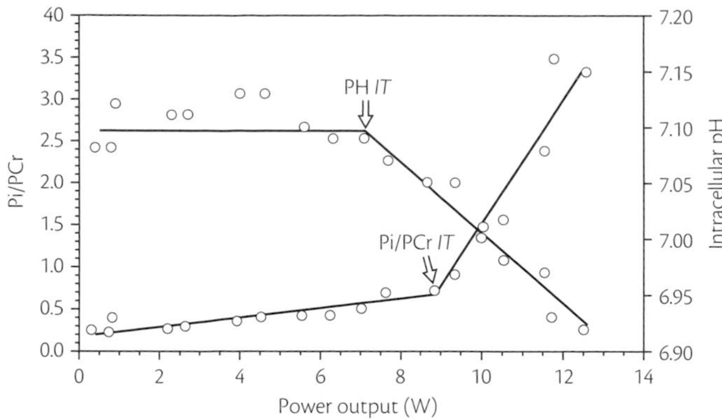

Fig. 16.2 Pi/PCr ratio and pH in relation to power output determined in the quadriceps muscle of a 9-year-old child during exercise in the magnet. The intracellular thresholds (ITs) are indicated. Reprinted from Armstrong and Welsman,[96] with permission.

methodology in a study of ^{31}P-MRS reliability with prepubertal children, Barker *et al.*[94] demonstrated a detection rate of 93% and 81% for the ITs of Pi/PCr ($IT_{Pi/PCr}$) and pH (IT_{pH}), respectively, and although the $IT_{Pi/PCr}$ and IT_{pH} did not always occur at exactly the same power outputs they were highly correlated (Fig. 16.2). Good test–retest reliability was observed with typical errors across three trials a week apart of about 10% for both $IT_{Pi/PCr}$ and IT_{pH}.[94]

Magnetic resonance studies during incremental exercise

Few ^{31}P-MRS studies have rigorously monitored children during incremental exercise but despite methodological limitations the findings are in general agreement. The first study to include child participants was reported by Zanconato *et al.*[98] and involved two girls and eight boys, aged 7–10 years, and three women and five men, aged 20–40 years, who carried out supine, incremental treadle plantar flexion exercise to voluntary exhaustion. Zanconato *et al.*[98] observed an increase in Pi/PCr and a decrease in pH in both children and adults with increasing exercise intensity. Intracellular thresholds were detected in 50% of the children and 75% of the adults and although the characteristics of the initial linear slopes in Pi/PCr and pH were similar regardless of age, following the ITs the incline in Pi/PCr and decline in pH were both steeper in adults than in children. The change in pH from rest to end-exercise was significantly greater in adults than in children, whose end-exercise Pi/PCr was, on average, only 27% of adult values. Zanconato *et al.* interpreted these findings as reflecting age-related differences in energy metabolism such that children rely less on anaerobic metabolism during high-intensity exercise than do adults.

Zanconato *et al.*'s research[98] was pioneering but the data raise several methodological concerns. For example, Zanconato *et al.* recruited small, mixed sex samples, pooled the data, and scaled data to body size (ratio scaling) without checking whether this process was appropriate (see Chapter 2). It is possible that the young participants may not have achieved true maximal values as an $IT_{Pi/PCr}$ was only detected in 50% of children whereas other researchers who followed the habituation procedures described earlier and rigorously monitored adherence to the exercise protocol observed an $IT_{Pi/PCr}$ in 100% of both children and adults.[99]

Finally, whereas Zanconato *et al.* noted end-exercise Pi/PCr values of 0.54 ratios in excess of 2.0 have been reported by others using a similar protocol.[94] Furthermore, the heterogeneity in calf muscle size between young children and adults may result in a disproportionate sampling of the gastrocnemius and soleus muscle compartments between groups, such that the soleus represents a greater portion of the ^{31}P-MRS signal in the children. As the soleus is composed mainly of type I muscle fibres and the gastrocnemius mainly of type II fibres, it is plausible that Zanconato *et al.*'s interrogation of the calf muscle might have biased the lower accumulation of Pi, breakdown of PCr, and fall in pH in child compared to adult muscle.

Nevertheless, Zanconato *et al.*'s observations were subsequently supported by a study of 14 trained and 23 untrained 12- to 15-year-old boys and six adults with an average age of 25 years.[100] Magnetic resonance spectra were collected from the quadriceps during supine, incremental exercise to exhaustion and higher values of intracellular pH, and the ratio PCr/(PCr + Pi) were noted in the boys at exhaustion. No significant differences were observed between the trained and untrained boys.

In a study of ageing effects on skeletal muscle, Taylor *et al.*[101] compared ^{31}P-MRS spectra at rest, during maximal calf muscle exercise and recovery from maximal exercise of fifteen 6–12 year olds with twenty 20–29 year olds, both groups consisted of unspecified numbers of males and females. The children had a higher pH during exercise, indicating a lower glycolytic contribution to metabolism and a faster resynthesis of PCr during recovery than adults. On the basis of the recovery data, Taylor *et al.* suggested that the oxidative capacity of skeletal muscle is highest in childhood. Taylor's work was subsequently supported by Ratel *et al.*,[102] who demonstrated that following maximal finger flexion exercise in a MR scanner the rate constant of PCr recovery was significantly faster in seven 11-year-old boys than in ten 35-year-old men. In contrast, Kuno *et al.*[100] observed no differences between boys and adults in the PCr time constant during recovery from maximal exercise and concluded that the invariant PCr kinetics were indicative of a comparable mitochondrial oxidative capacity between child and adult muscle. However, the experimental conditions (i.e. cellular acidosis) under which PCr recovery dynamics were determined in these three studies raise methodological concerns that preclude any firm conclusions being drawn.

Petersen *et al.*[103] investigated the effects of maturation on exercise metabolism by evaluating the responses of nine 10-year-old, 'prepubertal' and nine 15-year-old 'pubertal', trained girls swimmers to 2 min of calf exercise at light (40% of pre-determined maximal work capacity) followed by 2 min of 'supramaximal' (140% maximal work capacity) exercise using a plantar flexion ergometer. The girls self-assessed their stage of maturation from pubic hair and breast development using the techniques described by Tanner.[59] At the end of the exercise, intracellular pH was lower (6.66 vs. 6.76) and the Pi/PCr ratio was higher (2.18 vs. 1.31) in the 15 year olds but the differences were not statistically significant. Petersen *et al.*[103] concluded that glycolytic metabolism in physically active children is not maturity dependent. They commented, however, that this conclusion should be interpreted with caution. Scrutiny of the magnitude of the difference between the two groups in the Pi/PCr ratio (66%), the high variability, and the small sample sizes suggest that the observed differences might have biological meaning and deserve further study.

In a rigorous analysis of muscle phosphate and pH responses in relation to age and sex, Barker *et al.*[99] monitored 15 boys and 18 girls, aged 9–12 years, and eight men and eight women, aged 22–26 years, during a single legged quadriceps incremental test to exhaustion. They determined quadriceps muscle mass using MR imaging and used log-linear allometric regression models [power function ratios (see Chapter 2)] to normalize absolute power output measurements for quadriceps muscle mass. The participants were well habituated to exercising within a magnet and an $IT_{Pi/PCr}$ was detected in 100% of cases in both children and adults. Using the derived power function ratio to normalize power output at the $IT_{Pi/PCr}$ for muscle mass, no age- or sex-related differences in power output were identified between children and adults. The increase in Pi/PCr at the $IT_{Pi/PCr}$ was comparable between the boys and men, girls and women, boys and girls, and men and women, in fact, during exercise equal to or below the metabolic ITs, the muscle phosphate, and pH responses were observed to be remarkably similar between children and adults and boys and girls. However, above the ITs age- and sex-related differences in muscle phosphate and pH responses were readily apparent indicating that for a given increase in power output during exercise above $IT_{Pi/PCr}$, adults require a greater breakdown of PCr and accumulation of Pi compared to children (i.e. a greater anaerobic energy contribution). This was also observed to be the case when girls were compared to boys. Similarly, above the IT_{pH} pH changes were significantly less in boys compared to men and girls, possibly indicating a lower glycolytic energy contribution during high-intensity exercise. In girls, a number of significant relationships between the ^{31}P-MRS derived indices of anaerobic metabolism and maturation, which was estimated from the offset score from the age at peak height velocity[104] (see Chapter 12), were observed. In conflict with the conclusions of Petersen *et al.*,[103] the authors therefore suggested that the higher anaerobic energy contribution of the girls during exercise above the $IT_{Pi/PCr}$ might be attributable to their more advanced level of maturity than the boys who were largely prepubertal and early pubertal. The age- and sex-related responses to exercise observed by Barker *et al.*[99] are strikingly similar to those in studies comparing muscle phosphate and pH responses during exercise in muscles with different fibre type profiles.[105,106]

Magnetic resonance spectroscopy studies during constant intensity exercise

To date, only one study has investigated potential age- and sex-related differences in the kinetics of muscle PCr.[107] Eighteen 9-year-old children (eight boys and ten girls) and sixteen 23- to 25-year-old adults (eight men and eight women) initially completed an incremental exercise test to exhaustion to determine their $IT_{Pi/PCr}$. They then carried out repeat constant exercise intensity transitions corresponding to 80% of $IT_{Pi/PCr}$ (i.e. moderate intensity exercise) and consisting of 2 min rest, 6 min exercise, and 6 min recovery. In all cases, a single exponential model with no time delay provided an appropriate fit to the PCr response. The children completed 6 ± 2 and the adults 4 ± 1 repeat transitions which were subsequently averaged in order to achieve 95% confidence intervals of ±6 s. No significant age- or sex-related differences were found in the PCr kinetic τ either at the onset (boys, 21 ± 4 s; girls, 24 ± 5 s; men, 26 ± 9 s; women, 24 ± 7 s) or offset (boys, 26 ± 5 s; girls, 29 ± 7 s; men, 23 ± 9 s; women 29 ± 7 s) of exercise. It appears, on the basis of the findings of this study, that the kinetics of muscle PCr are unrelated to age and sex during the transition to and recovery from moderate intensity exercise. These findings are in accordance with $\dot{V}O_2$ kinetic data comparing boys and girls but in conflict with child–adult comparisons.[89] No published study to date has addressed age- and sex-related differences in the kinetics of muscle PCr during exercise above the $IT_{Pi/PCr}$.

Oxygen uptake kinetics and phosphocreatine kinetics

Studies with adult subjects have demonstrated that with the implementation of appropriate modelling techniques the phase 2 pulmonary $\dot{V}O_2$ response provides a close relationship with PCr kinetics at the onset of exercise both when $\dot{V}O_2$ kinetics are predetermined on a cycle ergometer[108] and when they are determined simultaneously with PCr kinetics using knee extensor exercise in a MR scanner.[73] Children display a lower $\dot{V}O_2$ signal amplitude than adults, which makes simultaneous assessment of $\dot{V}O_2$ and PCr kinetics in an MR scanner infeasible. To explore the strength of the association in children, Barker *et al.*[97] therefore determined the $\dot{V}O_2$ kinetic τ to moderate intensity exercise using cycle ergometry and the PCr kinetic τ to moderate intensity exercise using knee flexor exercise in a MR scanner. Using the techniques described earlier, six boys and six girls, aged 9.9 ± 0.3 years, completed, on average, six and seven constant intensity exercise transitions for the determination of the PCr and $\dot{V}O_2$ kinetics responses, respectively. The 95% confidence intervals were less than ±7 s for all estimated time constants. No significant differences were found between PCr and $\dot{V}O_2$ τs at either the onset (PCr, 28 ± 5 s; $\dot{V}O_2$ 29 ± 5 s) or offset (28 ± 5 s; $\dot{V}O_2$ 29 ± 5 s) of exercise, the mean difference between the PCr and $\dot{V}O_2$ τs was 4 s, a significant correlation ($r = 0.5$) between the PCr and $\dot{V}O_2$ τs was observed, and the 95% confidence intervals spanning the PCr and $\dot{V}O_2$ τs failed to overlap in only one child. The authors therefore concluded that children's PCr kinetics during prone quadriceps exercise and $\dot{V}O_2$ kinetics during upright cycling are similar, at least during moderate intensity exercise.

In summary, the use of ^{31}P-MRS in paediatric exercise science is in its infancy but the technique presents a huge untapped potential to examine exercise metabolism *in vivo* and to provide new insights into age-, maturation-, and sex-related differences. Rigorous studies are sparse but the extant evidence indicates that during exercise above the $IT_{Pi/PCr}$ (i.e. heavy intensity exercise) for a given increase in power output adults require a greater anaerobic contribution than children. This might also be the case when girls are compared to boys and there is some, albeit limited, evidence to suggest that the increased anaerobic energy contribution during heavy intensity exercise might be related to maturation. The kinetics of PCr breakdown during exercise below the $IT_{Pi/PCr}$ appear to be unrelated to age and sex but children's PCr kinetics during heavy intensity exercise remain to be explored.

Conclusion

Paediatric exercise scientists have investigated young people's exercise metabolism for over 70 years but research has been limited by ethical considerations and the lack, until recently, of non-invasive techniques of interrogating muscle *in vivo*. Much remains to be revealed but the weight of evidence from a wide range of techniques clearly indicates that during exercise there is an interplay of anaerobic and aerobic metabolism in which young people respond to an exercise challenge with higher oxidative activity than adults.

Glycolytic activity progressively increases with age at least into adolescence and possibly into young adulthood. An independent relationship (e.g. in addition to age) between maturation and exercise metabolism has been indicated by some studies but remains to be proven. Several studies have suggested the presence of intriguing sex differences in exercise metabolism but further research is required to tease out these differences, if they exist, and to explain the underlying mechanisms.

The rigorous application of non-invasive technologies such as ^{31}P-MRS and breath-by-breath determination of $\dot{V}O_2$ kinetics has the potential to provide new insights into paediatric exercise metabolism. However, the high cost of obtaining MR spectra, the time-consuming habituation of children to an exercise protocol confined within a tube and the restricted availability of MR scanners for research with healthy children may limit the development and application of the technique with the exercising child. More research using ^{31}P-MRS is urgently required but in the absence of ^{31}P-MRS data, the close relationship between PCr and $\dot{V}O_2$ kinetics in children encourages the use of more child-friendly and less expensive $\dot{V}O_2$ kinetics as an additional and valuable non-invasive window into muscle metabolism during growth and maturation.

Summary

- The well-documented age-related increases in aerobic and anaerobic fitness are not synchronous and young people experience a more marked increase in maximal measures of anaerobic fitness than aerobic fitness during adolescence. Metabolic profiles derived from maximal performance measures are useful indicators of metabolism during heavy intensity exercise but they are unable to provide the quality of data required to explore growth- and maturation-related changes in exercise metabolism.
- Muscle biopsy studies with children are sparse and data need to be treated with caution. However, the literature shows a clear age-related decline in the % of type I fibres from childhood to young adulthood and a consistent trend showing adolescent boys and young adult males to exhibit a higher % of type I fibres (8–15%) than females.
- Resting ATP stores appear to be invariant with age but PCr and glycogen stores progressively increase from childhood through adolescence into young adulthood.
- Young children have higher oxidative enzyme activity and lower glycolytic enzyme activity than adolescents and adults. Adolescents have an enhanced oxidative capacity compared to adults but the evidence indicating differences in the glycolytic activity of adolescents and adults is equivocal. A consistent finding is that the ratio of glycolytic/oxidative enzyme activity is higher in adults than in children or adolescents.
- Substrate utilization studies using RER and ^{13}C stable isotope methodology and investigations of plasma concentration of glucose and FFAs during submaximal steady-state exercise consistently indicate an age- and maturation-related effect with children relying more than adults on lipids as an energy source.
- Pulmonary $\dot{V}O_2$ kinetic responses to step changes in exercise intensity have been shown to provide a non-invasive window into muscle metabolism. Children's faster primary time constant during both moderate and heavy intensity exercise, greater O_2 cost of heavy (and possibly moderate) exercise, and smaller $\dot{V}O_2$ slow component suggest the presence of an enhanced oxidative function and/or greater % of type I muscle fibres during childhood. The sex difference in children's $\dot{V}O_2$ kinetic response to heavy but not moderate intensity exercise is consistent with boys having a higher % of type I fibres than girls.
- Although there are very few ^{31}P-MRS studies of the healthy, exercising child, this technique has the potential to revolutionize our understanding of muscle metabolism during growth and maturation. Current evidence indicates that during progressive exercise to exhaustion children and adults display a similar rate of mitochondrial oxidative metabolism below the $IT_{Pi/PCr}$ but adults exhibit superior glycolytic activity during exercise above the $IT_{Pi/PCr}$. Only one study has examined the kinetics of PCr breakdown during exercise below the $IT_{Pi/PCr}$ and no sex- or age-related differences were observed. Children's PCr kinetics above the $IT_{Pi/PCr}$ have not been investigated.
- Studies of exercise metabolism during growth and maturation are limited by ethical considerations. However, the weight of evidence from a wide range of investigative techniques clearly indicates that during exercise there is an interplay of anaerobic and aerobic metabolism in which young people exhibit higher oxidative activity than adults. There is a progressive increase in glycolytic activity with age, at least into adolescence and possibly into young adulthood. The sex differences in exercise metabolism during childhood and adolescence which have been identified in some studies require further exploration. Whether there is an independent influence of maturation on exercise metabolism remains to be proven but represents an intriguing avenue for future research.
- The development and rigorous application of relatively new non-invasive techniques such as ^{31}P-MRS and $\dot{V}O_2$ kinetics to interrogate muscles *in vivo* promises new insights into paediatric exercise metabolism. The research challenge is to explain the underlying mechanisms.

References

1. Armstrong N, Welsman JR, Chia M (2001). Short-term power output in relation to growth and maturation. *Br J Sports Med* **35**, 118–25.
2. Hebestreit H, Meyer F, Htay H, Heigenhauser GJ, Bar-Or O (1993). Recovery of muscle power after short-term exercise: Comparing boys and men. *J Appl Physiol* **74**, 2875–80.
3. Ratel S, Williams CA, Oliver J, Armstrong N (2004). Effects of age and mode of exercise on power output profiles during repeated sprints. *Eur J Appl Physiol* **92**, 204–10.
4. Ratel S, Williams CA, Oliver J, Armstrong N (2005). Effects of age and recovery duration on performance during multiple treadmill sprints. *Int J Sports Med* **26**, 1–8.
5. Chia M (2001). Power recovery in the Wingate anaerobic test in girls and women following prior sprints of short duration. *Biol Sport* **18**, 45–53.
6. Ratel S, Lazaar N, Williams CA, Bedu M, Duche P (2003). Age differences in human skeletal muscle fatigue during high-intensity intermittent exercise. *Acta Paediatr* **92**, 1248–54.
7. Ratel S, Duche P, Williams CA (2006). Muscle fatigue during high-intensity exercise in children. *Sports Med* **36**, 1031–65.
8. Falk B, Dotan R (2006). Child-adult differences in the recovery from high-intensity exercise. *Exerc Sport Sci Rev* **34**, 107–12.

9. Welsman JR, Armstrong N (2000). Statistical techniques for interpreting body size-related exercise performance during growth. *Pediatr Exerc Sci* **12**, 112–27.
10. Armstrong N, Welsman JR (1994). Assessment and interpretation of aerobic fitness in children and adolescents. *Exerc Sport Sci Rev* **22**, 435–76.
11. Armstrong N, Welsman JR (2001). Peak oxygen uptake in relation to growth and maturation. *Eur J Appl Physiol* **28**, 259–65.
12. Bergstrom J (1962). Muscle electrolytes in man determined by neutron activation analysis on needle biopsy specimens. *Scand J Clin Lab Invest* **14** (Suppl. 68), 1–110.
13. Bergstrom J (1975). Percutaneous needle biopsy of skeletal muscle in physiological and clinical research. *Scand J Clin Lab Invest* **35**, 609–16.
14. Astrand PO (1991). Influence of Scandinavian scientists in exercise physiology. *Scand J Med Sci Sports* **1**, 3–9.
15. Lexell J, Sjostrom M, Nordlund A-S, Taylor CC (1992). Growth and development of human muscle: A quantitative morphological study of whole vastus lateralis from childhood to adult age. *Muscle Nerve* **15**, 404–9.
16. Jansson, E (1996). Age-related fiber type changes in human skeletal muscle. In: Maughan TJ, Shirreffs SM (eds.), *Biochemistry of exercise IX*, pp. 297–307. Human Kinetics, Champaign, IL.
17. Elder GCB, Bradbury K, Roberts R (1982). Variability of fiber type distributions within human muscles. *J Appl Physiol* **53**, 1473–81.
18. Lexell J, Taylor C, Sjostrom M (1985). Analysis of sampling errors in biopsy techniques using data from whole muscle cross sections. *J Appl Physiol* **59**, 1228–35.
19. Boisseau N, Delamarche P (2000). Metabolic and hormonal responses to exercise in children and adolescents. *Sports Med* **30**, 405–22.
20. Komi PV, Karlsson J (1978). Skeletal muscle fibre types, enzyme activities and physical performance in young males and females. *Acta Physiol Scand* **103**, 210–18.
21. Jansson E, Hedberg G (1991). Skeletal muscle fibre types in teenagers: relationship to physical performance and activity. *Scand J Med Sci Sports* **1**, 31–44.
22. Van Praagh E, Dore E (2002). Short-term muscle power during growth and maturation. *Sports Med* **32**, 701–28.
23. Glenmark BC, Hedberg G, Jansson E (1992). Changes in muscle fibre type from adolescence to adulthood in women and men. *Acta Physiol Scand* **146**, 251–9.
24. Bell RD, MacDougall JD, Billeter R, Howald H (1980). Muscle fibre types and morphometric analysis of skeletal muscles in six year old children. *Med Sci Sports Exerc* **12**, 28–31.
25. Oertel G (1988). Morphometric analysis of normal skeletal muscles in infancy, childhood and adolescence. *J Neurol Sci* **88**, 303–13.
26. du Plessis MP, Smit PJ, du Plessis LAS, Geyer HJ, Mathews G (1985). The composition of muscle fibers in a group of adolescents. In: Binkhorst RA, Kemper HCG, Saris WHM (eds.), *Children and exercise XI*, pp. 323–4. University Park Press, Baltimore, MD.
27. Houmard JA, Smith R, Jendrasiak GL (1995). Relationship between MRI relaxation time and muscle fibre composition. *J Appl Physiol* **78**, 807–9.
28. Kuno S, Katsuta S, Inouye T, Anno I, Matsumoto K, Akisada M (1988). Relationship between MR relaxation time and muscle fiber composition. *Radiology* **169**, 567–8.
29. Eriksson BO, Karlsson J, Saltin B (1971). Muscle metabolites during exercise in pubertal boys. *Acta Paediatr Scand* **217**, 154–7.
30. Eriksson BO (1972). Physical training, oxygen supply and muscle metabolism in 11–13-year-old boys. *Acta Physiol Scand* **Suppl 384**, 1–103.
31. Eriksson BO, Gollnick PD, Saltin B (1973). Muscle metabolism and enzyme activities after training in boys 11–13 years old. *Acta Physiol Scand* **87**, 485–99.
32. Eriksson BO, Gollnick PD, Saltin B (1974). The effect of physical training on muscle enzyme activities and fiber composition in 11 year old boys. *Acta Paediatr Belg* **28**, 245–52.
33. Eriksson BO, Saltin B (1974). Muscle metabolism during exercise in boys aged 11 to 16 years compared to adults. *Acta Paediatr Belg* **28**, 257–65.
34. Eriksson BO (1980). Muscle metabolism in children—A review. *Acta Physiol Scand* **283**, 20–8.
35. Beneke R, Hutler M, Jung M, Leithauser RM (2005). Modeling the blood lactate kinetics at maximal short-term exercise conditions in children, adolescents and adults. *J Appl Physiol* **99**, 499–504.
36. Dotan R, Ohana S, Bediz C, Falk B (2003). Blood lactate disappearance dynamics in boys and men following exercise of similar and dissimilar peak-lactate concentrations. *J Pediatr Endocrinol Metab* **16**, 419–29.
37. Pfitzinger P, Freedson P (1997). Blood lactate responses to exercise in children: Part 1. Peak lactate concentration. *Pediatr Exerc Sci* **9**, 210–22.
38. Pfitzinger P, Freedson P (1997). Blood lactate responses to exercise in children: Part 2. Lactate threshold. *Pediatr Exerc Sci* **9**, 299–307.
39. Welsman J, Armstrong N (1998). Assessing postexercise blood lactates in children and adolescents. In Van Praagh E (ed.), *Pediatric anaerobic performance*, pp. 137–53. Human Kinetics, Champaign, IL.
40. Pianosi P, Seargeant L, Haworth JC (1995). Blood lactate and pyruvate concentrations, and their ratio during exercise in healthy children: Developmental perspective. *Eur J Appl Physiol* **71**, 518–22.
41. Beneke R, Hutler M, Leithauser RM (2007). Anaerobic performance and metabolism in boys and male adolescents. *Eur J Appl Physiol* **101**, 671–7.
42. Gollnick PD, Armstrong RB, Saubert CW, Piehl K, Saltin B (1972). Enzyme activity and fiber composition in skeletal muscle of untrained and trained men. *J Appl Physiol* **33**, 312–19.
43. Haralambie G (1979). Skeletal muscle enzyme activities in female subjects of various ages. *Bull Eur Physiopath Resp* **15**, 259–67.
44. Haralambie G (1982). Enzyme activities in skeletal muscle of 13–15 year old adolescents. *Bull Eur Physiopath Resp* **18**, 65–74.
45. Berg A, Keul J (1988). Biochemical changes during exercise in children. In: Malina RM (ed.), *Young athletes*, pp. 61–78. Human Kinetics, Champaign, IL.
46. Berg A, Kim SS, Keul J (1986). Skeletal muscle enzyme activities in healthy young subjects. *Int J Sports Med* **7**, 236–9.
47. Kaczor JJ, Ziolkowski W, Popinigis J, Tarnopolsky MA (2005). Anaerobic and aerobic enzyme activities in human skeletal muscle from children and adults. *Pediatr Res* **57**, 331–5.
48. Peronnet F (1991). Table of nonprotein respiratory quotient: An update. *Can J Appl Sport Sci* **16**, 23–9.
49. Foricher JM, Ville N, Gratas-Delamarche A, Delamarche P (2003). Effects of submaximal intensity cycle ergometry for one hour on substrate utilization in trained prepubertal boys versus trained adults. *J Sports Med Phys Fitness* **43**, 36–43.
50. Mahon AD, Duncan GE, Howe CA, Del Corral P (1997). Blood lactate and perceived exertion relative to ventilatory threshold: Boys versus men. *Med Sci Sports Exerc* **29**, 1332–7.
51. Montoye HJ (1982). Age and oxygen utilization during submaximal treadmill exercise in males. *J Gerontol* **37**, 396–402.
52. Rowland TW, Auchinachie JA, Keenan TJ, Green GM (1987). Physiologic responses to treadmill running in adult and prepubertal males. *Int J Sports Med* **8**, 292–7.
53. Rowland TW, Rimany TA (1995). Physiological responses to prolonged exercise in premenarcheal and adult females. *Int J Sports Med* **7**, 183–91.
54. Armstrong N, Kirby BJ, Welsman JR, McManus AM (1997). Submaximal exercise in prepubertal children. In: Armstrong N, Kirby BJ, Welsman JR (eds.), *Children and exercise X1X*, pp. 221–7. E & FN Spon, London.
55. Martinez LR, Haymes EM (1992). Substrate utilization during treadmill running in prepubertal girls and women. *Med Sci Sports Exerc* **24**, 975–83.

56. Friedlander AL, Casazza GA, Hornig MA, Huie MJ, Piacentini MF, Trimmer JK, Brooks GA (1998). Training-induced alterations of carbohydrate metabolism in women: Women respond differently from men. *J Appl Physiol* **85**, 1175–86.
57. D'Eon TM, Sharoff C, Chipkin SR, Grow D, Ruby BC, Braun B (2002). Regulation of exercise carbohydrate metabolism by estrogen and progesterone in women. *Am J Physiol Endocrinol Metab* **283**, 1046–55.
58. Stephens BR, Cole AS, Mahon AD (2006). The influence of biological maturation on fat and carbohydrate metabolism during exercise in males. *Int J Sport Nutr Exerc Metab* **16**, 166–79.
59. Tanner JM (1962). *Growth at adolescence* (2nd ed.). Blackwell Scientific, Oxford.
60. Timmons BW, Bar-Or O, Riddell MC (2003). Oxidation rate of exogenous carbohydrate during exercise is higher in boys than in men. *J Appl Physiol* **94**, 278–84.
61. Timmons BW, Bar-Or O, Riddell MC (2007). Energy substrate utilization during prolonged exercise with and without carbohydrate intake in preadolescent and adolescent girls. *J Appl Physiol* **103**, 995–1000.
62. Timmons BW, Bar-Or O, Riddell MC (2007). Influence of age and pubertal status on substrate utilization during exercise with and without carbohydrate intake in healthy boys. *Appl Physiol Nutr Metab* **32**, 416–25.
63. Delamarche PM, Monnier A, Gratas-Delamarche A, Koubi HE, Mayet MH, Favier R (1992). Glucose and free fatty acid utilization during prolonged exercise in prepubertal boys in relation to catecholamine responses. *Eur J Appl Physiol* **65**, 66–72.
64. Lehmann M, Keul J, Korsten-Reck U (1981). The influence of graduated treadmill exercise on plasma catecholamines, aerobic and anaerobic capacity in boys and adults. *Eur J Appl Physiol* **47**, 301–11.
65. Rowland TW, Maresh CM, Charkoudian N, Vanderburgh PM, Castellani JW, Armstrong LE (1996). Plasma norepinephrine responses to cycle exercise in boys and men. *Int J Sports Med* **17**, 22–6.
66. Mero A (1988). Blood lactate production and recovery from anaerobic exercise in trained and untrained boys. *Eur J Appl Physiol* **57**, 660–6.
67. Welsman JR, Armstrong N, Kirby BJ (1994). Serum testosterone is not related to peak $\dot{V}O_2$ and submaximal blood lactate in 12–16 year old males. *Pediatr Exerc Sci* **6**, 120–7.
68. Wirth A, Trager E, Scheele K, Mayer D, Diehm K, Reischle K, Weicker H (1978). Cardiopulmonary adjustment and metabolic response to maximal and submaximal physical exercise of boys and girls at different stages of maturity. *Eur J Appl Physiol* **39**, 229–40.
69. Delamarche P, Gratas-Delamarche A, Monnier M, Mayet MH, Koubi HE, Favier R (1994). Glucoregulation and hormonal changes during prolonged exercise in boys and girls. *Eur J Appl Physiol* **68**, 3–8.
70. Eriksson BO, Persson B, Thorell JI (1971). The effects of repeated exercise on plasma growth hormone, insulin, glucose, free fatty acids, glycerol, lactate and hydroxybutyric acid in 13-year-old boys and in adults. *Acta Paediatr Scand* **217** (Suppl.), 142–6.
71. Oseid S, Hermansen L (1971). Hormonal and metabolic changes during and after prolonged muscular work in prepubertal boys. *Acta Paediatr Scand* **217** (Suppl.), 147–53.
72. Tarnopolsky MA (2000). Gender differences in substrate metabolism during endurance exercise. *Can J Appl Physiol* **25**, 312–27.
73. Rossiter HB, Ward SA, Doyle VL, Howe FA, Griffiths JR, Whipp BJ (1999). Inferences from pulmonary O_2 uptake with respect to intramuscular (phosphocreatine) kinetics during moderate exercise in humans. *J Physiol (Lond)* **518**, 921–32.
74. Fawkner SJ, Armstrong N (2002). Modelling the kinetic response to moderate intensity exercise in children. *Acta Kinesiol Univ Tartuensis* **7**, 80–4.
75. Fawkner SJ, Armstrong N (2004). Modelling the $\dot{V}O_2$ kinetic response to heavy intensity exercise in children. *Ergonomics* **47**, 1517–27.
76. Fawkner SJ, Armstrong N (2007). Can we confidently study $\dot{V}O_2$ kinetics in young people? *J Sport Sci Med* **6**, 277–85.
77. Potter CR, Childs DJ, Houghton W, Armstrong N (1999). Breath-to-breath noise in the ventilatory gas exchange responses of children to exercise. *Eur J Appl Physiol* **80**, 118–24.
78. Fawkner SG, Armstrong N (2003). Oxygen uptake kinetic response to exercise in children. *Sports Med* **33**, 651–69.
79. Fawkner SG, Armstrong N, Childs D, Welsman J (2002). Reliability of the visually assessed ventilatory threshold and V-slope in children. *Pediatr Exerc Sci* **14**, 181–93.
80. Fawkner SG, Armstrong N (2002). Assessment of critical power in children. *Pediatr Exerc Sci* **14**, 259–68.
81. Fawkner SG, Armstrong N (2003). The slow component response of $\dot{V}O_2$ to heavy intensity exercise in children. In: Reilly T, Marfell-Jones M (eds.), *Kinanthropometry viii*, pp. 105–13. Routledge, London.
82. Fawkner SG, Armstrong N (2004). Longitudinal changes in the kinetic response to heavy-intensity exercise in children. *J Appl Physiol* **97**, 460–6.
83. Fawkner SG, Armstrong N (2004). Sex differences in the oxygen uptake kinetic response to heavy-intensity exercise in prepubertal children. *Eur J Appl Physiol* **93**, 210–16.
84. Obert P, Cleuziou C, Candau R, Courteix D, Lecoq A, Guenon P (2000). The slow component of O_2 uptake kinetics during high intensity exercise in trained and untrained prepubertal children. *Int J Sports Med* **21**, 31–6.
85. Armon Y, Cooper DM, Flores R, Zanconato S, Barstow TJ (1991). Oxygen uptake dynamics during high intensity exercise in children and adults. *J Appl Physiol* **70**, 841–8.
86. Williams CA, Carter H, Jones AM, Doust JH (2001). Oxygen uptake kinetics during treadmill running in boys and men. *J Appl Physiol* **90**, 1700–6.
87. Gaesser GA, Poole DC (1996). The slow component of oxygen uptake kinetics in humans. *Exerc Sport Sci Rev* **24**, 35–71.
88. Barstow TJ, Scheuermann BW (2006). Effects of maturation and aging on $\dot{V}O_2$ kinetics. In: Jones AM, Poole DC (eds.), *Oxygen uptake kinetics in sport, exercise and medicine*, pp. 332–52. Routledge, London.
89. Fawkner SG, Armstrong N, Potter CR, Welsman JR (2002). Oxygen uptake kinetics in children and adults after the onset of moderate-intensity exercise. *J Sport Sci* **20**, 319–26.
90. Koch G (1974). Muscle blood flow after ischemic work and during bicycle ergometer work in boys aged 12 years. *Acta Paediatr Belg* **28**, 29–39.
91. Koch G (1980). Aerobic power, lung dimensions, ventilatory capacity and muscle blood flow in 12–16 year old boys with high physical activity. In: Berg K, Eriksson BO (eds.), *Children and exercise IX*, pp. 99–108. University Park Press, Baltimore, MD.
92. Jones AM, Pringle JSM, Carter H (2006). Influence of muscle fibre type and motor unit recruitment on $\dot{V}O_2$ kinetics. In: Jones AM, Poole DC (eds.), *Oxygen uptake kinetics in sport, exercise and medicine*, pp. 261–93. Routledge, London.
93. Kent-Braun JA, Miller RG, Weiner MW (1995). Human skeletal muscle metabolism in health and disease: Utility of magnetic resonance spectroscopy. *Exerc Sports Sci Rev* **23**, 305–47.
94. Barker AR, Welsman JR, Welford D, Fulford J, Williams C, Armstrong N (2006). Reliability of ^{31}P-magnetic resonance spectroscopy during an exhaustive incremental exercise test in children. *Eur J Appl Physiol* **98**, 556–65.
95. Taylor DJ, Bore PJ, Styles P, Gadian DG, Radda GK (1983). Bioenergetics of intact human muscle: A ^{31}P nuclear magnetic resonance study. *Mol Biol Med* **1**, 77–94.
96. Armstrong N, Welsman JR (2006). Exercise metabolism. In: Armstrong N (ed.) *Paediatric exercise physiology*, pp. 71–97. Churchill Livingstone, Edinburgh.

97. Barker AR, Welsman JR, Fulford J, Welford D, Williams CA, Armstrong N (2008). Muscle phosphocreatine and pulmonary oxygen uptake kinetics in children at the onset and offset of moderate intensity exercise. *Eur J Appl Physiol* **102**, 727–38.
98. Zanconato S, Buchthal S, Barstow TJ, Cooper DM (1993). ^{31}P-magnetic resonance spectroscopy of leg muscle metabolism during exercise in children and adults. *J Appl Physiol* **74**, 2214–18.
99. Barker AR, Welsman JR, Fulford J, Welford D, Armstrong N (in press). Quadriceps muscle energetics during a step-incremental test to exhaustion in children and adults. *J Appl Physiol.*
100. Kuno S, Takahashi H, Fujimoto K, Akima H, Miyamaru M, Nemoto I, Itai Y, Katsuta S (1995). Muscle metabolism during exercise using phosphorus-31 nuclear magnetic resonance spectroscopy in adolescents. *Eur J Appl Physiol* **70**, 301–4.
101. Taylor DJ, Kemp GJ, Thompson CH, Raddar GK (1997). Ageing: Effects on oxidative function of skeletal muscle *in vivo*. *Mol Cell Biochem* **174**, 321–4.
102. Ratel S, Tonson A, Le Fur Y, Cozzone P, Bebdahan D (2008). Effects of age on skeletal muscle oxidative capacity: A ^{31}P-MRS study. In: Jurimae T, Armstrong N, Jurimae J (eds.), *Children and exercise XXIV*. pp. 225–8. Routledge, London.
103. Petersen SR, Gaul CA, Stanton MM, Hanstock CC (1998). Skeletal muscle metabolism during short-term high intensity exercise in prepubertal and pubertal girls. *J Appl Physiol* **87**, 2151–6.
104. Mirwald RL, Baxter-Jones AD, Bailey DA, Beunen GP (2002). An assessment of maturity from anthropometric measurements. *Med Sci Sports Exerc* **34**, 689–94.
105. Kushmerick MJ, Meyer RA, Brown TR (1992). Regulation of oxygen consumption in fast- and slow-twitch muscle. *Am J Physiol Cell Physiol* **263**, C598–606.
106. Minzo M, Secher NH, Quistorff B (1994). ^{31}P-NMR spectroscopy, EMG and histochemical fiber types of human wrist flexor muscles *J Appl Physiol* **76**, 531–8.
107. Barker AR, Welsman JR, Fulford J, Welford D, Armstrong N (in press). Muscle phosphocreatine kinetics in children and adults at the onset and offset of moderate intensity exercise. *J Appl Physiol.*
108. Barstow TJ, Buchthal SD, Zanconato S, Cooper DM (1994). Muscle energetics and pulmonary oxygen uptake kinetics during moderate exercise. *J Appl Physiol* **77**, 1742–9.

CHAPTER 17

Maximal intensity exercise

Craig A. Williams

Introduction

Most studies of paediatric maximal intensity exercise have been carried out using the Wingate anaerobic test (WAnT) devised by Cumming[1] and popularized by Ayalon *et al.*,[2] Bar-Or,[3] and Inbar *et al.*[4] from the Wingate Institute in Israel. This test, as explained more fully in Chapter 5, derives several indices of external mechanical power production: peak power (PP) usually over 1 or 5 s, mean power (MP) over 30 s, and the Fatigue Index (FI). Although other protocols such as the force–velocity test (F–V test) or isokinetic cycle sprint tests have emerged, the contribution of the Wingate Institute and the WAnT to the understanding of maximal intensity exercise should not be underestimated.

Despite a surge of interest over the past 10 years in young people's maximal intensity exercise, the growth and maturation of anaerobic performance is still poorly understood. This observation is interesting for a number of reasons. First, during the prepubertal years, children's physical activity patterns are characterized by short duration but high intensity bouts of effort.[5] Second, investigators are limited by the range of available methodologies, most of which are assessing external but indirect mechanical indices of maximal intensity so as to deduce metabolic changes. Third, there are few data available from females. Finally, due to the importance of maximal intensity efforts during team sports and the increasing emphasis on organized youth sport programmes, the differentiation between growth and maturation and training adaptations of maximal intensity performance need to be addressed. As a consequence of these four observations, important reliability and validity issues need to be resolved prior to paediatric exercise scientists determining which key factors influence maximal intensity exercise during childhood and adolescence. This chapter will therefore focus on the variables that have been most commonly measured and review the explanatory factors related to maximal intensity exercise during growth and maturation.

Definition of maximal intensity exercise

Throughout the paediatric exercise science literature there has been a plethora of terms used to describe exercise, that is, 'all-out'. This descriptor could conveniently be applied to peak or maximal oxygen uptake ($\dot{V}O_2$) but in the absolute sense of 'all-out' exercise, the mechanical power production during a peak $\dot{V}O_2$ test only represents 25–33% of the possible maximal intensity. For example, a child who produces a maximal power output of 200 W on a cycle ergometer when exhaustion sets in and who reaches the determination criteria for peak $\dot{V}O_2$ can produce two or three times as much power output during a 30-s sprint cycle ride. The power output during short maximal intensity sprints and peak $\dot{V}O_2$ have been examined between boys and men and adolescent boys and girls.[6,7] As predicted, both found significantly higher PP during a 90-s maximal sprint compared to maximal minute power obtained during a peak $\dot{V}O_2$ test. More interestingly, however, the adolescent boys and girls were able to attain $\dot{V}O_2$ values that were closer to their peak $\dot{V}O_2$ (~93%) than adults. These results demonstrate that the limits to the maximum sustainable adenosine triphosphate (ATP) turnover rate in the muscle are dependent on the maximum flux capacity for ATP production, in tandem with the duration of the required sprint. For short duration sprints, all three metabolic pathways will contribute to the sustainable rate. However, the important principle is the balance of the maximum flux capacities relative to each other and their differing elasticizes to calcium and net ATP hydrolysis.[8] The synchronous effect of the three pathways is represented by the power output profile in Fig. 17.1 where at the end of the 90-s test the maximum sustainable rate of exercise is becoming more dependent on oxidative phosphorylation than the glycolytic and high-energy phosphates. The misinterpretation of the synchrony between the three flux capacities has often led to a misconception that the aerobic system responds slowly to the energy demands of maximum intensity exercise, thereby playing little part in short duration exercise.[9]

To account for the discrepancy between the power output produced in peak $\dot{V}O_2$ tests compared to shorter duration sprint exercise tests, the descriptor 'supramaximal' has often been used to describe this intensity of all-out exercise. However, this descriptor is contradictory because it implies that a subject's maximal effort can be exceeded. Therefore, the appropriate term should not focus on the measurement variable *per se*, that is, power output, distance, speed, and impulse, but the metabolism that supplies the exercise demonstrates a higher anaerobic ATP yield than that of the metabolism of oxidative phosphorylation.[10]

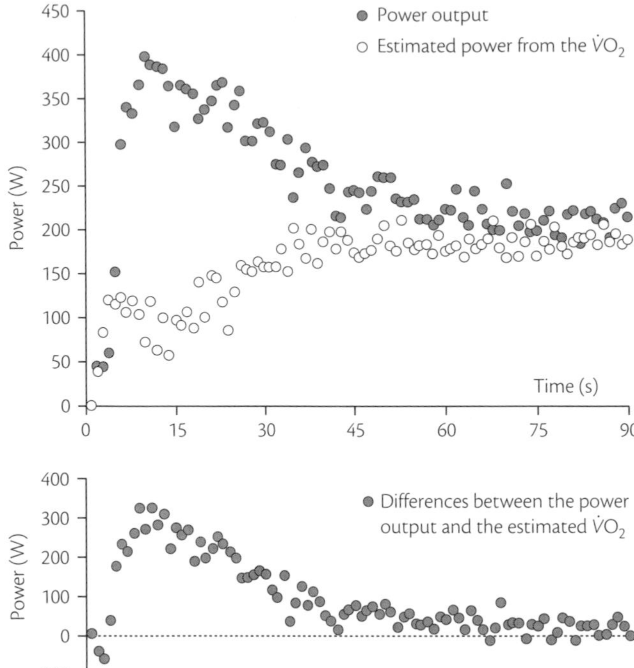

Fig. 17.1 Power output profile of a 90-s maximal isokinetic cycling sprint and estimated power from peak $\dot{V}O_2$ test for one adolescent boy (Williams, unpublished data).

Maximal intensity exercise and age

There is unequivocal evidence that maximal intensity exercise increases with age for both males and females. This observation has been confirmed whether the studies have been cross-sectional or longitudinal in design. There is less information provided beyond the age of 40 years, probably because maximal intensity exercise is largely regarded as a measure of performance rather than a health indicator. As illustrated in Fig. 17.2, the growth curves of some common sprinting events, which are indicative of maximal intensity performance, improve with age from childhood to adolescence and into adulthood.[11] Maximal intensity exercise typically plateaus for men in the third decade of life and for women in the second decade.

The athletic performance data also support data from laboratory testing.[12–14] In males, absolute PP increases from childhood to adolescence to adulthood with a typical surge in power output from the teenage years to adulthood. For females, PP also increases through childhood and adolescence although there appears to be more of a plateau in power output during the latter adolescent years into adulthood. However, some caution is warranted for two reasons. First, the lack of conformity of protocols, for example, duration of warm-up, differences in load, rolling or static start, and inertia uncorrected or corrected data have meant considerable variation during measurement. Second, there are considerably fewer female data available.

In a publication by Van Praagh[15] PP from force–velocity sprint protocols lasting less than 10 s were obtained across an age range of 7–21 years. In total, 1200 participants were tested and Figs. 17.3 and 17.4 show a significant increase in power with age. Interestingly, if the figures are examined carefully a number of observations can be made. First, there is less variance in the male data compared to the female data throughout the age range. In other words, the degree of heteroscedasticity, that is, the spread of the scores widening with age, is less for males than females. Second, there is a smaller linear increase for boys up to the age of 12–13 years before what appears to be a second and steeper linear increase is observed. For the females, the increase appears to be more consistently linear throughout the age range.

From maximal intensity cycling tests (i.e. the F–V test and WAnT), the average PP and MP scores for 10- to 12-year-old boys are approximately 43% and 47% compared to that of 25- to 35-year-old men. For similar aged girls, the scores are slightly higher for PP and MP at 44% and 55% compared to females aged between 18 and 25 years. Maximal intensity scores obtained from arm cranking, although fewer in number than data obtained from cycling, show that the upper limbs generate approximately 60–70% of the power generated by the legs.

Despite these concerns, it is possible to confirm that unlike peak aerobic power and no matter how maximal intensity exercise is standardized for size (see Chapter 2), children always have a significantly lower score than adolescents and adults, and adolescents' scores are significantly lower than those for adults. These findings have been interpreted as size-dependent (quantitative) factors which become less important with age whereas the size-independent (qualitative) factors, that is, neuromuscular, genetics, and hormonal factors become more important in explaining age differences. However, there is considerably less information on qualitative factors than quantitative ones and therefore qualitative factors should be focused upon in future studies.

Dore *et al.*[16] investigated the influence of age on PP in 506 males aged between 7.5 and 18 years using three maximal cycle sprints of less than 10 s duration to calculate the force, velocity, and power curves and to derive PP. Using allometric modelling procedures, a multiple stepwise regression equation predicted PP from age and fat-free mass. It was found that age (2.3%) contributed to a negligible part of the explanatory variable to PP and that other anthropometric variables were more predictive, for example, free fat mass and lean leg volume (LLV). Interestingly although the percentage contribution of age to the optimal velocity at PP was as low as 1.3%, it did provide a significant contribution to the prediction model. This small contribution of age might be a surrogate for other changes, which are occurring at the level of motor unit activation, or fibre type distribution, or hormonal influences, or a combination of all three factors. These three factors have all largely been ignored by paediatric exercise science researchers and more research is required to elucidate the influence of neuromuscular and hormonal factors.

In a study designed to examine the applicability of a regression model for PP and total mechanical work (TMW) for children, adolescents, and adults at the extremes of stature, mass, and hence body mass index (BMI), 454 participants between 6 and 20 years were studied.[17] All participants completed two unilateral WAnTs, one with each leg. The braking force was determined according to body mass equations and some modification based on practice tests. PP and TMW were averaged for the right and

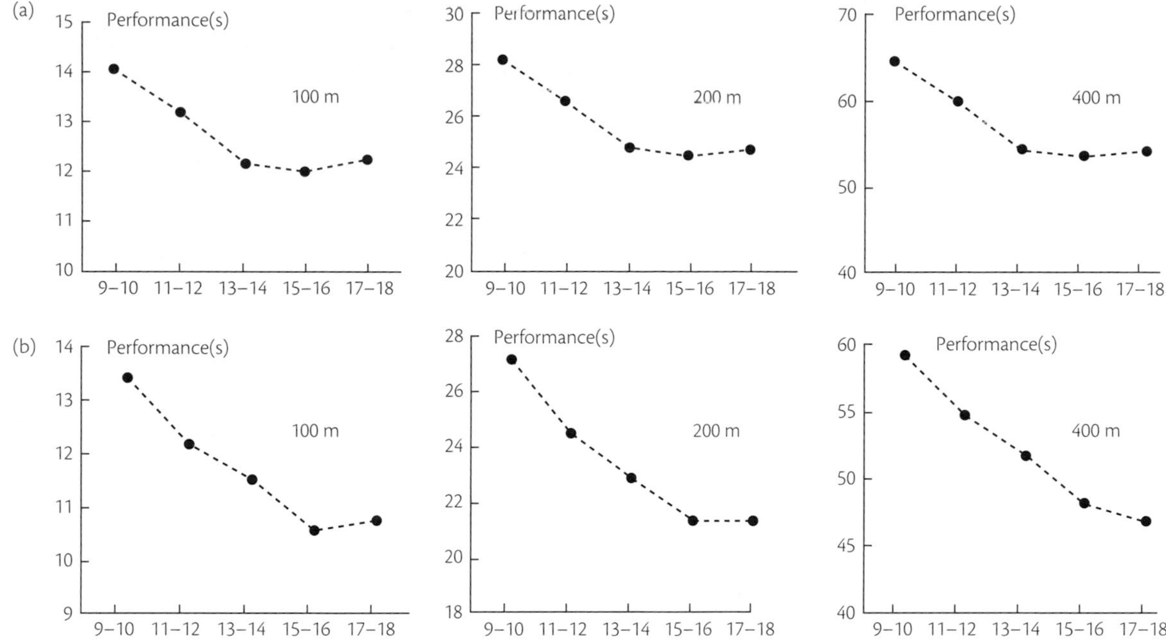

Fig. 17.2 Athletic performance of (a) girls and (b) boys in the United States Junior Olympic Championships (ages 9–18 years). Adapted from Van Praagh and Franca,[11] with permission.

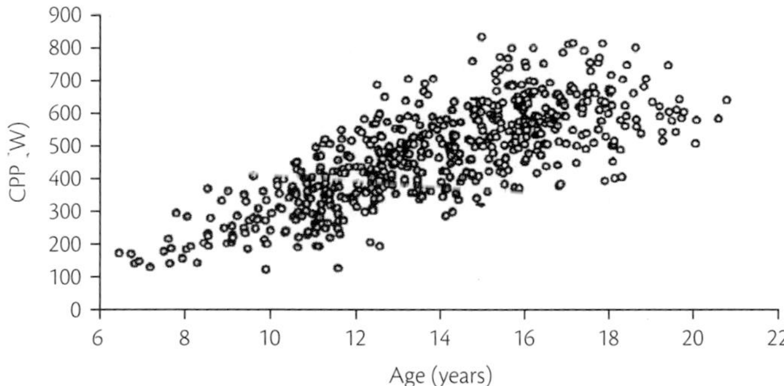

Fig. 17.3 Relationship between cycling peak power and age in females. Reprinted from Van Praagh,[15] with permission.

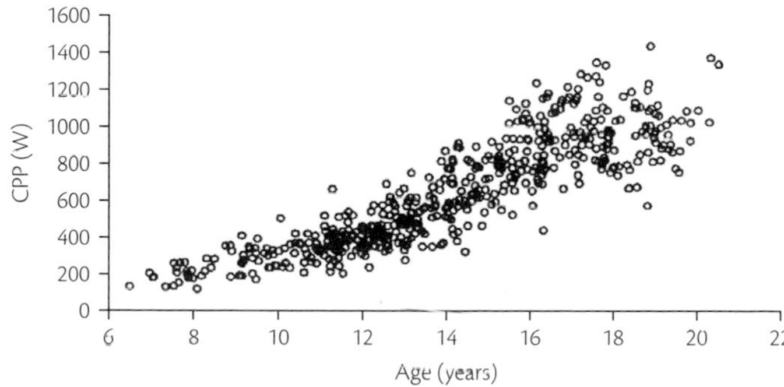

Fig. 17.4 Relationship between cycling peak power and age in males. Reprinted from Van Praagh,[15] with permission.

left leg of each participant. A total of 267 participants within the normal anthropometric range (defined as between 10th and 90th percentile for mass and stature) were then used to establish the log-transformed regression equation. The major finding of this study was that children, adolescents, and adults who were heavier than the reference group ($n = 267$) predictions for PP and TMW were overestimated compared to the reference group values on the WAnT. This observation also held true for those individuals who were taller than the reference group. However, the regression prediction equation worked adequately for those participants at the lower distribution of mass and stature. These results demonstrate the difficulties in adequately expressing mass to body fat and muscle ratios in extremely heavy participants. In particular, there is a potential to overestimate muscle mass in these participants. This finding was corroborated by Armstrong *et al.*,[12] who found a significant negative correlation between skinfold thickness and log-transformed PP and TMW. Regional distributions of fat, bone, and muscle are likely to be different in very heavy individuals and are likely to change with age. The observation of the 'wobble-gait' in overweight individuals when walking or running mean it is likely that body mass to bone–muscle–adiposity imbalances result in increased strain on tendons and joints, and therefore limit cycling performance. The authors also postulated that hypoactivity and muscle fibre recruitment might differ in overweight children resulting in a reduced anaerobic capacity. Although this inactivity recruitment paradigm might exist in the overweight individuals, it does not explain those individuals with greater stature. In addition, it is difficult to conclude that the capacity of the anaerobic system is deficient in these individuals as the WAnT cannot measure capacity of the anaerobic metabolism and it is more likely that the authors were implying mechanical power performance.

Maximal intensity exercise and sex

As stated previously there are both cross-sectional and longitudinal data available on males than females but it is often confined to a narrow age range typically 11–16 years of age. Comparisons between boys and girls using the WAnT have reported no sex differences for PP and MP,[18,19] higher PP and MP for girls, and higher MP in boys.[20] In fact, if Figs. 17.2 and 17.3 are examined carefully up to the age of 13 years there are no discernible absolute differences in power output between boys and girls. Hence, it is entirely possible that for PP and MP, girls could have higher performances in these later childhood years. In one of the first studies to examine the sex differences of anaerobic PP and MP in relation to body composition, it was found that absolute PP and MP were similar in both sexes.[21] Interestingly, when PP and MP scores were related to lean thigh volume (LTV), PP and MP were significantly higher in boys than girls. The girls had a higher mean LTV than boys, 6.0 ± 1.4 and 5.1 ± 1.7 L, respectively, but the difference was not statistically significant. Van Praagh *et al.*[21] explained part of these sex differences as due to qualitative factors, which might favour the higher relative power output in boys. Three lines of evidence supported their explanations. First, the lack of a significant difference in the LTV negated differences due to a quantitative factor. Second, it was noted that the boys developed more power than girls at the beginning of the exercise. Third, isometric evidence was presented to suggest a longer time rise of isometric force in adolescent girls than boys and thus a lower neuromotor efficiency and power output. However, each of these three explanations is not without repudiation. First, it has been established that the Jones and Pearson[22] anthropometric method of estimating LTV significantly underestimates volumes. Winsley *et al.*[23] reported that in 16 boys (mean age 9.9 years), the anthropometric technique underestimated the total, lean, and fat thigh volume by 36%, 31%, and 52% compared to magnetic resonance imaging (MRI). The size of this underestimation of LTV ranged from 0.4 to 1.3 L. It should not be forgotten that the original Jones and Pearson[22] method was validated against water displacement and x-ray techniques, a process unlikely to account for the differing quantities and distribution of fat and fat-free mass of growing children. In the Van Praagh *et al.*[21] study, although this under prediction is likely to be similar for both sexes, expressing the volume of the thigh as wholly indicative of muscle ignores intramuscular fat and other constituent tissues. This point is illustrated in Fig. 17.5, where the cross-sectional thigh MRIs are compared between an early maturing girl and a late maturing girl of the same chronological age. The images show the differing amounts of subcutaneous and intramuscular fat which although accounted for in the leg volume measure will not be aiding mechanical power production.

Second, if the development of total work output across time figure in the study of Van Praagh *et al.* is studied, although the maximum work achieved is higher in boys than girls it is not significantly different in its rate of development. In most instances across the abscissa, work and standard deviation lines appear to cross both sexes. Finally, the justification of isometric muscle actions for a concentric cycling action is not valid. Although Van Praagh *et al.* supported this observation by citing the significantly higher optimal braking force (F_{opt}) in boys compared to girls (F_{opt}, 0.085 ± 0.02 and 0.068 ± 0.01 kp/kg^{-1} body mass, respectively), they ignored the lack of significant differences in predicted unloaded

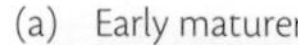
(a) Early maturer

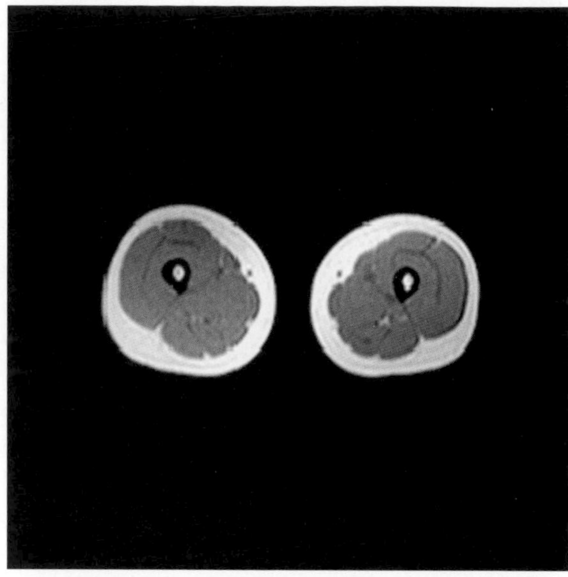

(b) Late maturer

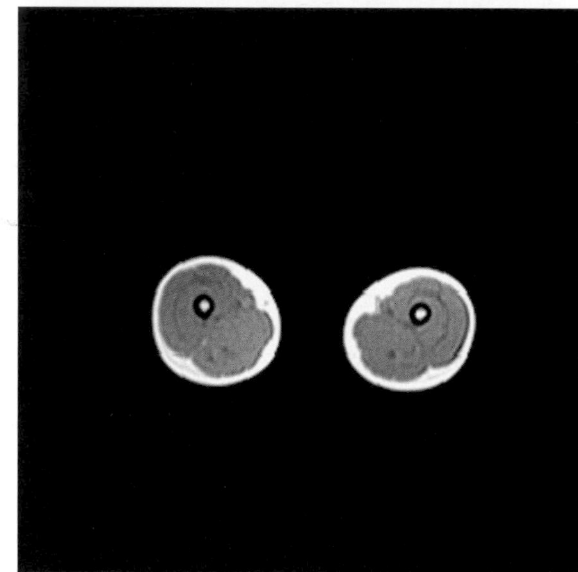

Fig. 17.5 MRI cross-sectional slice highlighting subcutaneous fat differences of the thigh between two same chronological age female child participants but different sexual maturational stages.

and maximal cycling (V_o, 228 ± 18 and 218 ± 21 rev·min^{-1}, respectively) and optimal velocity (V_{opt}, 114 ± 9 and 109 ± 11 rev·min^{-1}, respectively). These latter two variables would be more indicative of neuromuscular factors than either the optimal force variables or isometric muscle actions.

In a study by Armstrong *et al.*,[24] it was found that for absolute PP and MP derived from the WAnT with 100 boys and 100 girls aged 12 years, the girls had significantly higher PP and MP than the boys. This observation is, of course, the opposite of peak aerobic values where sex differences, in favour of the boys, have already significantly developed (see Chapter 20). This significant sex difference in maximal intensity exercise is likely due to the advanced biological maturation of girls who, despite being at the same chronological age, are on average 2 years ahead of the boys in maturation.[18,25] These findings reiterate the importance of the assessment of biological maturation alongside chronological age.

This potential sex difference in absolute PP and MP also highlights the difficulty of adequately controlling for body size differences between the girls and the boys. It is often common to report maximal intensity power standardized to body mass (W·kg^{-1}). However, this statistical technique fails to appropriately account for body size (see Chapter 2). In the study by Dore[26] examining PP relative to body mass (W·kg^{-1}) of 535 males and 510 females between the ages of 7 and 21 years, sex-related differences were found from as early an age as 10–11 years and continued to age 21 years. Although this study was cross-sectional in design and the statistical analyses can be criticized for not appropriately controlling the differences in body size, the inferences from the study for PP were confirmed later by a study which did appropriately account for body size. Armstrong *et al.*[12] appropriately controlled for body size using allometric scaling (log-linear model), and found that boys' PP and MP were significantly higher than the girls. This finding was despite the fact that their earlier analyses comparing absolute power output (W) had found girls to be significantly higher in PP and MP than the boys.[24] As expected for the analyses of PP, mass and stature were significant explanatory variables but maturity was found not to be significant and therefore excluded. The age by sex interaction was found to be non-significant but the age parameter was found to be positive and similar for both boys and girls. The negative parameter for sex (−0.057, SE 0.015) reflects girls' lower PP. The significant negative covariance between the level 2 random age/constant parameters indicates that there is a smaller rate of increase in PP for higher starting values of PP. However, when skinfolds were entered as an additional variable stature became non-significant. For MP, stature and age were once again significant explanatory variables. Similar to PP, girls' MP was significantly lower compared to boys but a significant and negative age by sex interaction was found. This result represents a smaller increase for MP in girls compared to boys. An additional parameter maturation effect (last two stages of the indices described by Tanner[27]) was also found to contribute to the explanation of MP. However, similar to PP, the addition of the skinfolds parameter removed both stature and maturation from the model. The two key findings from this study were first that age, mass and stature, as significant explanatory variables, revealed an incremental effect for early maturation on MP but not PP. Second, that stature which had previously been associated with a significant prediction of aerobic and strength performance measures was rendered non-significant by the skinfolds parameter.

In another study by the same group Santos *et al.*[28] investigated both age- and sex-related differences during the F–V test for optimal PP_{opt} in 41 participants aged 9–10 years (males = 21, females = 20), 45 participants aged 14–15 years (males = 23, females = 22), and 41 participants aged 21–22 years (males = 20, females = 21). As expected, absolute PP_{opt} was found to significantly increase with age in both boys and girls, whilst significant sex differences were only found between teenagers and adults but not pre-teens. For mass-related PP_{opt}, sex differences were non-significant between pre-teens but males obtained significantly higher scores than females in both teen and adult groups. The study by Santos and co-workers benefited from the fact that females were not disadvantaged by cycling against a fixed braking force. Fixed braking forces, commonly used during the WAnT, penalize females as the braking force cannot account for differences in body composition or muscularity between the sexes. In addition, the power output produced during a WAnT is usually lower than that achieved during a F–V test. Most importantly from this study, despite the observation of a mass-related PP_{opt} across the age ranges for males and an increase for females in the teenage years followed by a subsequent plateau into adulthood, allometric scaling revealed a different pattern for females. Using analysis of covariance (ANCOVA) on log-transformed data, which adjusted for differences in body mass, it was reported that PP_{opt} was found to significantly increase across all age groups for the females not just the males. Therefore, when body mass differences were appropriately adjusted, the age-related increases remained for both sexes, even though this effect was masked in females when only conventional ratio scaling (i.e. W·kg^{-1}) was utilized.

Santos *et al.*'s findings were largely confirmed in a later study by Martin *et al.*,[29] whose paper although entitled 'Longitudinal changes of maximal short-term peak power…' investigated cross-sectionally the influence of age, sex, and LLV on 100 girls and 109 boys aged 7.5–17.5 years. Using a variant of the F–V test with two randomized braking loads, individual power–velocity relationships determined maximal power, defined as the apex of the power–velocity relationship. Optimal force and pedalling frequency (V_{opt}) were also determined. Using multilevel modelling procedures which included allometric approaches to describe the developmental changes in maximal power, mass, LLV, and age proved to be significant explanatory variables. Martin *et al.* found a 273% increase for girls in PP from age 7 to 16 years with a plateau between 16 and 17 years. Boys' PP increased by 375% from 7 to 17 years. More interestingly, the difference between the sexes did not emerge until after 14 years of age, an observation supported by the negative age by sex interaction reflecting a smaller increase of maximal power with age in girls. Although all three independent variables, age, sex, and LLV, were significant explanatory variables, for girls LLV was the best predictor (68%) as was age for boys (57%). Both leg length (LL) (83%) and LLV (48%) were significant explanatory variables for V_{opt} and F_{opt}, respectively, for boys and girls combined as one group. For the V_{opt} data, it was shown that for the same LL, boys had a significantly higher V_{opt}. Hautier *et al.*[30] had previously shown a strong relationship between muscle fibre type and V_{opt}. Therefore, Martin and his co-authors concluded that sex differences of V_{opt} might be due to differences in glycolytic ability, proportion, and recruitment of type II muscle fibres and/or motor co-ordination differences. They also concluded that children should develop their neuromuscular determinants of contraction velocity rather than LLV but did not say how or indeed what the training effect is on such systems. Consequently, more focus should be on the velocity determinant of the power equation.

Maximal intensity exercise and maturation

It is well recognized that age and sex differences are important differentiators of maximal intensity exercise. Another important variable, which must also be considered alongside age and sex, is maturation. The most appropriate research design to investigate the role of maturation in explaining PP and MP differences is longitudinal studies. However, these are limited in number. To date, there have only been five paediatric longitudinal studies (defined as retesting on three or more occasions) investigating maximal intensity exercise, with three of these studies from the same group of researchers (see Table 17.1).

The first study by Duché *et al.*[31] investigated the bioenergetic profiles of boys aged from 9 to 14 years. In total, 13 prepubertal boys were studied for 3 years at ages 9, 10.5, and 11.5 years, with 11 more boys being studied at ages 12 years (prepubertal stage) and 14 years (pubertal stage). Significant increases in PP and MP over 30 s were observed between 9–10.5 and 12–14 years. The authors commented that the most important increases related to anaerobic performance appeared to occur at the time of puberty. Although the relatively small sample numbers and simplistic statistical analyses restricted more detailed explanations of the data set, this study highlights the importance of accounting for growth via a longitudinal design in examining the evolution of anaerobic performance.

The second longitudinal study was carried out by Falk and Bar-Or,[32] who reported PP and MP of 27 boys over an 18-month

Table 17.1 Summary of published longitudinal maximal intensity exercise studies of children and adolescents

Citation	Sample size	Age (in years)	Sex	Duration	Dependent measures analyses	Statistical
Duché *et al.*[32]	13	9	M	Once a year for 3 years	Max power by F–V test and mean 30-s WAnT power	Conventional power-to-body mass ratios
		10.5	M			
		11.5	M			
Falk and Bar-Or[32]	11 (prepubertal)	10.9	M	Four times at 6-month intervals for 18 months	Peak power over 3 s and mean 30 s WAnT power	MANOVA with repeated measures
	11 (midpubertal)	13.2	M			
	5 (pubertal)	16.2	M			
Armstrong *et al.*[18]	97	12.2	M	Once a year for 2 years then once 4 years later	Peak power over 1 s and mean 30-s WAnT power	Multilevel modelling
	95	13.2	M			
	28	17	M			
	100	12.2	F			
	80	13.2	F			
	17	17	F			
De Ste Croix *et al.*[34]	20	10.1	M	Eight times over 4 years	Peak extension and flexion torque	Multilevel modelling
	20	10.9	M			
	20	11.4	M			
	20	11.9	M			
	16	12.3	M			
	20	12.7	M			
	17	13.2	M			
	19	13.7	M			
	21	9.9	F			
	20	10.6	F			
	21	11.1	F			
	21	11.6	F			
	17	12.2	F			
	17	12.7	F			
	13	13.3	F			
	13	13.7	F			
Santos *et al.*[35]	17	12.4	M	Four times at approximately 6-month intervals	Optimized peak power, force, and velocity	Multilevel modelling
	22	12.8	M			
	20	13.3	M			
	20	13.8	M			
	18	12.2	F			
	18	12.6	F			
	15	13.2	F			
	16	13.6	F			

period and found that mass-related PP appeared to increase at each stage of maturation. Indeed 2 years later these findings were confirmed by Williams,[33] who similarly found mass-related increases at increasing stages of maturational development. However, both of these studies were restricted in their interpretations of the results as statistical analyses were confined to ratio standard and ANCOVA methods, respectively.

The third longitudinal study investigated maximal intensity exercise in relation to age, sex, and maturation.[18] The study by Armstrong *et al.* is probably the most complete study to date. Using a large sample size, inertia corrected measurements of the WAnT and appropriate statistical analyses, that is, multilevel modelling, participants were measured on three occasions at 12, 13, and 17 years. It was found that males' absolute PP and MP increased by 121% and 113%, respectively. However, for females, PP and MP increased only by 66% and 60%, respectively. Using multilevel regression models on log-transformed data, it was found that boys generated higher PP and MP than girls even when body mass and fatness were appropriately and concurrently controlled. Age showed a positive effect on PP and MP but was non-linear (see Table 17.2). The negative age by sex interaction for MP only illustrates a smaller increase in MP with age for the girls over the 5-year time span (see Table 17.3). However, unlike the earlier studies of Duché *et al.*[31] and Bar-Or and Falk,[32] once age, body size, and composition were controlled, sexual maturation (assessed by the indices of pubic hair development described by Tanner[27]) did not exert an independent effect on PP and MP.

In a study by the same group which was initiated with younger children commencing at 10 years of age, changes in peak extension (PET) and flexion torque (PFT) were investigated over a 48 month period.[34] Similar to the Armstrong *et al.*[18] study multilevel modelling was utilized and found, albeit in a narrower age range

Table 17.2 Multilevel regression analyses for peak power (n = 417)

Parameter	Model 1 Estimate (SE)	Model 2 Estimate (SE)
Fixed		
Constant	2.358 (0.169)	1.884 (0.165)
Log_e mass	0.878 (0.054)	1.232 (0.050)
Log_e stature	0.946 (0.187)	NS
Log_e skinfolds	NE	−0.159 (0.024)
Age	0.135 (0.010)	0.134 (0.002)
Age^2	−0.035 (0.002)	−0.034 (0.002)
Sex	−0.068 (0.016)	−0.054 (0.015)
Age·sex	NS	NS
Random		
Level 2		
Constant	0.007 (0.001)	0.006 (0.001)
Level 1		
Constant	0.011 (0.001)	0.011 (0.001)
−2·loglikelihood	−513.683	−530.243

Adapted from Armstrong *et al.*[18]

NE, not entered; NS, not significant.

Table 17.3 Multilevel regression analyses for mean power (n = 417)

Parameter	Model 1 Estimate (SE)	Model 2 Estimate (SE)
Fixed		
Constant	2.971 (0.172)	2.268 (0.165)
Loge mass	0.607 (0.055)	1.118 (0.051)
Loge stature	1.357 (0.196)	NS
Loge skinfolds	NE	−0.228 (0.024)
Age	0.111 (0.016)	0.097 (0.015)
Age^2	−0.013 (0.002)	−0.012 (0.002)
Sex	−0.087 (0.016)	−0.066 (0.015)
Age·sex	−0.046 (0.017)	−0.031 (0.017)
Random		
Level 2		
Constant	0.011 (0.001)	0.008 (0.001)
Level 1		
Constant	0.007 (0.001)	0.008 (0.001)
−2·loglikelihood	−565.784	598.498

Adapted from Armstrong *et al.*[18]

NE, not entered; NS, not significant.

that neither sex nor maturation exhibited a significant explanatory variable, although a significant negative sum of skinfolds effect was found for PFT. De Ste Croix *et al.*[34] incorporated MRI measures of extensor and flexor muscles cross-sectional areas into the model and demonstrated a non-significant covariate effect on both PET and PFT.

The final longitudinal study by Santos *et al.*[35] conducted over a 2-year period with four test occasions investigated the F–V test derived PP_{opt} in boys and girls aged 12–14 years. As with previous longitudinal studies age increased PP_{opt} but was not significantly different between the sexes. Similar to the study of De Ste Croix *et al.*,[34] even with body size controlled for, TMV was shown to be a significant and independent explanatory variable of PP_{opt}.

Determinants of maximal intensity exercise

A major methodological obstacle in assessing maximal intensity exercise via the production of mechanically measured power output on ergometers is the multitude of variables, which comprise the resultant muscle performance (see Fig. 17.6). These variables include the length–force relationship, the force–velocity and power–velocity relationships, muscle fibre composition, muscle size and geometry, muscle force, and dimensions. In addition, given the complexities of muscle geometry, that is, pennation angles, the unknown degrees of activation and contribution of different muscles acting around a joint, the length of the lever arm, fibres, and their tension, the intrinsic speed of active muscle fibres, and how mechanical output is modulated during growth, it should not be surprising that without improvements in technology, further advancement is unlikely. *In vitro* experiments have allowed some of these factors to be investigated using a controlled and standardized animal model,[36] but the examination of whole-body performance

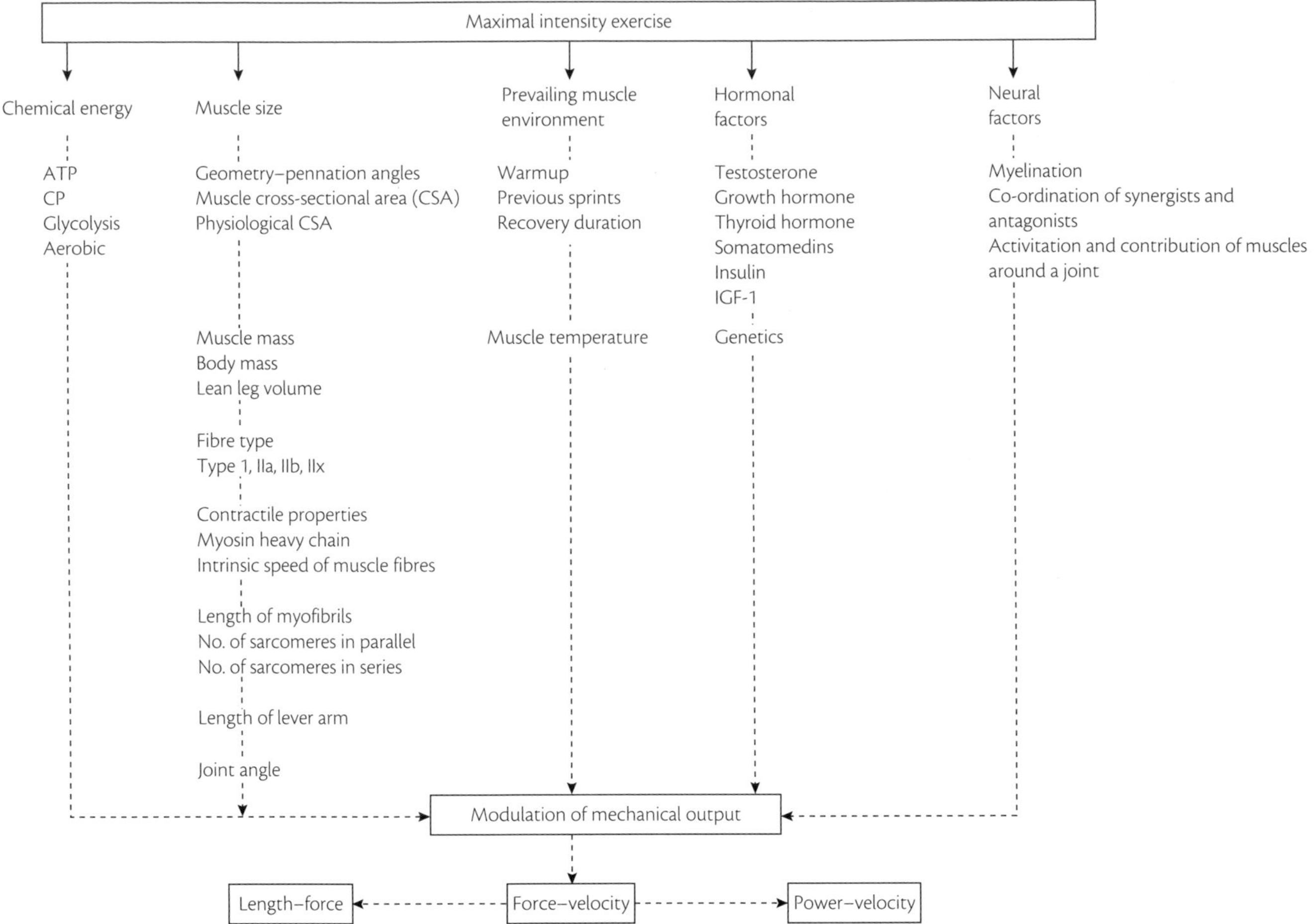

Fig. 17.6 Determinants of maximal intensity exercise.

to examine differences in force between children and adults is too blunt an experimental tool to definitively establish differences. However, despite these technical difficulties and providing the methodological limitations are acknowledged and results correctly interpreted, there is still much to infer from the published paediatric literature.

The use of the F–V test to infer relationships between power, velocity, and neuromuscular performance has found similar optimal cadences for maximal power production between boys and girls and between children and adults. Optimal cadences range from 114 to 109 rev·min^{-1} for 12.8-year-old boys and girls[21]; from 116 to 118 rev·min^{-1} for 15-year-old girls and 21-year-old women; 110 rev·min^{-1} [37] and 119.5 rev·min^{-1} [38] for female adults; 122 and 126 rev·min^{-1} for 14-year-old boys and 29-year-old men.[39] Even though there are some subtle differences between studies, which all used either isokinetic or friction braked ergometers, there does not appear to be any significant difference for optimal cadence (optimal velocity) for maximal power production.

These findings could explain similar evidence from the electrically evoked twitch and titanic tension method. Although the results from electrically stimulated methods must be interpreted carefully because the implication that failure to initiate muscle action under electrically stimulated isometric action translates directly to dynamic muscle actions is not supported. Using the electrical stimulation technique, Davies *et al.*[40] found no differences in relaxation time, specific muscle force per cross-sectional area (CSA), fatiguability or contraction velocity between pubescent boys and girls. It has also been reported that corticospinal tract maturity in conduction velocity increases to approximately 15 years of age, thus reaching maturity in the second decade of life.[10] Hence, maximal intensity power differences between adolescents and adults do not appear to be related to the influence of the contractile properties.

However, there may appear to be an age or maturation effect. Prepubertal boys have been reported as possessing significantly higher ratios of twitch peak force to maximal voluntary force of the plantar flexor muscles compared to pubertal boys and men.[41] The inference from these findings is that the demonstrated increase in isometric voluntary muscle strength during and after puberty is correlated with an increase in motor unit activation. The earlier findings of Blimkie[42] found that 16-year-old boys could voluntarily activate a greater available percentage of knee extensor motor units during a MVC trial compared to 11 year olds. In the same year, Belanger and McComas[43] also confirmed the difficulty of some prepubertal 11-year-old boys compared to pubertal 16.5-year-old boys, in being able to fully and optimally voluntarily activate the motor neuron pool of the plantar flexor muscles during an isometric trial. However, there was no significant age difference for the percentage motor unit activation. Although the area of neuromuscular activation has been ignored as a possible contributor to child and adult differences, care is warranted when transferring the inferences from isometric contractions to dynamic protocols. However, if there is a lower ability in prepubertal boys this would result in a low voluntary activation of muscle groups and result in a lower muscle force and power production.

Although it is extremely difficult to conclude that there are differences in intrinsic force and power production capabilities between children and adults using whole-body exercise, animal models may help. In one study to determine isometric force and power in rat muscle, muscle mass, physiological CSA, and fibre CSA were carefully standardized.[36] In young rats whose fibre differentiation was complete, but whose muscle fibre length was still lengthening, the specific force was approximately 30% less than young mature rats, whose muscle fibre length had ceased changing. It is still unclear why these differences exist but de Haan *et al.*[36] suggest possible factors as the increased density of myofibrillar packing; connective tissue changes in the muscle; more effective cross bridge kinetics; or a compromise of the force transmission related to growth processes.

During skeletal muscle growth from childhood to adulthood there are important changes in muscle mass and increases in protein content. It is known that between the 14th week of gestation and adulthood there is a four-fold increase in myofibrillar fraction, accompanied by a two-fold increase in sarcoplasmic protein.[44] These changes in myofibrillar proteins, particularly during maturation, have often been proposed to explain the differences during maximal intensity exercise between children and adults. However, even taking into account these muscle growth changes and appropriate normalization for power output, differences still remain between children and adults. This is despite the fact that there is a five-fold increase in muscle mass (7.5 to ~37 kg) in 5- to 18-year-old males or a three-fold increase (7 to ~24 kg) for similar aged females.

In association with the increase in muscle mass, there is an accompanying increase in muscle size. The early work of Saltin and Gollnick[45] in the 1980s demonstrated that growth in muscle circumference is associated with increases in fibre CSA and there is a positive correlation between age and fibre area. The moderate to strong correlation ($r = \sim 0.85$) between age and fibre area has long been associated with the relationship between CSA and force production. Correlations between CSA and maximal voluntary contractions in children are moderate to strong across a variety of muscle groups and in both sexes despite a variety of methods to assess muscle CSA. It is not until mid-puberty that the muscle size differences between the sexes begin to emerge. These differences are more marked in the upper limbs compared to the lower, where adolescent females have only 50% of the upper limb size but 70% of the lower limb size compared to similar aged males. However, as described by Blimkie and Sale,[46] if absolute force is normalized by CSA age and sex differences disappear, highlighting the importance of muscle CSA rather than age and sex as the more important factor influencing force production during growth.

One scientific method to isolate quantitative factors such as body mass and leg volume is to compare the same chronological aged children with similar body mass and volume values. This experimental design was utilized by Martin *et al.*[47] when they compared similar aged boys ($n = 132$, aged 9.5–16.5 years) who possessed similar LLV, % body fat (% BF), and LL so as to highlight the qualitative determinants of maximal peak power (P_{max}). By completing a modified F–V test,[48] P_{max}, F_{opt}, and V_{opt} values were obtained. As expected, the P_{max} increased with age and was statistically significant at the time of the adolescent growth spurt (around 14 years in this study). The V_{opt} in this study increased significantly in boys classified as prepubertal ($n = 37$), a finding explained by the possible development of motor co-ordination providing a basis for skill improvement. There were no significant differences for V_{opt} found between the older boys. This finding has been confirmed by other V_{opt} studies which have found no differences in adolescent boys or girls compared to adults.[39,49] Therefore, it would appear that V_{opt} changes in cycling sprint performance appear during the period of prepubescence. Optimal braking force, however, showed significant increases after the prepubertal period, a factor explained by the increase in ability to activate the motor units of the muscles. Therefore, this study provided evidence that the increasing P_{max} with age demonstrated by the boys was the result of differing components of the power equation. Similar groups for LLV, % BF, and LL increased PP by 17.2%, 19.8%, and 14.2% between the ages 10–12, 12–14, and 14–16 years, respectively. When grouped according to maturation, prior to puberty the increase in P_{max} was associated with an increase in V_{opt} of 9.3%, whereas the pubertal and post-pubertal boys showed increased P_{max} with a F_{opt} increase of 12.2% and 13.2%, respectively. Therefore, these results demonstrate that further investigations exploring qualitative factors which influence F_{opt} and V_{opt} are needed.

In adult studies, the optimal velocity for maximal power production has been related to muscle fibre type composition. Hautier *et al.*[30] determined force, velocity, and power averaged over each down pedal stroke of a friction-loaded ergometer in 10 subjects (eight men and two women). Muscle fibre composition of the vastus lateralis was determined using a Bergstrom biopsy needle. The relative proportion of fast twitch fibres correlated to optimal velocity was found to be high ($r = 0.88$, $p < 0.001$) as was squat jump performance ($r = 0.78$, $p < 0.01$) but was not significantly correlated to maximal anaerobic power relative to body mass ($r = 0.60$, $p > 0.06$). The authors suggested that the strong correlation between optimal velocity and fibre composition supported the proposition that optimal velocity in maximal sprint cycling is related to muscle fibre composition. At present, it is difficult to equate high optimal velocity with high maximal intensity scores thereby implying a high proportion of fast twitch fibres in children. However, the interpretation of these inferences is sound. A participant having a large proportion of fast twitch fibres should produce more power and greater force at high shortening velocities than a participant with a greater proportion of slow twitch fibres. This inference should equally apply to the participant who possesses more fast twitch fibres being able to accelerate their body mass during sprint running to a greater extent than another participant. Currently, no biopsy work coupled with force–velocity testing has established this association in children, but the use of MRI to measure fibre type could be a future possibility.

The limited muscle biopsy data from children show that children have a higher proportion of type I and thus less fatiguable fibres than adults.[49–52] Both Lexell *et al.*[52] and Oertel[53] have shown that the proportion of type I fibres decreases with age from childhood to adulthood. Declines of between 65% and 54% of type I fibres at age 5–6 years to between 50% and 42% at age 20 years were reported. Interestingly, in a review by Jansson[51] on the percentage of type I fibres, an inverted U-shaped curve was found for males from birth to 9 years and a decrease, which was significantly lower at 19 years compared to the 9-year-old age group. However, this relationship was not found for females. The majority of studies have in fact reported a higher percentage of type II fibres in adolescent females than in males[54–56] (and see chapter 16). Bell *et al.*[50] found that by 6 years of age histochemical analyses compared to adults were similar. In agreement with the higher proportion of type I fibres were the findings of Colling-Saltin,[57] Fournier *et al.*,[58] and Hedberg and Jansson,[59] who reported lower proportions of type II fibres in early childhood compared to adults. It is not clear if there is a greater prevalence of type IIa versus type IIX fibres during childhood and adolescence compared to adulthood as studies have found both for[54] and against this proposition.[50]

Other biopsy studies by Eriksson *et al.*,[60,61] Haralambie,[62] Fournier *et al.*,[58] and Berg *et al.*[63] have all examined biochemical changes following strenuous cycling exercise but not necessarily after maximal intensity exercise. Therefore, inferences from biopsy studies must be examined carefully because of the differing exercise protocols, the sample of muscle examined and the training status of the participants.

The pioneering work of Eriksson *et al.*[60,61] in the 1970s in examining muscle metabolism and children's exercise performance led to the suggestion that glycolytic activity is lower in children than in adults and was dependent on maturational status. The frequent citing of this work in the literature has led to these results appearing to be established as an accepted tenet. However, the acceptance of this principle is despite the fact that Eriksson's studies were not designed to test the effects of maturation and employed very small sample sizes.

Eriksson[64] found phosphofructokinase (PFK) levels to be threefold lower in 11- to 13-year-old boys compared to adult men despite an aerobic enzyme succinate dehydrogenase not being significantly different between age groups. Although this finding was supported by another study,[63] other groups have found similar enzymatic activity in similar aged children 13–15 years compared to adults.[62] Allied to the lower glycolytic enzymatic capacity and lower maximal intensity exercise of children is the reported lower blood lactate concentration after maximal exercise (see chapters 8 and 16). By investigating other enzymes, Kaczor *et al.*[65] examined the effects of age on creatine kinase (CK), adenylate kinase (AK), lactate dehydrogenase (LDH), carnitine palmitoyl-transferase (CPT), and 2-oxoglutarate dehydrogenase (OGDH) in 20 children (3–11 years) and 12 adults (29–54 years). All measurements were collected at rest and from participants who had been admitted to hospital for hernia surgery. Muscle samples were taken of the obliquus internus abdominis muscle. Significantly lower values for CK, AK, and LDH enzyme activity were found for children compared to adults. The enzyme LDH remained significantly lower even when the concentration was expressed relative to milligrams of total protein. The authors suggested 'the significantly lower LDH is likely to be a major factor of decreased anaerobic performance' (p. 334). This assertion is despite the fact that these measures were taken at rest and no indication was given of the maturity of the children's group or any activity status. The authors, however, concluded at the end of the paper that 'mechanisms behind the enzymatic differences reported here in children and adults are not clear' (p. 334).

Other researchers have also hypothesized that maximal intensity exercise differences between children and adults are due to hormonal changes during puberty.[66] It is well established that during puberty there are substantial increases in growth hormone and testosterone in males and oestradiol in females.[67] It has also been speculated that the anabolic effect of physical activity is somehow mediated by increases in insulin-like growth factor-1 (IGF-1), which is independent of growth hormone.[68] Levels of IGF-1 certainly appear to increase both in the lead up to and after peak height velocity (PHV) and tend to occur in advance of significant increases in sex hormones.[69] In the longitudinal study of Round *et al.*,[69] who investigated muscle strength and power related to circulating IGF-1 and testosterone, for girls' quadriceps muscle strength was proportional to height and total body mass. In boys, the additional factor of testosterone was found to explain the quadriceps strength. Testosterone in the boys was found to increase 1 year prior to PHV, then continued to increase and attained adult values 3 years post-PHV.

Recent investigations of maximal intensity exercise

The challenge for paediatric exercise scientists is to understand mechanistic aspects during maximal intensity exercise. This will undoubtedly require scientists to make creative use of methodological protocols to infer mechanisms. However, advances in technology will also undoubtedly play a significant part in furthering our understanding. Already some in-roads are being acquired through the use of magnetic resonance spectroscopy (MRS) and molecular biology. It is to this end that researchers should continue to utilize maximal intensity exercise to further our understanding of physiological responses to exercise, for example, the investigation of fatigue on performance or the recovery of muscle function following fatiguing maximal intensity exercise.

Fatigue

Studies have traditionally modelled fatigue from a mechanical viewpoint either during the course of cycling or running.[70,71] One interesting observation between the fatigue observed by children and adults is that children are considered to be able to resist fatigue better than adults.[72] Although the proposed mechanisms are still poorly understood many of the factors cited have commonality with previously discussed factors to explain the differences between children and adults during maximal intensity exercise. These include the recruited muscle during exercise, muscle morphology, energy metabolism, and neuromuscular activation. One such study investigated the differences in neuromuscular activation of agonist and antagonist muscles between men and prepubertal boys during a maximal isokinetic fatigue test. It was found that during a fatiguing knee extensor and flexor test adults were more fatigable than children. By recording EMG activity, the authors attributed the differences to agonist and antagonist activation, with children exhibiting either an increased inhibition or reduced facilitation of their agonist muscle drive.[73] More work is needed to examine the mechanisms controlling agonist (e.g. neuronal inhibition and metabolic concentrations) and antagonistic activity (e.g. reciprocal innervation and presynaptic inhibition) in children.

Factors during the recovery periods include differences in phosphocreatine (PCr) resynthesis, clearance of metabolic by-products, intracellular space, and diffusion of lactate and H^+ ions from muscle into blood. For further discussion of these topics, the reader is referred to a review by Ratel *et al.*[71] on muscle fatigue during high-intensity exercise in children.

Repeated-sprint ability tests

Maximal, but intermittent, intensity exercise either using treadmill or cycle ergometry has been used consistently to investigate the rate of recovery, the effect of prior bouts of exercise, and performance on subsequent bouts in adults.[74–77] Invariably, these protocols have employed a series of sprints, often as many as 10 of between 6 and 30 s in duration. Recovery duration during each successive sprint has also varied from 30 to 240 s. A variety of dependent measures have been utilized including muscle metabolites extracted from biopsy studies[74] to changes in peak and MP.[76] Although muscle biopsies are normally outside the ethical remit of the paediatric exercise scientist, repeated-sprint ability (RSA) research is a promising area to investigate the effects of successive bouts of maximal intensity exercise and the ensuing consequences of fatigue on performance. A variety of publications have sought to combine these protocols with children as participants using both cycling and running modalities.

Running

Repeated-sprint ability is usually defined as the ability to perform repeated short-duration sprints over a brief period of time.[78] Under laboratory conditions, there is limited information on the effects of age and recovery duration on repeated-sprint performance. To address this problem, Ratel *et al.* [79] compared the effects of 10 consecutive 10-s sprints on a non-motorized treadmill (NMT) separated by 15-s and 180-s passive recovery between 12 boys (mean age 11.7 years) and 13 men (mean age 22.1 years). Results showed that boys decreased their performance less than men during the 10 repeated sprints with 15-s recovery intervals. The lower decrease in running velocity of the boys was related to a lower decline in their relative step rate because the shortening in their relative step length was similar to the men. With 180-s recovery, boys were able to maintain running performance over the 10-s sprints. However, the men decreased their power and force outputs significantly, although they were able to maintain running velocity by increasing the relative step length to counteract the decline of the relative step rate.

Repeated-sprint ability tests are most associated with multi-team sprint sports such as football, hockey, and rugby, as the sprint is considered a crucial moment of match play.[80] Tests of RSA are either completed during field sessions or in a laboratory. Recent work has assessed the reliability and validity of a RSA test during field conditions and on a NMT.[81] Results showed high reliability between the two methods. Further reliability and validity work using the RSA during a soccer- specific test on a NMT with adolescent football players have been established.[82] Twelve youth soccer players completed two trials of the soccer-specific tests 3 months apart. The soccer test replicated the demands of competing in one half of a soccer match whilst sprint performance was monitored. In this test protocol, a 5-s sprint was included every 2 min. Reliability assessments included the calculation of typical error of performances as a percentage change of the mean coefficients of variation.[83] The mean coefficient of variation for total distance covered during the test was 2.5% and 3.8% for total distance sprinted but measures of MP were less reliable (≥5.9%). A significant reduction in sprint performance was observed over the course of the test (see Fig. 17.7). Physiological variables measured during the test including heart rate, blood lactate, and $\dot{V}O_2$ indicated a successful replication of the match demands often experienced in youth soccer. One of the advantages of the running RSA is the more acceptable face and ecological validity when inferences are drawn related to multi-team sprint performance. Further work using the RSA applicable to team sports includes the differentiation between young players of differing standards, the identification of limiting factors to RSA over 80 or 90 min and the assessment of intervention strategies, for example, nutritional feeding.

Cycling

Repeated-sprint ability protocols have also been applied to sprint cycling and children. Hebestreit *et al.* [84], using a WAnT protocol on three different occasions, had subjects complete two consecutive 30-s maximal intensity cycle sprints separated by a 1-, 2-, and 10-min recovery. Eight prepubertal boys (9–12 years) and 8 young men (19–23 years) completed the protocol, which was devised to determine the difference in ability to recover from the sprint cycling bouts. It was found that boys' MP reached 89.9 ± 3.6% of the first sprint value after 1-min recovery, 96.4 ± 2.3% after 2-min recovery, and 103.5 ± 1.3% after 10-min recovery. For the men, the values were 71.2 ± 2.6%, 77.1 ± 2.4%, and 94.0 ± 1.3%, respectively. It was concluded by the authors that boys recovered faster than men from the sprint cycling exercise. Possible explanations for this difference

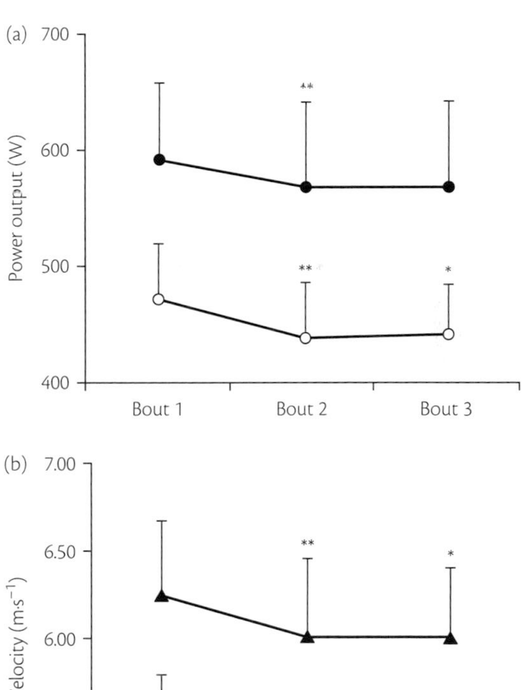

Fig. 17.7 (a) Peak power output (PPO) and mean power output (MPO) and (b) peak velocity (PV) and mean velocity (MV) during sprints in each bout of the SSIET. Asterisk denotes significantly different to bout 1, $p \leq 0.01$. Reprinted from Oliver *et al.*,[82] with permission.

included a lower reliance on glycolysis during the WAnT leading to lower acidosis and/or a faster post-exercise removal of metabolites. Using this RSA protocol other researchers have continued this line of investigation. Ratel *et al.*[85] investigated the acid–base balance during repeated cycling sprint bouts in 11 boys (9.6 ± 0.7 years) and 10 men (20.4 ± 0.8 years). Each participant performed ten 10-s sprints on a cycle ergometer separated by 30 s of passive recovery. Arterialized capillary blood samples were drawn from the earlobe at rest and before the first and then after the second, fourth, sixth, eighth, and tenth sprints to measure the time course of [La], [H^+], [HCO_3^-], base excess, and $PaCO_2$. Minute ventilation and carbon dioxide production were also measured breath-by-breath throughout each sprint. Significantly, lower blood [La] for boys compared to men was found from the third sprint to the tenth. Blood [H^+] was also significantly lower in boys than men after the second sprint to the tenth one. It was also found that for the same [La^+], blood [H^+] was lower in boys compared to men; similarly for the same [HCO_3], $PaCO_2$ was lower in boys. The main outcome of this study revealed that during repeated sprints children regulated their [H^+] better than adults, possibly due to a greater ventilation and exhalation of CO_2 thus reducing $PaCO_2$. Similar conclusions were drawn by the same researchers[86] when investigating the effects of age and recovery duration on PP during RSA in cycling. Eleven prepubescent (9.6 ± 0.7 years) and nine pubescent boys (15.0 ± 0.7 years) and 10 men (20.4 ± 0.8 years) completed ten 10-s cycling sprints separated by 30 s, 1 min, or 5 min of passive recovery. For the prepubescent boys whatever recovery duration was chosen, PP remained unchanged during the 10-s sprints. In the pubescent boys, PP decreased significantly by 18.5% during the 30-s recovery, by 15.3% during the 1-min recovery, and was unchanged by the 5-min recovery. For the men, PP significantly decreased by 28.5%, 1.3%, and decreased slightly but non-significantly during the 30-s, 1-min, and 5-min recovery periods. Lactate measurements were found to be significantly lower in the prepubescent groups of boys compared to the pubescent and adult men. It was concluded that prepubescent boys recover quicker than the other two groups possibly due to a lower glycolytic activity and higher muscle oxidative capacity that allows for faster PCr resynthesis. A practical interpretation of these research findings is that during sprint exercise lasting less than 10 s prepubescent children may need shorter rest periods than adults.

Ratel *et al.*[87] utilized both sprint cycling and running to examine any possible difference in fatigue due to the mode of exercise for both men and boys. As hypothesized, the extent of the fatigue was greater in MP output during sprint running for both adult men and boys compared to cycling. This contrasted to the decline in PP output for all participants, which was not dependent on the mode of exercise. The authors concluded that as PP was obtained within similar time periods for cycling and running that the maximal utilization of PCr stores was similar. The greater fall in MP for both boys and men in running indicated a more stressful situation indicated by the higher perceived exertion and blood lactate and glucose concentrations. In addition, the higher recruitment of body balance and weight bearing muscles during running will have an impact on contractile force production. Further work is required to investigate children's recovery from sprints, particularly applied to the sporting context.

In conclusion, systematic data on the development of maximal intensity exercise performance in children and adolescents have increased significantly over the past 10 years. Although many of the data are cross-sectional rather than longitudinal and are more focused on quantitative determinants in contrast to qualitative ones, they have allowed researchers to further interpret findings in respect of changes to growth, maturation, and sex. Although it is currently not possible to directly obtain measures of maximal intensity exercise during whole-body exercise, this should not act to deter future studies in this area.

Researchers in this area are faced with two main challenges. First, continued investigations of the determinants of maximal intensity exercise as determined by sex, growth, maturation, and by mode and different durations of exercise are still required. There is still much to be understood with respect to muscle dimension and geometry, the biomechanical aspects of force and power production, the stretch-shortening events that precede dynamic movement and neuromuscular changes to name but a few. The second challenge and more applied one is to utilize maximal intensity exercise as a protocol to examine potential mechanisms which differentiate children from adults. These types of experiments could include manipulating different muscle actions during exercise bouts, for example, isometric versus dynamic between children and adults, affecting the end exercise pH values or influencing different fatigue profiles to investigate recovery patterns. By using maximal intensity exercise as a method to examine underlying physiological change, researchers will advance current knowledge rather than merely focus on descriptive studies of differences between children and adults. This second challenge not only requires consideration of the physiological and psychological demands expected of the child but also requires creativity from the researcher in terms of experimental design.

Summary

- Definitions of maximal intensity exercise for children and adolescents, as in the adult literature, are numerous. Although it is easier to focus on a measurement variable, that is, power or speed, it is better to opt for the particular metabolism supplying the exercise, that is, a higher anaerobic ATP yield than oxidative metabolism to determine the definition.
- During childhood sex differences in maximal intensity exercise scores are minimal but become significantly different during the teenage years.
- Conventional usage of watts per body mass between the sexes will result in the masking of a 'true' age-related increase for females for PP_{opt}, an effect revealed when allometric scaling is performed to show age-related increases for both males and females from 10 to 21 years.
- A fixed braking force, as commonly used during the WAnT, can reduce the magnitude of age and sex differences in maximal intensity power output.
- Unlike previous cross-sectional studies, which have shown a significant effect of sexual maturation in explaining maximal intensity exercise, longitudinal studies have indicated that once the effects of age, body size, and composition have been accounted for, maturation is not a significant independent explanatory variable.
- The determinants for quantitative factors have been more systematically studied than qualitative ones. Muscle mass, muscle

volume, and lean leg volume are important determinants of power production but their relative importance can only be evaluated when such factors as geometric influences, length of lever arms, and interaction of tendon–bone–muscle have been investigated.

- The determinants of the qualitative factors need to be investigated more thoroughly. As velocity of movement forms one half of the power production equation, more studies in this area would make a significant contribution. Current information suggests that prepubertal children have a lower ability to voluntary activate muscle groups. This evidence has been used to explain lower power scores and a greater resistance to fatigue. However, these studies need to be replicated.
- The different modes of exercise such as running and cycling have allowed researchers to investigate power profiles between children and adults. In both cases, prepubertal children were found to have lower but more consistent power output in repetitious sprint running and cycling.
- An application of the lower and more consistent repeated power output of children is that children may cope better with intermittent type training. Consequently, the permutations of the training volumes, sets, and recovery times should be a function of age and body size of the child not just as a function of the training session. More work is needed in the field to translate these maximal intensity findings to competitive and training situations.
- The decline in maximal intensity power output with increasing duration of time is a natural consequence of fatigue. Fatigue profiles in children are inherently different to adults and little is known in this area. The lower muscle mass and absolute power production has consequences for lower accumulation of muscle by-products which might be suggestive of a reduced metabolic signal. Factors such as a faster resynthesis of PCr have been proposed as well as a greater oxidative capacity, a better acid–base balance, a faster readjustment of initial cardiorespiratory parameters and a higher removal of metabolic by-products.
- New instruments which can investigate maximal intensity exercise *in vivo* and which are ethically acceptable for use with children will undoubtedly advance knowledge in this area, but until that time, the challenge for paediatric researchers is to creatively manipulate maximal intensity protocols and infer underlying physiological mechanisms.

References

1. Cumming GR (1973). Correlation of athlete performance and aerobic power in 12- to 17-year-old children with bone age, calf muscle, total body potassium, heart volume, and two indices of anaerobic power. In: Bar-Or O (ed.), *Pediatric work physiology*, pp. 109–34. Wingate Institute, Natanya.
2. Ayalon A, Inbar O, Bar-Or O (1974). Relationships between measurements of explosive strength and anaerobic power. In: Nelson RC, Morehouse CA (eds.), *International series on sports sciences: Vol. 1, Biomechanics IV*, pp. 527–32. University Park Press, Baltimore, MD.
3. Bar-Or O (1983). *Pediatric sports medicine for the practitioner*. Springer, New York.
4. Inbar O, Bar-Or O, Skinner JS (1996). *The Wingate anaerobic test*. Human Kinetics, Champaign, IL.
5. Bailey RC, Olson J, Pepper SL, Porszasz J, Barstow TJ, Cooper, DM (1995). The level and tempo of children's physical activities: An observational study. *Med Sci Sports Exerc* **27**, 1033–41.
6. Carter H, Dekerle J, Brickley G, Williams CA (2005). Physiological responses to 90 s all out isokinetic sprint cycling in boys and men. *J Sports Sci Med* **4**, 437–45.
7. Williams CA, Ratel S, Armstrong N (2005). The achievement of peak $\dot{V}O_2$ during a 90 s maximal intensity cycle sprint in adolescent children. *Can J Appl Physiol* **30**, 157–71.
8. Meyer RA, Wiseman RW (2006). The metabolic systems: Control of ATP synthesis in skeletal muscle. In: Tipton CM, Sawka MN, Tate CA, Terjung RL (eds.), *ACSM's advanced exercise physiology*, pp. 370–84. Lippincott Williams and Wilkins, Philadelphia, PA.
9. Gastin PB (2001). Energy system interaction and relative contribution during maximal exercise. *Sports Med* **31**, 725–41.
10. Sargeant AJ (2000). Anaerobic performance. In: Armstrong N, Van Mechelen W (eds.), *Pediatric exercise science and medicine*, pp. 143–51. Oxford University Press, Oxford.
11. Van Praagh E, Franca N (1998). Measuring maximal short-term power output during growth. In: Van Praagh E (ed.), *Pediatric anaerobic performance*, pp. 155–89. Human Kinetics, Champaign, IL.
12. Armstrong N, Welsman JR, Williams CA, Kirby BJ (2000). Longitudinal changes in young people's short-term power output. *Med Sci Sport Exerc* **32**, 1140–5.
13. Bar-Or O (1996). Anaerobic performance. In: Docherty D (ed.), *Measurement in pediatric exercise science*, pp. 161–82. Human Kinetics, Champaign, IL.
14. Inbar O, Bar-Or O (1986). Anaerobic characteristics in male children and adolescents. *Med Sci Sports Exerc* **18**, 264–9.
15. Van Praagh E (2000). Development of anaerobic function during childhood and adolescence. *Pediatr Exerc Sci* **12**, 150–73.
16. Dore E, Diallo O, Franca NM, Bedu M, Van Praagh E (2000). Dimensional changes cannot account for all differences in short-term cycling power during growth. *Int J Sports Med* **21**, 360–5.
17. Unnithan VB, Nevill A, Lange G, Eppel J, Fischer M, Hebestreit H (2006). Applicability of an allometric power equation to children, adolescents and young adults of extreme body size. *J Sports Med Phys Fitness* **46**, 202–8.
18. Armstrong N, Welsman JR, Chia M (2001). Short term power output in relation to growth and maturation. *Br J Sports Med* **35**, 118–24.
19. Sutton NC, Childs DJ, Bar-Or O, Armstrong N (2000). A non-motorised treadmill test to assess children's short-term power output. *Pediatr Exerc Sci* **12**, 91–100.
20. Docherty D, Gaul CA (1991). Relationship of body size, physique, and body composition to physical performance in young boys and girls. *Int J Sports Med* **12**, 525–32.
21. Van Praagh E, Fellmann N, Bedu M, Falgairette G, Coudert J (1990). Gender difference in the relationship of anaerobic power output to body composition in children. *Pediatr Exerc Sci* **2**, 336–48.
22. Jones PRM, Pearson J (1969). Anthropometric determination of leg fat and muscle plus bone volumes in young male and female adults. *J Physiol* **204**, 63P–6P.
23. Winsley R, Armstrong N, Welsman J (2003). The validity of the Jones and Pearson anthropometric method to determine thigh volumes in young boys: A comparison with magnetic resonance imaging. *Portuguese J Sport Sci* **3**, 94–5.
24. Armstrong N, Welsman JR, Kirby BJ (1997). Performance on the Wingate anaerobic test and maturation. *Pediatr Exerc Sci* **9**, 253–61.
25. Armstrong N, Welsman JR (1996). *Young people and physical activity*. Oxford University Press, Oxford.
26. Dore E (1999). *Evolution de la puissance maximale anaérobie dans une population non-selectionnée de filles et de garçons agés de 7 à 21 ans*. Unpublished PhD Thesis, Blaise Pascal University, Clermont-Ferrand II, France.
27. Tanner JM (1962). *Growth at adolescence* (2nd ed.). Blackwell, Oxford.

28. Santos AMC, Welsman JR, De Ste Croix MBA, Armstrong N (2002). Age- and sex-related differences in optimal peak power. *Pediatr Exerc Sci* **14**, 202–12.
29. Martin RJF, Dore E, Twisk J, Van Praagh E, Hautier CA, Bedu E (2004). Longitudinal changes of maximal short-term peak power in girls and boys during growth. *Med Sci Sports Exerc* **36**, 498–503.
30. Hautier CA, Linnossier MT, Belli A, Lacour JR, Arsac LM (1996). Optimal velocity for maximal power production in non-isokinetic cycling is related to muscle fibre type composition. *Eur J Appl Physiol* **74**, 114–18.
31. Duché P, Falgairette G, Bedu M, Fellmann N, Lac G, Robert A, Coudert J (1992). Longitudinal approach of bio-energetic profile in boys before and during puberty. In: Coudert J, Van Praagh E (eds.), *Pediatric work physiology*, pp. 43–5. Masson, Paris.
32. Falk B, Bar-Or O (1993). Longitudinal changes in peak aerobic and anaerobic mechanical power of circumpubertal boys. *Pediatr Exerc Sci* **5**, 318–31.
33. Williams CA (1995). *Anaerobic performance of prepubescent and adolescent children*. Unpublished doctoral dissertation, University of Exeter, United Kingdom.
34. De Ste Croix MBA, Armstrong N, Welsman JR, Sharpe P (2002). Longitudinal changes in isokinetic leg strength in 10–14-year-olds. *Ann Hum Biol* **29**, 50–62.
35. Santos AMC, Armstrong N, De Ste Croix MBA, Sharpe P, Welsman JR (2003). Optimal peak power in relation to age, body size, gender and thigh muscle volume. *Pediatr Exerc Sci* **15**, 406–18.
36. de Haan A, de Rutier CJ, Lind A, Sargeant AJ (1992). Growth-related change in specific force but not in specific power of fast rat skeletal muscle. *Exper Physiol* **77**, 505–8.
37. Sargeant AJ, Dolan P, Thorne A (1984). Isokinetic measurement of leg force and anaerobic power output in children. In: Ilmarinen J, Valimaki I (eds.), *Children and sport*, pp. 93–8. Springer-Verlag, Berlin.
38. Sargeant AJ, Dolan P (1986). Optimal velocity of muscle contraction for short-term (anaerobic) power output in children and adults. In: Rutenfranz J, Mocellin R, Klimt F (eds.), *Children and exercise XII*, pp. 39–42. Human Kinetics, Champaign, IL.
39. Williams CA, Keen P (2001). Isokinetic measurement of maximal muscle power during leg cycling: a comparison of adolescent boys and adult men. *Pediatr Exerc Sci* **13**, 154–66.
40. Davies CTM, White MJ, Young K (1983). Muscle function in children. *Eur J Appl Physiol* **52**, 111–14.
41. Paasuke M, Ereline J, Gapeyeva H (2000). Twitch contraction properties of plantar flexor muscles in pre- and post-pubertal boys and men. *Eur J Appl Physiol* **82**, 459–64.
42. Blimkie CJR (1989). Age- and sex-associated variation in strength during childhood: Anthropometric, morphologic, neurologic, biomechanic, endocrinologic, genetic and physical activity correlates. In: Gisolfi CV, Lamb DR (eds.), *Perspectives in exercise science and sport medicine: Youth, exercise and sport*, Vol. 2, pp. 99–163. Benchmark Press, Indianapolis, IN.
43. Belanger AY, McComas AJ (1989). Contractile properties of human skeletal muscle in childhood and adolescence. *Eur J Appl Physiol* **58**, 563–7.
44. Dickerson JWT, Widdowson EM (1960). Chemical changes in skeletal muscle during development. *J Biochem* **74**, 247.
45. Saltin B, Gollnick PD (1983). Skeletal muscle adaptability: significance for metabolism and performance. In: Peachy LD (ed.), *Handbook of physiology*, pp. 555–631. Physiological Society, Bethesda, MD.
46. Blimkie JR, Sale DG (1998). Strength development and trainability during childhood. In: Van Praagh E (ed.), *Pediatric anaerobic performance*, pp. 193–224. Human Kinetics, Champaign, IL.
47. Martin RJF, Dore E, Hautier CA, Van Praagh E, Bedu M (2003). Short-term peak power changes in adolescents of similar anthropometric characteristics. *Med Sci Sports Exerc* **35**, 1436–40.
48. Arsac LM, Belli A, Lacour JR (1996). Muscle function during brief maximal exercise: accurate measurements on a friction-loaded cycle ergometer. *Eur J Appl Physiol* **74**, 100–6.
49. Williams CA, Hammond A, Doust JH (2003). Short term power output of females during isokinetic cycling. *Iso Exerc Sci* **11**, 123–31.
50. Bell RD, MacDougall JD, Billeter R, Howald H (1980). Muscle fibre types and morphometric analysis of skeletal muscle in six-year old children. *Med Sci Sports Exerc* **12**, 28–31.
51. Jansson E (1996). Age-related fiber type changes in human skeletal muscle. In: Maughan RJ, Shireffs SM (eds.), *Biochemistry of exercise IX*, pp. 297–307. Human Kinetics, Champaign, IL.
52. Lexell J, Sjostrom M, Nordlund AS, Taylor CC (1992). Growth and development of human muscle: A quantitative morphological study of whole vastus lateralis from childhood to adult age. *Muscle Nerve* **15**, 404–9.
53. Oertel G (1988). Morphometric analysis of normal skeletal muscles in infancy, childhood, and adolescence. An autopsy study. *J Neurolog Sci* **88**, 303–13.
54. Jannson E, Hedberg G (1991). Skeletal muscle fibre types in teenagers: relationship to physical performance and activity. *Scand J Med Sci Sports* **1**, 31–44.
55. du Plessis MP, Smit PJ, du Plessis LAS, Geyer HJ, Mathews G, Louw HNJ (1985). The composition of muscle fibers in a group of adolescents. In: Binkhorst RA, Kemper HCG, Saris WHM (eds.), *Children and exercise XI*, pp. 323–8. Human Kinetics, Champaign, IL.
56. Glenmark B, Hedberg G, Kaijser L, Jansson E (1994). Muscle strength from adolescence to adulthood-relationship to muscle fibre types. *Eur J Appl Physiol* **68**, 9–19.
57. Colling-Saltin AS (1980). Skeletal muscle development in human fetus and during childhood. In: Berg K, Eriksson BO (eds.), *Children and exercise IX*, pp. 193–207. University Park Press, Baltimore, MD.
58. Fournier M, Ricca J, Taylor AW, Ferguson RJ, Montpetit RR (1982). Skeletal muscle adaptation in adolescent boys: sprint and endurance training and detraining. *Med Sci Sports Exerc* **14**, 453–6.
59. Hedberg G, Jansson E (1976). Skeletal muscle fibre distribution, capacity and interesting different physical activities among students in high school. *Pedagogiska Rapporter* (English abstract) 54.
60. Eriksson BO, Karlsson J, Saltin B (1971). Muscle metabolites during exercise in pubertal boys. *Acta Paediatr Scand* **217** (Suppl.), 154–7.
61. Eriksson BO, Gollnick PD, Saltin B (1973). Muscle metabolism and enzyme activities after training in boys 11–13 years old. *Acta Physiol Scand* **87**, 485–97.
62. Haralambie G (1982). Enzyme activities in skeletal muscle of 13–15 years old adolescents. *Bull Eur Physiopathol Respir* **18**, 65–74.
63. Berg A, Kim SS, Keul J (1986). Skeletal muscle enzyme activities in healthy young subjects. *Int J Sports Med* **7**, 236–9.
64. Eriksson BO (1980). Muscle metabolism in children—a review. *Acta Paediatr Scand* **283**, 20–7.
65. Kaczor JJ, Ziolkowski W, Popinigis J, Tarnopolsky MA (2005). Anaerobic and aerobic enzyme activities in human skeletal muscle from children and adults. *Pediatr Res* **57**, 331–5.
66. Ferretti G, Narici MV, Binzoni T, Gariod L, Le Bas JF, Reutenauer H, Cerretelli P (1994). Determinants of peak muscle power: effects of age and physical conditioning. *Eur J Appl Physiol* **68**, 111–15.
67. Costin G, Kaufman FR, Brasel J (1989). Growth hormone secretory dynamics in subjects with normal stature. *J Pediatr* **115**, 537–44.
68. Cooper DM (1995). New horizons in pediatric exercise research. In: Blimkie CJR, Bar-Or O (eds.), *New horizons in pediatric exercise science*, pp. 1–24. Human Kinetics, Champaign, IL.
69. Round JM, Jones DA, Honor JW, Nevill AM (1999). Hormonal factors in the development of differences in strength between boys and girls during adolescence: a longitudinal study. *Ann Hum Biol* **26**, 49–62.

70. Vollestad NK (1997). Measurement of human muscle fatigue. *J Neurosci Meth* **74**, 219–27.
71. Ratel S, Duché P, Williams CA (2006). Muscle fatigue during high-intensity exercise in children. *Sports Med* **36**, 1031–65.
72. Ratel S, Lazaar N, Williams CA, Bedu M, Duche P (2003). Age differences in human skeletal muscle fatigue during high-intensity intermittent exercise. *Acta Paediatr* **92**, 1–7.
73. Paraschos I, Hassani A, Bassa E, Hatzikotoulas K, Patikas D, Kotzamanidis C (2007). Fatigue differences between adults and prepubertal males. *Int J Sports Med* **28**, 958–63.
74. Bogdanis GC, Graham C, Louis G, Lakomy HKA, Nevill ME (1994). Effects of resistive load on power output during repeated maximal sprint cycling. *J Sports Sci* **12**, 128–9.
75. Gaitanos GC, Williams C, Boobis LH, Brooks S (1993). Human muscle metabolism during intermittent maximal exercise. *J Appl Physiol* **75**, 712–19.
76. McCartney N, Spriet LL, Heigenhauser GJF, Kowalchuk JM, Sutton JR, Jones JL (1986). Muscle power and metabolism in maximal intermittent exercise. *J Appl Physiol* **60**, 1164–9.
77. Spriet LL, Lindinger MI, McKelvie RS, Heigenhauser GJF, Jones NL (1989). Muscle glycogenolysis and H^+ concentration during maximal intermittent cycling. *J Appl Physiol* **66**, 8–13.
78. Spencer M, Lawrence S, Rechichi C, Bishop D, Goodman C (2004). Time-motion analysis of elite hockey, with special reference to repeated-sprint activity. *J Sports Sci* **22**, 843–50.
79. Ratel S, Williams CA, Oliver J, Armstrong N (2006). Effects of age and recovery duration on performance during multiple treadmill sprints. *Int J Sports Med* **27**, 1–8.
80. Reilly T (1997). Energetics of high-intensity exercise (soccer) with particular reference to fatigue. *J Sports Sci* **15**, 257–63.
81. Oliver JL, Williams CA, Armstrong N (2006). The reliability and validity of running tests of repeated sprint ability. *Pediatr Exerc Sci* **18**, 339–50.
82. Oliver J, Armstrong N, Williams CA (2007). Reliability and validity of a soccer-specific test of prolonged repeated-sprint ability. *Int J Sports Physiol Perform* **2**, 137–49.
83. Hopkins WG (2000). Measures of reliability in sports medicine and science. *Sports Med* **30**, 1–15.
84. Hebestreit H, Mimura KI, Bar-Or O (1993). Recovery of muscle power after high-intensity short-term exercise: Comparing boys and men. *J Appl Physiol* **74**, 2875–80.
85. Ratel S, Duché P, Hennegrave A, Van Praagh E, Bedu M (2002). Acid-base balance during repeated cycling sprints in boys and men. *J Appl Physiol* **92**, 479–85.
86. Ratel S, Bedu M, Hennegrave A, Dore E, Duche P (2002). Effects of age and recovery duration on peak power output during repeated cycling sprints. *Int J Sports Med* **23**, 397–402.
87. Ratel S, Williams CA, Oliver J, Armstrong N (2004). Effects of age and mode of exercise on power output profiles during repeated sprints. *Eur J Appl Physiol* **92**, 204–10.

CHAPTER 18

Pulmonary function

Samantha G. Fawkner

Introduction

The primary purpose of the pulmonary system is to maintain blood–gas homeostasis under all conditions—from the prenatal state through to advanced years, under conditions ranging from rest to extreme environments and scenarios. In order to achieve this, the pulmonary system functions to maintain arterial partial pressure of oxygen (P_aO_2) and carbon dioxide (P_aCO_2) at all times, a requirement that is demanding, not least under exercising conditions.

The fundamental pulmonary response to an increase in metabolic demand is on face value very similar in the child and in the adult. Minute ventilation ($\dot{V}_E$) rises to accommodate the increase in carbon dioxide (CO_2) production, arrival of deoxygenated mixed venous blood to the lungs, and to minimize metabolic acidosis. Children display both a ventilatory threshold (T_{VENT}) and a ventilatory compensation point in response to an incremental exercise test, and maximal $\dot{V}_E$ ($\dot{V}_E$ max) is well below (~60–70%) maximum voluntary ventilation (MVV) at rest, similar to adults (see section on Maximal ventilation).

However, what is fascinating about the pulmonary response to exercise during the growth process is that these responses are managed despite obvious contradictions in structural and functional needs of prenatal life and adult life, which instigate that during the growing years considerable structural change to the pulmonary system must occur. Indeed, on closer examination, there are a number of intriguing differences between the adult and child ventilatory response to exercise that reflect changes in the mechanical properties of the pulmonary system and the changes in the metabolic capacities and competencies of the growing child.

There is an obvious need to understand the intricate details of the ventilatory response to exercise and its control during growth so that we can begin to unravel pathophysiological states that are increasingly prevalent in children. Despite this, there is an overwhelming dearth of concise and coherent literature from which it is possible to explore underlying mechanisms and, specifically, developmental changes in the control of ventilation. Maybe this is not surprising since despite its importance, the precise nature of the control of hyperpnoea in humans remains elusive. However, the advent of technology that has enabled us to examine the ventilatory response during exercise in more detail has encouraged a more recent focus in developmental research on modern concepts in pulmonary exercise science, such as the kinetics of ventilation and exercise-induced arterial hypoxaemia (EIAH). Although relatively little is known with regard to these physiological phenomena, even in adults, they hold a great deal of opportunity for further insight into the developmental aspects of pulmonary function.

There are also notable sex differences in the ventilatory response to exercise that are underpinned by two fundamental concepts: first, males on average have larger lungs than females and second, males on average have a higher percentage lean body mass and greater cardiovascular capacity such that they generate a higher metabolic demand, and thus demand for ventilation. This however is a simplistic view, and there are several nuances regarding sex differences in the response to exercise that are worthy of discussion.

Finally, the plasticity of the ventilatory response to exercise has important implications not only with regard to training elite athletes, but also with regard to the potential impact of low-activity levels on the basic functioning of the pulmonary system. Most endurance athletes demonstrate superior lung function to their age- and size-matched counterparts, but why is this? Is it a true training adaptation, or are these athletes simply selected into their respective sports due to genetic endowment?

The purpose of this chapter is therefore to

(i) describe important developmental changes in pulmonary structure and function that contribute to changes in the ventilatory response to exercise during growth,

(ii) describe age and sex differences in the ventilatory response to exercise,

(iii) provide insights into the developmental aspects of the control of exercise hyperpnoea,

(iv) explore current issues regarding the ventilatory response to exercise in children, and

(v) discuss the potential for training adaptations of pulmonary function during growth.

Structure and mechanics

Of primary influence on the change in the nature and magnitude of the ventilatory response to exercise with increasing age is the growth of the lung, the growth and number of its airways and alveoli, and changes in the inflation mechanics of the lung.

The lung increases in both its length and width with age, closely related to the timing and pattern of the growth velocity curves of height and weight. The age of peak velocity of lung width occurs at about 12.2 years and 13.8 years in girls and boys, respectively, and coincides closely with peak height velocity. Peak velocity of lung length, however, occurs some 6–8 months later[1] and may coincide with the peak velocity of chest depth. In parallel with changes in lung width and length, thoracic width as a percentage of thoracic height decreases with age.[2] However, whereas in boys, the height of the thorax increases about twice as fast as thorax width, in girls the increase in thoracic width is minimal, and between the ages of 11.5 and 18.5 years, the increase in thoracic height in males is twice that of females.[2] As the lung and thorax increase in size, so too does total lung capacity (TLC) and the various subdivisions of lung volume and function (see below). The TLC is well correlated with height[3] and increases from approximately 2 L at 120 cm to 3 L at 140 cm and to 6 L at 180 cm. However, as a volume that has three-dimensional properties, TLC is more closely related to the cube of height (height^3).[4]

At birth the number and branching pattern of the bronchial system are finalized, but subsequently both the diameter and length of the airways increase with age. Conversely, the number of alveoli in the lung only begin to noticeably increase after birth, multiplying exponentially from approximately 24 million to near maximal numbers by the 8th year (280 million).[5] Concurrently, alveolar surface area increases from 2.8 m^2 at birth to 12.2 m^2 at 13 months, 32 m^2 at 8 years, and 75 m^2 in adulthood[5] and, similar to the TLC, correlates closely with the cube of height. From around 2 years of age, alveoli enlargement coincident with the increasing size of the airways makes the most substantial contribution to the increasing volume of the lung. However, whereas some authors have suggested that the growth of the airways and air spaces is isotropic,[6] others consider that the rate of the increase in air spaces exceeds that of the airways.[7,8]

As airways change in size, so too does the resistance to flow. Resistance is increased by the power of 4 for any reduction in radius; therefore, there is an absolute reduction in airway resistance with age. Respiratory system resistance is closely related to height by an exponent of –1.7.[9] Owing to an increase in lung volume and number and volume of alveoli, there is also a reduction in the surface area to volume ratio and alveolar surface forces. As a result, absolute compliance increases with age and is related to height by the exponent 1.76.[9] However, at birth, the lungs are extremely flaccid and until late adolescence become increasingly more rigid with an increase in the density of connective tissue. As a result, specific compliance is thought to either decrease or remain stable with age.[9,10] Coincident with the increased density of connective tissue, lung recoil pressure increases throughout childhood until the age of about 18 years,[11] after which it declines into late adulthood and whereas the elastic recoil of the thorax is extremely low in the new born, it increases throughout childhood. It is not known whether the increase in elastic recoil of the lung and thorax are uniform, but there is some evidence that the ratio of functional residual capacity (FRC) to TLC and residual volume (RV) to vital capacity (VC) increases with age,[2,11] which may be due to the thoracic elasticity advancing more rapidly than that of the lung.

When matched by height, prepubertal boys tend to have higher TLC than girls, and thereafter, the volumes of the lung in boys exceed those in girls and boys have been shown to have a greater number of alveoli and a larger alveolar surface area than girls for a given age and height.[12] Despite this, girls have been shown to demonstrate higher maximum expiratory flows than boys[13] and superior airflow per unit lung volume.[14] Since there does not appear to be any sex differences in static elastic recoil,[10] this has been interpreted to infer that girls have shorter, but wider, airways in relation to lung size than boys.[13,14] Subsequently, the growth rate of airways relative to volume is greater in males such that by late adolescence, airways are equal to or relatively larger than in girls.[15] In addition, sex differences in the mechanical properties of the lung relating to tone of the airways have been reported[16] as has lower specific airway resistance in girls than boys,[17] although more recent work has failed to support these findings.[9]

Resting values

In absolute terms, lung volumes increase with growth. In line with TLC, the increases in the subdivisions of the lung are well correlated with height and more appropriately with height[3,4]. However, due to the various changes in the mechanical properties of the lung the rate at which they increase is not necessarily proportional. As stated above, the ratio of FRC to TLC is thought to be lower in children than in adults and between the ages of 11.5 and 18.5 years the ratio of RV to VC increases by about 1% per year (i.e. RV increases more rapidly than VC[2]). The ratio of tidal volume (V_T) to VC, on the other hand, declines with age. Tidal volume has most frequently been reported relative to either body weight (kg) or body surface area, but irrespective of the normalization procedure (see Chapter 2), relative V_T declines slightly with age. For example, in a group of 58 children, V_T was reported as 11.3 mL·kg^{-1} for children 6–8 years of age and 10.1 mL·kg^{-1} for children 8–16 years of age.[18] Coincident with a relative reduction in V_T, breathing frequency (f_R) decreases with age and body size. During early childhood, resting f_R will be as high as 25–30 breath·min^{-1}, but falls to around 10–15 breath·min^{-1} in adulthood. The fall in f_R is due to proportional increases in both the inspiratory (T_I) and expiratory (T_E) durations and is accompanied by a reduction in mean inspiratory flow relative to body weight.[18] As a result of both, a reduced number of breaths and relative volume of air inspired per breath, minute ventilation ($\dot{V}_E$·kg^{-1}) is quite dramatically lower in children than in adults, and mirrors via some as yet unidentified causative mechanism, the lower metabolic rate demonstrated by adults at rest.

Measures of dynamic lung function, forced VC (FVC), forced expiratory volume in 1 s (FEV_1), MVV, and peak expiratory flow rate (PEFR) map closely changes in lung size and somatic growth patterns during growth. In prepuberty stage, a linear increase in dynamic lung function with height is evident, with a divergence from linearity during the pubertal growth spurt which is likely related to thoracic growth.[14] Dynamic lung function is also related to changes with age in muscle strength, since this contributes to forced manoeuvres. Given that peak changes in muscle strength occur some time after peak height velocity, as does peak velocity of thoracic length, it stands to reason that maximum changes in lung function also lag behind peak height velocity from between 6 months to a year. This also contributes to sex differences in measures of dynamic lung function. FEV_1, FVC, and FEV_1/FVC are greater in height matched boys during prepuberty, but during the pubertal growth spurt, all measures of lung function apart from FVC are higher in females than males. Following the growth spurt, discontinuity in lung function is evident, and males outperform females in all parameters of lung function due to both greater lung and thoracic size as well as muscle strength.[14]

Ventilatory response to exercise

At the onset of progressive exercise, $\dot{V}_E$ rises to regulate the arterial partial pressure of carbon dioxide through the manipulation of both f_R and V_T (although see Kinetics section for further detail on the $\dot{V}_E$ response at the actual onset of exercise), and changes in $\dot{V}_E$ closely parallel changes in carbon dioxide output ($\dot{V}CO_2$) and oxygen uptake ($\dot{V}O_2$) up to intensities equating to the ventilatory threshold (T_{VENT}). Above the T_{VENT}, $\dot{V}CO_2$ is augmented by bicarbonate buffering of lactic acid, and $\dot{V}_E$ rises more quickly than $\dot{V}O_2$. Subsequently, as exercise approaches maximal intensity, ventilatory compensation for metabolic acidosis results in a rise in $\dot{V}_E$ disproportionate to both $\dot{V}O_2$ and $\dot{V}CO_2$. As stated above, the qualitative nature of the $\dot{V}_E$ response does not essentially differ between children and adults, but how it is achieved, and the quantitative nature of the $\dot{V}_E$ response does.

Hyperventilation

Children display a higher $\dot{V}_E$ per kilogram body mass ($\dot{V}_E \cdot kg^{-1}$) and a higher $\dot{V}_E$ for a given metabolic demand ($\dot{V}_E/\dot{V}O_2$) than do adults. This age-related improvement in ventilatory efficiency at submaximal levels has been confirmed through cross-sectional studies[18–23] and also longitudinal studies; Rowland and Cunningham[24] reported a decline in $\dot{V}_E/\dot{V}O_2$ of 5.11 and 3.23 during submaximal treadmill walking, in boys and girls, respectively, between the ages of 9 and 13 years (Fig. 18.1). In essence, children hyperventilate.

The control of ventilation

The origin of this ventilatory inefficiency is still not entirely understood. Some authors have suggested that mechanical limitations may play a role. Gratas-Delamarche *et al.*[20] considered that the more rapid and shallow breathing in children (see later) imposes an increase in the mechanical work involved in achieving a given $\dot{V}_E$ and also a limitation to alveolar wash out compared with adults.

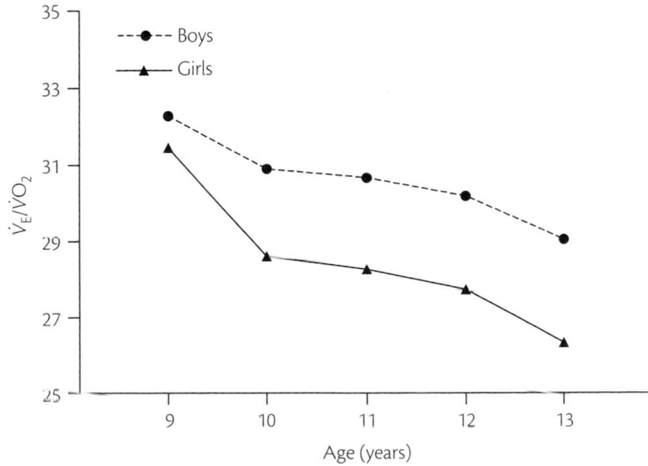

Fig. 18.1 Changes in ventilatory equivalent for oxygen ($\dot{V}_E/\dot{V}O_2$) during submaximal treadmill walking between the age of 9 and 13 years in boys and girls. Data from Rowland and Cunningham.[24]

Although this might be the case and is certainly intuitive, there is limited evidence to support this contention.

On the contrary, there is a larger body of evidence to support a causal relationship between this hyperventilation and a lower P_aCO_2 'set point' in children compared with adults. An age-related increase in exercise P_aCO_2 [usually estimated in paediatric populations from end-tidal partial pressures of CO_2 ($P_{ET}CO_2$) but see Chapter 6] has been demonstrated by a number of authors at rest and during exercise[19,25–27] (see also Fig. 18.5). For example, during steady-state moderate intensity exercise Cooper *et al.*[19] reported $P_{ET}CO_2$ to be 2.9 mmHg lower in eleven 9 year olds than in eleven 18 year olds, suggesting that P_aCO_2 is regulated at a lower 'set point'.

Cooper *et al.*[19] also demonstrated a steeper slope of the $\dot{V}_E/\dot{V}CO_2$ relationship during submaximal exercise, which has been confirmed elsewhere.[20,26,27] This relationship between $\dot{V}_E$ and $\dot{V}CO_2$ is defined by the interaction of the P_aCO_2 'set point' and the physiological dead space fraction (V_D) of the breath [see Eqn (18.1)]. Since the evidence suggests that the ratio of dead space volume to tidal volume (V_D/V_T) does not change with age,[27–30] it stands to reason that for conditions where the $\dot{V}O_2$ and $\dot{V}CO_2$ relationship is linear (i.e. moderate intensity) that an elevated $\dot{V}_E$ and steeper rise in $\dot{V}_E$ for a given $\dot{V}CO_2$ (and $\dot{V}O_2$) may indeed be due to a lower set point for P_aCO_2 in young people.

$$\dot{V}_E\,(\text{BTPS}) = \frac{863 \cdot \text{VCO}_2\,(\text{STPD})}{P_a\text{CO}_2(1 - V_D/V_T)} \qquad (18.1)$$

where $\dot{V}_E$ is ventilation, BTPS is body temperature and pressure, saturated with water vapour; 863 is the constant to correct standard temperature and pressure, dry (STPD) for transformation to BTPS; P_aCO_2 is the arterial partial pressure of carbon dioxide; V_D is dead space fraction of breath and V_T is tidal volume.

Thus, the evidence strongly suggests that this lower 'set point' in children does exist. However, why there should be an age-related increase in the P_aCO_2 'set point' is not understood, but it has been suggested that this is indicative of greater sensitivity of the respiratory drive centres and/or greater respiratory neural drive.

With respect to sensitivity of the respiratory drive centres, Gratas-Delamarche *et al.*[20] examined the $P_{ET}CO_2$ threshold above which $\dot{V}_E$ increased above its steady-state level in a group of ten men (24.9 ± 0.8 years) and nine boys (10.3 ± 0.1 years). There was a significant difference between the groups in the $P_{ET}CO_2$ threshold during exercise (54.2 ± 0.9 and 50.4 ± 0.6 mmHg for adults and boys, respectively), and thus, the authors concluded that children have greater sensitivity of the respiratory centres than adults. Other than cross-sectional observations of a lower $P_{ET}CO_2$ level in children compared with adults (see above), there is little additional evidence that sensitivity of the respiratory drive *per se* is the prevailing influencing factor.

On the other hand, respiratory neural drive has been assessed in children during both rest[18] and exercise.[22,31–33] Gaultier *et al.*[18] assessed mouth occlusion pressure ($P_{0.1}$; pressure recorded 100 ms after the onset of inspiration against a closed airway) and mean inspiratory flow (tidal volume/duration of inspiration, $V_T \cdot T_I^{-1}$), both of which are variables that are related to inspiratory neural drive. In 62 children, 4–16 years of age and at rest, both $P_{0.1}$ and

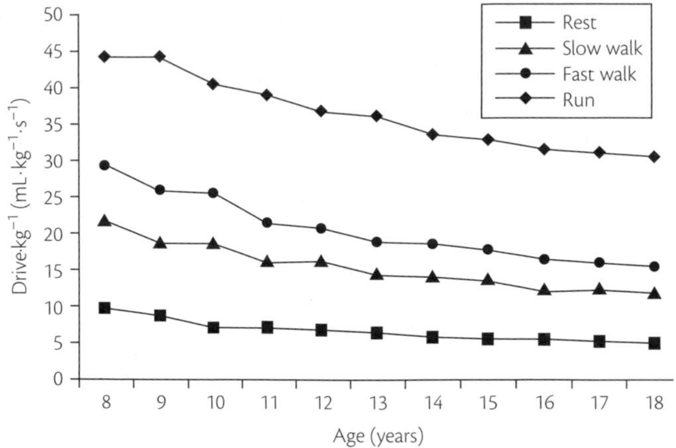

Fig. 18.2 Change in inspiratory drive (drive·kg^{-1}; V_T·kg^{-1}·T_I^{-1}) with age and exercise intensity. From Ondrak and McMurray,[33] with permission.

$V_T \cdot T_I^{-1}$ normalized for body weight declined with age in a similar manner, with power functions $P_{0.1} = 8.51\text{age}^{-0.62}$ and $V_T \cdot \text{kg}^{-1} \cdot T_I^{-1} = 46.3\text{age}^{-0.76}$. Similarly, Ondrak and McMurray[33] identified that $V_T \cdot \text{kg}^{-1} \cdot T_I^{-1}$ declined with age at a range of exercise intensities (Fig. 18.2). These authors, however, also reported that the relationship between ventilatory drive and $P_{ET}CO_2$ was substantially (three times) stronger at rest than during exercise, and concluded that during exercise, the relationship between $P_{ET}CO_2$ and ventilatory drive was only marginal. It seems, therefore, that respiratory drive may have an independent role to play in the hyperventilatory response in children under the influence of some, as yet unknown, feed forward or feedback mechanism that alters with age.

Breathing pattern

Minute ventilation is not a one-dimensional variable, and although it describes the total output of the respiratory system, its components are of equal interest when considering age-related changes in the ventilatory response to exercise.

In order to achieve a given $\dot{V}_E$ in response to changes in metabolic demand, as with adults, children alter their V_T and f_R subsidiary to which are changes in respiratory drive (or mean inspiratory flow) (see above) and changes in respiratory timing [inspiratory (T_I), expiratory (T_E), total time (T_{TOT}), and the duty cycle ($T_I \cdot T_{TOT}^{-1}$)].

As with at rest, the ratio of f_R to V_T during steady-state exercise declines with age due to a reduction in f_R and increase in absolute V_T (although V_T relative to body size either declines slightly[33] or remains stable[24]). Recently, it has been suggested that respiratory timing ($T_I \cdot T_{TOT}^{-1}$) might decline slightly with age at rest and during treadmill exercise, due to increases in T_I that are greater than increases in T_E.[33] However, in this study, the difference between an 8 and 18 year old was equated to be only ~5% and since $T_I \cdot T_{TOT}^{-1}$ has also been reported to remain unchanged with age at both rest and during exercise,[18,22,31] this would suggest that the decline in f_R with age is a function of relative increases in both T_I and T_E, that is, that respiratory timing might not change as a function of growth.

However, in response to an increasing exercise intensity, the pattern of change in f_R and V_T may differ between children and adults. In adults, at the onset of incremental exercise, the initial increase in $\dot{V}_E$ is achieved by increases in V_T and to a lesser extent f_R. At higher exercise intensities, the increase in V_T is attenuated and plateaus (at about 50–60% of VC) and increases in $\dot{V}_E$ are predominantly met by increases in f_R. Although some authors have proposed that this pattern is similar in children,[34] in contrast, it has also been suggested that during progressive submaximal exercise, children first rely more heavily on increases in f_R than V_T[35] and at high intensities, increases in $\dot{V}_E$ are primarily met by changes in V_T whilst f_R projects towards or reaches a plateau.[32,35]

Reasons behind age-related changes in respiratory control are, as stated above, not well understood. However, it is likely that in respect to the changing ratio of f_R to V_T that the mechanical properties of the pulmonary system play a significant role. The ratio of f_R to V_T is fundamentally governed by the requirement to maximize the mechanical efficiency of breathing. In this respect, the plateauing of the V_T response in adults at exercise intensities above 60% of maximum reflects a limit above which the effort involved in inflating the lungs further is more 'expensive' than substantially increasing the rate of inflation. With growth, the diameter of the respiratory airways increase, and increases in lung volume and respiratory recoil pressures also act to decrease resistance further as the airways are mechanically opened at high lung volumes,[9] thus airway resistance declines with age. In terms of mechanical efficiency, high resistance to flow favours low f_R and high V_T. However, small lungs and poorer compliance in children (see above) favour a high f_R and low V_T. Although there is no evidence to suggest that proportionally the change in lung size and lung compliance is greater than the change in airway resistance, it might be considered that there is a greater cost to overcoming the small lung size and compliance than the airway resistance in children. Irrespective of the precise limiting factor, the different breathing pattern observed in children compared with adults reflects a shift in the compromise between the cost of increasing f_R and V_T for a given relative exercise intensity.

Sex differences

Some authors have suggested that significant sex differences in the hyperneic, response to exercise exist. Godfrey[30] suggested that girls ventilate more relative to $\dot{V}O_2$ at maximal exercise than boys, and Rowland and Cunningham[24] in their longitudinal study reported a significantly higher $\dot{V}_E/\dot{V}O_2$ in girls than boys from the ages of 10 (boys, 28.61 ± 3.11; girls, 30.90 ± 2.47) to 13 years (boys, 26.34 ± 2.66; girls, 29.05 ± 2.34). In addition, Armstrong *et al.*[34] demonstrated that at maximum and at equal absolute or relative exercise intensities, prepubertal boys (n = 101) demonstrated a higher absolute and body size corrected $\dot{V}_E$ and V_T than prepubertal girls (n = 76). This latter finding was, however, attributable to the boys' significantly higher absolute and relative $\dot{V}O_2$ at each exercise intensity and more pertinently, these authors found no significant sex difference in f_R, V_T/FVC, $\dot{V}_E/\dot{V}O_2$, or $\dot{V}_E/\dot{V}O_2$ at all exercise intensities. Thus, the data are conflicting and whether sex differences in the response to exercise exist is presently not known.

Ventilation kinetics

Although it is appealing to the exercise scientist to examine the response to steady-state exercise in the laboratory environment, exercise and the response to exercise are dynamic. Therefore, studying the response to changes in metabolic states is not only more applicable to exploring the body's ability to cope with every day stresses, but also contains essential information regarding control and limitations.

In this respect, $\dot{V}_E$ kinetics represent the change in $\dot{V}_E$ at the onset of exercise, and is well described in adults.[36] Minute ventilation responds to the onset of constant load exercise with three temporal phases. During phase 1, $\dot{V}_E$ increases in virtual synchrony with the onset of exercise for approximately 20 s, after which it rises exponentially [with a time constant (τ) of ~70 s], and at moderate intensity achieves a steady state by the third minute of exercise. The rapid increase in $\dot{V}_E$ at the onset of exercise is accompanied by a rapid increase in cardiac output which causes $\dot{V}O_2$ measured at the mouth to rise, whilst $P_{ET}CO_2$ and $P_{ET}O_2$ remain constant. The precise control mechanisms responsible for this phase 1 response are not entirely understood but due to the speed of the response, neurogenic mechanisms, originating from the exercising limbs and/or the central motor areas[37] or cardiodynamic control[38] are considered to be most probable sources of the rapid hyperpnoea. During phase 2, the kinetics of $\dot{V}O_2$, $\dot{V}CO_2$, and $\dot{V}_E$ adopt first-order behaviour, that is, the magnitude of the response is dependent on the signal (exercise intensity) whereas the exponentiality is maintained. Oxygen uptake rises with a time constant of 30–45 s due to the exponentiality of the $\dot{V}O_2$ of the muscle and $\dot{V}CO_2$ and $\dot{V}_E$ follow this pattern of response in order to maintain normoxia. However, the kinetics of $\dot{V}CO_2$ lag behind those of $\dot{V}O_2$ due to tissue storage of $\dot{V}CO_2$, as do the kinetics of $\dot{V}_E$, with time constants in adults of some 20 and 25 s slower, respectively. As a result, there is a noticeable fall in $P_{ET}O_2$ during this stage (Fig. 18.5). The control of the close coupling of $\dot{V}CO_2$ and $\dot{V}_E$ remains an issue of some debate, although there is a possible, though unlikely to be isolated, involvement of chemosensory mechanisms.[39]

The kinetic response of $\dot{V}_E$ to a change in exercise intensity is very similar in character in children as it is in adults (Fig. 18.3), although to date, few have explored the components of the $\dot{V}_E$ kinetic response of children in any detail.

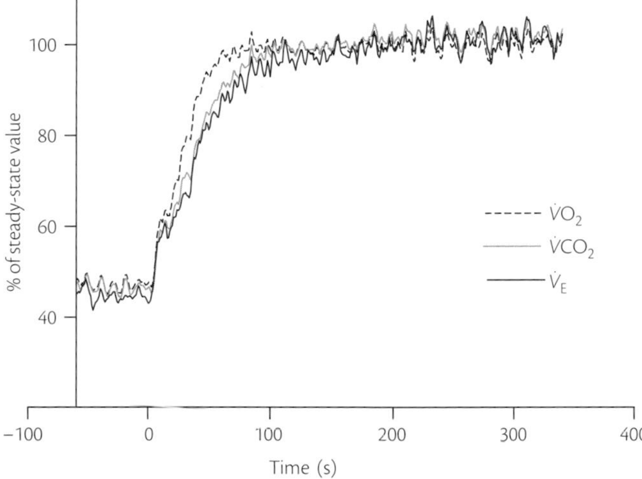

Fig. 18.3 Mean $\dot{V}O_2$, $\dot{V}CO_2$, and $\dot{V}_E$ response of 24 children (11–12 years of age) from baseline pedalling to 80% of ventilatory threshold, imposed as a square wave forcing function at $t = 0$ s. Each child completed at least four exercise transitions, which were time aligned and averaged. The averaged response was normalized to give a percentage of the moderate intensity steady state before time aligning and averaging the group data. (Unpublished data, Children's Health and Exercise Research Centre, University of Exeter)

The phase 1 response is inherently difficult to assess in children. This is due in part to the breath-by-breath noise which masks the true $\dot{V}_E$ response[40] and in part due to the possibility of situation response hyperventilation at the onset of exercise which is likely to occur with children who are not accustomed to the exercise tests. As a result, few authors have attempted to quantify the pattern, or the magnitude, or the time of response in young people. Recently, however, Sato *et al.*[41] have reported data concerning the inspiratory minute ventilation ($\dot{V}_I$), V_T and f_R response to 20 s of knee extensions in ten 11-year-old and ten 25-year-old males. They identified that the children responded to the exercise with a lower percentage change in both $\dot{V}_I$ and V_T with a higher, though non-significant, change in f_R (Fig. 18.4). These authors tentatively speculated that this might have been due to either lower central command and/or afferent signals arising from the exercising limbs, or age differences in respiratory resistance and compliance. However, without further

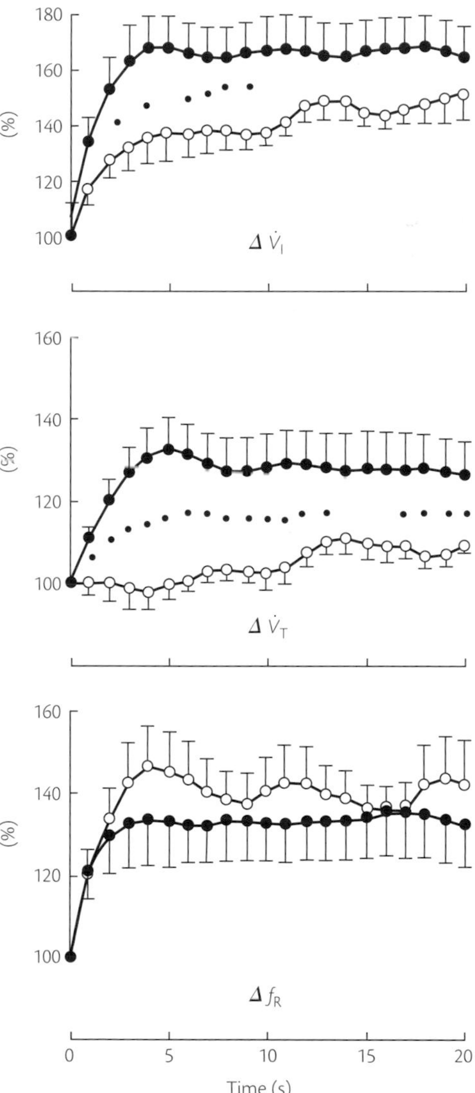

Fig. 18.4 Percentage changes from rest (100%) in inspiratory minute ventilation ($\Delta\dot{V}_I$), tidal volume (ΔV_T), and respiratory frequency (Δf_R) during flexion–extension of the lower leg. Asterisks indicate significant difference ($p < 0.05$) between children (○) and adults (●). From Sato *et al.*,[41] with permission.

research, the nature and the control mechanisms of the phase 1 response in children are not well understood.

The phase 2 response has also attracted little attention, but the body of evidence to date suggests that $\dot{V}_E$ rises towards its steady state more rapidly in children than it does in adults.[19,26,42] Cooper *et al.*[19] identified shorter $\dot{V}_E$ time constants in response to moderate intensity exercise in 8- to 10-year-old boys and girls (41.3 ± 12.5 s) than in 16- to 18-year-old males and females (52.4 ± 9.2 s) and Welsman *et al.*[26] identified shorter $\dot{V}_E$ time constants in 11- to 12-year-old boys (37.9 ± 5.9 s) and girls (41.9 ± 8.4 s) than in 19- to 27-year-old males (60.1 ± 16.3 s) and females (52.8 ± 9.5 s). A shorter $\dot{V}_E$ time constant in children than adults has also been confirmed using a sinusoidal forcing function.[42]

Although it is intuitive to suggest that this may be due to a greater chemosensory sensitivity to $\dot{V}CO_2$ in children than adults, in both adults and children, the time constant for $\dot{V}_E$ lags behind $\dot{V}CO_2$ by little more than a couple of seconds (Fig. 18.3), with no apparent age effect.[26] Therefore, the key to age-related differences in $\dot{V}_E$ kinetics is most probably to lie with the age differences in the kinetics of $\dot{V}CO_2$ at the onset of exercise. The time constant for $\dot{V}CO_2$ lags behind that of $\dot{V}O_2$ due to the storage capacity for CO_2 in haemoglobin and body tissues. This storage capacity for CO_2 during exercise is considered to be smaller in children than adults,[43] and hence metabolically produced CO_2 is detected earlier in the response, with a proportional effect on the rate of the rise in $\dot{V}_E$. The result of this is that at the onset of exercise, there is a closer coupling of $\dot{V}_E$ to $\dot{V}O_2$ in children, which is also made evident by a smaller disruption of $P_{ET}O_2$ during phase 2 (Fig. 18.5).

The third phase of the kinetic response at moderate intensity represents a period, theoretically, of homeostatic balance, such that oxidative phosphorylation is able to support ATP demand and $\dot{V}O_2$ and $\dot{V}CO_2$ remain stable. Contrary to this, $\dot{V}_E$ rises steadily during sustained steady-state exercise by about 10% over a 60-min period, due to an increase in f_R and a small fall in V_T. The precise mechanisms responsible for this ventilatory drift are not known, but may be related to increases in core temperature. When exercise is above the anaerobic threshold, that is, heavy or very heavy intensity, the ventilatory drift is exaggerated further due to increasing lactic acidosis and the release of CO_2. During sustained heavy intensity exercise in adults, $\dot{V}_E$ may increase 50% above the values

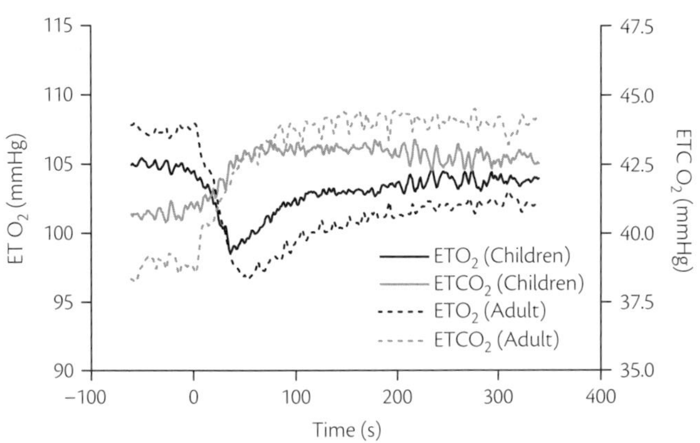

Fig. 18.5 Mean $P_{ET}O_2$ and $P_{ET}CO_2$ response of 24 children (11–12 years of age) and 22 adults (19–26 years of age) from baseline pedalling to 80% of ventilatory threshold, imposed as a square wave forcing function at t = 0 s. (Unpublished data, Children's Health and Exercise Research Centre, University of Exeter)

predicted by the subthreshold relationship between work rate and $\dot{V}_E$. There are limited data regarding children's $\dot{V}_E$ responses to prolonged steady-state exercise, and no published data regarding the nature of $\dot{V}_E$ during the phase 3 response to heavy intensity exercise in this population. Rowland and Rimany[44] compared the ventilatory response of premenarcheal girls and young adult females whilst cycling for 40 min at 63% of $\dot{V}O_2$ max. Minute ventilation and f_R rose and V_T fell in both groups (girls, +7.1%, +15%, and −6%; women, +11.7%,+14%, and −2%, $\dot{V}_E$, f_R, and V_T, respectively) with no significant differences between the groups. Thus, it could be concluded that the mechanisms controlling the $\dot{V}CO_2$ drift do not undergo maturation during growth. However, since at 63% $\dot{V}O_2$ max, it is most probable that some of the participants would have been exercising above, and some below their anaerobic threshold, it is not possible to extrapolate these results to make implications regarding subthreshold responses. In addition, lower blood lactates in children in response to heavy intensity exercise compared to adults may result in an abbreviated $\dot{V}_E$ response during heavy intensity exercise in children. Therefore, whether or not the magnitude of the $\dot{V}_E$ drift is age dependent at any exercise intensity is not currently known.

Maximum ventilation

The term maximum $\dot{V}_E$ (or $\dot{V}_E$ max) is inherently misleading, since the term suggests it to be the maximum $\dot{V}_E$ that the body is able to achieve. However, two issues contest the common use of this phrase. First, $\dot{V}_E$ at maximum exercise tolerance is usually significantly smaller than MVV and thus factors other than ventilation are limiting exercise tolerance, and second, $\dot{V}_E$ max is highly protocol dependent.[45] Thus, although $\dot{V}_E$ at the limit of tolerance ($\dot{V}_E$ max) might be the situation specific maximum $\dot{V}_E$, it is difficult to make valid interstudy comparisons. Despite this, it is important to consider the literature that explores the relationship between $\dot{V}_E$ max and growth, but this needs to be interpreted with the above concerns in mind.

During an incremental exercise test, the $\dot{V}_E$ max depends on the maximum level of aerobic metabolism achieved, the CO_2 by-product of anaerobic metabolism, and the level of ventilatory drive due to arterial acidosis. During growth, it is well established that peak $\dot{V}O_2$ increases, that end exercise lactate levels increase and end exercise pH levels decline with age (see Chapters 8 and 20). Thus, an increase in $\dot{V}_E$ max with age is a necessity, and is suitably achieved through an increase in the size of the lungs and the change in pulmonary mechanics, and has been shown longitudinally to increase between the ages of 9 and 13 years by 8.8 ± 1.9 L·min^{-1} per year.[24] However, although changes in lung size have been shown to relate closely to changes in body dimensions, there is less consensus with regard to the relationship between body size and $\dot{V}_E$ max.

Mercier *et al.*[31] examined the relationship between anthropometrical measurements and $\dot{V}_E$ max in 76 untrained boys, aged 10.5–15.5 years. They reported that lean body mass explained the greatest variance in $\dot{V}_E$ max (62.1%), and identified allometric exponents for height, body mass, and lean body mass of 2.06, 0.68, and 0.79, respectively. Similarly, Rowland and Cunningham[24] identified in 20 children over a 5-year period exponents of 2.50 and 0.92 for height and body mass, respectively. With a more homogenous sample of 177 boys and girls aged 11.1 ± 0.4 years, Armstrong *et al.*[34] identified exponents of 0.69 for height and 0.48 for body mass. The cause for the discrepancy in the height exponent is a function of the latter study combining both anthropometric measures in a single allometric analysis, whereas the former studies computed the exponents with single covariates. Irrespective of this, the evidence suggests that $\dot{V}_E$ max does not increase in direct proportion with body size, and thus the use of simple ratio scaling (i.e. $\dot{V}_E \cdot kg^{-1}$) is not appropriate.

Limitations to maximal ventilation

Since $\dot{V}_E$ max is repeatedly reported to be less than MVV, the suggestion that ventilation is not limiting to exercise tolerance has been easily adopted. However, the past 20 years has seen an increase in the awareness of and investigation into exercise induced arterial hypoxaemia (EIAH), a condition due to imperfect pulmonary ventilation which is apparent in both humans and animals and that can in fact be limiting to O_2 transport and utilization during maximal exercise.[46]

EIAH is most commonly evidenced by a significant fall in arterial P_aO_2 during exercise, but more specifically by a fall in O_2 saturation (SaO_2) and increase in the alveolar–arterial difference for O_2 (A–aDO_2). Dempsey and Wagner[47] suggest that when considering EIAH as a threat to O_2 transport (and thus peak $\dot{V}O_2$), mild cases should be defined as an absolute SaO_2 of 93–95% and severe cases as <88%. When considering EIAH as an indicator of inadequacies in ventilation and gas exchange, an A–aDO_2 in the range of 25–30 Torr might be considered excessive, and 35–40 Torr is indicative of severe inefficiencies. The use of the latter two indicators of EIAH allows for a closer examination of the causes of EIAH—these being an inadequate compensatory hyperventilation and inefficient gas exchange. The precise details regarding why the pulmonary system might become limited in these ways are still being explored. Inadequate compensatory hyperventilation suggests that $\dot{V}_E$ is not appropriate for the given metabolic demand, and may be due to poor sensitivity and stimulus responsiveness[48] or mechanical limitations.[49] Inefficient gas exchange seems most probably due to ventilation perfusion ($\dot{V}_A/\dot{Q}$) inequalities, which become more pronounced at high exercise intensities, but might also be contributed to by diffusion limitation and intrapulmonary and extrapulmonary shunts.

Evidence for EIAH has been found predominantly in young, highly fit males and whilst within this group there is considered a significant positive relationship between $\dot{V}O_2$ max and incidence of EIAH (~50% of male athletes in one study with a $\dot{V}O_2$ max > 68 mL·kg^{-1}·min^{-1} developed a significant reduction in SaO_2),[50] the relationship is neither able to predict nor discount an individual from either low P_aO_2 or a high A-aDO_2 at maximal exercise.[51] EIAH has also been demonstrated in females of average to high fitness levels, and in the fit and active elderly,[47] but despite the growing body of literature concerned with EIAH in adults, the prevalence of the condition, and its implications on exercise tolerance, is still not entirely understood.

It is, therefore, not surprising that very little is known with regard to the incidence of EIAH in children, or whether it is in any way limiting to maximal exercise tolerance in this population. Laursen *et al.*,[52] in the first of only two studies available on this topic in children, examined the incidence of EIAH in 19 healthy active prepubescent females (11.1 ± 1.6 years of age) during incremental exercise to exhaustion. The focus on female athletes was particularly pertinent since unlike in male adults, EIAH had been demonstrated in female adults with normal levels of $\dot{V}O_2$ max. This had been suggested to be due to their smaller lung size and airway diameters causing mechanical limitation at lower relative exercise intensities,[53] and thus it might have been hypothesized that EIAH would also be prevalent in young females. However, these authors reported no incidents of significant arterial oxyhaemoglobin desaturation in the 19 girls (mean % SaO_2 96.6 ± 1.2) and no relationship between peak $\dot{V}O_2$ and SaO_2, and therefore concluded that EIAH does not occur in prepubescent females. Despite this, closer examination of the results indicated that in three of the girls (with peak $\dot{V}O_2$ between 40 and 45 mL·kg^{-1}·min^{-1}) SaO_2 values fell to 94% or 95% SaO_2. This actually suggests that as with adult females, mild EIAH may occur in this population.

More recently, Nourry *et al.*[54] explored the incidence of EIAH (defined as a drop in SaO_2 of at least 4% from resting levels) in 16 prepubescent boys and 8 prepubescent girls (10.3 ± 0.2 years of age) during a maximal incremental test. Seven of the children (five boys and two girls) demonstrated EIAH, four in mild form (93–95% SaO_2) and three in moderate form (88–93% SaO_2). Separating the children into either a hypoxic group (H, n = 7) or non-hypoxic group (NH, n = 17), a significant difference in SaO_2 was evident at both submaximal and maximal exercise intensities (Fig. 18.6). There were also group differences in $\Delta\dot{V}_E/\Delta\dot{V}CO_2$ at submaximal exercise intensities (27.8 ± 2.4 vs. 35.7 ± 1.6, $p < 0.05$, H and NH, respectively), FVC and breathing reserve were lower and V_T/FVC was higher in H compared with NH at maximum. There were no group differences in physical activity levels, anthropometric variables or peak $\dot{V}O_2$ (50.6 ± 2.7 and 46.4 ± 1.7 mL·kg^{-1}·min^{-1}).

This study was a useful contributor to the study of EIAH in humans, but why some children might display EIAH at this stage can only be speculated upon. At submaximal levels, a lower $\Delta\dot{V}_E/\Delta\dot{V}CO_2$ in hypoxaemic children might have indicated inadequate compensatory ventilation due to lower chemoresponsiveness, but the authors also demonstrated no difference between the groups for $P_{ET}CO_2$ or $P_{ET}O_2$ and therefore suggested that relative hypoventilation in this group might not be a determining factor as it might be in adults. From the currently available literature, it is not possible to comment on any possible limitations due to $\dot{V}_A/\dot{Q}$

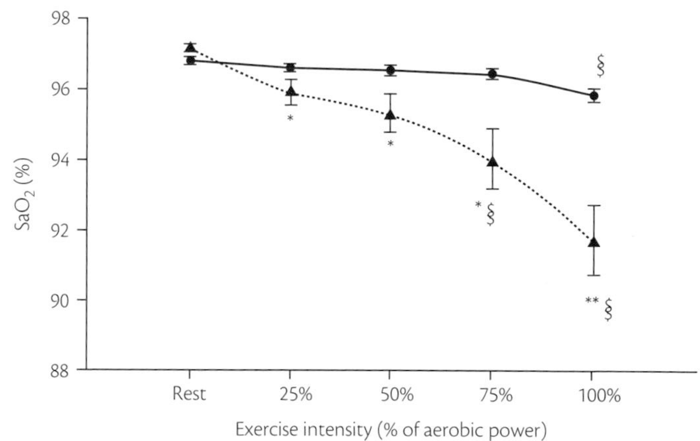

Fig. 18.6 Change in SaO_2 during incremental exercise in hypoxaemic children (▲) and non-hypoxaemic children (●). Significant differences between groups: *$p < 0.05$; **$p < 0.01$. Significant difference from rest in hypoxaemic group: §$p < 0.05$. From Nourry *et al.*,[74] with permission.

inequalities, diffusion capacity, or pulmonary shunts, and thus whether inefficient gas exchange plays a significant role in lower SaO_2 levels at either submaximal and maximal exercise intensities in this population is not known.

The most convincing suggestion for differences between hypoxaemic and non-hypoxaemic children at maximal levels is that the size of the lungs caused mechanical limitation in the hypoxaemic group, evidenced by the smaller breathing reserve and higher V_T/FVC at maximal exercise in this group. Since EIAH occurred as it does with adult females even at relatively low fitness levels, this contributes to the argument that mechanical limitation due to the proportional size of the lungs and the airways is most probably a significant contributor to the incidence of EIAH.

It must be noted that both of these studies reporting on the incidence of EIAH in children involved maximal exercise on a cycle ergometer. Recent evidence with adults has suggested that the severity of EIAH is greater during treadmill running than cycle ergometry even when relative exercise intensities are equated[55] and so whether the incidence of EIAH is greater in children during treadmill running than is currently thought for cycle ergometry, requires investigation.

Training adaptations

Despite a number of studies that have tried to identify changes in static and dynamic lung functions and exercise hypernoea in response to training in young people, surprisingly little can be concluded confidently. Training studies with young people are inherently difficult, and cross-sectional studies are unable to argue a case for training adaptation over and above genetic predisposition. In addition, much of the literature concerned with children has focussed heavily upon swim training, a training condition that imposes quite a different physical environment on the pulmonary system than is experienced on land. Thus, trying to elicit the precise mechanisms of training adaptations are beyond the current body of knowledge. Nevertheless, some common themes are apparent in the literature.

A number of studies have reported larger lung volumes in trained swimmers than in untrained children.[56–59] Andrew *et al.*[57] assessed static and functional lung volumes in male and female swimmers (8–18 years of age) and a non-trained reference group over a 3-year period. Relative to height, the swimmers had greater VC, TLC, and expiratory flow rates and the difference was more evident in the older children. These authors suggested that this was due to a training adaptation of the respiratory muscles and was either due to the training load *per se* and/or immersion during the respiratory cycle which, since this requires greater pulmonary pressures in order to inflate the lung than on land, invoked an overload response.

In order to examine whether in fact this training adaptation might be due to improvements in respiratory muscle force, Zinman and Gaultier[59] compared maximal static pressures (P_{max}) in 38 competitively trained female swimmers and 59 controls aged 7–13 years, and subsequently supplemented this with a 1-year follow-up study.[60] As expected, the authors demonstrated greater lung volumes (VC, TLC, and FRC) for height in the swimmers, which was more marked in the older children but absolute measures of P_{max} showed no significant difference between groups. The authors, therefore, suggested an alternative hypothesis for adaptive growth that should be based on the increased O_2 demand during training, rather than a mechanical adaptation *per se*.

Although these authors included a 1-year follow-up in their studies, there have been few well-controlled swim training studies from which to help define the differences between genetic predisposition and true training adaptations in this group of athletes. Although Zauner and Benson[61] noted increases in FVC over a 3-year period in trained swimmers compared with predicted values (109% in the third year), other early studies have been unable to detect increases in lung volumes in child swimmers following half a year of swim training.[62,63] Of note, despite the small subject numbers, is the study of Courteix *et al.*,[64] which followed five prepubertal girls (9.3 ± 0.5 years) who completed 12 hours a week of swim training and 11 matched controls over a 1-year period. These authors confirmed the findings of cross-sectional studies, reporting that despite no differences between the groups at baseline, VC, TLC, and FRC were significantly larger in the swimmers than the controls after 1 year, with no differences between the groups in height or weight. They also reported improvements in the conductive properties of the large and small airways in the swimmers but not the controls (through the assessment of airway resistance, $FEV_{1.0}$, and FEV_{25-75}), which led the authors to speculate that swim training led to not only increases in static and dynamic lung growth, but also the promotion of isotropic lung growth.

There is some evidence that swim training may also enhance other aspects of pulmonary function during growth. Yost *et al.*[65] compared the diffusion capacity for carbon monoxide (DL_{CO}) in a group of highly trained competitive swimmers (5 male and 7 females) and a group of age-, sex-, and size-controlled 9–17 year olds. At an exercise intensity corresponding to a heart rate of 170 beats·min^{-1}, DL_{CO} at rest and exercise was significantly higher for the swimmers. The swimmers were also reported to show a significantly greater increase in DL_{CO} over a 10-month period than would have been predicted by growth alone, and thus the authors proposed a training effect on diffusion capacity. To this effect, the authors accepted that the mechanism involved in the training adaptation could not be concluded. However, since there was no difference between the groups in body size or FVC, the authors suggested that differences in pulmonary capillary blood volume, rather than increases in alveolar surface area, might be responsible. Andrew *et al.*[57] also found that DL_{CO} was higher in swim-trained boys compared to non-trained counterparts, but these authors were also able to report no significant difference between the groups in stroke volume, and therefore suggested that changes in pulmonary capillarity may be more likely to explain these differences.

It seems that swim training may well induce training adaptations, but how much of this is due to adaptations to increases in metabolic requirements and exercise overload, and how much is due to a conditioning stimulus of breathing whilst immersed in water and breath holding procedures are difficult to determine.

There are a few direct comparisons in pulmonary function or training adaptations between swim athletes and land-based athletes, but they are non-conclusive. Doherty and Dimitriou[66] compared lung volumes in a large cross-sectional sample of male and female swimmers (n = 160), land-based athletes (n = 162), and sedentary (n = 156) 10–21 year olds. Using allometric scaling techniques, the swimmers were demonstrated to have superior FRV_1 independent of age and stature compared with both sedentary and land-based athletes. However, in this cross-sectional study, the authors were not able to conclude that the differences between land- and water-based trained athletes were not simply a function of genetic predisposition. Indeed, a 3-year longitudinal study following a large sample of young athletes in a variety of sports has demonstrated that on entry into the study, the FVC and FEV_1 of the swimmers was significantly higher than the other athletes and that subsequently these differences did not change with training, that is, training had no discernible impact on these parameters of pulmonary function.[67]

Further to this, cross-sectional and longitudinal studies exploring the effect of land-based training on pulmonary function might suggest that land-based training has less impact on lung size and function, contrary to the body of evidence regarding swimming.

Hamilton and Andrew[68] found no significant differences in static and dynamic lung functions or DL_{CO} between prepubertal and postpubertal boys undertaking intense hockey training and matched controls, and no such differences were also found by Vaccaro and Poffenbarger[69] between eight female track team athletes (10–14 years old) and matched controls. Koch and Eriksson[70] found no difference in DL_{CO}, VC, FRC, and FEV_1 after 16 weeks of training in nine 11- to 13-year-old boys, and subsequently, a 4-year longitudinal study demonstrated no additional effect of physical activity on lung volumes over and above those expected due to growth.[71] This was later supported by a further longitudinal investigation by Andersen *et al.*[72] who found no relationship between physical performance capacity and lung function in children between the ages of 8 and 18 years, and other studies have also supported the concept that growth in lung volumes parallels normal growth in both athletes and non-athletes.[73,74] It is quite probable, however, that the land-based training involved in these studies was simply not sufficient in intensity or duration to stress the pulmonary system to the same degree as during swim training, and that this might contribute to the relatively consistent differential trend in the literature between swim and land-based training effects. In fact, recently, a well-controlled training study identified pulmonary adaptations to high-intensity intermittent run training in nine children (three girls and six boys).[74] Eight weeks of training induced significant improvements in FVC and maximal expiratory flows compared with a control group who showed no changes. Therefore, this sort of training might provide the respiratory stimulus to impose adaptations not otherwise experienced through normal land-based training or by highly active children.

Nourry *et al.*[74] also investigated the effect of training on breathing pattern, a topic which had also been explored previously by other authors. As a response to the 8 weeks of training, there was an increase in peak $\dot{V}O_2$ (+15.5 ± 4.0%) and an increase in $\dot{V}_E$ (+16 ± 5%) and V_T (+15 ± 5%) at peak, but no change in f_R.

Increases in maximum $\dot{V}_E$ with training and in correlation with peak $\dot{V}O_2$ are consistent with longitudinal and cross-sectional studies[34,75–77] and this increase in maximum $\dot{V}_E$ seems to be entirely due to changes in V_T rather than f_R.[34,74,76] This suggests that in order to facilitate additional gas exchange, mechanical efficiency dictates an increase in V_T rather than f_R, which is in line with the understanding that in children f_R plateaus during incremental exercise at about 60% peak $\dot{V}O_2$ such that V_T then supports increases in $\dot{V}_E$ (see above).

At submaximal exercise intensities, Nourry *et al.*[74] demonstrated no changes in $\dot{V}_E$, f_R, or V_T. This was consistent with Ramonatxo *et al.* (77) who had also shown that swimmers (aged 11–16 years) with a high $\dot{V}O_2$ max (57.6 mL·kg^{-1}·min^{-1}, n = 10) used the same V_T and f_R for a given $\dot{V}_E$ as those with a lower $\dot{V}O_2$ max (43.8 mL·kg^{-1}·min^{-1}, n = 10). Conversely, Rowland and Green (35) have reported a lower f_R and higher V_T for a given $\dot{V}_E$ in trained child runners than non-trained children, and whereas Gratas *et al.* (78) also demonstrated lower f_R in trained children, this was for an equated work load rather than an equated $\dot{V}_E$ (which was lower in the trained group) and thus it is more difficult to meaningfully interpret.

Thus, whether training induces a change in breathing pattern at sub-maximal levels is not known, and equally, the evidence concerning any training adaptation on ventilatory efficiency in children is not presently conclusive. Ramonatxo *et al.*[77] have shown a significantly lower $\dot{V}_E/\dot{V}O_2$ in children with a high $\dot{V}O_2$ max, which was most apparent at high levels of $\dot{V}O_2$, and Rowland and Green[35] reported lower $\dot{V}_E/\dot{V}O_2$ in trained child runners (25.1 ± 2.1) compared with normal children (27.6 ± 3.5) , although this difference was not significant. Nourry *et al.*,[74] on the other hand, reported no such difference in $\dot{V}_E/\dot{V}O_2$ before and after training, but there was a significant reduction in $P_{ET}O_2$ and increase in $P_{ET}CO_2$ at a given submaximal work load after training. These data supported those of Gratas *et al.*[78] who also demonstrated lower $P_{ET}O_2$ and higher $P_{ET}CO_2$ in trained versus untrained boys, but both of these studies have potential flaws in their use of comparative absolute work loads rather than relative exercise intensities. Nevertheless, Nourry *et al.*[74] also reported a reduction in $\Delta\dot{V}_E/\Delta\dot{V}CO_2$ with training, and thus the data might indicate that training induces an improvement in ventilatory efficiency, possibly due to a higher $P_{ET}CO_2$ set point and/or mechanical efficiency.

Summary

- Despite discrepant growth patterns of the lung and its various components, the pulmonary system appears to achieve proportional relationships that optimize the pulmonary response, and thus support nearly all natural metabolic demands placed upon it throughout growth.
- The study of the pulmonary system and the ventilatory response to exercise in children is by no means complete, and a number of questions remain unanswered, specifically with regard to the control of exercise hypernoea, and other more recent research themes.
- Increases in lung and thorax size, airways and alveoli number, changes in the mechanical properties of the pulmonary system, and increases in muscle strength contribute to increases in lung volumes and static and dynamic lung function with age. Although these are closely related to the timing and tempo of increases in height and weight, their growth patterns are not isotropic. Since girls begin their adolescent growth spurt earlier than boys, with respect to chronological age there is a period when girls' lung volumes and dynamic lung function are superior to boys'. At all other times, boys outperform girls in all measures of lung function.
- Children's fundamental ventilatory response to exercise is similar to adults. However, children hyperventilate for a given metabolic demand. Although the exact reasons for this are not understood, it is likely that there is a significant association between this hyperventilatory response and a low exercise P_aCO_2, which is frequently reported in this population, and may infer that neural drive and/or sensitivity of the respiratory centres is age dependent.

- Most probably due to the changing mechanical properties of the lung and thorax, the ratio of f_R to V_T declines with age, but respiratory timing appears to be age independent.
- Few investigators have considered the $\dot{V}_E$ kinetic response to the onset of exercise in children, and therefore there is little known regarding the phase 3 response. As with adults, at the onset of exercise, $\dot{V}_E$ responds rapidly, after which it rises exponentially towards a steady state, with a time course about 25 s slower than $\dot{V}O_2$. This is substantially quicker than adults, and is most probably due to the greater tissue storage capacity for $\dot{V}CO_2$ in adults than children, and the tight coupling of $\dot{V}_E$ to $\dot{V}CO_2$ during this transient period.
- $\dot{V}_E$ max is a slightly misleading term, but infers the maximum $\dot{V}_E$ that can be achieved during a specific exercise test. $\dot{V}_E$ max increases with age with height and body weight as important explanatory variables.
- Whilst ventilation is generally considered not to be limiting to exercise tolerance, the incidence of exercise-induced arterial hypoxaemia has been demonstrated in both boys and girls of normal levels of fitness. Whether children are more susceptible to EIAH than adults due to their smaller lungs and airways is not currently known.
- Whether or not training adaptations of the pulmonary system occur has been traditionally difficult to define in the absence of well-controlled longitudinal studies. However, there is a body of evidence that suggests that swim training may impose a training effect, as might high intensity land-based training.

References

1. Simon G, Reid L, Tanner JM, Goldstein H, Benjamin B (1972). Growth of radiologically determined heart diameter, lung width, and lung length from 5–19 years, with standards for clinical use. *Arch Dis Child* **47**, 373–81.
2. DeGroodt EG, van Pelt W, Borsboom GJ, Quanjer PH, van Zomeren BC (1988). Growth of lung and thorax dimensions during the pubertal growth spurt. *Eur Respir J* **1**, 102–8.
3. Lyons HA, Tanner RW (1962). Total lung volume and its subdivisions in children: normal standards. *J Appl Physiol* **17**, 601–4.
4. Cook CD, Hamann JF (1961). Relation of lung volumes to height in healthy persons between the ages of 5 and 38 years. *J Pediatr* **59**, 710–14.
5. Dunnill MS (1962). Postnatal growth of the lung. *Thorax* **17**, 329–33.
6. Zapletal A, Motoyama EK, Van De Woestijne KP, Hunt VR, Bouhuys A (1969). Maximum expiratory flow-volume curves and airway conductance in children and adolescents. *J Appl Physiol* **26**, 308–16.
7. Mansell AL, Bryan AC, Levison H (1977). Relationship of lung recoil to lung volume and maximum expiratory flow in normal children. *J Appl Physiol* **42**, 817–23.
8. De Troyer A, Yernault JC, Englert M, Baran D, Paiva M (1978). Evolution of intrathoracic airway mechanics during lung growth. *J Appl Physiol* **44**, 521–7.
9. Lanteri CJ, Sly PD (1993). Changes in respiratory mechanics with age. *J Appl Physiol* **74**, 369–78.
10. Zapletal A, Paul T, Samanek M (1976). Pulmonary elasticity in children and adolescents. *J Appl Physiol* **40**, 953–61.
11. Mansell AL, Bryan AC, Levison H (1977). Relationship of lung recoil to lung volume and maximum expiratory flow in normal children. *J Appl Physiol* **42**, 817–23.
12. Thurlbeck WM (1982). Postnatal human lung growth. *Thorax* **37**, 564–71.
13. Hibbert ME, Couriel JM, Landau LI (1984). Changes in lung, airway, and chest wall function in boys and girls between 8 and 12 yr. *J Appl Physiol* **57**, 304–8.
14. Rosenthal M, Bain SH, Cramer D, Helms P, Denison D, Bush A, Warner JO (1993). Lung function in white children aged 4 to 19 years: I-Spirometry. *Thorax* **48**, 794–802.
15. Merkus PJ, Borsboom GJ, Van Pelt W, Schrader PC, Van Houwelingen HC, Kerrebijn KF, Quanjer PH (1993). Growth of airways and air spaces in teenagers is related to sex but not to symptoms. *J Appl Physiol* **75**, 2045–53.
16. Taussig LM, Cota K, Kaltenborn W (1981). Different mechanical properties of the lung in boys and girls. *Am Rev Respir Dis* **123**, 640–3.
17. Doershuk CF, Fisher BJ, Matthews LW (1974). Specific airway resistance from the perinatal period into adulthood. Alterations in childhood pulmonary disease. *Am Rev Respir Dis* **109**, 452–7.
18. Gaultier C, Perret L, Boule M, Buvry A, Girard F (1981). Occlusion pressure and breathing pattern in healthy children. *Respir Physiol* **46**, 71–80.
19. Cooper DM, Kaplan MR, Baumgarten L, Weiler-Ravell D, Whipp BJ, Wasserman K (1987). Coupling of ventilation and CO_2 production during exercise in children. *Pediatr Res* **21**, 568–72.
20. Gratas-Delamarche A, Mercier J, Ramonatxo M, Dassonville J, Prefaut C (1993). Ventilatory response of prepubertal boys and adults to carbon dioxide at rest and during exercise. *Eur J Appl Physiol* **66**, 25–30.
21. Astrand PO (1952). *Experimental studies of physical working capacity in relation to sex and age*. Munksgaard, Copenhagen.
22. Ramonatxo M, Mercier J, el-Fassi-Ben Abdallah R, Vago P, Prefaut C (1986). Breathing pattern and occlusion pressure during exercise in pre- and peripubertal swimmers. *Respir Physiol* **65**, 351–64.
23. Andersen KL, Seliger V, Rutenfranz J, Messel S (1974). Physical performance capacity of children in Norway. III. Respiratory responses to graded exercise loadings-population parameters in a rural community. *Eur J Appl Physiol* **33**, 265–74.
24. Rowland TW, Cunningham LN (1997). Development of ventilatory responses to exercise in normal white children. A longitudinal study. *Chest* **111**, 327–32.
25. Ohuchi H, Kato Y, Tasato H, Arakaki Y, Kamiya T (1999). Ventilatory response and arterial blood gases during exercise in children. *Pediatr Res* **45**, 389–96.
26. Welsman JR, Fawkner SG, Armstrong N (2001). Respiratory response to non-steady state exercise in children and adults (abstract). *Pediatr Exerc Sci* **13**, 263–4.
27. Nagano Y, Baba R, Kuraishi K, Yasuda T, Ikoma M, Nishibata K, Yokota M, Nagashima M (1998). Ventilatory control during exercise in normal children. *Pediatr Res* **43**, 704–7.
28. Gadhoke S, Jones NL (1969). The responses to exercise in boys aged 9–15 years. *Clin Sci* **37**, 789–801.
29. Shephard RJ, Bar-Or O (1970). Alveolar ventilation in near maximum exercise. Data on pre-adolescent children and young adults. *Med Sci Sports Exerc* **2**, 83–92.
30. Godfrey S (1974). *Exercise testing in children*. Saunders, London.
31. Mercier J, Varray A, Ramonatxo M, Mercier B, Prefaut C (1991). Influence of anthropometric characteristics on changes in maximal exercise ventilation and breathing pattern during growth in boys. *Eur J Appl Physiol* **63**, 235–41.
32. Boule M, Gaultier C, Girard F (1989). Breathing pattern during exercise in untrained children. *Respir Physiol* **75**, 225–33.
33. Ondrak KS, McMurray RG (2006). Exercise-induced breathing patterns of youth are related to age and intensity. *Eur J Appl Physiol* **98**, 88–96.
34. Armstrong N, Kirby BJ, McManus AM, Welsman JR (1997). Prepubescents' ventilatory responses to exercise with reference to sex and body size. *Chest* **112**, 1554–60.
35. Rowland TW, Green GM (1990). The influence of biological maturation and aerobic fitness on ventilatory responses to treadmill exercise. In: Dotson CO, Humphrey JH (eds.), *Exercise physiology: Current selected research*, pp. 51–9. AMS Press, New York.

36. Ward SA (2007). Ventilatory control in humans: Constraints and limitations. *Exp Physiol* **92**, 357–66.
37. Mitchell JH (1990). Neural control of the circulation during exercise. *Med Sci Sports Ex* **22**, 141–54.
38. Wasserman K, Whipp BJ, Castagna J (1974). Cardiodynamic hyperpnea: Hyperpnea secondary to cardiac output increase. *J Appl Physiol* **36**, 457–64.
39. Dempsey JA (2006). Challenges for future research in exercise physiology as applied to the respiratory system. *Exerc Sport Sci Rev* **34**, 92–8.
40. Potter CR, Childs DJ, Houghton W, Armstrong N (1999). Breath-to-breath 'noise' in children's ventilatory and gas exchange responses to exercise. *Eur J Appl Physiol* **80**, 118–24.
41. Sato Y, Katayama K, Ishida K, Miyamura M (2000). Ventilatory and circulatory responses at the onset of voluntary exercise and passive movement in children. *Eur J Appl Physiol* **83**, 516–23.
42. Haouzi P, Fukuba Y, Peslin R, Chalon B, Marchal F, Crance JP (1992). Ventilatory dynamics in children and adults during sinusoidal exercise. *Eur J Appl Physiol* **64**, 410–18.
43. Zanconato S, Cooper DM, Barstow TJ, Landaw E (1992). $^{13}CO_2$ washout dynamics during intermittent exercise in children and adults. *J Appl Physiol* **73**, 2476–82.
44. Rowland TW, Rimany TA (1995). Physiological responses to prolonged exercise in premenarchal and adult females. *Pediatr Exerc Sci* **7**, 183–91.
45. Armstrong N, Welsman J, Winsley R (1996). Is peak $\dot{V}O_2$ a maximal index of children's aerobic fitness? *Int J Sports Med* **17**, 356–9.
46. Powers SK, Lawler J, Dempsey JA, Dodd S, Landry G (1989). Effects of incomplete pulmonary gas exchange on $\dot{V}O_2$ max. *J Appl Physiol* **66**, 2491–5.
47. Dempsey JA, Wagner PD (1999). Exercise-induced arterial hypoxemia. *J Appl Physiol* **87**, 1997–2006.
48. Harms CA, Stager JM (1995). Low chemoresponsiveness and inadequate hyperventilation contribute to exercise-induced hypoxemia. *J Appl Physiol* **79**, 575–80.
49. Johnson BD, Saupe KW, Dempsey JA (1992). Mechanical constraints on exercise hyperpnea in endurance athletes. *J Appl Physiol* **73**, 874–86.
50. Powers SK, Dodd S, Lawler J, Landry G, Kirtley M, McKnight T, Grinton S (1988). Incidence of exercise induced hypoxemia in elite endurance athletes at sea level. *Eur J Appl Physiol* **58**, 298–302.
51. Hopkins SR (2006). Exercise induced arterial hypoxemia: The role of ventilation-perfusion inequality and pulmonary diffusion limitation. *Adv Exp Med Biol* **588**, 17–30.
52. Laursen PB, Tsang GC, Smith GJ, van Velzen MV, Ignatova BB, Sprules EB, Chu KS, Coutts KD, McKenzie DC (2002). Incidence of exercise-induced arterial hypoxemia in prepubescent females. *Pediatr Pulmonol* **34**, 37–41.
53. Harms CA, McClaran SR, Nickele GA, Pegelow DF, Nelson WB, Dempsey JA (1998). Exercise-induced arterial hypoxaemia in healthy young women. *J Physiol* **507** (**Pt 2**), 619–28.
54. Nourry C, Fabre C, Bart F, Grosbois JM, Berthoin S, Mucci P (2004). Evidence of exercise-induced arterial hypoxemia in prepubescent trained children. *Pediatr Res* **55**, 674–81.
55. Galy O, Le Gallais D, Hue O, Boussana A, Prefaut C (2005). Is exercise-induced arterial hypoxemia in triathletes dependent on exercise modality? *Int J Sports Med* **26**, 719–26.
56. Astrand PO, Eriksson BO, Nylander I, Engstroem L, Karlberg P, Saltin B, Thoren C (1963). Girl swimmers. With special reference to respiratory and circulatory adaptation and gynaecological and psychiatric aspects. *Acta Paediatr* **147** (Suppl.), 1–75.
57. Andrew GM, Becklake MR, Guleria JS, Bates DV (1972). Heart and lung functions in swimmers and nonathletes during growth. *J Appl Physiol* **32**, 245–51.
58. Engstrom I, Eriksson BO, Karlberg P, Saltin B, Thoren C (1971). Preliminary report on the development of lung volumes in young girl swimmers. *Acta Paediatr Scand* **217** (Suppl.), 73–6.
59. Zinman R, Gaultier C (1986). Maximal static pressures and lung volumes in young female swimmers. *Respir Physiol* **64**, 229–39.
60. Zinman R, Gaultier C (1987). Maximal static pressures and lung volumes in young female swimmers: one year follow-up. *Pediatr Pulmonol* **3**, 145–8.
61. Zauner CW, Benson NY (1981). Physiological alterations in young swimmers during three years of intensive training. *J Sports Med Phys Fitness* **21**, 179–85.
62. Vaccaro P, Clarke DH (1978). Cardiorespiratory alterations in 9 to 11 years old children following a season of competitive swimming. *Med Sci Sports Exerc* **10**, 204–7.
63. Gibbons JA, Cunningham DA, Shaw DB, Eynon RB (1972). The effect of swimming training on selected aspects of pulmonary function in young girls: A preliminary report. In: Taylor AW (ed.), *Training: scientific basis and application; a symposium conducted by the Canadian Association of Sports Sciences*, pp. 139–43. Thomas, Springfield, IL.
64. Courteix D, Obert P, Lecoq AM, Guenon P, Koch G (1997). Effect of intensive swimming training on lung volumes, airway resistance and on the maximal expiratory flow-volume relationship in prepubertal girls. *Eur J Appl Physiol* **76**, 264–9.
65. Yost LJ, Zauner CW, Jaeger MJ (1981). Pulmonary diffusing capacity and physical working capacity in swimmers and non-swimmers during growth. *Respiration* **42**, 8–14.
66. Doherty M, Dimitriou L (1997). Comparison of lung volume in Greek swimmers, land based athletes, and sedentary controls using allometric scaling. *Br J Sports Med* **31**, 337–41.
67. Baxter-Jones ADG, Helms PJ (1996). Effects of training at a young age: a review of The Training of Young Athletes (TOYA) Study. *Pediatr Exerc Sci* **8**, 310–27.
68. Hamilton P, Andrew GM (1976). Influence of growth and athletic training on heart and lung functions. *Eur J Appl Physiol Occup Physiol* **36**, 27–38.
69. Vaccaro P, Poffenbarger A (1982). Resting and exercise respiratory function in young female child runners. *J Sports Med Phys Fitness* **22**, 102–7.
70. Koch G, Eriksson BO (1973). Effect of physical training on anatomical R-L shunt at rest and pulmonary diffusing capacity during near-maximal exercise in boys 11–13 years old. *Scand J Clin Lab Invest* **31**, 95–103.
71. Koch G (1980). Aerobic power, lung dimensions, ventilatory capacity, and muscle blood flow in 12–16-year-old boys with high physical activity. In: Berg K, Eriksson BO (eds.), *Children and exercise IX*, pp. 99–108. University Park Press, Baltimore, MD.
72. Andersen KL, Rutenfranz J, Seliger V, Ilmarinen J, Berndt I, Kylian H, Ruppel M (1984). The growth of lung volumes affected by physical performance capacity in boys and girls during childhood and adolescence. *Eur J Appl Physiol* **52**, 380–4.
73. Lakhera SC, Kain TC, Bandopadhyay P (1994). Changes in lung function during adolescence in athletes and non-athletes. *J Sports Med Phys Fitness* **34**, 258–62.
74. Nourry C, Deruelle F, Guinhouya C, Baquet G, Fabre C, Bart F, Berthoin S, Mucci P (2005). High-intensity intermittent running training improves pulmonary function and alters exercise breathing pattern in children. *Eur J Appl Physiol* **94**, 415–23.
75. Ekblom B (1969). Effect of physical training in adolescent boys. *J Appl Physiol* **27**, 350–5.
76. Rowland TW, Boyajian A (1995). Aerobic response to endurance exercise training in children. *Pediatrics* **96**, 654–8.
77. Ramonatxo M, Mercier J, Prefaut C (1989). Relationship between aerobic physical fitness and ventilatory control during exercise in young swimmers. *Respir Physiol* **78**, 345–56.
78. Gratas A, Dassonville J, Beillot J, Rochcongar P (1988). Ventilatory and occlusion-pressure responses to exercise in trained and untrained children. *Eur J Appl Physiol Occup Physiol* **57**, 591–6.

CHAPTER 19

Cardiovascular function

Thomas W. Rowland

Introduction

A consideration of the circulatory responses to exercise in children can begin with the obvious: sustained motor activity is critically dependent on effective adaptations of the cardiovascular system. Without an adequate rise in blood circulation, exercising muscle would be deprived of the requisite oxygen supply for aerobic energy metabolism. Core temperature would rise rapidly to dangerous levels, tissue pH would plummet as lactic acid remained unbuffered, and increasing carbon dioxide levels would rapidly lead to somnolence and central nervous depression. Circulating fatty acids and glucose, counted on by the muscle fibres to replenish local substrate supplies, would fail to arrive, nor would important hormonal responses to exercise (catecholamines, cortisol, glucagon). In short, without an adequate circulatory response, exercise for more than a very brief period would be impossible. It is not surprising, then, that endurance exercise capacity is couched in terms of 'cardiovascular fitness'.

This conclusion is clearly as true for children as for adults. The difference between the two lies in the fact that as young people grow these cardiovascular responses are in a continuous state of evolution. Over time, children's circulatory adaptations to exercise follow inherent and predictable patterns of growth and development, reflecting increases in size and, at least potentially, in system function as well. Between the ages of 8 and 18 years, the volume of the heart more than doubled[1]; hence, increases in size-dependent factors such as stroke volume (SV) can be expected to contribute significantly to the development of circulatory responses to exercise as children grow. Responses of variables supposedly independent of body size (e.g. heart rate, blood pressure) also become modified during the course of childhood. Others, such as myocardial contractility, do not seem to be altered by biological maturation.

This chapter will serve to (i) describe the characteristics of the cardiovascular responses to exercise in youth and (ii) delineate the evolution of these adaptations as the child matures towards the adult state. Considerable pragmatic interest in this information has developed surrounding a number of issues. Only with an understanding of normal cardiovascular adaptations to exercise in this age group can insights be made into the safety and proper training of elite child athletes. Heart function in youth with cardiovascular disease needs to be accurately assessed relative to population norms. Similarly, such information is necessary in evaluating the effectiveness and feasibility of cardiac rehabilitation programmes. It will be apparent, too, that cardiovascular changes with exercise in children presented in the chapter may provide useful information to those investigators seeking an understanding of the basic anatomic and physiologic determinants of these responses.

While the critical nature of blood perfusion during exercise is well recognized, many questions remain incompletely answered. What are the mechanisms by which circulation of blood is increased during exercise? By what means is circulatory flow tightly linked to tissue metabolic demands? What limits increases in circulatory flow during exhaustive exercise? By what mechanism does repeated exercise (i.e. fitness training) improve cardiovascular capacity? And—germane to the present discussion—are the answers to any or all of these questions different in children than adults?

This chapter will consider these issues, summarizing available information in the paediatric population from the perspectives of three different exercise models: progressive treadmill or cycle ergometer exercise to exhaustion, sustained constant-load submaximal exercise (cardiovascular drift), and isometric or resistance exercise. For the most part, the information presented will pertain to youth who are in good health, ignoring important issues surrounding trained athletes as well as those with chronic disease. For these topics the reader is referred to other sources.[2,3] By the nature of exercise testing, cardiovascular features have been reported only from about age 8 years onwards. This discussion will include data into the teen years. Where possible, gender differences will be considered, although direct boy–girl comparisons have been infrequent.

Progressive exhaustive exercise

Cardiovascular responses to exercise have most commonly been assessed during cycle or treadmill testing with progressively increasing work loads (watts, slope, speed) to the point of subject exhaustion. Performance on such tests generally lasts 10–15 min and the findings are considered indicative of aerobic, or endurance, fitness.

The strength of this approach is that patterns of change in cardiovascular variables can be assessed relative to increasing levels of work intensity. Importantly, too, this model demonstrates 'peak' values at the point of subject exhaustion (although whether these can be considered truly 'maximal' can be conjectural). At the same time, it should be noted that the progressive nature of this model is anomalous in that it does not imitate any form of usual physical exercise nor sports activity.

Heart rate

As children age, their resting heart rate (HR) progressively falls. (HR here is that measured in basal conditions, rather than values determined immediately before exercise testing, which are obviously influenced by anxiety and pre-exercise anticipation.) Cross-sectional studies indicate that from age 4 years, when mean basal value is approximately 85 beats·min^{-1}, HR falls to 60 beats·min^{-1} at age 18 years.[4] Mean rates are typically 2–3 beats·min^{-1} faster in girls at all ages.

The decline in resting HR with age appears to reflect a true maturational decrease in the intrinsic firing rate of the sinus node rather than alteration of autonomic influence. Marcus *et al.*[5] found that under autonomic blockade resting HR in children (with a history of sinus node dysfunction) rose from an average of 89 beats·min^{-1} to 128 beats·min^{-1}, a magnitude of change similar to that observed in similar studies of adults, whose intrinsic rate was only approximately 100 beats·min^{-1}. The explanation for age-related decline in resting sinus node firing rate is unknown. Alterations in nodal membrane ion flux or changes in position of pacemaker cells within the node have been suggested.

The progressive fall in resting HR with age is linked to parallel declines in size-relative basal metabolic rate (BMR). As expected, absolute basal caloric expenditure increases as children grow in size. However, when adjusted for body size by expressing values relative to body surface area (BSA), BMR declines by approximately 23% between ages 6 and 16 years. This trend occurs concomitant with a fall in resting HR of similar magnitude (~20%) over the same age span.

During a progressive exercise test, the rise in HR is relatively linear until high intensities are reached (~75% peak $\dot{V}O_2$), when values retard to a slow taper. As in adults, this flattening of the HR–work load curve is observed in most, if not all, children. Rowland and Cunningham[6] described a tapering of HR above 60% peak $\dot{V}O_2$ in all 11- to 13-year-old children during treadmill walking. In 38% of the subjects, a plateau (defined as less than a three-beat increase in the final stage) was observed.

The explanation for this tapering of HR at high work loads remains obscure. Several investigators have described a coincidence of the point of HR deflection (HRD) in children with ventilatory anaerobic or lactate threshold.[7–9] However, no clear explanations for an effect of anaerobic metabolism on changes in HR have been forthcoming. Other suggested aetiologies for the HRD have included changes in venous return or baroreceptor sensitivity.

Peak HR during a progressive exercise in children depends on modality of testing (cycle, treadmill) and type of exercise (running, walking). During a treadmill running test, peak HR is expected to be, on the average, approximately 200 beats·min^{-1}, but 5 beats·min^{-1} slower with walking.[10–13] Cycle tests provoke lower peak HRs than treadmill running, with peak values of 190–195 beats·min^{-1}[14]. There appears to be no differences in peak HR in youth related to gender or level of aerobic fitness.

Considerable interindividual variability is observed in peak HRs in children, an important consideration when using the above values to predict peak rates or to define an exhaustive effort. In their evaluation of several treadmill and cycle testing protocols, Cumming and Langford[11] described standard deviations for all protocols ranging from 5 to 7 beats·min^{-1}. In the report by Sheehan *et al.*,[13] the standard deviations for peak HR were 12 beats·min^{-1} for treadmill walking and 9 beats·min^{-1} for running. This variability does not appear to simply reflect differences in subject motivation, as similar standard deviations have been described in testing of elite prepubertal athletes.[15]

It is important, as well, to recognize that cross-sectional and longitudinal studies indicate that peak HR on a progressive test remains stable throughout the paediatric years, at least until the late teen years.[10,14,16] This means that formulae utilized to predict maximal HR in adults subjects, such as 220-age, are not applicable to children.

As resting HR declines during childhood while peak HR is stable, the difference between the two, or the HR reserve, enlarges with age. Bar-Or[17] suggested that this trend, which parallels that of mass-relative $\dot{V}O_2$, might have bearing on performance differences between children and adults. However, possible implications of maturational differences in HR or metabolic reserve have not been elucidated.

Stroke volume

As noted above, considerations of SV require adjustment for body size, as blood expelled per beat is closely related to ventricular size, and, by extension, to somatic growth. Limited data suggest that expressing values of both SV and cardiac output ($\dot{Q}$) relative to BSA (the traditional stroke index and cardiac index) are an appropriate means of 'normalizing' values for interindividual or group comparisons or when assessing subjects longitudinally. Armstrong and Welsman[18] reported that changes in $\dot{Q}$ and SV increased in direct proportion to BSA in both boys and girls performing a submaximal treadmill run. However, Turley and Wilmore[19] found that stroke index and cardiac index did not completely eliminate the effects of values on body dimensions during submaximal exercise in 7- to 9-year-old children. For example, they reported a correlation coefficient of $r = 0.29$ between stroke index and BSA at a 60-W cycling workload. Rowland and co-workers[20] described an allometric exponent of 1.05 in premenarcheal girls and 1.03 in prepubertal boys for BSA relative to peak SV. On the basis of this information, most investigators have elected to express exercise SV as well as $\dot{Q}$ values relative to BSA (Table 19.1).

During upright exercise, SV rises initially by approximately 30–40% above pre-exercise values, but beyond light intensities (>50% peak $\dot{V}O_2$), SV plateaus and remains essentially stable to the point of subject exhaustion (Fig. 19.1). Supporting its validity, this pattern has been consistently demonstrated in children by Doppler echocardiography,[20–24] thoracic bioimpedance,[25–26] carbon dioxide rebreathing,[27] dye dilution,[28] and acetylene breathing methods,[29] and is no different from that observed in adult subjects.[23,24]

The initial rise in SV during progressive exercise appears to reflect mobilization of blood pooled in the legs upon assuming the sitting position. When an adult sits upright, central blood volume falls as 500–1000 mL of blood is drawn by gravity to the lower extremities, resulting in a decline in SV and $\dot{Q}$ by 20–40%. At the beginning of upright exercise, this dependent blood is mobilized by the contracting muscle, and central volume, SV, and $\dot{Q}$ increase.[30]

Supporting this concept, most studies have indicated that an early rise in SV is not observed when subjects (both adults and children) perform progressive supine exercise.[31,32] For example, Rowland *et al.*[31] compared SV changes during supine and upright

Table 19.1 Studies assessing peak cardiac output and stroke volume (SV) (mean values) in untrained healthy youth during upright cycle exercise

Citation	N	Age	Sex	Method	$\dot{Q}$ index (L·min^{-1}·m^{-2})	SV index (mL·m^{-2})
Nottin *et al.*[23]	17	10–13	M	Dopp	11.3	59
Nottin *et al.*[56]	13	10–12	M	Dopp	10.6	56
Nottin *et al.*[101]	14	9–11	M, F	Dopp	11.4	59
Obert *et al.*[72]	17	10–11	F	Dopp	9.4	46
	18	10–11	M	Dopp	10.1	51
Vinet *et al.*[35]	14	10–11	M, F	Dopp	12.9	66
Rowland and Blum[21]	10	10–12	M	Dopp	11.6	62
Rowland *et al.*[24]	15	9–12	M	Dopp	11.3	59
Rowland *et al.*[34]	24	11–13	F	Dopp	10.5	53
Rowland *et al.*[69]	39	11–13	M	Dopp	12.0	61
Rowland *et al.*[45]	14	7–12	M	Dopp	11.4	58
Welsman *et al.*[102]	11	10–11	F	imped	9.6	49
	9		M		9.5	49
Pianosi[26]	60	7–19	M	imped	9.8	51
	55		F		10.0	52
Rowland and Popowski[25]	15	9–12	M	imped	9.2	46
Eriksson and Koch[28]	9	11–13	M	dye	9.1	49
Miyamura and Honda[103]	16	9–10	M	CO_2	11.8	62
	16		F		10.0	54
	21	11–12	M		12.2	64
	17		F		11.5	61
Yamaji and Miyashita[104]	8	10–12	M	CO_2	10.4	
Gilliam *et al.*[105]	22	6–8	M, F	CO_2	11.8	61
	36	9–10	M, F		10.5	54
	24	11–13	M, F		10.0	52
Nottin *et al.*[101]	14	9–11	M, F	CO_2		
Cyran *et al.*[29]	17	8–15	M, F	acetyl	10.8	62

acetyl = acetylene rebreathing; CO_2 = carbon dioxide rebreathing; Dopp = Doppler echocardiography; dye = dye dilution; imped = thoracic bioimpedance.

cycle exercise in 13 boys aged 10–15 years. At rest, values for stroke index were 71 ± 15 and 51 ± 12 mL·m^{-2} in the supine and upright positions, respectively ($p < 0.05$). With progressive work loads, no significant change was observed in supine stroke index, while values rose initially by 29% during upright pedalling before plateauing. Above a work load of 50 W, there was no significant difference in stroke index between the sitting and supine exercise trials.

By this explanation, then, the early rise in SV at initiation of upright exercise can be interpreted as positional 're-filling' phenomenon and not part of the basic process by which circulation increases in response to the metabolic demands of exercise. Furthermore, it can be concluded that changes in SV do not contribute substantially to increases in $\dot{Q}$ during a progressive exercise test.

As indicted in Table 19.1, peak stroke index in youth during upright cycling has generally been reported to be 50–60 mL·m^{-2}. Values are higher in boys than girls. As will be discussed below, this sex difference can be explained principally by variations in body composition.[20,33]

No developmental data regarding stroke index during the paediatric years are available. However, no differences in peak values have been observed in studies directly comparing prepubertal children and young (20–30 years) adult males and females.[23,24,34,35] These limited data would suggest that values of stroke index in a given healthy, non-trained individual remain stable from age 10 years to at least the early adult years.

Cardiac output

In children, as well as adults, the rise in $\dot{Q}$ with progressive exercise is closely linked to the metabolic demands ($\dot{V}O_2$) of contracting muscle. In adults, the slope of the relationship between $\dot{Q}$ and $\dot{V}O_2$, or the exercise factor, is typically about 6.0 (a rise in $\dot{Q}$ of 6 L·min^{-1}

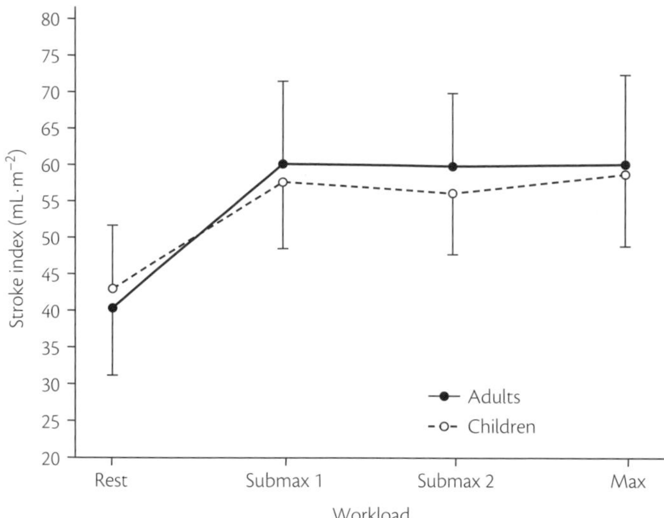

Fig. 19.1 Stroke index at rest, submaximal exercise, and exhaustion during progressive cycle exercise in young men and boys. From Rowland *et al.*,[24] reprinted with permission.

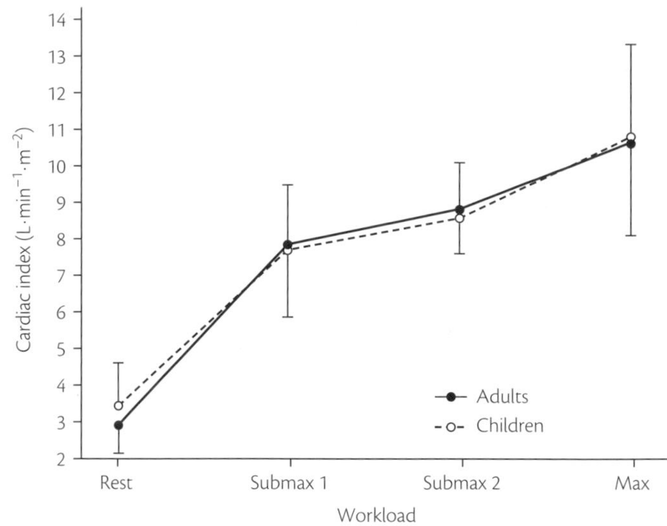

Fig. 19.2 Cardiac index at rest, comparable submaximal intensities, and maximal exercise during cycling in young men and boys. From Rowland *et al.*,[24] reprinted with permission.

is observed for each 1 L·min^{-1} increase in $\dot{V}O_2$).[36] Reduced values are seen in patients with depressed myocardial function.

Similar findings are observed in children. In five studies involving a variety of measurement techniques, the exercise factor in healthy subjects ranged from 5.7 to 7.1.[27,33,37–40] In a direct comparison of children and adults, Vinet *et al.*[35] described an exercise factor of 6.63 and 6.58, respectively. Similarly, Nottin *et al.*[23] could find no significant difference in slope of the submaximal $\dot{Q}$ – $\dot{V}O_2$ regression lines in 11- to 12-year-old boys and young men (4.54 and 4.58, respectively).

The relationship between $\dot{Q}$ and $\dot{V}O_2$ during a progressive test is not entirely linear. Several authors have demonstrated instead a curvilinear relationship in adults with declining values of $\dot{Q}/\dot{V}O_2$ at higher work levels.[41–43] Rowland[44] reported similar findings in 39 boys, with a $\dot{Q}$–$\dot{V}O_2$ relationship best described by the cubic equation $\dot{Q} = 3.6\,(\dot{V}O_2)^3 + 5.2\,(\dot{V}O_2)^2 + 2.4\,(\dot{V}O_2) - 0.94$. The $\%\Delta\,\dot{Q}/\%\Delta\,\dot{V}O_2$ fell from 0.70 between the first two workloads to 0.50 at peak exercise. The explanation for this trend is uncertain. The decline in the exercise factor at higher workloads has been viewed by some as an indicator of decreasing circulatory efficacy, perhaps reduced skeletal muscle pump performance.

When one plots absolute cardiac output against oxygen uptake in a progressive exercise test, values of $\dot{Q}/\dot{V}O_2$ for children cluster at the lower end of the normal range for adults.[17,24] While this has been viewed as evidence of a 'hypokinetic' cardiac response in youth,[17] there exists no evidence that circulatory variables, once related appropriately to body size, are any different either quantitatively or qualitatively during exercise in children than adults. As reviewed in this chapter, compared to young adults, children have similar values of peak cardiac index and stroke index, markers of ventricular systolic and diastolic function, exercise factor, cardiovascular drift, patterns of SV, and alterations in chamber size. The low absolute $\dot{Q}/\dot{V}O_2$ in children appears to be a reflection of the smaller SVs in young subjects; as such, this finding can be interpreted as biologically irrelevant, since children and adults do not typically exercise at the same absolute oxygen uptake.

Average reported peak cardiac index in children using various techniques are outlined in Table 19.1. Values in boys are typically 10–12 L·min^{-1}·m^{-2}. Limited studies suggest that values using thoracic bioimpedance are consistently 1–2 L·min^{-1}·m^{-2} lower. Peak cardiac index is approximately 10% greater in boys than girls, consistent with gender differences in $\dot{V}O_2$ max. Direct comparisons of maximal cardiac index between children and young adults have indicated no maturational differences (Fig. 19.2).[23,24,34,35]

The lower average values of SV, $\dot{Q}$, and $\dot{V}O_2$ max in girls compared to boys have been generally recognized to be related to sex difference in body composition. Vinet *et al.*[33] examined the relative contributions of body composition, blood haemoglobin concentration, and cardiac dimensions and function to sex differences in $\dot{V}O_2$ max in thirty-five 10- to 12-year-old children. Mean $\dot{V}O_2$ max values were 47.9 mL·kg^{-1}·min^{-1} in the boys and 40.9 mL·kg^{-1}·min^{-1} in the girls, but the sex difference disappeared when values were allometrically related to lean body mass (19.0 and 18.9 mL·kg·LBM$^{-1.33}$·min^{-1}, respectively). No differences were observed between boys and girls in maximal HR or arteriovenous oxygen difference. Maximal SV was greater in the boys, but the sex difference became insignificant when values were expressed related to lean body mass.

Rowland *et al.*[34] reported average maximal stroke index values of 62 ± 9 and 55 ± 9 mL·m^{-2} in boys and girls, respectively. When related to lean body mass the sex effect was lessened, but a 5% difference remained. Armstrong and Welsman[18] used multilevel regression modelling to examine sex difference to submaximal treadmill exercise in children tested annually from age 11 to 13 years. With body size and composition considered, SV was greater in the boys, but the difference was statistically significant only in the second test.

Ventricular function

Both myocardial contractility (systolic function) and ventricular relaxation properties (diastolic function) improve during an acute bout of progressive cycle exercise. Exactly what triggers these adaptations, as well as their role in the cardiovascular responses to exercise, has not been fully resolved. Understanding myocardial functional changes during dynamic exercise remains an intriguing challenge to the cardiac exercise physiologist.

Systolic function

During ventricular systole, myocardial contractility improves with increasing work load. 'Contractility' in this response can be identified as a greater rate of contraction (as manifest by greater acceleration of muscle shortening) and higher peak force of contraction (measured as increase in peak velocity of blood flow), both occurring in a progressively shortening ejection time. The resulting decrease in ventricular end-systolic volume reflects primarily circumferential fibre shortening, although contraction of the longitudinal axis also contributes. These vectors of augmented contractility can be measured, respectively, by (i) increases in left ventricular shortening fraction [(diastolic dimension – systolic dimension)/diastolic dimension × 100] or ejection fraction, and (ii) changes in longitudinal myocardial wall velocity [tissue Doppler imaging (TDI)].

All of these markers of increased systolic function have been illustrated in children during progressive cycle exercise. The magnitude of these changes appears to mimic that observed in adult subjects. Rowland *et al.*[45] described a decrease in acceleration time (from onset to peak aortic flow velocity) from 73 ± 9 ms at rest to 51 ± 10 ms at peak exercise in 7- to 12-year-old boys using Doppler echocardiography. In another study, mean acceleration from onset to peak of aortic flow velocity rose from 1490 ± 411 cm·s^{-2} at rest to 4007 ± 851 cm·s^{-2} at peak exercise in 12-year-old boys.[46] The rise in peak aortic velocity in that study from 109 ± 19 to 211 ± 13 cm·s^{-1} is typical of other reports. In a direct comparison study, 10-year-old boys and 30-year-old men had average peak aortic velocity values at exhaustive cycle exercise of 142 and 150 cm·s^{-1}, respectively (Fig. 19.3).[24]

Ventricular ejection time shortens by approximately 30% as HR increases to peak exercise in children.[22,45] This decline in ejection time is similar to that observed in adults (Fig. 19.4).[24]

Echocardiographic studies have consistently documented a rise in left ventricular shortening fraction during the course of a progressive test in children.[21–23,47] Nottin *et al.*[23] reported no group differences when shortening fraction responses to progressive cycle exercise were directly compared in boys and men. Among these studies, increases in shortening fraction have generally been from approximately 35% at rest to 50% at peak exercise.

Information regarding variations in ejection fraction, measured by radionuclide angiography, is limited due to ethical considerations in healthy children. In maximal testing of a group of 8- to 18-year-old subjects with hyperlipidaemia (but no clinical heart disease), DeSouza *et al.*[48] reported a rise in ejection fraction from 63% to 81%, mimicking the magnitude of responses observed in adults using the same technique.

Rowland *et al.*[45] reported that S wave velocity with Doppler tissue imaging, a marker of rate of longitudinal myocardial fibre shortening, rose from 3.8 ± 1.2 to 10.0 ± 2.5 cm·s^{-1} at peak exercise in 7- to 12-year-old boys. Increase in S velocity paralleled that of other markers of systolic function, and peak values were significantly associated with peak aortic velocity. This response is comparable to that described by DeSouza *et al.*[49] in 8- to 12-year-old subjects during semisupine exercise.

Determinants of myocardial systolic function are multiple, and each contributes to improved contractility during progressive exercise. A rise in HR by itself improves myocardial contractility (Bowditch effect), as does reduced systolic vascular resistance, sympathetic neural stimulation, and circulating catecholamines. In addition, improved function from myocardial fibre stretching (Frank–Starling mechanism) contributes to increases in contractility during the initial phases of upright exercise. The indicators of systolic function outlined above (i.e. shortening fraction, ejection fraction) are affected by different combinations of these determinants of contractility, and studying each in isolation becomes problematic. Consequently, a clear picture of the relative importance of individual determinants on increases in systolic function during exercise remains elusive.

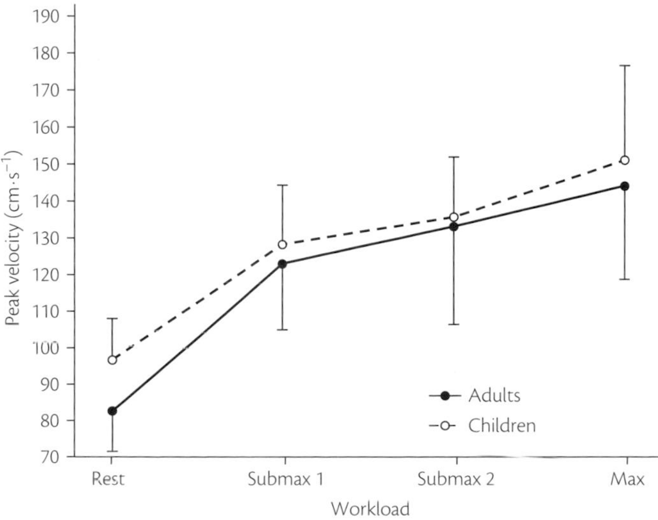

Fig. 19.3 Peak aortic velocity in young men and boys during progressive cycle exercise. From Rowland *et al.*,[24] reprinted with permission.

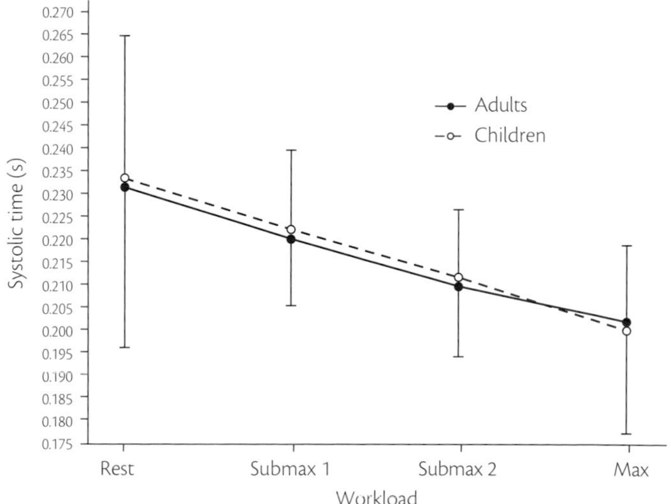

Fig. 19.4 Systolic ejection time as determined by Doppler echocardiography in boys and young men during progressive cycle exercise. From Rowland *et al.*,[24] reprinted with permission.

What is the role of this increase in systolic function during progressive exercise? Although improvements in contractility have been assumed to augment SV, empiric findings indicate that beyond the initial phase of upright exercise, SV is stable. As will be reviewed in the Synthesis section, increase in contractility appears to act instead to maintain SV as ventricular ejection time shortens with increasing HR.

Not surprisingly, measures of myocardial metabolism and energetics in normal children during exercise have not been performed. Onouchi *et al.*[50] made direct determinations of resting myocardial oxygen consumption ($M\dot{V}O_2$) and myocardial efficiency (heart work/$M\dot{V}O_2$) during cardiac catheterization in 58 children aged 1–19 years with a history of Kawasaki disease (but with normal coronary findings). As would be expected, absolute values of $M\dot{V}O_2$ progressively rose with increasing age. However, when expressed relative to BSA, $M\dot{V}O_2$ and cardiac efficiency remained essentially unchanged, indicating no maturational effects on resting myocardial energetics.

Diastolic filling

Filling of the left ventricle during diastole depends on the gradient established between the pressure head 'upstream' (left atrial volume and contractile force) and that 'downstream' (from end-systolic ventricular pressure and rate of myocardial relaxation). By measuring peak velocity of merged mitral E and A waves by echocardiography, it has been estimated that the left atrial–ventricular gradient increases four-fold in children from rest to peak exercise.[51] Findings with the TDI technique have shed some light on the determinants of this pressure gradient. The E′ wave velocity with TDI, an indicator of rate of myocardial relaxation, doubled during progressive exercise.[45] At the same time, the ratio of E′ to E, considered a load-independent marker of left ventricular end-diastolic (i.e. left atrial) pressure, does not change. This information, which has been evident in both paediatric and adult studies,[51,52] suggests that the transmitral gradient responsible for rate of ventricular filling is a manifestation of decrease in 'downstream' pressure. This left ventricular suction effect is, in turn, a reflection of both degree of systolic contractility (i.e. end-systolic pressure) and ventricular relaxation properties.[53]

The increases in diastolic function with exercise, which parallel those of systolic contractility, serve to facilitate transmitral flow of a stable volume as diastolic filling period progressively shortens. Rowland *et al.*[22] described these intervals using Doppler echocardiography in a group of 7- to 17-year-old children performing semisupine cycling exercise. At rest, the diastolic filling time greatly exceeded the systolic ejection period (0.487 and 0.260 s, respectively). As exercise intensity rose, both values progressively fell, and at peak exercise estimated diastolic filling time (0.149 s) was less than that of systolic ejection (0.181 s).

Systemic blood pressure and vascular resistance

Progressive dynamic exercise is characterized by a rise in systolic blood pressure with slight fall in diastolic pressure. Value of mean arterial pressure (MAP), calculated as 1/3 (systolic − diastolic) + diastolic, generally rises from rest to peak exercise by 20–30 mmHg. Resting blood pressure rises throughout the lifespan. Hence, since systolic pressure at peak exercise is related to that at rest, maximal systolic blood pressure increases as children grow.

Normal values for blood pressure measurements during exercise in children and adolescents have been published elsewhere.[54] These indicate that, besides age, greater systolic pressure is observed at maximal exercise in respect to larger body size, race (Blacks > Caucasians), athleticism (trained > untrained), and gender (males > females). Values of diastolic pressure, being more difficult to measure, are more variable in the published literature.

Systemic vascular resistance (R) during exercise has been estimated indirectly via Poiseuille's equation $R = \text{MAP}/\dot{Q}$. Studies in both children and adults have consistently demonstrated a progressive decline as work load increases, generally by approximately 60% from rest to maximal work.[22,23,45] These values reflect the combined effect of variations in vascular tone in multiple vascular beds (mesenteric, muscular, cutaneous), but the principal influence on the decline in resistance during exercise has been considered arteriolar vasodilatation within contracting muscle in response to local vasoactive agents and neural influences.[55]

The absolute values as well as magnitude of decline in calculated systemic vascular resistance during progressive exercise in children have been similar to those in adults. In a direct comparison of cardiovascular responses to maximal cycle exercise in 17 boys (mean age 11.7 year) and 23 men (mean age 21.2 year), Nottin *et al.*[23] found a fall in average systemic vascular resistance from 15 units at rest to 7 units at exhaustion in the boys and from 15 units to 6 units in the men.

Chamber dimensions

Since the volume of blood passing through the heart each minute from rest to exhaustion increases five-fold, progressive exercise has been considered to impose a ventricular volume overload. In fact, however, the end-diastolic size of the left ventricle does not enlarge as work load increases. Five studies have examined ventricular dimensions by two-dimensional echocardiography with progressive upright cycle exercise in children, and all have demonstrated the same pattern (Fig. 19.5).[21,31,47,56] With initiation of pedalling, a slight (~2 mm) rise is often observed, consistent with mobilization of dependent blood and re-filling of the ventricles in the sitting position described above. After this, a very slight but persistent decline is observed to the point of exhaustion. Reported values for resting and peak end-diastolic dimensions have generally not been significantly different. These data consistently indicate that as minute volume output of the heart rises with increasing workload, ventricular preload (end-diastolic volume) is essentially stable.

End-systolic dimension, on the other hand, progressively declines with increasing exercise intensity. For example, Rowland and Blum[21] reported a fall in systolic dimension from 28.3 ± 3.4 at rest to 20.0 ± 2.1 mm at peak exercise, while values for end-diastolic dimension were 39.9 ± 3.2 and 37.5 ± 1.9 mm, respectively. This explains the described increase in left ventricular shortening fraction.

The patterns of left ventricular diastolic and systolic dimension changes with upright progressive exercise in children are no different from those described in adults.[57] In a study directly comparing dimensional changes in 10- to 12-year-old boys and 19- to 24-year-old men, Nottin *et al.*[23] reported rest-maximal exercise declines of end-diastolic dimension from 44.4 ± 3.8 to 41.0 ± 5.1 mm and from 51.9 ± 3.6 to 49.7 ± 3.8 mm in the two groups, respectively. Average shortening fraction rose from 37% at rest to 50% at peak exercise in the boys and from 36% to 49% in the men.

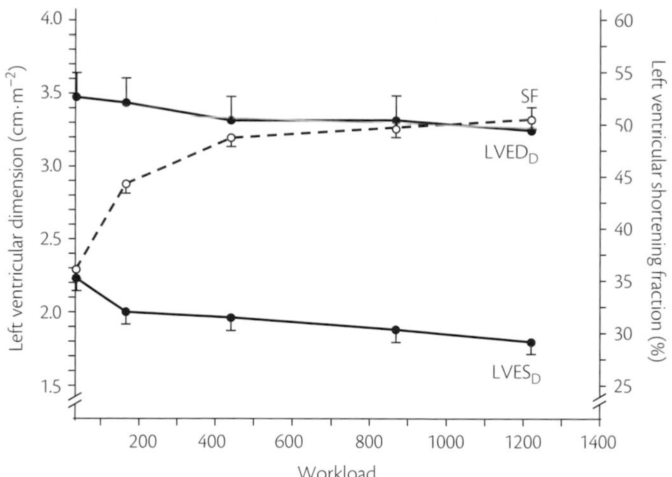

Fig. 19.5 Changes in left ventricular end-diastolic dimension (LVED), left ventricular end-systolic dimension (LVES), and shortening fraction (SF) during progressive cycling in 11 children (age 12.1 ± 3.3 years). Dimensions are indexed to body surface area. From Rowland *et al.*,[106] reprinted with permission.

Dynamic exercise synthesis

Any proposed mechanistic construct for the facilitation and control of circulatory responses to progressive exercise should conform to the empirically derived data outlined above. In summary, during the course of an acute bout of progressive exercise to subject exhaustion, (i) SV remains stable (other than a small initial postural-related rise); (ii) left ventricular end-diastolic volume (preload) does not change; (iii) ventricular contractility improves; and (iv) a substantial decline is observed in systemic vascular resistance.

These findings are predicted by a schema by which peripheral factors, most particularly the fall in vascular resistance with arteriolar dilatation, serve to regulate circulatory flow during exercise in response to metabolic demands. Guyton,[58] Rushmer and Smith,[59] and other researchers reached the same conclusion based on studies of both dogs and humans in the 1950s: 'the primary cause of augmented cardiac output is believed to be local vasodilatation in the skeletal muscle' and 'the heart has little effect on the normal regulation of cardiac output'.[58]

Exercise blood flow is defined by Poiseuille's law, exercise blood flow Pressure/Resistance, whereby the fall in resistance reflects skeletal muscle arteriolar dilatation triggered by local humoral factors. These vasoactive agents, in turn, are an expression of tissue metabolic demands. From a cardiac perspective, then, the pumping demands of the heart exercise are governed specifically by the augmented volume returning to the right atrium.

The empiric findings outlined above are consistent with this construct. First, if systemic venous return to the heart during the course of a progressive exercise test increases by a factor of 5, and ventricular preload is stable, the rise in HR must by necessity match the increasing volume of blood entering into the heart to maintain a constant diastolic ventricular size. This, in fact, defines the Bainbridge reflex, which proposed nearly a century ago that 'when venous filling is increased, the circulation can be maintained by the more rapid transference of blood from the venous to the arterial system and the risk of excessive dilatation is lessened'.[60] The reflex rise in HR, then, 'defends' left ventricular filling size. If it failed to do so, an increased left ventricular diameter would result in greater wall tension and decline in myocardial mechanical efficiency (in accordance with the law of LaPlace).[61]

As exercise intensity rises, increasing myocardial contractility (with decreasing systolic dimension) is evident without change in SV. This apparent paradox can be explained by the necessity for increased contractile force to eject the same volume of blood with each beat in an increasingly shorter ejection time. For example, citing values in a study of 10- to 13-year-old boys,[22] at light exercise average SV was 71 mL with HR 132 beats·min^{-1} and ejection time of 0.220 s. At peak exercise, stroke index had changed little (73 mL·m^{-2}) with mean HR of 193 beats·min^{-1} and ejection time shortened to 0.197 s. To eject the similar SV at the two work loads in the shorter ejection time required an increased flow rate from 323 mL·s^{-1} to 372 mL·s^{-1}, which must be met with increased contractile force and velocity. Indeed this magnitude of requisite increase in flow rate (15%) is consistent with that of typical rises observed in peak aortic blood velocity and left ventricular shortening fraction in this exercise model.[21–23] Thus, improved myocardial contractility with rising work intensity serves to maintain rather than increase SV. As would be predicted, then, patients with depressed ventricular function in whom myocardial contractile responses to exercise are impaired demonstrate a fall in SV with exercise.[22]

The empiric data are consistent with a central pump (the heart) functioning in a responsive manner to peripheral factors (principally arteriolar dilatation) that determine the volume of systemic venous return during exercise. This model supposes that the circulatory responses to exercise are similar to those of an arteriovenous fistula, an anatomic clinical condition in which the high resistance arterioles are by-passed, and $\dot{Q}$ increases in response to low systemic vascular resistance.[62] This concept was supported by Binak *et al.*,[63] who described similar circulatory responses to exercise and the effect of opening of a peripheral arteriovenous fistula in the same adult patients.

Other peripheral factors besides arteriolar dilatation may be involved, particularly the functioning of the contracting skeletal muscle as a circulatory pump.[64] Indeed, the functional characteristics of the skeletal muscle pump mimic those of the heart, with preload (arteriolar supply), contractile force of muscle compressing a blood volume, afterload (venous tone and right atrial pressure), one-way valves, and a nerve supply governing contractile rate (pedalling cadence) and strength of contraction. Blood flow can be effected by the skeletal muscle pump either via direct compression of venous vessels or by providing a suction effect to augment muscle blood inflow. Indeed, Rowell *et al.*[65] considered that 'the muscle pump can be viewed as a second heart on the venous portion of the circuit, having the capacity to generate blood flow rivaling that of the left ventricle'.

The characteristics of the skeletal muscle as a circulatory pump and its role in controlling or limiting blood flow during exercise have not, however, been well-clarified.[64] Particularly, it is not clear whether rapid contractile rates and/or increased muscle force might not occlude blood flow at high exercise intensities and negate pumping function. Some evidence suggests that the rise in circulatory response to metabolic demands near maximal exercise in both children and adults is blunted, supporting that possibility. Rowland and Lisowski[66] reported that $\dot{Q}$ fell by only 16% in the first 15 s after maximal exercise in 12-year-old boys, suggesting that the skeletal muscle pump does not play a major role in facilitating blood flow at high exercise intensities. Studies in adults have demonstrated similar findings.[67,68]

Explaining differences in aerobic fitness

Since $\dot{V}O_2$ max closely reflects maximal cardiac output ($\dot{Q}$ max), the factors responsible for individual differences in maximal aerobic power can be sought among the determinants of cardiac functional capacity. This issue has been examined in the paediatric population with studies of physiologic correlates of $\dot{Q}$ max among non-trained youth, cross-sectional comparisons of child endurance athletes and non-athletes, and in cardiovascular response to a period of endurance training. These reports have consistently reached the same conclusion: individual differences in $\dot{Q}$ max are accounted for entirely by maximal SV (as peak HR is not influenced by aerobic fitness). Maximal SV, in turn, reflects resting SV. Factors explaining variations in resting SV, most particularly ventricular filling volume or end-diastolic size, are thus critical to explaining maximal values. Ventricular contractility and systemic vascular resistance are not associated with the level of aerobic fitness. Consequently, factors influencing ventricular preload, such as plasma volume, autonomic influences on resting HR, and inherent left ventricular size, have been suggested as potential critical determinants of individual variations in $\dot{V}O_2$ max.

Normal population. Rowland *et al.*[69] examined cardiac physiologic correlates to $\dot{V}O_2$ max in 39 healthy boys (mean age 12.2 years) with a wide range of aerobic fitness. Maximal oxygen uptake in ratio with body mass correlated with maximal stroke index (r = 0.52, $p < 0.05$) but not with maximal HR or arteriovenous oxygen difference. Maximal stroke index, in turn, was related to values at rest (r = 0.67). The pattern of SV response (early small rise, then plateau) with increasing exercise intensity was identical in high and low fit boys, with greater values in the former group (Fig. 19.6).

Obert *et al.*[70] found that resting values of left ventricular end-diastolic dimension and SV were independent correlates of $\dot{V}O_2$ max in 142 healthy 10- to 11-year-old boys and girls. No relationship was observed between $\dot{V}O_2$ max and ventricular shortening fraction at rest.

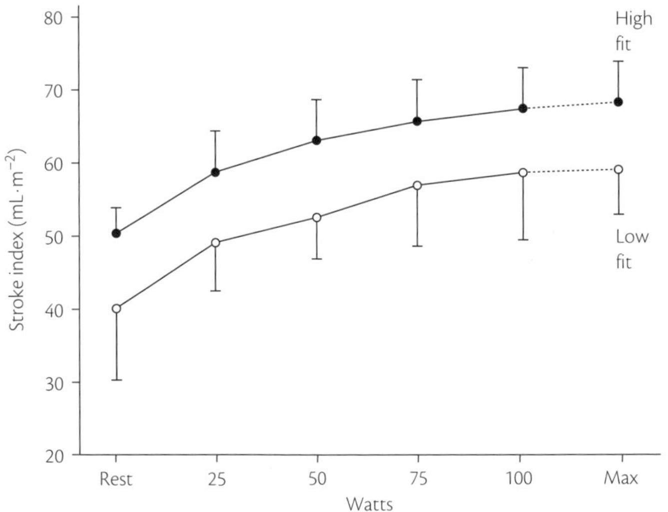

Fig. 19.6 Pattern of stroke index responses to progressive cycle exercise in high fit ($\dot{V}O_2$ max 54.8 ± 1.2 mL·kg^{-1}·min^{-1}) versus low fit ($\dot{V}O_2$ max 38.8 ± 2.5 mL·kg^{-1}·min^{-1}) 12-year-old boys. From Rowland *et al.*,[69] reprinted with permission.

Comparisons between athletes and non-athletes. Nottin *et al.*[56] compared echocardiographic findings during a maximal cycle test in 10 well-trained child cyclists ($\dot{V}O_2$ max 58.5 mL·kg^{-1}·min^{-1}) and 13 untrained children ($\dot{V}O_2$ max 45.9 mL·kg^{-1}·min^{-1}). There were no group differences in maximal HR or arteriovenous oxygen difference. Rest and exercise stroke index was significantly higher in the cyclists, but with parallel patterns of SV response to increased work loads. Similarly, left ventricular end-diastolic size was greater in the athletes at rest and all levels of exercise, with no significant change during exercise. Shortening fraction responses to exercise were similar between the two groups (rising from 41% at rest to 51% at peak exercise in the untrained boys and from 37% to 48% in the athletes. Values and increase in MAP and decline in systemic vascular resistance were similar in the athletes and non-athletes.

Rowland *et al.*[46] demonstrated similar findings in a study of highly trained young cyclists (mean age 13.7 ± 1.0 years) and age-matched non-trained boys. The cyclists demonstrated greater resting and exercise cardiac diastolic dimensions as well as SV, but there were no differences in maximal HR or arteriovenous oxygen difference. The plateauing pattern of SV response was the same in the cyclists and untrained boys. No group differences were seen in shortening fraction response.

Obert *et al.*[71] described greater resting values of left ventricular internal diameter and SV in 10- to 11-year-old trained swimmers compared to age-matched non-athletes. No group differences were observed in resting shortening fraction or ejection fraction.

Effects of endurance training. Obert et al.[72] examined the effect of a 13-week endurance training programme on resting and maximal exercise cardiovascular measures in 19 children (10 girls, 9 boys) compared to untrained control subjects. As a result of the training, $\dot{V}O_2$ max rose by 15% in the boys and 8% in the girls. The increase in $\dot{V}O_2$ was accounted for entirely by rise in maximal SV, as maximal HR and arteriovenous oxygen difference did not change. The plateau response of SV was unaffected by training. Change in maximal SV was closely linked to that of resting SV (r = 0.73), and both were significantly related to resting left ventricular end-diastolic dimension (r = 0.51, 0.35, respectively). Shortening fraction was not altered by training. In this study, a significant fall was observed in systemic vascular resistance following the training period.

The nine boys aged 11–13 years trained by Eriksson and Koch[28] for 4 months demonstrated a 16.7% rise in $\dot{V}O_2$ max (mL·kg^{-1}·min^{-1}). The increase was accounted for entirely by a greater SV, while maximal arteriovenous oxygen difference as well as the decline in total peripheral resistance were unchanged. Radiographic heart volume rose as a result of training from 499 ± 113 to 548 ± 137 mL. Blood volume rose by an estimated 12%.

George *et al.*[73] reported no 'biologically meaningful' increases in peak $\dot{V}O_2$ after a 12-week aerobic training programme in 11 girls aged 10.5 ± 0.7 years. Predictably, then, these subjects demonstrated no alterations in left ventricular morphology at rest compared to non-training controls.

Summary

The qualitative and quantitative features of the cardiovascular responses to an acute bout of progressive exercise are similar in adults in children. Certain age-related variations in absolute values (HR, blood pressure) do not translate into any observed maturational differences in cardiovascular capacity to response in this model of exercise. When appropriately related to body size, changes in cardiac volumes are not different between children and adults, and patterns of SV and indices of ventricular systolic and diastolic function are not maturation-related. Limited data (i.e. at rest) would suggest as well that myocardial metabolism and efficiency is not influenced by biological maturation. Exercise data obtained in children mimic those in adults which suggest that peripheral factors (arteriolar dilatation, skeletal muscle pump) serve to 'drive' the circulatory responses to acute dynamic exercise.

Sustained constant-load exercise (cardiovascular drift)

The previous section addressed circulatory responses to exercise that taxed the cardiovascular system with progressively intense work loads to exhaustion. In the real world, of course, one engages rarely, if ever, in such forms of physical activity. Instead, dynamic endurance exercise is typically performed in the setting of sustained submaximal work (as in a 1-mile run test in physical education class, or a 5 km road race). Thus, considerable interest has focused on the cardiovascular adaptations to constant-load, submaximal exercise performed at an intensity equivalent to a certain percentage of peak $\dot{V}O_2$.

During such exercise, changes in both metabolic rate ($\dot{V}O_2$) and circulatory measures are well-recognized, termed aerobic and cardiovascular drift, respectively.[74,75] It might be anticipated that the two should be related, since (i) although work load is not increased, metabolic rate is expected to rise over time with increase in muscle temperature (the Q_{10} effect)[76] and (ii) increases in blood circulation should respond to augmented metabolic demands of aerobic exercise. The traditional findings in this exercise model, however, have not supported this association.

A slow rise in $\dot{V}O_2$ typically accompanies steady load cycle exercise performed at 50–75% peak $\dot{V}O_2$ for 30–60 min. Concomitantly, a pattern described as 'classic' cardiovascular drift is observed consisting of (i) progressive fall in SV and MAP, (ii) rise in systemic vascular resistance, and (iii) no increase in $\dot{Q}$.[74] Given these discordant changes in $\dot{V}O_2$ and $\dot{Q}$, a cause-and-effect relationship between the two has generally been discounted, and other factors have been considered important in causing cardiovascular drift (such as dehydration, increased cutaneous blood flow, and/or sympathetic stimulation of HR).[75,77,78]

Studies of circulatory response to sustained submaximal exercise in children have indicated no important differences in classic cardiovascular drift from those described in adults. Cheatham *et al.*[79] compared cardiovascular responses in eight 10- to 13-year-old boys and ten 18- to 25-year-old men during 40 min of cycle exercise at approximately 65% peak $\dot{V}O_2$. Between 10 and 40 min of exercise, HR increased by 9.5% and 13.6% in the boys and men, respectively, while MAP fell by 4.2% in men (but was stable in the boys). No significant change was observed in $\dot{Q}$ or calculated arteriovenous oxygen difference over time in either group.

Similar findings were reported by Asano and Hirakoba[80] in their study of 11 boys aged 10–12 years and 12 men aged 20–34 years. During 1 hour of cycling at 60% peak $\dot{V}O_2$, mean $\dot{Q}$ was unchanged in both groups, while HR rose from 152 to 166 beats·min^{-1} in the boys and from 134 to 154 beats·min^{-1} in the men. SV declined from 58 to 54 mL and from 98 to 86 mL in the two groups, respectively.

Studies in euhydrated subjects

Subjects in these reports demonstrating classic cardiovascular drift did not consume fluids during exercise and were presumably (or documented to be) significantly underhydrated. Studies in adults have indicated that if dehydration is avoided (by subject drinking), the pattern of response to constant-load exercise differs from that seen with classic cardiovascular drift.[81–83] These reports indicate that in euhydrated subjects, SV and MAP do not change over time, while HR and $\dot{Q}$ progressively rise. Moreover, the magnitude of increase in $\dot{Q}$ in these studies mimics that of $\dot{V}O_2$. These findings suggest, then, that (i) aerobic and cardiovascular drift are, in fact, causally related, and (ii) patterns of change seen in classic cardiovascular drift reflect the effects of dehydration superimposed on direct circulatory responses to increases in metabolic demand during sustained exercise.

Similar findings have been observed in children who have remained euhydrated during sustained submaximal exercise.[84,85] Rowland *et al.*[84] examined characteristics of aerobic and cardiovascular drift in eight prepubertal boys (mean age 11.7 ± 0.4 years) who pedalled at 63% peak $\dot{V}O_2$ to exhaustion (mean 41.4 ± 6.3 min). Subjects drank water voluntarily and at end-exercise were not significantly dehydrated (mean 0.28%). Mean $\dot{V}O_2$ rose from 1.25 ± 0.20 L·min^{-1} at 10 min to 1.35 ± 0.24 L·min^{-1} at maximum (+8.0%). During the same time, cardiac index increased from 10.19 ± 1.82 to 11.25 ± 2.13 L·min^{-1}·m^{-2} (+10.4%). No change was observed in SV, MAP, or arteriovenous oxygen difference, while systemic vascular resistance fell by 10.5%.

Rowland and Rimany[85] found similar cardiovascular responses during 40 min of cycling at 63% peak $\dot{V}O_2$ in groups of premenarcheal girls and adult women who drank *ad libitum* during the test. Cardiac output and HR increased, while SV remained stable. The women demonstrated a greater magnitude of rise in HR than the girls.

A primary role of aerobic drift in causing cardiovascular drift is thereby supported by these observations in children as well as adults. The failure of $\dot{Q}$ to rise during sustained exercise in the scenario of classic cardiovascular drift appears to reflect the influence of dehydration, masking the link between parallel changes in $\dot{Q}$ and $\dot{V}O_2$. Current evidence indicates that the cardiovascular responses to sustained constant-load exercise as well as the perturbations affected by hydration status are independent of biological maturation.

Cardiac fatigue

Adult endurance athletes participating in ultramarathon events and untrained adults performing extended submaximal cycling (170 min) demonstrate evidence of mild depression of both systolic and diastolic ventricular function immediately post-exercise.[86,87] Changes in markers such as left ventricular shortening fraction and wall-stress are transient, returning to normal in 24–48 hours without apparent clinical significance. Animal studies have supported the idea that intense exercise can cause myocardial fatigue, with findings of depressed contractility, possibly related to alterations in calcium transport capacity of the sarcoplasmic reticulum.[88]

The question of possible myocardial fatigue during extended exercise in children has not been systematically investigated. In a study of nine trained child runners (ages 9–14 years), no significant changes were observed in left ventricular shortening fraction or electrocardiogram findings immediately after a 4-km road race.[89] Maximal exercise testing performed 24 hours post-race demonstrated similar peak work capacity and values of maximal SV and $\dot{Q}$ compared to pre-race findings.

Rost[90] described the growth of cardiac volume and chamber size in a 10-year longitudinal assessment of child swimmers, which was greater than that observed in untrained children. The author noted that 'there was no evidence to suggest that the early start of high-performance training had any bearing on the development of cardiac damage'. These limited data, then, support the clinical experience in the childhood population which fails to indicate evidence of cardiac dysfunction as a consequence of high-intensity sports training among elite-level child athletes.

Isometric exercise

During dynamic activities such as running or cycling, peripheral vasodilatation and increased pumping action of the heart and skeletal muscle dramatically increase circulatory flow to contracting muscles. Such cardiovascular responses are critical, since these forms of exercise, being dependent on aerobic metabolism, rely on an increased availability of circulating oxygen. Isometric, or static, exercise is different. In this case muscles are called upon to provide a short continuous force against a fixed, non-moveable resistance, resulting in high intramuscular pressures, and compression of blood vessels. The increased isometric muscle force generated by wrestlers, weight lifters, and skiers is sustained, relatively brief, and for the most part does not draw upon aerobic metabolic pathways for its energy supply. Not unexpectedly, then, cardiovascular responses are more modest. Indeed, an explanation for the specific pattern of circulatory changes during isometric exercise, which differ from those with dynamic activities, is not entirely clear.

Interest in the physiological responses to isometric exercise in youth has grown with the documentation of strength gains with resistance exercise training that occur in children and adolescents. The limited body of research data indicates that the pattern and magnitude of cardiovascular responses to static exercise in the paediatric age group are similar to those in adults.

Circulatory responses to isometric exercise have generally been assessed with a testing model whereby cardiovascular variables are measured during performance of muscle contractions at a certain percent of previously determined maximal voluntary contraction (MVC). These studies have typically involved handgrip or knee extension exercise at 30–50% MVC for up to 3 min in duration. Breath-holding is to be avoided, as a Valsalva manoeuvre during such efforts may alter cardiovascular responses.

The typical pattern of cardiovascular response to isometric exercise has been well characterized.[91] The principal finding, consistent to all studies, is a sharp rise in both systolic and diastolic pressure. This increase in blood pressure is typically accompanied by a modest rise in HR, stable or small fall in SV, and minor increase in $\dot{Q}$. Since calculated systemic vascular resistance is unchanged, the small rise in circulatory flow has been attributed to a primary increase in HR.

These circulatory changes occur in the milieu of increased sympathetic nervous activity.[92] This pressor stimulation reflects a reflex response involving the interplay of central neurologic drive (central command), muscle contractile pressure (mechanoreflex), and local metabolic factors (metaboreflex or chemoreflex).

Studies describing direct child–adult comparisons of cardiovascular responses to isometric exercise have demonstrated little group differences. Smith *et al.*[93] compared responses to supine handgrip exercise at 30% MVC for 3 min in premenarcheal girls and college-aged women. Average values for MAP rose from 75 to 82 mmHg in the girls and from 77 to 87 mmHg in the women. Average HR increased by 8% and 13% in the girls and women, respectively. SV declined by 13% in the girls and 12% in the women, with no significant change in $\dot{Q}$ in either group.

Turley *et al.*[94] evaluated cardiovascular responses to handgrip exercise at 10%, 20%, and 30% MVC in 7- to 9-year-old boys and 18- to 26-year-old men. No group differences in HR or blood pressure was seen except that at 30% MVC the men demonstrated a greater rise in blood pressure than the boys (35% vs. 24%, respectively). Mathews and Stoney[95] and Palmer *et al.*[96] found that children had a greater HR response but identical blood pressure changes to 30% MVC compared to adults.

In a later study, Turley[97] compared chemoreflex-related changes in cardiovascular variables during isometric exercise in 7- to 9-year-old boys and girls and 18- to 25-year-old adults. Four minutes of limb ischaemia were induced by blood pressure cuff occlusion immediately after 3 min of handgrip at 30% MVC. During contractions, average systolic pressure rose more in the men than the boys (23% vs. 18%) and by a greater degree in the women than girls (21% vs. 15%). No group or gender differences were seen in the magnitude of rise in diastolic pressure.

During the limb-occlusion phase, both children and adults had a decrease in HR back to baseline. In the first minute, both systolic and diastolic pressure fell in all groups but remained above baseline. In recovery, blood pressure fell back to baseline in the adults but remained elevated in the children for 1–2 min. These findings suggest that children might possess a more active chemoreflex than adults.

Rowland and Fernhall[98] noted that several aspects of the traditional picture of cardiovascular responses to isometric exercise were not consistent with certain expectations, particularly (i) compression of intramuscular blood vessels during isometric contractions should be expected to raise peripheral vascular resistance, yet stable values are reported, and (ii) while the rise in blood pressure has been considered secondary to increased $\dot{Q}$, isometric exercise under beta-blockade eliminates the $\dot{Q}$ response, yet the rise in MAP persists. They contended that these inconsistencies reflected an inappropriate calculation of systemic vascular resistance as MAP/$\dot{Q}$ when $\dot{Q}$ was expressed over an extended period (i.e. per minute) rather than during the systolic ejection time, when blood was actually flowing through the arterioles.

They reported findings in 14 prepubertal boys who performed leg extension at 30% MVC for 3 min.[99] As expected, average value of MAP increased by 23 mmHg, HR rose from 77 to 106 beats·min^{-1}, and SV declined from 59 to 52 mL. A small increase was observed in average $\dot{Q}$ (4.58–5.62 L·min^{-1}). Systemic vascular resistance calculated in the traditional manner as MAP/$\dot{Q}$ was not significantly changed (18.8 and 19.4 units at rest and exercise, respectively).

When flow rate per beat during systolic ejection (F) was substituted for $\dot{Q}$ in the calculation of resistance as MAP/F, however, a different picture emerged. Systemic vascular resistance was observed to increase significantly by 28%. The authors concluded that the findings from this approach are 'more intuitively attractive and conform more closely to expected haemodynamic events. By this analysis, an abrupt rise in systemic vascular resistance serves as the fundamental response to static exercise. The acute rise in MAP by this interpretation is accounted for by the increased vascular resistance rather than by a rise in $\dot{Q}$ assumed by the traditional model'.

Summary

- The current body of research information indicates that the morphological and functional responses of the cardiovascular system to dynamic and static exercise are no different in growing children than mature adults. Thus, early concerns that circulatory adaptations to exercise in youth are 'hypokinetic'[17] or might represent risk[100] have not been supported.
- Certain gaps in the current understanding of cardiac responses to exercise in children need to be filled:
  - (i) Little information is available regarding possible myocardial fatigue from extended exercise in young athletes.
  - (ii) Whether gender differences in cardiac characteristics exist independent of the effects of body composition remain to be clarified.
  - (iii) The most appropriate and feasible means of assessing myocardial contractile responses to exercise needs to be determined as a baseline for evaluating patients with ventricular dysfunction.
  - (iv) Factors which define the limitations of circulatory responses to dynamic exercise need to be characterized, particularly the role of variations in arteriolar dilatation and the functional capacity of the skeletal muscle pump.

References

1. Bouchard C, Malina RM, Hollman W, Leblanc C (1997). Submaximal working capacity, heart size and body size in boys 8 to 18 years. *Eur J Appl Physiol* **36**, 115–26.
2. Bar-Or O, Rowland TW (2004). *Pediatric exercise medicine. From physiologic principles to health care application.* Human Kinetics, Champaign, IL.
3. Rowland TW (2008). Cardiorespiratory responses during endurance exercise: Maturation and growth. In: Hebestreit H (ed.), *The child and adolescent athlete*, Vol. 2. pp. 39–49. Blackwell Science, London.
4. Malina RM, Roche AF (1983). *Manual of physical status and performance in childhood*, Vol. 2. Plenum, New York.
5. Marcus B, Gillette PC, Garson A (1990). Intrinsic heart rate in children and young adults: An index of sinus node function isolated from autonomic control. *Am Heart J* **119**, 911–16.
6. Rowland T, Cunningham L (1993). Heart rate deceleration during treadmill exercise in children (abstract). *Pediatr Exerc Sci* **5**, 463.
7. Conconi F, Ferrari M, Ziglio PG, Droghetti P, Codeca L (1982). Determination of the anaerobic threshold by a noninvasive field test in runners. *J Appl Physiol* **52**, 869–73.
8. Baraldi E, Zancanato S, Santuz PA, Zachello F (1989). A comparison of two noninvasive methods in the determination of the anaerobic threshold in children. *Int J Sports Med* **10**, 132–4.
9. Mahon AD, Vaccaro P (1991). Can the point of deflection from linearity of heart rate determine ventilatory threshold in children? *Pediatr Exerc Sci* **3**, 256–62.
10. Cumming GR, Everatt D, Hastman L (1978). Bruce treadmill tests in children: Normal values in a clinic population. *Am J Cardiol* **41**, 69–75.
11. Cumming GR, Langford S (1985). Comparison of nine exercise tests used in pediatric cardiology. In: Binkhorst RA, Kemper HCG, Saris WHM (eds.), *Children and exercise XI*, pp. 58–68. Human Kinetics, Champaign, IL.
12. Riopel DA, Taylor AB, Hohn AR (1979). Blood pressure, heart rate, pressure-rate product, and electrocardiographic changes in healthy children during treadmill exercise. *Am J Cardiol* **57**, 697–704.
13. Sheehan JM, Rowland TW, Burke EJ (1987). A comparison of four treadmill protocols for determination of maximal oxygen uptake in 10–12 year old boys. *Int J Sports Med* **8**, 31–4.
14. Washington RL, van Gundy JC, Cohen C, Sondheimer HM, Wolfe RR (1988). Normal aerobic and anaerobic exercise data for North American school-aged children. *J Pediatr* **112**, 223–33.
15. Mayers N, Gutin B (1979). Physiologic characteristics of elite prepubertal cross country runners. *Med Sci Sports* **11**, 172–6.
16. Bailey DA, Ross WD, Mirwald RL, Weese C (1978). Size dissociation of maximal aerobic power during growth in boys. *Med Sport* **11**, 140–51.
17. Bar-Or O (1983). *Pediatric sports medicine for the practitioner*, pp. 1–65. Springer-Verlag, New York.
18. Armstrong N, Welsman JR (2002). Cardiovascular responses to submaximal treadmill running in 11- to 13 year olds. *Acta Paediatr Scand* **91**, 125–31.
19. Turley KR, Wilmore JH (1997). Cardiovascular responses to submaximal exercise in 7- to 9 year old boys and girls. *Med Sci Sport Exerc* **29**, 824–32.
20. Rowland T, Goff D, Martel L, Ferrone L (2000). Influence of cardiac functional capacity on gender differences in maximal oxygen uptake in children. *Chest* **17**, 629–35.
21. Rowland T, Blum JW (2000). Cardiac dynamics during upright cycle exercise in boys. *Am J Hum Biol* **12**, 749–57.
22. Rowland T, Potts J, Potts T, Song-Hing J, Harbison G, Sandor G (1999). Cardiovascular responses to exercise in children and adolescents with myocardial dysfunction. *Am Heart J* **137**, 126–33.
23. Nottin S, Agnes V, Stecken N, Nguyen L-D, Ounissi F, Lecoq A-M, Obert P (2002). Central and peripheral cardiovascular adaptations during maximal cycle exercise in boys and men. *Med Sci Sport Exerc* **33**, 456–63.
24. Rowland T, Popowski B, Ferrone L (1997). Cardiac responses to maximal upright cycle exercise in healthy boys and men. *Med Sci Sport Exerc* **29**, 1146–51.
25. Rowland T, Popowski B (1997). Comparison of bioimpedance and Doppler cardiac output during exercise in children. *Pediatr Exerc Sci* **9**, 188.
26. Pianosi PT (2004). Measurement of exercise cardiac output by thoracic impedance in healthy children. *Eur J Appl Physiol* **92**, 425–30.
27. Bar-Or O, Shephard RJ, Allen CL (1971). Cardiac output of 10–13 year old boys and girls during submaximal exercise. *J Appl Physiol* **30**, 219–23.
28. Eriksson BO, Koch G (1973). Effect of physical training on hemodynamic response during submaximal and maximal exercise in 11–13 year old boys. *Acta Physiol Scand* **87**, 27–39.
29. Cyran SE, James FW, Daniels S, Mays W, Shukala R, Kaplan S (1988). Comparison of the cardiac output and stroke volume response to upright exercise in children with valvular and subvalvular aortic stenosis. *J Am Coll Cardiol* **11**, 651–8.
30. Notarius CF, Magder S (1996). Central venous pressure during exercise: Role of the muscle pump. *Can J Physiol Pharmacol* **74**, 647–51.
31. Rowland TW, Garrison A, DeIulio A (2003). Circulatory responses to progressive exercise: Insights from positional differences. *Int J Sports Med* **24**, 512–7.
32. Bevegard S, Holmgren A, Jonsson B (1960). The effect of body position on the circulation at rest and during exercise, with special reference to the influence on stroke volume. *Acta Physiol Scand* **49**, 279–98.

33. Vinet A, Mandigout S, Nottin S, Nguyen L-D, Lecoq A-M, Courteix D, Obert P (2003). Influence of body composition, hemoglobin concentration, and cardiac size and function on gender differences in maximal oxygen uptake in prepubertal children. *Chest* **124**, 1494–9.
34. Rowland T, Miller K, Vanderburgh P, Goff D, Martel L, Ferrone L (1999). Cardiovascular fitness in premenarcheal girls and young women. *Int J Sports Med* **20**, 117–21.
35. Vinet A, Nottin, S, Lecoq A-M, Obert P (2002). Cardiovascular responses to progressive cycle exercise in healthy children and adults. *Int J Sports Med* **23**, 242–6.
36. Epstein SE, Besier GD, Stampfer N, Robinson BF, Braunwald E (1967). Characterization of the circulatory response to maximal upright exercise in normal subjects and patients with heart disease. *Circulation* **35**, 1049–62.
37. Marx GR, Hicks RW, Allen HD (1987). Measurement of cardiac output and exercise factor by pulsed Doppler echocardiography during supine bicycle ergometry in normal young adolescent boys. *J Am Coll Cardiol* **10**, 430–4.
38. Edmunds AT, Godfrey S, Tooley M (1982). Cardiac output measured by transthoracic bioimpedance cardiography at rest, during exercise, and at various lung volumes. *Clin Sci* **63**, 107–13.
39. Godfrey S, Davies HTM, Wozniak E, Barnes CA (1971). Cardiorespiratory response to exercise in normal children. *Clin Sci* **40**, 419–31.
40. Locke JE, Einzig S, Moller JH (1978). Hemodynamic response to exercise in normal children. *Am J Cardiol* **41**, 1278–85.
41. Grimby G, Nilsson NJ, Saltin B (1966). Cardiac output during submaximal and maximal exercise in active middle-aged athletes. *J Appl Physiol* **21**, 1150–6.
42. Vella CA, Robergs RA (2005). Non-linear relationship between central cardiovascular variables and $\dot{V}O_2$ during incremental cycle exercise in endurance-trained athletes. *J Sports Med Phys Fitness* **45**, 452–9.
43. Yamaguchi I, Komatsu E, Miyazawa K (1986). Intersubject variability in cardiac output-O_2 uptake relation of men during exercise. *J Appl Physiol* **61**, 2168–74.
44. Rowland TW (2007). Circulatory 'efficacy' during progressive aerobic exercise in children: Insights from the $\dot{Q}:\dot{V}O_2$ relationship. *Eur J Appl Physiol* 101, 61–6.
45. Rowland T, Heffernan K, Jae SY, Echols G, Fernhall B (2006). Tissue Doppler assessment of ventricular function during cycling in 7- to 12-yr-old boys. *Med Sci Sport Exerc* **38**, 1216–22.
46. Rowland T, Unnithan V, Fernhall B, Baynard T, Lange C (2002). Left ventricular response to dynamic exercise in young cyclists. *Med Sci Sport Exerc* **34**, 637–42.
47. Kimball TR, Mays WA, Khoury PR, Mallie R. Claytor RP (1993). Echocardiographic determination of left ventricular preload, afterload, and contractility during and after exercise. *J Pediatr* **122**, S89–94.
48. DeSouza M, Schaffer MS, Gilday DL, Rose V (1984). Exercise radionuclide angiography in hyperlipidemic children with apparently normal hearts. *Nucl Med Comment* **5**, 13–17.
49. DeSouza AM, Potts JE, DeSouza ES (2001). Feasibility and results of using tissue Doppler imaging to assess ventricular function during exercise. *Med Sci Sport Exerc* **37** (Suppl.), 1221.
50. Onouchi Z, Hamaoka K, Sakata K, Liu Y, Suto F, Nakagawa Y, Teramachi S (1996). Myocardial oxygen consumption, cardiac work, and myocardial efficiency in children. *Eur J Pediatr* **155**, 436–9.
51. Rowland T, Mannie E, Gawle L (2001). Dynamics of left ventricular diastolic filling during exercise. *Chest* **120**, 145–50.
52. Ha J-W, Oh PA, Pellikka WA, Ommen SR, Stussy VL, Bailey KR, Seward JB, Tajik AJ (2005). Diastolic stress echocardiography: A novel noninvasive diagnostic test for diastolic dysfunction using supine bicycle exercise Doppler echocardiography. *J Am Soc Echocardiogr* **18**, 63–8.
53. Wang Z, Jalali F, Sun YH, Wang JJ, Parker KH, Tyberg JV (2005). Assessment of left ventricular diastolic suction in dogs using wave-intensity analysis. *Am J Physiol* **288**, H1641–51.
54. Alpert BS, Fox MF (1993). Blood pressure response to dynamic exercise. In: Rowland TW (ed.), *Pediatric laboratory exercise testing. Clinical guidelines*, pp. 67–90. Human Kinetics Publishers, Champaign, IL.
55. Boushel R (2003). Metabolic control of muscle blood flow during exercise in humans. *Can J Appl Physiol* **28**, 754–73.
56. Nottin S, Vinet A, Stecken F, N'Guyen L-D, Ounissi F, Lecoq A-M, Obert P (2002). Central and peripheral cardiovascular adaptations to exercise in endurance trained children. *Acta Physiol Scand* **175**, 85–92.
57. Pokan R, von Duvillard SP, Hofman P, Smekal G, Frohwald FM, Gasser R, Tschan H, Baron R, Schmid P, Bachl N (2000). Change in left atrial and ventricular dimensions during and immediately after exercise. *Med Sci Sport Exerc* **32**, 1713–18.
58. Guyton AC (1967). Regulation of cardiac output. *N Engl J Med* **277**, 805–12.
59. Rushmer RF, Smith OA (1959). Cardiac control. *Physiol Rev* **39**, 41–68.
60. Bainbridge FA (1915). The influence of venous filling upon the rate of the heart. *J Physiol* **50**, 65–84.
61. Linden RJ (1994). The size of the heart. *Cardioscience* **5**, 225–33.
62. Braunwald E, Ross J (1979). Control of cardiac performance. In: Berne RM (ed.), *Handbook of physiology. The cardiovascular system*, pp. 533–80. American Physiological Society, Bethesda, MD.
63. Binak K, Regan TJ, Christensen RC (1960). Arteriovenous fistula: Hemodynamic effects of occlusion and exercise. *Am Heart J* **60**, 495–502.
64. Rowland TW (2001). The circulatory response to exercise: Role of the peripheral pump. *Int J Sports Med* **22**, 558–65.
65. Rowell LB, O'Leary DS, Kellogg DL (1996). Integration of cardiovascular control systems in dynamic exercise. In: Rowell LB, Shepherd JT (eds.), *Handbook of physiology. Regulation and integration of multiple systems*, pp. 771–81. American Physiological Society, Bethesda, MD.
66. Rowland T, Lisowski R (2003). Determinants of diastolic filling during exercise. *J Sports Med Phys Fitness* **43**, 380–5.
67. Lutjemeier BJ, Miura A, Scheuermann BW (2005). Muscle contraction-blood flow interactions during upright knee extension exercise in humans. *J Appl Physiol* **98**, 1575–83.
68. Takayashi T, Miyamoto Y (1998). Influence of light physical activity on cardiac responses during recovery from exercise in humans. *Eur J Appl Physiol* **77**, 305–11.
69. Rowland T, Kline G, Goff D, Martel L, Ferrone L (1999). Physiological determinants of maximal aerobic power in healthy 12 year old boys. *Pediatr Exerc Sci* **11**, 317–26.
70. Obert P, Mandigout S, Vinet A, Nottin S, N'Guyen LD, Lecoq AM (2005). Relationships between left ventricular morphology, diastolic function and oxygen carrying capacity and maximal oxygen uptake in children. *Int J Sports Med* **26**, 122–7.
71. Obert P, Stecken F, Courteix D, Lecoq A-M, Guenon P (1998). Effect of long-term intensive endurance training on left ventricular structure and diastolic function in prepubertal children. *Int J Sports Med* **19**, 149–54.
72. Obert P, Mandigout S, Nottin S, Vinet A, N'Guyen LD, Lecoq AM (2003). Cardiovascular responses to endurance training in children: Effects of gender. *Eur J Clin Invest* **33**, 199–208.
73. George KP, Gates PE, Tolfrey K (2005). The impact of aerobic training upon left ventricular morphology and function in pre-pubescent children. *Ergonomics* **48**, 1378–89.
74. Raven PB, Stevens GHJ (1988). Cardiovascular function and prolonged exercise. In: Lamb DR, Murray R (eds.), *Perspectives in exercise science and sports medicine*. Vol. 1. Prolonged exercise, pp. 43–71. Benchmark Press, Indianapolis, IN.

75. Rowell LB (1986). *Human circulation during physical stress*, pp. 365–74. Oxford Press, New York.
76. Blaxter K (1989). *Energy metabolism in animals and man*. Cambridge University Press, Cambridge.
77. Coyle EF, Gonzalez-Alonso J (2001). Cardiovascular drift during prolonged exercise: New perspectives. *Exerc Sport Sci Rev* **29**, 88–92.
78. Fritzche RG, Switzer TW, Hodgkinson BJ, Coyle EF (1999). Stroke volume decline during prolonged exercise is influenced by the increase in heart rate. *J Appl Physiol* **86**, 799–805.
79. Cheatham CC, Mahon AD, Brown JD, Bolster DR (2000). Cardiovascular responses during prolonged exercise at ventilatory threshold in boys and men. *Med Sci Sport Exerc* **32**, 1080–7.
80. Asano K, Hirakoba K (1984). Respiratory and circulatory adaptation during prolonged exercise in 10–12 year old children and adults. In: Ilmarinen J, Valimaki I (eds.), *Children and sport*, pp. 119–28. Springer-Verlag, Berlin.
81. Ganio MS, Wingo JE, Carroll CE, Thomas MK, Cureton KJ (2006). Fluid ingestion attenuates the decline in $\dot{V}O_2$ peak associated with cardiovascular drift. *Med Sci Sport Exerc* **38**, 901–9.
82. Hamilton MT, Gonzalez-Alonso J, Montain SJ (1991). Fluid replacement and glucose infusion during exercise prevent cardiovascular drift. *J Appl Physiol* **71**, 871–7.
83. Montain SJ, Coyle EF (1992). Influence of graded hydration on hyperthermia and cardiovascular drift during exercise. *J Appl Physiol* **73**, 1340–50.
84. Rowland T, Pober D, Garrison A (2005). Determinants of cardiovascular drift in euhydrated prepubertal boys. *Med Sci Sport Exerc* **37**, S216.
85. Rowland TW, Rimany TA (1995). Physiological responses to prolonged exercise in premenarcheal and adult females. *Pediatr Exerc Sci* **7**, 183–91.
86. Douglas PS, O'Toole ML, Hiller WD (1987). Cardiac fatigue after prolonged exercise. *Circulation* **76**, 1206–13.
87. Seals DR, Rogers MA, Hagberg JM (1988). Left ventricular dysfunction after prolonged strenuous exercise in healthy subjects. *Am J Cardiol* **61**, 876–9.
88. Maher JT, Goodman AL, Francesconi R, Bowers WD, Hartley LH, Angelakos ET (1972). Responses of rat myocardium to exhaustive exercise. *Am J Physiol* **22**, 207–12.
89. Rowland T, Goff D, DeLuca P, Popowski B (1997). Cardiac effects of a competitive road race in trained child runners. *Pediatrics* **100**, e2.
90. Rost R (1987). *Athletics and the heart*. Year Book Medical Publishers, Chicago, IL.
91. Nutter DO, Schlant RC, Hurst JW (1972). Isometric exercise and the cardiovascular system. *Mod Concept Cardiovasc Dis* **41**, 11–15.
92. Mitchell JH (1990). Neural control of the circulation during exercise. *Med Sci Sport Exerc* **22**, 141–54.
93. Smith DL, Kocher BE, Kolesnikoff AL, Rowland TW (2000). Cardiovascular responses to isometric contractions in girls and young women (abstract). *Med Sci Sport Exerc* **32**, S95.
94. Turley KR, Martin DE, Marvin ED, Cowley KS (2002). Heart rate and blood pressure responses to static handgrip exercise of different intensities: Reliability and adult versus child differences. *Pediatr Exerc Sci* **14**, 45–55.
95. Mathews KA, Stoney CM (1988). Influence of sex and age on cardiovascular responses during stress. *Psychosom Med* **50**, 46–56.
96. Palmer GJ, Ziegler MG, Lake CR (1978). Responses of norepinephrine and blood pressure to stress increase with age. *J Gerontol* **33**, 482–7.
97. Turley KR (2005). The chemoreflex: Adult versus child comparison. *Med Sci Sport Exerc* **37**, 418–25.
98. Rowland T, Fernhall B (2007). Cardiovascular responses to static exercise: A re-appraisal. *Int J Sports Med* 28, 905–8.
99. Rowland T, Heffernan K, Jae SY, Echols G, Krull G, Fernhall B (2006). Cardiovascular responses to static exercise in boys: Insights from tissue Doppler imaging. *Eur J Appl Physiol* **97**, 637–42.
100. Karpovich V (1991). Textbook fallacies regarding the development of the child's heart. (Originally published in *Research Quarterly* vol. 8, 1937). Reprinted in *Pediatr Exerc Sci* **3**, 278–82.
101. Nottin S, Vinet A, Lecoq A-M, Guenon P, Obert P (2001). Test-retest reproducibility of submaximal and maximal cardiac output by Doppler echocardiography and CO_2 rebreathing in prepubertal children. *Pediatr Exerc Sci* **13**, 214–24.
102. Welsman J, Bywater K, Farr C, Welford D, Armstrong N (2005). Reliability of peak $\dot{V}O_2$ and maximal cardiac output assessed using thoracic bioimpedance in children. *Eur J Appl Physiol* **94**, 228–34.
103. Miyamura M, Honda Y (1973). Maximum cardiac output related to sex and age. *Jap J Physiol* **23**, 645–56.
104. Yamaji K, Miyashita M (1977). Oxygen transport during exhaustive exercise in Japanese boys. *Eur J Appl Physiol* **36**, 93–9.
105. Gilliam TB, Sady S, Thorland WG, Weltman AC (1977). Comparison of peak performance measures in children ages 6 to 8, 9 to 10, and 11 to 13 years. *Res Q* **48**, 695–702.
106. Rowland T, Potts J, Potts T, Sandor G, Goff D, Ferrone L (2000). Cardiac responses to progressive exercise in normal children: A synthesis. *Med Sci Sport Exerc* **32**, 253–9.

CHAPTER 20

Aerobic fitness

Neil Armstrong, Alison M. McManus, and Joanne R. Welsman

Introduction

Aerobic fitness may be defined as the ability to deliver oxygen to the exercising muscles and to utilize it to generate energy during exercise. Aerobic fitness therefore depends on the pulmonary, cardiovascular, and haematological components of oxygen delivery and the oxidative mechanisms of exercising muscle.

Maximal oxygen uptake ($\dot{V}O_2$ max), the highest rate at which an individual can consume oxygen during exercise, limits the capacity to perform aerobic exercise and is well established as the best single measure of adults' aerobic fitness.[1,2] Maximal $\dot{V}O_2$ is traditionally determined in the laboratory through an incremental exercise test to exhaustion. During the test $\dot{V}O_2$ rises with increasing exercise intensity up to a point beyond which no additional increase in $\dot{V}O_2$ takes place, despite a well-motivated subject being able to increase further the intensity of the exercise. As the test progresses lactate gradually accumulates in the muscles and leaks into the blood where it can be measured. However, exercise above the point where $\dot{V}O_2$ plateaus is assumed to be supported exclusively by anaerobic re-synthesis of adenosine triphosphate (ATP) resulting in a rapid accumulation of muscle and blood lactate, acidosis, and eventually termination of exercise. The conventional criterion for the attainment of $\dot{V}O_2$ max during a progressive exercise test is therefore a levelling-off or plateau in $\dot{V}O_2$ despite an increase in exercise intensity.[3,4] However, both the theoretical[5,6] and the methodological bases[7,8] of the $\dot{V}O_2$ plateau concept have been challenged and the validity of this traditional model is a topic of lively debate.[9,10]

Astrand[11] was the first to document that only a minority of children and adolescents terminate a progressive exercise test to exhaustion with a levelling-off in $\dot{V}O_2$ and subsequent studies have confirmed that a $\dot{V}O_2$ plateau is not a prerequisite for the valid determination of young people's aerobic fitness.[12,13] It has therefore become widely recognized that the appropriate term to use with young people is peak oxygen uptake (peak $\dot{V}O_2$), the highest $\dot{V}O_2$ elicited during an exercise test to exhaustion, rather than $\dot{V}O_2$ max which conventionally implies the existence of a $\dot{V}O_2$ plateau.[14–16] If a child or adolescent has been habituated to the laboratory environment and shows clear signs of intense effort supported by objective criteria peak $\dot{V}O_2$ can be accepted as a maximal index of aerobic fitness (see Chapter 8).

Peak $\dot{V}O_2$ limits the child's capacity to perform aerobic exercise but it does not describe fully all aspects of aerobic fitness. Exercise of the intensity and duration required to elicit peak $\dot{V}O_2$ is rarely experienced by many young people.[17,18] The vast majority of habitual physical activity is submaximal and of short duration and, under these circumstances, it is the transient kinetics of $\dot{V}O_2$ which reflect the integrated response of the oxygen delivery system and the metabolic requirements of the exercising muscle.[19–21] Furthermore, peak $\dot{V}O_2$ is neither the best measure of a child's ability to sustain submaximal aerobic exercise nor the most sensitive means to detect improvements in aerobic fitness after a training programme. Despite its origins in anaerobic metabolism, blood lactate accumulation is a valuable indicator of aerobic fitness and it can be used to monitor improvements in muscle oxidative capacity with exercise training in the absence of changes in peak $\dot{V}O_2$.[16,22] However, as $\dot{V}O_2$ kinetics is comprehensively reviewed in Chapter 22 and blood lactate accumulation during exercise is analysed in Chapter 8, we will focus herein on aerobic fitness as described by peak $\dot{V}O_2$.

Peak oxygen uptake

It is 70 years since Robinson[23] published the first laboratory investigation of boys' aerobic fitness and over 50 years since Astrand[11] reported his studies of the aerobic fitness of both sexes. The publication of these pioneering studies stimulated such interest in children's peak $\dot{V}O_2$ that it has become the most researched variable in paediatric exercise science but the interpretation of peak $\dot{V}O_2$ during growth and maturation remains shrouded in controversy. In this chapter, we will briefly examine the components of peak $\dot{V}O_2$ with reference to other more focused chapters in this book (e.g. Chapters 16, 18, and 19), scrutinize the increase in peak $\dot{V}O_2$ with age, challenge the traditional interpretation of peak $\dot{V}O_2$ during growth (with reference to Chapter 2), demonstrate the independent contribution of maturation to peak $\dot{V}O_2$, and address the progressive divergence of girls' and boys' peak $\dot{V}O_2$ during childhood and adolescence. We will also comment on the evidence suggesting that there have been secular changes in peak $\dot{V}O_2$.

Components of peak oxygen uptake

Pulmonary function

The assessment and interpretation of pulmonary function during growth and maturation is comprehensively reviewed in Chapters 6 and 18 and we will only summarize the salient issues here.

During progressive exercise minute ventilation $\dot{V}_E$ reflects increases in $\dot{V}O_2$ and carbon dioxide output ($\dot{V}CO_2$) and it is closely matched to the increase in exercise intensity until the ventilatory threshold (T_{VENT}) is reached. Beyond the T_{VENT}, which generally occurs at a higher relative exercise intensity and peak $\dot{V}O_2$ in children than in adults, the bicarbonate buffering of hydrogen ions accompanying lactic acid dissociation to lactate causes $\dot{V}CO_2$ and therefore $\dot{V}_E$ to rise relatively faster than $\dot{V}O_2$. As peak $\dot{V}O_2$ is approached, a further reduction in blood pH causes $\dot{V}_E$ to compensate by increasing at a disproportionately higher rate than $\dot{V}CO_2$.

The general pattern of the $\dot{V}_E$ response to progressive exercise is similar in children and adults but there are clear age[11,24] and growth and maturation[25–27] differences in the quantitative and relative responses of the components of $\dot{V}_E$. Data on sex differences in the pulmonary response to exercise are equivocal.[28–30] Children have a higher ratio of respiratory frequency (f_R) to tidal volume (V_T) than adults and during maximal exercise a f_R greater than 60 breaths·min^{-1} is not uncommon compared with about 40 breaths·min^{-1} in adults. Children display a higher $\dot{V}_E$ and therefore a less efficient response to a given metabolic demand (i.e. higher $\dot{V}_E/\dot{V}O_2$) than adults, which suggests that there is some maturation of the ventilatory control mechanisms during childhood and adolescence. However, gas exchange in the alveoli is determined by alveolar rather than pulmonary ventilation and young people's alveolar ventilation is more than adequate to optimize gas exchange. Although at peak $\dot{V}O_2$, $\dot{V}_E/\dot{V}O_2$ is generally lower in adults than in children, $\dot{V}_E$ at peak $\dot{V}O_2$ seldom exceeds values greater than 70% of maximal voluntary ventilation. With healthy children and adolescents, $\dot{V}_E$ does not therefore appear to limit peak $\dot{V}O_2$ and will not be considered further in this chapter. However, interested readers are directed to Chapter 18 for a discussion of recent evidence concerning the effects of exercise-induced arterial hypoxaemia on children's maximal ventilation.

Cardiovascular function

The Fick equation establishes that $\dot{V}O_2$ can be expressed as the product of cardiac output ($\dot{Q}$) and arteriovenous oxygen difference (a-v O_2 dif). Cardiac output is a function of heart rate (HR) and stroke volume (SV) but, as its assessment and interpretation during exercise is reviewed in detail in Chapters 7 and 19, it will only be briefly addressed here.

Heart rate

During a progressive exercise test, HR rises in an almost linear manner and then from about 75% of peak $\dot{V}O_2$ it gradually levels off to a value at peak $\dot{V}O_2$, which varies with the ergometer used[14,31,32] and the exercise protocol.[12,33,34] Progressive, incremental treadmill running protocols elicit the highest HRs with typical mean and standard deviation values for children and adolescents of 200 ± 7 beats·min^{-1}.[35–37] Both cross-sectional and longitudinal data are consistent and demonstrate that, during childhood and adolescence, heart rate at peak $\dot{V}O_2$ is independent of age,[38–40] maturation,[40–42] and sex.[36,43,44]

Stroke volume

Our understanding of the response of young people's SV and $\dot{Q}$ to exercise is subject to methodological limitations (see refs 45,46 and Chapter 7). Nevertheless, data for both adults and children are consistent and indicate that during exercise in the upright position SV rises progressively to values 30–40% greater than resting and reaches this level at 40–60% of peak $\dot{V}O_2$. Stroke volume then demonstrates a plateau despite a further increase in exercise intensity, with subsequent rises in $\dot{Q}$ relying exclusively on HR (see refs 47–49 and Fig. 19.1). Stroke volume is generally expressed in relation to body surface area as the stroke index[50–52] and data suggest that peak values of stroke index remain stable from age 10 years into young adulthood.[23,52,53] Data on young people's peak stroke index are sparse (see Table 19.1) but are generally reported to be about 50–60 mL·m^{-2}. Boys' peak stroke index has consistently been shown to be higher than girls' although this may be related to differences in lean body mass (LBM).[54–56]

Cardiac output

During a progressive exercise test $\dot{Q}$ increases with $\dot{V}O_2$ but not in an entirely linear manner.[49,57] As HR at peak $\dot{V}O_2$ is independent of age, body size, maturation, and sex, it follows that during childhood and adolescence $\dot{Q}$ at peak $\dot{V}O_2$ reflects changes in SV. In absolute values (L·min^{-1}) $\dot{Q}$ at peak $\dot{V}O_2$ increases with age[54,58] but children's peak cardiac index is similar to that of adults. Values vary with measurement technique but boys' peak cardiac index is about 10–12 L·min^{-1}·m^{-2} and about 10% higher than girls' values (see refs 59,60 and Table 19.1). Few studies have addressed the topic but maturity-related differences in the cardiac response to exercise are not evident in the extant literature (see refs 48,50 and Fig. 19.2).

Arteriovenous oxygen difference

Arteriovenous oxygen difference is a manifestation of a range of factors including blood haemoglobin concentration, blood volume, muscle blood flow, aerobic enzyme activity, and mitochondrial density. It therefore serves as an index of the haematological components of oxygen delivery and the oxidative mechanisms of exercising muscle. Ethical considerations and methodological problems have clouded our understanding of a-v O_2 dif during childhood and adolescence and few secure data are available.

Cardiac catheterization has been used to determine resting a-v O_2 dif and data indicate wide individual variations around a mean value of about 44 mL of O_2 per L of blood (mL·L^{-1}) with no relationship between resting a-v O_2 dif and age during the period from birth to 20 years.[61,62]

Arteriovenous oxygen difference during exercise is estimated from measurements of $\dot{V}O_2$ and estimates of $\dot{Q}$ via the Fick equation (i.e. $\dot{V}O_2 = Q \cdot$ a-v O_2 dif). Within the limitations of this methodology, it appears that a-v O_2 dif increases with progressive exercise[63] and it has been reported both to have a linear relationship with exercise intensity[64] and to plateau at near-maximal exercise.[65] Data on young people's a-v O_2 dif at peak $\dot{V}O_2$ are limited and the available evidence is equivocal. Yamaji and Miyashita[58] observed no relationship between a-v O_2 dif at peak $\dot{V}O_2$ and age in 77 boys aged 10–18 years whereas others have demonstrated age-related increases.[48,54,56] Reported mean values of a-v O_2 dif over the age range 6–18 years have been reported to vary between 103 and 147 mL·L^{-1}.[56,58,64] Data on girls' a-v O_2 dif at peak $\dot{V}O_2$ are sparse but a recent report, in which $\dot{Q}$ max was determined using thoracic bioelectrical impedance (see Chapter 7 for a review of this method), reported boys to have a significantly higher a-v O_2 dif than girls (147 vs. 126 mL·L^{-1}) at age 10 years.[66]

Although data showing an age-related increase in a-v O_2 dif at peak $\dot{V}O_2$ must be treated cautiously, the lower blood haemoglobin concentration in children than in adults supports the premise that adults have a greater arterial oxygen content. Blood haemoglobin concentration rises from 125 $g \cdot L^{-1}$ at age 2 years to 135 $g \cdot L^{-1}$ at 12 years and is independent of sex.[67] During the teen years, boys experience a marked increase in haemoglobin concentration to about 152 $g \cdot L^{-1}$ at 16 years whereas girls' values tend to plateau and only rise to perhaps 137 $g \cdot L^{-1}$ by 16 years.[67] As 1 g of fully saturated haemoglobin will hold 1.34 mL oxygen, the oxygen-carrying capacity of blood haemoglobin for girls rises from 168 $mL \cdot L^{-1}$ at 2 years to 184 $mL \cdot L^{-1}$ at 16 years, an increase of 9.5%, whereas boys' values rise by 21.4% over the same period. Children's mixed venous oxygen content at peak $\dot{V}O_2$ is unknown but as adults can lower their mixed venous oxygen content to 20–30 $mL \cdot L^{-1}$ during heavy exercise children inevitably have a lower a-v O_2 dif reserve than adults.

Haemoglobin is essential for oxygen transport[68] and blood haemoglobin concentration has been demonstrated to be significantly correlated with peak $\dot{V}O_2$ in 11–16 year olds.[35] Blood volume rises through childhood and adolescence[69] and therefore total haemoglobin also increases and has been shown to be linearly related to peak $\dot{V}O_2$ across all age levels and in both sexes.[11] The dissociation of oxygen from haemoglobin is, however, quite complex and influenced by factors such as temperature, acidity, carbon dioxide content, and concentration of 2,3 diphosphoglycerate (2,3 DPG).[70] A greater facility for oxygen unloading at the tissues has been observed in young people compared with adults[71] and, as 2,3 DPG reduces haemoglobin's affinity for oxygen, this may be due to the decline in 2,3 DPG with age.[72] Females have been reported to have significantly higher 2,3 DPG:haemoglobin ratios than males of similar fitness[73] and differing levels of 2,3 DPG may partially compensate for age and sex differences in haemoglobin concentration.

Arteriovenous oxygen difference is dependent on muscle blood flow and exercise results in a marked redistribution of blood away from non-exercising vascular beds to the muscles. The scale of blood redistribution may be different in young people[74] and lower noradrenaline levels at peak $\dot{V}O_2$[75,76] may be indicative of diminished sympathetic activity in children, which may result in less shunting of blood to exercising muscles. However, a study of nine 12-year-old trained boys[77] examined muscle blood flow during exercise and indicated that the boys had a higher muscle blood flow immediately following exercise than adults studied using comparable techniques (i.e. dye dilution; see Chapter 7 for a review of this method). The child–adult differences diminished when the same boys were tested 1 year[70] and 4 years[78] later.

Muscle oxygen utilization

Aerobic exercise is not only a function of oxygen delivery to muscles but also of oxygen utilization by exercising muscles. This topic is reviewed in Chapter 16 and only relevant aspects will be outlined here.

Data are equivocal but, on balance, they suggest that the activity of aerobic enzymes in children's muscle is significantly higher than in adult muscle.[79–81] Muscle biopsy data from children are sparse but there is evidence to suggest that the percentage of type 1 fibres decreases with age.[82–84] The slightly greater mitochondrial volume, ratio of mitochondria to myofibrillar volume, and intramuscular lipid storage observed in 6-year-old children compared with typical values from untrained adults[85] provides additional indications that children may have an enhanced ability to generate energy from aerobic metabolism. Recent investigations of $\dot{V}O_2$ kinetics in relation to age have revealed children to have a faster time constant, greater oxygen cost of exercise and a smaller slow component of $\dot{V}O_2$ than adults which suggests the presence of an enhanced oxidative function and/or a greater percentage of type 1 muscle fibres during childhood (see refs 86–88 and Chapters 16 and 22).

Research is limited by ethical and methodological constraints but evidence drawn from several methodologies indicates an interplay between aerobic and anaerobic exercise metabolism in which children have a relatively higher contribution from oxidative energy pathways than adolescents or adults. Current research using magnetic resonance spectroscopy (MRS) has a huge untapped potential to provide further insights in this field (see ref. 89 and Chapter 16).

Peak oxygen uptake and age

The peak $\dot{V}O_2$ of children and adolescents has been extensively documented[16,90,91] with data available from children as young as 3 years of age.[92] The validity of peak $\dot{V}O_2$ determinations in children younger than 8 years has been questioned[16,93] as young children typically have short attention spans, poor motivation, and lack sufficient understanding of experimental procedures therefore making it difficult to elicit genuine maximal efforts.[94] Equipment and protocols designed for adults make testing with young children problematic and the smaller the child the greater the potential problem (see Chapter 8). Reports of peak $\dot{V}O_2$ in very young children are difficult to interpret. Small sample sizes are common[95,96] and several studies have pooled data from boys and girls.[91,97,98] Whether the children exhibited maximal values is unclear in some reports in the absence of explicit exercise termination criteria[23,99,100] and there is a tendency to report only mass-related data.[98,101] In one large study of 592 6- to 7-year-old Danish children, data were rigorously collected and analysed and boys were reported to have peak $\dot{V}O_2$ values ($L \cdot min^{-1}$), on average, 10.9 % higher than girls.[102] There are, however, few secure data from young people aged less than 8 years and we will therefore focus on the age group 8–18 years.

Armstrong and Welsman[16] reviewed the extant literature and generated graphs representing over 10,000 peak $\dot{V}O_2$ determinations of untrained subjects, aged 8–16 years. Because of the ergometer dependence of peak $\dot{V}O_2$ (see Chapter 8) data from treadmill and cycle ergometry were graphed separately and the treadmill determined peak $\dot{V}O_2$ scores ($n = 4937$) are reproduced here as Fig. 20.1. The data must be interpreted cautiously, as means from both longitudinal and cross-sectional studies with varying sample sizes are included. No information is available on randomly selected groups of young people, and since participants are generally volunteers selection bias cannot be ruled out. Nevertheless, Fig. 20.1 clearly illustrates an almost linear increase in boys' peak $\dot{V}O_2$ in relation to age. Girls' data demonstrate a similar but less consistent trend, with several cross-sectional studies indicating a tendency to plateau at about 14 years of age.[103–105] The regression equations indicate that peak $\dot{V}O_2$ increases by about 80% from 8 to 16 years in girls and by 150% in boys over the same time period.

Longitudinal studies provide a more secure analysis of peak $\dot{V}O_2$ in relation to age but few studies of untrained young people have coupled rigorous determination of peak $\dot{V}O_2$ with substantial sample sizes (Table 20.1). Studies of German,[106] Norwegian,[106] Dutch,[107] and Canadian[108] children as well as Czech[109] and Canadian[110] boys were initiated in the 1970s. Rutenfranz *et al.*[106] determined the peak $\dot{V}O_2$ of Norwegian children from 8 to 15 years and German children from 12 to 16 years on a cycle ergometer. Cunningham *et al.*[110] mon-

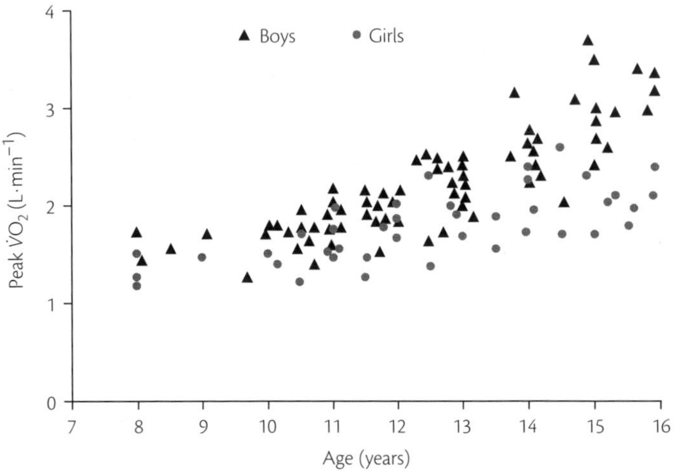

Fig. 20.1 Peak oxygen uptake by age and sex. Reprinted from Armstrong and Welsman,[16] with permission.

itored the cycle ergometer peak $\dot{V}O_2$ of Canadian boys from 10 to 14 years and another Canadian study used a treadmill to determine the peak $\dot{V}O_2$ of boys from 8 to 16 years and girls from 8 to 13 years.[108] Sprynarova *et al.*[109] determined the peak $\dot{V}O_2$ of 90 Czech boys annually from 11 to 15 years and then followed 36 of the boys for a further 3 years. The Amsterdam Growth and Health Study,[107] a 23 year study of young people aged 13 at the start of the project, provides annual peak $\dot{V}O_2$ data from 13 to 16 years. More recently in England, Armstrong *et al.*[111] reported annual peak $\dot{V}O_2$ measures on about 200 children from 11 to 13 years with a follow-up on a subsample at age 17 years.[42]

The boys' data are consistent and show a >120% increase in peak $\dot{V}O_2$ from 8 to 16 years[106,108] and a doubling of peak $\dot{V}O_2$ from 11 to 17/18 years[42,109] with the largest annual increases occurring between 13 and 15 years. It has been suggested that the greatest increase in boys' peak $\dot{V}O_2$ accompanies the attainment of peak height velocity (PHV)[108,112] but others[113] have noted a consistent growth in peak $\dot{V}O_2$ from 3 years before to 2 years after PHV.

Table 20.1 Longitudinal studies of peak $\dot{V}O_2$

Citation	Country	Age (years)	N	Mode of exercise	Peak $\dot{V}O_2$ (L·min⁻¹)
Boys					
Rutenfranz *et al.*[106]	Germany	12.7	28	CE	2.33 ± 0.32
		13.7	27	CE	2.50 ± 0.46
		14.7	26	CE	2.83 ± 0.49
		15.8	27	CE	3.05 ± 0.54
		16.7	23	CE	3.00 ± 0.34
		17.8	26	CE	3.11 ± 0.48
Rutenfranz *et al.*[106]	Norway	8.4	28	CE	1.44 ± 0.19
		9.4	29	CE	1.59 ± 0.24
		10.4	31	CE	2.03 ± 0.30
		11.4	29	CE	2.07 ± 0.30
		12.3	30	CE	2.31 ± 0.34
		13.3	29	CE	2.70 ± 0.51
		14.5	27	CE	2.82 ± 0.41
		15.3	27	CE	3.14 ± 0.38
Cunningham *et al.*[110]	Canada	10.8	62	CE	1.72 ± 0.38
		11.8	62	CE	1.90 ± 0.28
		12.8	62	CE	2.16 ± 0.40
		13.8	62	CE	2.58 ± 0.55
		14.8	62	CE	2.88 ± 0.51
Mirwald and Bailey[108]	Canada	8	75	TM	1.42 ± 0.21
		9	75	TM	1.60 ± 0.20
		10	75	TM	1.77 ± 0.22
		11	75	TM	1.93 ± 0.25
		12	75	TM	2.12 ± 0.29
		13	75	TM	2.35 ± 0.38
		14	75	TM	2.66 ± 0.46
		15	75	TM	2.98 ± 0.48
		16	75	TM	3.22 ± 0.45
Sprynarova *et al.*[109]	Czechoslovakia	11	90	TM	1.74 ± 0.23
		12	90	TM	2.02 ± 0.31
		13	90	TM	2.20 ± 0.35
		14	90	TM	2.76 ± 0.45
		15	90	TM	3.24 ± 0.47
		16	39	TM	3.38 ± 0.47
		17	39	TM	3.38 ± 0.48
		18	39	TM	3.53 ± 0.48

Table 20.1 *Continued*

Citation	Country	Age (years)	N	Mode of exercise	Peak $\dot{V}O_2$ (L·min^{-1})
Amsterdam Growth and Health Study (Van Mechelen, unpublished data)	The Netherlands	13	83	TM	2.66 ± 0.39
		14	80	TM	3.07 ± 0.48
		15	84	TM	3.37 ± 0.43
		16	79	TM	3.68 ± 0.52
Armstrong *et al.*[111] Armstrong and Welsman[42]	United Kingdom	11.2	119	TM	1.81 ± 0.26
		12.1	94	TM	2.11 ± 0.34
		13.1	93	TM	2.39 ± 0.44
		17.0	37	TM	3.55± 0.55
Girls					
Rutenfranz *et al.*[106]	Germany	12.7	24	CE	2.19 ± 0.30
		13.7	24	CE	2.20 ± 0.22
		14.7	22	CE	2.26 ± 0.26
		15.7	22	CE	2.18 ± 0.29
		16.7	17	CE	1.97 ± 0.31
		17.8	19	CE	2.06 ± 0.33
Rutenfranz *et al.*[106]	Norway	8.2	33	CE	1.25 ± 0.20
		9.3	33	CE	1.48 ± 0.19
		10.3	34	CE	1.79 ± 0.23
		11.2	34	CE	1.88 ± 0.22
		12.2	34	CE	2.26 ± 0.32
		13.3	33	CE	2.48 ± 0.46
		14.2	32	CE	2.35 ± 0.26
		15.2	30	CE	2.44 ± 0.30
Mirwald and Bailey[108]	Canada	8	22	TM	1.27 ± 0.14
		9	22	TM	1.39 ± 0.15
		10	22	TM	1.53 ± 0.20
		11	22	TM	1.72 ± 0.28
		12	22	TM	1.97 ± 0.36
		13	22	TM	2.20 ± 0.39
Amsterdam Growth and Health Study (Van Mechelen, unpublished data)	The Netherlands	13	97	TM	2.45 ± 0.31
		14	97	TM	2.60 ± 0.35
		15	96	TM	2.58 ± 0.34
		16	96	TM	2.65 ± 0.33
Armstrong *et al.*[111] Armstrong and Welsman[42]	United Kingdom	11.2	115	TM	1.63 ± 0.28
		12.2	88	TM	1.89 ± 0.29
		13.1	93	TM	2.10 ± 0.30
		17.0	26	TM	2.39 ± 0.40

Mode: CE is cycle ergometer, TM is treadmill. Peak $\dot{V}O_2$ values are mean ± standard deviation.

Girls' data are less clear and peak $\dot{V}O_2$ appears to progressively rise from 8 to 13 years and then level-off from about age 14 years. The English girls exhibited a 47% rise in aerobic fitness from 11 to 17 years whereas the German girls' peak $\dot{V}O_2$ declined from age 14.7 years through to 17.8 years where scores were below those 6 years earlier. This 'decrease' in aerobic fitness needs to be interpreted cautiously as it have might been an artefact of the motivation of the participants as the authors noted that some of the girls refused to take part in the tests at age 16 and 17 years. Dutch girls observed from 13 to 16 years exhibited a levelling-off, but not a reduction in aerobic fitness with only a 2% increase from 14 to 16 years. This is generally consistent with findings from cross-sectional studies.

Peak oxygen uptake and growth

Peak $\dot{V}O_2$ is strongly correlated with body size and coefficients describing its relationship with body mass or stature typically exceed $r = 0.70$ (see refs 16,114,115 and Chapter 2). Thus, much of the age-related increase in peak $\dot{V}O_2$ illustrated in Fig. 20.1 reflects the overall increase in body size during the transition from childhood through adolescence into young adulthood. Traditionally, researchers have attempted to control for body size differences by dividing peak $\dot{V}O_2$ by body mass and expressing it as the simple ratio mL·kg^{-1}·min^{-1} (ratio scaling). When peak $\dot{V}O_2$ is expressed in this manner a different picture emerges from that apparent when absolute values (L·min^{-1}) are used. Boys' mass-related peak $\dot{V}O_2$ remains essentially unchanged (at about 48–50 mL·kg^{-1}·min^{-1}) from 8 to 18 years, whilst in girls a progressive decline, from approximately 45 to 35 mL· kg^{-1}·min^{-1}, is apparent over this age range. Boys demonstrate higher mass-related peak $\dot{V}O_2$ than girls throughout childhood and adolescence with the sex difference being reinforced by the greater accumulation of body fat by girls during puberty.

The conventional use of mass-related values, however, might have clouded our understanding of peak $\dot{V}O_2$ during growth. Rather than removing the influence of body mass, ratio scaling 'overscales' favouring light children and penalizing heavy children. The underlying theory is addressed in detail in Chapter 2 where compelling arguments are presented to question the validity of simple ratio scaling to adequately remove the influence of body mass from size-dependent performance measures such as peak $\dot{V}O_2$.

Several studies have generated data illustrating how inappropriate ratio scaling has led to misplaced interpretation of physiological variables whereas studies in which the use of more appropriate means of controlling for body size have provided new insights into peak $\dot{V}O_2$ during growth. For instance, in an early exploration of scaling children's peak $\dot{V}O_2$, Williams *et al.*[116] used a linear regression model to investigate changes in peak $\dot{V}O_2$ with chronological age in two groups of boys aged 10 and 15 years. The mean values for peak $\dot{V}O_2$ were 1.73 L·min^{-1} and 3.12 L·min^{-1}, respectively, but when expressed as mass-related peak $\dot{V}O_2$ (i.e. ratio scaled) the two groups had identical values at 49 mL·kg^{-1}·min^{-1}. However, the regression lines for the relationship between peak $\dot{V}O_2$ and body mass described two clearly different populations with the older boys' peak $\dot{V}O_2$ when controlled for body mass higher than the younger boys' peak $\dot{V}O_2$. Intuitively, this appears appropriate and is in accordance with the observed differences in 11 and 15 year olds' performance in events dependent on aerobic fitness.

In a more sophisticated analysis, Welsman *et al.*[117] used both ratio and allometric (log-linear analysis of covariance) scaling to partition size effects from peak $\dot{V}O_2$ data in groups of males and females spanning the age range 11–23 years (see Table 20.2). The results of the traditional analyses conformed to the conventional interpretation described above, with mass-related peak $\dot{V}O_2$ consistent among the three male groups (11, 14, and 23 years) whilst in the females mass-related peak $\dot{V}O_2$ did not change from 11 to 13 years but there was a significant decrease in peak $\dot{V}O_2$ from 13 to 22 years. In direct contrast, allometric scaling revealed significant, progressive increases in peak $\dot{V}O_2$ across male groups suggesting that, relative to body size, aerobic fitness is, in fact, improving during growth rather than remaining static. In females, peak $\dot{V}O_2$ increased significantly from 11 to 13 years, subsequently remaining consistent with no decline into adulthood evident. These data clearly challenge the conventional interpretation of peak $\dot{V}O_2$ during growth in both boys and girls.

The application of allometry to longitudinal data is complex but its use is increasing and evidence to support the cross-sectional findings described above is accumulating. Multilevel modelling techniques (see ref. 118 and Chapter 2) represent a sensitive and flexible approach to the interpretation of longitudinal exercise data which enable body size, age, and sex effects to be partitioned concurrently within an allometric framework. Armstrong *et al.*[111] applied multilevel regression modelling to the interpretation of peak $\dot{V}O_2$ in 11- to 13-year-old boys and girls and founded the analysis on 590 peak $\dot{V}O_2$ determinations over three annual occasions. A multiplicative, allometric model was adopted based on the model originally proposed by Nevill *et al.*[119]:

$$\text{Peak } \dot{V}O_2\ (Y) = \text{mass}^{k_1} \cdot \text{stature}^{k_2} \cdot \exp(\alpha_j + b_j \cdot \text{age} + c \cdot \text{age}^2)\ \varepsilon_{ij}$$

where all parameters are fixed, with the exception of the constant (α, intercept term) and age parameters that were allowed to vary randomly at level 2 (between individuals), and the multiplicative

Table 20.2 Peak oxygen uptake in females and males in relation to body mass

	Prepubertal girls (Tanner stage 1) (n = 33)	Circumpubertal girls (Tanner stage 3/4) (n = 34)	Adult women (n = 16)
Females			
Age (years)	10.7 (0.2)†	13.0 (0.2)††	21.7 (2.8)
Body mass (kg)	32.7 (4.6)†	46.5 (9.6)††	60.5 (6.3)
Peak $\dot{V}O_2$ (L·min^{-1})	1.48 (0.2)†	2.14 (0.32)††	2.58 (0.26)
Ratio scaled peak $\dot{V}O_2$ (mL·kg^{-1}·min^{-1})	45 (3)	47 (4)†††	43 (3)
Allometrically adjusted peak $\dot{V}O_2$ (L·min^{-1})	1.99†	2.19††††	2.13
	Prepubertal boys (Tanner stage 1) (n = 29)	**Circumpubertal boys (Tanner stage 3/4) (n = 26)**	**Adult men (n = 18)**
Males			
Age (years)	10.7 (0.2)*	14.1 (0.3)**	22.8 (2.9)
Body mass (kg)	34.9 (5.4)*	49.5 (8.9)**	78.6 (8.7)
Peak $\dot{V}O_2$ (L·min^{-1})	1.76 (0.28)*	2.60 (0.47)**	4.18 (0.47)
Ratio scaled peak $\dot{V}O_2$ (mL·kg^{-1}·min^{-1})	50 (4)	53 (4)	53 (3)
Allometrically adjusted peak $\dot{V}O_2$ (L·min^{-1})	2.25*	2.50**	2.80

Values are mean (standard deviation). Level of significance $p < 0.05$.

†Significantly different from circumpubertal girls and adult women.

††Significantly different from prepubertal girls and adult women.

†††Significantly different from adult women.

††††Significantly different from prepubertal girls.

*Significantly different from circumpubertal boys and adult men.

**Significantly different from prepubertal boys and adult men.

Data from Welsman *et al.*[117]

error ratio ε that varies randomly at level 1, describing the error variance between occasions. The subscripts *i* and *j* denote this random variation at levels 1 and 2, respectively. The variable *age* was centred on the group mean age of 12.0 years.

In order to allow the unknown parameters to be solved using multilevel regression, the model was linearized by logarithmic transformation and multilevel regression analysis on $\log_e y$ used to solve for the unknown parameters. Once transformed, the equation above becomes

$$\text{Log}_e \text{ peak } \dot{V}O_2 (\log_e y) = k_1 \cdot \log_e \text{mass} + k_2 \cdot \log_e \text{stature} + \alpha_j + b_j \cdot \text{age} + c \cdot \text{age}^2 + \log_e(\varepsilon_{ij})$$

From this baseline model, the additional explanatory variable *sex* was incorporated as an indicator variable (i.e. sex, boys = 0; sex, girls = 1), which sets the boys' constant as the baseline from which the girls' parameter may deviate. The interaction term *age × sex* was constructed to investigate whether age effects on peak $\dot{V}O_2$ differed for boys and girls. Age was allowed to vary randomly at level 1 to investigate within individual variation around the individual growth trajectory. The need to allow each individual their own mass exponent was examined by letting body mass vary at level 2. The model is presented in Table 20.3.

The multilevel regression model reveals stature and body mass as significant covariates with an additional significant positive effect for age, which is larger for boys than girls as reflected by the significant age by sex interaction term. Girls' peak $\dot{V}O_2$ is significantly lower than boys' peak $\dot{V}O_2$, as indicated by the negative term for sex. These findings confirm the cross-sectional data and show that, in conflict with the (ratio scaling) conventional interpretation, there is a progressive increase in peak $\dot{V}O_2$ in both sexes independent of the influence of body size. With body size appropriately controlled, peak $\dot{V}O_2$ is higher in boys than in girls and sex differences increase during growth.

Table 20.3 Multilevel regression model for peak $\dot{V}O_2$ in 11- to 13-year-old boys and girls

Parameters	Estimate (SE)
Fixed	
Constant	−1.3903 (0.0970)
Log_e mass	0.5011 (0.0322)
Log_e stature	0.9479 (0.1162)
Age	0.0585 (0.0111)
Sex	−0.1378 (0.0093)
Age · sex	−0.0134 (0.0068)
Random	
Level 2	
Constant	0.0042 (0.0005)
Age	0.0007 (0.0003)
Covariance	NS
Level 1	
Constant	0.0030 (0.0004)

N = 590. NS = not significant.
Data from Armstrong *et al.*[111]

Peak oxygen uptake and maturation

As young people grow they also mature and the physiological responses of adolescents must be considered in relation to biological as well as chronological age. Relatively few studies have investigated peak $\dot{V}O_2$ in relation to maturation, perhaps because of the problems associated with the assessment of maturation. In paediatric exercise science, maturation is usually assessed using indicators of skeletal, sexual or somatic maturation or serum hormone concentrations. No single assessment gives a complete description of the tempo of maturation but there is reasonably high concordance between them (see refs 120,121 and Chapter 3).

Some studies indicate an adolescent growth spurt in peak $\dot{V}O_2$ in boys, with the spurt reaching a maximum gain near the time of PHV, but secure data are insufficient to offer any generalization for girls.[111] Several studies have reported that peak $\dot{V}O_2$ increases with maturation markers such as skeletal age or serum testosterone concentration but subsequent multiple regression analyses have revealed that chronological age, stature, and body mass explain most of the variation in peak $\dot{V}O_2$ with indicators of maturation not making a significant additional contribution.[122–124] Similarly, with stage of maturation classified as described by Tanner,[125] more mature subjects have been reported to have a higher peak $\dot{V}O_2$ in $\text{L}\cdot\text{min}^{-1}$ than less mature subjects but mass-related peak $\dot{V}O_2$ ($\text{mL}\cdot\text{kg}^{-1}\cdot\text{min}^{-1}$) has been reported to be unrelated to stage of maturation, indicating no additional effect of maturation on peak $\dot{V}O_2$ above that due to growth.[40,126]

Armstrong *et al.*[41] argued that the true relationship between peak $\dot{V}O_2$ and maturation may have been obscured through an inappropriate means of controlling for body mass. They determined the peak $\dot{V}O_2$ of one hundred and seventy-six 12 year olds and classified them according to the stages of maturation described by Tanner. In accordance with the extant literature, mass-related peak $\dot{V}O_2$ ($\text{mL}\cdot\text{kg}^{-1}\cdot\text{min}^{-1}$) was not significantly different across stages of maturation in both boys and girls whereas when body mass was controlled using allometry (log-linear analysis of covariance with mass as the covariate) peak $\dot{V}O_2$ was demonstrated to significantly increase with maturation in both sexes. None of the children was classified as stage 5, but boys in maturation stage 4 exhibited peak $\dot{V}O_2$ values 14% higher than similarly aged boys in stage 1. The corresponding difference in girls was 12%, thus demonstrating that in both boys and girls there is a significant additional effect of maturation on peak $\dot{V}O_2$ above that due to age and growth.

Armstrong and Welsman[42] introduced the same criterion of maturation into their multilevel regression model of 11–17 year olds and confirmed their earlier findings on 11–13 year olds[110] by showing incremental effects of stage of maturation on peak $\dot{V}O_2$ independent of chronological age and body mass (Table 20.4). The positive effect of maturation on aerobic fitness was consistent for both boys and girls. When skinfold thicknesses were introduced into the model, the stage of maturation remained a significant covariate, in all but stage 5, but the magnitudes of the effect were reduced, indicating the relationship between maturation and LBM. With body mass, skinfold thicknesses, and maturation accounted for peak $\dot{V}O_2$ was shown to increase with age throughout the age range studied in both sexes. The girls' data are noteworthy as earlier longitudinal studies suggested little change in females' peak $\dot{V}O_2$ from about age 14 years. Armstrong and Welsman concluded that fat-free mass was the predominant influence in the increase in peak

Table 20.4 Multilevel regression model for peak $\dot{V}O_2$ in 11- to 17-year-old boys and girls

Fixed	Estimate (SE)
Fixed	
Constant	−1.9005 (0.1400)
Log_e mass	0.8752 (0.0432)
Log_e stature	NS
Log_e skinfolds	−0.1656 (0.0174)
Age	−0.0470 (0.0094)
Sex	−0.1372 (0.0121)
Age · sex	−0.0214 (0.0053)
Maturity 2	0.0341 (0.0094)
Maturity 3	0.0361 (0.0102)
Maturity 4	0.0537 (0.0116)
Maturity 5	NS
Random	
Level 2	
Constant	0.0030 (0.0005)
Age	0.0004 (0.0001)
Level 1	
Constant	0.0032 (0.0004)

N = 388. NS = not significant.

Data from Armstrong and Welsman.[42]

$\dot{V}O_2$ through adolescence but both chronological age and stage of maturation were additional explanatory variables, independent of body size and fatness.

The results of the studies described herein provide convincing evidence that, with body size appropriately controlled, peak $\dot{V}O_2$ increases progressively in boys throughout childhood and adolescence into young adulthood and in girls peak $\dot{V}O_2$ increases at least into puberty and possibly into young adulthood. The maturational process itself induces increases in aerobic fitness over and above those explained by body size, body composition, and age. These patterns of change, although contrasting with the conventional interpretation of peak $\dot{V}O_2$ appear wholly consistent with the growth of the underlying physiological processes described in Chapters 12, 16, 18, and 19.

Peak oxygen uptake and sex

Boys' peak $\dot{V}O_2$ values are consistently higher than those of girls by late childhood and the sex difference becomes more pronounced as young people progress through adolescence. The data presented in Fig. 20.1 indicate that peak $\dot{V}O_2$ is 12% higher in boys than in girls at age 10 years, increasing to 23% higher at 12, 31% higher at 14, and 37% higher at 16 years of age. Longitudinal data (see Table 20.1) support this trend although with relatively small samples there is some variation in reported sex differences within the age range 12–14 years, which is most probably due to individual variations in rate of growth and maturation. These sex differences in peak $\dot{V}O_2$ during adolescence have been attributed to a combination of factors including differences in habitual physical activity, body composition, and blood haemoglobin concentration.

Boys are generally more physically active than girls,[17,18,127] but the evidence relating habitual physical activity to young people's peak $\dot{V}O_2$ is weak[128–130] and the issue is confounded by problems with accurately assessing children's and adolescents' physical activity patterns (see refs 17,21,131 and Chapter 10). However, both boys' and girls' current physical activity patterns demonstrate that they rarely experience the intensity, frequency, and duration of physical activity associated with increases in peak $\dot{V}O_2$ (e.g. compare habitual physical activity data reported in refs 132,133 with the volume of exercise required to increase peak $\dot{V}O_2$ as reviewed in refs 134,135 and see Chapters 10 and 39). Habitual physical activity is therefore unlikely to contribute to sex differences in peak $\dot{V}O_2$.

Muscle mass increases through childhood and adolescence but although boys generally have more muscle mass than girls marked sex differences do not become apparent until the adolescent growth spurt. Girls experience an adolescent growth spurt in muscle mass but it is less dramatic than that of boys. Between 5 and 16 years boys' relative muscle mass increases from 42% to 54% of body mass whereas in girls muscle mass increases from 40% to 45% of body mass between 5 and 13 years and then, in relative terms, it declines due to an increase in fat accumulation during adolescence. Girls have slightly more body fat than boys during childhood but during the adolescent growth spurt, girls' body fat increases to about 25% of body mass while boys decline to about 12–14% of body fat (see ref. 92 and Chapter 12). These dramatic changes in body composition during puberty contribute to the progressive increase in sex differences in peak $\dot{V}O_2$ over this period. Boys' greater muscle mass not only facilitates the use of oxygen during exercise but also supplements the venous return to the heart, and therefore augments stroke volume, through the peripheral muscle pump (see ref. 136 and Chapter 19). Armstrong and Welsman's[42] multilevel regression model (Table 20.4) demonstrated that the introduction of sum of triceps and subscapular skinfold thicknesses to the baseline model, incorporating body mass, stature, and age, reduced the sex difference in peak $\dot{V}O_2$ but could not explain fully the greater increase in boys' peak $\dot{V}O_2$ with growth. However, the authors concluded that sex, age, and maturational differences in the increase in fat-free mass relative to body mass are the predominant influences on the differential growth of boys' and girls' peak $\dot{V}O_2$ during the age range 11–17 years.[42]

During puberty, there is a marked increase in haemoglobin concentration and hence oxygen-carrying capacity in boys whereas girls' values plateau in their mid-teens.[67] It might therefore be expected that differences in haemoglobin levels between boys and girls, which are about 11% at 16 years, would be a contributory factor to the observed sex difference in peak $\dot{V}O_2$ during the late-teens.[40,122,137] However, when haemoglobin concentration was investigated longitudinally as an additional explanatory variable, to body mass, stature, skinfold thicknesses, age, and maturity, in a multilevel regression model of peak $\dot{V}O_2$ a non-significant parameter estimate was obtained with 11–17 year olds.[42]

Before puberty, there are only small sex differences in muscle mass and haemoglobin concentration, but even with body size controlled for, prepubertal boys have consistently been demonstrated to have higher peak $\dot{V}O_2$ than prepubertal girls.[36,138,139] For example, in a large, representative sample (n = 164) of 11-year-old prepubertal children, a 21.9% higher peak $\dot{V}O_2$ in boys than in girls was observed.[36] With the removal of the influence of body mass using a log-linear adjustment model, the boys' peak $\dot{V}O_2$ remained significantly higher than the girls' (16.2%) despite there being no sex difference in either skinfold thicknesses or haemoglobin concentration.

Why prepubertal boys have significantly higher values of peak $\dot{V}O_2$ than girls is not readily apparent but the explanation might lie in the Fick equation. There is no evidence to indicate sex differences in maximal HR but boys have been observed to have higher maximal SV[140] and therefore higher $\dot{Q}$ max, although there are conflicting data.[66] The trend for boys to have higher stroke volumes during exercise has been attributed to their greater heart mass (or size) in relation to body mass or size[141–143] but conflicting data indicating no sex differences in relative heart size are available.[144–146] Exercise stroke volume is, however, not just a function of ventricular size and it is difficult to distinguish between the complex and interrelated effects of ventricular preload, myocardial contractility, and ventricular afterload.

Two recent studies have addressed the topic using Doppler echocardiography (see Chapter 7) but although there were common findings the authors' interpretation of their data is conflicting. Rowland *et al.*[52] determined the maximal SV (SVmax) of 25 prepubertal boys and 24 premenarcheal girls aged 12 years. The girls were taller and fatter than the boys but there were no significant differences in LBM. No significant sex differences in maximal a-v O_2 dif or HR were reported but the boys demonstrated significantly higher SVmax (4.9%) than the girls. Stroke volume expressed in ratio with LBM was 5.2% higher in boys and when allometrically normalized to LBM the sex difference was 5.1%. On the basis of these findings, the authors suggested that factors such as systemic vascular resistance, adrenergic responses, and skeletal muscle pump function are most probably responsible for sex differences in SVmax than intrinsic ventricular size differences.

Vinet *et al.*[44] determined the SVmax of 18 boys and 17 girls, mean age 10.5 years. They observed no significant sex differences in stature, body mass, or haemoglobin concentration but LBM was higher in the boys. No significant sex differences in maximal a-v O_2 dif or HR were observed but the boys had significantly higher SVmax (18.9%) than the girls. When SVmax was controlled for LBM using allometry, the sex difference of 4.8% was no longer significant. Vinet *et al.*, therefore, concluded that cardiac size rather than function explains boys' greater SVmax.

There are few secure data on young children's a-v O_2 dif at peak $\dot{V}O_2$ but a recent exploratory study,[66] which used thoracic bioelectrical impedance to determine the $\dot{Q}$ at peak $\dot{V}O_2$, of 18 male and 13 female 10 year olds has provided some interesting insights into prepubertal differences in peak $\dot{V}O_2$. The boys had a significantly higher mean peak $\dot{V}O_2$ than the girls (18.7%) but no significant sex difference in stature, body mass, LBM, body fat %, body mass index, body surface area, blood haemoglobin concentration, HR at peak $\dot{V}O_2$, RER at peak $\dot{V}O_2$, SV at peak $\dot{V}O_2$, or $\dot{Q}$ at peak $\dot{V}O_2$ (mean values, 10.0 $L \cdot min^{-1}$ for both sexes) was observed. Furthermore, heart size variables determined at rest using magnetic resonance imaging (MRI) revealed no significant sex differences in left ventricular muscle mass, left ventricular muscle volume, posterior wall thickness, septal wall thickness, left ventricular end-diastolic chamber volume, or left ventricular end-systolic chamber volume. The only significant sex difference was in a-v O_2 dif at peak $\dot{V}O_2$ where the boys' values were, on average, 16.7% higher than those of the girls.

Secular trends in peak oxygen uptake

No studies have specifically addressed secular trends in directly determined peak $\dot{V}O_2$ but scrutiny of children's peak $\dot{V}O_2$ values from Europe and North America over the past 50–70 years reveals a remarkable consistency in aerobic fitness over time despite wide interstudy variation in the determination of peak $\dot{V}O_2$ (see ref. 16 and Table 20.1).

Eisenmann and Malina[147,148] examined secular change in the peak $\dot{V}O_2$ of samples of US children and adolescents using available data from a wide range of studies in the twentieth century. They concluded that from the 1930s to 2000, values (in $L \cdot min^{-1}$) have remained stable amongst boys aged 6–11 years and increased in boys aged 12–18 years. Corresponding data for girls indicate no change from the 1970s in girls aged 6–11 years and no change from the 1960s in girls aged 12–14 years. Amongst girls aged 15–18 years peak $\dot{V}O_2$ appears to have increased from the early 1960s to the late 1970s and then declined into the late 1990s. However, published values of peak $\dot{V}O_2$ are not necessarily population representative values and the data could be interpreted as suggesting that the peak $\dot{V}O_2$ of boys and girls volunteering for exercise tests has not changed much over the past 5–7 decades.

In contrast, data from performance tests have consistently indicated a secular decrease in aerobic performance (see refs 149–151 and Chapter 9). For example, Tomkinson *et al.*[152] analysed 55 studies of young people's 20-m shuttle run performance (see Chapter 9) in 11 countries, over the period 1980–2000. There was a great deal of variability between countries but when sample-weighted, mean rates of change were calculated for age groups rather than for countries, a more consistent trend was revealed with a reduction in aerobic performance of about 0.5% per year in children and 1% annually in adolescents. The authors noted, however, that running performance can be reduced by increases in body fatness independent of aerobic fitness and that children and adolescents were fatter in 2000 than in 1980.

Three recently published studies from Scandinavia[153–155] used laboratory tests to predict young people's peak $\dot{V}O_2$ rather than directly determine it and investigated changes over time in the predicted variable. Ekblom *et al.*[153] used the Astrand–Ryhming nomogram[1] to predict the peak $\dot{V}O_2$ ($mL \cdot kg^{-1} \cdot min^{-1}$) of Swedish 10, 13, and 16 year olds in 1987 and 2001. The initial study included 538 boys and 415 girls and the second observation involved 503 boys and 408 girls. The boys' peak $\dot{V}O_2$ was reported to decline by 12% but no significant change was observed in girls' predicted peak $\dot{V}O_2$.

Wedderkop *et al.*[154] analysed secular trends in predicted peak $\dot{V}O_2$ through two cross-sectional surveys, performed 12 years apart, of representative samples of 9-year-old children from Odense, Denmark. In 1985–1986, 670 girls and 699 boys participated and in 1997–1998, 310 girls and 279 boys participated. On both occasions fitness was determined by a maximal work test (watt-max test) which involved exercising to exhaustion on a cycle ergometer. The watt-max test was validated against directly determined peak $\dot{V}O_2$ and regression equations were used to predict peak $\dot{V}O_2$ in $mL \cdot kg^{-1} \cdot min^{-1}$ from watt-max data. The boys in 1997–1998 had a lower fitness level and a higher fat percentage than those in 1985–1986, whereas no overall differences in fitness or fatness were found between girls in 1997–1998 and 1985–1986. The same group[155] extended the study by testing 259 girls and 199 boys in 2003–2004 and reported no further change in boys' predicted peak $\dot{V}O_2$ but a significant 2.8% decline in girls' values.

Wedderkop *et al.*[154] split their sample into deciles and observed that in 1997–1998, the fittest boys had the same level of fitness as the fittest boys in 1985–1986, and the fittest girls had a significantly higher level of fitness in 1997–1998 than the fittest girls in 1985–1986. Whereas, both the boys and girls with the lowest fitness levels in 1997–1998 had significantly lower fitness than the least fit children in 1985–1986. The authors noted that the difference between the least fit and the most fit increased over time in both girls and boys. In boys, the difference between the top 10% and the lowest 10% was 38% in 1985–1986 and 45% in 1997–1998. The same polarization was found in girls, with a difference between the upper and lower deciles of 37% in 1985–1986 and 44% in 1987–1988. However, the decrease in predicted peak $\dot{V}O_2$ (mL·kg^{-1}·min^{-1}) from 1985–1986 to 1997–1998 in the least fit was partly explained by a higher body mass.

Secular trends in predicted peak $\dot{V}O_2$ expressed in ratio with body mass need to be interpreted cautiously as they may be a reflection of the rise in body mass and fatness over the past 20 years[156] rather than a true decline in peak $\dot{V}O_2$. However, it appears that the secular increase in body mass is not being accompanied by a corresponding increase in peak $\dot{V}O_2$, with the inevitable result that in high intensity activities which require moving body mass young people's aerobic performance is declining.

Summary

- Aerobic fitness can be defined as the ability to deliver oxygen to the exercising muscles and to utilize it to generate energy during exercise. The best single indicator of young people's aerobic fitness is peak $\dot{V}O_2$.
- Boys' peak $\dot{V}O_2$ expressed in L·min^{-1} increases in an almost linear manner from childhood, through adolescence and into young adulthood. Girls' data demonstrate a similar but less consistent trend with several (but not all) cross-sectional and longitudinal studies indicating a tendency for peak $\dot{V}O_2$ to plateau from about 14 years of age. Prepubertal boys' peak $\dot{V}O_2$ is higher than those of girls and the sex difference increases with age.
- Peak $\dot{V}O_2$ is strongly correlated with body size and much of the age-related increase in aerobic fitness reflects the increase in body size during growth. To control for body size, researchers have conventionally divided peak $\dot{V}O_2$ by body mass and expressed it in mL· kg^{-1}·min^{-1}. When peak $\dot{V}O_2$ is expressed in this manner a different picture emerges from that apparent when absolute values (L·min^{-1}) are used. Boys' mass-related peak $\dot{V}O_2$ is remarkably consistent from 8 to 18 years whilst in girls a progressive decline is often apparent over this age range. This outcome is a result of simply dividing peak $\dot{V}O_2$ by body mass which 'overscales' and therefore favours light subjects and penalizes heavy subjects.
- The use of ratio scaling (mL ·kg^{-1}·min^{-1}) has clouded our understanding of peak $\dot{V}O_2$ during growth. Allometrically scaled data have demonstrated that with age there is a progressive increase in peak $\dot{V}O_2$ in both sexes independent of the influence of body size. Even with body size appropriately controlled, peak $\dot{V}O_2$ is higher in boys than in girls and the sex difference increases with growth.
- As young people grow they also mature and recent data have demonstrated that maturation exerts a significant and positive effect on peak $\dot{V}O_2$ above that due to age, body composition, and body mass.
- Regardless of how it is expressed peak $\dot{V}O_2$ is higher in boys than in girls, at least from about 10 years of age, and the sex difference becomes more pronounced as young people progress through adolescence. Prior to puberty boys appear to benefit from a higher SVmax than girls, but whether this is due to differences in heart size or function remains to be proven, and there is evidence to suggest that boys may also have greater a-v O_2 dif at peak $\dot{V}O_2$ than girls although this requires further substantiation. As boys move through adolescence they are advantaged further by an increasingly greater muscle mass than girls. Greater haemoglobin concentration might augment boys' peak $\dot{V}O_2$ from mid- to late-teens but empirical evidence is equivocal.
- The directly determined peak $\dot{V}O_2$ of young people, particularly boys, who volunteer for exercise tests appears to have remained relatively stable over 50–70 years. However, less secure data from aerobic performance tests and predictions of peak $\dot{V}O_2$ (in mL·kg^{-1}·min^{-1}) indicate a secular decline in aerobic fitness and an emerging polarization with the difference between the fittest and the least fit children increasing over time. These findings generally reflect the secular increase in children's body fatness and indicate that peak $\dot{V}O_2$ is not increasing in line with body fatness and that young people's performance in aerobic activities involving the transport of body mass is therefore declining.

References

1. Astrand PO, Rodahl K (1986). *Textbook of work physiology*. McGraw-Hill, New York.
2. American College of Sports Medicine (1995). *ACSM's guidelines for exercise testing and prescription*. Williams and Wilkins, Baltimore, MD.
3. Shephard RJ (1984). Tests of maximum oxygen intake. A critical review. *Sports Med* **1**, 99–124.
4. Howley ET, Bassett DR, Welch HG (1995). Criteria for maximal oxygen uptake: Review and commentary. *Med Sci Sports Exerc* **27**, 1292–301.
5. Noakes TD (1988). Implications of exercise testing for prediction of athletic performance: A contemporary perspective. *Med Sci Sports Exerc* **20**, 319–30.
6. Noakes TD (1997). Challenging beliefs: Ex Africa semper aliquid novi. *Med Sci Sports Exerc* **29**, 571–90.
7. Myers J, Walsh D, Buchanan N, Froelicher VF (1989). Can maximal cardiopulmonary capacity be recognised by a plateau in oxygen uptake? *Chest* **96**, 1312–16.
8. Myers J, Walsh D, Sullivan M, Froelicher V (1990). Effect of sampling on variability and plateau in oxygen uptake. *J Appl Physiol* **68**, 404–10.
9. Bassett DR, Howley ET (1997). Maximal oxygen uptake: 'Classical' versus 'contemporary' viewpoints. *Med Sci Sports Exerc* **29**, 591–603.
10. Noakes TD (1998). Maximal oxygen uptake: 'Classical' versus 'contemporary' viewpoints: A rebuttal. *Med Sci Sports Exerc* **30**, 1381–98.
11. Astrand PO (1952). *Experimental studies of physical working capacity in relation to sex and age*. Munksgaard, Copenhagen.

12. Armstrong N, Welsman J, Winsley R (1996). Is peak $\dot{V}O_2$ a maximal index of children's aerobic fitness? *Int J Sports Med* **17**, 356–9.
13. Rowland TW (1993). Does peak $\dot{V}O_2$ reflect $\dot{V}O_2$ max in children? Evidence from supramaximal testing. *Med Sci Sports Exerc* **25**, 689–93.
14. Armstrong N, Davies, B (1981). An ergometric analysis of age group swimmers. *Br J Sports Med* **15**, 20–6.
15. Armstrong N, Davies B (1984). The metabolic and physiological responses of children to exercise and training. *Phys Educ Rev* **7**, 90–105.
16. Armstrong N, Welsman JR (1994). Assessment and interpretation of aerobic fitness in children and adolescents. *Exerc Sport Sci Rev* **22**, 435–76.
17. Armstrong N, Welsman JR (2006). The physical activity patterns of European youth with reference to methods of assessment. *Sports Med* **36**, 1067–86.
18. Riddoch CJ, Boreham CA (1995). The health-related physical activity of children. *Sports Med* **19**, 86–102.
19. Fawkner SG, Armstrong N (2003). Oxygen uptake kinetic response to exercise in children. *Sports Med* **33**, 651–69.
20. Barstow TJ, Scheuermann BW (2005). Effects of maturation and ageing on $\dot{V}O_2$ kinetics. In: Jones AM, Poole DC (eds.), *Oxygen uptake kinetics in sport, exercise and medicine*, pp. 331–52. Routledge, London.
21. Fawkner SG, Armstrong N (2006). Oxygen uptake kinetics. In Armstrong N (ed.), *Paediatric exercise physiology*, pp. 189–212. Churchill Livingstone, Edinburgh.
22. Armstrong N, Welsman JR (1996). *Young people and physical activity*. Oxford University Press, Oxford.
23. Robinson S (1938). Experimental studies of physical fitness in relation to age. *Arbeitsphysiologie* **10**, 251–323.
24. Morse M, Schlutz FW, Cassels DE (1949). Relation of age to physiological responses of the older boy to exercise. *J Appl Physiol* **1**, 683–709.
25. Rutenfranz J, Andersen KL, Seliger V, Klimmer F, Ilmarinen J, Ruppel M, Kylian H (1981). Exercise ventilation during the growth spurt period: Comparison between two European countries. *Eur J Pediatr* **136**, 135–42.
26. Mercier J, Varray A, Ramonatxo M, Mercier B, Prefaut C (1991). Influence of anthropometric characteristics on changes in maximal exercise ventilation and breathing pattern growth in boys. *Eur J Appl Physiol* **63**, 235–41.
27. Rowland TW, Green GM (1990). The influence of biologic maturation and aerobic fitness on ventilatory responses to treadmill exercise. In: Dotson CO, Humphrey JH (eds.), *Exercise physiology. Current selected research*, pp. 51–9. AMS Press, New York.
28. Armstrong N, Kirby BJ, McManus AM, Welsman JR (1997). Prepubescents' ventilatory responses to exercise with reference to sex and body size. *Chest* **112**, 1554–60.
29. Armstrong N, Kirby BJ, Mosney JR, Sutton NC, Welsman JR (1997). Ventilatory responses to exercise in relation to sex and maturation. In: Armstrong N, Kirby BJ, Welsman JR (eds.), *Children and exercise XIX: Promoting health and well-being*, pp. 204–10. E and FN Spon, London.
30. Rowland TW, Cunningham LN (1997). Development of ventilatory responses to exercise in normal caucasian children: A longitudinal study. *Chest* **111**, 337–42.
31. Boileau RA, Bonen A, Heyward VH, Massey BH (1977). Maximal aerobic capacity on the treadmill and bicycle ergometer of boys 11–14 years of age. *J Sports Med Phys Fitness* **17**, 153–62.
32. Bloxham SR, Welsman JR, Armstrong N (2005). Ergometer-specific relationships between peak oxygen uptake and short-term power output in children. *Pediatr Exerc Sci* **17**, 136–48.
33. Cumming GR, Langford S (1985). Comparison of nine exercise tests used in pediatric cardiology. In Binkhorst RA, Kemper HCG, Saris WHM (eds.), *Children and exercise XI*, pp. 58–68. Human Kinetics, Champaign, IL.
34. Sheehan JM, Rowland TW, Burke EJ (1987). A comparison of four treadmill protocols for determination of maximal oxygen uptake in 10 to 12 year old boys. *Int J Sports Med* **8**, 31–4.
35. Armstrong N, Balding J, Gentle P, Williams J, Kirby B (1990). Peak oxygen uptake and physical activity in 11 to 16 year olds. *Pediatr Exerc Sci* **2**, 349–58.
36. Armstrong N, Kirby BJ, McManus AM, Welsman JR (1995). Aerobic fitness of pre-pubescent children. *Ann Hum Biol* **22**, 427–41.
37. Turley KR, Rogers DM, Harper KM, Kujawa KI, Wilmore JH (1995). Maximal treadmill versus cycle ergometry testing in children: Differences, reliability, and variability of responses. *Pediatr Exerc Sci* **7**, 49–60.
38. Bailey DA, Ross WD (1978). Size dissociation of maximal aerobic power during growth in boys. *Med Sport* **11**, 140–51.
39. Bale P (1981). Pre- and post-adolescents' physiological response to exercise. *Br J Sports Med* **15**, 246–9.
40. Armstrong N, Williams J, Balding J, Gentle P, Kirby B (1991). The peak oxygen uptake of British children with reference to age, sex and sexual maturity. *Eur J Appl Physiol* **62**, 369–75.
41. Armstrong N, Welsman JR, Kirby BJ (1998). Peak oxygen uptake and maturation in 12-year-olds. *Med Sci Sports Exerc* **30**, 165–9.
42. Armstrong N, Welsman JR (2001). Peak oxygen uptake in relation to growth and maturation. *Eur J Appl Physiol* **28**, 259–65.
43. Andersen KL, Seliger V, Rutenfranz J, Skrobak-Kaczynski J (1976). Physical performance capacity of children in Norway. Part IV—The rate of growth in maximal aerobic power and the influence of improved physical education of children in a rural community. *Eur J Appl Physiol* **35**, 49–58.
44. Vinet A, Mandigout S, Nottin S, Nguyen L-D, Lecoq A-M, Courteix D, Obert P (2003). Influence of body composition, hemoglobin concentration, and cardiac size and function on gender differences in maximal oxygen uptake in prepubertal children. *Chest* **124**, 1494–9.
45. Washington RL (1993). Measurement of cardiac output. In: Rowland TW (ed.), *Pediatric exercise testing*, pp. 131–40. Human Kinetics, Champaign, IL.
46. Driscoll DJ, Staats BA, Beck KC (1989). Measurement of cardiac output in children during exercise: A review. *Pediatr Exerc Sci* **1**, 102–15.
47. Eriksson BO, Grimby G, Saltin B (1971). Cardiac output and arterial blood gases during exercise in pubertal boys. *J Appl Physiol* **31**, 348–52.
48. Rowland T, Popowski B, Ferrone L (1997). Cardiac responses to maximal upright cycling exercise in healthy boys and men. *Med Sci Sport Exerc* **29**, 1146–51.
49. Nottin S, Agnes V, Stecken N, Nguyen L-D, Ounissi F, Lecoq A-M, Obert P (2002). Central and peripheral cardiovascular adaptations during maximal cycle exercise in boys and men. *Med Sci Sports Exerc* **33**, 456–63.
50. Armstrong N, Welsman JR (2002). Cardiovascular responses to submaximal treadmill running in 11–13 year olds. *Acta Paediatr Scand* **91**, 125–31.
51. Turley KR, Wilmore JH (1997). Cardiovascular responses to submaximal exercise in 7- to 9 year old boys and girls. *Med Sci Sports Exerc* **29**, 824–32.
52. Rowland T, Goff D, Martel L, Ferrone L, (2000). Influence of cardiac functional capacity on gender differences in maximal oxygen uptake in children. *Chest* **17**, 629–35.
53. Rowland T, Miller K, Vanderburgh P, Goff D, Martel L, Ferrone L (1999). Cardiovascular fitness in premenarchael girls and young women. *Int J Sports Med* **20**, 117–21.
54. Miyamura M, Honda Y (1973). Maximum cardiac output related to sex and age. *Japanese J Physiol* **23**, 645–56.
55. Vinet A, Nottin S, Lecoq A-M, Obert P (2002). Cardiovascular responses to progressive cycle exercise in healthy children and adults. *Int J Sports Med* **23**, 242–6.

56. Gilliam TB, Sady S, Thorland WG, Weltman AL (1977). Comparison of peak performance measures in children ages 6 to 8, 9 to 10, and 11 to 13 years. *Res Quart* **48**, 695–702.
57. Rowland TW (2007). Circulatory 'efficacy' during progressive aerobic exercise in children: Insights from the $\dot{Q}:\dot{V}O_2$ relationship. *Eur J Appl Physiol* **101**, 61–6.
58. Yamaji K, Miyashita M (1977). Oxygen transport system during exhaustive exercise in Japanese boys. *Eur J Appl Physiol* **36**, 93–9.
59. Obert P, Mandigout S, Nottin S, Vinet A, N'Guyen LD, Lecoq A-M (2005). Relationships between left ventricular morphology, diastolic function and oxygen carrying capacity and maximal oxygen uptake in children. *Int J Sports Med* **26**, 122–7.
60. Nottin S, Vinet A, Lecoq A-M, Guenon P, Obert P (2001). Test-retest reproducibility of submaximal and maximal cardiac output by Doppler echocardiography and CO_2 rebreathing in prepubertal children. *Pediatr Exerc Sci* **13**, 214–24.
61. Krovetz LJ, McLoughlin TG, Mitchell MB, Schiebler GL (1967). Hemodynamic findings in normal children. *Pediatr Res* **1**, 122–30.
62. Sproul A, Simpson E (1964). Stroke volume and related hemodynamic data in normal children. *Pediatrics* **33**, 912–18.
63. Potter CR, Armstrong N, Kirby BJ, Welsman JR (1997). An exploratory study of cardiac output responses to submaximal exercise. In: Armstrong N, Kirby BJ, Welsman JR (eds.), *Children and exercise XIX: Promoting health and well-being*, pp. 440–5. E and FN Spon, London.
64. Eriksson BO (1972). Physical training oxygen supply and muscle metabolism in 11–13 year old boys. *Acta Physiol Scand* **384**, 1–48.
65. Rowland TW, Staab J, Unnithan V, Siconolfi S (1988). Maximal cardiac responses in prepubertal and adult males. *Med Sci Sports Exerc* **20**, S332.
66. Winsley RJ, Armstrong N, Fulford J, Roberts A, Welsman JR (2007). Heart size, lean body mass and the sex difference in peak oxygen uptake in prepubertal children. *Acta Kinesiol Universit Tartu* **12** (Suppl.), 205–6.
67. Dallman PR, Siimes MA (1979). Percentile curves for hemoglobin and red cell volume in infancy and childhood. *Pediatrics* **94**, 26–31.
68. Hsia CCW (1998). Respiratory function of hemoglobin. *N Engl J Med* **338**, 239–46.
69. Koch G (1978). Muscle blood flow in prepubertal boys. *Med Sport* **11**, 39–46.
70. McArdle WD, Katch FI, Katch VL (1996). *Exercise physiology*. Williams and Wilkins, Baltimore, MD.
71. Cassels DE, Morse M (1962). *Cardiopulmonary data for children and young adults*. Thomas, Springfield, IL.
72. Kalafoutis A, Paterakis S, Koutselinis A, Spanos V (1976). Relationship between erythrocyte 2, 3-diphosphoglycerate and age in a normal population. *Clin Chem* **22**, 1918–19.
73. Pate RR, Barnes C, Miller W (1985). A physiological comparison of performance matched female and male distance runners. *Res Quart Exerc Sport* **56**, 245–50.
74. Macek M (1986). Aerobic and anaerobic energy output in children. In: Rutenfranz J, Mocellin R, Klimt F (eds.), *Children and exercise XII*, pp. 3–10. Human Kinetics, Champaign, IL.
75. Berg A, Keul J (1988). Biochemical changes during exercise in children. In: Malina RM (ed.), *Young athletes*, pp. 61–78. Human Kinetics, Champaign, IL.
76. Lehmann M, Keul J, Korsten-Reck U (1987). The influence of graduated treadmill exercise on plasma catecholamines, aerobic and anaerobic capacity in boys and adults. *Eur J Appl Physiol* **47**, 301–11.
77. Koch G (1974). Muscle blood flow after ischemic work and during bicycle ergometer work in boys aged 12 years. *Acta Paediatr Belg* **28**, 29–39.
78. Koch G (1980). Aerobic power, lung dimensions, ventilatory capacity and muscle blood flow in 12–16 year old boys with high physical activity. In: Berg K, Eriksson BO (eds.), *Children and exercise IX*, pp. 99–108. University Park Press, Baltimore, MD.
79. Eriksson BO, Gollnick PD, Saltin B (1973). Muscle metabolism and enzyme activities after training in boys 11–13 years old. *Acta Physiol Scand* **87**, 485–99.
80. Haralambie G (1982). Enzyme activities in skeletal muscle of 13–15 year old adolescents. *Bull Euro Physiopathol Resp* **18**, 65–74.
81. Berg A, Kim SS, Keul J (1986). Skeletal muscle enzyme activities in healthy young subjects. *Int J Sports Med* **7**, 236–9.
82. Lexell J, Sjostrom M, Nordlund A-S, Taylor AC (1992). Growth and development of human muscle: A quantitative morphological study of whole vastus lateralis from childhood to adult age. *Muscle Nerve* **15**, 404–9.
83. Oertel G (1988). Morphometric analysis of normal skeletal muscles in infancy, childhood and adolescence. An autopsy study. *J Neurol Sci* **88**, 303–13.
84. Glenmark B, Hedberg C, Jansson E (1992). Changes in muscle fibre type from adolescence to adulthood in women and men. *Acta Physiol Scand* **146**, 251–9.
85. Bell RD, MacDougall JD, Billeter R, Howald H (1980). Muscle fibre types and morphometric analysis of skeletal muscles in six year old children. *Med Sci Sports Exerc* **12**, 28–31.
86. Fawkner SG, Armstrong N (2004). Longitudinal changes in the kinetic response to heavy intensity exercise. *J Appl Physiol* **97**, 460–6.
87. Fawkner SG, Armstrong N, Potter CR, Welsman JR (2002). Oxygen uptake kinetics in children and adults after the onset of moderate intensity exercise. *J Sports Sci* **20**, 319–26.
88. Williams CA, Carter H, Jones AM, Doust JH (2001). Oxygen uptake kinetics during treadmill running in boys and men. *J Appl Physiol* **90**, 1700–6.
89. Armstrong N, Fawkner SG (2008). Non-invasive methods in paediatric exercise physiology. *Appl Physiol Nutr Metab* **33**, 402–10.
90. Krahenbuhl GS, Skinner JS, Kohrt WM (1985). Developmental aspects of maximal aerobic power in children. *Exerc Sport Sci Rev* **13**, 503–38.
91. Léger L (1996). Aerobic performance. In: Docherty D (ed.), *Measurement in pediatric exercise science*, pp. 183–223. Human Kinetics, Champaign, IL.
92. Shuleva KM, Hunter GR, Hester DJ, Dunaway DL (1990). Exercise oxygen uptake in 3-through 6 year old children. *Pediatr Exerc Sci* **2**, 130–9.
93. Malina RM, Bouchard C, Bar-Or O (2004). *Growth, maturation and physical activity*. Human Kinetics, Champaign, IL.
94. Bar-Or O, Rowland TW (2004). *Pediatric exercise medicine*. Human Kinetics, Champaign, IL.
95. Davies CTM, Barnes C, Godfrey S (1972). Body composition and maximal exercise performance in children. *Hum Biol* **44**, 195–214.
96. Saris WHM (1982). *Aerobic power and daily physical activity in children*. Kripps Repro, Meppel, The Netherlands.
97. Krahenbuhl GS, Pangrazi RP, Stone WJ, Morgan DW, Williams T (1989). Fractional utilization of maximal aerobic capacity in children 6 to 8 years of age. *Pediatr Exerc Sci* **1**, 271–7.
98. Fenster J, Freedson P, Washburn RA, Ellison RC (1989). The relationship between physical activity and peak $\dot{V}O_2$ in 6 to 8 year old children. *Pediatr Exerc Sci* **1**, 127–36.
99. Cumming GR (1967). Current levels of fitness. *Can Medl Assoc J* **88**, 351–5.
100. Yoshizawa S, Ishizaki T, Honda H (1977). Physical fitness of children aged 5 and 6 years. *J Hum Erg* **6**, 41–51.
101. Forster MA, Hunter GR, Hester DJ, Dunaway D, Shuleva K (1994). Aerobic capacity and grade-walking economy of children 5–9 years old: A longitudinal study. *Pediatr Exerc Sci* **6**, 31–8.
102. Eiberg S, Hasselstrom H, Gronfeldt V, Froberg K, Svensson J, Andersen LB (2005). Maximum oxygen uptake and objectively measured physical activity in Danish children 6–7 years of age: The Copenhagen school child intervention study. *Br J Sports Med* **39**, 725–30.
103. Chatterjee S, Banerjee PK, Chatterjee P, Maitra SR (1979). Aerobic capacity of young girls. *Indian J Med Res* **69**, 327–33.

104. Nakagawa A, Ishiko T (1970). Assessment of aerobic capacity with special reference to sex and age of junior and senior high school students in Japan. *Japanese J Physiol* **20**, 118–29.

105. Yoshizawa S (1972). A comparative study of aerobic work capacity in urban and rural adolescents. *J Hum Erg* **1**, 45–65.

106. Rutenfranz J, Andersen KL, Seliger V, Klimmer F, Berndt I, Ruppel M (1981). Maximum aerobic power and body composition during the puberty growth period: Similarities and differences between children of two European countries. *Eur J Pediatr* **136**, 123–33.

107. Kemper HCG (2004). Amsterdam growth and health longitudinal study. *Med Sport* **47**, 1–198.

108. Mirwald RL, Bailey DA (1986). *Maximal aerobic power*. Sports Dynamics, London, Ontario.

109. Sprynarova S, Parizkova J, Bunc V (1987). Relationships between body dimensions and resting and working oxygen consumption in boys aged 11 to 18 years. *Eur J Appl Physiol* **56**, 725–36.

110. Cunningham DA, Paterson DH, Blimkie CJR, Donner AP (1984). Development of cardiorespiratory function in circumpubertal boys: A longitudinal study. *J Appl Physiol* **56**, 302–7.

111. Armstrong N, Welsman JR, Nevill AM, Kirby BJ (1999). Modeling changes in peak $\dot{V}O_2$ in 11–13 year olds. *J Appl Physiol* **87**, 2230–6.

112. Beunen G, Malina RM (1988). Growth and physical performance relative to the timing of the adolescent spurt. *Exerc Sport Sci Rev* **16**, 503–40.

113. Cunningham DA, Paterson DH, Blimkie CJR (1984). The development of the cardiorespiratory system with growth and physical activity. In: Boileau RA (ed.), *Advances in pediatric sport sciences*, Vol. 1, pp. 85–116. Human Kinetics, Champaign, IL.

114. Welsman JR, Armstrong N (2000). Statistical techniques for interpreting body size-related exercise performance during growth. *Pediatr Exerc Sci* **12**, 112–27.

115. Welsman JR, Armstrong N (2006). Interpreting performance in relation to body size. In: Armstrong N (ed.), *Paediatric exercise physiology*, pp. 27–46. Churchill Livingstone, Edinburgh.

116. Williams JR, Armstrong N, Winter EM, Crichton N (1992). Changes in peak oxygen uptake with age and sexual maturation in boys: Physiological fact or statistical anomaly? In: Coudert J, Van Praagh E (eds.), *Pediatric work physiology*, pp. 35–7. Masson, Paris.

117. Welsman JR, Armstrong N, Kirby BJ, Nevill AM, Winter EM (1996). Scaling peak $\dot{V}O_2$ for differences in body size. *Med Sci Sports Exerc* **28**, 259–65.

118. Goldstein H, Rasbash J, Plewis I, Draper D, Browne W, Yang M, Woodhouse G, Healy M (1998). *A user's guide to MlwiN*. University of London, Institute of Education, London.

119. Nevill AM, Holder RL, Baxter-Jones A, Round JM, Jones DA (1998). Modeling developmental changes in strength and aerobic power in children. *J Appl Physiol* **84**, 963–70.

120. Beunen GP (1989). Biological age in pediatric exercise research. In: Bar-Or O (ed.), *Advances in pediatric sport sciences*, Vol. 3, pp. 1–40. Human Kinetics, Champaign, IL.

121. Malina RM (1988). Biological maturity status of young athletes. In: Malina R (ed.), *Young athletes*, pp. 121–40. Human Kinetics, Champaign, IL.

122. Kemper HCG, Verschuur R (1981). Maximal aerobic power in 13 and 14 year old teenagers in relation to biologic age. *Int J Sports Med* **2**, 97–100.

123. Shephard RJ, Lavallee H, Jecquier JC, LaBarre R, Rajic M, Beaucage C (1978). In: Shephard RJ, Lavellee H (eds.), *Physical fitness assessment—Principles, practice and application*, pp. 194–210. Thomas, Springfield, IL.

124. Welsman JR, Armstrong N, Kirky B (1994). Serum testosterone is not related to peak $\dot{V}O_2$ and submaximal blood lactate responses in 12–16 year old males. *Pediatr Exerc Sci* **6**, 120–7.

125. Tanner JM (1962). *Growth at adolescence* (2nd ed.). Blackwell, Oxford.

126. Fahey TD, Del Valle-Zuris A, Oehlsen G, Trieb M, Seymour J (1979). Pubertal stage differences in hormonal and hematological responses to maximal exercise in males. *J Appl Physiol* **46**, 823–7.

127. Armstrong N, Van Mechelen W (1998). Are young people fit and active? In Biddle S, Sallis J, Cavill N (eds.), *Young and active*, pp. 69–97. Health Education Authority, London.

128. Morrow JR, Freedson PS (1994). Relationship between habitual physical activity and aerobic fitness in adolescents. *Pediatr Exerc Sci* **6**, 315–29.

129. Armstrong N (1998). Physical fitness and physical activity during childhood and adolescence. In: Chan KM, Micheli L (eds.), pp. 50–75. *Sports and children*. Williams and Wilkins, Hong Kong.

130. Armstrong N (2006). Aerobic fitness. In: Armstrong N (ed.), *Paediatric exercise physiology*, pp. 161–88. Churchill Livingstone, Edinburgh.

131. Trost SG (2001). Objective measurement of physical activity in youth: Current issues and future directions. *Exerc Sport Sci Rev* **29**, 32–6.

132. Armstrong N, Balding J, Gentle P, Kirby B (1990). Patterns of physical activity among 11 to 16 year old British children. *BMJ* **301**, 203–5.

133. Bailey RC, Olsen J, Pepper SL, Porszasz J, Barstow TT, Cooper DM (1995). The level and tempo of children's physical activities: An observational study. *Med Sci Sports Exerc* **27**, 1033–41.

134. Armstrong N, Barrett, LA, Welsman JR (2007). Cardiorespiratory training during childhood and adolescence. *J Exerc Sci Physiotherapy* **3**, 67–75.

135. Rowland TW (1992). Trainability of the cardiorespiratory system during childhood. *Can J Sport Sci* **17**, 259–63.

136. Rowell LB, O'Leary DS, Kellogg DL (1996). Integration of cardiovascular control systems in dynamic exercise. In: Rowell LB, Shephard JT (eds.), *Handbook of physiology, exercise: Regulation and integration of multiple systems*, pp. 778–81. American Physiological Society, Bethesda, MD.

137. Cunningham DA, Paterson DH (1988). Physiological characteristics of young active boys. In: Brown EW, Branta CF (eds.), *Competitive sports for children and youth*, pp. 159–70. Human Kinetics, Champaign, IL.

138. Dencker M, Thorsson O, Karlsson MK, Linden C, Eiberg S, Wollmer P, Andresen LB (2007). Gender differences and determinants of aerobic fitness in children aged 8–11 years. *Eur J Appl Physiol* **99**, 19–26.

139. Washington RL, van Gundy JC, Cohen C, Sondheimer HM, Wolfe RR (1988). Normal aerobic and anaerobic exercise data for North American school-age children. *J Pediatr* **112**, 223–33.

140. Turley KR (1997). Cardiovascular responses to exercise in children. *Sports Med* **24**, 241–57.

141. Scholz DG, Kitzman DW, Hagen PT, Ilstrup DM, Edwards WD (1998). Age-related changes in normal human hearts during the first 10 decades of life. Part 1 (Growth): A quantitative anatomic study of 200 specimens from subjects birth to 19 years old. *Mayo Clin Proc* **63**, 126–36.

142. Nagasawa H, Arakaki Y, Yamada O, Nakajima T, Kamiya T (1996). Longitudinal observations of left ventricular end-diastolic dimension in children using echocardiography. *Pediatr Cardiol* **17**, 169–74.

143. Daniels SR, Meyer RA, Liang Y, Bove K (1988). Echocardiographically determined left ventricular mass index in normal children, adolescents and young adults. *J Am Coll Cardiol* **12**, 703–8.

144. Maresh MM (1948). Growth of the heart related to bodily growth during childhood and adolescence. *Pediatrics* **2**, 382–404.

145. Nidorf SM, Picard MH, Triulzi MO, Thomas JD, Newell J, King ME, Weyman AE (1992). New perspectives in the assessment of cardiac chamber dimensions during development and adulthood. *J Am Coll Cardiol* **19**, 938–88.

146. Gutin B, Owens S, Trieber F, Mensah G (1997). Exercise haemodynamics and left ventricular parameters in children. In: Armstrong N, Kirby B, Welsman J (eds.), *Children and exercise XIX: Promoting health and well-being*, pp. 460–4. E and FN Spon, London.

147. Eisenmann JC, Malina RM (2002). Secular trend in peak oxygen consumption among United States youth in the 20th century. *Am J Hum Biol* **14**, 699–706.

148. Malina RM (2007). Physical fitness of children and adolescents in the United States: Status and secular change. *Med Sport Sci* **50**, 67–90.

149. Westerstahl M, Barnekow-Bergkvist M, Hedberg G, Jansson E (2003). Secular trends in body dimensions and physical fitness among adolescents in Sweden from 1974 to 1985. *Scand J Med Sci Sports* **13**, 128–37.
150. Przeweda R, Dobosz J (2003). Growth and physical fitness of Polish youths in two successive decades. *J Sports Med Phys Fitness* **43**, 465–74.
151. Strel J, Kovac M, Jurak G (2004). *Study on young people's lifestyle and sedentariness and the role of sport in the context of education and as a means of restoring the balance*, pp. 3–38. University of Ljubjana, Ljubjana, Slovakia.
152. Tomkinson GR, Leger LA, Olds TS, Cazonia G (2003). Secular trends in the performance of children and adolescents (1980–2000). *Sports Med* **33**, 285–300.
153. Ekblom O, Oddson K, Ekblom B (2004). Health-related fitness in Swedish adolescents between 1987–2001. *Acta Paediatr* **93**, 681–6.
154. Wedderkop N, Froberg K, Hansen HS, Andresen LB (2004). Secular trends in physical fitness and obesity in Danish 9-year-old girls and boys: Odense School Child Study and Danish substudy of the European Youth Heart Study. *Scand J Med Sci Sports* **14**, 150–55.
155. Moller NC, Wedderkop N, Kristensen PL, Andersen LB, Froberg K (2006). Secular trends in cardiorespiratory fitness and body mass index in Danish children: The European Youth Heart Study. *Scand J Med Sci Sports* **16**, 1–6.
156. Livingstone MBE (2001). Childhood obesity in Europe: A growing concern. *Pub Health Nutr* **4**, 109–16.

CHAPTER 21

Locomotor economy

Don W. Morgan

Introduction

Mobility is a quintessential human activity that promotes health, well-being, and independence. Because nearly all locomotor activities are performed at less than maximal intensity, a useful index of the energy expenditure associated with movement is locomotor economy, defined as the mass-related oxygen consumption ($\dot{V}O_2$) for a given submaximal speed. To the extent that economy can be optimized, the ability to engage in locomotor activities without becoming unduly fatigued is improved, thus leading to better endurance performance in children and adults.[1–15] From a clinical standpoint, knowledge of variables known to influence locomotor economy would also be useful in designing and implementing therapeutic regimens aimed at reducing the metabolic cost of transport in physically challenged individuals.[16–22]

The intent of this review is to present and synthesize research findings related to various aspects of locomotor economy during the childhood and adolescent years. Because the majority of research has been conducted on walking and running, the material presented in this chapter will focus exclusively on these modes of gait. The review will conclude by proposing future research directions to guide sport scientists, coaches, and clinicians in their quest to understand the factors responsible for efficient locomotion in children, improve the athletic performance of youngsters, and enhance the functional mobility and quality of life of physically challenged youth.

Economy differences among children, adolescents, and adults

Tables 21.1 and 21.2 display cross-sectional and longitudinal comparisons of mass-based walking and running economy values among children, adolescents, and adults.[4,8,9,23–44] Data found in Table 21.1 reveal that children and adolescents are less economical than adults. Relative differences in walking economy, which are substantive when children and adults are compared, are more muted when $\dot{V}O_2$ values for adolescents and adults are examined. As shown in Table 21.2, younger children are also less economical than older children, with economy differences becoming more pronounced as the disparity in age widens.

The higher metabolic costs of paediatric locomotion may be attributable to a variety of factors. These include

(i) less efficient ventilation (as evidenced by a higher ventilatory equivalent for oxygen)[35,45];

(ii) faster stride rates[24,31,34,41,46,47];

(iii) immature gait patterns (e.g. shorter strides, greater stride-to-stride variability, less-developed temporal structure of gait fluctuations, less stable pattern of coordination of the arms and legs, greater displacement of the centre of mass, less extension of the hip, knee, and ankle during take-off, a greater distance between the heel and the buttock during the forward swing phase, lower height of the forward knee during take-off, a longer relative distance of the support foot in front of the centre of mass, less single-leg stance time, higher relative peak vertical ground reaction forces, higher total and net vertical impulses, and greater co-activation of lower extremity muscles)[36,48–56];

(iv) larger surface area to body mass ratio[24,31,57];

(v) shorter height[37,41];

(vi) decreased ability to store and recoil elastic energy in the legs[47,58];

(vii) an imbalance between body mass and leg muscle contraction speed[47,59];

(viii) more distal distribution of mass in the lower extremities[60,61]; and

(ix) a greater dependence on fat as a metabolic substrate and a diminished ability to utilize anaerobic energy sources.[54,62,63]

There are consistent levels of experimental support for the notion that differences in body size contribute to child–adult disparities in locomotor economy. For example, since each gram of muscle uses a set amount of energy for each step taken,[51,64,65] children would be expected to consume more oxygen than adolescents or adults at any walking or running speed, because their shorter legs would be required to turn over at a faster rate to cover a given distance. Support for this hypothesis is found in a number of human studies, wherein comparable economy values have been obtained for adults and children, as well as for younger and older children, when $\dot{V}O_2$ is expressed per stride ($mL{\cdot}kg^{-1}{\cdot}stride^{-1}$).[24,31,34,41,46,47] Similar

Table 21.1 Comparison of walking and running economy values between children and adults

Authors (references)	Age (years)		Sex	W/R	Speed ($m \cdot s^{-1}$)	$\dot{V}O_2$ ($mL \cdot kg^{-1} \cdot min^{-1}$)		% Diff
	Child	Adult				Child	Adult	
Armstrong *et al.*[23]	11.0	21.7	F	R	2.50	38.2	36.3	5.2
Ebbeling *et al.*[24]	9.5	20.0	M	W	75% of mean walk speed in 1-mile walk	19.7	15.0	31.3
Krahenbuhl *et al.*[25]	8.0	Y&M	M	R	2.90	45.5	35.3–40.2	13–29
Van Mechelen *et al.*[26]	13.0	21.0	M	R	2.22	37.6	30.3	24.1
	13.0	21.0	F	R	2.22	36.5	29.8	22.5
Maliszewski and Freedson[27]	9.8	25.0	M	R	2.67	40.6	34.9	16.3
Martinez and Haymes[28]	9.1	24.4	F	R	2.00	32.9	27.6	19.2
McCann and Adams[29]*	9.2	40.7	M/F	W	1.1	237	163	45.4
	15.5	40.7	M/F	W	1.1	182	163	11.7
McCann and Adams[30]**	10.3	35.4	M/F	R	2.23	35.5	30.5	16.4
	15.7	35.4	M/F	R	2.23	33.5	30.5	9.8
Rowland *et al.*[31]	11.6	29.2	M	R	2.67	49.5	40.0	23.8
Rowland *et al.*[32]	11.3	28.7	F	R	2.03	35.8	30.9	15.9
Turley and Wilmore[33]	7–9	18–26	M/F	W	1.34	19.3	12.8	50.8
	7–9	18–26	M/F	R	2.23	39.3	30.3	29.7
Unnithan and Eston[34]**	10.4	20.8	M	R	2.67	47.5	40.0	18.8

% diff = absolute percentage difference from adult value; W/R = walking or running trials; M/F = male and female; Y&M = young and middle-aged adults.

*$\dot{V}O_2$ in $mL \cdot kg^{-1} \cdot km^{-1}$.

**Data estimated from figures provided in the cited publication.

results have been reported when gait transport costs for children and adults are expressed relative to body surface area (BSA) (e.g. $mL \cdot min^{-1} \cdot m^2$).[24,31,57] This latter finding is a reflection of both the need to maintain internal heat production to offset heat loss from the surface of the body and the progressive age-related decrease in the ratio of BSA to body mass. The BSA/body mass ratio hypothesis, therefore, predicts that children require a higher rate of oxygen use to move a unit of body mass because of their large relative surface area.[57]

Matching youngsters and adults on key structural components is another paradigm that has been used by researchers to evaluate the importance of body size and structure in accounting for child–adult disparities in locomotor economy. The essence of this argument is that if morphological variation is important, age-related differences in $\dot{V}O_2$ should be minimal or non-existent if the groups being compared display similar anthropometric profiles. To test this hypothesis, Allor *et al.*[66] measured submaximal $\dot{V}O_2$ in adolescent girls (age = 13.3 ± 0.9 years) and young adult women (age = 21.0 ± 1.5 years) who walked and ran at 1.33 and 2.45 $m \cdot s^{-1}$, respectively. While no group differences were observed in a host of structural (e.g. height, body mass, leg length, BSA, skinfold sum), metabolic [e.g. pre-exercise $\dot{V}O_2$, submaximal respiratory exchange ratio (RER), maximal aerobic power], and biomechanical (e.g. stride frequency) parameters, the adolescent girls displayed significantly higher walking and running $\dot{V}O_2$ values (16.4 ± 1.7 $mL \cdot kg^{-1} \cdot min^{-1}$ and 38.1 ± 3.7 $mL \cdot kg^{-1} \cdot min^{-1}$) compared to the women (14.4 ± 1.1 $mL \cdot kg^{-1} \cdot min^{-1}$ and 33.9 ± 2.4 $mL \cdot kg^{-1} \cdot min^{-1}$). Although heart rate and ventilation values were slightly elevated in the adolescent group, the predicted increase in locomotor energy cost was considered trivial.

Viewed collectively, the findings of Allor *et al.*[66] are provocative, because they imply that variation in body size is relatively unimportant in explaining age-related variation in walking and running economy. This assertion was challenged recently by Grossner and co-workers,[67] who quantified walking and running economy in female adolescents (13.7 ± 0.6 years) and young adult women (22.8 ± 3.2 years) who were matched on relevant anthropometric features (height, leg length, body mass, BSA, percent body fat, and lean body mass), $\dot{V}O_2$ peak, and stride frequency. Using the same speeds employed by Allor *et al.*,[66] Grossner and co-workers[67] found no significant difference in walking (W) or running (R) $\dot{V}O_2$ between the adolescent and adult participants [adolescent $\dot{V}O_2$ = 12.3 ± 1.7 $mL \cdot kg^{-1} \cdot min^{-1}$ (W) and 30.5 ± 3.5 $mL \cdot kg^{-1} \cdot min^{-1}$ (R); adult $\dot{V}O_2$ = 10.9 ± 1.4 $mL \cdot kg^{-1} \cdot min^{-1}$ (W) and 29.0 ± 2.0 $mL \cdot kg^{-1} \cdot min^{-1}$ (R)]. Although it is unclear why two investigations featuring nearly identical research designs produced such contradictory outcomes, the findings from the Grossner *et al.*[67] study reinforce the importance of body structure in accounting for variation in locomotor economy between children and adults.

Table 21.2 Comparison of walking and running economy values between younger and older children

Authors	Age (years)		Sex	Speed (m·s^{-1})	$\dot{V}O_2$ (mL·kg^{-1}·min^{-1})		% Diff	W/R
	YC	OC			YC	OC		
Astrand[35]***	4–6	16–18	M	2.78	47.0	38.0	23.7	R
	7–9	16–18	M	2.78	43.0	38.0	13.2	R
	10–11	16–18	M	2.78	42.0	38.0	10.5	R
	12–13	16–18	M	2.78	41.0	38.0	7.9	R
	14–15	16–18	M	2.78	39.0	38.0	2.6	R
	4–6	17	F	2.78	45.0	37.0	21.6	R
	7–9	17	F	2.78	43.0	37.0	16.2	R
	10–11	17	F	2.78	40.0	37.0	8.1	R
	12–13	17	F	2.78	40.0	37.0	8.1	R
	14–15	17	F	2.78	37.0	37.0	0.0	R
Cureton *et al.*[4]	7–10	15–17	M	2.22	39.3	32.6	20.6	R
	11–14	15–17	M	2.22	34.9	32.6	7.1	R
	7–10	15–17	F	2.22	36.9	30.2	22.2	R
	11–14	15–17	F	2.22	31.9	30.2	5.6	R
Daniels *et al.*[8]	10	12	M	3.37	53.9	45.7	17.9	R
	12	17	M	3.37	52.8	42.2	25.1	R
Donkervliet *et al.*[36]**	10	15	M/F	2.22	36.0	33.5	7.5	R
Forster *et al.*[37]	5.2	9.3	M/F	1.12, 10% grade	29.0	22.6	28.3	W
Frost *et al.*[38]	7–8	10–12	M/F	1.34	17.1	12.6	35.7	W
	10–12	15–16	M/F	1.56	15.6	14.0	11.4	W
	7–8	10–12	M/F	2.19	37.1	31.9	16.3	R
	10–12	15–16	M/F	2.32	33.2	29.5	12.5	R
Harrell *et al.*[39]	8–12	15–18	M/F	1.12	18.3	12.8	43.0	W
	12–15	15–18	M/F	1.12	15.2	12.8	18.8	W
Kanaley *et al.*[40]	<8.99	13–15	M	1.61, 10% grade	35.1	31.9	10.0	W
	9–10.99	13–15	M	1.61, 10% grade	34.0	31.9	6.6	W
	11–12.99	13–15	M	1.61, 10% grade	33.2	31.9	4.1	W
Krahenbuhl *et al.*[9]	9.9	16.8	M	2.23–2.90 (YC) 2.68–3.57 (OC)	234	203	15.3	R
MacDougall *et al.*[41]**	7–9	15–16	M/F	2.83	44.7	37.9	17.9	R
	10–12	15–16	M/F	2.83	41.8	37.9	10.3	R
	13–14	15–16	M/F	2.83	39.1	37.9	3.2	R
McCann and Adams[29]	9.2	15.5	M/F	1.1	237	182	30.2	W
McCann and Adams[30]**	10.3	15.7	M/F	2.23	35.5	33.5	6.0	R
McMurray *et al.*[42]**	8	18	M/F	2.22	39.5	31	27.4	R
Morgan *et al.*[43]	6.2	10.3	M/F	1.34	18.5	14.8	25.0	W
	7.2	10.3	M/F	1.34	17.0	14.8	14.9	W
	8.2	10.3	M/F	1.34	16.0	14.8	8.1	W
	9.3	10.3	M/F	1.34	15.4	14.8	4.1	W
Shuleva *et al.*[44]	3–4	5–6	M/F	1.12, 10% grade	31.1	26.1	19.2	W

% diff = absolute percentage difference from OC value; YC = younger children; OC = older children; W/R = walking or running trials; M/F = male and female.

*$\dot{V}O_2$ in mL·kg^{-1}·km^{-1}.

**Data estimated from figures or regression equations provided in the cited publication.

***Data from Krahenbuhl and Williams.[141]

The potential influence of muscle activity in contributing to age-linked differences in locomotor energy costs has also been examined. In three studies by Frost and co-workers,[38,53,68] locomotor economy, muscle co-activation, and total body mechanical power were measured in three groups of children (7–8 year olds, 10–12 year olds, and 15–16 year olds) who performed submaximal treadmill exercise. Data from these studies indicated that when the younger and next-older age groups were compared, walking and running $\dot{V}O_2$ values were significantly higher in the younger group. Mean co-activation indexes derived for the thigh and lower leg were also higher for the younger aged children, reaching statistical significance in some cases. However, mechanical power and energy transfer rates were not significantly different between older and younger age groups. On the basis of the results of this study, the authors suggested that the lower muscle co-activation values displayed by older youth may be a function of a more mature musculoskeletal system and a greater length of time spent in practising and refining walking and running skills.

In summary, the mass-related aerobic demands of walking and running are higher in children compared to adults and are elevated in younger children compared to older children. A number of physiological, biomechanical, and structural factors have been hypothesized to explain age-related differences in locomotor economy. The few data available indicate that a faster stride frequency, a higher body surface to body mass ratio, and greater muscle co-activation of the leg muscles may be key contributors to the inefficient metabolic responses displayed by children and adolescents when $\dot{V}O_2$ is expressed relative to total body mass.

Scaling of locomotor economy

The typical approach to scaling walking or running $\dot{V}O_2$ has been to divide absolute $\dot{V}O_2$ (mL·min^{-1}) by body mass. This ratio standard method of adjusting locomotor aerobic demand has been questioned by some researchers, who have suggested that allometric scaling may be more suitable for normalizing $\dot{V}O_2$ to body size in children.[69–71] The allometric scaling method expresses the relationship between $\dot{V}O_2$ and body mass according to the formula:

$$Y = a(x^b)$$

where y is $\dot{V}O_2$, x is body mass, b is the allometric coefficient (or scaling factor), a is a proportionality coefficient, and a and b are derived by linear regression after logarithmic transformation of x and y variables is performed to yield the equation:

$$\log y = log\ a + b\ (\log x)$$

Recently, a size-independent cost (SIC) index has been proposed as an alternative to ratio and allometric-based methods of controlling for body size differences when comparing locomotor economy among humans. This index, defined by McCann and Adams,[29] as the net amount of oxygen used to move a mass of 1 kg a distance equal to stature, is based on the 'dimensional relationships required for geometric, kinematic, and biological similarity' (p. 1010). As such, the SIC index is a size-independent expression of energy cost that represents a shift from a purely statistical paradigm to normalizing $\dot{V}O_2$. When these researchers used the SIC to adjust for standing metabolic rate, body mass, and stature, the aerobic demand of walking at 1.1 m·s^{-1} was similar for children (0.180 mL·kg^{-1}), adolescents (0.195 mL·kg^{-1}), and adults (0.180mL·kg^{-1}).[29] However, when age-related differences in the oxygen cost of running were scaled using this index,[30] children (0.323 ± 0.034 mL·kg^{-1}) and adults (0.338 ± 0.035 mL·kg^{-1}) displayed similar economy values, but both groups were more economical than adolescents (0.360 mL·kg^{-1}).

Given the number of metabolic scaling approaches that can be selected to control for differences in body size, it is important for researchers and clinicians to be familiar with the advantages and drawbacks of various adjustment procedures. For example, while the ratio standard method has been criticized because it may not yield a completely mass-independent measure of submaximal energy demand,[23,70,71] it enjoys widespread acceptance among exercise scientists because it is easy to calculate and is conceptually appealing, insofar as the total body mass is lifted, lowered, and supported with each step.[63,72,73] Similarly, while the use of allometric scaling has been touted as a valid means of removing the influence of body size on aerobic power, the lack of consistency in scaling factors, the narrow range of body mass values found in childrens' studies, and the use of single-cause allometric scaling models may obscure the relationship between submaximal $\dot{V}O_2$ and body mass.[30,73,74] Finally, despite the fact that the SIC index is based on the principles of dimensional analysis and similarity theory, it cannot be used to identify and measure the specific qualitative factors that might explain child–adolescent or child–adult economy differences.[30]

Because there is no unanimity of agreement as to which scaling method is most appropriate, it is recommended that investigators select a particular scaling technique to scale locomotor economy that is best suited to address the research or clinical question being asked. While an in-depth discussion of various scaling models and their applicability is beyond the scope of this review, the reader is referred to a number of excellent papers on the subject[29,30,69–73,75,76] (and see Chapter 2).

Inter- and intraindividual variability in locomotor economy

Little is known regarding the magnitude of interindividual variability in locomotor economy among youth. In a recent longitudinal study by Morgan *et al.*,[43] walking $\dot{V}O_2$ was measured at speeds ranging from 0.67 to 1.79 m·s^{-1} in boys and girls who were evaluated annually from ages 6 to 10 years. Before testing each year, participants received 60 min of treadmill walking practice. When $\dot{V}O_2$ variability [(highest individual $\dot{V}O_2$ – lowest individual $\dot{V}O_2$)/mean group $\dot{V}O_2$] at each age/speed combination was calculated and averaged across age, interindividual differences in walking economy ranged from 32% to 41%. A similar range in $\dot{V}O_2$ variability (30–44%) was documented when $\dot{V}O_2$ variability at each age/speed combination was averaged across walking speeds. No discernable trend in mean $\dot{V}O_2$ variability was observed with increases in either age or walking speed. This relatively large intersubject variation in walking energy costs is probably unrelated to motor skill deficiency, as most children exhibit mature walking patterns by 4–5 years of age.[48,74] Although speculative, differences in physical maturity and development may be a more probable explanation for the between-subject variability in walking $\dot{V}O_2$ documented in this group of children. As noted by

Morgan and co-workers,[43] factors known or postulated to account for economy differences among youth, such as step frequency, ventilatory efficiency, BSA to body mass ratio, and the balance between body mass and leg muscle contraction speed, have been tied to variation in body size and structure.

As a prelude to assessing the impact of treatments designed to improve locomotor economy in youth, it is essential to first establish that stable, pre-treatment $\dot{V}O_2$ data have been acquired. In this regard, recent studies have documented the stability of gait transport costs in youth. From a clinical perspective, data from two studies[77,78] have shown that acceptably stable within-day and between-day stability of treadmill walking $\dot{V}O_2$ can be achieved in children with mild cerebral palsy (CP) after a short period (5–15 min) of treadmill accommodation. Similarly, no mean between-trial or between-day group differences in $\dot{V}O_2$ were reported by Frost and co-workers[79] in 24 healthy children (age = 9.1 ± 1.4 years) who completed six 6 min bouts of treadmill walking or running on 2 days following a minimal amount (<1 min) of treadmill walking practice. Individual economy responses, however, varied considerably across trials. In another study, Unnithan and co-workers[80] demonstrated that a single exercise session yielded valid group measures of running economy in healthy prepubertal boys (age = 10.7 ± 0.71 years). Conversely, in a study of 42 able-bodied children (age = 8.9 ± 0.7 years) who were provided varying time periods (5–15 min) to practice treadmill walking or running on each of 2 days, Rogers *et al.*[81] found that running $\dot{V}O_2$ values at 5 and 6 miles·h^{-1} (8.0 and 9.6 km·h^{-1}) were lower on the second day of testing. In this study, between-day reliability estimates for $\dot{V}O_2$ were moderate to high in magnitude [range of intraclass correlation coefficients (ICC) = 0.71–0.94] and the coefficient of variation (CV) in $\dot{V}O_2$ ranged from 7.4% to 8.4% across the two running speeds.

In considering the issue of economy stability in children, it is possible that younger children, being less physically mature, might exhibit greater daily variation in submaximal exercise $\dot{V}O_2$ compared to older, physically mature children. With respect to this question, work conducted in our laboratory[82,83] has shown that after 10–15 min of treadmill accommodation, 6-year-old children walking at 3 miles·h^{-1} (4.8 km·h^{-1}, n = 41) and running at 5 miles·h^{-1} (8.0 km·h^{-1}, n = 30) displayed stable within-day walking economy values (mean CV = 2.0%; mean ICC = 0.96) and stable within-day and between-day running economy values (mean within-day CV = 2.2%; mean between-day CV = 2.4%; mean ICC = 0.96). Parenthetically, in our investigations, average CV values for $\dot{V}O_2$ were considerably lower (<3%) than those cited previously in the literature.[81]

An interesting question which has received little attention is the extent to which the relative ordering of individual gait economy values remains stable with increasing age. In an attempt to address this issue, the stability of locomotor $\dot{V}O_2$ values was assessed in young, normally active, but non-run-trained children who were tested annually from ages 6 to 10 years.[84] For both walking (W) and running (R), 27% of subjects displayed a mean change in $\dot{V}O_2$ rankings of ≤2 positions, 64% (W) and 61% (R) of participants exhibited an average yearly shift in $\dot{V}O_2$ rank order of ≤4 positions, and 85% of the children demonstrated a mean annual fluctuation of ≤6 positions in the rank order of walking and running $\dot{V}O_2$. High coefficient alpha values were observed for both walking (r = 0.91) and running (r = 0.94) over the testing span of 5 years. Secondary analyses also revealed moderate to high reliability coefficients for ventilatory equivalent for oxygen, BSA to body mass ratio, and RER (range = 0.50–0.95) from ages 6 to 10 years. Taken together, these findings suggest that both size-dependent and size-independent factors may account for the tracking of walking $\dot{V}O_2$ in young, healthy children.

The tendency for young, untrained children to express a bias towards good, average, or below-average locomotor economy during the mid-childhood years raises the intriguing possibilities that walking and running $\dot{V}O_2$ may be partially influenced by heredity or may reflect a more global expression of exercise economy across other physical activities. Relative to this point, data collected on eight male monozygotic twin pairs and eight male dizygotic twin pairs (age = 21 years) with similar familial and environmental influences and comparable patterns of habitual physical activity yielded low heritability indexes for submaximal $\dot{V}O_2$ (range = 0.02–0.35) at speeds varying from 5 to 8 km·h^{-1} [85]. Daniels *et al.*[86] have also reported that in trained adult distance runners, the degree of economy displayed while running does not seem to be consistently expressed across a variety of exercise tasks.

In summary, size-related differences in physiological, structural, and biomechanical factors may help explain the large variability in walking economy observed among able-bodied youth. If some degree of treadmill accommodation is provided, stable group responses in submaximal walking and running $\dot{V}O_2$ values can be secured in a relatively short time period in able-bodied and physically challenged children. The relative ordering of individual gait $\dot{V}O_2$ values within a group tends to be quite stable in normally developing boys and girls who have been exposed to a variety of physical activity experiences.

Sex differences in locomotor economy

Studies addressing the issue of sex differences in locomotor economy have produced equivocal findings, with some investigators reporting poorer running economy in boys[4,35,36,61] and others finding no sex disparity in either walking or running economy.[41,59,71,87–91] In some studies, economy differences between boys and girls varied as a function of running speed[23,92] or age.[93] This lack of consensus among studies may be related to differences in the age of subjects, the absence of equal numbers of males and females, the running speeds chosen for testing, or the use of small sample sizes. It is curious to note that none of the studies reviewed indicated that boys were more economical than girls while walking or running on a treadmill.

In one study in which submaximal running $\dot{V}O_2$ was generally lower in girls compared to boys, the girls (mean age = 11.0 years) were working at a higher percentage of $\dot{V}O_2$ max and displayed higher RER values particularly at faster running speeds, compared to identically aged boys.[23] Consequently, it is possible that girls may rely to a greater degree on anaerobic metabolism to fuel locomotor energy demands while running. Donkervliet *et al.*[36] also reported that among prepubertal (mean age = 10 years) and post-pubertal (mean age = 15 years) youth, girls exhibited better walking and running economy values compared to boys. In this study, a more stable movement coordination pattern of the arms and legs was observed in females and may have contributed to their lower gait energy costs. With respect to younger children, the influence of body composition and resting energy use on locomotor economy was examined in thirty-five 6 year olds (15 boys and 20 girls) following 30 min of treadmill running practice.[94] Results demonstrated that both sexes were comparable in height, body mass, and leg length, but the girls displayed a higher percentage of body fat and a lower fat-free mass (FFM). Analysis of sex differences in running economy demonstrated that absolute gross $\dot{V}O_2$ (L·min^{-1}) and mass-related gross and net $\dot{V}O_2$ (the latter calculated by subtracting resting $\dot{V}O_2$ from gross $\dot{V}O_2$) were higher in boys. However, when absolute gross $\dot{V}O_2$ was expressed relative to FFM, no sex difference in $\dot{V}O_2$ was present. On the basis of these findings, it was concluded that the greater leanness displayed by the boys was responsible for their higher absolute and mass-related running $\dot{V}O_2$ values.

Distance-running performance and running economy

Since better running economy has been linked to distance-running success in adults,[1–3,5,6,10,11,14] a logical question is to ask whether the same relationship exists in children. Early cross-sectional work conducted by Krahenbuhl and co-workers demonstrated that the $\dot{V}O_2$ of submaximal running at 2.23, 2.57, and 2.90 m·s^{-1} was similar among 8-year-old boys[25] and 10-year-old boys[95] stratified by distance covered in 5, 7, and 9 min runs or by time recorded for a 1.6-km run. The lack of a significant relationship between running economy and performance in various endurance-racing events (1500 m, 3 miles, and 5 km) has also been observed among older, endurance-trained adolescent boys and girls.[90,91,96] Conversely, descriptive data collected by Cureton *et al.*[4] on a large (n = 145), age-diverse (7–17 years) sample of males and females indicated that running economy improved by 1.0 mL·kg^{-1}·min^{-1}·year^{-1} and was significantly associated with 1-mile run/walk time in both boys (r = 0.48) and girls (r = 0.34). Using multiple regression analyses, these authors noted that when peak $\dot{V}O_2$ and % peak $\dot{V}O_2$ were held constant, the chronological improvement in running economy explained an additional 31% of the age-related decrease in 1-mile run/walk time. In addition, findings from recent studies of older (16–17 year olds), endurance-trained, male adolescent runners have revealed significant correlations (0.62 and 0.55, respectively) between running $\dot{V}O_2$ and performance times for shorter (800 m) and longer (5 km) running events.[13,91] Similarly, non-significant trends suggesting a positive association between middle- and long-distance running run time and submaximal $\dot{V}O_2$ have been noted for competitive adolescent male and female runners.[12,90]

Although few in number, longitudinal studies have established a stronger link between distance-running performance and running economy in children. Daniels and co-workers,[7,8] for instance, showed that marked decrements in submaximal $\dot{V}O_2$ were accompanied by significant reductions in 1 and 2 mile run times among 10 and 12 year olds who participated in middle- and long-distance run training for 2 and 5 years. Since mass-related $\dot{V}O_2$ max remained unchanged over time, it was speculated that improvements in running economy contributed to better running performance in their trained subjects. Using a different methodological approach, Krahenbuhl *et al.*[9] documented changes in 9-min run performance and running economy in six young boys (mean age = 9.9 years) who were tested initially and 7 years later (mean age = 16.8 years). During the intervening time span, none of the subjects engaged in formal distance-run training, but all had been active in recreational or high school sports. Congruent with the findings of Daniels and co-workers,[7,8] mass-related $\dot{V}O_2$ did not change over the 7-year period, but running economy and distance-running performance improved by 16% and 29%, respectively, and the estimated percentage of $\dot{V}O_2$ max incurred during the 9-min run rose by 13%. Overall, results from the Krahenbuhl *et al.*[9] study provide evidence showing that childhood distance-running performance can improve in the absence of run training. Since maximal lactate values and glycolytic enzyme activity increase with age,[35,54,97–101] the higher relative workload generated by the teenaged boys may be due to a greater contribution of anaerobic energy mechanisms to the total exercise energy requirement. Alternatively, it is possible that the older boys exhibited more mental toughness, which would also enable them to exercise at a higher percentage of $\dot{V}O_2$ max.

Malleability of locomotor economy: Effects of instruction and training

A topic of obvious practical importance to coaches and young athletes is whether children can be taught or trained to adopt a more economical running style. Petray and Krahenbuhl[102] addressed this issue by randomly selecting fifty 10 year olds and assigning them to one out of the five treatment groups. These groups were (i) a no-treatment control group, (ii) a control group in which subjects received instruction on a topic (namely, throwing) unrelated to running, (iii) a running technique instruction group which received 5 min of weekly instruction on various aspects of running form for 11 weeks, (iv) a run training group which has been trained 3–30 min per day for 3 days per week for 11 weeks, and (v) a group which combined both running instruction and run training. Data from their study were not encouraging, as none of the experimental manipulations produced a change in running economy, stride rate, stride length, or vertical displacement of the body. Lussier and Buskirk[103] also reported no change in the running economy of 10-year-old boys and girls who completed a 4 days · week^{-1}, 12-week programme featuring running games and continuous running.

While the previously cited studies imply that economy in children is not easily perturbed by short-term training regimens or instruction on running technique, some researchers have demonstrated enhanced gait economy among boys involved in middle- and long-distance running programmes. Sjodin and Svedenhag,[104] for instance, found that over an 8-year period, mass-related $\dot{V}O_2$ measured at 4.17 m·s^{-1} decreased in eight young male runners (mean age = 12.5 years) who ran an average of 48–60 km·week^{-1}. Submaximal $\dot{V}O_2$ values for the trained boys were also consistently lower compared to values obtained on age- and sex-matched controls. In addition, work by Daniels and co-workers[7,8] has shown that extended periods (2–5 years) of middle- and long-distance run training can improve running economy in 10- to 13-year-old boys. In their studies, absolute measures of $\dot{V}O_2$ max rose linearly across the yearly testing periods, but remained stable when expressed relative to body mass. Submaximal $\dot{V}O_2$, though, dropped by 15% in 10 year olds who were studied for 2 years and by 19% in 12 year olds followed for 5 years. Since participants were tracked over a number of years, improvement in running economy may have been partly due to physical growth and maturation. However, because the relative decrease in $\dot{V}O_2$ in the 12 year olds was greater than that observed in non-run-trained boys who were tested when they were 10 and 17 years of age,[9] run training may have exerted an influence on economy over and above that produced solely by variables affected by growth and physical maturity.

Physical growth and locomotor economy

Numerous cross-sectional investigations have demonstrated that older children display better locomotor economy compared to younger children.[4,35,40,41] However, longitudinal studies are better able to quantify the relationship between physical growth and locomotor economy because they yield accurate measures of change in submaximal $\dot{V}O_2$ over time and provide a clearer view of inter-individual variation in $\dot{V}O_2$ at a particular age. As noted earlier, longitudinal decreases in submaximal $\dot{V}O_2$ (16%) among boys aged 10–17 years have been attributed to physical growth.[9] While comparable reductions in graded walking economy (~21–22%) have been reported for children tested at 5 and 9 years of age,[37] pertinent factors underlying this relationship have not been systematically examined in a large, mixed-sex sample of children. To address this issue, our group has just completed a 5-year tracking study aimed at documenting yearly changes in walking and running $\dot{V}O_2$ among healthy untrained boys and girls who were tested annually, beginning at age 6 years, following an extensive period of treadmill walking and running practice. We hypothesized that mass-specific locomotor economy would improve with age and be accompanied by growth-related changes in selected physiological, structural, and biomechanical variables. Analysis of walking economy data collected on 23 participants (14 girls, 9 boys) at six speeds (0.67, 0.89, 1.12, 1.34, 1.56, and 1.79 $m \cdot s^{-1}$) has shown that mass-related $\dot{V}O_2$ was 27% higher for the 6 year olds compared with the 10 year olds.[43] Analysis of year-to-year changes in $\dot{V}O_2$ revealed a significant decrease in walking $\dot{V}O_2$ across all speeds between the ages of 6 and 8 years. Once the ages of 8 or 9 years were attained, improvements in walking economy were generally less pronounced, suggesting that factors affecting walking energy use may exert more of an impact during early childhood. Preliminary results indicate that this reduction in walking energy demand was associated with decreases in the ventilatory equivalent for oxygen, BSA to body mass ratio, and the normalized moment of inertia of the leg about the hip during the swing phase of gait. Step length (SL) and stance time also increased and average vertical ground reaction force (normalized to body weight) decreased over time. Although data continue to be processed, our initial findings suggest that physical growth is an important stimulus for improving locomotor economy in young boys and girls.

Prediction of locomotor economy

Because children are less economical than adults,[4,35,40,41] the use of adult prediction equations to estimate locomotor energy in youth will lead to an underestimation of walking and running $\dot{V}O_2$. Therefore, a need exists to develop metabolic equations that accurately predict movement energy costs in younger and older children. To address this issue, Walker *et al.*[105] derived generalized equations to predict relative $\dot{V}O_2$ ($mL \cdot kg^{-1} \cdot min^{-1}$) and caloric expenditure ($kcal \cdot kg^{-1} \cdot min^{-1}$) during level walking and running (speed range = 67–215 $m \cdot min^{-1}$) in 82 male and female adolescents varying in age from 12 to 18 years. While the group relationship between walking speed and $\dot{V}O_2$ was quadratic in nature, a linear relationship best described the association between running speed and $\dot{V}O_2$ in this sample. Multiple regression analysis indicated that speed and mode of locomotion were the primary sources of variation in predicting mass-related walking and running energy costs. While inclusion of skinfold sum (triceps and medial calf) produced a small, but significant, enhancement in the estimation of walking and running $\dot{V}O_2$, the addition of sex, age, and height did not significantly improve the prediction of walking and running $\dot{V}O_2$. Cross-validation conducted on a sample of 76 separate random observations yielded high correlations (0.95 and 0.94) between predicted and direct measures of $\dot{V}O_2$ and caloric expenditure, respectively, and prediction errors were 3.58 $mL \cdot kg^{-1} \cdot min^{-1}$ for $\dot{V}O_2$ and 0.019 $kcal \cdot kg^{-1} \cdot min^{-1}$ for caloric expenditure. More recently, Morgan and co-workers[106] measured walking $\dot{V}O_2$ at a variety of speeds (0.67–1.79 $m \cdot s^{-1}$) in 23 boys and girls who were tested annually from ages 6 to 10 years after receiving 1 hour of treadmill walking practice each year. A regression equation featuring speed and age as independent variables was deemed best suited to predict walking $\dot{V}O_2$, based on a strong correlation between predicted and measured $\dot{V}O_2$ ($r = 0.95$) and a low standard error of the estimate (1.74 $mL \cdot kg^{-1} \cdot min^{-1}$). In addition, results from Bland–Altman plots documented a 95% level of agreement between actual and predicted $\dot{V}O_2$ that ranged between ±1 MET.

The development and application of new motion-sensing devices to quantify physical activity in free-living environments has encouraged researchers to examine whether these devices can accurately predict locomotor energy use in children. To evaluate this possibility, Trost and co-workers[107] compared the accuracy of three equations (e.g. Freedman,[108,109] Puyau,[110] and Trost[111]) developed for the uniaxial Actigraph accelerometer in estimating walking and running economy in 45 children and adolescents (age = 13.7 ± 2.6 years) who performed overground walking and running trials. Data from their investigation revealed that no single equation accurately predicted energy use in all of the locomotor activities that were evaluated (e.g. normal walking, brisk walking, easy running, and fast running). However, each equation was able to accurately predict energy expenditure for at least one of the overground walking and running tasks. The potential influence of body size as a factor affecting the predictive validity of the Freedman equation was also examined by Wickel *et al.*[112] in 67 children (age = 9.4 ± 2.1 years) who completed five walking trials (1.6, 3.2, 4.0, 4.8, and 6.4 $km \cdot h^{-1}$) on a treadmill. Before testing, participants were stratified into small, medium, or large body size categories on the basis of their BSA. Results from this study indicated that the measured metabolic equivalent (MET) values and MET values predicted from Actigraph data were similar at the slowest walking speed, but at faster speeds, measured MET values were lower than predicted MET values. Moreover, the average difference between measured and predicted MET values was significantly greater for smaller children (those in the two lowest BSA groups) compared to larger children (those in the highest BSA group). Another new motion device that combines temperature, heat flux, and galvanic sensors with a biaxial accelerometer is the SenseWear Armband (SWA). Using activity-specific algorithms, the SWA integrates sensor and accelerometer data with sex, age, height, and weight to predict energy expenditure for different physical activities. However, in a recent validation study[113] involving 20 healthy boys and girls (age = 12.1 ± 0.9 years), the SWA was found to significantly underestimate energy costs for running (8–10 km·h^{-1}) and at walking speeds ranging from 4 to 7 km·h^{-1}.

Obesity and locomotor economy

With the increasing prevalence of childhood obesity, there is renewed interest in identifying factors that contribute to the higher energy costs of weight-bearing exercise observed in obese children and adolescents. In a recent study by Ekelund *et al.*[114] comparing walking economy in 18 obese adolescents and 18 normal-weight adolescents matched on age and sex, $\dot{V}O_2$ expressed relative to FFM was higher in the obese group. When absolute $\dot{V}O_2$ was expressed as a function of total body mass, though, submaximal $\dot{V}O_2$ was similar for the obese and normal-weight group, despite group differences of 29 kg in fat mass and more than 40 kg in total body mass. On the basis of this evidence, it was concluded that body mass is a major contributor to differences in absolute walking energy expenditure observed between obese and non-obese youth.

In another investigation, the degree to which total body mass and adiposity account for variation in walking $\dot{V}O_2$ among obese youngsters and their non-obese peers was examined by Ayub and Bar-Or.[115] Employing an innovative study design, these investigators measured seated resting $\dot{V}O_2$ and walking energy expenditure at 4, 5, and 6 km·h^{-1} in nine pairs of 11- to 18-year-old boys (one who was lean and one who was obese) matched on body mass. Expressed relative to body mass, net $\dot{V}O_2$ was similar between the lean (9% body fat) and obese (37%) boys at the two slowest speeds, but was 12% higher in the obese boys at the fastest walking speed. It was speculated that the higher energy demands measured at 6 km·h^{-1} in the obese group may have been due to greater ventilatory effort or uneconomical gait mechanics. When all subjects were considered as a single group and the contribution of age, height, body mass, and adiposity to variance in net walking economy was assessed, body mass accounted for 62–89% of the variance in net $\dot{V}O_2$, depending on walking speed. Adiposity, on the other hand, explained only 2–16% of the variation in net $\dot{V}O_2$ across speeds. Interestingly, when data for the lean and obese subjects were pooled, there was no discernable within- or between-group relationship between percentage of fat in the legs (the most active limbs during walking) and net $\dot{V}O_2$. Hence, the authors concluded that the aerobic demand of walking in obese boys is influenced primarily by total body mass and not by total or regional adiposity. From a clinical standpoint, this finding emphasizes the fundamental importance of weight loss as a practical means of improving the energetic ease of locomotion in the overweight or obese child.

Basic gait patterns and locomotor economy

In adults, minimization of aerobic demand has typically been thought to serve as the 'trigger' to switch from a walking to a running gait.[116,117] However, some evidence suggests that the preferred transition speed (PTS) in adults may actually be lower than the energetically optimal transition speed.[118] Currently, little is known regarding whether minimization of $\dot{V}O_2$ is a central principle underlying the selection of gait transition speed in youth. This is a potentially interesting question, given that children exhibit metabolic, structural, and biomechanical profiles that differ substantially from those displayed by adults. In a recent investigation, Tseh *et al.*[119] determined the PTS in a mixed-sex group of adolescents (ten 11 year olds, ten 13 year olds, and ten 15 year olds) by averaging transition speeds derived from five walk–run trials and five run–walk trials. Energetically optimal transition speed (EOTS) was subsequently identified by measuring $\dot{V}O_2$ while participants walked at 70%, 80%, 90%, 100%, and 110% and ran at 90%, 100%, 110%, 120%, and 130% of their respective PTS. Results indicated that for each age grouping, the mean EOTS was significantly faster than the mean PTS. In addition, when participants transitioned from a walk to a run, the $\dot{V}O_2$ needed to run at the PTS was not lower than the $\dot{V}O_2$ measured while walking at the PTS. On the basis of these findings, it was concluded that in older youth, the transition from a walk to a run does not occur to reduce energy expenditure. In view of a moderately strong association between leg length and the PTS ($r = 0.71$), it is possible that kinematic and kinetic features of leg movement may control the walk-to-run transition in adolescent boys and girls.

Walking speeds typically selected by young and older adults (~1.3 m·s^{-1}) are similar to speeds at which $\dot{V}O_2$ per unit distance travelled is lowest.[120,121] Little is known, however, regarding the extent to which locomotor economy is a primary determinant governing the choice of walking speed and other basic gait parameters in children. In this regard, DeJaeger *et al.*[122] reported that the speed at which the minimum mass-related cost of transport (C_{gross}) occurs increased from ~1.2 m·s^{-1} in 3–4 year olds to 1.5 m·s^{-1} in young adults. In our laboratory, we have observed no significant difference between preferred walking speed (mean = 1.30 ± 0.14 m·s^{-1}) and the most economical walking speed (mean = 1.28 ± 0.07 m·s^{-1}) in 6-year-old boys and girls.[123] Similarly, in this same age group, the mean absolute variation in SL between the freely chosen SL and the energetically optimal SL was associated with an average $\dot{V}O_2$ difference of only 0.1 mL·kg^{-1}·min^{-1}[124]. The importance of optimizing energy expenditure during walking also appears to extend to physically challenged youth, insofar as children with CP appear to select walking speeds and SL patterns that minimize $\dot{V}O_2$.[125,126] In summary, this close affinity between preferred and metabolically optimal conditions suggests that minimizing energy demand is a key factor regulating the choice of basic gait parameters in able-bodied children and children with neuromuscular disease.

Locomotor economy in youth with physical disabilities

The assessment of paediatric gait efficiency is important, not only with regard to the general health and sport performance of able-bodied children, but also for children with physical disabilities. From a clinical perspective, energetic penalties resulting from inefficient locomotion patterns may limit the functional capabilities of children with neuromuscular disease or lower extremity injuries, thus restricting their physical independence and involvement in family, school, and recreational activities.

While limited research has shown that children with below-knee amputations and spina bifida display elevated walking energy demands compared to control or expected population values,[127,128] the most studied developmental disorder linked to excessive paediatric locomotor energy demands is CP. This neurological condition refers to a collection of non-progressive motor impairment syndromes, which stem from brain anomalies occurring early in development.[129–131] The higher energy cost associated with CP has been ascribed to a variety of factors, including a lower leg strength to body mass ratio,[19] higher mechanical power output,[132] and excess lower limb muscle co-activation,[20] although the latter may be dependent on the topographical distribution of CP.[133] Descriptive studies have also indicated that walking energy expenditure rises with advancing age in children with CP,[134] a trend that runs counter to the improvement in economy with age seen in able-bodied youth.[43] It has been hypothesized that this age-related rise in walking $\dot{V}O_2$ is due to increases in body mass and adiposity that are not compensated for by offsetting gains in leg muscle strength. Because $\dot{V}O_2$ max values are substantially lower in children with CP compared to able-bodied controls,[20,135] the child with CP incurs a higher relative exercise intensity at any given walking speed.[19] From a clinical standpoint, this observation has important functional relevance for children with spastic CP, who may complain of activity-related fatigue, rely more often on assistive devices (such as crutches or wheelchairs) to traverse long distances, or participate less frequently in free-living physical activity. A link between gait economy and community mobility has been established by Maltais *et al.*,[18] who demonstrated a strong inverse relationship between physical activity levels and walking economy in children with mild CP. It has also been demonstrated that in children with CP, the energy cost of walking rises with an increase in the severity of gross motor function impairment.[136]

While a number of rehabilitative strategies have been employed to improve gait function in children with CP, surprisingly few studies have documented their impact on locomotor economy. Results from these investigations have been mixed, with some demonstrating no change in $\dot{V}O_2$ or heart rate measures of energy expenditure following short-term periods of lower extremity strength training[137,138] and others reporting a lower physiological cost index[19] (walking heart rate–resting heart rate divided by walking speed) following electrical stimulation of lower extremity muscles[139] and improved walking and arm cranking economy with the use of hinged ankle–foot orthoses,[17] partial body weight support,[140] and combined strength and aerobic training.[21]

Future directions

Since the initial publication of this chapter, some progress has been made in identifying and better understanding the factors that affect locomotion economy in youth. However, a number of important issues still remain unresolved. Against this backdrop, it should be noted that many studies have featured relatively small samples with a narrow range of participant characteristics. Consequently, larger, age-diverse samples of boys and girls are needed to confirm, refute, or refine current thinking and approaches.

There is a large body of evidence indicating that variability in locomotor energy demands in children and adolescents is related to differences in body structure and size. However, the investigation by Allor *et al.*,[66] who reported significantly different walking and running economy in female adolescents and adults who were matched on a variety of size-related factors, clearly deserves replication using adolescent–adult and younger–older child comparisons that allow for matching of critical size-related variables. More longitudinal studies are needed to evaluate the relative contribution of physiological, structural, and biomechanical variables to locomotor economy at different chronological ages and stages of physical maturity in boys and girls. The use of non-invasive techniques, such as magnetic resonance spectroscopy (MRS) and near-infrared spectroscopy, may also prove useful in monitoring age-related differences or changes in oxidative skeletal muscle metabolism resulting from physical growth and maturation, training, or clinical interventions (see Chapter 16).

From a performance standpoint, relatively little is known regarding the types of training regimens best suited to improve running economy in child athletes. Are there time periods in a child's life that are most optimal in eliciting positive changes in economy? Does pubertal status influence the ability to reduce locomotor energy use? While good potential exists for new motion-sensing devices to accurately estimate walking and running economy in children, there is a continuing need to develop and cross-validate energy prediction equations on youngsters differing in age, sex, and body size. Finally, more studies are needed to evaluate the short- and long-term impact of clinical and applied interventions (e.g. gait training, partial body weight support, aquatic therapy, surgery, pharmacological treatment, physical therapy, sport programmes) on the locomotor economy and functional mobility of physically challenged children.

Summary

- Locomotor economy is defined as the mass-related aerobic demand for a given submaximal walking or running speed. Children are less economical than adults and older children are more economical than younger children. Primary explanations for the higher walking and running $\dot{V}O_2$ values displayed by children include a higher stride frequency, a larger body surface area to mass ratio, and greater muscle co-activation in the legs.
- A variety of methods exist to scale absolute measures of submaximal $\dot{V}O_2$ to body size and each adjustment procedure has strengths and limitations. It is recommended that investigators select a scaling approach that is appropriate to the research question or clinical issue being addressed.
- At a given age, children exhibit notable interindividual differences in locomotor economy. Stable group responses in walking and running economy, however, can be obtained following a minimal amount of treadmill accommodation.
- As a group, normally active boys and girls tend to display a predisposition towards good, average, or sub-average economy that is reasonably maintained during the mid-childhood years. Little is known regarding the extent to which this tendency is manifested during adolescence and into adulthood.
- Girls display lower walking and running energy costs compared to boys. This sex difference in economy may be due to a greater reliance on anaerobic metabolism, more stable limb movement coordination patterns, and less fat-free mass.
- Results from descriptive studies present a mixed picture regarding the link between submaximal running $\dot{V}O_2$ and distance-running performance in youth. Limited longitudinal research, however, has demonstrated a positive relationship between performance in endurance runs and running economy.
- Extended periods of distance-running training have been shown to improve running economy in older children and adolescents. Growth-related improvements in walking economy have been tied to changes in selected physiological, structural, and

biomechanical variables known or hypothesized to influence locomotor energy use.

- Differences in walking energy cost between obese and non-obese youth are influenced primarily by body mass variation and not by overall body fat levels or fat percentage in the legs.
- In both able-bodied children and children with CP, the selection of basic gait parameters, such as walking speed and step length–step frequency patterns, appears to be tied to the minimization of aerobic demand.
- Youth with physical disabilities often display elevated walking energy demands that increase the relative exercise intensity of walking. In children with CP, reduced locomotor economy is associated with greater motor dysfunction and less mobility in free-living environments. Emerging research suggests that a variety of physical activity interventions, such as partial body weight support, aquatic therapy, and combinations of strength and endurance training, may improve economy and overall fitness in youth with CP and other physical disabilities.

Acknowledgement

The writing of this paper was supported by grants from the National Institute of Child Health and Human Development (HD 30749 and HD 48742).

References

1. Bransford DR, Howley ET (1977). Oxygen cost of running in trained and untrained men and women. *Med Sci Sports Exerc* **9**, 41–4.
2. Conley DL, Krahenbuhl GS (1980). Running economy and distance running performance of highly trained athletes. *Med Sci Sports Exerc* **12**, 357–60.
3. Conley DL, Krahenbuhl GS, Burkett LN (1981). Training for aerobic capacity and running economy. *Phys Sportsmed* **9**, 107–15.
4. Cureton KJ, Sloniger MA, Black DM, McCormack WP, Rowe DA (1997). Metabolic determinants of the age-related improvement in one-mile run/walk performance in youth. *Med Sci Sports Exerc* **29**, 259–67.
5. Daniels JT (1974). Physiological characteristics of champion male athletes. *Res Q* **45**, 342–8.
6. Daniels JT (1985). A physiologist's view of running economy. *Med Sci Sports Exerc* **17**, 332–8.
7. Daniels J, Oldridge N (1971). Changes in oxygen consumption of young boys during growth and running training. *Med Sci Sports Exerc* **3**, 161–5.
8. Daniels J, Oldridge N, Nagle F, White B (1978). Differences and changes in $\dot{V}O_2$ among young runners 10 to 18 years of age. *Med Sci Sports* **10**, 200–3.
9. Krahenbuhl GS, Morgan W, Pangrazi RP (1989). Longitudinal changes in distance in young males. *Int J Sports Med* **10**, 92–6.
10. Morgan D, Baldini F, Martin P, Kohrt W (1989). Ten kilometer performance and predicted velocity at $\dot{V}O_2$ max among well-trained male runners. *Med Sci Sports Exerc* **21**, 78–83.
11. Morgan DW, Craib MW (1992). Physiological aspects of running economy. *Med Sci Sports Exerc* **24**, 456–61.
12. Abe D, Yanagawa K, Yamanobe K, Tamura K (1998). Assessment of middle-distance running performance in sub-elite young runners using energy cost of running. *Eur J Appl Physiol* **77**, 320–5.
13. Cole AS, Woodruff ME, Horn MP, Mahon AD (2006). Strength, power, and aerobic exercise correlates of 5-km cross-country running performance in adolescent runners. *Pediatr Exerc Sci* **18**, 374–84.
14. Morgan DW, Bransford DR, Costill DL, Daniels JT, Howley ET, Krahenbuhl GS (1995). Variation in the aerobic demand of running among trained and untrained subjects. *Med Sci Sports Exerc* **27**, 404–9.
15. Paavolainen L, Hakkinen K, Hamalainen I, Nummela A, Rusko H (1999). Explosive-strength training improves 5-km running time by improving running economy and muscle power. *J Appl Physiol* **86**, 1527–33.
16. Durstine JL, Painter P, Franklin BA, Morgan D, Pitetti KH, Roberts SO (2000). Physical activity for the chronically ill and disabled. *Sports Med* **30**, 207–19.
17. Maltais DB, Bar-Or O, Galea V, Pierrynowski M (2005). Use of orthoses lowers the O_2 cost of walking in children with spastic cerebral palsy. *Med Sci Sports Exerc* **33**, 320–5.
18. Maltais DB, Pierrynowski MR, Galea VA, Bar-Or O (2005). Physical activity level is associated with the O_2 cost of walking in cerebral palsy. *Med Sci Sports Exerc* **37**, 347–53.
19. Rose J, Morgan DW, Gamble JG (2006). Energetics of walking. In: Rose J, Gamble JG (eds.), *Human walking*, pp. 77–102. Lippincott Williams and Wilkins, Philadelphia, PA.
20. Unnithan VB, Dowling JJ, Frost G, Bar-Or O (1996). Role of cocontraction in the O_2 cost of walking in children with cerebral palsy. *Med Sci Sports Exerc* **28**, 1498–504.
21. Unnithan VB, Katsimanis G, Evangelinou C, Kosmas C, Kandrali I, Killis E (2007). Effect of strength and aerobic training in children with cerebral palsy. *Med Sci Sports Exerc* **39**, 1902–9.
22. Waters RL, Mulroy S (1999). The energy expenditure of normal and pathologic gait. *Gait Posture* **9**, 207–31.
23. Armstrong N, Kirby BJ, Welsman JR, McManus AM (1997). Submaximal exercise in prepubertal children. In: Armstrong N, Kirby BJ, Welsman JR (eds.), *Children and exercise XIX*, pp. 221–7. E&FN Spon, London.
24. Ebbeling CJ, Hamill J, Freedson PS, Rowland TW (1992). An examination of efficiency during walking in children and adults. *Pediatr Exerc Sci* **4**, 36–49.
25. Krahenbuhl GS, Pangrazi RP, Chomokos EA (1979). Aerobic responses of young boys to submaximal running. *Res Q* **50**, 413–21.
26. Van Mechelen W, Kemper HCG, Twisk J (1994). The development of running economy from 13–27 years of age. *Med Sci Sports Exerc* **26** (Suppl.), S205.
27. Maliszewski AF, Freedson PS (1996). Is running economy different between adults and children? *Pediatr Exerc Sci* **8**, 351–60.
28. Martinez LR, Haymes EM (1992). Substrate utilization during treadmill running in prepubertal girls and women. *Med Sci Sports Exerc* **24**, 975–83.
29. McCann DJ, Adams W (2002). A dimensional paradigm for identifying the size-independent cost of walking. *Med Sci Sports Exerc* **34**, 1009–17.
30. McCann DJ, Adams WC (2003). The size-independent oxygen cost of running. *Med Sci Sports Exerc* **35**, 1049–56.
31. Rowland TW, Auchinachie JA, Keenan TJ, Green GM (1987). Physiologic responses to treadmill running in adult and prepubertal males. *Int J Sports Med* **8**, 292–7.
32. Rowland TW, Green GM (1988). Physiological responses to treadmill exercise in females: Adult-child differences. *Med Sci Sports Exerc* **20**, 474–8.
33. Turley KR, Wilmore JH (1997). Cardiovascular responses to treadmill and cycle ergometer exercise in children and adults. *J Appl Physiol* **83**, 948–57.
34. Unnithan VB, Eston RG (1990). Stride frequency and submaximal treadmill running economy in adults and children. *Pediatr Exerc Sci* **2**, 149–55.
35. Astrand P-O (1952). *Experimental studies of physical working capacity in relation to sex and age*. Munksgaard, Copenhagen.
36. Donkervliet E, Smits T, Ziemba AW, Kemper HCG, Wagenaar RC (2000). Can sex and puberty-related differences in walking and running economy be explained by the differences in coordination patterns? *Biol Sport* **17**, 243–54.

37. Forster MA, Hunter GR, Hester DJ, Dunaway D, Shuleva K (1994). Aerobic capacity and grade-walking economy of children 5–9 years old: A longitudinal study. *Pediatr Exerc* Sci **6**, 31–8.
38. Frost G, Dowling J, Dyson K, Bar-Or O (1997). Cocontraction in three age groups of children during treadmill locomotion. *J Electromyogr Kinesiol* **7**, 179–86.
39. Harrell JS, McMurray RG, Baggett CD, Pennell ML, Pearce PF, Bangdiwala SI (2005). Energy costs of physical activities in children and adolescents. *Med Sci Sports Exerc* **37**, 329–36.
40. Kanaley JA, Boileau RA, Massey BH, Misner JE (1989). Muscular efficiency during treadmill walking: The effects of age and workload. *Pediatr Exerc Sci* **1**, 155–62.
41. MacDougall JD, Roche PD, Bar-Or O, Moroz JR (1983). Maximal aerobic capacity of Canadian schoolchildren: Prediction based on age-related oxygen cost of running. *Int J Sports Med* **4**, 194–8.
42. McMurray RG, Harrell JS, Bangdiwala SI, Deng S, Baggett C (2003). Factors contributing to the energy expenditure of youth during cycling and running. *Pediatr Exerc Sci* **15**, 67–82.
43. Morgan DW, Tseh W, Caputo JL, Keefer DK, Craig IS, Griffith KB, Akins MB, Griffith GE, Martin PE (2001). Longitudinal profiles of oxygen uptake during treadmill walking in able-bodied children: The locomotion energy and growth study. *Gait Posture* **15**, 230–5.
44. Shuleva KM, Hunter GR, Hester DJ, Dunaway DL (1990). Exercise oxygen uptake in 3- through 6-year-old children. *Pediatr Exerc Sci* **2**, 130–9.
45. Anderson KL, Seliger V, Rutenfranz J, Messel S (1974). Physical performance capacity of children in Norway. Part III. Respiratory responses to graded exercise loadings-population parameters in a rural community. *Eur J Appl Physiol* **33**, 265–74.
46. Waters RL, Hislop HJ, Thomas L, Campbell J (1983). Energy cost of walking in normal children and teenagers. *Dev Med Child Neurol* **25**, 184–8.
47. Thorstensson A (1986). Effects of moderate external loading on the aerobic demand of submaximal running in men and 10 year-old boys. *Eur J Appl Physiol* **55**, 569–74.
48. Wickstrom RL (1983). *Fundamental motor patterns*. Lea and Febiger, Philadelphia, PA.
49. Kram R, Taylor CR (1990). Energetics of running: A new perspective. *Nature* **346**, 265–7.
50. Alexander RMcN, Ker RF (1990). Running is priced by the step. *Nature* **346**, 220–1.
51. Taylor CR (1985). Force development during sustained locomotion: A determinant of gait, speed and metabolic power. *J Exp Biol* **115**, 253–62.
52. Greer NL, Hamill J, Campbell KR (1989). Ground reaction forces in children's gait. *Pediatr Exerc Sci* **1**, 45–53.
53. Frost G, Bar-Or O, Dowling J, Dyson K (2002). Explaining differences in the metabolic cost of locomotion among three age groups of children. *J Sports Sci* **20**, 451–61.
54. Rowland TW (1996). *Developmental exercise physiology*. Human Kinetics, Champaign, IL.
55. Hausdorff JM, Zemany L, Peng C-K, Goldberger AL (1999). Maturation of gait dynamics: stride-to-stride variability and its temporal organization in children. *J Appl Physiol* **86**, 1040–7.
56. Heise GD, Martin PE (2001). Are variations in running economy in humans associated with ground reaction force characteristics? *Eur J Appl Physiol* **84**, 438–42.
57. Rowland TW (1989). Oxygen uptake and endurance fitness in children: A developmental perspective. *Pediatr Exerc Sci* **1**, 313–28.
58. Moritani T, Oddsson L, Thorstensson A, Astrand P-O (1989). Neural and biomechanical differences between men and young boys during a variety of motor tasks. *Acta Physiol Scand* **137**, 347–55.
59. Davies CTM (1980). Metabolic cost of exercise and physical performance in children with Some observations on external loading 1980). *Eur J Appl Physiol* **45**, 95–102.
60. Martin PE, Morgan DW (1992). Biomechanical considerations for economical walking and running. *Med Sci Sports Exerc* **24**, 467–74.
61. Ariens GAM, Van Mechelen W, Kemper HCG, Twisk JWR (1997). The longitudinal development of running economy in males and females aged between 13 and 27 years: The Amsterdam Growth and Health Study. *Eur J Appl Physiol* **76**, 214–20.
62. Martinez LR, Haymes EM (1992). Substrate utilization during treadmill running in prepubertal girls and women. *Med Sci Sports* **24**, 975–83.
63. Bar-Or O (1983). *Pediatric sport medicine for the practitioner*. Springer Verlag, New York.
64. Taylor CR, Heglund NC, Maloiy GMO (1982). Energetics and mechanics of terrestrial locomotion. I. Metabolic energy consumption as a function of speed and body size in birds and mammals. *J Exp Biol* **97**, 1–21.
65. Heglund NC, Taylor CR (1988). Speed, stride frequency and energy cost per stride: How do they change with body size and gait? *J Exp Biol* **138**, 301–18.
66. Allor KM, Pivarnik JM, Sam LJ, Perkins CD (2000). Treadmill economy in girls and women matched for height and weight. *J Appl Physiol* **89**, 512–16.
67. Grossner CM, Johnson EM, Cabrera ME (2005). Effect of body size on treadmill economy in female adolescents and adults. *Pediatr Exerc Sci* **17**, 301–10.
68. Frost G, Dowling J, Bar-Or O, Dyson K (1997). Ability of mechanical power estimations to explain differences in metabolic cost of walking and running among children. *Gait Posture* **5**, 120–7.
69. Armstrong N, Welsman JR (1994). Assessment and interpretation of aerobic fitness in children and adolescents. *Exerc Sport Sci Rev* **22**, 435–75.
70. Welsman JR, Armstrong N, Nevill AM, Winter EM, Kirby BJ (1996). Scaling peak $\dot{V}O_2$ for differences in body size. *Med Sci Sports Exerc* **28**, 259–65.
71. Rogers DM, Turley KR, Kujawa KI, Harper KM, Wilmore JH (1995). Allometric scaling factors for oxygen uptake during exercise in children. *Pediatr Exerc Sci* **7**, 12–25.
72. Krahenbuhl GS, Skinner JS, Kohrt WM (1985). Developmental aspects of maximal aerobic power in children. *Exerc Sport Sci Rev* **13**, 503–38.
73. Rowland TR (1998). The case of the elusive denominator. *Pediatr Exerc Sci* **10**, 1–5.
74. Malina RM, Bouchard C, Bar-Or O (2004). *Growth, maturation, and physical activity*. Human Kinetics, Champaign, IL.
75. Cooper DM, Berman N (1994). Ratios and regressions in body size and function: A commentary. *J Appl Physiol* **77**, 2015–17.
76. Darveau CA, Suarez RK, Andrews R, Hochachka PW (2002). Allometric cascade as a unifying principle of body mass effects on metabolism. *Nature* **417**, 166–70.
77. Keefer DJ, Tseh W, Caputo J, Apperson K, McGreal S, Morgan DW (2005). Within- and between-day stability of treadmill walking $\dot{V}O_2$ in children with hemiplegic cerebral palsy. *Gait Posture* **21**, 80–4.
78. Maltais D, Bar-Or O, Pierrynowski M, Galea V (2003). Repeated treadmill walks affect physiologic responses in children with cerebral palsy. *Med Sci Sports Exerc* **35**, 1653–61.
79. Frost G, Bar-Or O, Dowling J, White C (1995). Habituation of children to treadmill walking and running: Metabolic and kinematic criteria. *Pediatr Exerc Sci* **7**, 162–75.
80. Unnithan VB, Murray LA, Timmons JA, Buchanan D, Paton JY (1995). Reproducibility of cardiorespiratory measurements during submaximal and maximal running in children. *Brit J Sports Med* **29**, 66–71.
81. Rogers DM, Turley KR, Kujawa KI, Harper KM, Wilmore JH (1994). The reliability and variability of running economy in 7-, 8-, and 9-year-old children. *Pediatr Exerc Sci* **6**, 287–96.
82. Keefer DJ, Tseh W, Caputo JL, Craig IS, Martin PE, Morgan DW (2000). Stability of running economy in young children. *Int J Sports Med* **21**, 583–5.

83. Tseh W, Caputo JL, Craig IS, Keefer DJ, Martin PE, Morgan DW (2000). Metabolic accommodation of young children to treadmill walking. *Gait Posture* **12**, 139–42.
84. Morgan DW, Tseh W, Caputo JL, Keefer DJ, Craig IS, Griffith KB, Akins MB, Griffith GE, Krahenbuhl GS, Martin PE (2004). Longitudinal stratification of gait economy in young boys and girls: The locomotion energy and growth study. *Eur J Appl Physiol* **91**, 30–4.
85. Rodas G, Calvo M, Estruch A, Garrido E, Ercilla G, Arcas A, Segura R, Ventura J (1998). Heritability of running economy: A study made on twin brothers. *Eur J Appl Physiol* **77**, 511–16.
86. Daniels JT, Scardina NJ, Foley P (1984). $\dot{V}O_2$ submax during five modes of exercise. In: Bachl N, Prokop L, Sucket R (eds.), *Proceedings of the World Congress on Sports Medicine*, pp. 604–15. Urban & Schwartzenberg, Vienna.
87. Maffeis C, Schutz Y, Schena F, Zaffanello M, Pinelli L (1993). Energy expenditure during walking and running in obese and nonobese prepubertal children. *J Pediatr* **123**, 193–9.
88. Turley K, Wilmore JH (1997). Cardiovascular responses to submaximal exercise in 7- to 9-yr-old boys and girls. *Med Sci Sports Exerc* **29**, 824–32.
89. Rowland T, Cunningham L, Martel L, Vanderburgh P, Manos T, Charkoudian N (1997). Gender effects on submaximal energy expenditure in children. *Int J Sports Med* **18**, 420–5.
90. Almarwaey OA, Jones AM, Tolfrey K (2003). Physiological correlates with endurance running performance in trained adolescents. *Med Sci Sports Exerc* **35**, 480–7.
91. Fernhall B, Kohrt W, Burkett LN, Walters S (1996). Relationship between the lactate threshold and cross-country run performance in high school male and female runners. *Pediatr Exerc Sci* **8**, 37–47.
92. Freedson PS, Katch VL, Gilliam TB, MacConnie S (1981). Energy expenditure in prepubescent children: Influence of sex and age. *Am J Clin Nutr* **34**, 1827–30.
93. McMurray RG, Harrell JS, Bangdiwala SI, Deng S, Baggett C (2003). Factors contributing to the energy expenditure of youth during cycling and running. *Pediatr Exerc Sci* **15**, 67–82.
94. Morgan DW, Tseh W, Caputo JL, Craig IS, Keefer DJ, Martin PE (1999). Sex differences in running economy of young children. *Pediatr Exerc Sci* **11**, 122–8.
95. Krahenbuhl GS, Pangrazi RP (1983). Characteristics associated with running performance in young boys. *Med Sci Sports Exerc* **15**, 486–90.
96. Cunningham L (1990). Relationship of running economy, ventilatory threshold, and maximal oxygen consumption to running performance in high school females. *Res Q Exerc Sport* **61**, 369–74.
97. Morse M, Schultz FW, Cassels DE (1949). Relation of age to physiological responses of the older boy (10–17 years) to exercise. *J Appl Physiol* **1**, 683–709.
98. Eriksson BO, Gollnick PD, Saltin B (1973). Muscle metabolism and enzyme activities after training in boys 11–13 years old. *Acta Physiol Scand* **87**, 485–97.
99. Eriksson BO, Karlsson J, Saltin B (1971). Muscle metabolites during exercise in pubertal boys. *Acta Paediatr Scand* **217** (Suppl.), 154–7.
100. Cumming GR, Hastman L, McCort J, McCullough S (1980). High serum lactates do occur in young children after maximal work. *Int J Sports Med* **1**, 66–9.
101. Zanconato S, Buchtal S, Barstow TJ, Cooper DM (1993). ^{31}P-magnetic resonance spectroscopy of leg muscle metabolism during exercise in children and adults. *J Appl Physiol* **74**, 2214–18.
102. Petray CK, Krahenbuhl GS (1985). Running training, instruction on running technique, and running economy in 10-year-old males. *Res Q Exerc Sport* **56**, 251–5.
103. Lussier L, Buskirk ER (1977). Effects of an endurance training program on assessment of work capacity in prepubertal children. *Ann NY Acad Sci* **301**, 734–41.
104. Sjodin B, Svedenhag J (1992). Oxygen uptake during running as related to body mass in circumpubertal boys: A longitudinal study. *Eur J Appl Physiol* **65**, 150–7.
105. Walker JL, Murray TD, Jackson AS, Morrow JR, Michaud TJ (1999). The energy cost of horizontal walking and running in adolescents. *Med Sci Sports Exerc* **31**, 311–22.
106. Morgan DW, Tseh W, Caputo JL, Keefer DJ, Craig IS, Griffith KB, Akins MB, Griffith GE, Krahenbuhl GS, Martin PE (2002). Prediction of the aerobic demand of walking in children. *Med Sci Sports Exerc* **34**, 2097–102.
107. Trost SG, Way R, Okely AD (2006). Predictive validity of three Actigraph energy expenditure equations for children. *Med Sci Sports Exerc* **38**, 380–7.
108. Trost SG, Kerr LM, Ward DS, Pate RR (2001). Physical activity and determinants of physical activity in obese and non-obese children. *Int J Obes Relat Metab Disord* **25**, 822–9.
109. Trost SG, Pate RR, Sallis JF, Freedson PS, Taylor WC, Dowda M, Sirard J (2002). Age and gender differences in objectively measured physical activity in youth. *Med Sci Sports Exerc* **34**, 350–5.
110. Puyau MR, Adolph AL, Vohra FA, Butte NF (2002). Validation and calibration of physical activity monitors in children. *Obes Res* **10**, 150–7.
111. Trost SG, Ward DS, Moorehead SM, Watson PD, Riner W, Burke JR (1998). Validity of the computer science and applications (CSA) activity monitor in children. *Med Sci Sports Exerc* **30**, 629–33.
112. Wickel EE, Eisenmann JC, Welk GJ (2007). Predictive validity of an age-specific MET equation among youth of varying body size. *Eur J Appl Physiol* **101**, 555–63.
113 Arvidsson D, Slinde F, Larsson S, Hulthen L (2007). Energy cost of physical activities in children: Validation of SenseWear Armband. *Med Sci Sports Exerc* **39**, 2076–84.
114. Ekelund U, Franks PW, Wareham NJ, Aman J (2004). Oxygen uptakes adjusted for body composition in normal-weight and obese adolescents. *Obes Res* **12**, 513–20.
115. Ayub BV, Bar-Or O (2003). Energy cost of walking in boys who differ in adiposity but are matched for body mass. *Med Sci Sports Exerc* **35**, 669–74.
116. Falls H, Humphrey L (1976). Energy cost of running and walking in young women. *Med Sci Sports* **8**, 9–13.
117. Menier D, Pugh L (1968). The relation of oxygen intake and velocity of walking and running, in competition walkers. *J Physiol (Lond)* **197**, 717–21.
118. Hreljac A (1993). Preferred and energetically optimal gait transition speeds in human locomotion. *Med Sci Sports Exerc* **25**, 1158–62.
119. Tseh W, Bennett J, Caputo JL, Morgan DW (2002). Comparison between preferred and energetically optimal transition speeds in adolescents. *Eur J Appl Physiol* **88**, 117–21.
120. Corcoran PJ, Brengelmann GL (1970). Oxygen uptake in normal and handicapped subjects, in relation to speed of walking beside velocity-controlled cart. *Arch Phys Med Rehab* **51**, 78–87.
121. Ralston HJ (1958). Energy-speed relation and optimal speed during level walking. *Arbeitsphysiol* **17**, 277–83.
122. DeJaeger D, Willems PA, Heglund NC (2001). The energy cost of walking in children. *Eur J Physiol* **441**, 538–43.
123. Morgan DW, Martin PE, Tseh W, Caputo JL, Craig IS, Keefer DJ (1997). Relationship between preferred and energetically optimal walking speed in young children. *Med Sci Sports Exerc* **29** (Suppl.), S16.
124. Morgan D, Tseh W, Caputo J, Craig I, Keefer D, Martin P (1999). Effect of step length manipulation on the aerobic demand of walking in young children. *Proceedings of the 20th meeting of the European Group of Pediatric Work Physiology*, Sabaudia, Italy.
125. Morgan D, Tseh W, Caputo J, Keefer D, Craig I, Griffith K, Griffith G, Vint P (1999). Comparison of freely-chosen and energetically-optimal walking speeds in children with cerebral palsy. *Pediatr Exerc Sci* **11**, 181–2.

126. Morgan D, Tseh W, Caputo J, Keefer D, Craig I, Griffith K, Griffith G, Vint P (2003). Metabolic cost and preferred step length in children with spastic cerebral palsy. *Revista portuguesa de ciencias do desporto* **3** (Suppl.), 62–3.
127. Evans EP, Tew B (1981). The energy expenditure of spina bifida children during walking and wheelchair ambulation. *Zeitschrift Kinderchir* **34**, 425–7.
128. Herbert LM, Engsberg JR, Tedford KG, Grimston SK (1994). A comparison of oxygen consumption during walking between children with and without below-knee amputations. *Phys Ther* **74**, 943–50.
129. Gage JR (1991). *Gait analysis in cerebral palsy*. MacKeith Press, London.
130. Unnithan VB, Maltais D (2004). Pediatric cerebral palsy. In: LeMura L, von Duvillard SP (eds.), *Clinical exercise physiology*, pp. 285–99. Lippincott Williams & Wilkins, Philadelphia, PA.
131. Nelson KB (1996). Epidemiology and etiology of cerebral palsy. In: Capute AJ, Accardo PJ (eds.), *Developmental disabilities in infancy and childhood*, pp. 73–94. Paul H. Brookes Publishing Co, Baltimore, MD.
132. Unnithan VB, Dowling JJ, Frost G, Bar-Or O (1999). Role of mechanical power estimates in the O_2 cost of walking in children with cerebral palsy. *Med Sci Sports Exerc* **31**, 1703–8.
133. Keefer DJ, Tseh W, Caputo JL, Apperson K, McGreal S, Vint P, Morgan DW (2004). Interrelationships among thigh muscle co-contraction, quadriceps muscle strength and the aerobic demand of walking in children with cerebral palsy. *Electromyogr Clin Neurophysiol* **44**, 103–10.
134. Campbell J, Ball J (1978). Energetics of walking in cerebral palsy. *Orthop Clin N Am* **9**, 74–7.
135. Hoofwijk M, Unnithan V, Bar-Or O (1995). Maximal treadmill performance of children with cerebral palsy. *Pediatr Exerc Sci* **7**, 305–13.
136. Johnston TE, Moore SE, Quinn LT, Smith BT (2004). Energy cost of walking in children with cerebral palsy: Relation to the gross motor function classification system. *Dev Med Child Neurol* **46**, 34–8.
137. Wiley ME, Damiano DL (1998). Lower-extremity strength profiles in spastic cerebral palsy. *Dev Med Child Neurol* **40**, 100–7.
138. MacPhail HEA, Kramer JF (1995). Effect of isokinetic strength-training on functional ability and walking efficiency in adolescents with cerebral palsy. *Dev Med Child Neurol* **37**, 763–75.
139. Carmick J (1993). Clinical use of neuromuscular electrical stimulation for children with cerebral palsy, Part 1: Lower extremity. *Phys Ther* **73**, 505–13.
140. Unnithan VB, Kenne EM, Logan L, Collier S, Turk M (2006). The effect of partial body weight support on the oxygen cost of walking in children and adolescents with spastic cerebral palsy. *Pediatr Exerc Sci* **17**, 11–21.
141. Krahenbuhl GS, Williams TJ (1992). Running economy: Changes with age during childhood and adolescence. *Med Sci Sports Exerc* **24**, 462–6.

CHAPTER 22

Oxygen uptake kinetics

Samantha G. Fawkner and Neil Armstrong

Introduction

Aerobic metabolism is the most efficient process by which the body is able to generate energy for movement. Understanding its role in supporting energy demand under various conditions and being able to comprehend its adaptive contribution to changing metabolic demands is therefore of critical importance to the exercise physiologist.

Hill and Lupton[1] were amongst the first to identify that oxygen uptake ($\dot{V}O_2$) rose in an exponential fashion in response to an increase in exercise intensity but only in the past 20 or 30 years has there been a substantial progress towards understanding the true nature of the dynamics of the $\dot{V}O_2$ response to exercise. This has been partly due to the relatively recent advancement in the technology available for gas and ventilation analysis, which allows the $\dot{V}O_2$ response to be studied on a breath-by-breath basis and also due to the availability and accessibility of automated statistical modelling procedures. Together these allow demonstration of the dynamic properties of the $\dot{V}O_2$ response with relative ease.

The term $\dot{V}O_2$ kinetics has been embraced by the exercise scientist in order to define the changing contribution of oxidative phosphorylation to energy turnover, and pertains not only to the non-steady state at the immediate onset of exercise as described by Hill and Lupton[1] but also to transient changes in $\dot{V}O_2$ during constant load exercise—specifically the slow component of $\dot{V}O_2$. With adults, there have been a plethora of studies examining the $\dot{V}O_2$ kinetic response to exercise, exploring issues from the most basic rudimentary muscle physiology to the exercise response in clinical populations. Conversely, there is a scarcity of published work examining and interpreting the $\dot{V}O_2$ kinetic response in children. This is surprising because one of the fundamental utilities of the kinetic model is that it provides information pertaining to the integrated response of the pulmonary, cardiovascular, and metabolic systems to an exercise stress whilst also being essentially non-invasive; an obvious advantage when wishing to understand the physiology of the growing and maturing child.

Probably, the main reasons for the dearth of interest in this area are the perceived methodological barriers to collecting and interpreting the transient $\dot{V}O_2$ response of children. The sporadic breathing patterns and small response amplitudes of children infer that demanding testing schedules and careful data handling are required to obtain meaningful results, and also suggest that there may be flaws in much of the data that have been published to date.

Despite this, there is a body of literature that provides intriguing contributions to understanding developmental changes of the $\dot{V}O_2$ response to exercise and which may hold important information pertaining to developmental changes in metabolic activity at the muscular level.

The two main purposes of this chapter are therefore to (i) explore the methodological issues involved in assessing the $\dot{V}O_2$ kinetic response to exercise in children, and (ii) explain the $\dot{V}O_2$ kinetic response to exercise in children and review the literature regarding changes with age and sex and with respect to conventional markers of aerobic fitness.

Overview of the oxygen uptake kinetic response to exercise

With adults, and to an extent with children, the nature of the kinetic response has been identified to depend on the relative exercise intensity set. At the onset of moderate intensity exercise (below the anaerobic threshold, T_{AN}; ref. 2), a cardiodynamic phase (phase 1), which is independent of oxygen uptake at the muscle ($\dot{Q}O_2$), is followed by an observable exponential rise in $\dot{V}O_2$ (phase 2) towards a steady state (phase 3), and an oxygen (O_2) cost relative to work rate in adults of approximately 10 $mL \cdot min^{-1} \cdot W^{-1}$. When the exercise intensity is above T_{AN} but below critical power (CP),[3] in the heavy intensity domain, the steady state in $\dot{V}O_2$ is delayed, and an additional slow component of $\dot{V}O_2$ causes an eventual and elevated steady state, and an elevation in the oxygen cost of exercise.[4] Above CP, in the very heavy intensity domain, $\dot{V}O_2$ continues to rise almost linearly, and the slow component causes the eventual attainment of peak $\dot{V}O_2$. In severe intensity exercise, where the projected $\dot{V}O_2$ is greater than peak $\dot{V}O_2$, the response is truncated with the rapid attainment of peak $\dot{V}O_2$ within minutes (see ref. 5 and Fig. 22.1).

The rise in $\dot{V}O_2$ during phase 2 is thought to closely represent the rise in $\dot{Q}O_2$ and is considered to be a linear function of exercise intensity, certainly within the moderate domain. That is, the magnitude of the response is proportional to the stimulus, but the rate change is constant across exercise intensities. It is the rate of this change that is of considerable interest, since the more rapid is the rise to steady state, the smaller is the O_2 deficit, and the less is the

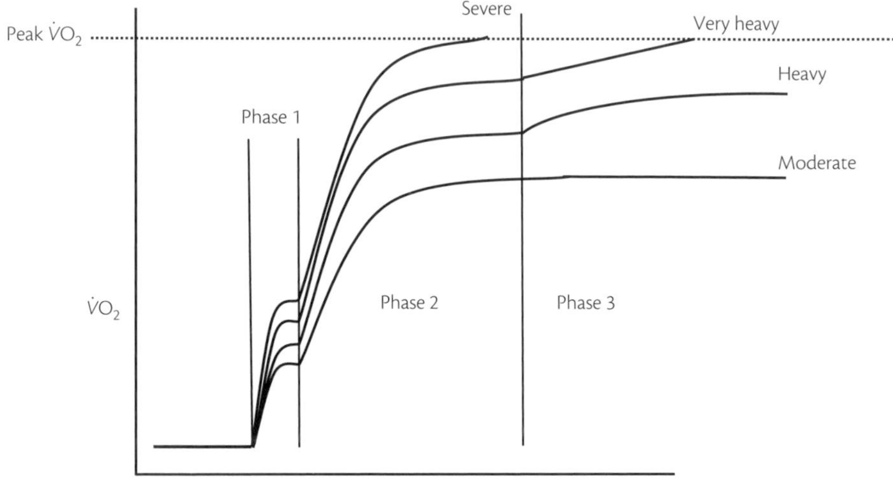

Fig. 22.1 The three phases of the kinetic rise in $\dot{V}O_2$ in response to a step change in exercise in four different exercise intensity domains. Reprinted from Fawkner and Armstrong,[6] with permission.

drain on exhaustible sources. The mechanism(s) controlling this response have been an issue of some contention, and will be considered later. With exercise intensities above T_{AN}, the exponential nature of phase 2 is maintained, but the true nature of the ensuing slow component of $\dot{V}O_2$ is yet to be determined. The source of the additional O_2 cost of exercise in phase 3 at intensities above T_{AN} remains equivocal, but has clear implications regarding efficiency.

Quantifying the oxygen uptake kinetic response

The aim of quantifying $\dot{V}O_2$ kinetics is to evaluate the speed and the magnitude of the $\dot{V}O_2$ response to a given metabolic demand. This is achieved in the laboratory by imposing an exercise stress of known relative intensity, collecting the breath-by-breath response data, and subsequently interpreting it. More often than not, investigators choose to impose a square-wave exercise stress and then use non-linear regression and iterative fitting procedures with the response data to fit a specified model to return the rate of the exponential rise (time constant, τ) and the amplitude of the response. Although some authors have alternatively used pseudo random binary sequence tests and Fourier techniques (which returns the phase delay and amplitude ratio, physiological correlates of the τ, and amplitude following a square-wave transition), the focus here is on the more commonly applied square-wave transition.

There are a number of factors that must be taken into account if the quantification process is to be meaningful. As will become clear, these are particularly pertinent when dealing with children and indicate limitations with a number of published studies reporting the $\dot{V}O_2$ kinetic response in this population.

(i) The relative exercise intensity must be known, and equal between subjects.

The amplitude and pattern of the $\dot{V}O_2$ kinetic response differs according to the exercise intensity domain (see Fig. 22.1), which means that making valid intrastudy and interstudy comparisons requires that subjects are exercising at the same exercise intensity relative to the domain demarcators. For moderate intensity, this is T_{AN}, or one of its derivatives, the lactate threshold (T_{LAC}) or ventilatory threshold (T_{VENT}). For heavy intensity, the demarcator is CP or maximum lactate steady state (MLSS) (see Chapter 8).

Despite this, in order to study the response to moderate intensity exercise, a number of studies with children have set exercise intensities relative to peak $\dot{V}O_2$ alone or have enforced a single exercise intensity across individuals.[7–10] This is problematic since T_{AN} has been shown in children to vary considerably as to the percentage of peak $\dot{V}O_2$ at which it occurs, not least due to the method by which T_{AN} is detected and the method's reliability and validity. More appropriately, setting the exercise intensity as a percentage of T_{AN} provides some assurance that subjects are at least within the same intensity domain, which due to the linearity of the response, is sufficient in order to make valid comparisons.

The kinetic response to exercise intensities above T_{AN} with children has rarely been studied within carefully defined exercise intensity domains. The majority of studies have assessed the response to maximal and 'supramaximal' exercise intensities[7,9,11–14] and few studies have attempted to assess the existence or magnitude of the slow component of $\dot{V}O_2$ with children.[15–20] This is most probably because the assessment of the threshold of heavy intensity exercise, CP or MLSS, is especially demanding in terms of both subject effort and testing time. MLSS is especially invasive involving multiple blood samples over extended periods, whereas CP, which can in theory be estimated from as few as three exhaustive exercise bouts, has only once to the authors' knowledge been attempted and reported with children.[21] As a result, investigators intending to explore the response to heavy intensity exercise have set exercise intensities as a percentage of the difference between T_{AN} and peak $\dot{V}O_2$. To this end, Fawkner and Armstrong[21] identified that CP occurred at between 70% and 80% of peak $\dot{V}O_2$ in 10- to 12-year-old children, similar to values reported for adults, and that 40% of the difference (40% Δ) between T_{AN} and peak $\dot{V}O_2$ was below CP and did indeed fall within the heavy intensity domain.[22]

(ii) The basic pattern of the response must be known so that an appropriate model can be applied for quantification purposes.

A number of models have been proposed to represent the pattern of the kinetic response, both generically and within well-defined exercise intensity domains. Originally, it was considered that the speed of the response to any exercise intensity could be assessed by measuring the time it took to reach half of the peak $\dot{V}O_2$ achieved during the exercise test (i.e. $t^{1/2}$). This method, however, failed to observe the exponential nature of the response, and subsequently

$$\Delta\dot{V}O_2(t) = \Delta\dot{V}O_2(ss)\cdot\left(1-e^{-t/\tau}\right) \qquad \text{[model 1]}$$

$$\Delta\dot{V}O_2(t) = \Delta\dot{V}O_2(ss)\cdot\left(1-e^{-(t-\delta)/\tau}\right) \qquad \text{[model 2]}$$

$$\Delta\dot{V}O_2(t) = A_1\cdot\left(1-e^{-(t-\delta_1)/\tau_1}\right) + A_2\cdot\left(1-e^{-(t-\delta_2)/\tau_2}\right) \qquad \text{[model 3]}$$

$$\Delta\dot{V}O_2(t) = A_1\cdot\left(1-e^{-(t-\delta_1)/\tau_1}\right) + S_2\cdot(t-\delta_2) \qquad \text{[model 4]}$$

Fig. 22.2 Models used for the estimation of kinetic parameters. t, time in seconds; $\Delta\dot{V}O_2$ (t), increase in $\dot{V}O_2$ at time *t* above the prior control level; $\Delta\dot{V}O_2$ (ss), steady-state increment in $\dot{V}O_2$; τ, time constant which is the time to achieve 63% of the $\Delta\dot{V}O_2$ (ss); A_1, A_2, and A_3, τ_1, τ_2, and τ_3; and δ_1, δ_2, and δ_3 represent amplitudes; time constants; and time delays of each exponential, respectively.

the time constant (τ), which represents the moment in time of the exponential function that represents 63% of the change in $\dot{V}O_2$ from baseline to steady state ($\Delta\dot{V}O_2$), has been used in its place and is solved using model 1 in Fig. 22.2.

This model allows a monoexponential to be fit to data from the onset of exercise (i.e. when time = 0 s), and the time constant is usually referred to as the mean response time (MRT). However, the phase 1 response that lasts 10–20 s is independent of $\dot{Q}O_2$, which only becomes evident at the mouth after the muscle to lung transit delay. Therefore, there is a delay in time before $\dot{V}O_2$ is representative of the exponential increase in $\dot{Q}O_2$. Acknowledging this, Whipp *et al.*[23] advocated that the most suitable approach to modelling the response to moderate intensity exercise required the inclusion of a delay term (δ) within the model as well as the model being fit to data following phase 1 only (Fig. 22.2, model 2). It should be noted that although the MRT does not necessarily allow for the accurate determination of the $\dot{V}O_2$ kinetics, it does provide a useful parameter with which to assess the O_2 deficit in the moderate intensity domain, which is the product of the increase in $\dot{V}O_2$ during the transition ($\Delta\dot{V}O_2$) and the MRT.[23]

A number of different models have been used to analyse the response to moderate intensity exercise with children, which makes interstudy comparisons difficult. To illustrate this, in an investigation into different modelling techniques used with children, Fawkner and Armstrong[24] identified that four models used on the same children's data returned time constants that differed by as much as 15 s. They also demonstrated that a single exponential and delay term following phase 1 (model 2) provided a better description of the response during the exponential rise in $\dot{V}O_2$ than did other model connotations (Fig. 22.3) and concluded that as with adults, this is the model of choice to use with children's response data.

The situation becomes more complex when dealing with heavy intensity exercise. The true nature of the response, specifically the slow component, is not entirely understood. Despite this, some authors have chosen to model the slow component as an additional exponential (Fig. 22.2, model 3), suggesting that it represents a delayed and slowly emerging component rather than the one that emerges in synchrony with the initial phase 2 primary component. Thus, the model includes two exponentials each with an independent

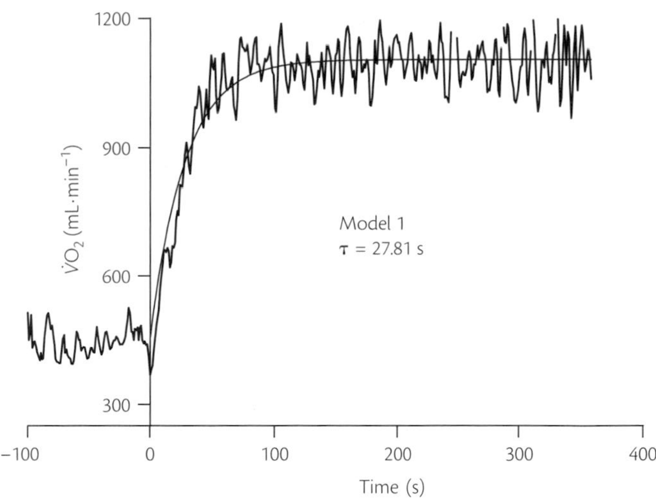

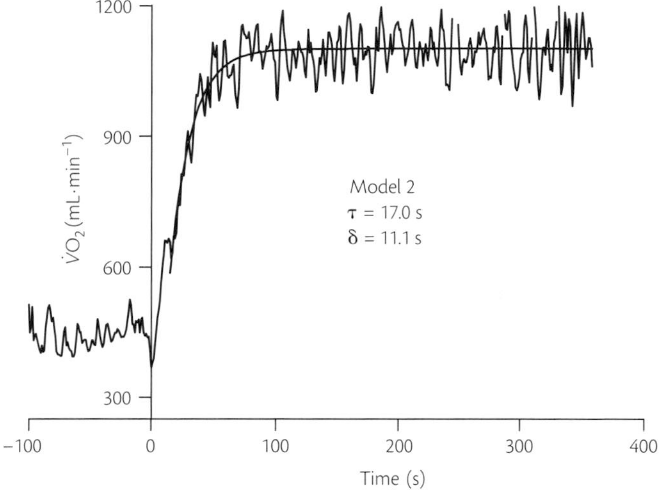

Fig. 22.3 A typical trace of a 12-year-old child's response to moderate intensity exercise. Shown are the best fit curves superimposed for model 1 (the MRT) and model 2 (a single exponential with delay term from 15 s after the onset of exercise) and the returned parameters for the time constant (τ) and delay term (δ). The better description of the response by model 2 is clearly visible during the initial rise in phase 2, and model 1 subsequently results in an underestimation of the $\dot{V}O_2$ as the exponential rises to its asymptotic value.

delay term and two amplitudes, which represent the amplitude of the primary and slow components. With this model, the secondary delay (δ_2) has been interpreted as the time of the onset of the slow component. Other authors have chosen to model the slow component as a linear term (Fig. 22.2, model 4), which has some justification at exercise intensities above CP since at these intensities $\dot{V}O_2$ rises rapidly towards peak $\dot{V}O_2$. Alternative methods of measuring the magnitude of the slow component, such as the change in $\dot{V}O_2$ between the third and sixth minute have also been used, but provide arbitrary analysis of this process, since the time of the onset of the slow component varies widely between individuals.[25]

Despite the widespread use of these models (with adults and to an extent with children), unlike the primary phase 2 component, modelling the slow component with either an exponential or a linear term does not have any confirmed physiological rationale. In fact, attempts to combine models of both the primary and slow components into one model can negate the accuracy with which the primary time constant and amplitude are estimated. This concern is paramount when a model is forced to fit a data set for which the basic pattern of response does not comply. In the case of fitting a double exponential, this is frequently the case if there is either no clear slow component or its rise more closely resembles a linear function than an exponential one.

As a result, more recently, authors have adopted the process of attempting to objectively identify the onset of the slow component, model the data of the primary component independently, and report the amplitude of the slow component with respect to the end exercise $\dot{V}O_2$.[15–17,26] Until a model with a sound physiological basis with which to paramaterize the slow component is identified, it has been suggested that this is the model of choice.[16]

In severe intensity exercise the slow component of $\dot{V}O_2$ does not have time to develop (although investigators must be assured that the exercise intensity is severe enough such that this is the case), and the monoexponentiality of the response is therefore not distorted,[27] and can be modelled as such (Fig. 22.2, model 2). However, only a few early studies have attempted to investigate the kinetic response to severe intensity exercise with children, and they adopted more simple methods to characterize the response.[9,11–14] This was possibly due to the poor temporal resolution of the data collected which would have prevented more complex model parameterization (see below).

(iii) The data must have high temporal resolution.

Early studies with children examining the $\dot{V}O_2$ kinetic response to exercise relied on traditional mixing chamber systems, whereby measures of mixed expired samples were drawn off mixing chambers with measurement intervals of typically 15–30 s. However, since the $\dot{V}O_2$ kinetic response is dynamic and a function of time, it is crucial to carefully preserve the temporal nature of the $\dot{V}O_2$ response during the exercise test and therefore gas and respiratory data must be collected with a much higher temporal resolution, that is, on a breath-by-breath basis. Online metabolic carts have developed significantly since the pioneering work of Beaver *et al.*[28] and although the combination of mass spectrometry and turbine flow meters is possibly still the ultimate tool for assessing true 'breath-by-breath' responses at the mouth, most commercially available metabolic carts with rapidly responding oxygen and carbon dioxide analysers now have the facility to generate breath-by-breath data. Despite this, there are still few studies that have employed these techniques with children.

(iv) The signal-to-noise ratio must be high enough to be able to report response parameters with confidence.

One of the disadvantages of assessing gas and ventilatory variables on a breath-by-breath basis is that the response data reflect not only the true physiological signal of interest, but also breath-by-breath fluctuations in breathing patterns (see Fig. 22.3). Traditionally, of course, the use of mixing chambers dampens this effect, as does averaging a number of breaths together. The source of this 'noise' is mostly due to breath-by-breath variance in minute ventilation (caused by variation in both tidal volume and breathing frequency) and is probably physiological in origin. It does, however, mask the underlying signal that is of interest. Unfortunately for the paediatric exercise physiologist, the magnitude of these fluctuations (the noise) seems to be larger during exercise with children than it is with adults.[29] Since the signal ($\dot{V}O_2$ amplitude in this case) is also smaller with children, the resulting signal-to-noise ratio is often so poor that fitting complex mathematical models requires serious consideration if the investigator is to be at all confident that the model fit is a true reflection of the physiological signal. This is particularly so when models involve a number of parameters, all of which are interdependent (such as in Fig. 22.2, models 3 and 4). It is also a serious issue when dealing with clinical populations, whose tolerance of exercise stresses may be restricted such that the stimulus must be low and thus the response signal disproportionately small.

There are two main procedures that the investigator might carry out to improve confidence in their reported response parameters; reducing the signal-to-noise ratio and reporting the 95% confidence intervals of the response parameters.

The latter of these procedures is now relatively simple to achieve, as many iterative fitting programmes also return the 95% confidence intervals for the response parameters. Ideally, a confidence interval of no more than ±5 s for the primary τ, and ±5% for the primary amplitude should be achieved. Reducing the signal-to-noise ratio to achieve this can however place a substantial practical demand upon the study design. By carrying out a number of repeat transitions, time aligning, and averaging the responses, the magnitude of the noise may be reduced, whilst theoretically the signal remains unaltered.[30] Therefore, whilst a single transition does not allow suitable confidence in estimating response parameters, averaging a series of data sets may do so. The number of transitions that are required to achieve suitable confidence is directly proportional to the amount of data being fit, the variability of the data and the magnitude of the signal, and thus will vary from one individual to another. With children's data that are inherently noisy, as many as 10 transitions at moderate intensity might be required. At heavier intensities, fewer transitions are required because the signal is greater. This concept also allows the investigator to estimate the number of repeat transitions required to achieve a given 95% confidence interval using the amplitude and standard deviation of the steady-state $\dot{V}O_2$ following a single transition for each individual. This technique has proved useful when investigating the $\dot{V}O_2$ kinetic response in children[31] but might be especially effective when dealing with young children with cardiorespiratory or metabolic disorders. In these instances, a number of repeat bouts of exercise might be particularly demanding and practically difficult to achieve, yet may also be meaningless if the responses are still too noisy after averaging for use.[32] For example, a recent study examining $\dot{V}O_2$ kinetics in cystic fibrosis patients (mean age 15.8 ± 6.1 years) had to exclude 6 out of the 24 patients due to noise magnitude, despite averaging up to four transitions.[33]

Unfortunately, few investigations of children to date have incorporated either of these procedures, and where they may have averaged a number of transitions together in order to reduce the signal-to-noise ratio, this is relatively meaningless unless confidence intervals are also reported.

The three phases of the oxygen uptake kinetic response

Phase 1

Characteristics of phase 1

Following the onset of exercise, $\dot{V}O_2$ as measured at the mouth is dissociated temporally from $\dot{Q}O_2$ by the muscle–lung transit delay. As a result, the rise in $\dot{V}O_2$ that is evidenced at the mouth during this transitional phase is independent of absolute changes in mixed venous partial pressures arising from the working muscles. In keeping with the Fick equation, the consequent assumption of constant arteriovenous partial pressures at the lung has provided the basic understanding that immediate changes in $\dot{V}O_2$ are dependent on the circulation of blood through the lungs.[34,35] This is in direct accordance with studies that have shown a rapid increase in heart rate (HR), increases in stroke volume (SV), and total cardiac output ($\dot{Q}$) following the onset of work, and thus this transitional phase has been termed 'cardiodynamic'.[23]

In parallel to the cardiovascular response, exercise hyperpnoea is found to increase at a synchronous rate; hence, this transitional phase is characterized by stable end tidal partial pressures of both oxygen and carbon dioxide, and respiratory exchange ratio (RER) due to close coupling of pulmonary blood flow and alveolar ventilation (see also Chapter 18).

Thus, the end of phase 1 may theoretically be identified as the time at which these ventilatory variables change from their baseline values.[23] However, accurately identifying the precise nature and time of the phase 1 response is made difficult due to breath-by-breath variations and noise superimposed upon the physiological response, and this is particularly so with children's responses (see also Chapter 18). Even if the noise element has been reduced by averaging a number of transitions together, the results of studies which have attempted to define the end of phase 1 visually from response profiles[7,8] must be interpreted cautiously. Where it has not been possible to identify the end of phase 1 with some degree of integrity, and for the purposes of modelling phase 2, phase 1 has also been assumed to be constant amongst individuals (usually 15–20 s).[31,36,37]

Phase 1 responses

Only two studies have examined the magnitude of the phase 1 response between different aged subjects. Springer *et al.*[37] in comparing the response of 6–10 and 18–33 year olds reported that 15 s following a transition from rest to 80% $\dot{V}O_2$, the mass-related phase 1 $\dot{V}O_2$ was similar between groups, although representing a greater percentage of the steady-state response [%$\Delta\dot{V}O_2$(ss)] in the adult group. This was in contrast to an earlier study[36] which found no difference in the %$\Delta\dot{V}O_2$(ss) between 7–10 year olds and 15–18 year olds, the reasons for these discrepancies possibly being related to the more narrow age differences in this latter study. Cooper *et al.*[36] also compared the phase 1 response of an adult group to both 80% T_{AN} and 20 W, which was approximately a 300% difference in exercise intensity. At 20 W, the phase 1 response represented a greater %$\Delta\dot{V}O_2$(ss) in all the subjects, but there was either no difference or only a marginal (25%) absolute increase in the phase 1 amplitude at 80% T_{AN}. Thus, the authors suggested that the phase 1 response may be only moderately dependent on the magnitude of the exercise intensity. Work with adults supports this contention,[38] whereby increases in the phase 1 response to different exercise intensities were small compared with the increase in total $\Delta\dot{V}O_2$(ss).

Hebestreit *et al.*[7] considered the change in the duration of the phase 1 response in adults and children with changing exercise intensities. They documented that the length of phase 1 in 9- to 12-year-old children varied little with the different work rate transitions, whereas it was significantly reduced with increasing exercise intensities with the adult group. In addition, the adult phase 1 response was significantly longer following the 50% peak transition than was found with the children. In the only study to date to consider sex differences in the phase 1 response, phase 1 was found to be significantly shorter in prepubertal boys than girls following the onset of heavy intensity exercise.[15]

Whether, physiologically, we might expect age or sex differences in the phase 1 amplitude and duration is difficult to speculate upon. There are few data illustrating the change in $\dot{Q}$, SV, or HR immediately following the onset of exercise in children, but steady-state data have suggested that children have smaller SVs than adults during submaximal exercise. Effectively, the larger the change in SV and HR, the larger the contribution to steady-state $\dot{V}O_2$ that can be made during phase 1; therefore, it could be expected that the $\dot{V}O_2$ amplitude would be equal between adults and children when expressed relative to body surface area (therefore, removing the effect of differing SV) but in absolute terms represent a higher %$\Delta\dot{V}O_2$(ss) in adults. This hypothesis is supported by Springer *et al.*[37] and may also explain the results of Cooper *et al.*[36] who by indirectly quantifying the change in SV using the Fick equation and values for $\dot{V}O_2$ and HR, older children responded with a greater SV increase during phase 1 than the younger group.

Phase 2

Characteristics of phase 2

The rise in $\dot{V}O_2$ during phase 2 is also disassociated from the rise in $\dot{Q}O_2$ in magnitude due to the muscle utilization of O_2 stores, and in its rate of change, due to an increase in $\dot{Q}$ during the transit delay.[39] Despite this, within the moderate domain, the rate of the exponential increase in $\dot{V}O_2$ when modelled appropriately (see above) has been shown to correlate closely (within 10%) with the exponential rise in $\dot{Q}O_2$.[40–42] During both phases 1 and 2, adenosine triphosphate (ATP) resynthesis cannot be entirely met by the availability of inspired O_2, and energy requirements are primarily met by the breakdown of phosphocreatine via the creatine kinase reaction as well as contributions via anaerobic glycolysis, and from usable O_2 stores including muscle venous O_2 content, tissue PO_2 in the contracting muscles, and oxymyoglobin desaturation.[27] The O_2 equivalent of these alternative sources of energy has been termed the O_2 deficit, and thus, the rate by which aerobic metabolism can adjust to the change in exercise demand influences the depletion of energy reserves.

The mechanism(s) controlling the rate of this response have been an issue of some contention, and also huge interest. The literature suggests that it is primarily governed by the muscles' potential for O_2 utilization, with a number of additional contributory factors involved (see ref. 43 for an in depth review of this topic). With exercise intensities above T_{AN}, although the exponential nature of phase 2 is maintained, the influence of exercise intensity upon the rate change within the heavy and very heavy domains is not confirmed. Although there is conflicting evidence,[44,45] it is possible that at these higher exercise intensities, O_2 delivery may play a greater contributory role in the adaptation of $\dot{V}O_2$.[46]

Phase 2 response to moderate intensity exercise

A few studies have used cross-sectional designs to attempt to identify whether or not the phase 2 $\dot{V}O_2$ time constant (τ) is dependent on age. Early studies were contradictory, but also methodologically flawed due to long sampling intervals and crude modelling techniques[9,10] or no attempt to reduce the noise element in the response.[47] The first study to set exercise intensities relative to T_{AN}, collect breath-by-breath data, and attempt to improve the signal-to-noise ratio by using multiple transitions was that of Cooper *et al.*[36]

Five boys and five girls aged 7–10 years, and five boys and five girls aged 15–18 years completed six square-wave transitions from rest to 75% of T_{VENT}. The data were modelled from 20 s, using model 1. There was no difference in τ between the younger boys (26.5 ± 3.0 s) and the older boys (24.3 ± 2.3 s) but a significant difference between the younger girls (26.5 ± 4.0 s) and older girls (31.6 ± 6.2 s). The older girls also had a lower $\dot{V}O_2$ max [expressed relative to body mass (i.e. $mL{\cdot}kg^{-1}{\cdot}min^{-1}$)] than any of the other groups, and thus the authors concluded that the longer τ in the older girls was a function of their lower fitness rather than age- or sex-related differences in $\dot{V}O_2$ dynamics *per se*. However, the use of simple ratio scaling for the determination of a size-free measure of aerobic fitness is known to artificially lower the 'relative' peak $\dot{V}O_2$ of older and heavier females (see Chapter 2). Indeed, more recent data have identified no relationship between appropriately scaled peak $\dot{V}O_2$ and τ in boys, girls, and women[31] or differences in τ between trained and untrained prepubertal boys and girls.[19] Thus, this explanation seems unlikely.

Using similar protocols, Springer *et al.*[37] examined $\dot{V}O_2$ kinetics in response to a square-wave transition to 80% T_{VENT} during normoxic and hypoxic (15% O_2) conditions. Nine children (five boys and four girls) and nine adults (five males and four females) completed five rest to constant exercise intensity transitions. In this study, a single exponential and delay term were fit to averaged data following the first 15 s (model 2). The time constant (τ) was not significantly longer in the adults than the children during normoxic breathing. During hypoxia, τ was significantly increased in both the children and adults, but the difference between the groups remained non-significant (30.1 ± 4.2 s in children and 37.3 ± 9.9 s in adults). Springer *et al.*'s conclusion was that the control of oxidative metabolism during exercise is mature in childhood, which might also be assumed from more recent data.[7,18] Hebestreit *et al.*[7] assessed the dynamic response from cycling at 20 W to 50% peak $\dot{V}O_2$ in nine boys and eight men. Four 3-min steady-state transitions were averaged and modelled using model 2, following a visually identified phase 1. Mean τ was not significantly different between the boys and men. Williams *et al.*[18] compared the kinetic response to 80% T_{LAC} in treadmill running in boys and men. Eight boys (12.0 ± 0.2 years) and eight men (30.0 ± 7.3 years) took part in the study, which involved four transitions from rest. The averaged response profiles were fit using a double exponential from $t = 0$ s (model 3). There was no significant difference in the mean τ and delay between the boys (10.2 ± 1.0 and 24.7 ± 2.6 s), and the men (14.7 ± 2.8 and 26.8 ± 3.3 s, τ, and delay, respectively).

In this latter study, the authors chose to model the entire response using a double exponential from $t = 0$ s (i.e. they modelled the phase 1 with an exponential process). As has been explained above, over parameterizing the response in this way can introduce substantial error in the response variables, and in this example, an arbitrary adoption of an exponential to model the phase 1 had no physiological rationale and with what was probably noisy data, leaves questions over the confidence in the estimates for τ. In fact, the MRT in this study was significantly different between the boys and men (19.8 ± 1.2 s and 27.2 ± 2.4 s). Similarly, when Hebestreit *et al.*[7] re-analysed their data, they found significant differences in the MRT between the boys (27.3 ± 7.7 s) and men (51.3 ± 10.9 s).

Armon *et al.*[20] also reported faster MRTs in children than men. Six 6- to 12-year-old boys and girls and seven 27- to 40-year-old men completed a single transition from baseline pedalling to 80% of T_{VENT}. The MRT for the children and men was 26 ± 8 s and 44 ± 7 s, respectively. Thus, it seems that the MRT is age-dependent and slows with age. Nevertheless, none of the studies discussed above have provided the methodological rigour required to make substantiated statements with regard to the control of $\dot{V}O_2$ response dynamics. In order to achieve this, Fawkner *et al.*[31] carried out an investigation into the $\dot{V}O_2$ kinetic response to 80% T_{VENT} in 11 boys and 12 girls (11–12 years) and 12 men and 13 women (19–25 years), whilst adopting the techniques of Lamarra *et al.*[30] to maximize the signal-to-noise ratio, using model 2 from $t > 15$ s, and reporting the 95% confidence interval for τ to be less than ±5 s for all subjects. This required some children to complete as many as 10 repeat exercise transitions. These authors found significantly shorter τs for boys (19.0 ± 2.0 s) than men (27.9 ± 8.6 s) and girls (21.0 ± 5.5 s) than women (26.0 ± 4.5 s), and suggested that this might be indicative of enhanced potential for oxidative metabolism in children. Longitudinal studies are required to substantiate fully this hypothesis.

As has been alluded to above, it is not only the speed of the $\dot{V}O_2$ kinetic response, but also the magnitude of the response that provides some indications as to the efficiency of the integrated systems. This is referred to as the gain, or oxygen cost, of the primary component. A higher O_2 cost in younger subjects when expressed as a $\Delta\dot{V}O_2{\cdot}mass^{-1}$ has been reported (12.8 ± 3.5 and 14.3 ± 3.5 $mL{\cdot}min^{-1}{\cdot}kg^{-1}$, older and younger subjects, respectively[36]) and similarly a higher mass-related O_2 cost in children compared with adults was found by Springer *et al.* (10.7 ± 2.0 and 15.1 ± 3.3 $mL{\cdot}min^{-1}{\cdot}kg^{-1}$ in adults and children, respectively[37]) and Williams *et al.* (167.7 ± 3.4 and 239.1 ± 7.5 $mL{\cdot}kg^{-1}{\cdot}km^{-1}$ in adults and children, respectively[18]). However, it has been illustrated from steady-state measures that such differences in the O_2 cost between adults and children are accentuated by the inappropriate normalization procedure of the simple body mass ratio. In fact, when steady-state data are scaled appropriately for body mass, these differences disappear (see ref. 48 and Chapter 2).

Alternatively, O_2 cost (or gain) can be assessed by dividing the $\Delta\dot{V}O_2$ by the change in work rate. Using this parameter of gain, a significant difference between children (11.92 ± 1.12 $mL{\cdot}min^{-1}{\cdot}W^{-1}$) and adults (9.34 ± 1.77 $mL{\cdot}min^{-1}{\cdot}W^{-1}$) exercising at 80% T_{VENT} has been reported,[20] but in another study this difference was not significant (10.9 ± 2.2 and 9.7 ± 0.9 $mL{\cdot}min^{-1}{\cdot}W^{-1}$ boys and men, respectively see ref. 7). Although, in general, the gain in adults is approximately 10 $mL{\cdot}min^{-1}{\cdot}W^{-1}$ (see ref. 49), studies have reported a gain in adults exercising below T_{AN} of 11.2 $mL{\cdot}min^{-1}{\cdot}W^{-1}$ (see ref. 50). Whether or not there is an age-dependent effect on the gain of the primary component during moderate intensity transitions is therefore not known, but remains to be examined further.

Phase 2 response to exercise intensities above the anaerobic threshold

Data relating to the kinetic response to exercise intensities above T_{AN} are restricted to a handful of studies. These include some of the earliest studies regarding the kinetic response to exercise in children, and despite limitations in methodologies and analyses these studies were the first to suggest that children's dynamic response to exercise might be faster than adults. Robinson[12] and Mácek and Vavra[13] identified that during treadmill running, children achieved a greater percentage of their peak exercise response after 30 s of exercise compared with adults. This was later supported using cycle ergometry[14] whereby boys exercising at 100% $\dot{V}O_2$ max achieved 56.4 ± 7.0% $\dot{V}O_2$ max after 30 s compared with 35.5 ± 7.0% $\dot{V}O_2$ max in men. The children also had smaller O_2 deficits and lower end exercise blood lactates. These data were interpreted as evidence of a faster adaptation of aerobic metabolism in children. There has, however, been some contradictory evidence, since both Hebestreit *et al.*[7] and Zanconato *et al.*[11] did not identify any age-related changes to the speed of the response to maximal and supramaximal exercise (100%, 125%, and 130% peak $\dot{V}O_2$). However, despite both of these studies adopting breath-by-breath methodologies, the exercise durations were truncated, and thus parameterization of the system limited response may not have been appropriate to make valid intersubject comparisons.

More recent data examining the response to heavy intensity exercise further supports the contention that the kinetic response to exercise undergoes developmental change. Williams *et al.*[18] and Fawkner and Armstrong[17] have modelled multiple transitions of treadmill running at 50% Δ and cycle ergometry at 40% Δ, respectively. Williams *et al.*[18] reported significantly faster primary components in boys (14.9 ± 1.1 s) than men (19.0 ± 1.6 s) and Fawkner and Armstrong[17] demonstrated a significant slowing of the primary component over a 2-year period in 13 boys and 9 girls aged 10 years at the onset of the study (Table 22.1). This latter study reported the first and, to date, only longitudinal data regarding the kinetic response to exercise in children, which also modelled the primary component independently from the slow component and was also able to demonstrate acceptable confidence intervals for the time constant and amplitude of the primary component. This study also demonstrated a higher O_2 cost of work during the primary component in the younger subjects (Table 22.1 and Fig. 22.4), which supported data previously described regarding the response to heavy intensity exercise.[11,20] This led the authors to further develop the concept that there is a developmental influence on O_2 utilization potential, as a possible function of mitochondrial enzyme activation or intracellular concentration of putative enzyme activation. Whether this is a possible function of fibre type recruitment (see below and Chapter 16), though an attractive explanation, requires substantial further investigation. In addition, it should not be ignored that there is evidence that O_2 delivery (muscle blood flow per unit tissue) may decrease from the ages of 12 through to 14 years.[51] However, the extent to which O_2 delivery limits the phase 2 response to heavy intensity exercise is clouded by contradictory literature, and it seems most probably that O_2 becomes limiting only when severely restricted by disease or old age. Whether poorer O_2 delivery develops during the transition from childhood into adulthood and limits the kinetic response to heavy intensity exercise remains to be proven.

Phase 3 and the slow component

Characteristics of phase 3

In the moderate intensity domain, a steady state in $\dot{V}O_2$ is achieved within approximately 2–3 min, and the amplitude of the response is a linear function of exercise intensity. This is not the case during exercise above T_{AN}, and the linear power–$\dot{V}O_2$ relationship appears to be disrupted resulting in an additional slow component of $\dot{V}O_2$ when exercise is in the heavy and very heavy intensity domains.[4] The source of the additional O_2 cost of exercise at these intensities is most likely to originate from the exercising muscle,[52] rather than the additional cardiac and ventilatory work associated with higher exercise intensities, and although the literature supports a greater phosphate cost of generating muscular force, rather than a greater O_2 cost of phosphate production[53] the precise cause of the reduction in muscle efficiency remains equivocal. Current consensus refutes a causative link with lactate production,[52,54] and favours a dependence on fibre type distribution and recruitment,[55,56] with a range of possible contributory factors (see Gaesser and Poole[57] for a review), particularly the matching of O_2 delivery to the active muscle fibres.[44,58,59]

The slow-component response

Before considering the slow-component response in children, it needs to be noted that discrete phases of the response are a rather

Table 22.1 Changes in the response to heavy intensity exercise over a 2-year period in 22 children

		Test occasion 1		Test occasion 2	
	RM ANOVA	Male (n = 13)	Female (n = 9)	Male (n = 13)	Female (n = 9)
Age (years)	‡	10.6 ± 0.3	10.9 ± 0.2	12.6 ± 0.3	12.9 ± 0.3
Phase 1 (s)	†	16.7 ± 3.3	20.7 ± 4.7	19.5 ± 3.0	24.3 ± 6.1
δ_1 (s)		13.2 ± 4.9	16.0 ± 6.2	13.0 ± 2.7	12.9 ± 3.5
τ_1 (s)	‡	16.8 ± 5.3	21.1 ± 8.1	21.7 ± 5.3	26.4 ± 8.4
A_1 (L·min^{-1})	‡	0.88 ± 0.15	0.79 ± 0.11	1.11 ± 0.11	1.02 ± 0.82
SC (%)	‡	9.4 ± 4.6	10.3 ± 2.4	13.8 ± 5.3	15.5 ± 2.8
G_1 (mL·min^{-1}·W^{-1})	†	11.7 ± 1.1	12.1 ± 0.9	11.6 ± 1.2	11.2 ± 1.3
G_2 (mL·min^{-1}·W^{-1})		12.9 ± 1.0	13.5 ± 1.0	13.3 ± 1.4	13.2 ± 1.3

Values are mean ± SD. RM ANOVA, repeated measures analysis of variance; n, number of subjects; δ and τ, time delay and time constant of the primary component (phase 2); A_1, amplitude of the primary component; SC, difference between the end exercise $\dot{V}O_2$ and A_1 expressed as a percentage of the total change in $\dot{V}O_2$; G_1, O_2 cost (gain) of the primary component; G_2, O_2 cost (gain) at the end of exercise.

† Significant difference between test occasions, $p < 0.05$.

‡ Significant difference between test occasions, $p < 0.01$.

Data taken from Fawkner and Armstrong.[17]

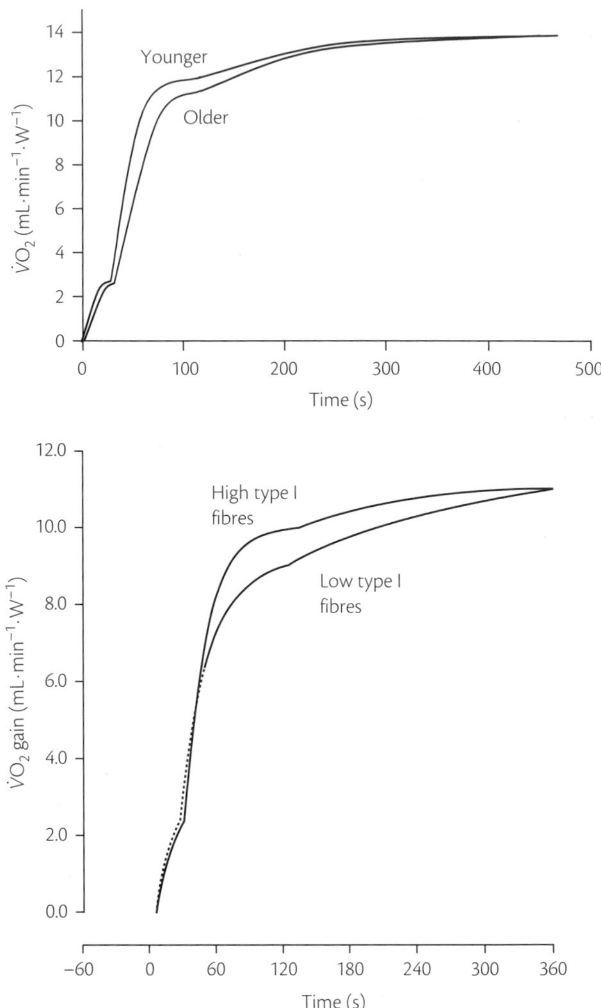

Fig. 22.4 Schematic representations of the gain of the primary component and oxygen cost at the end of a bout of heavy intensity exercise in (i) older and younger subjects (adapted from Fawkner and Armstrong,[17] with permission), and (ii) adults with high and low percentage of type I fibres (adapted from Pringle *et al.*,[59] with permission). Of note is the remarkably similar trend between younger and older subjects and adults with higher and lower percentage of type 1 fibres. Also of interest is the comparison between the two studies in the primary $\dot{V}O_2$ gain, which is substantially higher in the children than it is in the adults.

crude simplification of a complex physiological process. Although there is a sound rationale for the discrete separation of the first and second phases of the kinetic response, this is not the case for phase 3, certainly at exercise intensities above T_{AN}. This was alluded to under the discussion regarding the quantification of the slow component, and it is equally important to keep this in mind when considering the interpretation of the available data, especially since, as will become clear, the nature of the primary component seems inextricably linked to the slow component.

Although there are concerns with some of the methodology adopted by Armon *et al.*,[20] these authors made the first valuable contribution to identifying that, unlike at moderate intensity, not only the speed but also the pattern of the response to heavy intensity exercise might be different in children. These authors suggested that the response to heavy and very heavy intensity cycling in children could be suitably modelled using a single exponential. In other words, children did not display the slow-component response identified in adults. It was further suggested that this was due to children achieving a greater percentage of the final $\dot{V}O_2$ steady state during the primary component (phase 2), a greater O_2 gain during the primary component and a faster primary time constant (as we have seen above). This study was later supported during treadmill running, in which the contribution of the slow component (suitably quantified as the difference between the amplitude of the primary component and the end exercise $\dot{V}O_2$ as a percentage of the total change in $\dot{V}O_2$) was significantly smaller in boys compared with men.[18] Again, these authors suggested that the children's responses could be adequately modelled using the equivalent of just a single exponential.

In Fawkner and Armstrong's[17] study of children at age 10 and then 12 years, the response to 40% Δ was modelled by first identifying the onset of the slow component, and then modelling with a single exponential (model 2) only the primary component. The slow component was then quantified as in the study of Williams *et al.*[18] As with previous studies, when the children were younger, the relative slow component was smaller, the gain of the primary response was greater and the primary time constant was faster. Contrary to other authors, however, a slow component was clearly demonstrated in the children at both ages, and it has also been demonstrated empirically elsewhere[16] that in fact the slow component does exist in children and should not be modelled as a single exponential process.

Explanations for these age-related changes in the slow component are difficult to confirm but it is interesting that they mirror very closely differences between adults with high and low percentage of fast twitch muscle fibres (see Fig. 22.4 and refs 55, 60). These studies have identified a significant negative correlation between % type I fibres and the relative amplitude of the slow component and the primary time constant, and positive correlations with the primary gain. Also similar to the comparison across ages, these authors found no differences between those with a high and low % of slow twitch fibres in the gain at the end of a heavy intensity exercise bout. There is currently limited evidence suggesting that the fibre type profile of the muscle changes during growth and maturation, and whether changes in fibre type profiles and their activation contributes to observed changes in the parameters of the kinetic response to heavy intensity exercise remains a topic of great interest in both the adult and paediatric literature (see Chapter 16).

Oxygen uptake kinetics, sex differences, and the relationship with peak oxygen uptake

Two studies have addressed sex differences in the $\dot{V}O_2$ kinetic response to moderate intensity exercise. Cooper *et al.*[36] reported a significantly slower τ in five teenage (15–18 years) girls, then in five teenage boys, and in five younger (7–10 years) girls and boys, and as discussed above, attributed the sex and age difference to the teenage girls' significantly smaller mass-related $\dot{V}O_2$ max. Contrary to this study, Fawkner *et al.*[31] found no sex difference in τ in either children or adults, despite significant sex differences in peak $\dot{V}O_2$ expressed in traditional ratio form or when suitably scaled to body mass. This study also reported no significant relationship between peak $\dot{V}O_2$ and τ in the children or the women, but a significant negative relationship between the two variables in the men. To this effect, traditionally, it had been assumed that peak $\dot{V}O_2$ and τ were causally linked, but more recent data have contradicted this. Training studies completed with adults have identified independent training adaptations on peak $\dot{V}O_2$ and τ[61] and Obert *et al.*[19] have demonstrated significant differences in peak $\dot{V}O_2$ between a group of trained (51.1 ± 3.8 mL·kg^{-1}·min^{-1}) and untrained (38.3 ± 5.6 mL·kg^{-1}·min^{-1}) boys and girls, but no significant difference in τ.

Peak $\dot{V}O_2$ is considered to be predominantly limited by $\dot{Q}$, that is, O_2 delivery (see Chapter 20). Conversely, it is generally accepted that O_2 delivery plays a minor role in limiting the speed of the kinetic response to moderate intensity exercise which is limited by the aerobic potential of the exercising muscle. It is therefore not surprising that these two parameters of 'aerobic fitness' are not causally linked. In fact, sex differences in peak $\dot{V}O_2$ even in the prepubertal years are explained by sex differences in $\dot{Q}$, but to date there is limited evidence that sex differences in the metabolic profile of the exercising muscle exist (see Chapters 16 and 20). Thus, it appears that certainly in children, sex differences in the kinetic response to moderate intensity do not exist, and that τ is independent of peak $\dot{V}O_2$.

As with moderate intensity exercise, the relationships between parameters of the $\dot{V}O_2$ kinetic response to heavy intensity exercise and peak $\dot{V}O_2$ are not as close as one might expect and, in adults, a reduction in the amplitude of the slow component has been demonstrated following short periods of training without substantial increases in peak $\dot{V}O_2$.[62] There is no evidence to date to suggest that the response to heavy intensity exercise in children may equally respond to training. Obert *et al.*[19] identified no difference between their group of trained and untrained children in the percentage contribution of the slow component to the total change in $\dot{V}O_2$ when cycling at 90% of their maximal aerobic power. However, longitudinal training studies that are appropriately controlled and that are of sufficient length are required before training adaptations of the $\dot{V}O_2$ kinetic response to exercise in children might be identified.

There are some data to suggest that sex differences in the kinetic response to heavy intensity exercise might exist, independent of sex differences in peak $\dot{V}O_2$. A comparison of 25 prepubertal males and 23 prepubertal females identified that the boys had a faster primary time constant than the girls (17.6 ± 5.8 and 21.9 ± 8.2 s, respectively) and a smaller contribution of the slow component to the total change in $\dot{V}O_2$ (8.9 ± 3.7 and 11.8 ± 5.5%, respectively).[14] This was contrary to the same researchers' findings with respect to moderate intensity exercise. Since the response to heavy intensity exercise is thought more likely to be limited by O_2 delivery than at moderate intensity, it is reasonable to suggest that these sex differences might be due to the sex differences in SV that are known to exist in prepubertal years (see Chapter 19). The girls, however, had higher end exercise HR values, and as with steady-state exercise, this may have been sufficient to offset any sex difference in SV such that $\dot{Q}$ was equal between the boys and girls. As mentioned previously, there is only limited evidence to suggest that sex differences in the metabolic profile of the muscle, specifically fibre types, might exist and therefore explanations for these sex differences remain elusive. Nevertheless, these data support the concept that even in the prepubertal years, sex differences in the response to exercise do exist.

Summary

- The study of $\dot{V}O_2$ kinetics provides essential information regarding the efficiency of the cardiovascular, pulmonary, and metabolic systems via non-invasive methods, and therefore has a great deal of potential for use by the paediatric exercise physiologist.
- Critical to the effective interpretation of $\dot{V}O_2$ kinetics is the appropriate and careful application of exercise testing and data analysis methods. In the case of exercise testing with children, this requires additional methodological rigour in order to be confident in the model parameters on which the interpretation is based.
- Compared with the interest and available data regarding the $\dot{V}O_2$ kinetic response in adults, there are few studies that have considered age, sex, or training interactions with $\dot{V}O_2$ kinetics in young people, and a number of these can be questioned with regard to the rigour of the methodologies adopted.
- Despite this, the data do suggest that phase 2 of the $\dot{V}O_2$ kinetic response is faster in younger compared with older children and adults, and that children display a greater O_2 cost of exercise during phase 2. This trend is most consistently seen at exercise intensities above the anaerobic threshold.
- The slow-component response to exercise above the anaerobic threshold as typically seen in adults is demonstrated by children, but the evidence to date suggests that it is attenuated in younger children.
- Sex differences in the $\dot{V}O_2$ response to moderate intensity exercise do not appear to exist whereas in the response to heavy intensity, girls appear to have slower phase 2 $\dot{V}O_2$ kinetics and a larger relative slow component than boys. Whether this reflects sex differences in O_2 delivery or potential for aerobic metabolism is not known.
- Parameters of the $\dot{V}O_2$ kinetic response appear to be poorly correlated with peak $\dot{V}O_2$ in children, and there are no longitudinal data available to suggest whether or not training will impart a significant influence on $\dot{V}O_2$ kinetics in young people.
- Explanations for the apparent age-dependent effect on the $\dot{V}O_2$ kinetic response can only be speculative at this stage. Under the premises that the response to moderate intensity exercise is primarily governed by the muscles' potential for oxidative phosphorylation, and that differences in the response to heavy intensity exercise in younger and older children mirror closely the differences between adults with high and low percentage type 1 fibres, these data contribute to the body of evidence which suggests that children, compared with adults, have an enhanced potential for aerobic metabolism.

References

1. Hill AV, Lupton H (1923). Muscular exercise, lactic acid and the supply and utilization of oxygen. *Q J Med* **16**, 135–71.
2. Wasserman K, Hansen JE, Sue DY, Whip BJ, Casaburi R (1994). *Principles of exercise testing and interpretation* (2nd ed.). Lea and Febiger, Philadelphia, PA.
3. Moritani T, Nagata A, deVries HA, Muro M (1981). Critical power as a measure of physical work capacity and anaerobic threshold. *Ergonomics* **24**, 339–50.

4. Poole DC, Ward SA, Gardner GW, Whipp BJ (1988). Metabolic and respiratory profile of the upper limit for prolonged exercise in man. *Ergonomics* **31**, 1265–79.
5. Whipp BJ, Mahler M (1980). Dynamics of pulmonary gas exchange during exercise. In: West BJ (ed.), *Pulmonary gas exchange* (2nd ed.), pp. 33–96. Academic Press, New York.
6. Fawkner SG, Armstrong N (2003). Oxygen uptake kinetic response to exercise in children. *Sports Med* **33**, 651–69.
7. Hebestreit H, Kriemler S, Hughson RL, Bar-Or O (1998). Kinetics of oxygen uptake at the onset of exercise in boys and men. *J Appl Physiol* **85**, 1833–41.
8. Hamar D, Tkac M, Komadesl L, Kuthanová O (1991). Oxygen uptake kinetics at various intensities of exercise on the treadmill in young athletes. In: Frenkl R, Szmodis I (eds.), *Children and exercise pediatric work physiology xv*, pp. 187–201. National Institute for Health Promotion, Budapest.
9. Sady SP (1981). Transient oxygen uptake and heart rate responses at the onset of relative endurance exercise in prepubertal boys and adult men. *Int J Sport Med* **2**, 240–4.
10. Freedson PS, Gilliam TB, Sady SP, Katch VL (1981). Transient $\dot{V}O_2$ characteristics in children at the onset of steady-rate exercise. *Res Q Exerc Sport* **52**, 167–73.
11. Zanconato S, Cooper DM, Armon Y (1991). Oxygen cost and oxygen uptake dynamics and recovery with 1 min of exercise in children and adults. *J Appl Physiol* **71**, 993–8.
12. Robinson S (1938). Experimental studies of physical fitness in relation to age. *Int Z Angew Physiol* **10**, 251–323.
13. Mácek M, Vavra J (1977). Relation between aerobic and anaerobic energy supply during maximal exercise in boys. In: Lavallée H, Shephard RJ (eds.), *Frontiers of activity and child health*, pp. 157–9. Pelican, Quebec.
14. Mácek M, Vávra J (1980). The adjustment of oxygen uptake at the onset of exercise: A comparison between prepubertal boys and young adults. *Int J Sport Med* **1**, 70–2.
15. Fawkner SG, Armstrong N (2004). Sex differences in the oxygen uptake kinetic response to heavy-intensity exercise in prepubertal children. *Eur J Appl Physiol* **93**, 210–16.
16. Fawkner SG, Armstrong N (2004). Modelling the $\dot{V}O_2$ kinetic response to heavy intensity exercise in children. *Ergonomics* **47**, 1517–27.
17. Fawkner SG, Armstrong N (2004). Longitudinal changes in the kinetic response to heavy-intensity exercise in children. *J Appl Physiol* **97**, 460–6.
18. Williams CA, Carter H, Jones AM, Doust JH (2001). Oxygen uptake kinetics during treadmill running in boys and men. *J Appl Physiol* **90**, 1700–6.
19. Obert P, Cleuziou C, Candau R, Courteix D, Lecoq AM, Guenon P (2000). The slow component of O_2 uptake kinetics during high-intensity exercise in trained and untrained prepubertal children. *Int J Sports Med* **21**, 31–6.
20. Armon Y, Cooper DM, Flores R, Zanconato S, Barstow TJ (1991). Oxygen uptake dynamics during high-intensity exercise in children and adults. *J Appl Physiol* **70**, 841–8.
21. Fawkner SG, Armstrong N (2002). Assessment of critical power in children. *Pediatr Exerc Sci* **14**, 259–68.
22. Fawkner SG, Armstrong N (2003). The slow-component response of $\dot{V}O_2$ to heavy intensity exercise in children. In: Reilly T, Marfell-Jones M (eds.), *Kinanthropometry VIII*, pp. 105–13. Routledge, London.
23. Whipp BJ, Ward SA, Lamarra N, Davis JA, Wasserman K (1982). Parameters of ventilatory and gas exchange dynamics during exercise. *J Appl Physiol* **52**, 1506–13.
24. Fawkner SG, Armstrong N (2002). Modelling the $\dot{V}O_2$ kinetic response to moderate intensity exercise in children. *Acta Kinesiol Universit Tartu* **7**, 80–4.
25. Bearden SE, Moffatt RJ (2001). $\dot{V}O_2$ slow component: To model or not to model? *Med Sci Sports Exerc* **33**, 677–80.
26. Rossiter HB, Ward SA, Kowalchuk JM, Howe FA, Griffiths JR, Whipp BJ (2002). Dynamic asymmetry of phosphocreatine concentration and O_2 uptake between the on- and off-transients of moderate- and high-intensity exercise in humans. *J Physiol* **541**, 991–1002.
27. Whipp B, Özyener F (1998). The kinetics of exertional oxygen uptake: Assumptions and inferences. *Med Sport (Roma)* **51**, 139–49.
28. Beaver WL, Wasserman K, Whipp BJ (1973). On-line computer analysis and breath-by-breath graphical display of exercise function tests. *J Appl Physiol* **34**, 123–32.
29. Potter CR, Childs DJ, Houghton W, Armstrong N (1999). Breath-to-breath 'noise' in children's ventilatory and gas exchange responses to exercise. *Eur J Appl Physiol* **80**, 118–24.
30. Lamarra N, Whipp BJ, Ward SA, Wasserman K (1987). Effect of interbreath fluctuations on characterizing exercise gas exchange kinetics. *J Appl Physiol* **62**, 2003–12.
31. Fawkner SG, Armstrong N, Potter CR, Welsman JR (2002). $\dot{V}O_2$ kinetics in children and adults following the onset of moderate intensity exercise. *J Sports Sci* **20**, 319–26.
32. Potter CR, Unnithan VB (2005). Interpretation and implementation of oxygen uptake kinetics studies in children with spastic cerebral palsy. *Dev Med Child Neurol* **47**, 353–7.
33. Hebestreit H, Hebestreit A, Trusen A, Hughson RL (2005). Oxygen uptake kinetics are slowed in cystic fibrosis. *Med Sci Sports Exerc* **37**, 10–17.
34. Weissman ML, Jones PW, Oren A, Lamarra N, Whipp BJ, Wasserman K (1982). Cardiac output increase and gas exchange at start of exercise. *J Appl Physiol* **52**, 236–44.
35. Casaburi R, Daly J, Hansen JE, Effros RM (1989). Abrupt changes in mixed venous blood gas composition after the onset of exercise. *J Appl Physiol* **67**, 1106–12.
36. Cooper DM, Berry C, Lamarra N, Wasserman K (1985). Kinetics of oxygen uptake and heart rate at onset of exercise in children. *J Appl Physiol* **59**, 211–17.
37. Springer C, Barstow TJ, Wasserman K, Cooper DM (1991). Oxygen uptake and heart rate responses during hypoxic exercise in children and adults. *Med Sci Sport Exerc* **23**, 71–9.
38. Sietsema KE, Daly JA, Wasserman K (1989). Early dynamics of O_2 uptake and heart rate as affected by exercise work rate. *J Appl Physiol* **67**, 2535–41.
39. Whipp BJ, Ward SA (1990). Physiological determinants of pulmonary gas exchange kinetics during exercise. *Med Sci Sport Exerc* **22**, 62–71.
40. Barstow TJ, Molé PA (1987). Simulation of pulmonary O_2 uptake during exercise transients in humans. *J Appl Physiol* **63**, 2254–61.
41. Grassi B, Poole DC, Richardson RS, Knight DR, Erickson BK, Wagner PD (1996). Muscle O_2 uptake kinetics in humans: Implications for metabolic control. *J Appl Physiol* **80**, 988–98.
42. Rossiter HB, Ward SA, Doyle VL, Howe FA, Griffiths JR, Whipp BJ (1999). Inferences from pulmonary O_2 uptake with respect to intramuscular (phosphocreatine) kinetics during moderate exercise in humans. *J Physiol (Lond)* **518**, 921–32.
43. Jones AM, Poole DC (2005). *Oxygen uptake kinetics in sport, exercise and medicine.* Routledge, London and New York.
44. Burnley M, Jones AM, Carter H, Doust JH (2000). Effects of prior heavy exercise on phase II pulmonary oxygen uptake kinetics during heavy exercise. *J Appl Physiol* **89**, 1387–96.
45. Tschakovsky ME, Hughson RL (1999). Interaction of factors determining oxygen uptake at the onset of exercise. *J Appl Physiol* **86**, 1101–13.
46. Grassi B, Hogan MC, Kelley KM, Aschenbach WG, Hamann JJ, Evans RK, Patillo RE, Gladden LB (2000). Role of convective O_2 delivery in determining $\dot{V}O_2$ on-kinetics in canine muscle contracting at peak $\dot{V}O_2$. *J Appl Physiol* **89**, 1293–301.
47. Cooper DM, Weiler-Ravell D, Whipp BJ, Wasserman K (1984). Aerobic parameters of exercise as a function of body size during growth in children. *J Appl Physiol* **56**, 628–34.

48. Armstrong N, Kirby B, Welsman J (1997). Submaximal exercise in prepubertal children. In: Armstrong N, Kirby B, Welsman J (eds.), *Children and exercise XIX*, pp. 221–7. E & FN Spon, London.
49. Whipp BJ (1994). The slow component of O_2 uptake kinetics during heavy exercise. *Med Sci Sport Exerc* **26**, 1319–26.
50. Barstow TJ, Molé PA (1991). Linear and non-linear characteristics of oxygen uptake kinetics during heavy exercise. *J Appl Physiol* **71**, 2099–106.
51. Koch G (1977). Development of aerobic power, lung dimensions and muscle blood flow during the age period 12–14 years under the influence of intensive physical training. In: Lavallée H, Shephard R (eds.), *Frontiers of activity and child health*, pp. 169–78. Pelican, Quebec.
52. Poole DC, Schaffartzik W, Knight DR, Derion T, Kennedy B, Guy HJ, Prediletto R, Wagner PD (1991). Contribution of exercising legs to the slow component of oxygen uptake kinetics in humans. *J Appl Physiol* **71**, 1245–60.
53. Rossiter HB, Ward SA, Howe FA, Kowalchuk JM, Griffiths JR, Whipp BJ (2002). Dynamics of intramuscular ^{31}P-MRS Pi peak splitting and the slow components of PCr and O_2 uptake during exercise. *J Appl Physiol* **93**, 2059–69.
54. Womack CJ, Davis SE, Blumer JL, Barrett E, Weltman AL, Gaesser GA (1995). Slow component of O_2 uptake during heavy exercise: Adaptation to endurance training. *J Appl Physiol* **79**, 838–45.
55. Barstow TJ, Jones AM, Nguyen PH, Casaburi R (1996). Influence of muscle fiber type and pedal frequency on oxygen uptake kinetics of heavy exercise. *J Appl Physiol* **81**, 1642–50.
56. Poole DC, Barstow TJ, Gaesser GA, Willis WT, Whipp BJ (1994). $\dot{V}O_2$ slow component: Physiological and functional significance. *Med Sci Sport Exerc* **26**, 1354–8.
57. Gaesser GA, Poole DC (1996). The slow component of oxygen uptake kinetics in humans. *Exerc Sport Sci Rev* **24**, 35–71.
58. Bohnert B, Ward SA, Whipp BJ (1998). Effects of prior arm exercise on pulmonary gas exchange kinetics during high-intensity leg exercise in humans. *Exp Physiol* **83**, 557–70.
59. Gerbino A, Ward SA, Whipp BJ (1996). Effects of prior exercise on pulmonary gas-exchange kinetics during high-intensity exercise in humans. *J Appl Physiol* **80**, 99–107.
60. Pringle JS, Doust JH, Carter H, Tolfrey K, Campbell IT, Jones AM (2003). Oxygen uptake kinetics during moderate, heavy and severe intensity 'submaximal' exercise in humans: The influence of muscle fibre type and capillarisation. *Eur J Appl Physiol* **89**, 289–300.
61. Phillips SM, Green HJ, MacDonald MJ, Hughson RL (1995). Progressive effect of endurance training on $\dot{V}O_2$ kinetics at the onset of submaximal exercise. *J Appl Physiol* **79**, 1914–20.
62. Carter H, Jones AM, Barstow TJ, Burnley M, Williams C, Doust JH (2000). Effect of endurance training on oxygen uptake kinetics during treadmill running. *J Appl Physiol* **89**, 1744–52.

CHAPTER 23

Temperature regulation

Bareket Falk and Raffy Dotan

Introduction

Humans live in a broad range of environmental conditions, yet can maintain body temperature within a relatively narrow range (35–41°C). This is achieved behaviourally, technologically, and physiologically. This chapter will only deal with the latter. The physiological ability to regulate body temperature is essential for maintaining normal physiological function. During exercise, the metabolic heat produced by the working muscles can be up to ~20 times that produced during rest, depending on the intensity of exercise and the working muscle mass. In a hot environment, this heat production places an added stress on the thermoregulatory mechanisms, while in a cold environment, that extra heat may relieve some or all of the cold stress.

Heat is exchanged between the body and the environment via evaporation or via dry heat exchange (radiation, convection, conduction). In a hot environment, physiological means for heat dissipation include sweating, intended to enhance evaporative heat loss, cutaneous vein dilation, and increased skin blood flow to enhance heat transfer from the body's core to the periphery and from there to the environment. In the cold, physiological means of heat conservation include increased metabolic rate for enhancing heat production and peripheral vasoconstriction to minimize heat loss to the environment.

Thermoregulation is affected by environmental conditions as well as by physical and physiological characteristics of the body. Depending on the medium (e.g. air vs. water), environmental factors that affect thermoregulation include temperature, humidity, velocity, and density, and solar or other sources of radiation. Physical factors that can affect evaporative and dry heat exchange include body dimensions, composition, and proportions (e.g. body surface area to mass ratio). Physiological factors affecting thermoregulation include thermal sensitivity of various organ systems, level of acclimatization, aerobic fitness, and hydration state. These factors affect the thermoregulatory response to heat and to cold, although their unique effect in a particular environment is not always clear.

This chapter outlines the physical and physiological changes that occur during growth and maturation and the possible effects these changes can have on the nature and effectiveness of thermoregulation. The physiological responses to heat stress are discussed in terms of metabolic, circulatory, hormonal, and sweating responses, changes in body temperature, and in terms of heat tolerance. Also discussed is hydration status, which can affect thermoregulatory effectiveness in the heat. The physiological response to cold stress is considered in terms of the metabolic and circulatory responses and their possible influence on the effectiveness of thermoregulation. The discussion does not outline the thermoregulatory response *per se*, but rather emphasizes the differences in that response between children and adults. Finally, child–adult differences in the acclimatization- and training-induced adaptations to thermal stress are discussed.

Most studies characterize their subjects by chronological rather than maturational stage, although the latter may be more significant for thermoregulation. For the purpose of this discussion, the term '*children*' is used for girls and boys younger than 10 and 11 years, respectively. When maturational stage is not mentioned, children in this age category are considered '*prepubescents*'. The term '*adolescents*' is used for older children and, when not specifically mentioned, adolescents are considered '*mid- or late-pubescents*'.

Physical and physiological child–adult differences

Many of the physical and physiological characteristics that change during growth and maturation affect the ability to dissipate or preserve body heat. These changes occur at different rates and both their unique and combined thermoregulatory effects are, therefore, difficult to quantitatively evaluate. Table 23.1 summarizes these changes and their likely effects on thermoregulation. A short discussion of these changes follows.

Physical differences

Body surface area to mass ratio

Heat transfer between the body and the environment is related to the exposed body surface area. Metabolic heat production during exercise, on the other hand, is proportional to the active muscle mass, which in turn is related to body mass. The surface area to mass ratio of a 10 year old, 135 cm, and 30 kg child (SA = 1.07 m^2), would be 356 $cm^2 \cdot kg^{-1}$, or 32% greater than the 269 $cm^2 \cdot kg^{-1}$ of a 180 cm and 70 kg adult (SA = 1.89 m^2). During growth and maturation, there is a proportionally greater increase in body mass than in surface area. Therefore, the surface area to mass ratio decreases.

Table 23.1 Physical and physiological changes occurring during growth and maturation and their effect on thermoregulation

Change	Effect on thermoregulation	
	Heat	**Cold**
Physical		
Decrease in body surface area to mass ratio	Decrease in heat gain	Decrease in heat loss
Increase in adiposity (in girls vs. women)	Increase in insulation—impedes heat loss	Increase in insulation—enhance heat conservation
Increase in blood volume per unit body surface area	Decrease in the proportion of blood volume necessary for the perfusion of the periphery or the central nervous system	
Increase in sweat gland size	Increase in sweat gland output	
Physiological		
Decrease in the oxygen cost of locomotion	Decrease in metabolic heat production per unit body mass	Decrease in metabolic heat production per unit body mass
Increase in submaximal and maximal cardiac output	Possible increase in the perfusion of the periphery or the central nervous system	
Increase in sweat gland anaerobic metabolism	Increase in sweating rate	
Increase in prolactin response to exercise in the heat	Possible change in electrolyte composition	

In a thermoneutral or warm environment, children's greater surface area to mass ratio allows them to rely more on dry heat loss (radiation, convection, conduction) and less on evaporative cooling.[1–4] In more extreme hot or cold conditions, the skin to air temperature gradient is large, and more heat is exchanged between the body and the environment. In a hot environment, the child's greater surface area to mass ratio means elevated heat absorption from the surroundings. At some point, the child may no longer be able to compensate sufficiently with evaporative cooling. In the cold, on the other hand, the child's greater ratio results in a greater heat loss to the environment. At a certain stage, the child may not be capable of compensating via vasoconstriction or the limited extent to which metabolic heat production could be raised.

Body composition

The specific heat of fat is much lower than that of fat-free mass (1.67 vs. 3.35 $kJ \cdot kg^{-1} \cdot {}^{\circ}C^{-1}$, respectively). Thus, the body's specific heat depends, to a large extent, on its level of adiposity. Adiposity level is generally similar in prepubescent girls and boys and in men, which means that they all have similar specific heat characteristics. Women, on the other hand, have a body composition marked by a higher fat to lean mass ratio[5] and would therefore possess lower relative heat capacity. That is, under heat stress, prepubertal girls' core temperature would be expected to rise more slowly than that of women. The significance of the specific heat issue has, however, been exaggerated. A much more significant issue with adiposity is overweight, not fat to lean mass ratio. This means higher, not lower, total heat capacity of overweight/obese individuals.

The main significance of adiposity is the insulative properties of fat. Thus, overweight/obese individuals are less effective heat dissipaters—a severe burden and potential risk under heat stress, but a clear advantage in cold exposure.

Children are characterized by a lower proportion of muscle mass compared with adults.[6] This could be significant to the amount of heat produced by shivering in passive cold exposure and the amount of heat that can be produced by physical exercise to counter excessive heat loss in extreme cold.

Blood volume

Children have a smaller absolute blood volume compared with adults. Mean volumes of 2.4 and 4.0 L have been reported for 10- and 16-year-old boys, respectively.[7] The difference is also evident when blood volume is expressed relative to body surface area (e.g. 2.18 vs. 2.35 $L \cdot m^{-2}$).[8]

A smaller blood volume has two distinct effects: (i) it compromises venous return and lowers cardiac output, particularly during exercise and peripheral vasodilation (see Circulatory differences section); and (ii) it reduces the fluid reserve available for sweating (see Differences in the sweating mechanism section).

Physiological differences

Metabolic differences

The oxygen cost of bipedal locomotion (walking, running) per unit mass can be 15–20% higher in children compared with adults,[8–10] resulting in higher metabolic heat production. The decrease in the cost of locomotion takes place during adolescence, as persuasively demonstrated in the Amsterdam Growth, Health and Fitness Study that followed children from 13 years of age to adulthood (ref. 11 and see also Chapter 21). The additional energy expenditure is manifested as extrametabolic heat production constituting an added strain on the thermoregulatory system during walking/running in the heat.

In the cold, children's higher locomotive heat production may be advantageous in the short term but it might leave children with smaller energy reserves for long-term exercise.[12]

Circulatory differences

At any given exercise intensity, children are characterized by a lower cardiac output compared with adults.[13] In view of the larger proportion of blood volume which is routed to the periphery, this may hinder the transfer of body heat from the working muscles to the environment. This hindrance may be especially evident while exercising in a hot environment[14] when a larger proportion of a child's cardiac output must be routed to the periphery for adequate perfusion and heat transfer. Moreover, in light of children's higher surface area to mass ratio and their greater reliance on dry heat dissipation rather than on evaporative heat transfer, they actually require a much higher proportion of their cardiac output for peripheral circulation than do adults. Ultimately, therefore, under high heat stress, children would reach the point of circulatory insufficiency and thermoregulatory failure earlier than adults.

Haemoglobin concentration is lower in boys than in men.[15] This most probably compromises circulatory effectiveness and contributes to children reaching earlier circulatory insufficiency under high heat stress.

The lower cardiac output and lower haemoglobin concentration in children compared with adults do not present a disadvantage during cold exposure. That is, they are unlikely to contribute to an added heat loss and do not affect the extent of metabolic elevation in the cold.[12]

Hormonal differences

Basal activities of aldosterone and vasopressin, associated with fluid and electrolyte regulation, are not known to differ between children, adolescents, and adults.[16] In addition, there is no evidence to suggest that sensitivity to these hormones changes during maturation or growth.

Several hormones whose activity changes during growth and is associated with physical and sexual development have been implicated in thermoregulation—particularly in the sweating mechanism. These include testosterone, oestrogen, prolactin, and growth hormone (GH).

As early as 1960, Kawahata[17] argued that testosterone has a sudorific (sweat-releasing) effect. He based this argument on the observation of enhanced sweating rate in 70- to 81-year-old men following injections of testosterone propionate. Indeed, androgen receptors have been detected on the secretory coils of sweat glands.[18] However, Rees and Shuster[19] could not demonstrate any sudorific effect of testosterone in adult men and women. Thus, they suggested that androgens may initiate but not maintain the increase in sweating rate that takes place during maturation.

In women, the menstrual cycle has been shown to influence the thermoregulatory response to exercise in the heat.[20] Although an oestrogen receptor-related protein has been described in human sweat ducts,[21] the thermoregulatory differences between the menstrual phases have not been directly linked to any of the hormonal changes (mainly oestrogen and progesterone) that occur during these phases. Furthermore, it is unknown what if any effect concentration changes of these hormones during maturation may have on thermoregulation.

Prolactin has been associated with osmoregulation and is suggested to influence sweat electrolyte concentration among adults[22,23] as well as among adolescents.[24] However, its exact influence on sweat gland function and its possible differential role in children and adults is unclear.

Finally, several studies have described a reduced local sweating rate in patients with GH deficiency[24–26] and patients with Laron Syndrome [undetectable to low insulin growth factor 1 (IGF-1) levels with normal GH levels].[27] In addition, GH receptors and binding protein have been observed in the human sweat duct.[28,29] The mechanism by which the GH–IGF-1 axis may affect sweat gland function and the possible differential effect of this axis on thermoregulation during growth and maturation needs to be examined.

Differences in the sweating mechanism

When ambient temperature is equal to or higher than that of the skin, the only means of heat dissipation is sweat evaporation. A consistent finding at all levels or forms of heat load is that children sweat less than do adults not only in absolute but also in relative terms as well. Several changes occur in the sweating mechanism during growth and maturation that may play a role in the increased sweating response to environmental heat taking place between childhood and adulthood (see refs 20,30–34 for review).

Three types of sweat glands have been recognized—eccrine, apocrine, and apoeccrine,[35] of which eccrine glands are the most abundant and of thermoregulatory significance and the only ones to be discussed in this chapter. They are smaller in childhood[36,37] and their size then is directly related to age ($r = 0.77$) and stature ($r = 0.81$).[36] *In vitro* experiments in adults demonstrated that gland size was directly related to its sweating rate and to its cholinergic sensitivity.[38] Thus, the maturation-related increase in sweat gland size appears to be associated with the greater sweating response to heat stress observed in adults.

The total number of eccrine glands is determined by the age of 3 years[39] and due to growth, their population density (per unit skin area) decreases from that time on.[40,41] Thus, the observed increase in sweating rate during growth and maturation is largely attributable not to sweat gland number but rather to their size and possibly other changes at the level of the activated sweat glands.

Sweat production was shown to be directly related to the sweat gland's glycolytic metabolism and lactate excretion rate.[42] Indeed, lactate excretion rate has been used as an index of sweat gland metabolism (see refs 37,42,43 and Fig. 23.1). Much of the observed increase in sweat gland metabolism and sweating rate is a mere reflection of growth-related increase in gland size. It is not clear how much of the sweating rate increase can be attributed to a general, maturation-related, elevation of glycolytic capacity as evidenced during adolescence, in glycolytic muscle-enzyme activity[44] or the increase in anaerobic muscle power.[45]

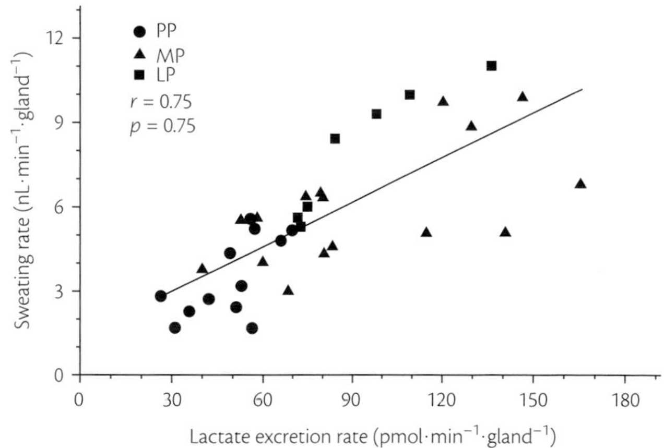

Fig. 23.1 The relationship between lactate excretion rate per gland and sweating rate per gland among pre-, mid-, and late-pubertal boys (PP, MP, and LP, respectively) cycling in the heat (50% $\dot{V}O_2$ max, 42°C, 20% relative humidity). Modified from Falk *et al.*[42]

Further research is needed to elucidate the exact contribution of sweat gland size and metabolic nature, as well as the possible effect of other factors, to the lower observed sweating rate of children.

The physiological response to thermal stress

Thermal stress, with or without exercise, is accompanied by changes in body temperature, metabolic, circulatory, and hormonal responses, as well as an activation of the sweating mechanism. This section focuses on the differences in the physiological responses to heat and to cold stress between children and adults, and the changes that may take place in this response during growth and maturation. Table 23.2 summarizes the available information on the differential physiological response to rest and exercise in the heat and in the cold between children and adults. It is clear that there still are wide gaps in our knowledge, especially with regard to cold stress.

The effectiveness of thermoregulation is reflected by heat and cold tolerance, and by the stability of core temperature (T_{re}) and the circulatory system, both at rest and while performing various tasks in the heat and cold. Ultimately, the question is whether the change in the physiological response that takes place with growth and maturation also results in a change in heat or cold tolerance. In other words, is children's physiological response to environmental heat or cold stress deficient, or is it simply different? This issue is also discussed in this section.

Physiological response to heat stress

Metabolic response

The higher cost of bipedal locomotion mentioned earlier implies that while walking/running at identical speeds children are under a greater metabolic strain than adults. This is the case in both thermoneutral and hot conditions.

The effect that heat stress has on the metabolic response at rest or during exercise is mainly reflected by changes in oxygen uptake ($\dot{V}O_2$). Most studies comparing child–adult physiologic responses standardize the metabolic load. That is, subjects exercise at the same load relative to peak $\dot{V}O_2$ and the same environmental conditions, while no comparison is normally made with thermoneutral conditions. Therefore, the differential effect that environmental heat may have on children's and adults' metabolic responses is difficult to gauge.

Two studies compared the metabolic response of children and adults in different environmental conditions. No $\dot{V}O_2$ change was seen in prepubertal girls or adult women walking for 1 h (30% peak $\dot{V}O_2$) in dry [48°C, 10% relative humidity (RH)] or humid (35°C, 65% RH) heat, compared with warm conditions (28°C, 45% RH).[14] However, a significant $\dot{V}O_2$ rise at the hot conditions in the girls but not in the women was observed during the second hour of exercise. Carlson and Le Rossignol[46] observed no $\dot{V}O_2$ effect of radiation (T_g = 37°C vs. 49°C) in 10-year-old boys, or in adults, cycling at 50% peak $\dot{V}O_2$ for 40 min in humid heat (31°C, 73% RH). Thus, it is clear that further research is needed to clarify the metabolic response to heat stress in children and in adolescents and to determine whether this response is different from that in adults.

Circulatory response

The circulatory response to thermal stress can be reflected by changes in cardiac output, stroke volume, and heart rate, and by changes in blood pressure and peripheral blood flow. Very limited information on the cardiovascular response to heat stress is available for children and adolescents.

Table 23.2 Differences in the physiological response to heat and cold exposure among children and adults

	Response	Children compared with adults	
		Heat	Cold
Body temperature	Rectal	Similar or higher	Similar or lower
	Skin	Higher	Lower
Metabolism	$\dot{V}O_2$	Higher (may be similar during exercise)	Higher
Circulation	Cardiac output	Similar or lower	?
	Stroke volume	Lower	?
	Heart rate	Higher	Lower
	Skin blood flow	Higher	Lower on the extremities (possibly higher on the trunk)
	Blood pressure	Lower	Lower
Endocrine system	Fluid and electrolyte regulation	Similar or lower	?
	Stress hormones	Similar or lower	?
Sweating rate	Per unit surface area	Lower	—
	Per gland	Lower	—
	Per unit body mass	Similar	—
Sweat composition	Sodium chloride	Lower	—
	Potassium	Higher	—
	Lactate	Higher	—
Fluid regulation	Rate of dehydration	Similar	—

? = unknown; — = not relevant.

Cardiac output during exercise of a given intensity is known to be lower in children compared with adults (see ref. 13 and Chapter 19). This, added to their smaller blood volume relative to body surface area, places an added strain on the cardiovascular system in children exercising in the heat. Walking (30% peak $\dot{V}O_2$) in various environmental heat conditions, prepubertal girls' cardiac output was consistently lower compared with that of women, even when corrected for body surface area. In addition, the girls' heart rate was consistently higher[14] (beyond age-dependent differences). Likewise, Jokinen *et al.*[47] reported that children younger than 5 years, resting for 10 min in a Finnish sauna (70°C, 20% RH), displayed higher heart rates and larger decreases in stroke volume compared with older children, adolescents, and adults. Cardiac output increased in the adults but not in the children.

On the other hand, Rowland *et al.*[48] recently reported that in non-acclimatized prepubertal boys cycling to exhaustion at 65% $\dot{V}O_2$ max, exercise tolerance was expectedly lower in the heat (31°C, 56% RH) than in cooler, thermoneutral conditions (20°C, 66% RH). Neither cardiac output nor stroke volume differed between the two conditions. In fact, no circulatory insufficiency was apparent, as cardiac output increased in the first 10 min and then stayed stable until exhaustion. Similarly, Rivera-Brown *et al.*[49] recently reported that among prepubertal, heat-acclimatized girls, there was no apparent cardiovascular insufficiency during cycling in humid heat (60% $\dot{V}O_2$ max 33°C, 55% RH). That is, cardiac output increased in the first 10 min of exercise but stayed stable for the next 50 min. Furthermore, when corrected for body surface area (cardiac index), the authors reported no differences between girls and women in the stroke or cardiac indices (Fig. 23.2). The discrepancy between the latter study and those of Drinkwater *et al.*[14] may have been due to several factors, including mode of exercise (walking vs. cycling), level of acclimatization (none vs. heat-acclimatized), or more importantly, to the rehydration regimen used (none vs. sports-drink equivalent to weight loss). It should be noted, however, that although differences in cardiovascular response between girls and women in the Rivera-Brown *et al.*[49] study did not reach statistical significance, stroke volume and cardiac output, even when corrected for body size, were consistently lower in the girls, as is evident in Fig. 23.2.

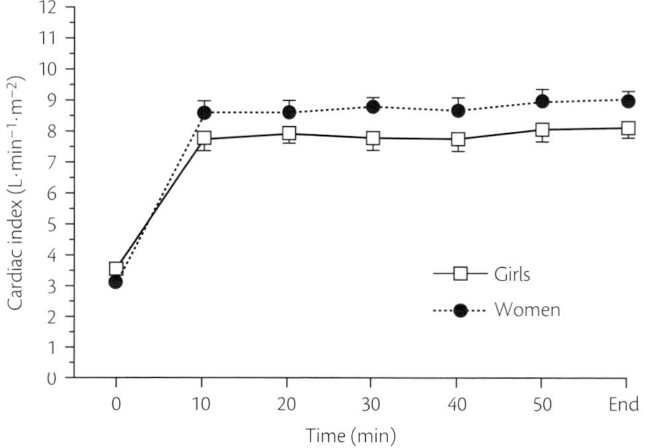

Fig. 23.2 Cardiac index in 11.3-year-old girls and 26.8-year-old-women cycling in the heat (60% $\dot{V}O_2$ max, 33°C, 55% relative humidity). Reproduced from Rivera-Brown *et al.*[49]

Hebestreit *et al.*[50] reported that children's heart rate at a given exercise intensity increased linearly with ambient temperature. No comparison was made with adults. Other studies[51] have reported higher heart rates during exercise in the heat in children compared with adults (beyond age-dependent differences). On the other hand, Falk *et al.*[52] reported no difference in the heart rate response to cycling in the heat (50% peak $\dot{V}O_2$, 42°C, 20% RH) in pre-, mid-, and late-pubertal boys. Similarly, Rivera-Brown *et al.*[49] reported no girl–woman heart rate differences while cycling in the heat (60% peak $\dot{V}O_2$, 43°C, 55% RH). The discrepancy may have been due to differences in exercise mode (walk/run vs. cycle) or intensity (30% vs. 50–60% peak $\dot{V}O_2$), as noted earlier.

Peripheral blood flow has been reported to be higher in children than in adults during, or immediately following, exercise in the heat in most studies[14,51–53] although not in all.[49] A greater skin blood flow was also demonstrated in prepubertal, compared with mid- and late-pubertal boys[52] and girls.[54] In support of children's higher cutaneous blood flow, a faster rise in skin temperature was observed in 6- to 11-year-old boys compared with adults during heat exposure.[4,55] Furthermore, Shibasaki *et al.*[53] reported that while exercising in the heat, boys had a greater increase of cutaneous blood flow for a given increase in T_{re} than did men. Owing to the boys' lower blood pressure, the differences were even more pronounced when cutaneous vascular resistance was calculated (dividing skin blood flow by mean arterial pressure). The higher peripheral blood flow means that a greater proportion of cardiac output is diverted to the periphery, imposing an added strain on the cardiovascular system. The higher strain may have been partly compensated for by a greater increase in plasma volume in girls compared with women exercising in the heat, as reported by Drinkwater *et al.*[14]

Shibasaki *et al.*[53] recently reported higher skin blood flow, as measured by laser Doppler flowmetry (LDF) (see Chapter 7), on the trunk but not the forearm of children compared with adults during moderate exercise in warm conditions (46% peak $\dot{V}O_2$, 30°C, 45% RH) (Fig. 23.3). Furthermore, no difference in regional skin blood flow was observed in the children, while in the men, skin blood flow in the forearm was higher than on the trunk. The authors suggested that regional differences exist in the maturation-related change in peripheral blood flow in response to exercise in the heat. The authors further suggested that these differences may be explained by structural changes in the cutaneous vasculature or by different sensitivity to vasoactive peptides.

It is suggested that the sometimes reported lower subjective exercise tolerance in children exercising in the heat[14,49,52,56] may be due to maladjustment of the cardiovascular system, resulting in reduced blood flow to the working muscles and to the central nervous system. In fact, Jokinen *et al.*[57] reported two cases of vasovagal collapse immediately following exposure to a Finnish sauna in children younger than 10 years, but not in older children, adolescents, or adults. The same group[58] also reported extrasystoles among children as well as a reversible sinus arrest in a 5-year-old girl during and following 10 min in a sauna. In both cases, the authors emphasized that extreme heat places an added demand on the cardiovascular system in young children.

Hormonal response

The hormonal response to exercise in the heat has traditionally been studied in relation to hormones associated with fluid and

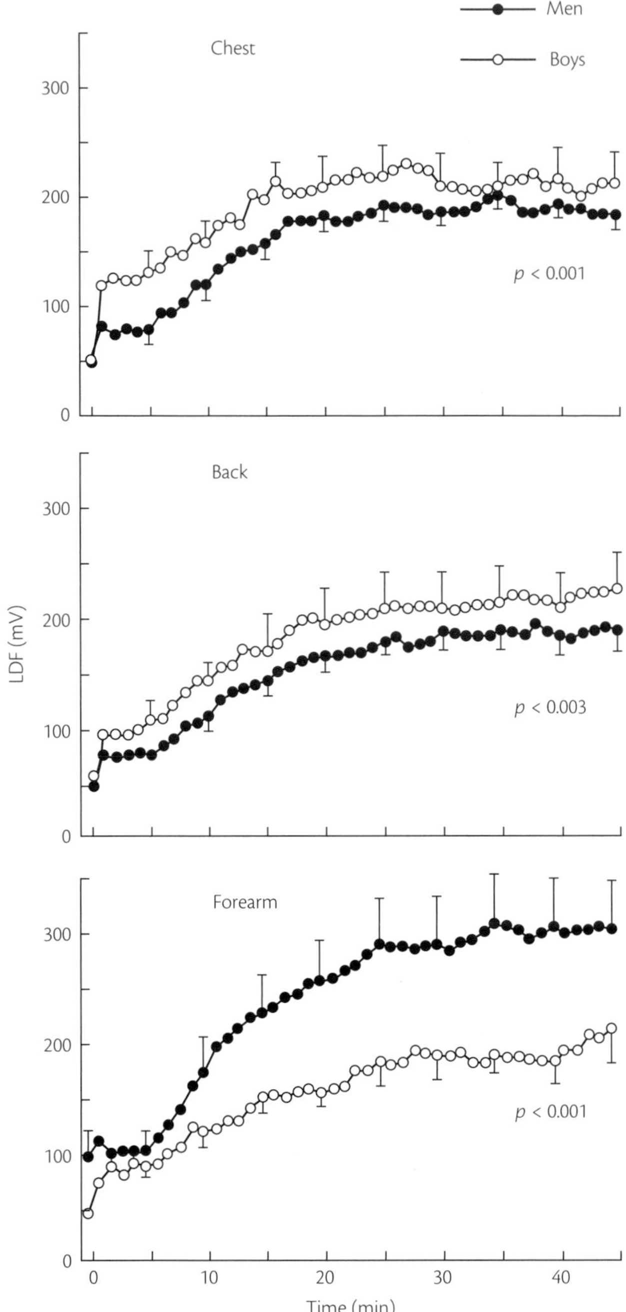

Fig. 23.3 Skin blood flow (LDF), as measured by laser Doppler flowmetry, on the chest, back, and forearm of 10- to 11-year-old prepubertal boys and 20- to 25-year-old men cycling in the heat (40% $\dot{V}O_2$ peak, 30°C, 45% relative humidity). *p*-values are for overall effect of age during exercise. Reprinted from Shibasaki *et al.*[53]

electrolytes balance. Few studies have examined this response in children. An increase in aldosterone has been reported in pre- to late-pubertal boys following rest and exercise in the heat.[24,47] This is similar to the response generally described in adults. No change in vasopressin, cortisol, or catecholamines concentration was observed in children following a 10-min exposure to a Finnish sauna, although an increase was observed among adults.[47]

Of the hormones associated with puberty, only the prolactin response to heat stress was investigated in children and adolescents, probably due to its association with osmoregulation. Heat stress, whether accompanied by exercise or not, has been reported to result in an increase in prolactin concentration in children and adolescents,[24,47] as well as in adults.[22,59] Prolactin has also been implicated in sweat electrolyte composition in adults[22,23] and adolescent boys.[24] However, its differential influence on sweat gland function in children and adults is unknown. To the authors' knowledge, no studies have examined the effect of thermal stress on other hormones associated with puberty or growth among children and adolescents. Therefore, it is unclear whether and how these hormones may modify the thermoregulatory response and what may be the differential response in children compared with adults.

The sweating response

As mentioned earlier, children's sweating apparatus and pattern is quantitatively and qualitatively different from that of adults. These dissimilarities are reflected in differences in the sweating rate, sensitivity, as well as in the sweat composition between children and adults.

Sweating rate

In any given environmental and metabolic load, the sweating rate in prepubertal boys is consistently and distinctly lower compared with men[20,30–33] even when expressed per body surface area.[1,14,17,27,51,53,60–63] Sweating response is also lower relative to a given rise in body temperature (T_{body}) or T_{re} (see refs 62,64). This difference between boys and men becomes more evident as exercise intensity or heat stress increase.[33] In contrast, the difference in the sweating rate between girls and women is much smaller[14,63] and sometimes non-existent.[27,49]

In an effort to temporally define the observed child–adult differences in sweating rate, Falk *et al.*[65] compared pre-, mid-, and late-pubertal boys, exercising at 50% $\dot{V}O_2$ max at 42°C, 20% RH. Sweating rate per body surface area and per gland increased with physical maturity. Inoue *et al.*[33] suggested that most of the sweating rate increase takes place at the onset of puberty. This was based on a report by Araki *et al.*,[60] who showed sweating rate to increase with age in 7- to 16-year-old boys, especially around 12–13 years of age, corresponding to the onset of puberty. The onset of puberty and the accelerated changes in bodily dimensions and hormonal function are temporally linked. Therefore, it is unclear whether the maturation-related change in sweating rate[66] is primarily due to the hormonal, or merely to the dimensional changes of the pubertal growth spurt. Tsuzuki-Hayakawa *et al.*[67] reported that 9 months to 4.5-year-old boys and girls, resting in a warm and humid environment (35°C, 70% RH), displayed a higher sweating rate compared with their mothers. Thus, differences between children and adults may not be so apparent at a very young age.

Most studies comparing children and adults have measured whole-body sweating rate. Some, however, investigated localized sweating rates in an attempt to shed more light on the seeming discrepancy of children's lower sweating rates.[14,53] However, site variations could not clarify the issue of children's lower sweating rate. Thus, as long as children do not drip their sweat to any appreciable extent, what matters is the cooling power associated with the total sweating and not any particular distribution of the latter.

Sweating rate per gland can be estimated given the sweating rate and the population density of the heat-activated eccrine sweat glands. The calculated sweating rate per gland has been shown to be much lower in children compared with adults during rest, as well as during exercise in the heat.[17,53,61,68] Similarly, Foster *et al.*[68]

estimated a three-fold lower sweating rate per gland in newborn babies compared with adults, when sweat was induced by an intradermal injection of acetylcholine.

The differences between children and adults described above were more closely examined by comparing pre-, mid-, and late-pubertal boys who exercised in the heat (50% peak $\dot{V}O_2$, 40°C, 20% RH).[65] The authors observed an increase in sweating rate per unit body surface area and per gland with increasing maturity (Fig. 23.4). Furthermore, within an 18-month follow-up of these boys, sweating rate increased with age.[66] However, it could not be determined whether the increase was progressive, or whether it coincided with the physical growth spurt and hormonal changes that take place during puberty.

Gender differences in sweating rate have been reported in adults,[69] but these differences are not so clear among prepubescents and adolescents. Several studies reported greater sweating rates in boys compared with girls in response to thermal[17,70] or pharmacological[27] stimuli. However, others reported similar sweating rates, or only a tendency towards a greater rate in boys compared with girls.[19,63,71–73]

Children's maximal sweating rate has not been determined. Rivera-Brown *et al.*,[49,74] for instance, measured twice the normal reported peak sweating rates in heat-acclimatized children (~500 vs. 200–300 mL·m^{-2}·h^{-1}). However, in many thermally stressing environments this might be a mute point due to sweat dripping. The latter is not normally reported but experience and anecdotal evidence suggests it to frequently occur in adults but hardly, if ever, in children. Dripped sweat is lost to both the evaporative cooling potential and to the body's fluid reserve.

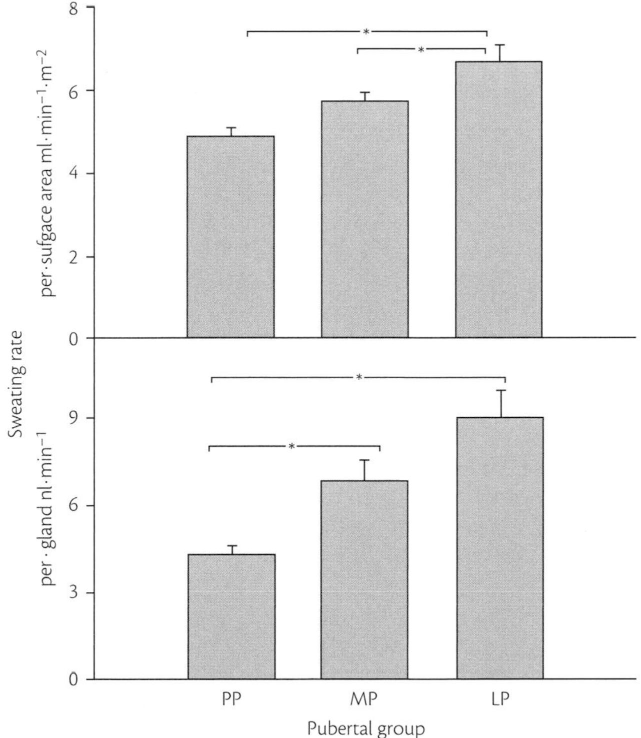

Fig. 23.4 Sweating rate per skin surface area and per gland among pre-, mid-, and late-pubertal boys (PP, MP, and LP, respectively) cycling in the heat (50% $\dot{V}O_2$ max, 42°C, 20% relative humidity). Modified from Falk *et al.*[65,66]

Bar-Or *et al.*[75] showed that for any given percentage loss of body mass, due to sweating, children's core temperature rose nearly 50% more than that of adults. That is, a similar relative fluid loss was much more detrimental to the children than to the adults. Thus, in this respect, children have a greater need to conserve fluids. Therefore, children's lower sweating rate should not be regarded as a disadvantage or a liability that has to be compensated for by other means. Rather, the lower sweating rate is part of a thermoregulatory strategy that takes advantage of unique characteristics (i.e. high surface to mass ratio) and avoids unique pitfalls (i.e. heightened susceptibility to the ill effects of fluid loss).

Sweating sensitivity

Sweating sensitivity is typically defined as the change in body temperature that elicits a given sweating response, or the sweating rate associated with each degree rise in rectal temperature. Under these definitions, children's sensitivity has been found to be lower than that of adults.[60,62] Araki *et al.*[60] demonstrated that during exercise in the heat, boys began to sweat only when their rectal temperature rose by 0.7°C, compared with adults who commenced sweating already at a 0.2°C rise. Inbar and co-workers[61,62] demonstrated a lower sweat production per degree rise in rectal temperature in 8- to 10-year-old children compared with adults. In addition, Wada[76] showed that the sweating response to intradermal adrenaline injection rose from prepubertal values and peaked at the age of 14 years.

It should be pointed out though that those definitions of sweating sensitivity have been founded on the premise that sweating is the predominant heat-dissipating mechanism under all heat stress conditions. Since children have a larger surface area to mass ratio they rely more on dry rather than evaporative cooling mechanisms and thus, the validity of both the premise and the definitions in the framework of child–adult comparisons should be questioned.

Sweating deficiency or a difference in sweating strategy?

There is no disputing the fact that for the reasons outlined above, under equivalent heat loads children sweat less than do adults per unit surface area. Historically, this has been viewed as a handicap and a manifestation of an immature thermoregulatory system, in general, and the sweating mechanism, in particular. This view should be reconsidered. In the array of available heat-dissipating venues, children possess a higher surface to mass ratio that under most common heat load conditions (when ambient temperature is lower than that of the skin) affords them an advantage in dry heat dissipation. Only under extreme conditions (higher than skin ambient temperature or high thermal radiation) does the larger relative skin area gradually become a liability.

Indeed, several studies have reported higher skin temperatures in children than in adults at similar thermal loads,[2,4,51,60,67] as could be anticipated from increased peripheral vasodilation and reliance on dry heat dissipation, along with lower and delayed sweating response. However, following the onset of sweating, Shibasaki *et al.*[53] showed that boys had lower skin temperatures while exercising in a warm environment, despite greater vasodilation and lower sweating rates, than their adult counterparts. The authors suggested this to reflect a more effective cooling. More recently, this suggestion was supported by Inbar *et al.*[62] who concluded that prepubertal boys were more efficient in their evaporative cooling. Namely, for the same cooling effect, boys needed to sweat less than adults.

From the vantage point of hindsight it seems surprising that sweating rate has, typically, been related to body surface area from which it evaporates rather than to the body mass that produced the heat that the sweat must dissipate. Indeed, when previously reported sweating rates in children and adults were related to metabolic load (originally standardized for peak $\dot{V}O_2$ and body mass), no clear age-related differences were observed (Falk and Dotan, unpublished data). Furthermore, Rivera-Brown *et al.*[49] reported a similar sweating rate per unit body mass in prepubertal, acclimatized girls and women. Similarly, Meyer and Bar-Or[77] could not ascertain differences in the sweat loss per unit body mass among children, adolescents, and adults in similar environmental conditions. It is possible that although children exhibit a lower sweating rate relative to their surface area, when considered in relation to the metabolic load, it is no different from adults.

Sweat composition

The concentration of sodium and chloride in children's sweat, while exercising in a hot environment, is lower than that of adults (30 vs. 60–90 mmol·L^{-1}, respectively). This difference is apparent in boys versus men[60] as well as in young children (boys and girls) compared with their mothers.[67] On the other hand, potassium[63] concentration appears to be higher in children's sweat compared with that of adults.

In both, children and adults, sweat chloride and sodium concentrations appear to increase with an increase in sweating rate, possibly due to the shorter time the secretory fluid spends in the sweat duct where electrolyte re-absorption takes place. However, a consistent finding is lower electrolyte concentration and osmolality of children's sweat compared with adults.[60,63,67]

Interesting to note is that proteins seen in pharmacologically induced sweat in men but not in women were observed in pubertal boys but not in prepubertal boys or girls.[78] It was suggested that the protein profile of sweat may be related to the degree of sexual maturity in young males and may shed light on the issue of gender and age differences in sweating rates.

While children's lower sweat concentration does not seem to advance our understanding of why they sweat less than adults, it does afford them two advantages: (i) it conserves electrolytes, particularly in prolonged and chronic heat exposures, thus improving retention of subsequent water intake and minimizing the likelihood of heat cramps; and (ii) it facilitates sweat evaporation and promotes cooling efficiency.

Differences in body temperature and heat tolerance

Environmental heat stress, especially when accompanied by physical exercise, brings about an increase in core and peripheral temperatures. In children and adolescents, T_{re} has been used to represent core temperature, but in adults, oesophageal or tympanic temperatures have also been used. Peripheral temperature has been approximated by averaging skin temperatures (T_{sk}) at various sites.

Theoretically, heat tolerance should be defined as either the highest core temperature prior to physiological collapse or that beyond which maintenance of body temperature and circulatory sufficiency within physiological limits is no longer possible. For ethical and safety reasons, neither criterion can serve in practice. Therefore, various alternatives have been used as criteria for terminating exposure or assessing relative thermal strain. These criteria have been both objective (e.g. T_{re}, T_{body}, total body heat storage) and subjective (e.g. dizziness, high rating of perceived exertion). The ingrained methodological difficulty, when comparing children with adults, is that the appropriateness of these criteria for different age groups is assumed but is not necessarily similarly applicable. For example, the subjective exhaustion criterion does not take into account known age-dependent differences in the subjective rating of perceived exertion and possibly motivation. Similarly, using a uniform T_{re} cut-off value does not take into account the possibility that the critical core temperature may change with growth or maturation. In addition, the use of the current T_{body} and heat storage formulae may result in an overestimation of these indices in children. T_{body} is calculated in most studies, as a weighted average of T_{re} and T_{sk} (e.g. $0.8T_{re} + 0.2T_{sk}$), based on estimated adult proportions of core versus periphery. Such a formula, even if imprecise, is satisfactory in dimensionally uniform populations. However, since children are smaller and have a relatively larger skin area, their periphery to core volume ratio should be higher than that of adults. That is, a higher T_{sk} proportion in the T_{body} and heat storage formulae. These methodological limitations should be borne in mind when considering the results and conclusions of the studies below. In light of these difficulties, and since the determining factor in heat tolerance is the critical core temperature, the justification for calculating T_{body} and total heat storage should be questioned in child–adult comparisons.

Studies investigating the thermoregulatory response to exercise in thermoneutral or warm environments, reported similar or even lower T_{re} in children compared with adults.[1–3,49,79] In warm conditions (30°C, 45% RH), Shibasaki *et al.*[53] found exercising boys and men to produce a similar rise in T_{re}. This agrees with previous findings comparing girls with women in similar conditions (28°C, 45% RH).[14] That is, under thermoneutral or warm conditions, the effectiveness of thermoregulation, as reflected by T_{re}, is similar in children and adults.

When ambient temperatures are high and particularly, when accompanied by high humidity, mean body temperature,[46,51,67,80] and heat storage per unit body mass[14,71,72] have been reported to be higher in children compared with adults. Two technical reservations to these findings should be raised: (i) all the above studies used walking—an exercise modality associated with higher energy cost and heat production, and therefore heat load in children, compared with adults (see Metabolic response section); and (ii) the inherent error in weighting T_{re} and T_{sk} for the calculation of T_{body} and heat storage, mentioned above, results in overestimating the children's values.

These problems notwithstanding, we question the use of these two parameters in cross-age comparisons because the physiological significance of both the T_{body} and heat storage criteria depends on the thermoregulatory strategy used, which is different in children and adults. A more fundamental question is the preference of using these criteria over core temperature (T_{re}), which is the ultimate criterion of heat tolerance and thermoregulatory failure. Indeed, when relying on T_{re} and using cycling as the exercise modality, different tolerance outcomes and conclusions are reached. Falk *et al.*[52] found similar T_{re} in children and adolescents of different ages and pubertal stages who cycled in hot, dry conditions (50% $\dot{V}O_2$ max 42°C, 20% RH). Furthermore, a longitudinal follow-up of these boys did not demonstrate any change in the rate of T_{re} rise.[66] Similarly, no T_{re} differences were observed between boys and men[62] or girls and women[49] cycling in hot conditions.

Fig. 23.5 schematically describes the effectiveness of thermoregulation in children versus adults in varying environmental stress conditions. In accordance with the above, in thermoneutral and warm conditions, children appear to thermoregulate as effectively as adults.[1,2,14] Under these conditions, children's higher relative skin area allows them to utilize relatively more dry rather than evaporative heat dissipation. However, when the heat stress becomes more extreme, thermoregulation in children appears to be somewhat deficient to that of adults[14, 40, 51, 72, 80, 81]. It has been suggested that this lower heat tolerance is due, at least in part, to children's cardiovascular insufficiency[52,57] and to their lower sweating rates,[51,63,72,80] and a consequently compromised evaporative cooling.

Nevertheless, at 41°C, Inbar *et al.*[62] found prepubertal boys the more efficient sweaters and the better thermoregulators compared with their adult counterparts. Thus, it is possible that even at ambient temperatures that exceed T_{sk}, possibly up to approximately 42°C, children's higher surface area to mass ratio may still provide them some thermoregulatory advantage in terms of evaporative cooling. That is, under these conditions, evaporative cooling could possibly still exceed the heat gain accrued by conduction, convection, or radiation.

Hydration during heat stress

During exercise in the heat, hypohydration may develop due to fluid losses through sweating. Studies have shown that when water is available *ad libitum*, neither children,[48,75,82] adolescents,[70] nor adults[83] sufficiently replace fluid losses. This phenomenon was initially labelled 'voluntary dehydration',[84] although the term 'involuntary dehydration' is commonly used in more recent years. We feel 'inadvertent dehydration' is a more appropriate term.

Chronic hypohydration in children may be present even with no particular exercise regimen. Nursery (2–6 years old) and elementary school (8–10 years old) children, living in a hot climate, were shown to be in a state of chronic hypohydration, reflected by high urine osmolality.[85,86] Among the nursery school children, urine osmolality increased with age.[85] Prolonged periods of hypohydration and concentrated urine are associated with heightened risks of thermoregulatory failure, as well as the eventual development of renal stones.

One way to enhance fluid consumption among children, especially while exercising in the heat, is to flavour the beverage.[74,87,88] In addition, when carbohydrates (~8%) and electrolytes (NaCl, 15–20 mmol·L^{-1}) are added to the flavoured beverage, as in most commercial sports drinks, fluid consumption is increased by as much as 90% in children.[88–90] In fact, when consuming a flavoured beverage, enriched with carbohydrates and electrolytes, inadvertent dehydration in children appears to be prevented.[74,88,91] Nevertheless, Wilk *et al.*[92] recently noted that among 12- to 15-year-old male athletes, a carbohydrate and electrolyte beverage did not prevent dehydration during exercise in the heat. The apparent incongruence between the latter and earlier studies is possibly due to the higher exercise intensity (65 vs. 50–60% $\dot{V}O_2$ max), presumably with more attendant sweating. Most probably, it is due to the much shorter rest intervals (5 vs. 25 min), with a limited opportunity for fluid consumption in the latter study. Thus, during training or competition in the heat, it is important not only to encourage fluid consumption to maintain proper hydration status, but also to provide the opportunity to do so.

The rise in heart rate and the reduction of stroke volume during exercise is directly related to the degree of hypohydration.[93] This places an added strain on the cardiovascular system. The cardiovascular strain, in turn, may result in reduced skin blood flow[94,95] and be accompanied by a lower sweating rate.[94,96] Although these phenomena have not been clearly demonstrated in children,[75] it should be noted that the added cardiovascular strain may be more detrimental in children than in adults. This is due to the fact that children rely more on dry heat loss, and therefore on higher cutaneous blood flow, than on evaporation for heat dissipation. In fact, as mentioned previously, Bar-Or *et al.*[82] demonstrated that, while exercising in the heat, the same degree (body mass percentage) of fluid loss will result in a considerably greater rectal temperature rise in children than in adults (Fig. 23.6). Thus, children's ability to thermoregulate effectively is more dependent on their body water and therefore, even a small reduction in body fluids can be detrimental.

In spite of the widely reported decrements in physical performance in adults as a result of dehydration, many athletes deliberately dehydrate before competition.[97,98] Walsh *et al.*[99] reported mild dehydration (2% body mass) to result in performance decrement in adults. In 12- to 15-year-old male basketball players,

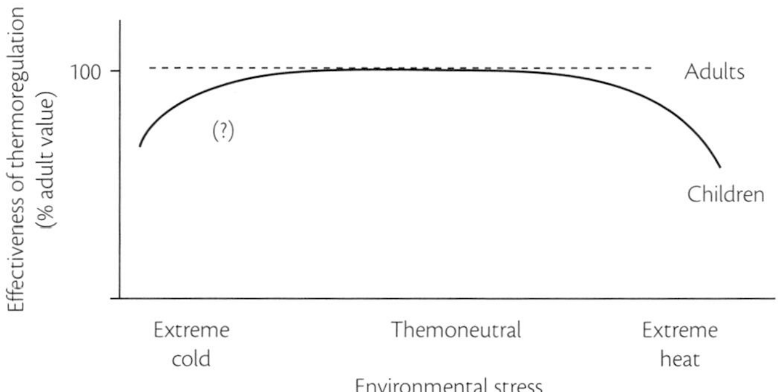

Fig. 23.5 Schematic representation of the effectiveness of thermoregulation among children, compared with adults, in relation to the environmental stress. Modified from Bar-Or.[31]

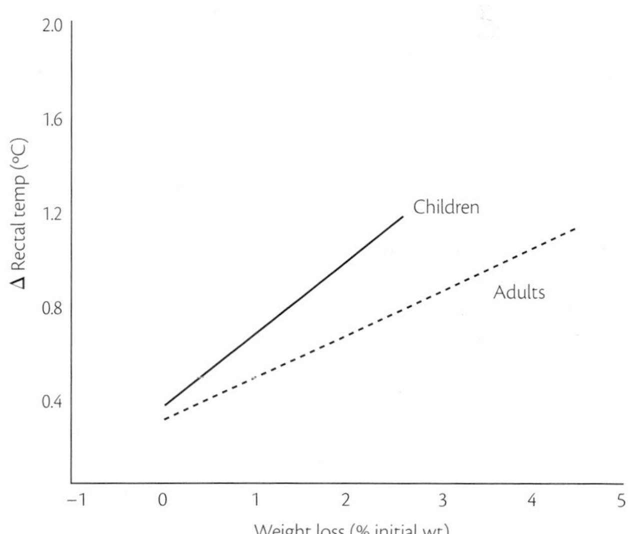

Fig. 23.6 The change in rectal temperature in relation to body mass loss in children and adults. Reproduced from Bar-Or.[30]

2% dehydration was shown to impair performance of basketball skills.[100] In 10- to 12-year-old children, a preliminary report suggested that even a 1% decrease in body mass could decrease aerobic performance (90% $\dot{V}O_2$ max to exhaustion).[101] In adults, carbohydrate and electrolyte solutions have been demonstrated to improve performance while exercising in the heat (see refs 102,103 for review). This was also demonstrated among adolescents,[100] but not in children.[104,105] Further studies are required to determine the level of dehydration critical to exercise capacity and heat tolerance in children and adolescents and its dependence on the type of exercise and heat load, and consumed beverage.

A state of hypohydration has also been identified in adolescent athletes upon arrival at practice sessions—a condition that was only exaggerated during the ensuing workout.[106–108] Moreover, wrestlers, boxers, judoka, and body builders commonly lose 3–5% of their body mass for 'making weight' before competition.[109] In fact, some wrestlers, mostly in the lightweight categories, lose as much as 10% or more of their body mass before competition.[110] Although the American National Collegiate Athletic Association has adopted rules intended to eliminate such acute weight loss procedures,[111] these practices continue. Sansone and Sawyer[112] recently reported on a 5-year-old boy who was pressured to lose weight in order to wrestle at a lower weight category.

Once hypohydration has set in it is very difficult to reverse during exercise. Thus, the above findings emphasize the need for sound hydration practices before, during, and following physical activity in children and adolescents, as well as in adults. The American College of Sports Medicine recently published a position stand[113] on exercise and fluid replacement in adults. Similar position stands for children were published earlier.[114,115] Specific fluid consumption recommendations for children include initiating fluid consumption even before (20–30 min) training or competition. During exercise, fluid consumption should be frequent (every 15–20 min) but in small volumes (2–3 $mL \cdot kg \cdot body\ mass^{-1}$).[116,117] In endurance events conducted in the heat, this frequency should likely be even higher. Also, to encourage fluid consumption, beverages should be flavoured (especially orange and grape[87]), enriched with carbohydrates (6–8%) and NaCl (18–20 $mmol \cdot L^{-1}$), cool, and non-carbonated.[88,91,118] Although not necessary for performance enhancements in most sporting events, commercial sports drinks are instrumental in encouraging fluid consumption, water absorption, and retention.[119]

Physiological response to cold stress

Environmental cold stress not countered by environmental modifications (seeking shelter, clothing) results in a peripheral temperature drop, often accompanied by a decrease in core temperature. To a limited extent this is countered by peripheral vasoconstriction and a rise in basal metabolism. However, in all but borderline cases this is not sufficient by itself. In such cases, preventing or attenuating continued heat loss necessitates further increase of the metabolic rate via piloerection, shivering, or exercise. Very few studies have addressed paediatric thermoregulation in cold, in general, and children's adaptations to cold environments, in particular.

Metabolic response

In adults, rest or submaximal exercise in the cold is accompanied by a marked increase in $\dot{V}O_2$ as a result of hormone-mediated rise in basal metabolism, piloerection ('goosebumps'), shivering, or a decrease in exercise efficiency. Increased $\dot{V}O_2$ has also been reported in children in most studies, both at rest and during exercise in the cold,[12,64,120–123] although not in all.[124,125] In fact, when compared with adults, $\dot{V}O_2$ increase was greater in children. Ueda *et al.*[122] comment that the increase in $\dot{V}O_2$ during swimming in cold water (20°C and 25°C) in 10- to 12-year-old boys was largely attributed to shivering, although it is unclear how this was measured. This is in line with children's higher subjective sensitivity to cold compared with adults.[12,64] Most studies do not report on shivering, or on mechanical efficiency. Therefore, it is impossible to determine the mechanisms responsible for the increase in metabolic rate and the possible differences between children and adults. Nevertheless, in view of children's greater body surface area to mass ratio, it is expected that at any given cold environment, children would have to elicit a higher metabolic rate to maintain core temperature.

Circulatory response

Very little is known about the cardiovascular response to cold in children. Lower skin temperatures or a faster decrease in skin temperature was reported in children than in adults resting or exercising in the cold.[12,55,120,124] The authors argue that the lower skin temperatures reflect a greater vasoconstriction in the children. However, only two studies actually measured peripheral blood flow in children during cold stress. Wagner *et al.*[120] reported lower finger blood flow in 10- to 13-year-old boys compared with adolescent and adult males, while resting in a cool environment (17°C). More recently, Inoue *et al.*[126] reported a greater decline in cutaneous vascular conductance (derived from blood flow and blood pressure) in the finger but a higher cutaneous conductance in the trunk in boys compared with men, while resting in progressively reduced ambient temperature (30–17°C). The authors suggested that lower skin temperatures generally reported in children in the cold may reflect anthropometric differences (body surface area, subcutaneous fat), and not only cutaneous vasoconstriction.

In adults, heart rate generally decreases in response to cold stress during rest or submaximal exercise, likely due to decreased cardiac output with decreasing peripheral demand. In children, several studies,[122,125,127] although not all,[121] also report decreased heart rate with lower environmental temperatures. Swimming at 32°C, 25°C, and 20°C, 12-year-old boys exhibited decreasing heart rates with decreasing temperatures.[122] Mackova *et al.*[125] showed the same effect, also in 12-year-old boys, cycling at effective temperatures of 10°C and 25°C. Their post-exercise heart rate decline was faster at the lower temperature. Similarly, 11- to 12-year-old boys cycling at 7°C and 13°C displayed a lower heart rate compared with that at 22°C.[127] Recovering in a thermoneutral environment, following the cold exposure, the children's T_{re} fell 0.10°C below cold exposure values and did not increase during the 30-min follow-up. There are no published observations of this phenomenon in adults. In a previous study in adults and in more extreme conditions (5°C vs. 7–13°C, shorts only vs. sweat suit)[128] smaller and shorter-lived rectal temperature drops were observed (unpublished observations). These observations may reflect the presumably greater vasoconstrictor cold response in children. In view of the limited number of studies, further research is needed to examine the various issues of children's cardiovascular response to exercise in the cold.

Changes in body temperature and cold tolerance

Among 8- to 18-year-old subjects, swimming in cool water (20.3°C, 30 m·min^{-1}), oral temperature was found to decrease at a slower rate with an increase in age.[129] That is, in spite of the fact that the younger children swam at a faster speed relative to their size and assumed potential, their rate of cooling was faster than that of the older children. Similarly, Klentrou *et al.*[123] demonstrated a greater drop in T_{re} in smaller, premenarcheal girls, compared with larger, postmenarcheal girls. In both studies, the greater surface area to body mass ratio was related to the greater drop in temperature. In fact, in the study by Klentrou *et al.*,[123] it was the surface area to body mass ratio which explained most of the variance in the T_{re} change (and not age or menarcheal status). These results demonstrate the importance of body dimensions, rather than age *per se*, for thermoregulation in the cold. The rate of cooling was inversely related to the level of adiposity, as recently also supported by Wakabayashi *et al.*,[130] who investigated the effect of cool water (23°C) immersion on body temperature in prepubertal children. These results indicate the importance of body dimensions, as well as body adiposity, in maintaining body temperatures in the cold.

The faster cooling rate in the younger children, reported above, is supported by Inoue *et al.*[124] They compared the thermoregulatory response to a linear decrease in ambient temperature (28–15°C) in prepubertal boys with that of young men, at rest. The boys' skin temperature was lower than the men's, presumably reflecting a greater extent of vasoconstriction. This is in line with other reports of lower T_{sk} in children and adults resting in cool conditions (15–20°C).[55,120] Nevertheless, T_{re} decreased in the boys while it remained stable in the men.

Different results were reported by Smolander *et al.*[12] who compared body temperature responses in children and adults during exercise in a cold environment (5°C). Pre- and early-pubescent boys were able to maintain their body temperature as effectively as adults while cycling (30% peak $\dot{V}O_2$) in the cold. In fact, the children's T_{re} even slightly (insignificantly) rose during exercise, compared with the adults. The children's skin temperature was significantly lower at several sites, indicating a greater peripheral vasoconstriction, than in the adults. The authors argued that the children were able to maintain their core temperature during exercise, by increasing their metabolic rate and constricting peripheral vessels to a greater extent than the adults. This age-related difference was observed when comparing two boys with two men of similar surface area to mass ratios. That is, thermoregulatory strategy in the cold is apparently determined by maturation and not only by body size.

We studied 11- to 12-year-old boys during rest and exercise (50 min rest, 10 min cycle, 50 min rest) in a cold (7°C), cool (13°C), and thermoneutral (22°C) environment.[127] T_{re} decreased during the first 50 min of rest and continued to decrease in the subsequent rest period, in spite of the fact that the boys were dressed in sweat pants and shirts (Fig. 23.7). Following the 10 min of exercise, T_{re} slightly increased in the cool and neutral but not in the cold conditions. It should be stressed that T_{re} did not return to pre-exposure levels even following 30 min of re-warming recovery in a thermoneutral environment (21–23°C). Skin temperature of the exposed hands decreased in the cold and cool environments, while there was no apparent change in chest temperature which was covered by two layers of clothing. While Smolander *et al.*'s[12] boys were able to maintain their body temperature while exercising in 5°C, wearing only shorts, our boys were unable to do so in

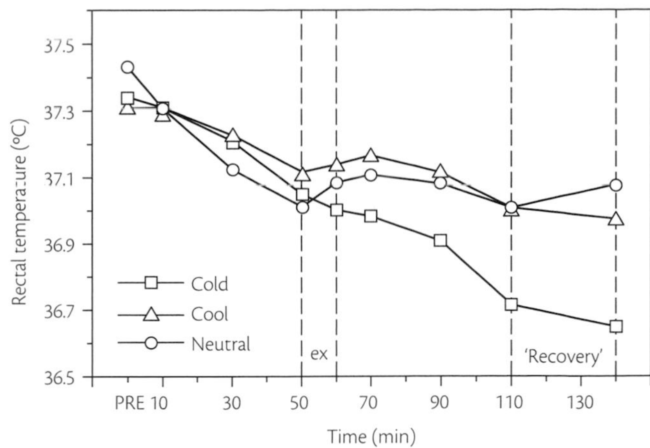

Fig. 23.7 Mean rectal temperature in 11- to 12-year-old boys resting and cycling (50 min rest, 10 min cycle, 50 min rest) in a cold (7°C), cool (13°C), and thermoneutral (22°C) environment. (ex = exercise). Modified from Falk *et al.*[127]

7°C with more clothing. This seeming discrepancy is accounted for by the much longer exercise duration (40 vs. 10 min) and much shorter rest duration (20 vs. 50 min) in Smolander *et al.*'s study. This observation demonstrates the importance of increasing metabolic rate during cold exposure of children for the maintenance of body temperature. The importance of the elevated metabolic rate during exercise in the cold was also demonstrated by the 0.5–0.6°C increase in T_{re} in 12-year-old boys exercising at 50% peak $\dot{V}O_2$ for 60 min in effective temperature of 10°C.[125]

The studies described above suggest that during rest, thermoregulatory effectiveness in the cold is lower in children compared with adults, as schematically illustrated in Fig. 23.5. During exercise, children may maintain their core temperature by increasing their metabolic rate. However, it is unclear how long this higher metabolic rate can be sustained.

Adaptation to thermal stress

Repeated exposures to heat stress result in an adaptation to heat, termed '*acclimatization*' or '*acclimation*', which is clearly evidenced in an array of parameters, both in adults and in children. Repeated cold exposures, on the other hand, result in a limited range of adaptations in adults. In children, cold adaptation has not been investigated. Thus, the following section discusses only child–adult differences in heat adaptation. In addition, physical exercise training, as such, induces adaptations that carry over to better coping with heat stress, but not necessarily with cold. A discussion of the effects of training and fitness, in children and adolescents, on the response to heat and cold stresses follows.

Heat acclimatization/acclimation

The process of heat acclimation (a controlled, regimented form of acclimatization) is similar in children, adolescents, and adults, although the rate of that process may differ. Children and adults were shown to reach a similar acclimation level following a 2 week, 3 times per week, acclimation protocol of exercise in the heat (43°C, 21% RH).[61] However, the rate of acclimation in the early stages was slower in the children than in the adults (Fig. 23.8).

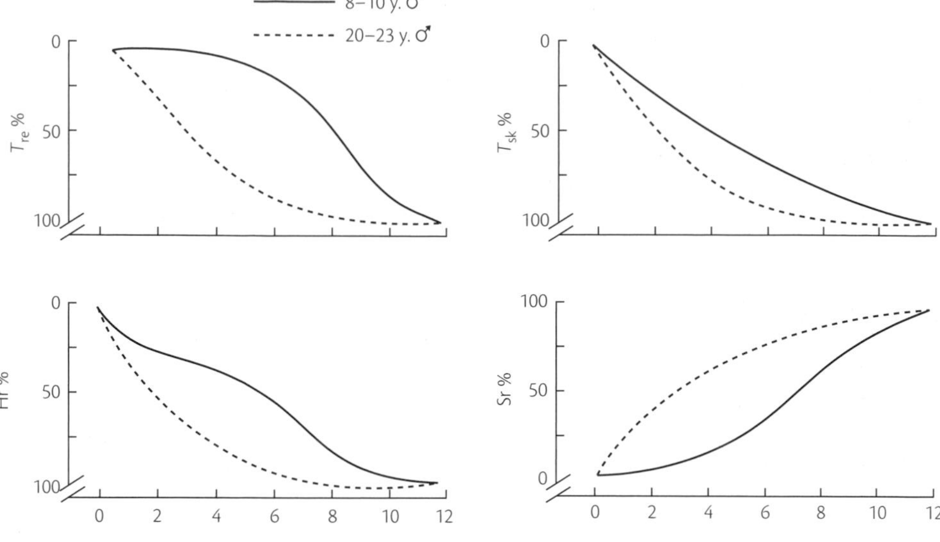

Fig. 23.8 Physiological adaptations during the course of heat acclimation among 8- to 10-year-old boys and 20- to 23-year-old men. Adaptations in rectal and skin temperatures, heart rate, and sweating rate are expressed as per cent of final acclimation value, where baseline values are 0%. Schematic representation from Bar-Or.[30]

These findings are in line with the lower level of acclimation found in 11- to 16-year-old boys, compared with men, following an 8-day acclimation protocol of exercise in the heat (48°C, 17% RH).[53]

One of the major changes characterizing the process of heat acclimation, is an increase in sweating rate. This has been demonstrated in children,[6,131] as well as in adults.[132] In adults, five daily exercise in heat sessions were found to provide only a minimal stimulus for sweating adaptation.[133] In children, six exercise in the heat sessions (50% $\dot{V}O_2$ max, 35°C, 55% RH) over a 2-week period did not have an effect on the total sweating rate during the exposure session, but exercise sweating rate increased, while resting sweating rate decreased.[134] Inbar,[61] on the other hand, did find an increased total sweating rate using the same acclimation protocol, most probably due to the difference in ambient conditions (43°C vs. 35°C, 21% vs. 55% RH). He also found most of the adaptation to take place during the later acclimation exposures. Thus, the exact nature of children's sweating response to different acclimation regimens has not been sufficiently elucidated. It is, however, worthwhile noting that children who were already well acclimatized demonstrated sweating rates which were nearly twice as high as those normally reported for children.[49,74] That is, it is likely that under various conditions full adaptation of the sweating rate response may not be realized in only 2 weeks.

From the above studies, it is clear that added precaution is warranted during the early days of summer or during sudden weather changes. This is true for all but especially for children. It is particularly warranted since, during heat acclimation, children's subjective rating of perceived strain was found to decrease faster than the rate of their physiological adaptation and faster than that in adults.[135] That is, children are less likely to match their behaviour to the actual physiological strain.

Although children appear to adapt more slowly to exercise-heat acclimation, it should be noted that in children, less severe acclimation regimens have been found effective as well. For example, exercise alone (in thermoneutral conditions) has been found as effective as the exercise-heat regimen in children but only partially so in adults.[131] Clearly, much more research is needed to elucidate the mechanism of acclimation in children.

Training-induced adaptations and the response to heat stress

Physical training results in numerous physiological adaptations, some of which bear direct relationships to the thermoregulatory response to heat stress. For example, enhanced cardiovascular function can improve heat tolerance by making more of the increased cardiac output available for peripheral flow. Presumably, this should be more pronounced in children who rely, to a greater extent, on peripheral blood flow and whose cardiac output is more heavily strained. However, while the relationship between physical training or aerobic fitness and heat tolerance has been clearly demonstrated in adults, it has not been as consistently shown in children.

In adults, peak $\dot{V}O_2$ has been associated with enhanced heat tolerance. On the other hand, in prepubertal boys, Delamarche *et al.*[2] could not demonstrate such a relationship. Similarly, peak $\dot{V}O_2$ was found to account for only 16% of the variance in the T_{re} response to exercise in the heat among prepubertal boys.[136]

Intervention training studies in children have demonstrated inconsistent effects on the body temperature response to heat load. For example, Araki *et al.*[55] found no effect of training on the body temperature response to passive heat stress. On the other hand, Inbar *et al.*[131] observed, in 8- to 10-year-old boys, that a 2-week cycling training (85% of maximal heart rate) in either hot or thermoneutral environment, resulted in similarly lower rectal temperature and heart rate responses to exercise in the heat.

Training has been shown to result in an increased sweating rate in adults. Cross-sectional comparisons of trained and untrained boys revealed a higher sweating rate at any given T_{re} in trained compared with untrained boys resting in a warm and humid environment (30°C, 70% RH).[137] However, a 2-week training programme did not result in any change in sweating rate.[131] Clearly, further research is needed to investigate the relationship between fitness and training-induced adaptations on the one hand, and the response to heat stress on the other hand.

Training-induced adaptations and the response to cold stress

Little is known about training-induced adaptations and the thermoregulatory response to cold stress in adults. We know of no study on children that investigated this issue in true cold exposure. Two studies investigated the effect of training on the response to relatively cool conditions (18–20°C), not far below the thermoneutral zone. During passive resting at 18°C, a smaller drop in T_{re} was observed in trained compared with untrained prepubertal boys.[137] In a different study[55] when ambient temperature was only 2°C higher (20°C), no difference in the resting T_{re} response was observed in four prepubertal boys following 40 days of physical training. Thus, very little is known about the possible training effects on the thermoregulatory response to cold in children, as in adults.

Summary

Thermoregulation during exposure to hot or cold environments differs between children and adults. Physiological but particularly physical differences between them may explain much of their dissimilarities in the response to thermal stress.

- The main physical child–adult differences that affect thermoregulation are the larger surface area to mass ratio and the smaller blood volume in the children. These affect children's thermoregulatory strategy, allowing them to rely more on dry heat loss and less on evaporative cooling in a warm environments. However, in extreme conditions, hot or cold, the greater surface area to mass ratio results in a higher rate of heat absorption or heat loss, respectively. The smaller blood volume in children, when normalized for body surface area, may compromise their exercise performance in the heat and exaggerate the circulatory effects of hypohydration.
- The main physiological difference between children and adults is the lower sweating rate characteristic of children. This has been shown to be due to a lower sweating rate of the prepubertal gland and not to a smaller number of sweat glands. The gland's lower sweating rate, in turn, appears to be the direct result of its smaller size, a higher threshold of sweating onset and possibly, to the gland's lower metabolic capacity.
- Metabolic, circulatory, and hormonal differences between children and adults may also affect thermoregulation. Children are characterized by a higher metabolic cost of bipedal locomotion which places an added strain on the thermoregulatory system during heat exposure but may be advantageous in cold exposures. The lower cardiac output at any given exercise intensity and the lower haemoglobin concentration in boys compared with men, contribute to an added cardiovascular strain during exercise in the heat. Finally, baseline concentrations of testosterone, oestrogen, prolactin, and GH differ between children and adults, which may account for some of the observed differences in sweat gland function and sweat composition.
- During exercise in thermoneutral or warm environments, children thermoregulate as effectively as adults. In extreme environmental conditions, children's thermoregulation appears to be somewhat deficient compared with that of adults.
- Heat stress elevates body temperatures, while cold stress lowers them, particularly skin temperatures, more in children than in adults. In children, the changes in body temperature are accompanied by a greater increase in the metabolic cost of exercise in the cold. The cardiovascular system appears to be strained more in children when compared with adults exposed to heat, possibly explaining the greater subjective intolerance to heat stress sometimes reported in children. On the other hand, relatively little is known about the circulatory response to cold stress in children and adolescents. The few reports on the endocrine response to heat stress demonstrate a similar or sometimes lower response in children, while the hormonal response to cold stress has not been investigated in either children or adolescents.
- Except under extreme heat stress children manage their core temperatures as well and sometimes, even better than adults. They do this with lower sweating rates while taking advantage of their higher relative surface area. Thus, relative to their surface area, children's sweating rate is lower than adults. When related to body mass, work load, and heat production, children appear to sweat as much as adults. Therefore, children cannot be regarded as 'immature', or inferior thermoregulators but rather as utilizing a different thermoregulatory strategy than that used by adults.
- Inadvertent dehydration ('involuntary dehydration') is a phenomenon occurring in both children and adults, while exercising in the heat. The ensuing state of hypohydration and the resulting extra cardiovascular strain are apparently more detrimental to children than to adults, probably because children rely more on increased skin blood flow for heat dissipation. Dehydration in children can be prevented or mitigated by providing a flavoured carbohydrate–electrolyte beverage.
- Much is yet to be learnt about children's thermoregulatory response:
  - (i) The fine interaction between the principal tools of thermoregulation (e.g. body surface area, cardiac output, peripheral blood flow, sweating rate and its threshold, sweat gland function, sweat composition, and heat load/strain perception).
  - (ii) How the thermoregulatory response changes during adolescence.
  - (iii) The determinants of effective acclimation and training-induced thermoregulatory adaptations to heat and particularly to cold, in children and adolescents.
  - (iv) Girl–woman thermoregulatory differences seem somewhat smaller than the corresponding male differences. Are there, indeed, gender differences and where do they manifest themselves most?

References

1. Davies CT (1981). Thermal responses to exercise in children. *Ergonomics* **24**, 55–61.
2. Delamarche P, Bittel J, Lacour JR, Flandrois R (1990). Thermoregulation at rest and during exercise in prepubertal boys. *Eur J Appl Physiol* **60**, 436–40.
3. Gullestad R (1975). Temperature regulation in children during exercise. *Acta Paediatr Scand* **64**, 257–63.

4. Tochihara Y, Ohnaka T, Nagai Y (1995). Thermal responses of 6- to 8-year-old children during immersion of their legs in a hot water bath. *Appl Hum Sci* **14**, 23–8.
5. Forbes GB (1986). Body composition in adolescence. In: Falkner F, Tanner JM (eds.), *Human growth*, pp. 119–45. Plenum Press, New York.
6. Malina RM, Bouchard C, Bar-Or O (2004). *Growth, maturation and physical activity.* Human Kinetics, Champaign, IL.
7. Koch G (1978). Muscle blood flow in prepubertal boys. *Med Sport* **11**, 39–46.
8. Astrand PO (1952). Experimental studies of physical work capacity in relation to sex and age. Mundsgaard, Copenhagen.
9. Robinson S (1938). Experimental studies of physical fitness in relation to age. *Int Z Ang Physiol Einschl Arbeitsphysiol* **10**, 251–323.
10. Unnithan VB, Eston RG (1990). Stride frequency and submaximal treadmill running economy in adults and children. *Pediatr Exerc Sci* **2**, 149–55.
11. Ariens GA, van Mechelen W, Kemper HC, Twisk JW (1997). The longitudinal development of running economy in males and females aged between 13 and 27 years: The Amsterdam Growth and Health Study. *Eur J Appl Physiol* **76**, 214–20.
12. Smolander J, Bar-Or O, Korhonen O, Ilmarinen J (1992). Thermoregulation during rest and exercise in the cold in pre- and early pubescent boys and in young men. *J Appl Physiol* **72**, 1589–94.
13. Turley KR, Wilmore JH (1997). Cardiovascular responses to treadmill and cycle ergometer exercise in children and adults. *J Appl Physiol* **83**, 948–57.
14. Drinkwater BL, Kupprat IC, Denton JE, Crist JL, Horvath SM (1977). Response of prepubertal girls and college women to work in the heat. *J Appl Physiol* **43**, 1046–53.
15. Dallman PR, Siimes MA (1979). Percentile curves for hemoglobin and red cell volume in infancy and childhood. *J Pediatr* **94**, 26–31.
16. Soldin SJ, Hicks JM (1995). *Pediatric reference ranges.* AACC Press, Washington, D.C.
17. Kawahata A (1960). Sex differences in sweating. In: Yoshimura H, Ogata K, Itoh S (eds.), *Essential problems in climate physiology*, pp. 169–84. Nankodo, Kyoto.
18. Choudhry R, Hodgins MB, Van der Kwast TH, Brinkmann AO, Boersma WJ (1992). Localization of androgen receptors in human skin by immunohistochemistry: Implications for the hormonal regulation of hair growth, sebaceous glands and sweat glands. *J Endocrinol* **133**, 467–75.
19. Rees J, Shuster S (1981). Pubertal induction of sweat gland activity. *Clin Sci (Lond)* **60**, 689–92.
20. Bar-Or O (1996). Thermoregulation in females from a life span perspective. In: Bar-Or O, Lamb DR, Clarkson PM (eds.), *Exercise and the female—A life span approach*, pp. 250–83. Cooper Publishing Group, Traverse City, MI.
21. Fraser D, Padwick ML, Whitehead M, Coffer A, King RJ (1991). Presence of an oestradiol receptor-related protein in the skin: Changes during the normal menstrual cycle. *Br J Obstet Gynaecol* **98**, 1277–82.
22. Kaufman FL, Mills DE, Hughson RL, Peake GT (1988). Effects of bromocriptine on sweat gland function during heat acclimatization. *Horm Res* **29**, 31–8.
23. Robertson MT, Boyajian MJ, Patterson K, Robertson WV (1986). Modulation of the chloride concentration of human sweat by prolactin. *Endocrinology* **119**, 2439–44.
24. Falk B, Bar-Or O, MacDougall JD (1991). Aldosterone and prolactin response to exercise in the heat in circumpubertal boys. *J Appl Physiol* **71**, 1741–5.
25. Juul A, Main K, Nielsen B, Skakkebaek NE (1993). Decreased sweating in growth hormone deficiency: Does it play a role in thermoregulation? *J Pediatr Endocrinol* **6**, 39–44.
26. Juul A, Hjortskov N, Jepsen LT, Nielsen B, Halkjaer-Kristensen J, Vahl N, Jorgensen JO, Christiansen JS, Skakkebaek NE (1995). Growth hormone deficiency and hyperthermia during exercise: A controlled study of sixteen GH-deficient patients. *J Clin Endocrinol Metab* **80**, 3335–40.
27. Main K, Nilsson KO, Skakkebaek NE (1991). Influence of sex and growth hormone deficiency on sweating. *Scand J Clin Lab Invest* **51**, 475–80.
28. Lobie PE, Breipohl W, Lincoln DT, Garcia-Aragon J, Waters MJ (1990). Localization of the growth hormone receptor/binding protein in skin. *J Endocrinol* **126**, 467–71.
29. Oakes SR, Haynes KM, Waters MJ, Herington AC, Werther GA (1992). Demonstration and localization of growth hormone receptor in human skin and skin fibroblasts. *J Clin Endocrinol Metab* **75**, 1368–73.
30. Bar-Or O (1980). Climate and the exercising child—A review. *Int J Sports Med* **1**, 53–65.
31. Bar-Or O (1989). Temperature regulation during exercise in children and adolescents. In: Gisolfi CV, Lamb DR (eds.), *Youth, exercise and sports*, pp. 335–62. Benchmark Press, Indianapolis, IN.
32. Falk B (1998). Effects of thermal stress during rest and exercise in the paediatric population. *Sports Med* **25**, 221–40.
33. Inoue Y, Kuwahara T, Araki T (2004). Maturation- and aging-related changes in heat loss effector function. *J Physiol Anthropol Appl Hum Sci* **23**, 289–94.
34. Falk B (1996). Physiological and health aspects of exercise in hot and cold climates. In: Bar-Or O (ed.), *The Child and adolescent athlete*, pp. 326–52. Blackwell Scientific, Oxford.
35. Sato K, Leidal R, Sato F (1987). Morphology and development of an apoeccrine sweat gland in human axillae. *Am J Physiol* **252** (1 Pt 2), R166–80.
36. Landing BH, Wells TR, Williamson ML (1968). Studies on growth of eccrine sweat glands. In: Cheek DB (ed.), *Human growth: Body composition, cell growth, energy and intelligence*, pp. 382–94. Lea & Febiger, Philadelphia, PA.
37. Wolfe S, Cage G, Epstein M, Tice L, Miller H, Gordon RS Jr (1970). Metabolic studies of isolated human eccrine sweat glands. *J Clin Invest* **49**, 1880–4.
38. Sato K, Sato F (1983). Individual variations in structure and function of human eccrine sweat gland. *Am J Physiol* **245**, R203–8.
39. Kuno Y (1956). *Human perspiration.* C.C. Thomas, Springfield, IL.
40. Bar-Or O, Magnusson LI, Buskirk ER (1968). Distribution of heat-activated sweat glands in obese and lean men and women. *Hum Biol* **40**, 235–48.
41. Szabo G (1962). The number of eccrine sweat glands in human skin. *Adv Biol Skin* **3**, 1–5.
42. Falk B, Bar-Or O, MacDougall JD, McGillis L, Calvert R, Meyer F (1991). Sweat lactate in exercising children and adolescents of varying physical maturity. *J Appl Physiol* **71**, 1735–40.
43. Fellmann N, Labbe A, Gachon AM, Coudert J (1985). Thermal sweat lactate in cystic fibrosis and in normal children. *Eur J Appl Physiol* **54**, 511–16.
44. Eriksson BO, Saltin B (1974). Muscle metabolism during exercise in boys aged 11 to 16 years compared to adults. *Acta Paediatr Belg* **28**, 257–65.
45. Falk B, Bar-Or O (1993). Longitudinal changes in peak aerobic and anaerobic mechanical power of circumpubertal boys. *Pediatr Exerc Sci* **5**, 318–31.
46. Carlson JS, Le Rossignol P (1995). Children and adults exercising in hot wet climatic conditions with different levels of radiant heat. *Pediatr Exerc Sci* **7**, 219–20.
47. Jokinen E, Valimaki I, Marniemi J, Seppanen A, Irjala K, Simell O (1991). Children in sauna: Hormonal adjustments to intensive short thermal stress. *Acta Physiol Scand* **142**, 437–42.
48. Rowland T, Garrison A, Pober D (2007). Determinants of endurance exercise capacity in the heat in prepubertal boys. *Int J Sports Med* **28**, 26–32.
49. Rivera-Brown AM, Rowland TW, Ramirez-Marrero FA, Santacana G, Vann A (2006). Exercise tolerance in a hot and humid climate in heat-acclimatized girls and women. *Int J Sports Med* **27**, 943–50.

50. Hebestreit H, Bar-Or O, McKinty C, Riddell M, Zehr P (1995). Climate-related corrections for improved estimation of energy expenditure from heart rate in children. *J Appl Physiol* **79**, 47–54.
51. Wagner JA, Robinson S, Tzankoff SP, Marino RP (1972). Heat tolerance and acclimatization to work in the heat in relation to age. *J Appl Physiol* **33**, 616–22.
52. Falk B, Bar-Or O, MacDougall JD (1992). Thermoregulatory responses of pre-, mid-, and late-pubertal boys to exercise in dry heat. *Med Sci Sports Exerc* **24**, 688–94.
53. Shibasaki M, Inoue Y, Kondo N, Iwata A (1997). Thermoregulatory responses of prepubertal boys and young men during moderate exercise. *Eur J Appl Physiol* **75**, 212–18.
54. Brien EK, Wilk B, Iwata M, Bar-Or O (2000). Forearm blood flow in pre/early-, mid, and late-pubertal girls exercising in the heat. *Med Sci Sports Exerc* **32**, S157.
55. Araki T, Tsujita J, Matsushita K, Hori S (1980). Thermoregulatroy responses of prepubertal boys to heat and cold in relation to physical training. *Hum Ergonomics* **9**, 69–80.
56. Mackie JM (1982). *Physiological responses of twin children to exercise under conditions of heat stress.* Unpublished MSc thesis, University of Waterloo, Canada.
57. Jokinen E, Valimaki I, Antila K, Seppanen A, Tuominen J (1990). Children in sauna: Cardiovascular adjustment. *Pediatrics* **86**, 282–8.
58. Jokinen E, Valimaki I (1991). Children in sauna: Electrocardiographic abnormalities. *Acta Paediatr Scand* **80**, 370–4.
59. Brisson GR, Audet A, Ledoux M, Matton P, Pellerin-Massicotte J, Peronnet F (1986). Exercise-induced blood prolactin variations in trained adult males: A thermic stress more than an osmotic stress. *Horm Res* **23**, 200–6.
60. Araki T, Toda Y, Matsushita K, Tsujino A (1979). Age differences in sweating during muscular exercise. *Jap J Fitness Sports Med* **28**, 239–48.
61. Inbar O (1978). *Acclimatization to dry and hot environments in young adults and children 8–10 years old.* Unpublished EdD thesis, Columbia University, USA.
62. Inbar O, Morris N, Epstein Y, Gass G (2004). Comparison of thermoregulatory responses to exercise in dry heat among prepubertal boys, young adults and older males. *Exp Physiol* **89**, 691–700.
63. Meyer F, Bar-Or O, MacDougall D, Heigenhauser GJ (1992). Sweat electrolyte loss during exercise in the heat: Effects of gender and maturation. *Med Sci Sports Exerc* **24**, 776–81.
64. Anderson GS, Mekjavic IB (1996). Thermoregulatory responses of circum-pubertal children. *Eur J Appl Physiol* **74**, 404–10.
65. Falk B, Bar-Or O, Calvert R, MacDougall JD (1992). Sweat gland response to exercise in the heat among pre-, mid-, and late-pubertal boys. *Med Sci Sports Exerc* **24**, 313–19.
66. Falk B, Bar-Or O, MacDougall D, Goldsmith C, McGillis L (1992). A longitudinal analysis of the sweating response of pre-, mid- and late-pubertal boys during exercise in the heat. *Am J Hum Biol* **4**, 527–35.
67. Tsuzuki-Hayakawa K, Tochihara Y, Ohnaka T (1995). Thermoregulation during heat exposure of young children compared to their mothers. *Eur J Appl Physiol* **72**, 12–17.
68. Foster KG, Hey EN, Katz G (1969). The response of the sweat glands of the newborn baby to thermal stimuli and to intradermal acetylcholine. *J Physiol* **203**, 13–29.
69. Shapiro Y, Pandolf KB, Avellini BA, Pimental NA, Goldman RF (1980). Physiological responses of men and women to humid and dry heat. *J Appl Physiol* **49**, 1–8.
70. Iuliano S, Naughton G, Collier G, Carlson J (1998). Examination of the self-selected fluid intake practices by junior athletes during a simulated duathlon event. *Int J Sport Nutr* **8**, 10–23.
71. Haymes EM, McCormick RJ, Buskirk ER (1975). Heat tolerance of exercising lean and obese prepubertal boys. *J Appl Physiol* **39**, 457–61.
72. Haymes EM, Buskirk ER, Hodgson JL, Lundegren HM, Nicholas WC (1974). Heat tolerance of exercising lean and heavy prepubertal girls. *J Appl Physiol* **36**, 566–71.
73. Dill DB, Horvath SM, Van Beaumont W, Gehlsen G, Burrus K (1967). Sweat electrolytes in desert walks. *J Appl Physiol* **23**, 746–51.
74. Rivera-Brown AM, Gutierrez R, Gutierrez JC, Frontera WR, Bar-Or O (1999). Drink composition, voluntary drinking, and fluid balance in exercising, trained, heat-acclimatized boys. *J Appl Physiol* **86**, 78–84.
75. Bar-Or O, Dotan R, Inbar O, Rotshtein A, Zonder H (1980). Voluntary hypohydration in 10- to 12-year-old boys. *J Appl Physiol* **48**, 104–8.
76. Wada M (1950). Sudorific action of adrenalin on the human sweat glands and determination of their excitability. *Science* **111**, 376–7.
77. Meyer F, Bar-Or O (1994). Fluid and electrolyte loss during exercise. The paediatric angle. *Sports Med* **18**, 4–9.
78. Sens DA, Simmons MA, Spicer SS (1985). The analysis of human sweat proteins by isoelectric focusing. I. Sweat collection utilizing the macroduct system demonstrates the presence of previously unrecognized sex-related proteins. *Pediatr Res* **19**, 873–8.
79. Bittel J, Henane R (1975). Comparison of thermal exchanges in men and women under neutral and hot conditions. *J Physiol* **250**, 475–89.
80. Sohar E, Shapiro Y (1965). The physiological reactions of women and children marching during heat. *Proceedings of the Israel Physiology and Pharmacology Society Annual Meeting*, p. 50. Israel.
81. Leppaluoto J (1988). Human thermoregulation in sauna. *Ann Clin Res* **20**, 240–3.
82. Bar-Or O, Blimkie CJ, Hay JA, MacDougall JD, Ward DS, Wilson WM (1992). Voluntary dehydration and heat intolerance in cystic fibrosis. *Lancet* **339**, 696–9.
83. Pugh LG, Corbett JL, Johnson RH (1967). Rectal temperatures, weight losses, and sweat rates in marathon running. *J Appl Physiol* **23**, 347–52.
84. Rothstein A, Adolph EF, Wills JH (1947). Voluntary dehydration. In: Adolph EF (ed.), *Physiology of man in the desert*, pp. 254–70. Interscience, New York.
85. Philip M, Chaimovitz C, Singer A, Golinsky D (1993). Urine osmolality in nursery school children in a hot climate. *Isr J Med Sci* **29**, 104–6.
86. Bar-David Y, Landau D, Bar-David Z, Pilpel D, Phillip M (1998). Voluntary dehydration among elementary school children living in a hot climate. *Child Ambulatory Health* **4**, 393–7.
87. Meyer F, Bar-Or O, Salsberg A, Passe D (1994). Hypohydration during exercise in children: Effect on thirst, drink preferences, and rehydration. *Int J Sport Nutr* **4**, 22–35.
88. Wilk B, Bar-Or O (1996). Effect of drink flavor and NaCl on voluntary drinking and hydration in boys exercising in the heat. *J Appl Physiol* **80**, 1112–17.
89. Bar-Or O, Wilk B (1996). Water and electrolyte replenishment in the exercising child. *Int J Sport Nutr* **6**, 93–9.
90. Hall EL, Bergeron MF, Brenner JS, Wang X, Ludwig DA (2005). Voluntary fluid intake and core temperature responses in children during exercise in the heat. *Med Sci Sports Exerc* **37**, S28.
91. Wilk B, Kriemler S, Keller H, Bar-Or O (1998). Consistency in preventing voluntary dehydration in boys who drink a flavored carbohydrate-NaCl beverage during exercise in the heat. *Int J Sport Nutr* **8**, 1–9.
92. Wilk B, Jae-Hyun L, Bar-Or O (2005). Drink composition, voluntary drinking and aerobic performance in heat-acclimated adolescent male athletes. *Med Sci Sports Exerc* **37**, S464.
93. Heaps CL, Gonzalez-Alonso J, Coyle EF (1994). Hypohydration causes cardiovascular drift without reducing blood volume. *Int J Sports Med* **15**, 74–9.
94. Fortney SM, Wenger CB, Bove JR, Nadel ER (1984). Effect of hyperosmolality on control of blood flow and sweating. *J Appl Physiol* **57**, 1688–95.
95. Kenney WL, Tankersley CG, Newswanger DL, Hyde DE, Puhl SM, Turner NL (1990). Age and hypohydration independently influence the peripheral vascular response to heat stress. *J Appl Physiol* **68**, 1902–8.
96. Sawka MN, Young AJ, Francesconi RP, Muza SR, Pandolf KB (1985). Thermoregulatory and blood responses during exercise at graded hypohydration levels. *J Appl Physiol* **59**, 1394–401.

97. Webster S, Rutt R, Weltman A (1990). Physiological effects of a weight loss regimen practiced by college wrestlers. *Med Sci Sports Exerc* **22**, 229–34.
98. Shirreffs SM (2005). The importance of good hydration for work and exercise performance. *Nutr Rev* **63** (6 Pt 2), S14–21.
99. Walsh RM, Noakes TD, Hawley JA, Dennis SC (1994). Impaired high-intensity cycling performance time at low levels of dehydration. *Int J Sports Med* **15**, 392–8.
100. Dougherty KA, Baker LB, Chow M, Kenney WL (2006). Two percent dehydration impairs and six percent carbohydrate drink improves boys basketball skills. *Med Sci Sports Exerc* **38**, 1650–8.
101. Wilk B, Yuxiu H, Bar-Or O (2002). Effect of hypohydration on aerobic performance of boys who exercise in the heat. *Med Sci Sports Exerc* **34**, S48.
102. Carter J, Jeukendrup AE, Jones DA (2005). The effect of sweetness on the efficacy of carbohydrate supplementation during exercise in the heat. *Can J Appl Physiol* **30**, 79–391.
103. Maughan RJ (2001). Food and fluid intake during exercise. *Can J Appl Physiol* **26**, S71–8.
104. Meyer F, Bar-Or O, MacDougall D, Heigenhauser GJ (1995). Drink composition and the electrolyte balance of children exercising in the heat. *Med Sci Sports Exerc* **27**, 882–7.
105. Meyer F, Bar-Or O, Wilk B (1995). Children's perceptual responses to ingesting drinks of different compositions during and following exercise in the heat. *Int J Sport Nutr* **5**, 13–24.
106. De Felix-Davila RA, Rivera-Brown AM, Lebron Le (2005). Hydration status and sweat electrolyte loss in adolescent judokas training in hot and humid conditions. *Med Sci Sports Exerc* **37**, S167–8.
107. Yeargin SW, Casa DJ, Decher NR, O'Connor CB (2005). Incidence and degree of dehydration and attitudes regarding hydration in children at summer football camp. *Med Sci Sports Exerc* **37**, S463.
108. Casa DJ, Yeargin SW, Decher NR, McCaffrey M, James CT (2005). Incidence and degree of dehydration and attitudes regarding hydration in adolescents at summer football camp. *Med Sci Sports Exerc* **37**, S463.
109. Tipton CM, Tcheng TK, Zambraski EJ (1976). Iowa wrestling study: Weight classification systems. *Med Sci Sports* **8**, 101–4.
110. Tipton CM, Tcheng TK (1970). Iowa wrestling study. Weight loss in high school students. *JAMA* **214**, 1269–74.
111. Oppliger RA, Steen SA, Scott JR (2003). Weight loss practices of college wrestlers. *Int J Sport Nutr Exerc Metab* **13**, 29–46.
112. Sansone RA, Sawyer R (2005). Weight loss pressure on a 5 year old wrestler. *Brit J Sports Med* **39**, e2.
113. Sawka MN, Burke LM, Eichner ER, Maughan RJ, Montain SJ, Stachenfeld NS (2007). American College of Sports Medicine position stand. Exercise and fluid replacement. *Med Sci Sports Exerc* **39**, 377–90.
114. Committee on Sports Medicine (1982). American Academy of Pediatrics Committee on Sports Medicine: Climatic heat stress and the exercising child. *Pediatrics* **69**, 808–9.
115. Committee on Sports Medicine and Fitness (2000). Climatic heat stress and the exercising child and adolescent. *Pediatrics* **106**, 158–9.
116. American College of Sports Medicine (1987). ACSM position statement: Prevention of thermal injuries during distance running. *Med Sci Sports Exerc* **19**, 529–33.
117. American College of Sports Medicine (1996). Position stand on heat and cold illnesses during distance running. *Med Sci Sports Exerc* **28**, i–x.
118. Horswill CA, Passe DH, Stofan JR, Horn MK, Murray R (2005). Adequacy of fluid ingestion in adolescents and adults during moderate-intensity exercise. *Pediatr Exerc Sci* **17**, 41–50.
119. Johnson HL, Nelson RA, Consolazio CF (1988). Effects of electrolyte and nutrient solutions on performance and metabolic balance. *Med Sci Sports Exerc* **20**, 26–33.
120. Wagner JA, Robinson S, Marino RP (1974). Age and temperature regulation of humans in neutral and cold environments. *J Appl Physiol* **37**, 562–5.
121. Marsh ML, Mahon AD, Naftzger LA (1993). Children's physiological responses to exercise in a cold and neutral temperature. *Pediatr Exerc Sci* **5**, 89–90.
122. Ueda T, Choi TH, Kurokawa T (1994). Ratings of perceived exertion in a group of children while swimming at different temperatures. *Ann Physiol Anthropol* **13**, 23–31.
123. Klentrou P, Cunliffe M, Slack J, Wilk B, Bar-Or O, De Souza MJ, Plyley M (2004). Temperature regulation during rest and exercise in the cold in premenarcheal and menarcheal girls. *J Appl Physiol* **96**, 1393–8.
124. Inoue Y, Araki T, Tsujita J (1996). Thermoregulatory responses of prepubertal boys and young men in changing temperature linearly from 28 to 15 degrees C. *Eur J Appl Physiol* **72**, 204–8.
125. Mackova J, Sturmova M, Macek M (1984). Prolonged exercise in prepubertal boys in warm and cold environments. In: Illmarinen J, Valimaki I (eds.), *Children and sports*, pp. 135–41. Springer-Verlag, Heidelberg.
126. Inoue Y, Nakamura S, Yonehiro K, Kuwahara T, Ueda H, Araki T (2006). Regional differences in peripheral vasoconstriction of prepubertal boys. *Eur J Appl Physiol* **96**, 397–403.
127. Falk B, Bar-Eli M, Dotan R, Yaaron M, Weinstein Y, Epstein S, Blumenstein B, Einbinder M, Yarom Y, Tenenbaum G (1997). Physiological and cognitive responses to cold exposure in 11–12 year-old boys. *Am J Hum Biol* **9**, 39–49.
128. Falk B, Bar-Or O, Smolander J, Frost G (1994). Response to rest and exercise in the cold: Effects of age and aerobic fitness. *J Appl Physiol* **76**, 72–8.
129. Sloan RE, Keatinge WR (1973). Cooling rates of young people swimming in cold water. *J Appl Physiol* **35**, 371–5.
130. Wakabayashi H, Kaneda K, Okura M, Nomura T (2007). Insulation and body temperature of prepubescent children wearing a thermal swimsuit during moderate-intensity water exercise. *J Physiol Anthropol* **26**, 179–83.
131. Inbar O, Bar-Or O, Dotan R, Gutin B (1981). Conditioning versus exercise in heat as methods for acclimatizing 8- to 10-yr-old boys to dry heat. *J Appl Physiol* **50**, 406–11.
132. Armstrong LE, Maresh CM (1991). The induction and decay of heat acclimatisation in trained athletes. *Sports Med* **12**, 302–12.
133. Cotter JD, Patterson MJ, Taylor NA (1997). Sweat distribution before and after repeated heat exposure. *Eur J Appl Physiol* **76**, 181–6.
134. Wilk B, Bar-Or O (1997). Heat acclimation and sweating pattern in prepubertal boys. *Pediatr Exerc Sci* **9**, 92.
135. Bar-Or O, Inbar O (1977). Relationship between perceptual and physiological changes during heat acclimatization in 8–10 year-old boys. In: Lavalee H, Shephard RJ (eds.), *Frontiers of activity and child health*, pp. 205–14. Pelican Press, Quebec.
136. Docherty D, Eckerson JD, Hayward JS (1986). Physique and thermoregulation in prepubertal males during exercise in a warm, humid environment. *Am J Phys Anthropol* **70**, 19–23.
137. Matsushita K, Araki T (1980). The effect of physical training on thermoregulatory responses of pre-adolescent boys to heat and cold. *Jap J Fitness Sports Med* **29**, 69–74.

PART III

Physical Activity, Physical Fitness, and Health

CHAPTER 24

Physical activity, physical fitness, and health: current concepts

Sean Cumming and Chris Riddoch

Introduction

With regard to children and physical activity, we live in a world of contrasts and contradictions. On one hand, children are specializing and participating in competitive sports at increasingly early ages.[1] Teenage world record holders in swimming are commonplace, many Olympic female gymnasts can be defined as prepubescent, a 7-year-old Indian boy has a training programme involving running a marathon a day, and a 13-year-old boy has run the marathon in 2 hours and 55 min. Similarly, an increasing number of leisure facilities now offer fitness programmes for children and child size exercise equipment. On the other hand, there appears to be a widespread decline in children's physical activity, both in and outside of school, a general perception that children's freedom to cycle, walk and play outdoors is being curtailed, and that too much time is spent watching television and playing video games. Such contrasts beg the questions: 'is there a happy medium of physical activity for the child that will ensure optimum growth and health (physical, psychological, and behavioural) into adulthood?' and, 'to what extent are children today achieving this level?'

These questions are difficult to answer. Despite the widespread acceptance that physical activity is generally beneficial for children's health and improvements in the quantity and quality of evidence supporting this position, our understanding remains limited. Methodological and conceptual discrepancies still exist, including a lack of clear consensus in how to define and assess physical activity in children,[2] a limited consideration of concurrent factors such as growth and maturation,[3] and a general failure to address the potential interactions of biological, psychological, and social variables. As such, it is difficult to distil the available information with a view to establishing absolute recommendations for activity and/or fitness levels that are optimal for health in children.

Nevertheless, a number of organizations have put forward physical activity guidelines for optimizing health and functional capacity in children.[2] The earliest recommendation was presented by the American College of Sports Medicine.[4] On the basis of the adult guidelines, they recommended that children should engage in at least 20 min of vigorous physical activity each day. Recognizing that children are not simply small adults, the International Conference on Physical Activity Guidelines for Adolescents (ICC) conducted a systematic review of the available literature to establish empirically based guidelines for physical activity.[5] The panel recommended that all adolescents should (i) be active on a daily basis, whether it be through work, play, physical education, sport, or active transport, and (ii) engage in at least 20 min of sustained moderate to vigorous activity at least three times per week. In 1997, the Health Education Authority of England commissioned guidelines for activity in children.[6] Recognizing individual differences in fitness and activity levels, the recommendations were that currently active children should achieve a minimum of 60 min of moderate activity per day, whereas less active children should strive for at least 30 min of moderate activity. Children should also engage at least twice per week in activities designed to promote bone growth, flexibility, and strength. These recommendations were restated in the Chief Medical Officer's 2004 report on physical activity and health in the United Kingdom.[7] Most recently, a systematic review conducted in the United States concluded that school children should engage in at least 1 hour of moderate to vigorous activity per day, emphasizing that activities should be enjoyable and developmentally appropriate.[8]

The lack of a clear consensus regarding optimal levels of physical activity in children is in stark contrast to available evidence relating to adults. In adults, we are now undoubtedly much clearer about the general strength and direction of the associations between activity, fitness, and health. In particular, there exists a large measure of consistency between the results of many large studies that lead us to conclude that virtually any increase in activity from a state of sedentariness is beneficial to health. We now know that sedentary living is an element of contemporary lifestyle that impacts significantly, and adversely, upon health. Given the current epidemic of lifestyle-related chronic diseases, contemporary lifestyles of developed nations have become a matter of concern.[9] The increasing prevalence of sedentary living has been documented in adults,[10,11] and more recently children.[12] Secular trends in children's activity mirror those observed in adults, with decreased activity in many different contexts including active transport, physical education, and freedom to play outside. The general decline in children's activity levels undoubtedly contributes to the escalating levels of childhood overweight and obesity seen in both the United States and the United Kingdom.[13–16] It is noteworthy that the increasing levels of obesity are occurring despite children having a lower daily caloric intake compared to previous generations.[13–17]

Reductions in the activity levels of children probably stem from social and environmental change, rather than a decreased interest in physical activity or decreased participation in sport. The opportunities for children to be active have become increasingly constrained by factors such as school policy or curricula, parental rules regarding safety and convenience, and a range of other environmental factors.[12] Accordingly, there is growing concern that children may now be at considerable risk as a result of sedentary living—both during childhood, in terms of adverse effects on growth and development, and later as an adult. There continues to be much current interest in children's levels of physical activity and fitness, and in their apparent decline.[18–20] Physical education teachers are concerned that fitness levels in children appear to be falling, and recruits to the armed forces are less aerobically fit than in previous times.[21]

Although it would appear that children are becoming less active, there has, until recently, been surprisingly little high-quality evidence to suggest that children's activity and/or fitness levels are so low as to compromise their current or future health.[2,22,23] However, the increasing use of objective motion sensors—most notably accelerometers—has greatly increased our ability to measure activity levels more accurately (see Chapter 10), and these more accurate data now clearly suggest that low activity levels are indeed compromising the health of children. This can be seen in terms of higher levels of overweight and obesity,[24–26] cardiovascular disease (CVD) risk factors,[27–29] and bone health.[30] There are, therefore, increasingly strong grounds to be very concerned about children's levels of physical activity. In this respect, Blair[31] has hypothesized a number of possible relationships between activity levels, health, and stage of life (Fig. 24.1).

The hypothesized relationships within this model suggest three main beneficial effects that might derive from adequate childhood activity:

- Enhancement of physiological and psychological development during childhood—directly improving childhood health status and quality of life (A).
- Delay in the onset, or retardation of the rate of development of health risk factors—directly improving adult health status (B).
- Improved likelihood of maintaining adequate activity levels into adulthood, thus indirectly enhancing adult health status (C).

Considering these possible relations, it is interesting to note that the majority of evidence we have relates to adult activity and adult health (D). Relations between child activity and either child health (A), or adult health (B), or adult activity (C) are still weak by comparison. Further, as a cautionary note, it is important to note that increased activity may also carry a measure of increased health risk, through trauma, overuse or burnout, which must be balanced against the potential benefits.[1]

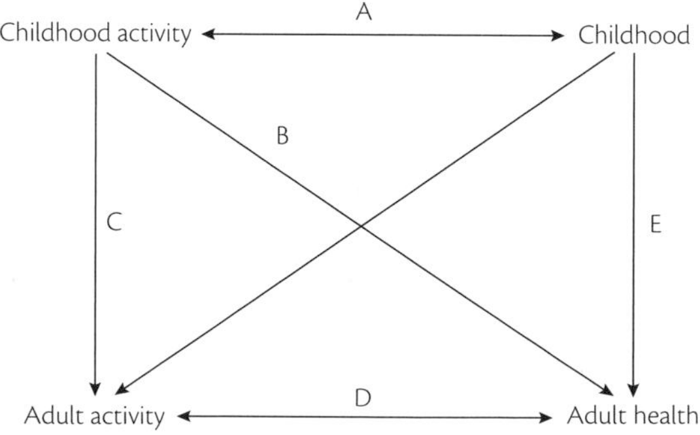

Fig. 24.1 Hypothetical relationships between physical activity and health in children and adults. Reproduced from Blair *et al*,[31] with permission from McGraw-Hill Companies, Inc., New York.

Defining physical activity and physical fitness

Physical activity is a behaviour, and indeed a very complex behaviour. Activity behaviour can vary within a range of dimensions—the type of activity, the duration of activity sessions, the intensity—both absolute (energy cost) and relative (proportion of maximal capacity)—and the frequency of sessions. We can also consider activity in terms of energy expenditure—in other words, the metabolic cost of performing all the day's physical activities. Physical activity also has a performance dimension that can be assessed in terms of functional or skill capacity.[3] We might additionally consider whether the activity is *unavoidable*—for example, for subsistence or work, or *voluntary*—for example, for sport and recreation. Finally, it is important to acknowledge that physical activity, as behaviour, is generally meaningful and purposeful and must be viewed within its cultural or social context if it is to be truly understood.[3]

Physical activity is even more complex when studied in children. All children are faced with three primary tasks that constitute the business of 'growing up',[3] namely, to grow (changes in body size, physique, and composition); to mature (progress towards a biologically mature state); and to develop (learn culturally appropriate cognitive, emotional, social, and motor behaviours). Although distinct, these processes interact with one another to govern the majority of children's experiences during the first two decades of their life and may confound relations between health and physical activity. Maturity-associated variability in physical characteristics (e.g. size, physique, body composition) and functional capacity (e.g. strength, speed, aerobic capacity) have already been documented as predictors of physical and psychological health[32,33] and involvement in physical activity and sport.[32,34] As a result, researchers interested in examining the health benefits of physical activity in children need to be aware of and/or control for individual variation in growth and maturation.[35]

Because activity behaviour is so complex (and variable), it is extremely difficult to measure. No valid method of measuring physical activity exists which accurately reflects all of its dimensions.[2] An obvious problem we have when a behaviour is so difficult to assess is that a high degree of misclassification of individuals is likely. For example, a questionnaire concentrating on sports and fitness training is likely to miss much activity performed through informal play, work, and travel. An individual who plays no sport, but who walks a lot and does large amounts of housework, can potentially be misclassified as a sedentary person. When assessing relations between activity levels and other parameters—for example, health status—misclassification in terms of activity will weaken the observed relations and limit the accuracy of estimated dose–response effects.[36]

The strength and limitations of various methods for assessing physical activity have been reported elsewhere (see refs 2,37 and Chapter 10. Doubly labelled water is considered the 'gold standard' when assessing energy expenditure in living subjects. (The term *doubly labeled water test* refers to a particular type of test of metabolic rate, in which average metabolic rate of an organism is measured over a period of time. This is done by administering a dose of doubly labeled water, and then tracking the loss of deuterium and O-18 in the subject, over time, through the use of regular sampling of saliva, urine, or blood. The test essentially measures the subject's carbon dioxide production over the interval, which is related to the amount of activity performed.) However, its practicality is limited by the financial costs required for its use and the need to collect accurate dietary records during the period of study. Accelerometers, and other motion sensitive devices (e.g. pedometers), are identified as objective, reasonably accurate, and less expensive alternative to doubly labelled water. Although currently considered the method of choice for assessing physical activity even in large-scale studies, accelerometers remain limited in some ways, as they are impractical when assessing certain activities, such as contact sports (e.g. rugby) or water-based activities (e.g. swimming). The development of accelerometers that simultaneously record movement and heart rate provide a more accurate assessment of the intensity of activity or individual exertion but still present a problem in terms of assessing activity in contact or water-based sports.[2,38,39] Self-report questionnaires, though lacking in precision, can provide informative overviews of children's activity in surveillance studies.

In contrast to physical activity, physical fitness is an attribute, and generally refers to one's capacity to undertake physical work. Similar to physical activity, there are many dimensions of fitness, for example, cardiovascular fitness, strength, flexibility, speed, power, and anaerobic endurance. Many of these dimensions are not only related to performance, but also to health. The component that is most strongly associated with health is cardiovascular (C-V) endurance, defined as 'the ability to sustain moderate intensity, whole-body activity for extended time periods' (ref. 40). It can be measured objectively in the laboratory setting using a variety of ergometers (cycle, treadmill, etc.) with or without respiratory gas analysis, or more simply in the field by maximal running tests or submaximal cycle or step tests (see Chapters 4, 5, 8, and 9). Fitness is partly genetically determined, but can also be improved by regular appropriate physical activity. In contrast to physical activity, physical fitness can be accurately measured, leading to less misclassification of individuals and observed relations that may be nearer to reality. Both fitness and activity are strongly and independently associated with health in adults, and similar associations can now be observed in children.

Activity and health in adults

Relations between activity and health

In order to understand activity/health relations in children, it is first necessary to look at the equivalent relations in adults, where the picture is much clearer. The question that arises is: 'What are the implications of the strong adult data—which clearly demonstrate that physical activity promotes improved health—to children?'

In adults, both physical activity and cardiorespiratory fitness levels are strongly and inversely related to both morbidity and mortality.[7,11,41,42] Prospective population studies of adults have shown that higher levels of physical activity lead to reduced risk of coronary heart disease (CHD), stroke, hypertension, non-insulin-dependent diabetes mellitus (NIDDM), osteoporotic fractures, some cancers, and clinical and non-clinical forms of anxiety and depression.[7,43,44] The level of individual risk attributed to low levels of physical activity is comparable to the risk associated with cigarette smoking.[7] Similar (and stronger) associations have been reported for cardiorespiratory fitness.[45]

From a public health perspective, it is important to note that whereas inactivity carries similar individual *risk* as the other major CVD risk factors, the *prevalence* of inactivity is far higher—may be up to three times as high.[46] This is of crucial importance, because it indicates that on a population basis, sedentary living may be the most significant adverse health behaviour because of the high level of individual risk combined with the large proportion of the population exposed to that risk. Expressed in a different way, the greatest *scope* for population health gain may lie in preventing and reversing sedentary living habits.

Dose–response relations

There appears to exist a graded dose–response relationship between activity level and mortality, with mortality being greatest at the lower end of the activity distribution, and lowest at the more active end.[42] Importantly, *increments* of risk reduction are greatest between activity groups at the low end of the activity distribution with a 'law of diminishing returns' as one moves along the distribution from low activity to high activity. There is also some evidence of a 'levelling off' of benefit at a certain point, which is suggestive of an *optimum* level of activity, above which few further health benefits can be gained. However, this level may vary—or not exist—depending on the health outcome selected. Similar relations can be identified between fitness and health, with the greatest difference in cardiovascular risk being observed between individuals in the least fit groups and those who are slightly fitter. Increments of benefit between these groups and subsequent (fitter) groups are smaller.[41]

At the higher end of the activity spectrum, where activity levels may be taken to the extreme, some body systems react adversely—even when the body has been conditioned gradually to these physical stresses—compared to more moderate levels of activity. For example, high levels of activity can cause musculoskeletal injuries, renal abnormalities, gastrointestinal disturbances, immune system suppression, menstrual irregularities, and psychological burnout. Although some of these conditions are not necessarily serious, they are undoubtedly troublesome, and may partly offset any health benefits accruing from higher levels of activity. They may also have an adverse effect on adherence to activity. This again leads us towards the conclusion that an optimal level of activity—for health purposes—may exist.

An optimal level for health?

From the above, we might conclude that there exists a level of activity, lying somewhere between the couch potato and the trained athlete, which is *optimal* for health. Indeed it is likely that in evolutionary terms we have developed the biological equipment necessary for the lifestyle of a hunter/gatherer—daylong intermittent activities of varying intensity—but we are now forced by cultural, technological, and environmental circumstances into a far more sedentary lifestyle.

Changing this propensity for a sedentary lifestyle will not be easy. To go some way towards returning people to a more active lifestyle, health-related activity guidelines have been formulated for adults. The central message of the recommendation is the accumulation of 30 min of moderate intensity activity (equating to brisk walking for the majority of people), on at least 5 days of the week.[7] The daily recommended level of activity can be achieved in a single bout or in three shorter, and perhaps more manageable and realistic, bouts of 10 min each.[47] A stepping-stone of 30 min on 1 day per week is suggested for those who are initially totally sedentary, and a more distant goal of taking three sessions of more vigorous activity per week—approximating cardiorespiratory fitness training guidelines—is provided for people who are more ambitious or more motivated. The health-enhancing properties of more vigorous activity have recently been reinforced.[48]

These guidelines balance what is known to be beneficial to health and what is likely to be *achievable* by the majority of people. It should be noted that the majority of health benefits should accrue with moderate intensity activity, but there is some evidence to suggest that more vigorous activity may be necessary for certain improvements to take place—most notably normalization of blood pressure.[48] However, such high levels of activity are probably not necessary to improve the majority of the dimensions of health,[49] and the widely held view that running three times a week is in some way a health-related *threshold* has now been rightly discarded.

We can therefore conclude that (i) avoiding the low end of the activity or fitness spectrum is the 'healthiest' scenario, and (ii) high levels of activity are probably unnecessary for the achievement of most health benefits. In this respect, examples of activities that have been shown to confer a significant reduction in the risk of CHD include gardening,[46] lawn mowing,[46] walking,[42,46] and stair climbing.[42] While such activities may not be so attractive for children, these data do support the view that total activity energy expenditure, irrespective of the type, intensity, duration, or frequency may be the key dimension of activity for the improvement of health. The important question is, however, do these adult data hold true for children?

Physical activity and health in children

It is clear that young children enjoy active play. Given a free choice, most young children will play or invent active ways of passing time which involve jumping, dancing, skipping, hopping, chasing, running, climbing, and cycling. Older children might play more organized sports—either formally, in clubs and teams, or informally, in parks and playgrounds. Generally speaking, these forms of play provide a large volume of activity incorporating a wide variety of movements, using many muscle groups, and promoting cardiorespiratory development, muscular strength, muscular endurance, speed, power, and flexibility. These activities also afford the opportunity for children to develop and apply various social and psychological skills (i.e. communication, cooperation, reasoning), enhancing psychosocial development. In the later teenage years, these relatively high levels of activity decline as more sedentary alternatives are chosen. This decline is not necessarily problematic, and is seen in many other animal species. However, if activity levels decline to levels that are too low—and we should remember that adult levels are undoubtedly too low—then this may constitute a 'problem in the making'.

The question is, therefore, 'do children's activity levels decline over the teenage years to such an extent that either their current or future health is compromised?' To answer this question, we must scrutinize the evidence relating activity to indicators of health status—or health risk factors—in children.

There is an emerging body of evidence suggesting associations between childhood physical activity and childhood health, reflected by more favourable overweight/obesity status or a healthier CVD risk profile.[26,27,29] We should therefore more closely examine the evidence relating to each of the three hypothesized relationships suggested by Fig. 24.1.

Activity and current health status

Overweight and obesity

Clear associations have been reported between children's activity levels and measures of overweight and obesity.[24–26] These strong associations tend to be seen in studies where activity has been measured more accurately (e.g. with accelerometers). There appear to be stronger associations with moderate and vigorous activity than with total activity.[26]

The limited effectiveness of obesity prevention and treatment programmes (both activity and nutrition based) has been highlighted.[50] A lack of tailoring of interventions to address the needs of specific subsamples of children (e.g. immigrants in industrialized countries, those aged 0–6 years, and males) was identified as a particular limitation of these programmes, as was the failure to integrate the strategies for healthy living or use evidence-based strategies.[51] The need to create change at the institutional level (e.g. provide opportunity for competitive and non-competitive forms of physical activity) and to educate parents about reducing TV and computer games use have also been identified as key factors in the fight against childhood obesity.[52] More holistic, multidimensional (i.e. activity, psychology, and nutrition-based) interventions are probably required in order to achieve real impacts on children's activity levels.

The importance of avoiding overweight during adolescence has been highlighted.[53] In a large, prospective study with 55 years of follow-up, being overweight in adolescence predicted a broad range of adverse health effects in adulthood that were independent of adult weight. Overweight during adolescence is therefore concluded to be a more significant predictor of a range of future diseases than being overweight as an adult. A review of 32 longitudinal studies tracking adiposity in youth in relation to physical activity or sedentary behaviour concluded that physical activity and decreased sedentary behaviour are protective against relative weight and fatness gains over childhood and adolescence.[54] This position is supported by results from large-scale epidemiological studies of European[27] and British youth.[26]

We can suggest three reasons why the increased prevalence of childhood obesity might be a major source of concern. First, obesity is a major risk factor in adults for insulin resistance and diabetes, hypertension, cancer, gallbladder disease, and atherosclerosis.[55,56] Second, obesity tends to track from childhood into adulthood,[57] and third, adults who were obese children have increased morbidity and mortality, irrespective of adult weight.[53] For these reasons, childhood obesity might be a major target for intervention from both primary prevention and treatment perspectives, and physical activity should feature strongly in this.

Metabolic syndrome

The principal features of metabolic syndrome are increased insulin resistance, hypertension, dyslipidaemia, and obesity (especially central obesity). Whereas the existence of clinical metabolic syndrome in children is debated, clustering of CVD risk factors can undoubtedly be detected in children.[27,58] Studies of associations between physical activity and single CVD risk factors in children[47,59,60] have reported only weak associations and in many cases evidence is equivocal. However, studies investigating clustering of CVD risk factors in children have produced much stronger associations. Data derived from the European Heart Study indicate a strong, negative association between physical activity (measured by accelerometry) and the clustering of CVD risk factors in a sample of over 1700 Estonian, Portuguese, and Danish youth. Time spent in moderate and vigorous forms of physical activity was 116 min in 9 year olds and 88 min in 15 year olds), for the most active (and least at risk) groups. This suggests that the recommendation of 60 min of moderate physical activity per day may not be sufficient to prevent the clustering of CVD risk factors in children. Although none of the children in the study presented symptoms of CVD, clustered risk factors have been shown to track from childhood into early adulthood.[27] In a related study with Danish youth, Brage *et al.*[61] observed an inverse relation between physical activity and clustered risk, even when potential confounders such as age, sex, maturation, ethnicity, socio-economic factors, and smoking behaviour were controlled for. In contrast, data collected from the Early Bird diabetes study suggest a lack of relation between objectively measured physical activity in children and metabolic health.[62]

Type 2 diabetes

The prevalence of Type 2 diabetes (T2DM), traditionally referred to as non-insulin-dependent diabetes, is increasing both in the American[63] and British[7] children, although incidences are relatively low (see Chapter 29). The increased prevalence of this disease in children is of particular concern in low socio-economic groups and minority populations. In the United States, almost 50% of African–American and Hispanic children are expected to develop T2DM as adults.

Analyses of children aged 10–12 years taken from the third NHANES study (1999–2000) revealed that although being overweight was associated with an increased risk of T2DM, fewer hours of active play is not.[63] Independent of physical activity, children's risk for T2DM was positively associated with time playing video games or watching TV. In a related study, using the NHANES 1999–2002 data, levels of physical activity and cardiovascular fitness were associated with increased insulin sensitivity in boys, but not girls.[64] In contrast, a study of Danish youth taken from the European Heart Study reported a positive association between activity (measured by accelerometry) and insulin resistance in females, but not males.[28] In lean and obese Greek children aged between 9 and 11.5 years, central adiposity and physical activity were positively and negatively, associated with insulin resistance, respectively.[65]

Bone health

Osteoporosis, and the fractures that are associated with it, are largely a feature of old age, the scale of the problem is certain to grow as life expectancy increases. It is estimated, for example, that the 6.26 million hip fractures currently recorded annually on a worldwide basis will increase four-fold by the year 2050.[66] Although osteoporosis is principally a condition of the elderly, attainment of a strong, dense skeleton during the growing years may be the best way to prevent osteoporosis in later life (see refs 67,68 and Chapter 27).

Peak bone mass, which is achieved in the majority of people by the third decade,[69,70] appears to be largely under the control of genetic influences. Approximately 70–85% of the interindividual variance in bone mass is genetically determined, with several candidate genes involved in the regulation and metabolism of collagen (*COLIA 1* gene), vitamin D (*VDR* gene), oestrogen (*ER* gene), and nitric oxide (*ec NOS* gene) being strongly implicated.[71] However, the residual variance in bone mass is under environmental influences which are amenable to early intervention. The most important environmental factors appear to be diet—notably calcium intake[72]—and the amount and type of physical activity taken throughout childhood and adolescence.

Investigations examining the relationship between physical activity in childhood and adolescence and bone mineral acquisition have been reviewed in detail by Bailey *et al.*[67] Studies of representative populations have, in the main, been conducted retrospectively,[73–75] although longitudinal or prospective studies have reported.[30,76–78] These studies indicate that weight-bearing physical activity in childhood and adolescence is an important predictor of bone geometry, mineral content, and density (IBS), while non-weight-bearing activity (such as swimming or cycling) is not.[79] The size of the effect of physical activity (difference in BMD between the high and low fitness or activity groups) is, typically, between 5% and 15%. Appropriate physical activity increases peak bone mass somewhat less than 1 SD, or 7–8% approximately.[68] This would be sufficient, if maintained into old age, to substantially reduce the risk of osteoporotic fracture.[80] However, more research on the optimal type and volume of physical activity required for bone health in young people is required. On the basis of the available information,[81] it is likely that activities which involve high strains, developed rapidly and distributed unevenly throughout the movement pattern, may be particularly osteogenic. Thus, activities such as aerobics, dancing, volleyball, basketball, and racket sports may be effective, and need not necessarily be of prolonged duration, as the osteogenic response to such movement appears to saturate after only a few loading cycles.[81] It is also interesting to note that the natural play activities of young children do provide a significant element of high impact movement, and may be optimal—in type—for health.

Questions for future examination include when is the optimal time to introduce physical activity for the purposes of enhancing bone development, and what dose responses are required to obtain these benefits. In adults, bone seems relatively unresponsive to all but the most vigorous of exercise regimes.[82–84] There is some evidence,[77] however, that physical activity during the immediate prepubescent and pubescent years may be crucial for maximizing peak bone mass. Data collected from the Avon Longitudinal Study of Parents and Children (ALSPAC) suggests that moderate and vigorous physical activity is positively associated with increased bone density and bone mineral content in 11-year-old boys and girls.[30,36] Further, evidence from the Iowa Bone Development Study[85] suggests that positive associations between physical activity and bone measures are present during early childhood, well in advance of the onset of peak bone mass. In the light of these observations, intervention strategies to optimize bone development in children might be most effective if introduced during childhood. Whether or not early or late childhood is the optimal time period in which activity promotes bone growth is as yet unknown.

In summary, physical activity is an essential stimulus for bone structure, and has the potential to increase peak bone mass in children and adolescents within the limits set by genetic, hormonal, and nutritional influences. Such enhanced bone mass has considerable potential to reduce risk of osteoporosis and associated fracture in later life, particularly if the increase can be maintained throughout adulthood by physical activity.

Psychological health

Evidence supporting the psychological benefits of physical activity has been well documented in adult samples.[86,87] However, the evidence supporting the existence of similar relations in children and adolescents is limited (see Chapter 28). Given the increased prevalence of children presenting psychological problems (an estimated 20% of all children in the United Kingdom[88]), there is a growing need to examine and understand the role that physical activity plays in the prevention and treatment of psychological problems in children. The majority of research supporting the psychological benefits of physical activity in children is cross-sectional in design. As such, it is not possible to infer cause and effect relations. Nevertheless, more active children tend to report higher levels of self-esteem, happiness, and life satisfaction[89] and lower levels of anxiety, depression,[90] stress,[91] and peer victimization.[92] Consistent with evidence from adult samples, it would appear that the psychological health benefits associated with physical activity can also be achieved through low to moderate intensity activities such as walking and jogging. Similarly, over involvement in intense, frequent, sustained bouts of activity can result in 'burnout', a special case of sport withdrawal in which child athletes cease to participate in sport due to chronic stress.[1,93] This is a particular concern for athletes who specialize and compete at an early age (see ref. 1 and see Chapter 37).

Other health issues

Asthma represents another leading form of chronic illness in children and adolescents. Although acute bouts of strenuous exercise have been identified as triggers for asthmatic attacks, moderate and low intensity exercise is often recommended as a complementary therapy in the treatment of asthma. Little is known, however, about the role that physical activity plays in the prevention and treatment of asthma (see Chapter 32). A cross-sectional study that included over 13,000 U.S. adolescents[94] revealed that sedentary behaviour (>3 hours computer use per day) and being overweight were associated with an increased prevalence of asthma. Surprisingly, levels of physical activity did not predict incidences of asthma.

From the above, it is apparent that there is an emerging body of evidence linking physical activity levels to various health parameters in children. To gain a more comprehensive understanding of these relations researchers must strive to develop and employ more sophisticated research designs and sensitive measurement tools. Researchers also needed to recognize that the absence of evidence does not indicate the evidence of absence. The failure of many previous studies to identify relations between activity and health parameters may result from limitations associated with research designs, methods, sampling procedures, the types of analysis used, or a failure to control for confounding factors, such as growth and maturation. In other words, subtle relations and effects may exist, but we may not have been able to detect them.

Activity and future health status

Direct effects

It has been hypothesized that degenerative biological processes are initiated during infancy and childhood that will manifest themselves as chronic disease in later life. In fact, there is evidence to suggest that adult health status may be determined, at least in part, by biological events that occur *in utero*.[95] It is argued that early biological events trigger a morphological and/or functional change that subsequently becomes a chronic and worsening condition, ultimately leading to overt signs and symptoms, chronic illness, and death. The individual is effectively 'programmed' for susceptibility to a disease through an early biological event. Crucially, the biological event may itself be triggered by an environmental influence (inadequate maternal nutrition, smoking) and it is in this respect that physical activity may be important. It should be stressed that these assertions are currently hypothetical—and remain to be fully tested—but nevertheless, we have one further argument that physical activity during the early part of the lifespan is important, despite the fact that morbidity and mortality are features of adult life.

Indirect effects

It seems reasonable to presume that if high activity as a child increases the likelihood of being a more active adult—which we know enhances health—then childhood activity can be considered to indirectly influence adult health status. It is often presumed that this link exists, but the evidence is again rather sparse. The persistence of a behaviour, or attribute, over time is called 'tracking', and refers to the short, medium, or long-term maintenance of a rank-order position compared to one's peers. Our main concern, therefore, might be whether inactivity in childhood would lead to inactivity in adulthood, and subsequent elevated risk of adult disease.[96] Conversely, does high activity as a child predict high activity as an adult ?

Levels of tracking through various stages of the lifespan have been comprehensively reviewed.[97] Activity tracks at weak to moderate levels during adolescence, from adolescence into adulthood, and across various ages during adulthood. Data from more recent studies[98,99] provide supporting evidence, indicating weak to moderate associations between childhood and adult levels of physical activity and health?

Tracking of activity from childhood to adulthood is therefore not strong. However, it might be the case that substantial tracking should not be expected in the case of physical activity. A multitude of factors can influence activity levels and patterns from day to day, between seasons of the year, and because of various 'life events'. Examples of life events that can disturb activity patterns include changing schools, school-to-work transition, leaving home, moving house, moving to a new neighbourhood, biological and psychological development (especially puberty and adolescence), illness, marriage, and child rearing. Any one of these can significantly affect activity habits, and therefore it is to be expected that activity levels will fluctuate greatly within any one individual over all stages of the lifespan. Linked with this is the fact that both active children and active adults are likely to change the dimension of activity they favour. As we grow older, we move from play, through sport, to social and recreational activities and the level of 'background' or lifestyle activity we do—for example, walking to work and housework confound the whole scenario. We might therefore expect tracking coefficients to be only weak or moderate.

The methodological and conceptual problems are therefore considerable in our quest to assess the stability of this complex and fundamentally changeable behaviour. Interestingly, there is some evidence to suggest[100] that how 'comfortable' an adult is about the concept of physical activity ('psychological readiness') is positively correlated with how active the adult is. For example, PE grade at the age of 15 years (a measure of competence) is positively associated with psychological readiness to participate in activity at age 30. This suggests that encouraging promoting actual and perceived competence in sports and physical recreation—which may not promote higher *childhood* activity levels—may nevertheless have long-lasting effects on adult attitudes towards activity and subsequently higher *adult* activity levels.

Prevalence of activity/inactivity

Whether children are 'active enough' to gain health benefits is one of the important outstanding questions. At this point data are equivocal—even confusing. Studies conducted on British children have been reviewed[101] and suggest that children seldom participate in activity at a level which would have a cardiovascular training effect, or a health benefit. Sallis[102] examined nine studies and concluded that the average child is sufficiently active to meet the adult recommendations for conditioning activities, with the exception of the average female in mid to late adolescence. It has been argued that young children are highly and spontaneously active.[103,104] 'Simple observation tells us that toddlers are constantly on the move, exploring the environment, playing, and moving apparently for the sheer joy of it'.[105] Blair[106] has noted that children are generally fitter and more active than adults, and most of them are active enough to receive important health benefits from their activity.

Saris *et al.*[107] have reported physical activity level (PAL) values (PAL = total energy expenditure/resting metabolic rate) of 1.95 in 9-year-old boys and 1.71 in 8-year-old girls, and Davies *et al.*[108] have reported PAL values of 1.84 for 9-year-old boys and 1.65 in 9-year-old girls. Using energy intake as an indirect measure of activity Boreham *et al.*[109] have reported energy intakes for 12- and 15-year-old British children equating to average daily PAL values of 1.8–1.9. These results compare favourably with defined PAL values of 1.7 (moderately active) and 1.9 (very active).[110] Research employing accelerometers to measure physical activity in British youth have presented conflicting results. Whereas Sleap and Tolfrey[111] suggest that British children, aged 9–12 years, engage in sufficient quantities of physical activity to meet U.S. and U.K. daily recommendations, evidence from the ALSPAC longitudinal study suggest that the great majority of children fail to meet international standards for physical activity.[112] European children appear to be more active than U.K. children,[113] although methodological discrepancies between studies probably account for this.

From the above, it is clear that we have a great deal of conflicting data, but that more precise measurement techniques employed in the more recent (and larger) studies are allowing a better under standing to emerge. We are not at the stage yet to definitively answer the question 'are children active enough to be healthy?' However, as obesity levels continue to rise, the answer for many children is probably 'no'.

Guidelines for physical activity

As noted previously, guidelines for health-related activity in children have been formulated despite a relative lack of supporting scientific evidence.[7,114,115] There are intuitive biological and behavioural arguments in favour of promoting physical activity to all children. Guidelines tend to reinforce the concept of a health-related threshold, yet the amount and type of physical activity during childhood which is appropriate for optimal health is probably impossible to ascertain. Relationships between the different dimensions of activity and the different health outcomes will vary, are probably dynamic, and subject to fluctuations depending on age, gender, and a broad range of socio-demographic and environmental variables. The concept of a single health-related activity threshold is probably misguided.

Earlier criteria, or thresholds, were generally based on the amount of activity required for the development of cardiovascular fitness. However, they may not only have been too stringent for the majority of children to achieve, but may also have been unrelated to the amount of activity necessary to achieve a health benefit. It has been suggested[116] that from a behavioural perspective physical activity needs to be seen by children as an achievable and positive experience, and that adult fitness training guidelines, emphasizing continuous bouts of vigorous exercise, do not fulfil this. In this respect, criteria[7,114,115] are based more on the existing evidence of activity/health relationships in children, the stronger adult data, and also take account of behavioural issues, in terms of activity adoption and maintenance. The most recent guidelines[7,114] propose the accumulation of 60 min of moderate intensity activity every day, including activities which promote strength, flexibility, and bone health.

Fitness and health

Many of the studies investigating associations between fitness and health have been large-scale, cross-sectional population surveys, using multivariate analysis to adjust for potential confounding variables. More powerful evidence for causal links between fitness and health come from rarer longitudinal population studies, or from training studies in which changes in the two or more variables can be compared over time. Irrespective of study design, one important distinction between adult and child studies is that the former have the advantage of examining associations between fitness and morbidity/mortality, whereas children's studies in this field are restricted to examining risk factors that are problematic to define and measure. Developing work on the genetics of fitness[117] may improve our understanding of how fitness and health are pre-determined and interrelated, and how independent it is of activity level.

Numerous adult population studies[41,118–122] have shown strong and consistent relationships between C-V fitness and mortality from CHD and all causes, independent of possible confounding variables. Even more compelling has been evidence from prospective studies,[123] which indicate that the risk of mortality may be reduced substantially in middle-aged men who improve their fitness over a number of years.

The situation with children appears to be less clear-cut, partly because the outcome measure—'health'—cannot, for obvious reasons, be judged by mortality statistics. Rather, the investigator must rely upon risk factors for CHD mortality, such as high blood pressure, elevated blood lipids, and fatness. However, such risk factors may only account for 50% of eventual coronary mortality and are therefore a relatively crude yardstick for cardiovascular health.[124] Furthermore, as a result of maturation, these biological risk factors are constantly changing through adolescence, and may or may not relate to adult values.[125] Despite these limitations, some population studies have shown an independent relation between C-V fitness and levels of risk factors.[27,61,126,127] Further evidence of a causal relationship between fitness and coronary risk status in children comes from long-term fitness training studies that report concomitant improvements in individual risk factors.[128,129]

One consistent finding in children's studies is the very strong relationship observed between C-V fitness and fatness.[130–132] It is thus not surprising that several studies indicate that fatness is a major confounding variable in the relationship between fitness and other CHD risk factors. In at least four population studies,[133–136] robust associations between C-V fitness and level of risk were abolished after accounting statistically for body fatness, while one other study[127] reported severely attenuated relationships. It is worth noting that this feature has also been observed in an adult study[137] investigating fitness and coronary risk factors, and so the confounding influence of body fatness on coronary risk does not seem to be confined to paediatric populations.

Therefore, although strong associations between cardiovascular fitness and CHD risk status exist in children, these may be partly mediated by the level of fatness. Thus, any initiative to improve the health of children should ideally involve measures that simultaneously improve fitness and lower fatness, namely increased physical activity and dietary control.

Which is more important—activity or fitness?

It has been argued[138–140] that physical training adaptations may not be directly related to, nor necessary for, good health. We have discussed the evidence regarding both activity and fitness in relation to health, but the interesting question of whether physical activity level, or fitness level, is most strongly related to health status remains open for discussion. For example, does an individual who has genetically high fitness, but who is inactive, achieve health benefits from his/her high fitness level? Conversely, can the genetically low-fit individual gain health benefits through being active? These questions are largely unanswered.

It may be that high fitness, especially C-V fitness, is directly related to improved health status. The morphological and functional condition of the heart and circulatory system may lead directly to a reduced risk of, for example, CHD. In this scenario, a genetically high-fit individual would automatically be blessed with better health status. Studies on the relationship between polymorphisms of the angiotensin-converting enzyme (ACE) and C-V fitness[117] give some credence to this hypothesis. An alternative explanation might be that fitness acts as a marker for high activity levels. This activity might not only produce an improved cardiovascular system, but might also promote other biochemical and haemodynamic changes (lower blood pressure, higher HDL cholesterol, lower triglycerides, improved glucose tolerance, modified clotting factors, and post-prandial lipidaemia) which are the 'real' mechanisms that promote improved health. What we are considering is, by common understanding, almost a 'spin-off' effect of activity that might be termed 'metabolic fitness'. It is entirely possible that this type of fitness is the true health-related dimension of the generic term 'fitness'.

Physical activity and risks to the child

Physical activity can carry its own inherent risk to both adults and children. Van Mechelen[141] has highlighted the potential for childhood injury when free play in various physical activities is replaced by competitive participation in just one or two sports. Whereas all activities carry increased risk of traumatic (acute) injury, too strong a focus on training for competition in a limited range of activities can result in the additional risk of overuse (chronic) injury. Whereas both types of injury normally heal without permanent disability, the costs must be considered in terms of activity time lost, school time lost, predisposition to re-occurrence, the risk of permanent damage, and the financial cost of treatment. Baxter-Jones *et al.*[142] have reported for elite child athletes an estimated 1 year incidence rate of 40 injuries per 100 children, equating to less than one injury per 1000 hours of training. In these elite child athletes, about one third of injuries were overuse injuries, which were in turn more severe than the traumatic injuries (20 days lay-off vs. 13 days, respectively). It is equally important to consider the psychological costs associated with overtraining injuries or burnout in competitive sports. Negative experiences during childhood may result in a decreased desire to engage in sport and exercise in adolescence or adulthood, potentially placing the child at greater risk for activity related illnesses.

It should be emphasized that all sports and active recreational pursuits carry increased injury risk. In both adults and children, the risks and benefits must be carefully balanced. However, we should not forget the moral issue of when, or at what age or stage of development, a child is capable of making such important judgements. The roles and responsibilities of teachers, parents, sports governing bodies, and coaches in this matter are considerable.

Summary

- The past decade has seen a noticeable increase in the quantity and quality of evidence linking physical activity/fitness with various health parameters in children.
- Nevertheless, our general understanding of how physical activity impacts on the current or future health of children remains limited. This is most likely due to a number of factors including (i) a lack of large-scale longitudinal studies and randomized control trials; (ii) difficulties inherent in measuring health, fitness, and activity over the adolescent period (e.g. naturally occurring shifts in blood pressure, lipids, activity patterns, adiposity); and (iii) a general failure to control for potential confounders (e.g. growth and maturation).
- Given the strong and consistent relations between activity/fitness and health in adults, it is highly likely that ensuring adequate activity and fitness in children will be of ultimate benefit. However, we must be clear that we are basing this judgement largely on limited (but developing) paediatric data, strong adult data, a good measure of common sense, and sound physiological and psychological principles.
- It is intuitively logical that preventive measures, that is, the fostering of active lifestyles, should begin early in life, and that 'the public health goal of physical education is to prepare children for a lifetime of regular physical activity'.[143] We must not forget that physical activity is our evolutionary heritage—we have evolved

as a species for an active lifestyle, and yet we are now living in an environment which is toxic to activity, where the opportunities for children—and adults—to be physically active are fast disappearing.

- Only enlightened public policy regarding school curricula, school transportation, safe play areas outside of the house, increased licence for children to 'roam', and enhanced sports opportunities can change this situation for tomorrow's adults.

References

1. American Academy of Pediatrics (2006). Intensive training and sports specialization in young athletes. *Pediatrics* **106**, 154–7.
2. Armstrong N, Welsman JR (2006). The physical activity patterns of European youth with reference to methods of assessment. *Sports Med* **36**, 1067–86.
3. Malina RM, Katzmarzyk PT (2006). Physical activity and fitness in an international growth standard for preadolescent and adolescent children. *Food Nutr Bull* **27**, S295–313.
4. American College of Sports Medicine (1988). Physical fitness in children and youth. *Med Sci Sport Exerc* **20**, 422–3.
5. Sallis JF, Patrick K (1988). Physical activity guidelines for adolescents: A consensus statement. *Pediatr Exerc Sci* **6**, 302–14.
6. Biddle SJH, Sallis JF, Cavill N (1998). *Young and active? Young people and health-enhancing physical activity—evidence and implications.* Health Education Authority, London.
7. Department of Health Physical Activity Health Improvement and Prevention (2004). *At least five a week: Evidence on the impact of physical activity and its relationship to health.* Department of Health, London.
8. Strong WB, Malina RM, Blimkie CJR, Daniels SR, Dishman RK, Gutin B, Hergenroeder AC, Must A, Nixon PA, Pivarnik JM, Rowland TW, Trost S, Trudeau FO (2005). Evidence based physical activity for school-age youth. *J Pediatr* **146**, 732–7.
9. Department of Health and Social Services (1992). *The health of the nation.* HMSO, London.
10. Department of Health and Social Services (1996). *Strategy statement on physical activity.* Department of Health, London.
11. U.S. Department of Health and Human Services (1996). *Physical activity and health: A report of the Surgeon General.* Department of Health and Human Services, Centers for Disease Control and Prevention, National Center for Chronic Disease Prevention and Health Promotion, Pittsburgh, PA.
12. Dollman J, Norton K, Norton L (2005). Evidence for secular trends in children's physical activity behaviour. *Br J Sport Med* **39**, 892–7.
13. Campaigne BN, Morrison JA, Schumann BC, Falkner F, Lakatos E, Sprecher D, Schreiber CB (1994). Indexes of obesity and comparisons with previous National Survey data in 9-year-old and 10-year-old black-and-white girls—the National Heart, Lung, and Blood Institute Growth and Health Study. *J Pediatr* **124**, 675–80.
14. Chinn S, Rona RJ (1994). Trends in weight-for-height and triceps skinfold thickness for English and Scottish children, 1972–1982 and 1982–1990. *Paediatr Perinat Epidemiol* **8**, 90–106.
15. Freedman DS, Srinivasan SR, Valdez RA, Williamson DF, Berenson GS (1997). Secular increases in relative weight and adiposity among children over two decades: The Bogalusa Heart Study. *Pediatrics* **99**, 420–6.
16. Troiano RP, Flegal KM, Kuczmarski RJ, Campbell SM, Johnson CL (1995). Overweight prevalence and trends for children and adolescents—the National-Health and Nutrition Examination Surveys, 1963 to 1991. *Arch Pediatr Adolesc Med* **149**, 1085–91.
17. Durnin JVGA (1992). Physical activity levels—past and present. In: Norgan NG (ed.), *Physical activity and health: Symposium of the Society for the Study of Human Biology*, pp. 20 7. Cambridge University Press, Cambridge.
18. Adams J (2006). Trends in physical activity and inactivity amongst US 14–18 year olds by gender, school grade and race, 1993–2003: Evidence from the youth risk behavior survey. *BMC Public Health* **6**, 1–7.
19. Armstrong N (1989). Children are fit but not active! *Educ Health* **7**, 28–32.
20. Reiff GG, Dixon WR, Jacoby D, Ye GX, Spain GG, Hunsicker PA (1986). *The President's Council on Physical Fitness and Sports national school population fitness survey.* University of Michigan, Ann Arbor, MI.
21. Knapik JJ, Sharp MA, Darakjy S, Jones SB, Hauret KG, Jones BH (2006). Temporal changes in the physical fitness of army recruits. *Sports Med Arthrosc* **36**, 613–34.
22. Armstrong N, Mechelen WV (1998). Are young people fit and active? In: Biddle SJH, Sallis JF, Cavill N (eds.), *Young and active? Young people and health-enhancing physical activity: Evidence and implications*, pp. 69–97. Health Education Authority, London.
23. Harris J, Cale L (2006). A review of children's fitness testing. *Eur Phys Educ Rev* **12**, 201–25.
24. Ekelund U, Sardhina LB, Anderssen SA, Harro M, Andersen LB, Riddoch C, Froberg K (2004). Associations between physical activity and body fatness in 9- to 10-year-old children: The European Youth Heart Study. *Med Sci Sport Exerc* **36**, S183.
25. Ekelund U, Sardinha LB, Anderssen SA, Harro M, Franks PW, Brage S, Cooper AR, Andresen LB, Riddoch C, Froberg K (2004). Associations between objectively assessed physical activity and indicators of body fatness in 9- to 10-y-old European children: A population-based study from 4 distinct regions in Europe (the European Youth Heart Study). *Am J Clin Nutr* **80**, 584–90.
26. Ness AR, Leary SD, Mattocks C, Blair SN, Reilly JJ, Wells J, Ingle S, Tilling K, Smoth GD, Riddoch C (2007). Objectively measured physical activity and fat mass in a large cohort of children. *Plos Med* **4**, 476–84.
27. Andersen LB, Harro M, Sardinha LB, Froberg K, Ekelund U, Brage S, Andersen SA (2006). Physical activity and clustered cardiovascular risk in children: A cross-sectional study (The European Youth Heart Study). *Lancet* **368**, 299–304.
28. Brage S, Wedderkopp N, Ekelund U, Franks PW, Wareham NJ, Andersen LB, Froberg K (2004). Objectively measured physical activity correlates with indices of insulin resistance in Danish children. The European Youth Heart Study (EYHS). *Int J Obes* **28**, 1503–8.
29. Ekelund U, Brage S, Froberg K, Harro M, Anderssen SA, Sardinha LB, Riddoch C, Andersen LB (2006). TV viewing and physical activity are independently associated with metabolic risk in children: The European Youth Heart Study. *Plos Med* **3**, 2449–57.
30. Tobias JH, Steer CD, Mattocks C, Riddoch C, Ness AR (2006). Habitual levels of physical activity influence bone mass in 11 year-old children from the UK: Findings from a large population-based cohort. *J Bone Miner Res* **21**, S206.
31. Blair SN, Clark DG, Cureton KJ, Powell KE (1989). Exercise and fitness in childhood: Implications for a lifetime of health. In: Gisolfi CV, Lamb DR (eds.), *Perspectives in exercise science and sports medicine*, pp. 401–30. McGraw-Hill, New York.
32. Malina RM, Bouchard C, Bar-Or O (2004). *Growth maturation and physical activity.* Human Kinetics, Champaign, IL.
33. Krahnstoever Davison K, Werder JL, Trost SG, Baker BL, Birch LL (2007). Why are early maturing girls less active? Links between pubertal development, psychological well-being, and physical activity among girls at ages 11 and 13. *Soc Sci Med* **64**, 2391–404.
34. Thompson AM, Baxter-Jones ADG, Mirwald RL, Bailey DA (2003). Comparison of physical activity in male and female children: Does maturation matter? *Med Sci Sport Exerc* **35**, 1684–90.
35. Baxter-Jones ADG, Eisenmann JC, Sherar LB (2005). Controlling for maturation in pediatric exercise science. *Pediatr Exerc Sci* **17**, 18–30.
36. Wareham NJ, Rennie KL (1998). The assessment of physical activity in individuals and populations: Why try to be more precise about how physical activity is assessed? *Int J Obes* **22**, S30–8.

37. Harro M, Riddoch CJ (2000). Physical activity. In: Armstrong N, Van Mechelen W (eds.), *Paediatric exercise science and medicine*, pp. 77–84, Oxford University Press, Oxford.
38. Loney T, Standage M (2007). Assessing physical activity in psychology research: Future directions. *Adv Psy Res* **52**, 1–3.
39. Standage M, Vallerand RJ (2007). Self-determined motivation in sport and exercise groups. In: Beauchamp MR, Eys MA (eds.), *Group dynamics in sport and exercise psychology: Contemporary themes*, pp. 179–99. Routledge, New York.
40. Baranowski T, Bouchard C, Bar-Or O, Bricker T, Heath G, Kimm SYS, Malina RM, Obarzanek E, Pate R, Strong WB, Truman B, Washington R (1992). Assessment, prevalence, and cardiovascular benefits of physical-activity and fitness in youth. *Med Sci Sport Exer* **24**, S237–47.
41. Blair SN, Kohl HW, Paffenbarger RS, Clark DG, Cooper KH, Gibbons LW (1989). Physical-fitness and all-cause mortality—a prospective-study of healthy-men and women. *JAMA* **262**, 2395–401.
42. Paffenbarger RS, Hyde RT, Wing AL, Hsieh C (1986). Physical activity, all-cause mortality, and longevity of college alumni. *N Engl J Med* **314**, 605–13.
43. Mutrie N (2000). The relationship between physical activity and clinically defined depression. In: Biddle SJH, Fox KR, Boutcher SH (eds.), *Physical activity and psychological well-being*, pp. 46–62. Routledge, London.
44. Taylor A (2000). Physical activity, anxiety and stress. In: Biddle SJH, Fox KR, Boutcher SH (eds.), *Physical activity and psychological well-being*, pp. 10–45. Routledge, London.
45. Blair SN, Kampert JB, Kohl HW, Barlow CE, Macera CA, Paffenbarger RS, Gibbons LW (1996). Influences of cardiorespiratory fitness and other precursors on cardiovascular disease and all-cause mortality in men and women. *JAMA* **276**, 205–10.
46. Leon AS, Connett J, Jacobs DR, Rauramaa R (1987). Leisure-time physical-activity levels and risk of coronary heart-disease and death—The multiple risk factor intervention trial. *JAMA* **258**, 2388–95.
47. Riddoch CJ (1998). Relationships between physical activity and physical health in young people. In: Biddle SJH, Sallis JF, Cavill N (eds.), *Young and active?*, pp. 17–48. Health Education Authority, London.
48. Haskell WL, Lee IM, Pate RR, Powell KE, Blair SN, Franklin BA, Macera CA, Heath GW, Thompson PD, Bauman A (2007). Physical activity and public health—Updated recommendation for adults from the American college of sports medicine and the American heart association. *Circulation* **116**, 1081–93.
49. Blair SN, Kohl HW, Gordon NF, Paffenbarger RS (1992). How much physical activity is good for health. *Annu Rev Publ Health* **13**, 99–126.
50. Wareham NJ, van Sluijs EMF, Ekelund U (2005). Physical activity and obesity prevention: A review of the current evidence. *P Nutr Soc* **64**, 229–47.
51. Stone EJ, McKenzie TL, Welk GJ, Booth ML (1998). Effects of physical activity interventions in youth—Review and synthesis. *Am J Prev Med* **15**, 298–315.
52. Sothern MS (2004). Obesity prevention in children: Physical activity and nutrition. *Nutrition* **20**, 704–8.
53. Must A, Jacques PF, Dallal GE, Bajema CJ, Dietz WH (1992). Long-term morbidity and mortality of overweight adolescents—a follow-up of the Harvard Growth Study of 1922 to 1935. *N Engl J Med* **327**, 1350–5.
54. Must A, Tybor DJ (2005). Physical activity and sedentary behavior: A review of longitudinal studies of weight and adiposity in youth. *Int J Obes* **29**, S84–96.
55. SchonfeldWarden N, Warden CH (1997). Pediatric obesity—An overview of etiology and treatment. *Pediatr Clin N Am* **44**, 339–61.
56. Vanhala M, Vanhala P, Kumpusalo E, Halonen P, Takala J (1998). Relation between obesity from childhood to adulthood and the metabolic syndrome: Population based study. *BMJ* **317**, 319–20.
57. Clarke WR, Lauer RM (1993). Does childhood obesity track into adulthood. *Crit Rev Food Sci* **33**, 423–30.
58. Andersen LB, Wedderkopp N (2003). Biological cardiovascular risk factors cluster in Danish children and adolescents: The European Youth Heart Study. *Prev Med* **37**, 363–7.
59. Alpert BS, Wilmore JH (1994). Physical activity and blood pressure in adolescents. *Pediatr Exerc Sci* **6**, 361–80.
60. Armstrong N, Simons-Morton B (1994). Physical activity and blood lipids in adolescents. *Pediatr Exerc Sci* **6**, 381–405.
61. Brage S, Wedderkopp N, Ekelund U, Franks PW, Wareham NJ, Andersen LB, Froberg K (2004). Features of the metabolic syndrome are associated with objectively measured physical activity and fitness in Danish children—the European Youth Heart Study (EYHS). *Diabetes Care* **27**, 2141–8.
62. Metcalf BS, Voss LD, Jeffery AN, Wilkin TJ (2005). Physical activity of young UK children does not impact on their metabolic health—an objective assessment. (The EarlyBird Diabetes Study). *Diabetologia* **48**, A74.
63. Urrutia-Rojas X, Menchaca J (2006). Prevalence of risk for type 2 diabetes in school children. *J School Health* **76**, 189–94.
64. Imperatore G, Cheng YLJ, Williams DE, Fulton J, Gregg EW (2006). Physical activity, cardiovascular fitness, and insulin sensitivity among US adolescents—The National Health and Nutrition Examination Survey, 1999–2002. *Diabetes Care* **29**, 1567–72.
65. Krekoukia M, Nassis GP, Psarra G, Skenderi K, Chrousos GP, Sidossis LS (2007). Elevated total and central adiposity and low physical activity are associated with insulin resistance in children. *Metabolism* **56**, 206–13.
66. Cooper C, Campion G, Melton LJ (1992). Hip-fractures in the elderly—A worldwide projection. *Osteoporos Int* **2**, 285–9.
67. Bailey DA, Faulkner RA, McKay HA (1996). Growth, physical activity and bone mineral acquisition. *Exerc Sports Sci Rev* **24**, 233–66.
68. Vuori I (1996). Peak bone mass and physical activity: A short review. *Nutr Rev* **54**, S11–14.
69. Lu PW, Brody JN, Ogle GD (1994). Bone mineral density of total body, spine and femoral neck in children and young adults: A cross-sectional and longitudinal study. *J Bone Miner Res* **9**, 1451–8.
70. Theintz G, Buchs B, Rizzoli R, Slosman D, Clavien H, Sizonenko PC, Bonjour JP (1992). Longitudinal monitoring of bone mass accumulation in healthy adolescents—Evidence for a marked reduction after 16 years of age at the levels of lumbar spine and femoral-neck in female subjects. *J Clin Endocr Metab* **75**, 1060–5.
71. Ralston SH (1997). Osteoporosis. *BMJ* **315**, 469–72.
72. Cadogan J, Eastell R, Jones N, Barker ME (1997). Milk intake and bone mineral acquisition in adolescent girls: randomised, controlled intervention trial. *BMJ* **315**, 1255–60.
73. Ruiz JC, Mandel C, Garabedian M (1995). Influence of spontaneous calcium intake and physical exercise on the vertebral and femoral bone-mineral density of children and adolescents. *J Bone Miner Res* **10**, 675–82.
74. Teegarden D, Proulx WR, Kern M, Sedlock D, Weaver CM, Johnston CC, Lyle RM (1996). Previous physical activity relates to bone mineral measures in young women. *Med Sci Sport Exerc* **28**, 105–13.
75. Tylavsky FA, Anderson JJB, Talmage RV, Taft TN (1992). Are calcium intakes and physical-activity patterns during adolescence related to radial bone mass of white college-age females. *Osteoporos Int* **2**, 232–40.
76. Gunnes M, Lehmann EH (1996). Physical activity and dietary constituents as predictors of forearm cortical and trabecular bone gain in healthy children and adolescents: A prospective study. *Acta Paediatr* **85**, 19–25.
77. Morris F, Naughton GA, Gibbs JL, Carlson J, Wark JG (1997). Prospective ten-month exercise intervention in premenarcheal girls: Positive effects on bone and lean mass. *J Bone Min Res* **12**, 1453–62.
78. Slemenda CW, Reister TK, Hui SL, Miller JZ, Christian JC, Johnston CC (1994). Influences on skeletal mineralization in children and adolescents—Evidence for varying effects of sexual-maturation and physical-activity. *J Pediatr* **125**, 201–7.

79. Grimston SK, Willows ND, Hanley DA (1993). Mechanical loading regime and its relationship to bone-mineral density in children. *Med Sci Sport Exerc* **25**, 1203–10.
80. Rubin K, Schirduan V, Gendreau P, Sarfarazi M, Mendola R, Dalsky G (1993). Predictors of axial and peripheral bone-mineral density in healthy-children and adolescents, with special attention to the role of puberty. *J Pediatr* **123**, 863–70.
81. Lanyon LE (1996). Using functional loading to influence bone mass and architecture: Objectives, mechanisms, and relationship with estrogen of the mechanically adaptive process in bone. *Bone* **18**, S37–43.
82. Friedlander AL, Genant HK, Sadowsky S, Byl NN, Gluer CC (1995). A 2-Year Program of aerobics and weight training enhances bone-mineral density of young-women. *J Bone Miner Res* **10**, 574–85.
83. Lohman T, Going S, Pamenter R, Hall M, Boyden T, Houtkooper L, Ritenbaugh C, Bare L, Hill A, Aickin M (1995). Effects of resistance training on regional and total bone-mineral density in premenopausal women—A randomized prospective-study. *J Bone Miner Res* **10**, 1015–24.
84. Skerry TM (1997). Mechanical loading and bone: What sort of exercise is beneficial to the skeleton? *Bone* **20**, 179–81.
85. Janz KF, Burns TL, Torner JC, Levy SM, Paulos R, Willing MC, Warren JJ (2001). Physical activity and bone measures in young children: The Iowa Bone Development Study. *Pediatrics* **107**, 1387–93.
86. Biddle SJH, Mutrie N (2008). *Psychology of physical activity: Determinants, well-being and interventions*. Routledge, London.
87. Faulkner GEJ, Taylor AH (2005). *Exercise and mental health: Emerging relationships*. Routledge, London.
88. Mutrie N, Parfitt G (1998). Physical activity and its link with mental, social and moral health in young people. In: Biddle SJH, Sallis JF, Cavill N (eds.), *Young and active*, pp. 49–68. Health Education Authority, London.
89. Stubbe JH, Moor MHM, Boomsma DI, Gues EJC (2007). The association between exercise participation and well-being: A co-twin study. *Prev Med* **24**, 148–52.
90. Parfitt G, Eston RG (2005). The relationship between children's habitual activity level and psychological well-being. *Acta Paediatr* **94**, 1791–7.
91. Yin ZN, Davis CL, Moore JB, Treiber FA (2005). Physical activity buffers the effects of chronic stress on adiposity in youth. *Ann Behav Med* **29**, 29–36.
92. Storch EA, Milsom VA, DeBraganza N, Lewin AB, Geffken GR, Silverstein JH (2007). Peer victimization, psychosocial adjustment, and physical activity in overweight and at-risk-for-overweight youth. *J Pediatr Psychol* **32**, 80–9.
93. Weinberg RS, Gould D (2007). *Foundations of sport and exercise psychology* (4th ed.). Human Kinetics, Champaign, IL.
94. Everett-Jones S, Merkle SL, Fulton JE, Wheeler LS, Mannino DM (2006). Relationship between asthma, overweight, and physical activity among US high school students. *J Comm Health* **31**, 469–78.
95. Barker DJP (1990). The fetal and infant origins of adult disease. *BMJ* **301**, 1111.
96. Riddoch C, Savage JM, Murphy N, Cran GW, Boreham C (1991). Long-term health implications of fitness and physical-activity patterns. *Arch Dis Child* **66**, 1426–33.
97. Malina RM (2001). Tracking of physical activity across the lifespan. *Res Digest* **3**, 1–7.
98. Matton L, Thomis M, Wijndaele K, Duvigneaud N, Beunen G, Claessens AL, Vanreusel B, Philippaerts R, Lefevre J (2006). Tracking of physical fitness and physical activity from youth to adulthood in females. *Med Sci Sport Exerc* **38**, 1114–20.
99. Yang X, Telama R, Viikar J, Raitakari OT (2006). Risk of obesity in relation to physical activity tracking from youth to adulthood. *Med Sci Sport Exerc* **38**, 919–25.
100. Engstrom LM (1986). The process of socialisation into keep-fit activities. *J Sport Sci Med* **8**, 89–97.
101. Cale L, Almond L (1992). Children's activity levels: A review of studies conducted on British children. *Phys Educ Rev* **15**, 111–18.
102. Sallis JF (1993). Epidemiology of physical-activity and fitness in children and adolescents. *Crit Rev Food Sci* **33**, 403–8.
103. Astrand PO (1994). Physical activity and fitness: evolutionary perspective and trends for the future. In: Bouchard C, Shephard RJ, Stephens T (eds.), *Physical activity, fitness, and health: international proceedings and consensus statement*, pp. 98–105. Human Kinetics, Champaign, IL.
104. Rowland TW (1990). *Exercise and children's health*. Human Kinetics, Champaign, IL.
105. Blair SN, Meredith MD (1994). The exercise-health relationship: Does it apply to children and youth? In: Pate RR, Hohn RC (eds.), *Health and fitness through physical education*, pp. 11–19. Human Kinetics, Champaign, IL.
106. Blair SN (1992). Are American children and youth fit? The need for better data. *Res Q Exerc Sport* **63**, 120–3.
107. Saris WHM, Emons HJG, Emons HJG, Westerterp KR (1990). Discrepancy between FAO/WHO energy requirements and actual energy expenditure levels in healthy 7–11 year old children. In: Beunen G, Ghesquiere J, Reybrouck T, Claessens AL (eds.), *Children and exercise*, p. 119. Enke, Stuttgart.
108. Davies PSW, Day JME, Lucas A (1991). Energy-expenditure in early infancy and later body fatness. *Int J Obes* **15**, 727–31.
109. Boreham C, Savage JM, Primrose D, Cran G, Strain J (1993). Coronary risk-factors in schoolchildren. *Arch Dis Child* **68**, 182–6.
110. Department of Health (1991). *Dietary reference values for food energy and nutrition for the United Kingdom. Report on health and social subjects n.41*. HMSO, London.
111. Sleap M, Tolfrey K (2001). Do 9- to 12 yr-old children meet existing physical activity recommendations for health? *Med Sci Sport Exerc* **33**, 591–6.
112. Riddoch C, Mattocks C, Deere K, Saunders J, Kirkby J, Tilling K, Blair SN, Ness A (2007). Objective measurement of levels and patterns of physical activity. *Arch Dis Child* **92**, 963–9.
113. Riddoch CJ, Andersen LB, Wedderkopp N, Harro M, Klasson-Heggebo L, Sardinha LB, Cooper AR, Ekelund U (2004). Physical activity levels and patterns of 9- and 15-yr-old European children. *Med Sci Sport Exerc* **36**, 86–92.
114. Biddle SJH, Cavill N, Sallis JF (1998). Policy framework for young people and health-enhancing physical activity. In: Biddle SJH, Sallis JF, Cavill N (eds.), *Young and active? Young people and health-enhancing physical activity—evidence and implications*, pp. 3–16. Health Education Authority, London.
115. Sallis JF, Patrick K (1994). Physical activity guidelines for adolescents: Consensus statement. *Pediatr Exerc Sci* **6**, 302–14.
116. Cale L, Harris J (1993). Exercise recommendations for children and young people. *Phys Educ Rev* **16**, 89–98.
117. Montgomery HE, Marshall R, Hemingway H, Myerson S, Clarkson P, Dollery C, Hayward M, Holliman DE, Jubb M, World M, Thomas EL, Brynes AE, Saeed N, Barnard M, Bell JD, Prasad K, Rayson M, Talmud PJ, Humphries SE (1998). Human gene for physical performance. *Nature* **393**, 221–2.
118. Cooper AR, Page A, Fox KR, Misson J (2000). Physical activity patterns in normal, overweight and obese individuals using minute-by-minute accelerometry. *Eur J Clin Nutr* **54**, 887–94.
119. Farrell SW, Kampert JB, Kohl HW, Barlow CE, Macera CA, Paffenbarger RS, Gibbons LW, Blair SN (1998). Influences of cardiorespiratory fitness levels and other predictors on cardiovascular disease mortality in men. *Med Sci Sport Exerc* **30**, 899–905.
120. Gibbons LW, Blair SN, Cooper KH, Smith M (1983). Association between coronary heart-disease risk-factors and physical-fitness in healthy adult women. *Circulation* **67**, 977–83.
121. Sandvik L, Erikssen J, Thaulow E, Erikssen G, Mundal R, Rodahl K (1993). Physical fitness as a predictor of mortality among healthy, middle-aged Norwegian men. *New Engl J Med* **328**, 533–7.
122. Van Saarse J, Noteboom WMP, Vandenbrouke JP (1990). Longevity of men capable of prolonged vigorous physical exercise: A 32 year follow-

up of 2259 participants in the Dutch eleven cities ice skating tour. *BMJ* **301**, 1409–11.

123. Blair SN, Kohl HW, Barlow CE, Paffenbarger RS, Gibbons LW, Macera CA (1995). Changes in physical fitness and all-cause mortality—a prospective study of healthy and unhealthy men. *JAMA* **273**, 1093–8.
124. Thompson GR, Wilson PW (1982). *Coronary risk factors and their assessment*. Science Press, London.
125. Raitakari OT, Porkka KVK, Rasanen L, Ronnemaa T, Viikari JSA (1994). Clustering and 6 year cluster-tracking of serum total cholesterol, HDL-cholesterol and diastolic blood-pressure in children and young-adults—The Cardiovascular Risk in Young Finns Study. *J Clin Epidemiol* **47**, 1085–93.
126. Hofman A, Walter HJ (1989). The association between physical fitness and cardiovascular disease risk factors in children in a five-year follow-up study. *Int J Epidemiol* **18**, 830–5.
127. Tell GS, Vellar OD (1988). Physical-fitness, physical-activity, and cardiovascular-disease risk-factors in adolescents—The Oslo Youth Study. *Prev Med* **17**, 12–24.
128. Eriksson BO, Koch G (1973). Effect of physical training on hemodynamic response during submaximal and maximal exercise in 11-year-old to 13-year-old boys. *Acta Physiol Scand* **87**, 27–39.
129. Hansen HS, Froberg K, Hyldebrandt N, Nielsen JR (1991). A controlled-study of 8 months of physical-training and reduction of blood-pressure in children—The Odense Schoolchild Study. *BMJ* **303**, 682–5.
130. Boreham CAG, Strain JJ, Twisk JWR, Van Mechelen W, Savage JM, Cran GW (1997). Aerobic fitness physical activity and body fatness in adolescents. In: Armstrong N, Kirby B, Welsman JR (eds.), *Children and exercise*, pp. 69–75. E & FN Spon, London.
131. Gutin B, Islam S, Manos T, Cucuzzo N, Smith C, Stachura ME (1994). Relation of percentage of body-fat and maximal aerobic capacity to risk-factors for atherosclerosis and diabetes in black-and-white 7-year-old to 11-year-old children. *J Pediatr* **125**, 847–52.
132. Hager RL, Tucker LA, Seljaas GT (1995). Aerobic fitness, blood lipids and body fat in children. *Am J Pub Health* **85**, 1702–6.
133. Bergstrom E, Hernell O, Persson LA (1997). Endurance running performance in relation to cardiovascular risk indicators in adolescents. *Int J Sports Med* **18**, 300–7.
134. Fripp RR, Hodgson JL, Kwiterovich PO, Werner JC, Schuler HG, Whitman V (1985). Aerobic capacity, obesity, and atherosclerotic risk-factors in male-adolescents. *Pediatrics* **75**, 813–18.
135. Hansen HS, Hyldebrandt N, Nielsen JR, Froberg K (1990). Blood-pressure distribution in a school-age population aged 8–10 years—The Odense Schoolchild Study. *J Hypertens* **8**, 641–6.
136. Sallis JF, Patterson TL, Buono MJ, Nader PR (1988). Relation of cardiovascular fitness and physical-activity to cardiovascular-disease risk-factors in children and adults. *Am J Epidemiol* **127**, 933–41.
137. Haddock BL, Hopp HP, Mason JJ, Blix G, Blair SN (1998). Cardiorespiratory fitness and cardiovascular disease risk factors in postmenopausal women. *Med Sci Sport Exerc* **30**, 893–8.
138. Cureton KJ (1987). Commentary on "children and fitness: A public health perspective". *Res Q* **58**, 315–20.
139. Haskell WL, Montoye HJ, Orenstein D (1985). Physical-activity and exercise to achieve health related physical-fitness components. *Pub Health Rep* **100**, 202–12.
140. Seefeldt V, Vogel P (1987). Children and fitness: A public health perspective. *Res Q* **58**, 331–3.
141. Van Mechelen W (1997). Etiology and prevention of sports injuries in youth. In: Froberg K, Lammert O, Steen Hansen H, Blimkie JR (eds.), *Children and exercise XVIII: Exercise and fitness—benefits and risks*, pp. 209–27. Odense University Press, Odense.
142. Baxter-Jones A, Maffulli N, Helms P (1993). Low injury rates in elite athletes. *Arch Dis Child* **68**, 130–2.
143. Sallis JF, McKenzie TL (1991). Physical Education's role in public health. *Res Q Exerc Sport* **62**, 124–37.

CHAPTER 25

Physical activity, physical fitness, and cardiovascular health

Jos Twisk and Isabel Ferreira

Introduction

Cardiovascular disease (CVD) is one of the greatest causes of death in Western societies, and this is likely to continue in the future, particularly in developing countries. It is now recognized that CVD is partly a paediatric problem; that is, the onset of CVD lies in early childhood, even though the clinical symptoms of this disease do not become apparent until much later in life. The ideal study to answer the question whether high levels of physical activity and physical fitness during childhood and adolescence lower the risk of developing CVD later in life is a randomized-controlled trial with a lifetime follow-up, in which a large group of children and adolescents are assigned to either a sedentary or an active lifestyle; a study that will probably never take place. The most classical and probably the only study investigating the relationship between physical activity in relatively young people and the occurrence of CVD at later age is the Harvard Alumni Study, performed by Paffenbarger.[1] In one part of this extensive observational study, physical activity levels during the student period (gathered from university archives) were related to the occurrence of CVD later in life. Students were divided into three groups according to their physical activity levels: (i) athletes, (ii) intramural sports play for more than 5 hours per week, and (iii) intramural sports play for less than 5 hours (usually none at all) per week. The three groups did not differ regarding the occurrence of CVD later in life. Student athletes who discontinued their activity levels after college encountered a CVD incidence similar to the risk of alumni classmates who never had been athletes. In fact, subjects who became physically active later in life had the same health benefits as the subjects who were active throughout the observation period.

The incidence of morbidity and mortality related to CVD is rather low in a paediatric population. Studies investigating the relationship between physical activity, physical fitness, and cardiovascular health in children and adolescents are therefore mostly limited to CVD risk factors as outcome measures. For this reason, this chapter will focus on the association of physical activity and physical fitness with CVD risk factors in children and adolescents. These risk factors can be divided into the so-called traditional CVD risk factors; that is, lipoproteins [total cholesterol, low-density lipoprotein (LDL) cholesterol, high-density lipoprotein (HDL) cholesterol, triglycerides (TG)], blood pressure, body fatness, and diabetes, and 'new' CVD risk factors; that is, other lipoproteins [lipoprotein(a) (Lp(a)), apolipoprotein (apo)B, and apoA-1], coagulation and inflammation markers [fibrinogen, C-reactive protein (CRP)], homocysteine, and heart rate variability.

Traditional cardiovascular disease risk factors

Lipoproteins

It is known that lipoprotein levels are directly related to the process of atherosclerosis and therefore to the occurrence of CVD. Although total serum cholesterol has been found to be related to CVD, its atherogenic effect merely depends on the structure of the cholesterol; or, in other words, on the ratio between LDL and HDL. It is assumed that LDL may act directly or indirectly to cause endothelial damage, with subsequent proliferation of arterial smooth muscle cells resulting in the accumulation of lipids and progression to atherosclerotic plaque formation. HDL, on the other hand, is assumed to be protective against CVD; HDL seems to be responsible for carrying cholesterol from peripheral tissue, including the arterial walls, back to the liver where it is metabolized and excreted. Besides HDL and LDL, also very low density lipoprotein (VLDL) cholesterol and plasma TG need to be considered, although the atherogenic effects of VLDL and TG are not firmly established. It is further assumed that during exercise, fatty acids are released from their storage sites to be burnt for energy production. Several studies suggest that human growth hormone may be responsible for this increased fatty acid mobilization. Growth hormone levels increase sharply with exercise and remain elevated for up to several hours in the recovery period. Other research has suggested that, with exercise, the adipose tissue is more sensitive either to the sympathetic nervous system or to the rising of circulating catecholamines. Either situation would increase lipid mobilization.

From epidemiological studies, among adults there is (some) evidence that physical activity and physical fitness are associated with favourable lipid profiles. However for children and adolescents, there is not much evidence that physical activity and physical fitness have beneficial effects on lipids (Table 25.1). From cross-sectional, longitudinal, as well as experimental studies, there is ambiguous evidence with regard to the beneficial effects physical activity and/or physical fitness may have on any of the lipid levels. For an extensive overview regarding this topic one is referred to Armstrong and Simons-Morton.[2]

One of the problems is that most of the studies in this field have a cross-sectional design. Sallis *et al.*,[3] for instance, did not find any relation between activity and HDL in children aged 11–12 years. In the Beaver County Lipid Study, a positive cross-sectional relation was found between daily physical activity and HDL in young adults.[4] However in multivariate analyses [correcting for smoking, alcohol consumption, and body mass index (BMI)], this positive relation disappeared.

There are only a few longitudinal studies investigating this problem. In the Amsterdam Growth and Health Study, an observational longitudinal study covering a period of 15 years from adolescence into young adulthood, the longitudinal development of daily physical activity (assessed by a structured interview covering 3 months prior to the interview; and expressed as a weighted activity score in METs·week^{-1}) was positively related to the development of HDL. No relations were, however, found between the development of daily physical activity on the one hand, and the development of TC and the TC:HDL ratio, on the other.[5] In the Cardiovascular Risk in Young Finns Study, boys with an initial age of 12 years who remained active over a period of 6 years showed lower values of the TC:HDL ratio at the age of 18 years than boys who had a sedentary lifestyle over that period.[6] However, in boys no differences were found in TC and HDL values when examined separately, and females did not show any significant differences for all three parameters. Changes in physical activity over the 6-year period were also not associated with the change in any of the lipoprotein levels in both boys and girls.

Intervention studies also show contradictory results. A limitation of these studies is the fact that most are carried out on very few subjects. An exception is the Child and Adolescent Trial for Cardiovascular Health (CATCH). In this large study including more than 4000 children and adolescents a multidisciplinary intervention was carried out (i.e. a 30-month diet, exercise, and non-smoking programme). No significant differences were found in TC and HDL after the intervention.[7] The same result was found in the Cardiovascular Health in Children Study after 8 months of aerobic training.[8] Casanovas *et al.*,[9] on the other hand, found an increase in TC and a decrease in HDL after a programme in which the daily physical activity was decreased. These relationships were shown in more than 400 young adults over a period of 8 months.

In conclusion, there is some evidence that physical activity and physical fitness are related to favourable HDL levels. This positive effect is probably caused by an increased activity of lipoprotein lipase (LPL) and lecithin:cholesterol acyltransferase (LCAT). Both activities are increased by high levels of cardiopulmonary work and both are known to increase the levels of HDL.[10,11]

Table 25.1 Overview regarding relationships between physical activity (PA) and physical fitness (PF) and total serum cholesterol (TC), high-density lipoprotein cholesterol (HDL), low-density lipoprotein cholesterol (LDL), the TC:HDL ratio, and serum triglycerides (TG) in normal populations of children and adolescents

			TC	HDL	LDL	TC:HDL	TG
Observational	Cross-sectional	PA	±	+	±	±	±
		PF	–	±	±	±	±
	Longitudinal	PA	–	±	±	±	±
		PF	±	–	±	±	±
Intervention			±	±	±	±	±

++, strong evidence; +, moderate evidence; ±, ambiguous evidence; –, no evidence.

Blood pressure

Endurance training can reduce both systolic (SP) and diastolic (DP) blood pressure by approximately 10 mmHg in adults with moderate essential hypertension, but exercise does not seem to have an effect on subjects with severe hypertension.[12] The mechanisms responsible for the decrease in blood pressure with physical activity and endurance training are yet to be determined. A reduced cardiac output has been suggested as a potential mechanism, although cardiac output reducing the effect of physical activity and fitness is not found in all the studies.[13] If there is no influence on cardiac output, then the blood pressure decreasing effect may be caused by a reduction in peripheral vascular resistance, which may be due to an overall reduction of sympathetic nervous system activity.[13] In addition, the relation between physical activity and blood pressure can be caused by the anxiety-reducing effect of physical activity.[14] It is questionable, however, if this mechanism is present in children and adolescents.

It appears that essential hypertension may begin early in life and that detection and treatment of possible blood pressure abnormalities at young ages is important. There is, however, no direct evidence that elevated blood pressure in children is related to CVD later in life. There is also not much evidence that physical activity and physical fitness have beneficial effects on blood pressure in children and adolescents. The studies analysing these relationships have been extensively reviewed by Alpert and Wilmore.[15] There are many cross-sectional studies investigating this relationship, but again the best evidence comes from longitudinal and well-controlled intervention studies. In the Amsterdam Growth and Health Study, daily physical activity during adolescence was not significantly related to both SP and DP at young adult age[5] and, in addition to that, the longitudinal development of physical activity was not related to either SP or DP (Twisk, unpublished results). The latter was also reported in the Cardiovascular Risk in Young Finns Study.[16] In the CATCH study, the 30-month multidisciplinary intervention among more than 4000 children and adolescents did not have any effect on blood pressure.[7] Baranowski *et al.*[17] argued that, as in adults, the possible lowering effect of physical activity on blood pressure only holds for children and adolescents with hypertension and not for youngsters with normal values of blood pressure. This implies that this effect is difficult to observe in population studies in children with low incidence of hypertension. Besides, this effect is probably confined to high-intensity aerobic type training and not for 'normal' habitual daily physical activity.[15] In Table 25.2, an overview of studies is given regarding

Table 25.2 Overview regarding relationships between physical activity (PA) and physical fitness (PF) and diastolic and systolic blood pressure (BP) in normal populations of children and adolescents

			Systolic BP	Diastolic BP
Observational	Cross-sectional	PA	–	–
		PF	±	±
	Longitudinal	PA	–	–
		PF	±	–
Intervention		–	–	–

++, strong evidence; +, moderate evidence; ±, ambiguous evidence; –, no evidence.

Table 25.3 Overview regarding relationships between physical activity (PA) and physical fitness (PF) and body fatness and body fat distribution in normal populations of children and adolescents

			Body fatness	Body fat distribution
Observational	Cross-sectional	PA	±	±
		PF	+	±
	Longitudinal	PA	±	–
		PF	±	–
Intervention			++	NA

++, strong evidence; +, moderate evidence; ±, ambiguous evidence; –, no evidence; NA, not applicable, that is, no studies available.

the relationships between physical activity and physical fitness and diastolic and systolic blood pressure in children and adolescents.

Body fatness and body composition

High body fatness (i.e. obesity) is known to be a risk factor for CVD in adults.[18] This effect has been shown to be at least partially mediated by and also independent of other CVD risk factors, such as lipoprotein levels and blood pressure. Prospective studies have also shown that, in adults, a central pattern of body fat is also associated with CVD morbidity and mortality.[19] Adolescence is a sensitive period for the development of a central pattern of body fat.[20] Therefore, adolescent body fat patterns may be of consequence for the development of CVD morbidity and mortality later in life. The aetiology of childhood obesity/body fat distribution is very complex. Besides heredity, which is regarded to be a major contributing factor, neuroendocrine and metabolic disturbances also contribute significantly to one's propensity for fatness. Environmental factors, such as cultural background, socio-economic status, nutrition, and physical activity, have also been recognized as causes for childhood obesity. In the light of energy balance, it is obvious that the relationships between physical activity, physical fitness, and body fatness and body fat distribution cannot be separated from the influence of food (i.e. energy) intake. There is a theory which states that a certain minimum level of physical activity is necessary for the body to precisely regulate energy intake to counterbalance energy expenditure. A sedentary lifestyle may reduce this regulatory ability, resulting in a positive energy balance and an increase in body fatness.[21] Another theory states that exercise is a mild appetite suppressant; this is based on research in which the total number of calories consumed did not change after a training programme was started, although an increase in energy expenditure was observed due to the training programme.[21] It is also suggested that resting metabolic rate increases as a result of physical activity and/or aerobic training but this has not been confirmed in all studies.[22,23]

Table 25.3 shows an overview of studies investigating the relationship between physical activity, physical fitness, and body fatness and body fat distribution in children and adolescents. In general, it can be concluded that there is some evidence for a relationship between physical activity, physical fitness, and body fatness in children and adolescents. This was also the conclusion of an extensive review performed by Bar-Or and Baranowski.[24] The evidence derives mainly from several cross-sectional studies[17,25] but longitudinal studies have shown similar results. In the Amsterdam Growth and Health Study, it was found that 'long-term exposure' to daily physical activity during adolescence was inversely related to the sum of four skinfolds at adult age.[5] In another study with data from the Amsterdam Growth and Health Study, it was shown that the longitudinal development (from 13 to 27 years of age) both daily physical activity and physical fitness (expressed as $\dot{V}O_2$ max) was strongly inversely related to the development of the sum of four skinfolds.[26]

The evidence for a positive effect of physical activity and/or physical fitness on body fat distribution is, in contrast to the results for body fatness, very weak and ambiguous. In the Amsterdam Growth and Health Study, the amount of daily physical activity during adolescence was positively related to the waist-to-hip ratio (WHR) at adult age, but this was only observed in females and not in males.[5] This finding is difficult to explain; first, because WHR is found to be primarily under genetic control[27] and second, if there is a relationship between physical activity and WHR, this relationship is expected to be inverse.[28,29] An explanation for this paradoxical finding might be that in females inactivity leads to a greater accumulation of fat in the thighs, which would result in a lower WHR.[5] However, another study conducted within the Amsterdam Growth and Health Study did not find a longitudinal relationship between physical activity and body fat distribution (expressed as the ratio between the thickness of the triceps skinfold and the subscapular skinfold and not as the WHR).[30]

A major problem in the investigation of the relationship between physical activity, physical fitness, and body fatness or obesity is the fact that it is not clear how to make a distinction between cause and effect (Fig. 25.1). Physical activity, physical fitness, and body fatness are closely intertwined and this cluster of factors is assumed to constitute a risk factor for CVD by itself. It is difficult to investigate what comes first. Another problem in the investigation of the relationship between physical activity and body fatness is the interpretation of body fatness. Most commonly, body fatness is expressed as BMI. BMI is easy to measure and therefore widely used as an indicator for body fatness. Another option is the use of the sum of two or more skinfold thicknesses. Although both methods are used as an indicator for the same parameter (i.e. body fatness), they reflect different aspects of body composition and, therefore, analyses using these different interpretations of body fat can lead to different results, especially when one is interested in the relationship between physical activity and/or physical fitness, and body fatness. Indeed, in the Amsterdam Growth and Health Study a highly

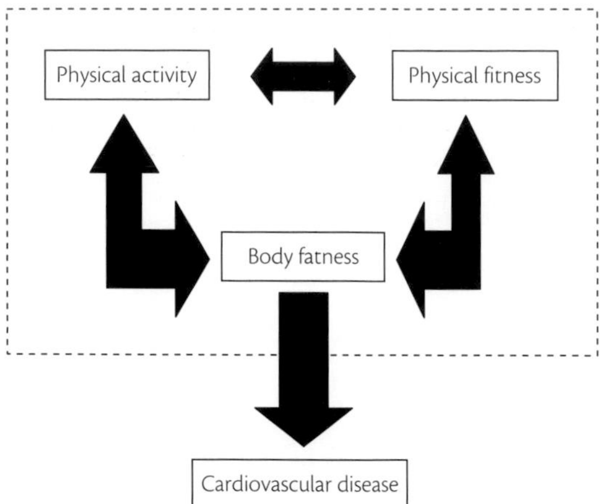

Fig. 25.1 Hypothetical relationships between physical activity, physical fitness, and body fatness.

significant inverse relationship was found between $\dot{V}O_2$ max (directly measured by a treadmill test) and the sum of four skinfolds but not with BMI.[26] Similarly, the amount of daily physical activity was found to be inversely related to the sum of four skinfolds, but not to BMI. These discrepancies may be explained by the fact that BMI is not only an indicator of fat mass, but also of lean body mass or muscle mass. Subjects with high muscle mass and moderate fat mass will have high values for BMI, but only moderate values for the sum of four skinfolds. When BMI is used as an indicator of body fatness, the negative relationships between body fatness and $\dot{V}O_2$ max, and between daily physical activity and body fatness can therefore be counterbalanced by the opposite relationships with lean body mass. The same phenomenon was observed by Bergström *et al.*[31] in an observational cross-sectional study in more than 1000 adolescents, where running performance (an indicator of physical fitness measured by a 3-km running test) was highly related to the sum of four skinfolds in both boys and girls; in addition, but only in girls (and with much lower levels of significance) was running performance associated with BMI. Taken together, these findings suggest that results obtained with BMI as indicator for body fatness should be interpreted cautiously; this is especially true in children and adolescents because in this particular population the variables concerned are also influenced by natural growth and biological development.

Diabetes

Diabetes mellitus is a disorder of carbohydrate metabolism characterized by high blood glucose levels. Diabetes is a very strong CVD risk factor. It develops when there is inadequate production of insulin by the pancreas, or inadequate utilization of insulin by the cells. A distinction must be made between immune-mediated (insulin-dependent) diabetes mellitus (type 1 diabetes) and non-immune-mediated diabetes mellitus (type 2 diabetes). Although type 1 diabetes remains the most prevalent form of the disease in children, recent reports indicate that 8–45% of the newly diagnosed cases of diabetes are of type 2.[32] The recent increase in the prevalence and incidence of type 2 diabetes (typically regarded as a disease of the middle-aged and elderly) among children has been attributed to the epidemic of paediatric obesity observed in the past decades.[33]

Table 25.4 Overview regarding relationships between physical activity (PA) and physical fitness (PF) and serum insulin and serum glucose concentrations in normal populations of children and adolescents

			Insulin	Glucose
Observational	Cross-sectional	PA	±	–
		PF	±	–
	Longitudinal	PA	NA	NA
		PF	NA	NA
Intervention			±	NA

++, strong evidence; +, moderate evidence; ±, ambiguous evidence; –, no evidence; NA, not applicable, that is, no studies available.

In adults physical activity has many desirable effects on people with diabetes, particularly those with type 2 diabetes.[34] Glycaemic control is improved, possibly due to the insulin-like effect of muscle contractions on translocating glucose from the plasma into the cell.[35] Exercise leads to an increase in muscle mass (lean body mass) and therefore to lower blood glucose levels, assisting in better glycaemic control and reduction of insulin resistance. Some researchers believe that regular physical activity can have an effect on glycaemic control in children with type 1 diabetes,[36] but this is yet to be confirmed.

The outcome variables most commonly used in studies relating physical activity and physical fitness to glucose metabolism disorders are glucose and insulin concentrations [and/or a combination of both—the homeostasis model assessment (HOMA) insulin resistance score] in blood serum. A brief review of the literature shows that there are not many studies investigating the relationships between physical activity, physical fitness, and serum insulin and glucose concentrations in children and adolescents (Table 25.4 gives an overview). For insulin levels the results are ambiguous. In the Cardiovascular Risk in Young Finns Study, for instance, an inverse cross-sectional relationship was observed between physical activity and insulin levels in males but not in females.[37] With regard to blood glucose levels the few studies carried out did not show any influence of physical activity and physical fitness in children and adolescents. More consistent results were found in (the even more limited number of) studies among obese children and adolescents. In these studies, a positive effect was found for physical activity on parameters related to insulin metabolism.[38] Interestingly, and similar to observations in adults, a recent aerobic exercise trial in obese girls showed improved insulin sensitivity, without any concomitant changes in body weight, fat, and inflammatory markers. Instead, exercise-related increases in lean body mass seemed to play a key mediating role.[39]

Multiple risk factors—the metabolic syndrome

The clustering of risk factors, notably (central) obesity, dyslipidaemia (i.e. elevated TG and decreased HDL-cholesterol), elevated blood pressure, and high fasting glucose levels, occurs more often than chance alone would dictate. This clustering has been named the Syndrome X, Insulin Resistance Syndrome, and, more recently, the Metabolic Syndrome (MetS).[40] The MetS raises the risk of CVD and even more of type 2 diabetes.[41] Body fatness and a sedentary lifestyle, in the setting of a genetic predisposition, are considered its prime aetiological factors. Therefore, the prevalence of the MetS (similar to that of type 2 diabetes) is increasingly important among the young.[42] Not surprisingly, the amount of studies around the MetS/risk factor clustering (e.g. definitions—a recent one has just been proposed for children and adolescents,[43] prevalence, determinants, complications, prevention, and treatment) have increased exponentially in recent years (not without many—still ongoing—debates and controversies).

Clustering of cardiovascular risk factors has been recognized in children long before this latest worldwide interest in the phenotype.[44–47] Several studies—mostly with a cross-sectional design—have addressed the extent to which physical activity and/or physical fitness are associated with the MetS/clustered risk factors. Their main findings can be summarized as follows: lower levels of self-reported physical activity are inversely (but not 'significantly') associated with the MetS.[48,49] In studies where physical activity was 'objectively' measured (i.e. with accelerometers), these inverse associations were stronger[50–53] but attenuated when further adjustments for physical fitness (and also fatness, though to a lesser extent) were considered.[50,51] Interestingly, a significant interaction with fitness has also been reported, suggesting that the beneficial effects of increasing physical activity levels (if any), in the setting of MetS prevention, may be highest among the less fit.[50] The studies mentioned above have argued that physical activity is more strongly associated with risk factor clustering than with each of the risk factors separately. Studies investigating the association between physical fitness and the MetS have all reported an inverse association that was only partially mediated by (but still independent of) body fatness.[54–57] Prospective studies examining the associations between physical activity and/or physical fitness during childhood/adolescence and the occurrence of the MetS later in life are scarce. In a small study of Danish adolescents, despite the inverse cross-sectional association observed between physical fitness and MetS, physical fitness levels during adolescence did not predict clustered risk 8 years later (when subjects' mean age was 23–27 years).[55] In the Amsterdam Growth and Health Study, we have recently shown that subjects, who had the MetS at the mean age of 36 years, when compared to their counterparts without the syndrome, were characterized by a steeper decrease in physical fitness levels from adolescence to the age of 36 years.[58] However, the differences between the two groups emerged around the age of 21–27 years (but not during adolescence), remaining present thereafter. In addition, this association was only partially mediated by body fatness. Differences in the time spent in (self-reported) vigorous physical activities have also emerged at the same age, but these disappeared after further adjustments for fitness and fatness levels. In the CARDIA Study, young adults (18–30 years) with low fitness levels (lowest quintile) were three-fold to six-fold (two-fold after adjustments for body fatness) more likely to develop diabetes and the MetS in a 15-year follow-up study.[59]

The extent to which changes in physical activity at a young age are associated with changes in clustered risk have only been investigated in three longitudinal studies. The Cardiovascular Risk in Young Finns Study[43] examined 'high risk cluster' (defined as higher age- and sex-specific tertiles of each of the following risk factors: elevated levels of total cholesterol, HDL-cholesterol, and diastolic blood pressure) in a large cohort (initial age between 3 and 18 years) followed for a period of 6 years. A shift from not belonging to this 'high risk cluster' at the initial measurement to belonging to this 'high risk cluster' at the follow-up was associated with a decrease in physical activity levels. In the Amsterdam Growth and Health Study, daily physical activity was strongly associated with risk factor clustering (which included the TC:HDL ratio, mean arterial blood pressure, the sum of four skinfolds, and $\dot{V}O_2$ max) throughout a 15-year period (between the ages of 13 and 27 years).[60] However, no such associations were found in the Northern Ireland Young Hearts Project where analyses were confined to a 3-year longitudinal period (between the ages of 12 and 15 years).[61]

Other lifestyles

Physical inactivity is, at least partially, an independent correlate of CVD risk factors. Physical inactivity is also often found to be associated with other unhealthy lifestyles such as smoking, alcohol consumption, and unhealthy dietary habits. This clustering of unhealthy lifestyles may introduce a health risk that is greater than one would expect from the individual unhealthy lifestyles.[62] It is unlikely that these unhealthy lifestyles are related to each other in a causal chain. Instead, it is more likely that there is one or more underlying mechanism(s) (e.g. genetic, psychosocial, socioeconomic, environmental factors, etc.) which underlie the construct of 'unhealthy behaviour' (i.e. inactivity, smoking behaviour, alcohol consumption, and unhealthy diet). In the Cardiovascular Risk in Young Finns Study, physical inactivity was found to be associated with smoking behaviour, alcohol consumption, and having a diet with an excessive intake of fat.[63] These findings were not confirmed in the Amsterdam Growth and Health Study where physical inactivity was not found to be associated with any of the other unhealthy lifestyles.[64] In a cross-sectional study among 18-year-old Australians (301 males and 282 females), smoking, drinking alcohol, and unhealthy dietary habits were related to each other in both males and females; in females low levels of physical activity were also associated with the other 'unhealthy' behaviours.[65] Terre *et al.*[66] also showed correlations between unhealthy behaviours and argued that a multidimensional view should be used in the prevention of chronic diseases in childhood. As a consequence there is nowadays the belief that prevention should not focus on a particular lifestyle, but that a multidisciplinary, healthy behaviour oriented preventive programme should be developed in order to prevent CVD. Such programmes would not only be beneficial for the prevention of CVD, but also for the prevention of many other chronic diseases.[67]

New cardiovascular risk factors

Lipoproteins [Lp(a), apoB, and apoA-1]

Owing to the progress in lipid biochemistry in the late 1970s and early 1980s, it was shown that it is not the lipoprotein levels *per se* but the protein parts of the lipoproteins (apolipoproteins) instead that are most deleterious with regard to the onset of CVD.[68] The two most important apolipoproteins (apos) are (i) apoA-1, the major protein content of HDL and which is therefore assumed to be protective against CVD; and (ii) apoB, the major protein content of LDL, and which is therefore assumed to be atherogenic.[69–71] Later, Lp(a) was also detected. Lp(a) is comparable to LDL and was found to be an independent risk factor for CVD.[72,73] Unlike LDL, Lp(a) is inherited as a quantitative genetic trait.[74]

There are not many studies investigating the relationships between physical fitness and physical activity and apoA-1, apoB, and Lp(a) among children and adolescents. Table 25.5 gives an overview of the results of different studies, which are ambiguous. In a cross-sectional study based on data from the Cardiovascular Risk in Young Finns Study including more than 2000 children, adolescents, and young adults, physical activity was inversely related to apoB in males, but not in females. No relationship was observed with apoA-1.[16] In a longitudinal study with the same data, however, subjects who remained active over a period of 6 years showed no different apoB and apoA-1 levels compared with subjects who remained inactive over the same time period.[6] In the previously mentioned CATCH study, the large multidisciplinary intervention had no effect on apoB levels 7. In a population-based study including more than 4000 young adults, aged between 23 and 35 years, Lp(a) was not associated with daily physical activity, suggesting that Lp(a) levels are largely genetically determined.[75] In the Cardiovascular Risk in Young Finns Study, however, an inverse cross-sectional relationship was observed between physical activity and Lp(a) levels, that is, high levels of Lp(a) (>25 mg·dL^{-1}) were less frequent in the physically most active subjects.[76]

C-reactive protein and fibrinogen

C-reactive protein (CRP) is a circulating acute-phase reactant that is increased manyfold during the inflammatory response to tissue injury. CRP is synthesized primarily in the liver and its release is stimulated by interleukin-6 and other proinflammatory cytokines. In recent years CRP has received great attention, particularly with regard to its role in the prediction of atherosclerotic disease.[77] This has resulted from the shift in thinking about the pathogenesis of atherosclerosis. Atherosclerosis was once considered to be primarily the result of lipid storage on the vascular walls, but inflammation is now known to play a key role in every stage of the atherosclerotic process (i.e. from its initiation to its progression to plaque rupture).[78] Fibrinogen is a circulating glycoprotein that acts in the final step in the coagulation response to vascular and tissue injury. Cleavage by thrombin produces soluble fibrin fragments which are the most abundant component in blood clots. In addition to its role in thrombosis, fibrinogen has many other functions, sustaining its likely involvement in vascular disease; these include the regulation of cell adhesion and proliferation, vasoconstriction at sites of vessel wall injury, stimulation of platelet aggregation, and determination of blood viscosity. Similar to CRP, fibrinogen is also an acute-phase reactant: hepatic synthesis of fibrinogen increases greatly in response to inflammatory triggers.[77] Both CRP and fibrinogen have been shown to be independent predictors of CVD and mortality even among apparently healthy individuals.[77,79]

A recent review of the literature in adults has shown that physical activity and/fitness is consistently associated with lower levels of CRP and in two thirds of the 40 observational studies reviewed, this inverse association was independent of body fatness; evidence from 12 randomized-controlled trials, however, did not support this hypothesis, suggesting that weight loss may instead be the key factor.[80] Another review focusing on coagulation and fibrinolysis markers showed that, although most cross-sectional studies show a consistent inverse association with physical activity, mixed results derive from training studies (which could be attributed to differences in type and intensity of exercise used and population characteristics such as age and health status).[81]

Compared to adults, there is a paucity of data on the younger population, however, in the Petah Tikva Project a low but statistically significant inverse relationship was observed between sports activity and plasma fibrinogen levels of 9- to 18-year-old boys and girls.[82] In the Ten Towns Children's Study, parent but not self-reported levels of children's physical activity were also inversely associated with CRP levels in 699 9–11 year olds, and this association remained even after further adjustment for ponderal index.[83] However, another study has shown that the inverse association between physical activity and CRP in apparently healthy children is greatly mediated by body fatness.[84] In The Columbia University Biomarkers Study, a study among children and young adults aged 6–24 years, physical fitness was also inversely associated with both fibrinogen and CRP levels, and these associations were at least partially independent of BMI.[85,86] All these studies had a cross-sectional design. The extent to which physical activity and/or fitness during youth predict levels of markers of coagulation and inflammation later in life is not known. In addition, there are few intervention studies examining the effects of physical activity on these markers among the young and these have been confined to studies of the obese. Interestingly, both after 4 and 8 months of exercise training no significant changes in fibrinogen and CRP levels were observed, despite favourable changes in adiposity and fitness.[87,88] In conclusion, and similar to many other CVD risk factors, the evidence for a possible inverse relationship between physical activity, physical fitness, and CRP and fibrinogen levels in children and adolescents is also rather weak.

Table 25.5 Overview regarding relationships between physical activity (PA) and physical fitness (PF) and apolipoprotein (apoA-1, apoB) and lipoprotein (a) [Lp(a)] in normal populations of children and adolescents

			apoB	apoA-1	Lp(a)
Observational	Cross-sectional	PA	±	±	±
		PF	–	–	–
	Longitudinal	PA	NA	NA	NA
		PF	NA	NA	NA
Intervention			±	±	NA

++, strong evidence; +, moderate evidence; ±, ambiguous evidence; –, no evidence; NA, not applicable, that is, no studies available.

Other risk factors (homocysteine and heart rate variability)

Recently it was recognized that hyperhomocysteinaemia is related to CVD morbidity and mortality. Homocysteine levels are assumed to be independent of the traditional risk factors (lipoproteins, age, gender, blood pressure, and smoking). In a large cross-sectional study of 16,000 middle-aged subjects, an inverse relation was found between homocysteine level and physical activity.[89] Until now no studies investigating the relationship between physical activity and physical fitness and homocysteine levels in children and adolescents have been reported in the literature.

Another CVD risk factor that has received a lot of attention recently is heart rate variability, which seems to be impaired in chronic artery disease. The biological mechanisms behind this phenomenon are not yet fully understood. The possible influence of physical activity and physical fitness on heart rate variability in children and adolescence has yet to be determined. It is assumed that the adaptive responses of the cardiovascular system to regular physical activity includes a reduction in sympathetic and an increase in parasympathetic activity during rest and at different absolute intensities of exercise. This assumption was not confirmed in a cross-sectional study in young subjects where it was shown that both sympathetic and parasympathetic activities were not different in trained versus non-trained subjects.[90] In adults, there is limited and conflicting evidence on the influence of physical activity and physical fitness on heart rate variability. In a cross-sectional study among 88 middle-aged subjects, no relationship could be shown between heart rate variability and physical activity (assessed by a 2-month diary follow-up).[91] In another study among 19 middle-aged subjects, it was found that after a training period of 30 weeks heart rate variability was increased in the training group compared to the control group.[92]

New developments

Gene–environment interactions

With the development of genetic epidemiology and the discovery of certain polymorphisms that are related to CVD risk factors (especially related to lipoproteins and body fatness), there is a lot of scientific interest in the so-called gene–environment interactions. In other words, the following question arises: is the relationship between physical activity, physical fitness, and CVD risk factors different for different genotypes? Up until now, to our knowledge, the only study investigating the interaction between physical activity and genetic predisposition in a young population is the Cardiovascular Risk in Young Finns Study, which focused on apolipoprotein (apo)E. Apolipoprotein (apo)E determines serum total cholesterol and LDL and is therefore associated with CVD. In plasma three major apoE isoforms can be determined (E2, E3, and E4) which are coded by three codominant alleles (ε2, ε3, and ε4), resulting in six major apoE phenotypes (E2/2, E3/2, E4/2, E3/3, E4/3, and E4/4). In a cross-sectional sample of 1498 boys and girls (aged between 9 and 24 years), the relationship between daily physical activity (a weighted activity score assessed by a questionnaire) and TC and LDL was analysed for different subgroups with different apoE phenotypes. It was shown that the influence of physical activity differed for the different subgroups. No associations were found in E4/4; moderate associations were found in E4/3 and E3/3, and much stronger associations were observed in E3/2 phenotype.[93] From these results, it appears that apoE phenotype partly determines the association between physical activity and TC and LDL, that is, there exists some degree of gene–environment interaction. However, much more research is this field is warranted.

Preclinical atherosclerosis and arterial stiffness

Atherosclerosis and arterial stiffness are main causes of CVD and reflect the impairment of the two major functions of the arterial system (which are distinct but often related): to deliver blood to the tissues and organs of the body according to their needs (i.e. a conduit function), and to smooth flow pulsations imposed by the intermittent contracting heart so that the blood is directed through the body organs and tissues in an almost steady stream (i.e. a cushioning function).[91] Atherosclerosis is a gradual process that leads to thickening and narrowing of major arteries locally, thereby impairing their *conduit function*, and leading to ischaemia or infarction of the organ or tissue downstream. Arterial stiffness is a generalized process that reflects the level of impairment of the *cushioning function* of arteries which increases cardiac workload and arterial stress in general by increasing systolic and pulse pressure, thereby leading to left ventricular hypertrophy and impaired coronary perfusion and ultimately to heart failure and stroke.[95] Both processes of arterial dysfunction are affected by the arterial degeneration that occurs with ageing and exposure to various risk factors.

Up until now, research regarding the relationship between physical activity and physical fitness among children and adolescents and CVD mortality and morbidity later in life has been limited to the analysis of the associations between physical activity and physical fitness and biological CVD risk factors. The development in the past two decades of non-invasive ultrasonography methods capable of imaging and quantifying arterial wall structure and function (motion) characteristics have enabled the study of vascular abnormalities (i.e. the degree of atherosclerosis and arterial stiffness) and its related risk factors in the earlier stages of disease (i.e. before clinical events occur).[96] These methods are currently of great aid in the study of the pathophysiology and treatment of arterial dysfunction. Arterial surrogate end points are therefore used to substitute a clinical end point. In the case of atherosclerosis, arterial wall thickness, in particular the intima-media thickness (IMT) of the carotid artery is widely recognized as such a surrogate end point.[96] Changes in brachial artery diameter after different stimuli are also assessed as a marker of endothelial (dys)function, a early precursor of the atherosclerotic process.[97] In the case of arterial stiffness, which is a construct, various types of information on arteries, such as their size, the change of their size during cardiac pulsation (i.e. at given pressure levels), and the speed of transmission of blood pulse waves, are combined to calculate stiffness estimates such as distensibility and compliance coefficients (locally) and pulse wave velocity (PWV) (regionally).[95] Given its non-invasive nature, ultrasound imaging methods have thus the advantage of being suitable not only in small clinical studies but also in large epidemiological studies at the population level, notably in children and young adults.[98,99]

Most of the studies examining the correlates of carotid IMT, endothelial function, and arterial stiffness in young subjects have been confined to clinical populations (e.g. severely obese, type 1 diabetes, familial hypercholesterolaemia). The best evidence so far obtained in apparently healthy populations has been derived from the prospective studies described below. Extending the pioneer findings of autopsy studies performed within the Pathobiological Determinants of Atherosclerosis in Youth Study (PDAY), and making use of non-invasive ultrasound imaging techniques, three large longitudinal studies (The Muscatine Study, The Bogalusa Heart Study, and The Cardiovascular Risk in Young Finns Study) have recently identified body fatness, elevated cholesterol and blood pressure levels during childhood as independent predictors of adult carotid IMT.[100–102] Studies using similar prospective data analyses conducted by us within the Amsterdam Growth and Health Longitudinal Study have identified low levels of physical fitness (and a central pattern of fat distribution rather than total adiposity) during adolescence (both variables not considered by the above mentioned studies) to be independent predictors of carotid IMT in adulthood.[103,104] Changes in physical fitness levels between adolescence and adulthood, however, were not associated with carotid IMT.[105] In the Cardiovascular Risk in Young Finns

Study, childhood body fatness, elevated blood pressure, and LDL-cholesterol, and smoking were associated with arterial stiffness in adulthood.[106] In the Amsterdam Growth and Health Longitudinal Study, fitness levels during adolescence were not clearly associated with arterial stiffness later in life.[103] Instead, we found that a central pattern of fat distribution (but not total fatness) during adolescence was adversely associated with arterial stiffness two decades later.[104] Changes in physical activity and fitness levels between adolescence and the age of 36 years, however, were inversely associated with stiffness estimates, particularly, of the brachial and femoral arteries (i.e. the muscular part of the arterial tree).[105]

In summary, several childhood/adolescent biological risk factors have been identified as precursors of preclinical atherosclerosis and/or arterial stiffness later in life. However, little is known with regard to the impact of lifestyles (e.g. physical activity) adopted at young age on vascular damage in childhood and later in life. More importantly, over time how the natural development of physical activity and fitness impact on arterial damage is not known, and needs to be further investigated.

General comments

Possible reasons for the lack of evidence

While analysing the effect of physical activity and physical fitness on CVD risk factors in children and adolescents one must realize that almost all risk factors have a (large) genetic component; therefore, the changes in CVD risk factors observed as a result of physical activity and/or physical fitness are generally small. Furthermore, it must be taken into account that the development of CVD risk factors during childhood and adolescence can also be the result of normal growth and development. Especially during adolescence the rate of maturation can be a very important factor. A nice example to illustrate the importance of this factor is the so-called adolescent dip in total serum cholesterol levels,[107] which can highly bias the results of studies investigating the relationship between physical activity and physical fitness and total serum cholesterol in adolescents. A third important issue is the problem of assessing the amount of physical activity. There are many different ways described to measure physical activity (see ref. 108 and Chapter 10). They vary from direct measurements (i.e. observation, diary, questionnaires, interview) to indirect measurements (i.e. physiological measurements, mechanical devices, 'doubly labelled' water). First, the use of different methods to assess physical activity in different studies can lead to ambiguous results. Second, the definition of physical activity is often different between studies. Sometimes physical activity is defined as total habitual physical activity, while in other studies physical activity is limited to sports activity. Also proxy measures such as the time an individual watches television are used (as a measure of physical inactivity). However, regardless of the method used, it is impossible to measure the amount of physical activity in children and adolescents exactly. The best one can do is to get a crude indication of habitual physical activity (probably achieved by a combination of different methods). The measurement error related to the assessment of physical activity is, in general, non-differential, that is, not related to the health outcome. This non-differential misclassification will lead to bias towards the null, which causes relationships to be underestimated; a phenomenon which exists both for under-reporting as for over-reporting. Another important issue concerns the intensity of different activities. One is often interested in the total energy expenditure of a certain individual. With questionnaires or interviews (the methods mostly used in large population-based studies) it is very difficult to assess the intensity of the different activities carried out by a particular subject. Data from questionnaires are often converted to an activity measure using standard tables in which a particular activity is related to a certain amount of energy expenditure. This certain amount of energy expenditure is often seen as an indicator of intensity. This method introduces a new source of bias: not only can the intensity of the same activity be extremely different for different individuals, but also different absolute levels of aerobic fitness between individuals can have important implications for the translation of certain activities into energy expenditure.

Finally when $\dot{V}O_2$ max is used as an indicator for physical fitness, there is the problem that $\dot{V}O_2$ max is highly related to body composition; that is, body weight. Therefore, $\dot{V}O_2$ max is often expressed per kg body weight or per kg body weight to the 2/3 power. It is, however, known that in children and adolescents the relationship between $\dot{V}O_2$ max and body weight is not that straightforward (see Chapter 2). Furthermore, the relationship with body weight changes over time; that is, it differs across different age groups. This can also be a possible reason for ambiguous results.

Cardiovascular health importance

To evaluate the importance of relationships between physical activity, physical fitness, and CVD risk factors in childhood and adolescence, it is important to realize that a high level of a risk factor during childhood and adolescence is not health threatening *per se*; that is, it is mostly not directly related to the disease. In fact the value of a particular CVD risk factor measured at an early age is a (less than perfect) predictor of that CVD risk factor in middle age, which is a (less than perfect) predictor of the occurrence of CVD events. In other words, 'high risk' values for CVD risk factors in childhood or adolescence are a risk factor for 'high risk' values for CVD risk factors in adulthood, which are a risk factor for the development of CVD. In Fig. 25.2 this problem

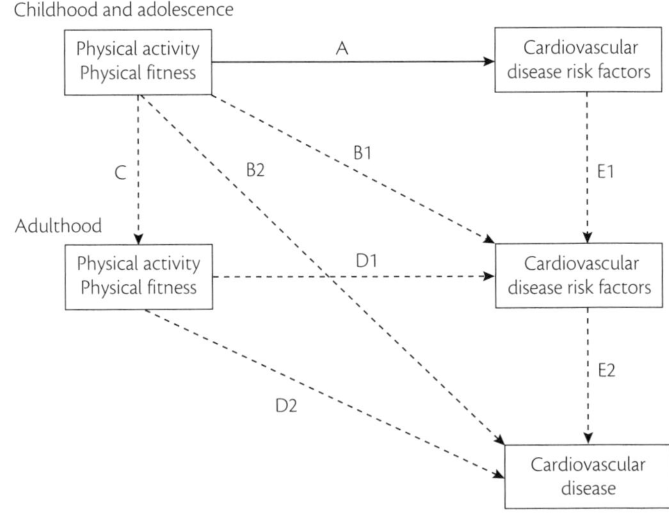

Fig. 25.2 Hypothetical relationships between physical activity, physical fitness, and cardiovascular disease risk factors, and cardiovascular disease throughout life [characters (A to E2) are explained in the text].

is illustrated, showing that the situation is much more complicated than just the analysis of the relationships between physical activity or physical fitness and CVD risk factors in childhood and adolescence. Figure 25.2 is an extension of the hypothesized relationships between activity, health, and stage of life by Blair *et al.*[109]

Summarizing the evidence depicted by the different arrows in Fig. 25.2: there is no evidence that physical activity and/or physical fitness during childhood and adolescence are related to CVD risk factors in adulthood (B1). There is no evidence that physical activity and/or physical fitness during childhood and adolescence are related to the occurrence of CVD in adulthood (B2). There is (as been shown earlier) weak evidence that physical activity and/or physical fitness in childhood and adolescence are related to CVD risk factors in childhood and adolescence (A) and there is (better) evidence that physical activity and/or physical fitness in adulthood are related to both CVD risk factors and to the occurrence of CVD (D1 and D2).[1,110] Therefore, in fact, the only two pathways involved in the potential benefits of physical activity and physical fitness for cardiovascular health concern the predictability of CVD risk factors in adulthood from the values of the same risk factors measured in childhood and adolescence (E1) and the predictability of physical activity and physical fitness in adulthood from the amount of physical activity and physical fitness measured in childhood and adolescence (C). The issue of the predictability of a certain variable measured at young age for the value of the same variable later in life is called tracking. For several CVD risk factors this predictability is rather high; especially for the lipoproteins and for body fatness. For blood pressure this predictability is quite low. This is also the case for the predictability of physical activity and physical fitness.[111] Figures 25.3 and 25.4 show data from the Amsterdam Growth and Health Study in which tracking was analysed for biological CVD risk factors as well as for physical activity and physical fitness from adolescence into young adulthood. A few remarks must be made regarding the interpretation of the results of studies investigating tracking. First of all many authors are satisfied with a tracking coefficient that is statistically significant.[112] However, a significant tracking coefficient does not mean that the predictive value of measurements during childhood or adolescence for values later in life is high. Suppose that tracking is calculated for subjects in a particular 'risk' quartile in a longitudinal study with two measurements in time and that 50% of the initial 'high risk' quartile maintain their position at the follow-up measurement. In this situation, the initial measurement had a predictive value of 50% and a highly significant odds ratio of 5.0 would be found (an OR of 5.0 calculated for 'risk' quartiles translates to a predictive value of the initial measurement of 50%). This method to assess tracking was applied to the dataset of the Amsterdam Growth and Health Study.[111] A summary of the results is shown in Fig. 25.4. From Fig. 25.4 it can be seen that odds ratios >5.0 were only observed for lipoproteins and body fatness, while for blood pressure and physical activity and physical fitness much lower values were found.[111] The second problem is that tracking concerns the relative position of a certain individual within a group of subjects over time. When tracking for a certain variable over time is high it does not necessarily mean that the absolute level of that variable does not change over time. Especially for daily physical activity it is known that the amount of physical activity in the total population is decreasing dramatically from childhood into adolescence and from adolescence into adulthood.[113] In other words, when everybody decreases levels to the same degree, tracking of physical activity will be high, while from a health perspective this is still an undesirable situation. Third, one must also take into account that tracking coefficients are highly influenced by measurement error. The assessment of physical activity for instance is not very accurate (i.e. the reproducibility of the measurement of physical activity is rather low). Consequently, the low tracking coefficients for physical activity are partly caused by this low reproducibility of the assessment method.

How much activity/fitness is good for cardiovascular health?

Although there is not much evidence for a strong relationship between physical activity and/or physical fitness during childhood and adolescence and cardiovascular health at adult age,

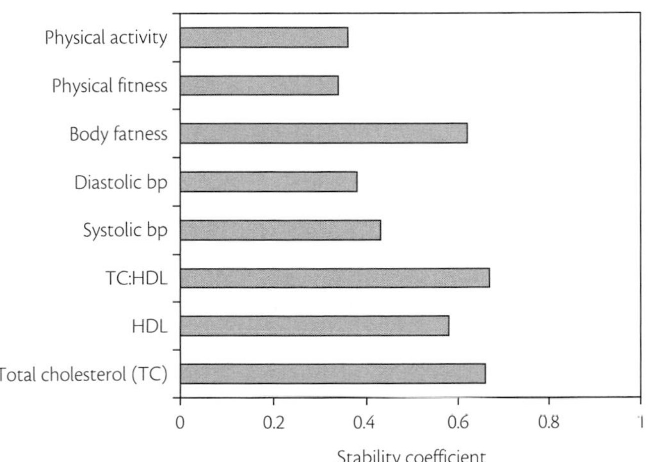

Fig. 25.3 Stability coefficients, which are interpretable as correlation coefficients varying between 0 and 1, calculated with generalized estimating equations over a period of 15 years from 13 to 27 years of age. Results from the Amsterdam Growth and Health Study.[76]

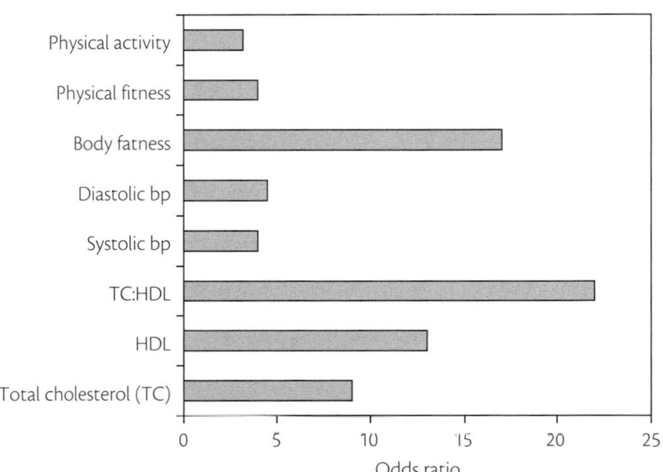

Fig. 25.4 Odds for subjects at risk at an initial measurement at the age of 13 years to stay at risk over a period of 15 years compared to the odds for subjects not at risk at the initial measurements. Results from the Amsterdam Growth and Health Study.[76]

there is much discussion about the amount of physical activity which should be recommended to young people from a health perspective. These guidelines vary from 30 min of light intensity physical activity most of the days to 1 hour of moderate intensity physical activity all days of the week.[114] When looking critically at these guidelines from the perspective of cardiovascular health, there is no direct scientific evidence for these guidelines. The argument against the 'old' guideline of 30 min of moderate physical activity on most days of the week is supported by the fact that although the majority of young people are currently meeting this old criterion, childhood overweight and obesity are increasing and that many young people have been shown to possess at least one modifiable CVD risk factor.[114] Although there is some rationale behind these two arguments, they ignore the fact that there is almost no evidence that physical activity is related to CVD risk factors in children and adolescents and ignore the fact that the aetiology of CVD is multidimensional. In other words, there is no real scientific rationale for these guidelines.

If there is a relationship between physical activity, physical fitness, and CVD risk factors in children and adolescents, this relationship will probably have some sort of S-shaped curve; that is, at least in a large range of physical activity levels this relationship will be more or less a continuum; however, even above and beyond the guidelines, an increase in physical activity will have beneficial effects. Probably, the proposed guidelines are equivalent with the sharpest increase in this S-shaped curve, which then can be seen as the optimal level of physical activity for cardiovascular health benefits. Although on a population level these guidelines can be of importance, at the individual level this importance is rather doubtful. Another issue related to these guidelines is the identification of so-called high risk individuals; that is, individuals who do not meet the physical activity criterion. These 'high risk' individuals are the primary focus of preventive strategies. However, on the basis of the lack of scientific evidence for the guidelines this is a debatable approach. Preventive strategies to improve physical activity in our young population should aim at the entire young population. If there are beneficial effects of physical activity and/or physical fitness in children and adolescents, these will be beneficial for all.

Summary

- There is only little evidence that physical activity and physical fitness are related to a healthy CVD risk profile in children and adolescents. The best evidence is found for a positive relationship with body fatness.
- One must bear in mind that most research is limited to the so-called traditional risk factors and that the outcome of most studies is hampered by the poor methods available to measure physical activity.
- With regard to new developments in CVD research (i.e. 'new' risk factors, gene–environment interaction, preclinical atherosclerosis, and arterial stiffness), the influence of physical activity and physical fitness in children and adolescents are yet to be determined.
- There is no scientific evidence to support the widely used guidelines for health-related physical activity.

References

1. Paffenbarger RS (1988). Contributions of epidemiology to exercise science and cardiovascular risk. *Med Sci Sports Exerc* **20**, 426–38.
2. Armstrong N, Simons-Morton B (1994). Physical activity and blood lipids in adolescents. *Pediatr Exerc Sci* **6**, 381–405.
3. Sallis JF, Patterson TL, Buono MJ, Nader PR (1988). Relation of cardiovascular fitness and physical activity to cardiovascular disease risk factors in children and adults. *Am J Epidemiol* **127**, 933–41.
4. Donahue RP, Orchard TJ, Becker DJ, Kuller LH, Drash AL (1988). Physical activity, insulin sensitivity, and the lipoprotein profile in young adults: The Beaver County Study. *Am J Epidemiol* **127**, 95–103.
5. Twisk JW, van Mechelen W, Kemper HC, Post GB (1997). The relation between 'long term exposure' to lifestyle during youth and young adulthood and risk factors for cardiovascular disease. *Adolesc Health* **20**, 309–19.
6. Raitakari OT, Porkka KV, Taimela S, Telama R, Räsänen L, Viikari JS (1994). Effects of persistent physical activity and inactivity on coronary risk factors in children and young adults: The Cardiovascular Risk in Young Finns Study. *Am J Epidemiol* **140**, 195–205.
7. Webber LS, Osganian SK, Feldman HA, Wu M, McKenzie TL, Nichaman M, Lytle LA, Edmunson E, Cutler J, Nader PR, Luepker RV (1996). Cardiovascular risk factors among children after a two and a half year intervention—The CATCH study. *Prev Med* **25**, 432–41.
8. Harrel JS, McMurray RG, Bangdiwala SI, Frauman AC, Gansky SA, Bradley CB (1996). Effects of a school-based intervention to reduce cardiovascular disease risk factors in elementary-school children: The Cardiovascular Health in Children (CHIC) Study. *J Pediatr* **128**, 797–805.
9. Casanovas JA, Lapetra A, Puzo J, Pelegrin J, Hermosilla T, De Vicente J, Garza F, Del Rio A, Giner A, Ferreira IJ (1992). Tobacco, physical exercise and lipid profile. *Eur Heart J* **13**, 440–5.
10. Nikkilä EA, Taskinen MR, Rehunen S, Harkonen M (1978). Lipoprotein lipase activity in adipose tissue and skeletal muscle of runners: Relation to serum lipoproteins. *Metabolism* **27**, 1661–71.
11. Berg A, Frey I, Baumstark MW, Halle M, Keul J (1994). Physical activity and lipoprotein lipid disorders. *Sports Med* **17**, 6–21.
12. Tipton CM (1991). Exercise training and hypertension: An update. *Exerc Sport Sci Rev* **19**, 447–505.
13. Hagberg JB (1990). Exercise, fitness and hypertension. In: Bouchard C, Sheppard RJ, Stephens T, Sutton JR, McPherson BD (eds.), *Exercise, fitness, and health.* pp. 455–66. Human Kinetics, Champaign, IL.
14. Petruzzello SJ, Landers SM, Hatfield BD, Kubitz KA, Salazar W (1991). A meta-analysis on the anxiety-reducing effects of acute and chronic exercise. Outcomes and mechanisms. *Sports Med* **11**, 143–82.
15. Alpert B, Wilmore JH (1994). Physical activity and blood pressure in adolescents. *Pediatr Exerc Sci* **6**, 361–80.
16. Raitakari OT, Taimela S, Porkka KV, Telama R, Välimäki I, Åkerblom HK, Viikari, JS (1997). Associations between physical activity and risk factors for coronary heart disease: The Cardiovascular Risk in Young Finns Study. *Med Sci Sports Exerc* **29**, 1055–61.
17. Baranowski T, Bouchard C, Bar-Or O, Bricker T, Heath G, Kimm SY, Malina R, Obarzanek E, Pate R, Strong WB (1992). Assessment, prevalence, and cardiovascular benefits of physical activity and fitness in youth. *Med Sci Sports Exerc* **24**, S237–47.
18. Hubert HB, Feinleib M, McNamara PM, Castelli WP (1983). Obesity as an independent risk factor for cardiovascular disease: A 26-year follow-up of participants in the Framingham Heart Study. *Circulation* **67**, 968–77.
19. Lapidus L, Bengtsson C, Larsson B, Pennert K, Rybo E, Sjöström L (1984). Distribution of adipose tissue and risk for cardiovascular disease and death: A 12 year follow-up of participants in the population study of women in Gotenburg, Sweden. *BMJ* **289**, 1257–61.
20. Donahue RP, Abbott RD, Bloom E, Reed DM, Yano K (1987). Central obesity and coronary heart disease in men. *Lancet* **8537**, 821–4.

21. Björntorp P, Brodoff BN (1992). *Obesity.* Lipincott, Philadelphia, PA.
22. Poehlman ET (1989). A review: Exercise and its influence on resting energy metabolism in man. *Med Sci Sports Exerc* **21**, 515–25.
23. Broeder CE, Burrhus KA, Svanevik LS, Wilmore JH (1992). The effects of either high intensity resistance or endurance training on resting metabolic rate. *Am J Clin Nutr* **55**, 802–10.
24. Bar-Or O, Baranowski T (1994). Physical activity, adiposity, and obesity among adolescents. *Pediatr Exerc Sci* **6**, 348–60.
25. Moussa MA, Skaik MB, Selwanes SB, Yaghy OY, Bin-Othman SA (1994). Factors associated with obesity in school children. *Int J Obes* **18**, 513–15.
26. Twisk JW, Kemper HC, van Mechelen W, Post GB, van Lenthe FJ (1998). Body fatness: Longitudinal relationship of body mass index and the sum of four skinfolds with other risk factors for coronary heart disease. *Int J Obes* **22**, 915–22.
27. Stern MP, Haffner SM (1986). Body fat distribution and hyperinsulinemia as risk factors for diabetes and cardiovascular disease. *Artheriosclerosis* **6**, 123–30.
28. Marti B, Tuomilehto J, Salomaa V, Kartovaara L, Korhonen HJ, Pietinen P (1991). Body fat distribution in the Finnish population: Environmental determinations and predictive power for cardiovascular risk factor levels. *J Epidemiol Comm Health* **45**, 131–7.
29. Seidell JC, Cigolini M, Deslypere JP, Charzewski J, Ellsinger BM (1991). Body fat distribution in relation to physical activity and smoking habits in 38-year old European man. *Am J Epidemiol* **133**, 257–65.
30. van Lenthe FJ, van Mechelen W, Kemper HC, Post GB (1998). Behavioral variables and development of body fat from adolescence into adulthood in normal-weight whites: The Amsterdam Growth and Health Study. *Am J Clin Nutr* **67**, 846–52.
31. Bergström E, Hernell O, Persson LA (1997). Endurance running performance in relation to cardiovascular risk indicators in adolescents. *Int J Sports Me* **18**, 300–7.
32. American Diabetes Association (2000). Type 2 diabetes in children and adolescents. *Diabetes Care* **23**, 381–9.
33. Goran MI, Ball GD, Cruz ML (2003). Obesity and risk of type 2 diabetes and cardiovascular disease in children and adolescents. *J Clin Endocrinol Metabol* **88**, 1417–27.
34. Helmrich SP, Ragland DR, Leung RW, Paffenbarger RS (1991). Physical activity and reduced occurrence of non-insulin-dependent diabetes mellitus. *N Engl J Med* **325**, 147–52.
35. Ivy JL (1987). The insulin-like effect of muscle contraction. *Exerc Sport Sci Rev* **15**, 29–51.
36. Vitug A, Schneider SH, Ruderman NB (1988). Exercise and Type I diabetes mellitus. *Exerc Sport Sci Rev* **16**, 285–304.
37. Raitakari OT, Porkka KV, Rasanen L, Viikari JS (1994). Relations of life-style with lipids, blood pressure and insulin in adolescents and young adults. The Cardiovascular Risk in Young Finns Study. *Atherosclerosis* **111**, 237–46.
38. Riddoch CJ (1998). Relationships between physical activity and health in young people. In: Biddle S, Sallis J, Cavill N (eds.), *Young and active? Young people and health-enhancing physical activity—evidence and implications*, pp. 17–48. Health Education Authority, London.
39. Nassis GP, Papantaku K, Skenderi K, Triandafillopoulou M, Kavouras SA, Yannakoulia M, Chrousos GP, Sidossis LS (2005). Aerobic exercise training improves insulin sensitivity without changes in body weight, body fat, adiponectin, and inflammatory markers in overweight and obese girls. *Metabolism* **54**, 1472–9.
40. Grundy SM (2006). Metabolic syndrome: Connecting and reconciling cardiovascular and diabetes worlds. *J Am Coll Cardiol* **47**, 1093–100.
41. Ford ES (2005). Risks for all-cause mortality, cardiovascular disease, and diabetes associated with the metabolic syndrome: A summary of the evidence. *Diabetes Care* **28**, 1769–78.
42. Duncan GE, Li SM, Zhou X-H (2004). Prevalence and trends of a metabolic syndrome phenotype among U.S. adolescents, 1999–2000. *Diabetes Care* **27**, 2348–443.
43. Jolliffe CJ, Janssen I (2007). Development of age-specific adolescent metabolic syndrome criteria that are linked to the adult Panel III and International Diabetes Federation Criteria. *J Am Coll Cardiol* **49**, 891–8.
44. Webber LS, Voors AW, Srinivasan SR, Frerichs RP, Berenson GS (1979). Occurrence in children of multiple risk factors for coronary heart disease: The Bogalusa Heart Study. *Prev Med* **8**, 407–18.
45. Khoury P, Morrison JA, Kelly K, Mellies M, Horvitz R, Glueck CJ (1980). Clustering and interrelationships of coronary heart disease risk factors in schoolchildren, ages 6–19. *Am J Epidemiol* **112**, 524–38.
46. Raitakari OT, Porkka KV, Räsänen L, Rönnemaa T, Viikari JS (1994). Clustering and six year cluster-tracking of serum total cholesterol, HDL-cholesterol and diastolic blood pressure in children and young adults. The Cardiovascular Risk in Young Finns Study. *J Clin Epidemiol* **47**, 1085–93.
47. Bao W, Srinivasan SR, Wattigney W, Berenson GS (1994). Persistence of multiple cardiovascular risk clustering related to syndrome X from childhood to young adulthood. The Bogalusa Heart Study. *Arch Int Med* **154**, 1842–7.
48. Ribeiro JC, Guerra S, Oliveira J, Teixeira-Pinto A, Twisk JW, Duarte JA, Mota J (2004). Physical activity and biological risk factors clustering in pediatric population. *Prev Med* **39**, 596–601.
49. Platat C, Wagner A, Klumpp T, Schweitzer B, Simon C (2006). Relationships of physical activity with metabolic syndrome features and low-grade inflammation in adolescents. *Diabetologia* **49**, 2078–85.
50. Brage S, Wedderkopp N, Ekelund U, Franks P, Wareham NJ, Andersen LB, Froberg K (2004). Features of the metabolic syndrome are associated with objectively measured physical activity and fitness in Danish children. *Diabetes Care* **27**, 2141–8.
51. Rizzo NS, Ruiz JR, Hurtig-Wennlof A, Ortega F, Sjöström M (2007). Relationships of physical activity, fitness, and fatness with clustered metabolic risk in children and adolescents: The European Youth Heart Study. *J Pediatr* **150**, 388–94.
52. Andersen LB, Harro M, Sardinha S, Froberg K, Ekelund U, Brage S (2006). Physical activity and clustered cardiovascular risk in children: A cross-sectional study (The European Youth Heart Study). *Lancet* **368**, 299–304.
53. Ekelund U, Brage S, Broberg K, Harro M, Anderssen AA, Sardinha LB, Riddoch C, Andersen LB (2006). TV viewing and physical activity are independently associated with metabolic risk in children: The European Youth Heart Study. *PLoS Med* **3**, e488.
54. Anderson LB, Wedderkopp N, Hansen HS, Cooper AR, Froberg K (2003). Biological risk factors cluster in Danish children and adolescents: The European Youth Heart Study. *Prev Med* **37**, 363–67.
55. Andersen LB, Hasselstrom H, Gronfeldt V, Hansen SE, Froberg K (2004). The relationship between physical fitness and clustered risk, and tracking from adolescence to young adulthood: Eight years follow-up in the Danish Youth and Sports Study. *Int J Behav Nutr Phys Act* **1**, 6.
56. Ruiz JR, Ortega FB, Meusel D, Harro M, Pekka O, Sjöström M (2006). Cardiorespiratory fitness is associated with features of metabolic risk factors in children. Should cardiorespiratory fitness be assessed in a European health monitoring system? The European Youth Heart Study. *J Pub Health* **14**, 94–102.
57. Torok K, Zselenyi Z, Porszasz J, Molnar D (2001). Low physical performance in obese adolescent boys with metabolic syndrome. *Int J Obes* **25**, 966–70.
58. Ferreira I, Twisk JW, van Mechelen W, Kemper HC, Stehouwer CD (2005). Development of fatness, fitness, and lifestyle from adolescence to the age of 36 years. Determinants of the metabolic syndrome in young adults: The Amsterdam Growth and Health Longitudinal Study. *Arch Int Med* **165**, 42–48.
59. Carnethon MR, Gidding SS, Nehgme R, Sidney S, Jacobs DR, Liu K (2003). Cardiorespiratory fitness in young adulthood and the development of cardiovascular disease risk factors. *JAMA* **290**, 3092–100.

60. Twisk JW, Kemper HC, van Mechelen W, Post GB (2001). Clustering of risk factors for coronary heart disease. The longitudinal relationship with lifestyle. *Ann Epidemiol* **11**, 157–65.
61. Twisk JW, Boreham C, Cran G, Savage JM, Strain J, van Mechelen W (1999). Clustering of biological risk factors for cardiovascular disease and the longitudinal relationship with lifestyle in an adolescent population: The Northern Ireland Young Hearts Project. *J Cardiovasc Risk* **6**, 355–62.
62. Hulshof KF, Wedel M, Löwik MR, Kok FJ, Kistemaker C, Hermus RJ, Hoor F ten, Ockhuizen Th (1992). Clustering of dietary variables and other lifestyle variables (Dutch Nutritional Surveillance System). *J Epidemiol Comm Health* **46**, 417–24.
63. Raitakari OT, Leino M, Räikkönen K, Porkka KV, Taimela S, Räsänen L, Viikari JS (1995). Clustering of risk habits in young adults, The Cardiovascular Risk in Young Finns Study. *Am J Epidemiol* **142**, 36–44.
64. Kilkens OJ, Gijtenbeek BA, Twisk JW, van Mechelen W, Kemper HC (1999). Clustering of lifestyle CVD risk factors and its relationship with biological CVD risk factors. *Pediatr Exerc Sci* **11**, 169–77.
65. Burke V, Milligan RA, Beilin LJ, Dunbar D, Spencer M, Balde E, Gracey MP (1997). Clustering of health-related behaviours among 18-year-old Australians. *Prev Med* **26**, 724–33.
66. Terre L, Drabman RS, Meydrech EF (1990). Relationships among children's health related behaviours: A multivariate developmental perspective. *Prev Med* **19**, 134–46.
67. Berenson GS, Arbeit ML, Hunter SM, Johnsson CC, Nicklas TA (1991). Cardiovascular health promotion for elementary school children. The Heart Smart Program. *Ann NY Acad Sci* **623**, 299–313.
68. Breslow JL (1985). Human apolipoprotein molecular biology and genetic variation. *Ann Rev Biochemics* **54**, 699–727.
69. Riesen WF, Mordasini R, Salzmann A, Theler A, Gurtner HP (1980). Apoproteins and lipids as discriminators of severity of coronary heart disease. *Atherosclerosis* **37**, 152–62.
70. De Backer G, Rosseneu M, Deslypere JP (1982). Discriminative value of lipids and apoproteins in coronary heart disease. *Atherosclerosis* **42**, 197–203.
71. Hamsten A, Walldius G, Dahlén G, Johansson B, Faire U de (1986). Serum lipoproteins and apolipoproteins in young male survivors of myocardial infarction. *Atherosclerosis* **59**, 223–35.
72. Armstrong VW, Cremer P, Eberle E, Manke A, Schulze F, Wieland H, Kreuzer H, Seidel A (1986). The association between serum Lp(a) concentrations and angiographically assessed coronary atherosclerosis: Dependence on serum LDL levels. *Atherosclerosis* **62**, 249–57.
73. Marai A, Miyahara T, Fujimoto N, Matsuda M, Kameyama M (1986). Lp(a) lipoprotein as a risk factor for coronary heart disease and cerebral infarction. *Atherosclerosis* **59**, 199–204.
74. Hasstedt SJ, Williams RR (1986). Three alleles for quantitative Lp(a). *Gen Epidemiol* **3**, 53–5.
75. Howard BV, Le NA, Belcher JD, Flack JM, Jacobs DR Jr, Lewis CE, Marcovina SM, Perkins LL (1994). Concentrations of Lp(a) in black and white young adults: Relations to risk factors for cardiovascular disease. *Ann Epidemiol* **4**, 341–50.
76. Taimela S, Viikari JS, Porkka KV, Dahlen GH (1994). Lipoprotein (a) levels in children and young adults: The influence of physical activity. The Cardiovascular Risk in Young Finns Study. *Acta Paediatr* **83**, 1258–63.
77. Hackman DG, Anand SS (2003). Emerging risk factors for atherosclerotic vascular disease. A critical review of the evidence. *JAMA* **290**, 932–40.
78. Ross R (1999). Atherosclerosis—an inflammatory disease. *N Eng J Med* **340**, 115–26.
79. Ridker PM (2003). High-sensitive C-reactive protein and cardiovascular risk: Rationale fro screening and primary prevention. *Am J Cardiol* **92** (Suppl.), 17K–22K.
80. Hamer M (2007). The relative influence of fitness and fatness on inflammatory factors. *Prev Med* **44**, 3–11.
81. Lee KW, Lip GY (2003). Effects of lifestyle on hemostasis, fibrinolysis, and platelet reactivity. A systematic review. *Arch Int Med* **163**, 2368–92.
82. Zahavi I, Yaari S, Salman H, Creter D, Rudnicki C, Brandis S, Ferrara M, Marom R, Katz M, Canetti M, Hart J, Goldbourt U (1996). Plasma fibrinogen in Israeli Moslem and Jewish school-children: Distribution and relation to other cardiovascular risk factors. The Petah Tikva project. *Israel J Med Sci* **32**, 1207–12.
83. Cook DG, Mendall MA, Whincup PH, Carey IM, Ballam L, Morris JE, Miller GJ, Strachan DP (2000). C-reactive protein concentration in children: Relationship to adiposity and other cardiovascular risk factors. *Atherosclerosis* **149**, 139–50.
84. Moran A, Lyn MS, Jacobs DR, Steinberger J, Pankowm JS, Hong C, Tracy RP, Sinaiko AR (2005). Relation of C-reactive protein to insulin resistance and cardiovascular risk factors in youth. *Diabetes Care* **28**, 1763–68.
85. Isasi CR, Starc TJ, Tracy RP, Deckelbaum R, Berglund L, Shea S (2000). Inverse association of physical fitness with plasma fibrinogen level in children: The Columbia University BioMarkers Study. *Am J Epidemiol* **152**, 212–18.
86. Isasi CR, Deckelbaum R, Tracy RP, Starc TJ, Berglund L, Shea S (2003). Physical fitness and C-reactive protein level in children and young adults: The Columbia University BioMarkers Study. *Pediatrics* **111**, 332–38.
87. Barbeau P, Litaker MS, Woods KF, Lemmon CR, Humphries MC, Owens S, Gutin B (2002). Hemostatic and inflammatory markers in obese youths: Effects of exercise and adiposity. *J Pediatr* **141**, 415–20.
88. Ferguson MA, Gutin B, Owens S, Barbeau P, Tracy RP, Litaker M (1999). Effects of physical training and its cessation in the hemostatic system of obese children. *Am J Clin Nutr* **69**, 1130–4.
89. Nygard O, Vollset SE, Refsum H, Stensvold I, Tverdal A, Nordrehaug JE, Ueland M, Kvale G (1995). Total plasma homocysteine and cardiovascular risk profile. The Hordaland Homocysteine Study. *JAMA*, **274**, 1526–33.
90. Gregoire J, Tuck S, Yamamoto Y, Highson RL (1996). Heart rate variability at rest and exercise: Influence of age, gender and physical training. *Can J Appl Physiol* **21**, 455–70.
91. Kupari M, Virolainen J, Koskinen P, Tikkanen MJ (1993). Short-term heart rate variability and factors modifying the risk of coronary heart disease in a population sample. *Am J Cardiol* **72**, 897–903.
92. Seals DR, Chase PB (1989). Influence of physical training on heart rate variability and baroflex circulatory control. *J Appl Physiol* **66**, 1886–95.
93. Taimela S, Lehtimaki T, Porkka KV, Rasanen L, Viikari JS (1996). The effect of physical activity on serum total and low-density lipoprotein cholesterol concentrations varies with apolipoprotein E phenotype in male children and young adults. The Cardiovascular Risk in Young Finns Study. *Metabol Clin Exper* **45**, 797–803.
94. O'Rourke M (1995). Mechanical principles in arterial disease. *Hypertension* **26**, 2–9.
95. Laurent S, Cockcroft J, Van Bortel L, Boutouyrie P, Giannattasio C, Hayoz D, Pannier B, Vlachopoulos C, Wilkinson I, Struijker-Boudier H (2006). European Network for Non-invasive Investigation of Large Arteries. Expert consensus document on arterial stiffness: Methodological issues and clinical applications. *Eur Heart J* **27**, 2588–605.
96. Reneman RS, Hoeks AP (2000). Noninvasive vascular ultrasound: An asset in vascular medicine. *Cardiovasc Res* **45**, 27–35.
97. Celermajer DS, Sorensen KE, Gooch VM, Spiegelhalter DJ, Miller OI, Sullivan ID, Lloyd JK, Deanfield JE (1992). Non-invasive detection of endothelial dysfunction in children and adults at risk of atherosclerosis. *Lancet* **340**, 1111–15.
98. Aggoun Y, Szezepanski I, Bonnet D (2005). Noninvasive assessment of arterial stiffness and risk of atherosclerotic events in children. *Pediatr Res* **58**, 173–8.
99. Charakida M, Tousoulis D, Stefanadis C (2006). Early atherosclerosis in childhood: Diagnostic approaches and therapeutic strategies. *Int J Cardiol* **109**, 152–9.

100. Davis PH, Dawson JD, Riley WA, Lauer RM (2001). Carotid intimal-medial thickness is related to cardiovascular risk factors measured from childhood through middle age: The Muscatine Study. *Circulation* **104**, 2815–19.
101. Li S, Chen W, Srinivasan SR, Bond MG, Tang R, Urbina EM, Berenson GS (2003). Childhood cardiovascular risk factors and carotid vascular changes in adulthood: The Bogalusa Heart Study. *JAMA* **290**, 2271–6.
102. Raitakari OT, Juonala M, Kahonen M, Taittonen L, Laitinen T, Maki-Torkko N, Jarvisalo MJ, Uhari M, Jokinen E, Ronnemaa T, Akerblom HK, Viikari JS (2003). Cardiovascular risk factors in childhood and carotid artery intima-media thickness in adulthood: The Cardiovascular Risk in Young Finns Study. *JAMA* **290**, 2277–83.
103. Ferreira I, Twisk JW, van Mechelen W, Kemper HC, Stehouwer CD (2002). Current and adolescent levels of cardiopulmonary fitness are related to large artery properties at age 36: The Amsterdam Growth and Health Longitudinal Study. *Eur J Clin Invest* **32**, 723–31.
104. Ferreira I, Twisk JW, van Mechelen W, Kemper HC, Seidell JC, Stehouwer CD (2003). Current and adolescent body fatness and fat distribution: Associations with carotid intima-media thickness and large-artery stiffness at the age of 36 years. *J Hypertension* **22**, 145–55.
105. Ferreira I, Twisk JW, van Mechelen W, Stehouwer CD, Kemper HC (2003). Longitudinal changes in $\dot{V}O_2$ max: Associations with carotid IMT and arterial stiffness. *Med Sci Sports Exerc* **35**, 1670–8.
106. Juonala M, Jarvisalo MJ, Maki-Torkko N, Kahonen M, Viikari JS, Raitakari OT (2005). Risk factors identified in childhood and decreased carotid artery elasticity in adulthood: The Cardiovascular Risk in Young Finns Study. *Circulation* **112**, 1486–93.
107. Twisk JW, Kemper HC, Mellenbergh GJ (1995). Longitudinal development of lipoprotein levels in males and females aged 12–28 years: The Amsterdam Growth and Health Study. *Int J Epidemiol* **24**, 69–77.
108. Montoye HJ, Kemper HC, Saris WH, Washburn RA (eds.) (1996). *Measuring physical activity and energy expenditure.* Human Kinetics, Champaign, IL.
109. Blair SN, Clark DG, Cureton KJ, Powell KE (1989). Exercise and fitness in childhood: Implications for a lifetime of health: In: Gisolfi CV, Lamb DR (eds.), *Perspectives in exercise science and sports medicine,* pp. 401–30. Benchmark Press, Indianapolis, IN.
110. Blair SN, Kohl HW, Barlow CE, Paffenbarger RS, Gibbons LW, Maccra CA (1995). Changes in physical fitness and all-cause mortality: A prospective study of healthy and unhealthy men. *JAMA* **273**, 1093–8.
111. Twisk JW, Kemper HC, van Mechelen W, Post GB (1997). Tracking of risk factors for coronary heart disease over a 14 year period: A comparison between lifestyle and biological risk factors with data from the Amsterdam Growth and Health Study. *Am J Epidemiol* **145**, 888–98.
112. Twisk JW, Kemper HC, Mellenbergh GJ (1994). The mathematical and analytical aspects of tracking. *Epidemiol Rev* **16**, 165–83.
113. Riddoch CJ, Boreham CAG (1995). The health related physical activity of children. *Sports Med* **19**, 86–102.
114. Biddle S, Sallis J, Cavill N (1998). Policy framework for young people and health-enhancing physical activity. In: Biddle S, Sallis J, Cavill N (eds.), *Young and active? Young people and health-enhancing physical activity—evidence and implications*, pp. 3–16. Health Education Authority, London.

CHAPTER 26

Gene–physical activity interactions and their role in determining cardiovascular and metabolic health

Paul W. Franks and Helen C. Looker

Introduction

Although cardiovascular and metabolic diseases such as hypertension, atherosclerosis, and type 2 diabetes have traditionally been deemed 'adult' diseases, their occurrence during childhood is becoming increasingly common.[1] The emergence of these diseases at a young age is almost certainly a consequence of the rapid corresponding increase in the prevalence of overweight and obesity in many industrialized societies during recent years.[2–7] The mechanisms for the causal relationship between obesity and cardiovascular and metabolic risk factors, which include gene–lifestyle interactions, are shown in Fig. 26.1.

Obesity occurs when chronic energy intake exceeds chronic energy expenditure. Thus, the epidemics of childhood obesity are likely to be caused by the decline in physical activity and the increased consumption of diets rich in animal fats and sugars that, in recent decades, have become commonplace in many societies. Despite the apparently simple explanation for the cause of obesity (i.e. a chronic positive energy balance), the long-term prevention or treatment of obesity is complex and often unsuccessful,[8] as evidenced by the progressive rise in the prevalence of childhood obesity in many of the world's industrialized nations. For example, between 2003 and 2004, 17.1% of U.S. children are estimated to have been overweight or obese[9] and similar prevalences have been

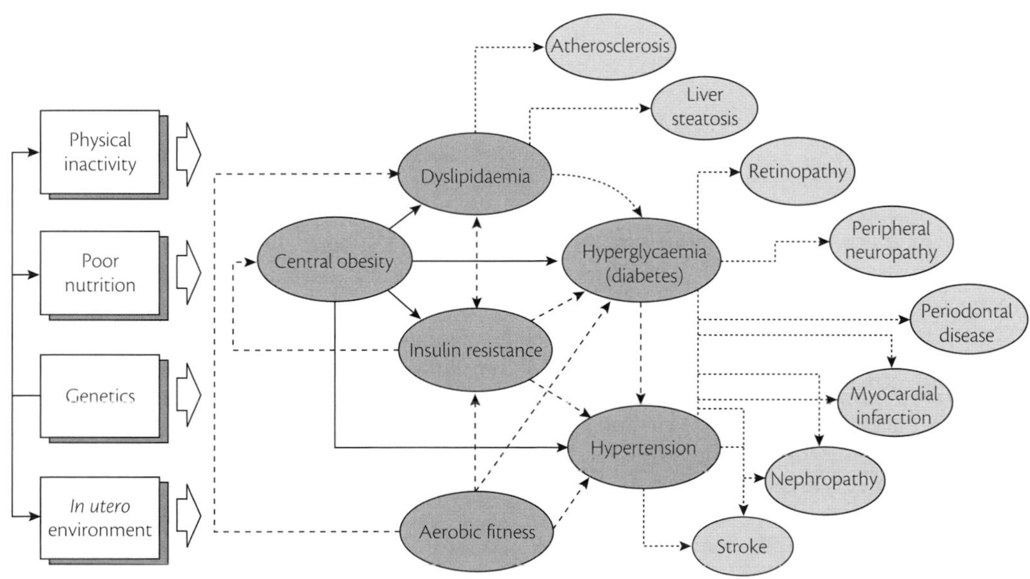

Fig. 26.1 Putative and known causal relationships between genetic and environmental exposures, features of the metabolic syndrome, and primary health outcomes. Reproduced from Huang *et al.*[1]

reported for contemporary European children.[3,4,7] Most projections conclude that these prevelances will increase dramatically during the next decade.

The difficulties in preventing obesity or sustaining weight loss indicate that obesity is a complex disease with intrinsic mechanisms of action that are resilient to an individual's often overwhelming desire to be lean. Thus, obesity most probably results from disturbances in the ability to regulate the intake and the expenditure of energy. This realization has prompted the search for genetic factors that regulate energetic behaviours.

The classic twin studies on overfeeding show that although weight gain is a natural consequence of short-[10] or long-term[11] overnutrition, the variance in the amount of weight gained within twin pairs is substantially less than the variance between twin pairs, suggesting that genetic factors influence the propensity for weight gain. The mechanisms through which genes might affect weight gain during childhood include behavioural drives (e.g. dietary nutrient preference[12,13] and the tendency to be physically active) and cellular mechanisms (e.g. energy uncoupling in the mitochondria[14,15]).

In modern, particularly Western, industrialized societies, a propensity for weight gain during childhood is generally disadvantageous owing to the negative impact on long-term health and longevity.[16,17] However, during human evolution, a propensity for weight gain was counterbalanced by environmental pressures for weight loss, such as famine, migration, or chronic exposure to cold environments. As argued by others, most notably Neel in his seminal paper on the thrifty genotype hypothesis,[18] those with a genetic predisposition to lay down energy reserves in the form of body fat may have gained a survival advantage during periods when food was scarce and energy demands were high. A survival advantage before and during the reproductive phase of life would be particularly important, because those with the highest level of reproductive fitness would be most likely to successfully pass on their genes to their offspring. Through this process, the selective pressures of physically demanding environments would have resulted in an enrichment of the genotypes associated with weight gain within certain populations. Hypothetically, populations that migrated furthest and which were exposed to the most energy demanding environments throughout evolution would have the greatest genetic propensity for weight gain. This is one possible explanation for the extreme levels of childhood obesity observed in populations such as Pima Indians[19] and the lower levels of obesity in European Caucasians.[20]

An important and largely unanswered question is whether genetic factors associated with common childhood obesity function by affecting behaviour. Although it is plausible, given what is known from animal models, that physical activity levels in children are under genetic control, genetic effects on behaviour are likely constricted or promoted by environmental factors.[21] Thus, even though, as is likely, genes exist that can directly influence activity-related behaviours, they may be difficult to detect during childhood when a child's behaviour is heavily influenced by his or her environment. The rationale for this argument becomes clearer when one considers that children in most societies are encouraged to attend school and participate in family and other social activities, and the decision on whether or not to do so is seldom that of the child alone. Restrictions on where, when and how children can play, because of safety or a lack of access to facilities, are also likely to affect the expression of genetically mediated behaviours in children. Thus, interactions between genes and lifestyle factors may be more relevant in the context of understanding children's health-related behaviours than the independent effects of genes and the environment.

Studies that seek to determine the mechanisms that underlie these behavioural defects and the way in which physical activity interacts with genetic factors may help improve our understanding of how and why children become obese and develop cardiovascular risk factors, how these children should be treated, and ultimately how the development of cardiovascular risk in childhood can be prevented.

Genetics of common disease—background and principles

The study of genetics has given rise to a number of terms and concepts and the following section is intended to provide a guide to the language of genetics, which when reading this chapter or other related material might be useful to those with little or no previous exposure to this sometimes convoluted field of research.

While environmental exposures vary through life our genes are with us unchanged from birth. Therefore, one important characteristic of a child's genotype is that it may indicate (predict) risk for later disease, even though no other pathology is evident. For example, identifying a marker for risk for cardiovascular disease could theoretically be done in infancy before any overt evidence of atheroma had developed. This is attractive in that it may allow us to identify people at risk of disease at a very early stage of the disease process. The caveat of genetic screening, which we will not discuss in this chapter, but is necessary to highlight, is that knowing one is at genetic risk may by some be perceived as a burden and thus adversely affect quality of life (see Khoury *et al.*[22] for an in depth discussion of this topic).

Genetic information is arranged on chromosomes and for autosomal chromosomes we inherit two copies of each chromosome, one from each parent. As a result we have two copies of all genes. A person's genotype is the genetic code for both gene copies whilst the haplotype specifically refers to the genetic code on a single chromosomal arm. During meiosis, genes can cross over from one chromosome arm to another and as a result mutations become separated and the chromosome inherited by the offspring is not necessarily an identical copy of the parental chromosome. These crossovers are termed translocations and they are the basis for the measurement of genetic distance as well as for linkage analysis and association studies. This is because due to translocations two markers that are originally on a single chromosome will not always remain on the same chromosome for subsequent generations. The probability of a translocation occurring between two loci depends, in part, on the distance between the two loci. The closer the loci are the less likely a translocation will occur and the greater the distance the more likely. The centiMorgan unit for genetic distance is defined as the distance between two points on a chromosome that is associated with a 1% chance of translocation. Translocations are not wholly dependent on distance as some areas of the genome experience far more translocations than others; the reason for this is not yet known. In addition to genetic distance, now that direct genotyping is possible, physical distance can be established and is given as the number of base pairs between two points. Linkage disequilibrium (LD) is a key concept in statistical genetics. Consider two loci, A and B on a chromosome both of which have two alleles

a_1 and a_2 and b_1 and b_2. We would expect that if the markers are transmitted independently the frequency of finding the a_1b_1 haplotype would depend entirely on the relative frequencies of the a_1 and b_1 alleles. However, if the observed frequency of the a_1b_1 haplotype is different from the predicted frequency it would suggest that the two loci were transmitted together more often than expected by chance and thus would be said to be in LD with each other. The degree of LD between two loci is often expressed as D′ (pronounced 'D-prime'), which is 1 for two loci in perfect LD and 0 when two loci are in perfect linkage equilibrium. The frequency for alleles at both loci is factored in to the calculation of D′, as unless the allele frequencies are identical, two loci will never be in perfect LD. However, when two alleles have a D′ of 1 knowing the genotype at one locus tells you what the allele at the other locus will be without needing to measure it. This has led to the identification of so-called haplotype blocks, which are regions of the genome containing markers in strong LD. Because of this, it is sufficient to genotype a single marker from a haplotype block rather than all the markers with each block. These single markers are called 'tagging single nucleotide polymorphisms (tag-SNPs)'. The use of tag-SNPs is not without limitations, but the method is financially economic.

So what constitute 'genetic markers'? Basically they represent any variation within the genetic code which can be a series of additional repeated sequences or a simple substitution of a nucleotide. The latter are termed single nucleotide polymorphisms (SNPs) and millions have been identified across the genome. The majority of SNPs found have not been seen to directly lead to a change in gene function (i.e. there is no change in the quality or amount of protein produced) and many are not located within a gene. Occasionally, a SNP will be functional and its presence results in for instance an amino acid substitution in the code for a protein or the production of a truncated protein. SNPs are important for genetic research primarily because they can be used as stable markers. The value of a SNP as a marker usually depends on its minor allele frequency being of at least 1% in the population being studied (not all SNPs are polymorphic in every population) and the SNP not being in complete LD with other SNPs that have been measured. While it is unknown at the outset, the most powerful marker in theory will be the one in strongest LD with the unknown functional SNP. More often, marker SNPs that are observed to be strongly associated with a disease phenotype are consequently assumed to be in high LD with the unknown functional variant, which may prompt more detail genotyping (sequencing) of the chromosomal regions proximal to the marker SNP in an attempt to discover the causal locus.

The phenotype is the physical measure of interest that results from the combination of genes and environment. Phenotypes include hair colour, height, blood glucose levels, and behaviours, for example. Most phenotypes are influenced by environmental as well as genetic factors. Thus, in contrast to a genotype, which does not change over time, a phenotype can change with time and environment. Phenotypes need to be well characterized in genetic studies as a poorly defined phenotype will limit any ability to identify genes associated with it. In some studies a dichotomous variable is required, for example, obese versus lean, while other studies can include a continuously distributed variable, for example, body mass index (BMI). In general, studies of continuously distributed traits are more powerful than studies that use dichotomous traits (see Ragland[23] for an extended discussion of this point). The models that test genetic associations with phenotypic variables may also be adjusted for other factors known to influence the relationship, such as age and ethnicity. The factors that one might select to adjust for should either by confounders or effect-mediators.

The rules of confounding that are applied to conventional tests of associations between two factors differ somewhat in genetic studies from non-genetic studies. This is because, for confounding to occur in a genetic association study, the confounder must influence the distribution of the genotypes. Age can indirectly influence the distribution of genotypes within a population if people with a risk genotype die younger than those without that genotype. This process can result in lower than expected risk genotype frequencies in the observed fraction of the population who have the disease phenotype, which can lead to an incorrect conclusion about the magnitude or even the direction of the association between the genotype and the disease trait. Ethnicity can also cause confounding in genetic association studies, because the haplotype structure and the frequencies of disease traits may simultaneously, but coincidently, differ between ethnic groups, giving the impression of association when no causal relationship exists. However, in large, normally distributed population samples, biologic, anthropometric, or behavioural traits are less likely to confound genetic associations with disease traits, because these factors cannot influence the genotype of an individual. When these traits fall on the causal pathway between the gene and the phenotype, they are termed effect-mediators, the meaning of which is discussed below. For a more detailed discussion on effect mediation and confounding in genetic association studies, see ref. 24.

Genetic studies in humans can be divided into family studies and population association studies. Family studies range from simple calculations of familial aggregation through to the more complex linkage studies. Using phenotype data alone and by comparing the segregation of the phenotype within and between family members, one can estimate the heritability of a disease trait. Although often defined as such, most classical estimates of heritability are not direct evidence of genetic involvement in the disease, as in addition to shared genes family members also share many environmental factors that may influence a phenotype. Twin studies are a specialized form of family study and allow a better separation of the environmental factors from the genetic factors. Monozygotic (identical) twins are genetically identical, whilst dizygotic (fraternal) twins share on average 50% of their genetic information. Therefore, in a condition wholly attributable to a genetic cause we would predict complete concordance between monozygotic twins but only 50% concordance for dizygotic twins. Using structural equation modelling in twin data the phenotypic variance can be apportioned to the genetic component, the shared environment component, and an individual environment component.

Linkage studies also require family data. These studies essentially involve the comparison of the genotype at a marker, the concordance for the phenotype, and the segregation of genotypes and phenotypes within and between family units. The theory being that if a marker loci is close to the functional mutation responsible for the phenotype there will be a lower rate of recombination between that marker loci and the functional mutation and so in family members concordant for the phenotype they will also be concordant at the marker loci. Results from linkage analyses are usually expressed in terms of a LOD score, which stands for 'logarithm of odds' and essentially represents the log of the ratio of the probability of the observed recombination rate at the marker and the probability of the recombination rate if there was no linkage—the null hypothesis. Logarithm of odds scores above three are considered as demonstrating statistically significant linkage, though lower values are often taken as suggestive of linkage. Linkage studies are used to identify areas on the genome that may contain genes responsible for the phenotype, but they do not have sufficient power to pin point the specific gene responsible for the linkage signal. When the phenotype is a continuum rather than a dichotomous trait (e.g. BMI as opposed to obesity) the area identified is termed a quantitative trait locus (QTL). Linkage studies are generally followed up by fine mapping studies (sequencing), which focus on the identified genomic region defined by the linkage signal. This requires a denser selection of markers and the use of association studies.

Association studies make use of population data from unrelated individuals. Association studies compare the frequency of a specific allele at a marker with the presence or absence of the phenotype (or the level of the phenotype if it is a continuous trait). Association studies can be done using markers within single genes or across the whole genome. Conventionally, association studies have primarily focused on the candidate gene approach, which makes use of existing biological evidence to select a specific gene to be studied. This evidence is often derived from animal, *in vitro,* or extreme phenotype human studies. The limitation of this approach is that genes are only selected if there is prior evidence that they might be involved in the disease process and thus truly novel discoveries are not possible. In contrast, the new approach to studying human disease genetics involves genotyping hundreds of thousands of SNPs located across the human genome; these studies are referred to as genome-wide association studies. The very recent first reports from the GWAS approach have proven highly successful in discovering genetic variations in common human diseases such as type 2 diabetes and obesity,[25–29] three of which extended their findings to paediatric cohorts.[30,31] The main caveat to the GWAS approach is that owing to the multiple hypothesis tests that are performed, many of the SNPs that are highly statistically significantly associated with a disease phenotype are false-positive (i.e. the association is due to chance, and no true biological relationship between the SNP and the disease exists). Thus, distinguishing between the highly significant, yet false-positive associations from the true positive associations has proven difficult. Moreover, because association tests assess the association between the alleles and a phenotype, it is not apparent how best to allow for the importance of being heterozygous for a 'risk allele' versus being homozygous for the 'risk allele'. By consequence, multiple models will often be run to compare combinations of alleles within a SNP. These combinations are referred to as 'additive', where each of the three genotypes at a locus are assumed to have a linear effect on the phenotype (i.e. XX vs. Xx vs. xx), 'recessive', where the carriers of the most common allele are compared with those carrying both copies of the minor allele (i.e. XX + Xx vs. xx), and 'dominant' where people who carry both copies of the most common allele are compared with those who carry at least one copy of the minor allele (i.e. XX vs. Xx + xx). Without knowing the effect of the unknown functional mutation on the phenotype it is impossible to determine the most biologically appropriate model *a priori.*

Genetic studies are not confined to studies of DNA. Gene expression studies are used to examine how expression of certain genes varies by phenotype under various conditions. These studies examine the transcription of genes by measuring the messenger RNA (mRNA) produced. Unlike a genotype which remains the same throughout life regardless of phenotypic changes and is present in all cells, gene expression varies between cell types and according to specific environmental stimuli. Gene expression studies can be used to examine the differences in mRNA levels between patients with a specific disease phenotype and healthy controls, and how these levels differ in each of the two groups in response to specific stimuli such as exercise training or pharmacotherapy. For example, we can measure basal gene expression in muscle cells for lean and obese subjects and also measure gene expression in the same subjects in response to weekly aerobic exercise training. These studies can help determine whether people who are characterized by different disease phenotypes respond differently at a genetic level to treatment. Such studies are extremely rare in children owing to the degree of invasiveness involved in tissue collection. Gene expression studies can be restricted to examine expression levels for a pre-selected set of genes which are related to a proposed mechanism. Alternatively, microarrays are often used as a hypothesis generating tool whereby the expression of hundreds of thousands of genes are tested simultaneously, with those showing the greatest difference in expression being prioritized for more detailed examination. As with GWAS, the results from studies that test differences in gene expression between sets of genes are prone to a high percentage of false-positive findings and thus require careful adjustment to account for multiple hypothesis testing.

Another valuable tool for genetic studies is the use of animal models. It is possible to create animals that lack the gene of interest (knockout animals) or alternatively overexpress the gene (transgenically overexpressing animals). This allows the study of the phenotype associated with the specific genetic intervention. These studies can be used to prove a gene has a causative role in the development of a phenotype.

Statistical tests of gene–lifestyle interactions in epidemiological data are intended to determine whether a genetic factor influences the relationship between a lifestyle exposure and a disease-related trait. The term gene–lifestyle interaction (or gene–environment interaction) is often used to describe slightly different concepts. In epidemiological studies, gene–lifestyle interactions are determined by testing the magnitude of the association between the environmental exposure (e.g. physical activity) and a disease outcome, and comparing the strength of this association between different genotypes at a given genetic locus. If the difference in the magnitude of the physical activity–disease association is statistically significant between genotypes, a gene–physical activity interaction is said to exist [see Figs. 26.2 (a) and (b)]. This concept is also referred to as effect-modification. In biology, however, an interaction is said to occur when, for example, two proteins combine to jointly influence the expression of phenotype. In this sense, the presence of interaction is evidence that the two proteins share the same biological pathway and act in a coordinated way to influence the phenotype. In epidemiology, this concept would usually be referred to as effect-mediation (as described above). In this chapter, we will use the first definition of interaction outlined above.

The paradox of genetically determined disease in childhood

Although the patterns of variation in the susceptibility to obesity and its sequelae indicate the involvement of genetic factors,[21]

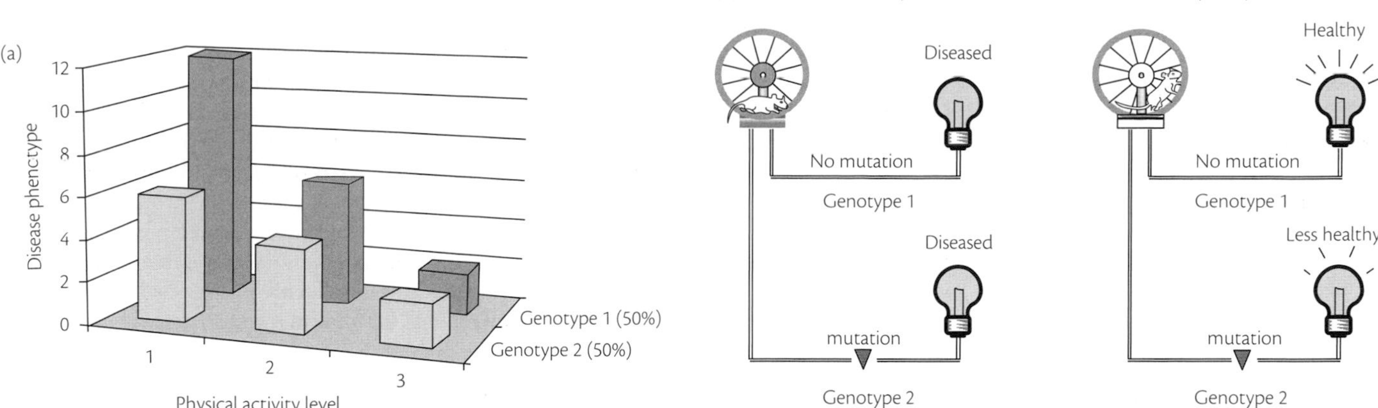

Fig. 26.2 (a) A gene–lifestyle interaction occurs when the relationships between lifestyle exposure and a disease phenotypic differ in magnitude when stratified by a genetic subgroup (genotype). (b) A model for gene–exercise interaction. Loss of function occurs when the genetic circuitry is disrupted and when the environmental triggers are absent. In this example, the phenotypic effects of exercise are blunted in carriers of the genetic mutation because the ability of the genetic circuitry to mediate the signal of exercise is impeded.

marked changes in the structure of the human genome require many, many generations of out-breeding which take many thousands of years to occur. Thus, the magnitude of change in genomic structure during the past 50 years is insufficient to explain the corresponding rise in the prevalences of most common diseases. This presents a paradox; how can diseases which were rare until relatively recently but that are now increasingly common have a strong genetic basis without changes having occurred in the structure of the human genome? One possible explanation for this paradox is that genetic and environment factors interact, such that genes which may have had little influence on survival throughout the majority of human evolution are now activated by modern environmental triggers to cause disease.

A test of this hypothesis would be to take people with a high genetic risk of disease and transport them back in time to an era when the environmental triggers were absent, and observe whether the symptoms of disease in these individuals and their offspring are reduced. A realistic alternative to the time travel experiment is to randomly assign individuals at high risk of disease to receive an intensive 'lifestyle' intervention, where physical activity and healthy diets are encouraged, and compare the progression to disease with a group of high-risk individuals who are assigned to a normal treatment 'control' group. If the genetic risk factors for the disease favourably interact with lifestyle factors, one would expect the rates of disease progression to differ significantly by genotype in the control group, but to be similar irrespective of genotype in the lifestyle intervention group. With this evidence, one might conclude that the recent shift away from our evolutionary environment, where physical inactivity and energy dense diets were rare, towards the modern industrialized environment, where these factors are common, has increased the risk of disease attributable to specific genotypes.

One example in adults where this experiment has been carried out is in the Diabetes Prevention Program (DPP). The DPP was a multi-centre randomized clinical trial in which the effects of anti-diabetic drugs and intensive lifestyle intervention on the incidence of type 2 diabetes were assessed. A total of 3500 non-diabetic individuals with impaired glucose regulation were randomized to receive normal treatment (control), the anti-diabetic drug metformin, or a lifestyle intervention programme aimed at ~7% reduction in body weight, ~150 min of physical activity per week, and a reduced consumption of dietary saturated fats and sugars. The principal end point was the development of diabetes within 4 years by confirmed oral glucose tolerance testing. In that study, the incidence of diabetes at 4 years post-randomization was 58% lower in the lifestyle intervention group than in the control group.[32] In a subsequent study within the DPP, individuals were genotyped for variants in the *TCF7L2* gene,[33] a gene that had previously been associated with type 2 diabetes in Danish, Icelandic, and American cohorts.[34] As in the initial study, the rarer form of this genotype (TT) was associated with a two-fold greater risk of developing diabetes compared with the common CC genotype in people assigned to the control group. However, in people assigned to the lifestyle intervention group, the risk of developing diabetes was similar irrespective of which *TCF7L2* genotype an individual had. These observations suggest that intensive lifestyle intervention may reduce the genetic risk of developing diabetes that is attributable to the *TCF7L2* TT genotype in people with 'normal' lifestyles.

Very few examples presently exist where gene–lifestyle interactions on cardiovascular risk factors have been assessed in children, and no clinical trials testing such hypotheses in children are presently available. This may be partly because of the ethical circumstances related to genetic studies in children, or that few large studies of children exist where lifestyle behaviours have been assessed using sufficiently precise and unbiased methods to permit meaningful assessments of gene–lifestyle interactions. One of the few studies published on this topic was undertaken in 1016 Greek adolescents aged 11–18 years.[35] In that study, Moran *et al.*[35] genotyped three angiotensin I-converting enzyme (ACE) polymorphisms and assessed them for association and interaction with lifestyle behaviours on obesity-related traits. No significant associations were observed for two of the variants (rs4424958, rs4311) in males or females. In females only, the authors found statistically significant associations with tricep and subscapular skinfolds for the third variant (an insertion/deletion polymorphism). The authors also undertook analyses stratified by self-reported activity levels, in which significant associations with obesity traits were observed in the inactive (n = 207), but not in physically active (n = 274) females. The authors concluded that these observations indicate the presence of gene–physical activity interaction, although no formal statistical test for interaction was reported to support that conclusion.

Genetic determinants of physical activity and aerobic fitness

Physical activity

Few studies in children have reported on the relationships between genetic factors and physical activity. One reason for this, aside from the specific ethical considerations when studying children, might be that heritability studies have traditionally used questionnaires to assess physical activity, and these methods are unsuitable for use with children due to unacceptable levels of error and bias,[36] whereas objective assessment methods, which are less prone to error and bias, are frequently perceived as infeasible for use in large studies.

To our knowledge, only three studies have been reported in which genetic determinants of physical activity were assessed. Two of these reports emanate from the Viva la Familia Study, which incorporated objective assessments of physical activity via uniaxial accelerometry in more than 1000 Hispanic children from 319 families aging from 4 to 19 years. In that study, 32–60% of the variance in physical activity was attributed to inherited factors (genetic variation and the family environment).[37] In the second report from the Viva la Familia Study using the classical linkage approach,[38] a region of chromosome 18 was identified as the putative locus for a gene(s) for physical inactivity; the LOD score for total physical activity was 2.28, and for time spent sedentary whilst awake, the LOD score was 4.07. Interestingly, the chromosomal region identified in that study flanks the melanocortin 4 receptor (*MC4R*) gene, the relevance of which we discuss below.

In the initial published study to report on the genetics of physical activity in children, we used the gold-standard method, doubly labelled water, to assess physical activity energy expenditure in 200 twins aged 4–10 years.[21] Owing to the design of that study, we were able to partition out the variance in physical activity attributable to genetic factors from the variance attributable to environmental factors. Although in our study, familial factors explained a large fraction of the variance in physical activity energy expenditure (mean variance 69%; 95% CI = 33–77%), no significant genetic effect was detectable (mean variance 0%; 95% CI = 0–32%). We concluded that the effects of the common environment, such as the attitudes and actions of parents and school teachers, and accessibility to facilities that promote physical activity (e.g. play areas) or sedentary behaviours (e.g. watching TV and playing computer games), constrict genetic influences on physical activity to the point where no association is detectable. We also suggested that the extent to which these environmental factors constrict the expression of genetic effects in childhood may diminish as the child ages and as environmental constraints relax. This hypothesis is supported by observations in Dutch adolescents. In a study of 821 monozygotic and 809 dizygotic twin pairs, Stubbe *et al.*[39] assessed the genetic and environmental influences on self-reported physical activity. The authors observed that between the ages of 13 and 16 years, shared environmental factors explained 78–84% of the individual differences in sport participation and genetic factors explained none of the variance in this phenotype; between 17 and 18 years of age, genetic influences had emerged and accounted for approximately one third of the variation in sports participation; in the oldest adolescents (18–12 years), genetic influences explained roughly 85% of the variance in sports participation.

Although genetic variation may have little detectable influence on activity-related behaviours in the presence of strong environmental factors, it is important to consider which genes and pathways of genes might influence the propensity for spontaneous physical activity in settings where environmental factors have less influence on behaviour. This is important so that one can begin to understand the molecular mechanisms that influence physical activity, particularly those also involved in gene–lifestyle interactions. Such mechanisms may involve the actions of neuroendocrine hypothalamic signalling hormones, for example, leptin, neuromodulin, and orexin-A.

The leptin hormone is secreted from adipose tissue and binds to receptors in the hypothalamus to control energy balance, reproductive function and maturation. Mice deficient in hypothalamic leptin receptors are hypoactive and develop features of the metabolic syndrome.[40] Selectively restoring leptin signalling in the arcuate nucleus of these animals markedly increased locomotor activity. A possible indirect pathway through which leptin influences the behaviour of physical activity is via activation of *MC4R* in the arcuate nucleus, a notion which is supported by animal and human studies.[41–44] Moreover, *MC4R* gene mutations cause childhood obesity, although this has largely been attributed to disturbances of appetite regulation[45] and not physical inactivity. In cross-sectional and prospective studies of adults, plasma leptin levels are, independently of obesity, associated with physical inactivity in adults[46,47] and children[48,49] and increased risk of cardiovascular and metabolic disease.[50] In the adult studies, higher leptin concentrations appear disadvantageous, which directly contrasts findings in leptin-deficient animals and humans where leptin infusion improves health and stimulates physical activity. These disparities may, analogous to other endocrine hormones such as insulin, result from a U-shaped relationship between leptin and health outcomes.

In contrast to the findings in adult studies, studies of leptin and physical activity in children, reported either no association or a positive association between leptin concentrations and physical activity.[48,49,51] Thus, it is possible that hormonal changes during puberty or other environmental factors associated with childhood influence the effects of leptin on behaviour.

Aerobic fitness

A low level of aerobic fitness is a strong predictor of type 2 diabetes, cardiovascular disease, and early mortality.[52,53] Aerobic fitness and physical activity levels correlate in children,[20] as they do in adults.[54] The mechanisms through which aerobic fitness influences disease risk involve decreases in the capacity to oxidize lipids and glucose due to defects in mitochondrial function (see Fig. 26.1). Numerous reports exist of rare genetic defects that influence aerobic fitness levels, several of which cause exercise intolerance via mitochondrial defects.[55–57] Although these rare cases may provide insight into the origins of common genetic risk factors for low aerobic fitness, the details of the genetic risk variants for common cases of low aerobic fitness (if they indeed exist) remain to be determined.

Given that exercise intervention increases aerobic fitness levels in children, some of the effects of low fitness levels on cardiovascular and metabolic disease traits can be modified by increasing physical activity levels.[58] In a study of around 400 Danish school children from the European Youth Heart Study (EYHS), we assessed the relationships between physical activity and aerobic fitness with a metabolic syndrome score.[59] In that study we observed an interaction between physical activity and fitness, which indicated that the children who were sedentary and had high aerobic fitness levels had similar levels of the metabolic syndrome score as the children who were physically active and unfit. As one might predict, the children who were unfit and sedentary had the highest levels of the metabolic syndrome score, and those who were active and fit, had the lowest levels. We observed similar relationships between physical activity and fitness with the metabolic syndrome score in adults,[60] and when Ekelund *et al.*[61] and Andersen *et al.*[20] extended our findings to children from across Europe, their conclusions were similar. These studies suggest that children who can maintain moderate to high levels of aerobic fitness when physically inactive are protected against cardiovascular and metabolic disease. Although our study was not designed to ascertain which factors might help preserve aerobic fitness in sedentary children, it suggests that some children are genetically predetermined to maintain moderate to high levels of aerobic fitness, irrespective of their activity levels.

A strong candidate gene for aerobic fitness and metabolic health *per se* is the peroxisome proliferator-activated receptor gamma, coactivator 1 alpha (*PPARGC1A*). We have examined the relationship between *PPARGC1A* and metabolic fitness in a number of studies. In one study of nearly 9000 adults, we confirmed that the minor serine allele (Ser) at the Gly482Ser genotype is associated with type 2 diabetes,[62] and that this allele is significantly less frequent in elite endurance runners and cyclists than in unfit non-diabetic population controls.[63] Only one study in adolescents on *PPARGC1A* genotypes has been reported to date, and that study from Argentina focused on associations with the features of the metabolic syndrome.[64]

The *PPARGC1A* gene is an exercise-responsive transcriptional coactivator of a complex pathway of genes involved in mitochondrial biogenesis, oxidative fibre formation, and oxidative phosphorylation.[65] Owing to our earlier observations, we hypothesized that the *PPARGC1A* gene and its downstream molecular targets might be involved in modulating the relationships between physical activity and metabolic fitness in children. Therefore, as described later in this chapter, we recently embarked on a project to assess the relationships between variants at the *PPARGC1A* locus and its downstream targets with aerobic fitness and the features of the metabolic syndrome in more than 3000 children from across Europe (the EYHS). We anticipate that the first results from that study will be available in 2008.

Biological and anthropometric markers of cardiovascular and metabolic risk during childhood

As cardiovascular disease rarely manifests clinically until adulthood studies of risk factors assessed during childhood are limited. In their place studies make use of tracking of known risk factors for cardiovascular or metabolic disease from childhood into adulthood, autopsy studies which can associate risk factors with autopsy evidence of early cardiovascular disease and, cross-sectional associations with subclinical evidence of early cardiovascular disease. Here we will consider the evidence in children for the commonly identified risk factors for cardiovascular disease in adults, which include obesity, hyperglycaemia, hypertension, and dyslipidaemia, as well as the metabolic syndrome. As with adults, each element is potentially modifiable by lifestyle changes, including alterations in the level of physical activity and physical fitness, though as yet evidence is scant to show-long term benefits from exercise interventions during childhood.

Obesity

The most commonly available early life measure of growth is birth weight, which has been studied extensively. Barker *et al.*[66] described an association between low birth weight and standardized mortality rates for coronary heart disease in British men and this finding has been confirmed in many populations.[67–69] In addition, low birth weight has been found to be associated with type 2 diabetes and insulin resistance, hypertension, and the metabolic syndrome.[70,71] However, at least within the Pima Indians where there is a high prevalence of diabetes during pregnancy there is a U-shaped relationship between birth weight and diabetes, with higher birth weight associated with exposure to diabetes *in utero*.[72]

Defining unhealthy weight in childhood is much less straightforward than it is in adults where the BMI categories for overweight and obesity are often used. Because children are growing, weight must be considered in relation to age and gender. Abnormal weight values are determined primarily by the distance from the population mean and are primarily given as *z*-scores or being above a specific percentile based on population growth charts.[73]

Weight 'tracks' through childhood, meaning that an overweight child is at high risk of becoming an overweight adult.[74,75] Childhood obesity is associated with a range of cardiovascular risk factors. For example, flow-mediated dilatation is impaired in obese children compared to non-obese children with obese children having similar results to children with type 1 diabetes.[76] Furthermore, excess adiposity in very young children is associated with early pathological evidence of cardiovascular disease,[77] and carotid intimal thickening measured in adults is associated with childhood BMI, though this may be mediated by adult BMI.[75]

Rapid weight gain in low birth weight children may also represent a particularly high risk group for future obesity.[78] Rapid weight gain in the first year of life is also associated with a higher risk for obesity in adulthood.[79] In contrast, a retrospective study of men with and without cardiovascular disease found that the men who went on to develop cardiovascular disease had both lower birth weight than their contemporaries without cardiovascular disease but also had poorer growth in the first year of life before rapid growth subsequently.[80] Poor early growth was also predictive of higher risk for type 2 diabetes in adulthood.[81]

Glucose

Type 1 diabetes is associated with premature cardiovascular disease in young adults and is associated with the usually observed lower prevalence of cardiovascular in women.[82,83] Tight glucose control in subjects with type 1 diabetes is associated with a reduction in risk for cardiovascular disease in adults[84] but it is unclear if the same is true in prepubertal children. However, in children and adolescents with type 1 diabetes flow-mediated vasodilatation, a marker of endothelial dysfunction, is associated with glucose concentrations.[85] Type 2 diabetes is becoming increasingly common in children but as yet no studies have reported the role of tight glucose control in young people with type 2 diabetes and cardiovascular disease. In the absence of diabetes, glucose concentrations in childhood along with weight are independent predictors of incident type 2 diabetes.[86] In non-diabetic children, glyceryl trinitrate mediated dilatation, a measure of vascular smooth muscle function, is negatively associated with fasting glucose concentrations.[76]

Blood pressure

Similar to weight, blood pressure tracks through childhood into adulthood.[87] Definitions of what constitutes high blood pressure in children are not clear but autopsy studies have found high blood pressure to be associated with the presence of early atheromatous lesions in childhood.[77] Blood pressure is highly correlated with BMI in children.[88] Elevated blood pressure in 5–7 year olds predicts hypertension in adults and elevated blood pressure in children aged 8–13 years is associated with a greater than two-fold risk of metabolic syndrome as an adult.[89] A single measure of systolic blood pressure in childhood is not associated with left ventricular mass after adjustment for BMI but the area under the curve for repeated measures of blood pressure in childhood is significantly positively associated with left ventricular mass.[90] In contrast, carotid intima-media thickness assessed in adults is associated with childhood systolic blood pressure after adjustment for age, sex, and childhood BMI, though only borderline significant after adjustment for adult systolic blood pressure.[75]

Lipids

The Bogalusa Heart Study reported good tracking of total cholesterol as well as the cholesterol subfractions from childhood into early adulthood.[91] In addition, children in the top quartile for low-density lipoprotein (LDL) or non-high-density lipoprotein (HDL) cholesterol were at increased risk for dyslipidaemia as adults independent of childhood BMI and change in BMI between measures.[92] Elevated concentrations of both were also associated with adult obesity while non-HDL cholesterol was additionally predictive of greater adult insulin resistance and hyperglycaemia. Autopsy studies show a positive association between serum LDL and triglycerides with aortic and coronary atheroma in children and young adults,[77] but as of yet no studies have reported a direct association between childhood cholesterol concentrations and later cardiovascular disease. However, the American Heart Association has now issued guidelines for the management of cholesterol in children already at high risk for cardiovascular disease due to the presence of conditions such as familial hypercholesterolaemia, diabetes, chronic kidney disease- and Kawasaki disease.[93]

Metabolic syndrome

As in adults, there is a tendency for the above risk factors to cluster in children and various groups have tried to define a paediatric 'metabolic syndrome' using age–sex appropriate cut points. Different studies have employed a variety of definitions and though all include a measure of adiposity (BMI or waist circumference), lipids (triglycerides and HDL-cholesterol), blood pressure, and glucose, the prevalence of metabolic syndrome reported is highly dependent on the definition used. Applying the different definitions to a single group provided prevalence estimates ranging from 0 to 26.3%.[94] Studies that compare the prevalence of metabolic syndrome in obese and non-obese children have consistently reported extremely low prevalence in normal weight children compared with obese children demonstrating the centrality of obesity to this syndrome in children.[95] In the Bogalusa Heart Study, clustering of metabolic syndrome variables measured in childhood tracked into adulthood.[96] In the same population clustering of the risk variables at the lowest quartile was also demonstrated with a frequency greater than predicted if the factors were not associated and there was a significant trend for greater carotid intima-media thickness in young adults and the fewer number of risk variables clustering at the lowest quartile in childhood.[97]

How might exercise influence these risk factors in children? At this time, there have been mixed results for improvement in obesity and other cardiovascular risk factors in childhood.[98–103] The interventions have come in many different forms and most include both an element of diet and lifestyle education as well as an exercise programme. In the most successful trials, changes have been observed in BMI, per cent body fat, blood pressure, glucose and insulin, and lipids. Why some trials have proven successful and others not may well depend on the quality and intensity of the programme as well as the population studied. At this time no study has been able to show benefits in cardiovascular outcomes. In contrast, as reviewed in detail elsewhere,[1] evidence from epidemiological studies suggests a strong inverse relationship between physical activity and cardiovascular risk factors. At this stage, no exercise intervention studies in children have assessed the effect modifying role of genetics on cardiovascular or metabolic outcomes.

The future of gene–lifestyle interaction studies in children

As outlined earlier in this chapter, very little direct evidence of gene–physical activity interaction on cardiovascular and metabolic traits in childhood exists. This is largely owing to a dearth of reports, rather than evidence suggesting the absence of gene–lifestyle interactions. There are, however, several initiatives in progress which should within the next few years help clarify whether gene–lifestyle interactions have an important role to play in childhood health and disease.

The National Health and Nutrition Examination Survey (NHANES) is a survey based on a representative sample of the U.S. population. Within NHANES, demographic, health history, and health behaviour characteristics and detailed nutritional and biochemical analyses were undertaken in several thousand children. In the most recent phase (2003–2004), physical activity was objectively assessed using uniaxial accelerometry. Whether DNA is available for genotyping in children from NHANES is less clear; only participants aged 20 years or older were asked specifically to consent to the use of their samples for genetic research. In younger participants, they and their parents were asked to consent to the storage of biological samples for other research projects, which presumably could include genetic research. Notwithstanding the uncertainty about DNA access in NHANES children, the assessment of gene–environment interactions is described as an objective of the study. Thus, assuming samples from children can be used for DNA extraction and genotyping, it is possible that reports on gene–lifestyle interactions will emerge from NHANES within the next few years.

The Viva la Familia Study, which we discussed earlier in this chapter incorporates objective assessments of physical activity in more than 1000 Hispanic children using the similar type of uniaxial accelerometer used in NHANES. The study is based on family pedigrees, which presents the opportunity to undertake linkage studies, DNA is available and detailed disease phenotyping has also been undertaken. At the time of writing, no reports of gene–lifestyle interaction have been published from the Viva la Familia Study.

In Europe, two large studies in children exist where objective assessments of physical activity have been made and biological material, including DNA, has been obtained. One of these studies is the Avon Longitudinal Study of Parents and Children (ALSPAC). In that study, DNA and measure of anthropology are available in more than 10,000 children, objective measures of obesity and physical activity (using the same uniaxial accelerometer as in NHANES) are available in 5500 children, and in more than 1000 children measures of insulin, glucose, and glycosylated haemoglobin (HbA1c) are also available. One attractive aspect of the ALSPAC study from the perspective of genetics is that DNA is also available in many of the parents of the children who took part in the project allowing allele phasing to be directly observed, an attribute that is useful when studying the role of genetic imprinting (i.e. the differential phenotypic effects attributable to inheriting an allele from either the mother or the father). Thus far, several genetics publications relating to cardiovascular or metabolic traits have emerged from the ALSPAC project,[104–108] one of the most notable of which reported on the relationship between variation at the *FTO* gene and obesity,[31] but no reports on gene–lifestyle interaction have emerged to date.

In a genetics study of 3200 children from Denmark, Estonia, and Portugal based within the EYHS, we have genotyped in detail several pathways of genes involved in lipid and glucose oxidation, appetite regulation, and obesity. Many of the genes are exercise-responsive, whilst others are activated by dietary nutrients, supporting their candidacy for gene–lifestyle interaction. In the EYHS, physical activity was assessed objectively (using the same model of uniaxial accelerometer as in NHANES) as was aerobic fitness, using a maximal exercise stress test on a bicycle ergometer.[20] Fasting blood samples were also collected, providing information on glucose, lipid, and insulin levels.

Summary

- As we report in this chapter, the field is wide open so far as the study of gene–lifestyle interactions in children is concerned.
- There is excellent published evidence illustrating the separate associations between genetic risk factors and physical activity with cardiovascular risk factors in childhood, but no compelling evidence supports gene–physical activity interactions in childhood cardiovascular health and disease. This is not because the available evidence points to an absence of gene–lifestyle interactions, but because no compelling evidence exists at all, to either support or refute such effects.
- The results from several recent genome-wide association studies point to a small number of candidate genes that may influence cardiovascular health via birth weight and/or childhood obesity.
- The results of a number of large studies of children in which objective assessments of physical activity have been made underscore the strong association that exists between physical inactivity in childhood and the development of cardiovascular risk factors.
- Whilst not all existing paediatric cohorts are large enough to be powered to detect gene–lifestyle interactions, and some do not have coincident objective measures of physical activity and DNA for genetic testing, at least four fairly large cohorts exist with these characteristics. Ideally, some or all of these cohorts will be combined to systematically test hypotheses of gene–lifestyle interactions; the emphasis in doing so should be on testing candidate genes with strong biological or statistical evidence underpinning their plausibility for gene–lifestyle interaction.
- As a simple guide to the selection of biologic candidate genes, the answer to the following questions should preferably be 'yes': (i) does the gene encode a protein important for the regulation of a relevant phenotype (or one that regulates the expression of other such genes)? (ii) is the gene responsive to changes in physical activity/exercise intervention? and (iii) is the gene characterized by functional variation within its nucleotide sequence?
- One might also focus on genes that control the activity of subsets of genes involved in diabetes, such as transcriptional coactivators, as functional variability at these loci may have the widest consequences on energy storage and metabolism.[65]
- An alternative and equally valuable approach to the candidate gene approach could involve the selection of genetic variants discovered using genome-wide scans. This approach, though largely untested, might also yield plausible candidate genes for studies of gene–lifestyle interaction, particularly when the disease phenotypes are evident at a young age and sufficiently developed to interfere with reproduction

References

1. Huang TT, Ball GD, Franks PW (2007). Metabolic syndrome in youth: Current issues and challenges. *Appl Physiol Nutr Metab* **32**, 13–22.
2. Hedley AA, Ogden CL, Johnson CL, Carroll MD, Curtin LR, Flegal KM (2004). Prevalence of overweight and obesity among US children, adolescents, and adults, 1999–2002. *JAMA* **291**, 2847–50.
3. Lioret S, Maire B, Volatier JL, Charles MA (2007). Child overweight in France and its relationship with physical activity, sedentary behaviour and socioeconomic status. *Eur J Clin Nutr* **61**, 509–16.
4. Maffeis C, Consolaro A, Cavarzere P, Chini L, Banzato C, Grezzani A, Silvagni D, Salzano G, De Luca F, Tato L (2006). Prevalence of overweight and obesity in 2- to 6-year-old Italian children. *Obesity (Silver Spring)* **14**, 765–9.
5. Malecka-Tendera E, Mazur A (2006). Childhood obesity: A pandemic of the twenty-first century. *Int J Obes (Lond)* **30** (**Suppl. 2**), S1–3.
6. Schokker DF, Visscher TL, Nooyens AC, van Baak MA, Seidell JC (2007). Prevalence of overweight and obesity in the Netherlands. *Obes Rev* **8**, 101–8.
7. Serra-Majem L, Aranceta Bartrina J, Perez-Rodrigo C, Ribas-Barba L, Delgado-Rubio A (2006). Prevalence and determinants of obesity in Spanish children and young people. *Br J Nutr* **96** (Suppl. 1), S67–72.
8. Whitlock EP, Williams SB, Gold R, Smith PR, Shipman SA (2005). Screening and interventions for childhood overweight: A summary of evidence for the US Preventive Services Task Force. *Pediatrics* **116**, e125–44.
9. Ogden CL, Carroll MD, Curtin LR, McDowell MA, Tabak CJ, Flegal KM (2006). Prevalence of overweight and obesity in the United States, 1999–2004. *JAMA* **295**, 1549–55.
10. Poehlman ET, Tremblay A, Despres JP, Fontaine E, Perusse L, Theriault G, Bouchard C (1986). Genotype-controlled changes in body composition and fat morphology following overfeeding in twins. *Am J Clin Nutr* **43**, 723–31.

11. Bouchard C, Tremblay A, Despres JP, Nadeau A, Lupien PJ, Theriault G, Dussault J, Moorjani S, Pinault S, Fournier G (1990). The response to long-term overfeeding in identical twins. *N Engl J Med* **322**, 1477–82.
12. Goldstein GL, Daun H, Tepper BJ (2007). Influence of PROP taster status and maternal variables on energy intake and body weight of pre-adolescents. *Physiol Behav* **90**, 809–17.
13. O'Connor TM, Yang SJ, Nicklas TA (2006). Beverage intake among preschool children and its effect on weight status. *Pediatrics* **118**, e1010–18.
14. Le Fur S, Le Stunff C, Dos Santos C, Bougneres P (2004). The common -866 G/A polymorphism in the promoter of uncoupling protein 2 is associated with increased carbohydrate and decreased lipid oxidation in juvenile obesity. *Diabetes* **53**, 235–9.
15. Kovacs P, Ma L, Hanson RL, Franks P, Stumvoll M, Bogardus C, Baier LJ (2005). Genetic variation in UCP2 (uncoupling protein-2) is associated with energy metabolism in Pima Indians. *Diabetologia* **48**, 2292–5.
16. Lawlor DA, Martin RM, Gunnell D, Galobardes B, Ebrahim S, Sandhu J, Sandhu J, Ben Shlomo Y, McCarron P, Davey Smith G (2006). Association of body mass index measured in childhood, adolescence, and young adulthood with risk of ischemic heart disease and stroke: findings from 3 historical cohort studies. *Am J Clin Nutr* **83**, 767–73.
17. Gunnell DJ, Frankel SJ, Nanchahal K, Peters TJ, Davey Smith G (1998). Childhood obesity and adult cardiovascular mortality: A 57-y follow-up study based on the Boyd Orr cohort. *Am J Clin Nutr* **67**, 1111–18.
18. Neel JV (1962). Diabetes mellitus: a "thrifty" genotype rendered detrimental by "progress"? *Am J Hum Genet* **14**, 353–62.
19. Salbe AD, Weyer C, Lindsay RS, Ravussin E, Tataranni PA (2002). Assessing risk factors for obesity between childhood and adolescence: I. Birth weight, childhood adiposity, parental obesity, insulin, and leptin. *Pediatrics* **110**, 299–306.
20. Andersen LB, Harro M, Sardinha LB, Froberg K, Ekelund U, Brage S, Anderssen SA (2006). Physical activity and clustered cardiovascular risk in children: A cross-sectional study (The European Youth Heart Study). *Lancet* **368**, 299–304.
21. Franks PW, Ravussin E, Hanson RL, Harper IT, Allison DB, Knowler WC, Tataranni PA, Salbe AD (2005). Habitual physical activity in children: The role of genes and the environment. *Am J Clin Nutr* **82**, 901–8.
22. Khoury MJ, Little J, Burke B (2003). *Human genome epidemiology: A scientific foundation for using genetic information to improve health and prevent disease.* Oxford University Press, New York.
23. Ragland DR (1992). Dichotomizing continuous outcome variables: Dependence of the magnitude of association and statistical power on the cutpoint. *Epidemiology* **3**, 434–40.
24. Franks PW (2006). Obesity, inflammatory markers and cardiovascular disease: Distinguishing causality from confounding. *J Hum Hypertens* **20**, 837–40.
25. Saxena R Voight BF, Lyssenko V Burtt NP, de Bakker PI, Chen H, Roix JJ, Kathiresan S, Hirschhorn JN, Daly MJ, Hughes TE, Groop L, Altshuler D, Almgren P, Florez JC, Meyer J, Ardlie K, Bengtsson, Bostrom K, Isomaa B, Lettre G, Lindblad U, Lyon HN, Melander O, Newton-Cheh C, Nilsson P, Orho-Melander M, Rastam L, Speliotes EK, Taskinen MR, Tuomi T, Guiducci C, Berglund A, Carlson J, Gianniny L, Hackett R, Hall L, Holmkvist J, Laurila E, Sjogren M, Sterner M, Surti A, Svensson M, Svensson M, Tewhey R, Blumenstiel B, Parkin M, Defelice M, Barry R, Brodeur W, Camarata J, Chia N, Fava M, Gibbons J, Handsaker B, Healy C, Nguyen K, Gates C, Sougnez C, Gage D, Nizzari M, Gabriel SB, Chirn GW, Ma,Q, Parikh H, Richardson D, Ricke D, Purcell S (2007). Genome-wide association analysis identifies loci for type 2 diabetes and triglyceride levels. *Science* **316**, 1331–6.
26. Sladek R, Rocheleau G, Rung J, Dina C, Shen L, Serre D, Boutin P, Vincent D, Belisle A, Hadjadj S, Balkau B, Heude B, Charpentier G, Hudson TJ, Montpetit A, Pshezhetsky AV, Prentki M, Posner BI, Balding DJ, Meyre D, Polychronakos C, Froguel P (2007). A genome-wide association study identifies novel risk loci for type 2 diabetes. *Nature* **445**, 881–5.
27. The Wellcome Trust Case Control Consortium (2007). Genome-wide association study of 14,000 cases of seven common diseases and 3,000 shared controls. *Nature* **447**, 661–78.
28. Scott LJ, Mohlke KL, Bonnycastle LL, Willer CJ, Li Y, Duren WL, Erdos MR, Stringham HM, Chines PS, Jackson AU, Prokunina-Olsson L, Ding CJ, Swift AJ, Narisu N, Hu T, Pruim R, Xiao R, Li XY, Conneely KN, Riebow NL, Sprau AG, Tong M, White PP, Hetrick KN, Barnhart MW, Bark CW, Goldstein JL, Watkins L, Xiang F, Saramies J, Buchanan TA, Watanabe RM, Valle TT, Kinnunen L, Abecasis GR, Pugh EW, Doheny KF, Bergman RN, Tuomilehto J, Collins FS, Boehnke M (2007). A genome-wide association study of type 2 diabetes in Finns detects multiple susceptibility variants. *Science* **316**, 1341–5.
29. Zeggini E, Weedon MN, Lindgren CM, Frayling TM, Elliott KS, Lango H, Timpson NJ, Perry JR, Rayner NW, Freathy RM, Barrett JC, Shields B, Morris AP, Ellard S, Groves CJ, Harries LW, Marchini JL, Owen KR, Knight B, Cardon LR, Walker M, Hitman GA, Morris AD, Doney AS, McCarthy MI, Hattersley AT (2007). Replication of genome-wide association signals in UK samples reveals risk loci for type 2 diabetes. *Science* **316**, 1336–41.
30. Dina C, Meyre D, Gallina S, Durand E, Korner A, Jacobson P, Carlsson LM, Kiess W, Vatin V, Lecoeur C, Delplanque J, Vaillant E, Pattou F, Ruiz J, Weill J, Levy-Marchal C, Horber F, Potoczna N, Hercberg S, Le Stunff C, Bougneres P, Kovacs P, Marre M, Balkau B, Cauchi S, Chevre JC, Froguel P (2007). Variation in FTO contributes to childhood obesity and severe adult obesity. *Nat Genet* **39**, 724–6.
31. Frayling TM, Timpson NJ, Weedon MN, Zeggini E, Freathy RM, Lindgren CM, Perry JR, Elliott KS, Lango H, Rayner NW, Shields B, Harries LW, Barrett JC, Ellard S, Groves CJ, Knight B, Patch AM, Ness AR, Ebrahim S, Lawlor DA, Ring SM, Ben Shlomo Y, Jarvelin MR, Sovio U, Bennett AJ, Melzer D, Ferrucci L, Loos RJ, Barroso I, Wareham NJ, Karpe F, Owen KR, Cardon LR, Walker M, Hitman GA, Palmer CN, Doney AS, Morris AD, Smith GD, Hattersley AT, McCarthy MI (2007). A common variant in the FTO gene is associated with body mass index and predisposes to childhood and adult obesity. *Science* **316**, 889–94.
32. The Diabetes Prevention Program Research Group (2002). Reduction in the incidence of type 2 diabetes with lifestyle intervention or metformin. *N Engl J Med* **346**, 393–403.
33. Florez JC, Jablonski KA, Bayley N, Pollin TI, de Bakker PI, Shuldiner AR, Knowler WC, Nathan DM, Altshuler D (2006). TCF7L2 polymorphisms and progression to diabetes in the Diabetes Prevention Program. *N Engl J Med* **355**, 241–50.
34. Grant SF, Thorleifsson G, Reynisdottir I, Benediktsson R, Manolescu A, Sainz J, Helgason A, Stefansson H, Emilsson V, Helgadottir A, Styrkarsdottir U, Magnusson KP, Walters GB, Palsdottir E, Jonsdottir T, Gudmundsdottir T, Gylfason A, Saemundsdottir J, Wilensky RL, Reilly MP, Rader DJ, Bagger Y, Christiansen C, Gudnason V, Sigurdsson G, Thorsteinsdottir U, Gulcher JR, Kong A, Stefansson K (2006). Variant of transcription factor 7-like 2 (TCF7L2) gene confers risk of type 2 diabetes. *Nat Genet* **38**, 320–3.
35. Moran CN, Vassilopoulos C, Tsiokanos A, Jamurtas AZ, Bailey ME, Wilson RH, Pitsiladis YP (2005). Effects of interaction between angiotensin I-converting enzyme polymorphisms and lifestyle on adiposity in adolescent Greeks. *Obes Res* **13**, 1499–504.
36. Sallis JF, Saelens BE (2000). Assessment of physical activity by self-report: Status, limitations, and future directions. *Res Q Exerc Sport* **71** (**Suppl**), S1–14.
37. Butte NF, Cai G, Cole SA, Comuzzie AG (2006). Viva la Familia Study: Genetic and environmental contributions to childhood obesity and its comorbidities in the Hispanic population. *Am J Clin Nutr* **84**, 646–54; quiz 73–4.
38. Cai G, Cole SA, Butte N, Bacino C, Diego V, Tan K, Goring HH, O'Rahilly S, Farooqi IS, Comuzzie AG (2006). A quantitative trait locus on chromosome 18q for physical activity and dietary intake in Hispanic children. *Obesity (Silver Spring)* **14**, 1596–604.

39. Stubbe JH, Boomsma DI, De Geus EJ (2005). Sports participation during adolescence: a shift from environmental to genetic factors. *Med Sci Sports Exerc* **37**, 563–70.
40. Coppari R, Ichinose M, Lee CE, Pullen AF, Kenny CD, McGovern RA, Tang V, Liu SM, Ludwig T, Chua SC Jr, Lowell BB, Elmquist JK (2005). The hypothalamic arcuate nucleus: a key site for mediating leptin's effects on glucose homeostasis and locomotor activity. *Cell Metab* **1**, 63–72.
41. Adage T, Scheurink AJ, de Boer SF, de Vries K, Konsman JP, Kuipers F, Adan RA, Baskin DG, Schwartz MW, van Dijk G (2001). Hypothalamic, metabolic, and behavioral responses to pharmacological inhibition of CNS melanocortin signaling in rats. *J Neurosci* **21**, 3639–45.
42. Loos RJ, Rankinen T, Tremblay A, Perusse L, Chagnon Y, Bouchard C (2005). Melanocortin-4 receptor gene and physical activity in the Quebec Family Study. *Int J Obes (Lond)* **29**, 420–8.
43. Marie M, Findlay PA, Thomas L, Adam CL (2001). Daily patterns of plasma leptin in sheep: effects of photoperiod and food intake. *J Endocrinol* **170**, 277–86.
44. Patel L, Cooper CD, Quinton ND, Butler GE, Gill MS, Jefferson IG, Kibirige MS, Price DA, Shalet SM, Wales JK, Ross RJ, Clayton PE (2002). Serum leptin and leptin binding activity in children and adolescents with hypothalamic dysfunction. *J Pediatr Endocrinol Metab* **15**, 963–71.
45. Farooqi IS, Keogh JM, Yeo GS, Lank EJ, Cheetham T, O'Rahilly S (2003). Clinical spectrum of obesity and mutations in the melanocortin 4 receptor gene. *N Engl J Med* **348**, 1085–95.
46. Franks PW, Farooqi IS, Luan J, Wong MY, Halsall I, O' Rahilly S, Wareham NJ (2003). Does physical activity energy expenditure explain the between-individual variation in plasma leptin concentrations after adjusting for differences in body composition? *J Clin Endocrinol Metab* **88**, 3258–63.
47. Holtkamp K, Herpertz-Dahlmann B, Mika C, Heer M, Heussen N, Fichter M, Herpertz S, Senf W, Blum WF, Schweiger U, Warnke A, Ballauff A, Remschmidt H, Hebebrand J (2003). Elevated physical activity and low leptin levels co-occur in patients with anorexia nervosa. *J Clin Endocrinol Metab* **88**, 5169–74.
48. Romon M, Lafay L, Bresson JL, Oppert JM, Borys JM, Kettaneh A, Charles MA (2004). Relationships between physical activity and plasma leptin levels in healthy children: The Fleurbaix-Laventie Ville Sante II Study. *Int J Obes Relat Metab Disord* **28**, 1227–32.
49. Salbe AD, Nicolson M, Ravussin E (1997). Total energy expenditure and the level of physical activity correlate with plasma leptin concentrations in five-year-old children. *J Clin Invest* **99**, 592–5.
50. Franks PW, Brage S, Luan J, Ekelund U, Rahman M, Farooqi IS, Halsall I, O'Rahilly S, Warehan NJ (2005). Leptin predicts a worsening of the features of the metabolic syndrome independently of obesity. *Obes Res* **13**, 1476–84.
51. Nagy TR, Gower BA, Shewchuk RM, Goran MI (1997). Serum leptin and energy expenditure in children. *J Clin Endocrinol Metab* **82**, 4149–53.
52. Wei M, Gibbons LW, Mitchell TL, Kampert JB, Lee CD, Blair SN (1999). The association between cardiorespiratory fitness and impaired fasting glucose and Type 2 diabetes mellitus in men. *Ann Intern Med* **130**, 89–96.
53. Astrand PO (1992). J.B. Wolffe Memorial Lecture. "Why exercise?" *Med Sci Sports Exerc* **24**, 153–62.
54. Boule NG, Kenny GP, Haddad E, Wells GA, Sigal RJ (2003). Meta-analysis of the effect of structured exercise training on cardiorespiratory fitness in Type 2 diabetes mellitus. *Diabetologia* **46**, 1071–81.
55. Lalani SR, Vladutiu GD, Plunkett K, Lotze TE, Adesina AM, Scaglia F (2005). Isolated mitochondrial myopathy associated with muscle coenzyme Q10 deficiency. *Arch Neurol* **62**, 317–20.
56. Mayr JA, Moslemi AR, Forster H, Kamper A, Idriceanu C, Muss W, Huemer M, Oldfors A, Sperl W (2006). A novel sporadic mutation G14739A of the mitochondrial tRNA(Glu) in a girl with exercise intolerance. *Neuromuscul Disord* **16**, 874–7.
57. Pulkes T, Liolitsa D, Eunson LH, Rose M, Nelson IP, Rahman S, Poulton J, Marchington DR, Landon DN, Debono AG, Morgan-Hughes JA, Hanna MG (2005). New phenotypic diversity associated with the mitochondrial tRNA(SerUCN) gene mutation. *Neuromuscul Disord* **15**, 364–71.
58. Carrel AL, Clark RR, Peterson SE, Nemeth BA, Sullivan J, Allen DB (2005). Improvement of fitness, body composition, and insulin sensitivity in overweight children in a school-based exercise program: a randomized, controlled study. *Arch Pediatr Adolesc Med* **159**, 963–8.
59. Brage S, Wedderkopp N, Ekelund U, Franks PW, Wareham NJ, Andersen LB, Froberg K (2004). Features of the metabolic syndrome are associated with objectively measured physical activity and fitness in Danish children: the European Youth Heart Study (EYHS). *Diabetes Care* **27**, 2141–8.
60. Franks PW, Ekelund U, Brage S, Wong MY, Wareham NJ (2004). Does the association of habitual physical activity with the metabolic syndrome differ by level of cardiorespiratory fitness? *Diabetes Care* **27**, 1187–93.
61. Ekelund U, Andersen LB, Froberg K, Sardinha LB, Anderssen SA, Brage S (2007). Independent associations between physical activity and aerobic fitness with metabolic risk factors in children: The European Youth Heart Study. *Diabetologia* **50**, 1832–40.
62. Barroso I, Luan J, Sandhu M, Franks PW, Crowley V, Schafer A, O'Rahilly S, Wareham NJ (2006). Meta-analysis of the Gly482Ser variant in PPARGC1A in type 2 diabetes and related phenotypes. *Diabetologia* **49**, 501–5.
63. Lucia A, Gomez-Gallego F, Barroso I, Rabadan M, Bandres F, San Juan AF, Chicharro JL, Ekelund U, Brage S, Earnest CP, Wareham NJ, Franks PW (2005). PPARGC1A genotype (Gly482Ser) predicts exceptional endurance capacity in European men. *J Appl Physiol* **99**, 344–8.
64. Sookoian S, Garcia SI, Porto PI, Dieuzeide G, Gonzalez CD, Pirola CJ (2005). Peroxisome proliferator-activated receptor gamma and its coactivator-1 alpha may be associated with features of the metabolic syndrome in adolescents. *J Mol Endocrinol* **35**, 373–80.
65. Franks PW, Loos RJ (2006). PGC-1 alpha gene and physical activity in type 2 diabetes mellitus. *Exerc Sport Sci Rev* **34**, 171–5.
66. Barker DJ, Winter PD, Osmond C, Margetts B, Simmonds SJ (1989). Weight in infancy and death from ischaemic heart disease. *Lancet* **2**, 577–80.
67. Frankel S, Elwood P, Sweetnam P, Yarnell J, Smith GD (1996). Birthweight, body-mass index in middle age, and incident coronary heart disease. *Lancet* **348**, 1478–80.
68. Stein CE, Fall CH, Kumaran K, Osmond C, Cox V, Barker DJ (1996). Fetal growth and coronary heart disease in south India. *Lancet* **348**, 1269–73.
69. Rich-Edwards JW, Stampfer MJ, Manson JE, Rosner B, Hankinson SE, Colditz GA, Willett WC, Hennekens CH (1997). Birth weight and risk of cardiovascular disease in a cohort of women followed up since 1976. *BMJ* **315**, 396–400.
70. Lithell HO, McKeigue PM, Berglund L, Mohsen R, Lithell UB, Leon DA (1996). Relation of size at birth to non-insulin dependent diabetes and insulin concentrations in men aged 50–60 years. *BMJ* **312**, 406–10.
71. Rich-Edwards JW, Colditz GA, Stampfer MJ, Willett WC, Gillman MW, Hennekens CH, Speizer FE, Manson JE (1999). Birthweight and the risk for type 2 diabetes mellitus in adult women. *Ann Intern Med* **130**, 278–84.
72. McCance DR, Pettitt DJ, Hanson RL, Jacobsson LT, Knowler WC, Bennett PH (1994). Birth weight and non-insulin dependent diabetes: Thrifty genotype, thrifty phenotype, or surviving small baby genotype? *BMJ* **308**, 942–5.
73. Center for Disease Control and Prevention (2000). CDC Growth Charts. Washington, DC, Department of Health and Human Services, National Center for Health Statistics, (U.S. publ. no. 314).
74. Clarke WR, Lauer RM (1993). Does childhood obesity track into adulthood? *Crit Rev Food Sci Nutr* **33**, 423–30.

75. Raitakari OT, Juonala M, Viikari JS (2005). Obesity in childhood and vascular changes in adulthood: insights into the Cardiovascular Risk in Young Finns Study. *Int J Obes (Lond)* **29** (**Suppl. 2**), S101–4.
76. Pena AS, Wiltshire E, MacKenzie K, Gent R, Piotto L, Hirte C, Couper J (2006). Vascular endothelial and smooth muscle function relates to body mass index and glucose in obese and nonobese children. *J Clin Endocrinol Metab* **91**, 4467–71.
77. Berenson GS, Srinivasan SR, Bao W, Newman WP, 3rd, Tracy RE, Wattigney WA (1998). Association between multiple cardiovascular risk factors and atherosclerosis in children and young adults. The Bogalusa Heart Study. *N Engl J Med* **338**, 1650–6.
78. Ong KK, Ahmed ML, Emmett PM, Preece MA, Dunger DB (2000). Association between postnatal catch-up growth and obesity in childhood: Prospective cohort study. *BMJ* **320**, 967–71.
79. Stettler N, Zemel BS, Kumanyika S, Stallings VA (2002). Infant weight gain and childhood overweight status in a multicenter, cohort study. *Pediatrics* **109**, 194–9.
80. Eriksson JG, Forsen T, Tuomilehto J, Osmond C, Barker DJ (2001). Early growth and coronary heart disease in later life: longitudinal study. *BMJ* **322**, 949–53.
81. Eriksson JG, Forsen T, Tuomilehto J, Osmond C, Barker DJ (2003). Early adiposity rebound in childhood and risk of Type 2 diabetes in adult life. *Diabetologia* **46**, 190–4.
82. Jensen T, Borch-Johnsen K, Kofoed-Enevoldsen A, Deckert T (1987). Coronary heart disease in young type 1 (insulin-dependent) diabetic patients with and without diabetic nephropathy: incidence and risk factors. *Diabetologia* **30**, 144–8.
83. Lloyd CE, Kuller LH, Ellis D, Becker DJ, Wing RR, Orchard TJ (1996). Coronary artery disease in IDDM. Gender differences in risk factors but not risk. *Arterioscler Thromb Vasc Biol* **16**, 720–6.
84. Nathan DM, Cleary PA, Backlund JY, Genuth SM, Lachin JM, Orchard TJ, Raskin P, Zinman B (2005). Intensive diabetes treatment and cardiovascular disease in patients with type 1 diabetes. *N Engl J Med* **353**, 2643–53.
85. Wiltshire EJ, Gent R, Hirte C, Pena A, Thomas DW, Couper JJ (2002). Endothelial dysfunction relates to folate status in children and adolescents with type 1 diabetes. *Diabetes* **51**, 2282–6.
86. McCance DR, Pettitt DJ, Hanson RL, Jacobsson LT, Bennett PH, Knowler WC (1994). Glucose, insulin concentrations and obesity in childhood and adolescence as predictors of NIDDM. *Diabetologia* **37**, 617–23.
87. Lauer RM, Clarke WR, Mahoney LT, Witt J (1993). Childhood predictors for high adult blood pressure. The Muscatine Study. *Pediatr Clin North Am* **40**, 23–40.
88. Paradisi G, Smith L, Burtner C, Leaming R, Garvey WT, Hook G, Johnson A, Cronin J, Steinberg HO, Baron AD (1999). Dual energy X-ray absorptiometry assessment of fat mass distribution and its association with the insulin resistance syndrome. *Diabetes Care* **22**, 1310–17.
89. Sun SS, Grave GD, Siervogel RM, Pickoff AA, Arslanian SS, Daniels SR (2007). Systolic blood pressure in childhood predicts hypertension and metabolic syndrome later in life. *Pediatrics* **119**, 237–46.
90. Li X, Li S, Ulusoy E, Chen W, Srinivasan SR, Berenson GS (2004). Childhood adiposity as a predictor of cardiac mass in adulthood: the Bogalusa Heart Study. *Circulation* **110**, 3488–92.
91. Webber LS, Srinivasan SR, Wattigney WA, Berenson GS (1991). Tracking of serum lipids and lipoproteins from childhood to adulthood. The Bogalusa Heart Study. *Am J Epidemiol* **133**, 884–99.
92. Srinivasan SR, Myers L, Berenson GS (2006). Changes in metabolic syndrome variables since childhood in prehypertensive and hypertensive subjects: The Bogalusa Heart Study. *Hypertension* **48**, 33–9.
93. Kavey RE, Allada V, Daniels SR, Hayman LL, McCrindle BW, Newburger JW, Parekh RS, Steinberger J (2006). Cardiovascular risk reduction in high-risk pediatric patients: A scientific statement from the American Heart Association Expert Panel on Population and Prevention Science; the Councils on Cardiovascular Disease in the Young, Epidemiology and Prevention, Nutrition, Physical Activity and Metabolism, High Blood Pressure Research, Cardiovascular Nursing, and the Kidney in Heart Disease; and the Interdisciplinary Working Group on Quality of Care and Outcomes Research: endorsed by the American Academy of Pediatrics. *Circulation* **114**, 2710–38.
94. Chi CH, Wang Y, Wilson DM, Robinson TN (2006). Definition of metabolic syndrome in preadolescent girls. *J Pediatr* **148**, 788–92.
95. Saland JM (2007). Update on the metabolic syndrome in children. *Curr Opin Pediatr* **19**, 183–91.
96. Bao W, Srinivasan SR, Wattigney WA, Berenson GS (1994). Persistence of multiple cardiovascular risk clustering related to syndrome X from childhood to young adulthood. The Bogalusa Heart Study. *Arch Intern Med* **154**, 1842–7.
97. Chen W, Srinivasan SR, Li S, Xu J, Berenson GS (2005). Metabolic syndrome variables at low levels in childhood are beneficially associated with adulthood cardiovascular risk: the Bogalusa Heart Study. *Diabetes Care* **28**, 126–31.
98. Reinehr T, Temmesfeld M, Kersting M, de Sousa G, Toschke AM (2007). Four-year follow-up of children and adolescents participating in an obesity intervention program. *Int J Obes (Lond)* **31**, 1074–7.
99. Reilly JJ, Kelly L, Montgomery C, Williamson A, Fisher A, McColl JH, Lo Conte R, Paton JY, Grant S (2006). Physical activity to prevent obesity in young children: cluster randomised controlled trial. *BMJ* **333**, 1041.
100. Sharma M (2006). School-based interventions for childhood and adolescent obesity. *Obes Rev* **7**, 261–9.
101. Monzavi R, Dreimane D, Geffner ME, Braun S, Conrad B, Klier M, Kaufman FR (2006). Improvement in risk factors for metabolic syndrome and insulin resistance in overweight youth who are treated with lifestyle intervention. *Pediatrics* **117**, e1111–18.
102. Carrel A, Meinen A, Garry C, Storandt R (2005). Effects of nutrition education and exercise in obese children: the Ho-Chunk Youth Fitness Program. *WMJ* **104**, 44–7.
103. Nassis GP, Papantakou K, Skenderi K, Triandafillopoulou M, Kavouras SA, Yannakoulia M, Chrousos GP, Sidossis LS (2005). Aerobic exercise training improves insulin sensitivity without changes in body weight, body fat, adiponectin, and inflammatory markers in overweight and obese girls. *Metabolism* **54**, 1472–9.
104. Dunger DB, Ong KK, Huxtable SJ, Sherriff A, Woods KA, Ahmed ML, Golding J, Pembrey ME, Ring S, Bennett ST, Todd JA (1998). Association of the INS VNTR with size at birth. ALSPAC Study Team. Avon Longitudinal Study of Pregnancy and Childhood. *Nat Genet* **19**, 98–100.
105. Heude B, Petry CJ, Pembrey M, Dunger DB, Ong KK (2006). The insulin gene variable number of tandem repeat: Associations and interactions with childhood body fat mass and insulin secretion in normal children. *J Clin Endocrinol Metab* **91**, 2770–5.
106. Petry CJ, Ong KK, Barratt BJ, Wingate D, Cordell HJ, Ring SM, Pembrey ME, Reik W, Todd JA, Dunger DB (2005). Common polymorphism in H19 associated with birthweight and cord blood IGF-II levels in humans. *BMC Genet* **6**, 22.
107. Petry CJ, Ong KK, Wingate DL, Brown J, Scott CD, Jones EY, Pembrey ME, Dunger DB (2005). Genetic variation in the type 2 insulin-like growth factor receptor gene and disparity in childhood height. *Growth Horm IGF Res* **15**, 363–8.
108. Tobias JH, Steer CD, Vilarino-Guell C, Brown MA (2007). Effect of an estrogen receptor alpha intron 4 polymorphism on fat mass in 11-year-old children. *J Clin Endocrinol Metab* **92**, 2286–91.

CHAPTER 27

Physical activity, physical fitness, and bone health

Han C.G. Kemper

Introduction

Most people think that the skeleton is a passive structure: when bone is formed and calcified the structure remains stable and even after death the remains of the skeleton can be found in graves hundreds to thousands of years later. However, bone is a vital, dynamic connective tissue, which can grow and continuously adapt its structure to its function.[1] To fulfil this structure–function relation adequately, bone is continuously being broken down and rebuilt in a process that is called 'bone remodelling'.

Bone mass increases at the same rate during growth and development in boys and girls, but at the beginning of puberty a sexual dimorphism occurs and bone mass increases faster in boys than girls. Maximal bone mass is reached in the late teens and early 20, thereafter it gradually declines, this decrease is accelerated in women after the menopause (Fig. 27.1).

The average woman has a higher risk of osteoporosis than the average man for at least two reasons: first, women reach a lower maximal bone mass in their youth and second, women loose bone at a higher rate after the menopause. This decrease in bone density leaves elderly individuals and particularly females, at risk for exaggerated bone thinning, or osteoporosis, with subsequent disability and death from bone fractures.

This chapter reviews (i) the different methods to measure bone mass, (ii) the growth and development of bone mass during

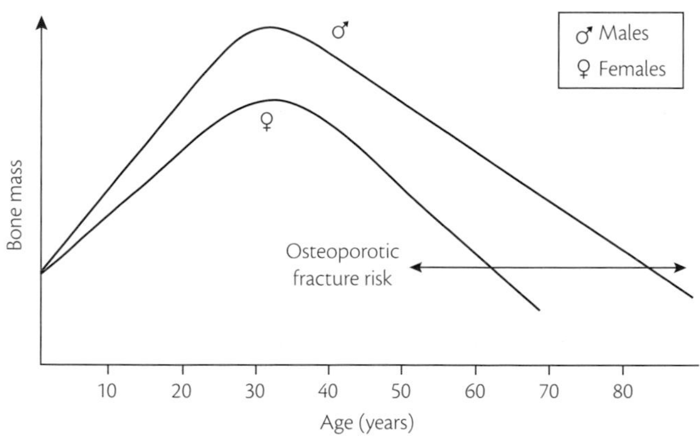

Fig. 27.1 The development of bone mass in males and females with age: the osteoporotic fracture risk is usually reached at an earlier age in females than in males. After Kemper,[22] with permission.

childhood and adolescence, (iii) the effects of physical activity and exercise on physical fitness and bone health during youth, and (iv) the most effective exercise regimens to strengthen the bone.

Because bone mass predicts fracture risk and peak bone mass, this knowledge can help us to understand the impact of physical activity as one of the important lifestyle factors during youth for the prevention of osteoporosis at older age.[2] Strategies that optimize bone strength and maximize peak bone mass are therefore required to counter the deleterious effects of age-related bone loss and the anticipated global epidemic in osteoporosis.[3–5]

Growth of bone

Physical growth and development have been extensively investigated from prenatal growth to birth and from postnatal growth to adulthood by many longitudinal studies all over the world. In 1955, J.M. Tanner published the first edition of his book *Growth at Adolescence*[6] and, in 1981, *A History of the Study of Human Growth*.[7] Since then both books have been used as state-of-the-art publications on human growth and development. The methods that are used in general to measure growth changes are mainly based on simple anthropometric measurements of the total body (body height, body mass) or of body segments (trunk height, limb lengths). Also breadth measurements (shoulder, hip, wrist, and knee), circumferences (head, trunk, hip, waist, and limbs), and skinfold measurements at different sites of the body are applied according to standard methods[8] (and see chapter 3). All of these measurements estimate different dimensions of the body but do not take into consideration changes in the composition of these body parts.

Radiographic methods are used to indicate calcified cartilage and ossificated bone and to estimate skeletal maturation. Different methods have been developed to assess the rate of maturation or biological age from X-rays at wrist and knee. From a comparison of skeletal age with calendar age the child can be characterized as an early or late maturer.[9]

In recent years new methods have been developed to measure the bone mass by energy absorption from gamma radiation by calcium in the bone. The methods mostly described in the literature are single photon absorptiometry (SPA), dual photon absorptiometry (DPA), dual energy X-ray absorptiometry (DEXA), and quantitative computed tomography (QCT).

In the reviewed literature, bone mass is measured in different parts of the human skeleton such as the arm, hip, spine, and heel or in the total body mass. The details of the method and place of measurement will only be mentioned here if necessary and if they have important consequences for the interpretation of the outcomes.

Since not much is known about the natural development of bone mass during youth, the literature will be reviewed on (i) the changes in bone mass during prepubertal, circumpubertal, and postpubertal development; (ii) the differences in bone development between boys and girls; and (iii) the point of time at which the maximal amount of bone mass, or the so-called peak bone mineral density (PBMD), is reached.

Most bone mineral density (BMD) studies are aimed at prevention and retardation of bone loss in postmenopausal women. An important question remains: whether is it possible to increase the bone mass during the growing years by exercise in order to attain higher maximal bone mass at young adult age?[10] There are to date several experimental studies published that have investigated the effects of physical activity programmes on bone health in youth.

Methods of measurements of bone mass

Anthropometrics

Von Döbeln[11] proposed a measure for the estimation of skeletal weight from height and four breadth measurements (left and right femur condyli and radioulnar width). This sounds good as long as it is used for estimating total weight of bone mass in comparison with estimates of muscle and fat mass estimated by skinfolds and circumferences in combination with height and weight. In the Netherlands, this concept is used to correct the body weight to body height relationship: The Dutch Heart Foundation constructed a reference scale (for ideal body weight) based on the Quetelet Index or body mass index [Ql or BMI (kg·m^{-2})] that included the possibility of calculating the ideal body weight taking the breadth of the femur condyle into consideration. However, this is a misuse of the skeletal component of this algorithm because an adjustment is made for the least variable of the three-component model of body composition, with lean and fat mass being the other components.

Radiographics

In November 1895, the German physicist Wilhelm Conrad Röntgen discovered gamma radiation and demonstrated a radiogram showing the bones of his own hand. He called this the X radiation. The anatomist Albert von Kölliker connected Röntgen's name to this kind of radiation. Since then, X rays have been widely used in medicine for the detection of infectious diseases, pathologic neoplasmata, and traumatology.

Another field in radiographics is its use as a measure of biological age with respect to skeletal growth and development. Skeletal maturation begins as a process when rudiments of bones appear during embryonic life and is completed when skeletal form becomes comparatively stable in young adulthood. During maturation there are increases in the types and numbers of specialized cells, including cartilage and fibrous tissue cells that form part of a bone.[12] In 1950, Greulich and Pyle published their radiographic atlas of skeletal development of the hand and wrist with a second edition in 1959. Roche *et al.*[13] in their longitudinal study used the knee joint as bones of interest for the determination of skeletal maturation [Roche-Wainer-Thissen (RWT) method] however, most assessments of skeletal maturity are made from radiographs of the hand–wrist because this site has considerable advantages over other parts of the skeleton. These advantages stem from the little irradiation required, the ease of radiographic positioning, and the large number of bones included in the area. Therefore, the RWT method using the knee joint as a biological indicator for growth was extended with the hand–wrist method. In Europe, Tanner *et al.*[14] from the Institute of Child Health in London published in 1975 their Tanner–Whitehouse II (TW2) method for the determination of growth also using X-ray photographs of the left hand including 20 bones of the hand and wrist.

All these skeletal maturity scales are used to estimate the developmental or biological age of children, correcting for children who mature faster or slower than the average child with the same calendar age. In paediatrics, it can be used to predict adult height of children (mostly girls) who or whose parents expect that they will end up very tall, and consider to intervene in their growth by using hormones to close their endplates earlier.

Dual energy X-ray absorptiometry

Radiographs cannot easily quantify changes in bone density, because 30% of it has to be lost before it can be detected by X-ray. However, recent technical advances have made it possible to measure bone mass by energy absorption from gamma radiation in the bone. DEXA is now the most precise and widely used method of assessing bone density, and the preferred method because scanning time is shorter than with DPA. Also resolution has been improved, and measurements can be made of the lumbar spine (LS), femoral neck (FN), and forearm and for the total body.

From the DEXA method, two measures are calculated: the bone mineral content (BMC) and the BMD. The BMC is the total amount of minerals in the selected bone in grams, and the BMD is the amount of grams of bone mineral divided by the area of the selected bone (g·cm^{-2}). The BMD, however, is not a real measure of bone density (g·cm^{-3}) and is therefore called area density or areal BMD. In growth bones not only increase their area but also their volume. These size changes influence the areal BMD. Therefore, attempts have been made to estimate the volume of the bone of interest and to correct for this bone size effect by an additional measure of bone mineral apparent density (BMAD).[15]

Quantitative computed tomography

QCT systems have been adapted for the estimation of BMC allowing cortical bone to be separated from trabecular bone. Furthermore, it provides us with a true measure of total, cortical, or trabecular bone mineral volumetric density (mg·mm^{-3}). However, the equipment is more expensive, and exposes patients to high radiation doses. A peripheral QCT system is now available for the forearm with a lower dose of radiation.

Quantitative ultrasound

Ultrasound measurements have been available since 1980s, and have the potential for widespread clinical applications because it does not use radiation. QUS measurements are made to assess broadband ultrasound attenuation (BUA in dB/MHz) and SOS (speed of sound in m·s^{-1}). One of the advantages is that it not only gives a quantitative measure of bone (mass) but also a qualitative aspect (structure). The validity of ultrasound for bone measurement has, however, still to be proven.

Mechanisms of bone formation

Movement is the result of electric impulses being passed from the central nervous system to the skeletal muscles. These muscles contract (shorten) in order to move body parts with respect to each other (arms, legs, head, and trunk) and/or the whole body with respect to the surroundings (walking, cycling, swimming). Exercise is not necessarily dynamic—sometimes muscles contract without causing movements but increase their tension as in static exercises such as standing, active sitting, or pushing against a wall.

Both the duration and intensity of exercise play a role in the physical load placed on the body. Low-intensity, long-lasting exercise increases ventilation and circulation to meet oxygen demand for delivery of energy to the active muscles. This is important for a better capillarization and oxygen delivery to the muscle. High-intensity, short-lasting exercise is important for the development of muscle and bone mass. Results show that of these two factors it is not the duration of exercise which is the key factor affecting bone health but the intensity of the forces that act upon the bones. Weight-bearing activities, such as walking, running, and dancing, have more effect on bone health of the legs and vertebrae of the lower back than have swimming and cycling, although all activities need approximately the same amount of energy when performed for identical lengths of time. This difference in effect on bone health is in contrast to the effects of these activities on the lungs, heart, and circulation: if performed with the same intensity and duration, swimming has the same effect as running on the oxygen transport system.

Two different mechanisms seem to act on bone mass: central hormonal factors, such as oestrogen production, and local mechanical factors, such as the muscle forces exerted on the bones of the skeleton during contraction and the forces of gravity that act on the entire body during standing and other weight bearing activities.[16]

Central hormonal factors maintain serum calcium concentrations within a limited range. Calcium is one of the most common ions in the human body, and almost 99% of body calcium is deposited in the skeleton. Oestrogens suppress the activity of osteoclasts, the bone-resorbing cells, and thus help to maintain bone mass. During exercise, serum concentrations of testosterone and oestrogen are elevated, influencing calcium homeostasis and the activity of osteoclasts and osteoblasts. Hormonal replacement therapy in women after the menopause makes use of this action of oestrogen.

The local mechanical forces of exercise cause (i) stress on the bone and calcium accumulation on the concave side of the bending bone, and (ii) microtraumata which are removed by osteoclasts and repaired by osteoblasts.

The supposed mechanisms behind the local mechanical forces are as follows:

First, during flexion the bone acts similar to a piezoelectric crystal while accumulating calcium at the concave (negative loaded) side. Second, mechanical demands, occurring by overload, are sensed in the bone by osteocytes via strain-derived flows of interstitial fluid. They stimulate the osteoclasts in removing the damaged structures and at the same time the osteoblasts repair the structure of the bone matrix.[17] In the case of a too strong or too often damaged bone, the process of repairing falls behind the process of removal and microfracture will occur. When the mechanical load falls below the fracture intensity, remodelling activities are stimulated and result in bone hypertrophy. Remodelling of the bone after a change in mechanical load by weight-bearing activities (including experiments with added extra weights) has been proved in experimental studies in a great number of animals.[18] Moreover, in some of these experiments it has been shown that the effects are proportional to the intensity of the (extra) load. The amount of hypertrophy also seems to depend on the difference between the extra load and the load to the bone before the extra load was added.

Not much is known about the interaction between central hormonal and local mechanical factors. However, physical activity leads to an increase of serum oestrogen levels; this diminishes the sensitivity of the bone for the parathyroid hormone and the activity of the osteoclasts; when bone mass thus increases, more calcium (Ca^{2+}) and phosphorus (P) are resorbed from the blood; this lowering of Ca^{2+} and P concentrations in the blood stimulates the parathyroid hormone; the latter inhibits vitamin D production, stimulates calcium absorption, and decreases calcium secretion.

As long as the forces exerted on the bones remain weaker than those needed to cause a macro fracture (referred to as the fracture limit), this remodelling process is able to adapt the bone to the external biomechanical stress and bring about bone thickening (hypertrophy). During long periods of inactivity, such as prolonged bed rest, the bone becomes atrophic as a result of relatively higher osteoclast activity compared to osteoblast activity. The central hormonal system and the local mechanical system interact to optimize the function of the skeletal system. In the case of exercise, mechanical factors seem to be most important for affecting bone mass.

Animal experiments[19] in an ulna-model of roosters have shown that loading of bone a few times (four times) a day can prevent bone loss, and that high frequency of loading (36 per day) results in an optimal increase in bone mass. Bone mass is not further increased by increasing the daily frequency of bone loading to 360 or even 1800 times per day. This suggests that bone tissue rapidly becomes desensitized to prolonged exercise. Others have replicated these findings.[20] Rats that were trained to jump multiple times increased tibial and femoral bone mass, but the anabolic response saturated after about 40 loading cycles. The results of both experiments are illustrated in Fig. 27.2.

Therefore in humans, short bursts of explosive exercise, such as skipping, stair climbing, and jumping, are supposedly more effective for bone development, than popular forms of exercise such as walking, jogging, bicycling, and swimming.

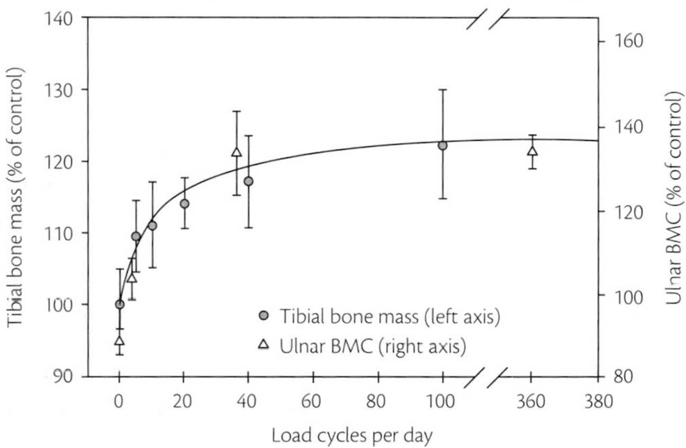

Fig. 27.2 Experiments in animals (roosters and rats) show that loading bones at a frequency more than 40 load cycles per day is an optimal rate to increase bone mass [open triangles, tibia of roosters (Rubin and Lanyon[19]); closed circles, ulna of rats (Umemura *et al.*[20])]. After Turner,[23] with permission.

Bone, therefore, appears to react best to exercise that is characterized by a pattern of unexpected and irregular high dynamic loads with a relatively low frequency and short duration.[21] Turner formulated three rules: (i) bone adaptation is driven by dynamic, rather than static, loading; (ii) only a short duration of mechanical loading is necessary to initiate an adaptive response, extending the loading duration has a diminishing effect on further bone adaptation; and (iii) bone cells accommodate to a customary mechanical loading environment, making them less responsive to routine loading signals.

This is quite different from endurance exercise aiming at the moving aerobic function, which needs a load of long duration (or high frequency) and low intensity. For comparison, Fig. 27.3 shows an example of a typical and effective exercise for loading bone (skipping) and an effective exercise for loading the oxygen transport system (jogging). Extrapolated from the results of animal studies, skipping for 1 min a day (six times for 10 s) seems effective for maintaining bone mass, whereas jogging for 1 hour a day (i.e. two times 30 min) is more effective for the development of the oxygen transport system. Exercise that is effective in maintaining bone mass seems to take a lot less time than endurance exercise![22]

From the available data on exercise regimens, Turner and Robling[23] constructed an osteoporotic index (OI) including intensity of load upon bone (times body weight), times the number of loading cycles, times the number of days per week. The OI increased by 30% if the number of day·week^{-1} were increased from 1–5 times per week and as much as 50% if daily exercise is divided in two shorter sessions separated by at least 8 hours and an increase of loading cycles from 150 to 600 resulted in a 20% increase.

Natural course of bone mass development

Although in Fig. 27.1 the general course of bone mass was outlined, not much is known about the exact timing of the age at which the maximal amount of bone mass is reached. Therefore, first, the literature is reviewed about bone development in boys and girls before puberty. Second, an estimation is made about the importance of the pubertal period in the total development of bone mass. Third, the question regarding the age at which maximal or PBMD occurs in males and females is answered.

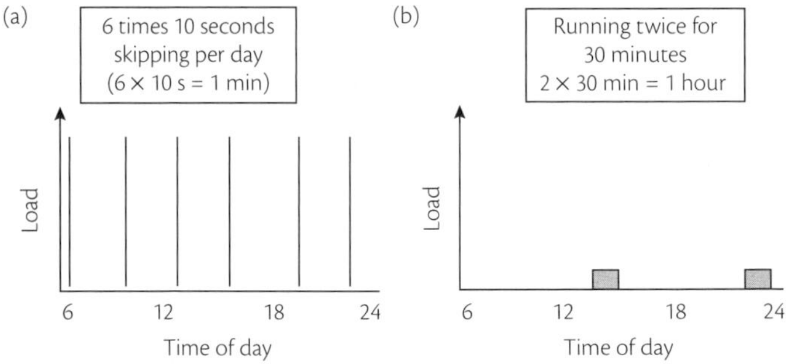

Fig. 27.3 Comparison of two types of exercise with different effects on the musculoskeletal and the cardiorespiratory system. Short explosive exercise (a), such as skipping six times a day for 10 s (total exercise time per day is 60 s), is effective for bone and muscle strength, whereas low-intensity exercise (b) of long duration, such as jogging two times a day for 30 min (total exercise time is 60 min), is more effective for the development of the oxygen transport system. After Kemper,[22] with permission.

Development of bone density before puberty

Six cross-sectional studies[24–29] and one longitudinal study[30] conclude that between boys and girls there is no significant difference between the BMD of the radius and the LS. This indicates that the development of BMD before puberty is not dependent on steroids.

Although there is a trend for a gradual increase from birth to puberty in bone mass, from seven reviewed publications it is not possible to make a quantitative estimation of the proportional contribution of this time window to the total (adult) bone mass. Before puberty there is no difference in BMD between boys and girls.

Development of bone density during puberty

Puberty is a relative short period of 3–5 years in the life of boys and girls. This short period seems to be a very important one for the development of bone mass, if we review the literature. The results of six cross-sectional studies[24–29] report increases of BMD in girls that vary between 17% and 70% and in boys between 11% and 75% of total adult values.

The high variation in these results can be attributed to several factors:

(i) Differences in the classification of puberty.

(ii) Confounding factors such as nutritional and/or activity patterns that are different for the populations studied.

(iii) The possible influence of early or late maturation: early maturation coincides with a relative but longer exposition to sex-specific hormones than late maturation; oestrogen levels in girls and testosterone levels in boys seem to be related to bone mass development.

These cross-sectional data suggest that in boys and girls the pubertal years add 50–75% to total bone mass of the LS and 30% to the radial bone mass.[31]

However, Bailey *et al.*[32] reported that the BMD changes should be interpreted with caution because of the methods used. Determination of BMD by projectional methods such as DEXA provide areal densities (g·cm^{-2}), which are confounded by the earlier mentioned size changes accompanying growth. Consequently, calculated volumetric BMD percentage increases are substantially less than the corresponding area BMD value increases.

This dimensional consideration explains why Gilsanz *et al.*[24] showed the lowest increase (15%) since they were the only ones that used the quantified computerized tomography (QCT) method to measure BMD and this method provides real volumetric BMDs.

The BMD changes during the growth period that are reported in the literature, indicating that around puberty 50% of BMD is accreted, are measured with DEXA and must therefore be doubted. The only study with QCT methodology reports a 15% volume BMD increase in pubertal girls, which seems to be a more realistic value.

The most convincing data regarding the normal pattern of bone mineral accrual around the ages 8–18 years comes from the University of Saskatchewan Pediatric Bone Mineral Accrual study.[33] The authors measured BMC in 200 boys and girls annually for 7 years at four anatomical regions (LS, FN, proximal femur, and total body). The velocity curves showed that the bone mineral accrual occurs about one and a half years earlier in girls than in boys and is 20% less in magnitude. The former is of clinical interest because the dissociation between peak linear growth and peak bone mineral accrual may constitute a period of relative bone fragility during the 4 years around peak height velocity (PHV).

Age at which maximal bone mass is reached

Most of the anatomical structures and physiological functions, such as muscle mass, cardio respiratory functions, immune system, and central nervous system, show a typical pattern over time. This is characterized by a steep increase during the growth period till the age of 20 years and thereafter a much slower decrease and gradual decline during ageing.[34] This pattern implies that there is a point or period in time where the human functions reach their maximal capacities. The question is, if there is a similar pattern observable in the development of bone mass, then at what point in time of life peak bone mineral density (PBMD) occurs.

Twelve cross-sectional studies have been published since 1981; seven were performed on girls and five on both boys and girls. In principle, a cross-sectional design is not adequate to indicate individual changes over time. It also has methodological constraints (such as cohort effects, secular trend, etc.). With these flaws in mind the results of six cross-sectional studies, with acceptable methodology and with sufficient information from the publication, are taken into account.[24,25,28,30,35,36]

They report an age period of reaching PBMD in girls between 16 and 23 years and in boys between 16 and 25 years. In Table 27.1, the results of estimated age of PBMD of each of the six valid studies are given separately for boys and girls.

Eight longitudinal studies have investigated the development of BMD and PBMD. All of them used female subjects. From a methodological point of view, the quality of the three studies can be questioned seriously. These studies tend to confirm the cross-sectional results that PBMD occurs before the age of 20 years. However two high-quality studies, from Davies *et al.*[37] with a follow up of 4 years and from Recker *et al.*[38] with a follow up of 5 years, show very clearly that at least in females the age of PBMD is reached much later than 20 years: both lumbar, radial, and total BMD reach their highest values around the age of 30 years.

In Table 27.2, the estimated age at PBMD of three low-quality[39–41] and two high-quality[35,38] longitudinal studies is summarized. Because no data are available from males it remains still unknown at what age PBMD is reached in males.

The discrepancies between the results of cross-sectional and longitudinal studies should be attributed to confounding factors. In general, high-quality cross-sectional studies tend to establish PBMD in females between 16 and 25 years of age and the high-quality longitudinal investigations much later, around the age of 30 years. Because longitudinal data are more valid to detect age changes, it is more likely that PBMD in females is occurring not in their late teens but in their mid- or late-20s.

To investigate how bone mineral at clinically important sites proceeds in relation to maturation and size in youth, distance and velocity curves for body height and BMC were made in both boys and girls based on the data from the Saskatchewan Pediatric Bone Mineral Accrual Study,[42] measured every 6 months during a follow-up of 6 years. Figure 27.4 shows the results: in both boys and girls over 35% of total body BMC was laid down during the 4-year circumpubertal period. This is 30% greater than cross-sectional estimates,[42] which demonstrates the 'blunting of values that occurs when cross-sectional data are used to represent longitudinal change'[43]

A subsequent report from this longitudinal study determined the amount of calcium that was added to the skeleton. To meet the demands of the skeleton during this rapid growth period, a mean dietary calcium intake of approximately 1100 mg·d^{-1} for boys at age 14 years and of 850 mg·d^{-1} for girls at age 12.5 years would be required. These values are comparable to the current recommended dietary allowances for calcium of 900–1200 mg·d^{-1} during the pubertal years of boys and girls.

Table 27.1 Estimated age at peak bone mineral density (PBMD) reported in six cross-sectional studies*

	Age at PBMD (years)	
Cross-sectional study	**Females**	**Males**
Gilsanz *et al.*[24]	16–17	—
Buchanan *et al.*[35]	15–23	—
Glastre *et al.*[25]	>15	>15
Geusens *et al.*[29]	16–20	21–25
Bonjour *et al.*[28]	14–15	17–18
Rico *et al.*[36]	15–19	—

*Twelve studies found between 1981 and 1992, six valid studies are considered.

Table 27.2 Estimated age at peak bone mineral density (PBMD) reported in three low-quality and two high-quality longitudinal studies in females*

Longitudinal studies	Age at PBMD (years)
Invalid studies	
Riggs *et al.*[39]	17
Moen *et al.*[40]	17–18
Slemenda *et al.*[41]	<20
Valid studies	
Davies *et al.*[37]	>26
Recker *et al.*[38]	29

*Eight studies found with females.

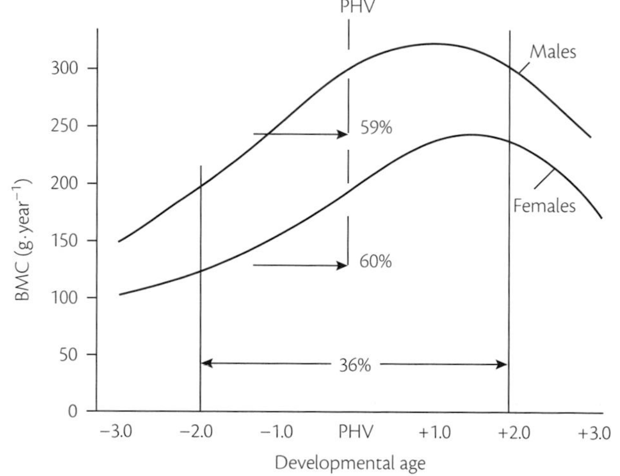

Fig. 27.4 Total body bone mineral content (BMC) velocity curves of boys and girls aligned around the 4 years of age at peak height velocity (PHV). After Bailey,[42] with permission.

Effects of physical activity and physical fitness on bone mass

Physical fitness (including neuromotor and cardiorespiratory fitness) is often used as a proxy measure of physical activity. In theory, however, physical fitness is the result of both genetic and environmental influences. For most physical fitness parameters, the genetic component is responsible for about 60–80% of the variance (e.g. maximal aerobic power, maximal muscle force, flexibility). Physical activity is the only one of several other environmental factors that can modify physical fitness. Therefore, in this chapter, the relationship between bone health and physical fitness is not considered further.

Randomized-controlled trials

Longitudinal studies that include interventions with extra physical activity are indispensable to prove that bone mass can be influenced by the daily activity pattern of the subjects involved. The majority of these so-called randomized-controlled trials (RCTs) are done in females older than 45 years in order to prevent postmenarcheal bone loss osteoporosis.

In a meta-analysis, the effects of exercise training programmes in pre- and postmenopausal women on BMD of the LS and the FN were studied by Wolff *et al.*[44] The study treatment effect was defined as the difference between the percentage change in BMD per year in the training and the control group. Seventeen articles were included. The summary treatment effects were in premenopausal women 0.9% (95% CI: 0.4–1.4) in LS and 0.9% (0.3–1.5) and in postmenopausal women 0.9 (0.4–1.3) in LS and 1.0 (0.4–1.5) in FN. It showed that exercise prevented almost 1% BMD loss per year in both pre- and postmenopausal women. The separate analysis for endurance and strength training type did not reveal large differences. The main reasons for this are two-fold: (i) small number of studies with specific strength training and (ii) the endurance programmes also might have included exercises with high strains.

The number of RCT studies in young subjects is scarce: in boys three studies are valid for review[45–47] and six studies in girls.[48–53]

The boys' study of Margulies[45] with 268 military recruits, age 18–21 years (intensive training 8 hours per day per week), however, had no control group and the period of follow-up was relatively short (14 weeks), but more importantly about 40% of the subjects could not comply because of stress fractures. In 1998, Bradney *et al.*[46] published a study in prepubertal boys comparing an 8 months, three times per week 30-min programme consisting of weight-bearing exercise with a control group matched for age, height, weight, and BMD. The increase in BMD was site-specific and twice that in controls in LS, legs, and total body. In the Copenhagen School Child Intervention Study, Hasselstrom *et al.*[47] demonstrated in 6- to 8- year old boys (n = 297) and girls (n = 265) that different intensities of physical activities, measured with accelerometers, both the amount of daily physical activity and the amount of vigorous physical activity are associated with significantly higher forearm and calcaneal BMD.

Gleeson *et al.*[48] performed a 1 year three times per week weight training programme of 30-min duration, with an intensity of 60% of the one repetition maximum in 34 postpubertal women (24–46 years). They compared the bone density in the LS and the calcaneus with 38 controls. No changes in BMD could be found in both groups. Blimkie *et al.*[49] also found non-significant changes in younger postpubertal girls (14–18 years) following a weight-training programme over a shorter period of 26 weeks.

A 10-month intervention in premenarcheal girls by Morris *et al.*[50] with high impact strength-building exercise showed a significant increase at all four bone sides of interest (proximal femur, neck of femur, LS, and total body). This increase was accompanied by a better physical fitness (decrease in fat mass, gain in lean mass, shoulder, knee, and grip strength).

Heinonen *et al.*[52] compared the effects of 9-month step aerobics intervention on BMD in pre- and postmenarcheal girls. Only in the premenarcheal girls significant more bone gain (in the LS and FN BMD) was found between exercisers and controls.

A 2-year prospective controlled exercise intervention trial in ninety-nine 7- to 9-year-old girls from the Pediatric Osteoporosis Prevention Study, evaluating a school curriculum-based training programme (5 days with 40 min vs. 2 days 30 min per week), showed that the annual gain in BMC, areal BMD, and bone size of LS, FN, and legs was greater in the intervention group than in the controls.[53]

A study from Witzke and Snow[54] in postpubescent girls intervening with a progressive programme of plyometric jumps over a period of 9 months also did not succeed in significant BMC at hip and spine, although knee extensor strength was improved.

McKay *et al.*[51] randomized 10 grade three and four classes (mean age 8.9 years) into exercise (tuck jumps, hopping, and skipping for 10–20 min within school physical education classes)

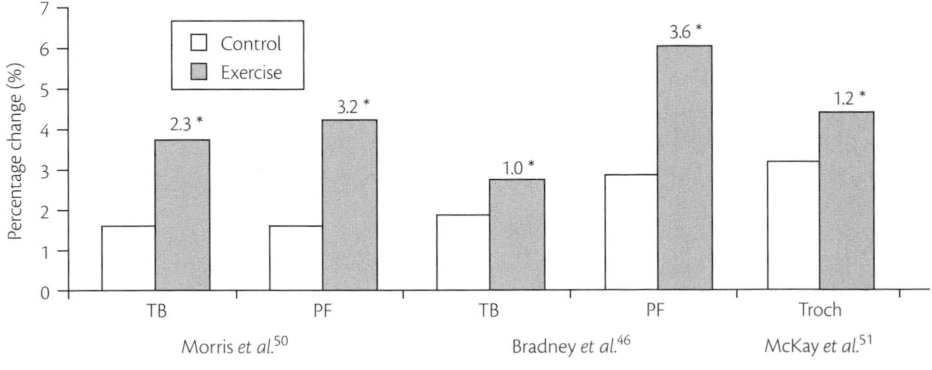

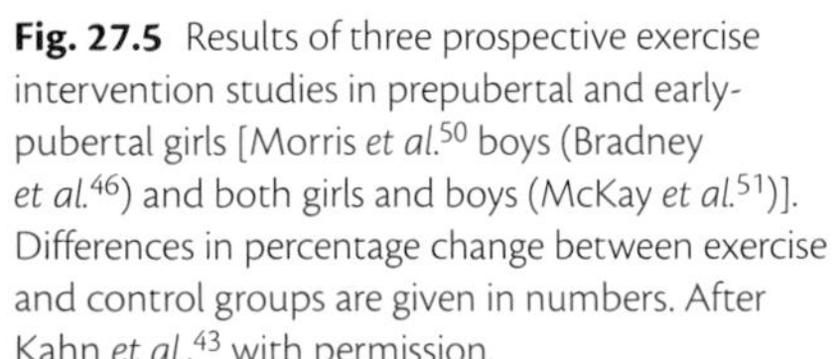
Fig. 27.5 Results of three prospective exercise intervention studies in prepubertal and early-pubertal girls [Morris *et al.*[50] boys (Bradney *et al.*[46]) and both girls and boys (McKay *et al.*[51])]. Differences in percentage change between exercise and control groups are given in numbers. After Kahn *et al.*,[43] with permission.

and control groups. The groups consisted of both boys and girls. After an 8-month intervention, the exercise group showed a significantly greater change in proximal femur and trochanter BMD compared to the control classes with regular physical education.

The outcome of the above mentioned studies seems to vary depending on the maturity level of the adolescents: studies in prepubescent and early-pubescent children report significant increases in BMC and BMD, but studies with postpubertal adolescents report no significant difference in bone mineral between control and intervention groups.

The results of three prospective exercise intervention studies in prepubertal and pubertal girls and boys are illustrated in Fig. 27.5.

Systematic review of randomized-controlled trials

Recently, a systematic review was published that evaluated 22 RCTs and non-RCTs on the effects on bone mineral accrual in children and adolescents.[55] All nine early-pubertal trials reported positive effects, measured as a mean increase over 6 months (0.9–4.9%), six prepubertal trials (1.1–5.5%), and two pubertal trials (0.3–1.9%).

Long-term effects of physical activity

Non-true-experimental results are available from the Amsterdam Growth and Health Longitudinal Study.[56] About 200 boys and 200 girls were measured longitudinally from age 13 to age 27 years. In this follow-up six measurements were taken of habitual physical activity and nutritional intake. At age 27 years the BMD of the lumbar region was measured by DEXA. The longitudinal information of weight-bearing activity and calcium intake were considered over three periods: the adolescent period from 13 to 18 years, the period between 13–22 years, and the total period between the ages of 13–27 years.

Results of multiple regression analysis showed that in both sexes weight-bearing activity and body mass were significant positive contributors in the prediction of BMD at age 27 years. Calcium intake never appeared to be a significant predictor of BMD in the three periods. From these results, it can be concluded that BMD in the LS at age 27 years may be influenced by body mass and a high level of weight-bearing physical activity carried out during youth.

To answer the question what the most important factor is for bone mass development during youth in the same study, the physical activity data were scored in two different ways: (i) by calculating the total weekly energy expenditure of all weight-bearing activities (expressed as the number of weight-bearing METs per week); and (ii) by calculating a score that takes into account the ground reaction forces of weight-bearing activities as multiples of body weight, irrespective of the frequency and the duration of the activity, that is, giving a weighted peak strain score. This is comparable with the bone loading history questionnaire from Dolan *et al.*[57] which proved to be a reproducible and valid measure of bone loading exposure in premenopausal women.

The two different habitual physical activity scores were again calculated for each subject over three time periods: the adolescent period (four annual measurements between 13 and 17 years of age), the young adult period (two measurements between 17 and 22 years of age), and the adult period (two measurements between 22 and 27 years of age).

Linear regression analysis was performed to analyse the relation between BMD at age 28 years and the physical activity scores over three foregoing periods. The physical activity scores were entered in the regression model as independent variables, and gender was added to the model as a covariate. In Fig. 27.6, the standard regression coefficients of lumbar BMD are given for the MET score and the peak strain score, and for the three different periods.

The results show that the time period, over which the physical activity scores were taken, came closer to the BMD measurement at age 27 years; the more important became the peak strain score of physical activity. For this biomechanical component of physical activity, the explained variance of BMD increased from 2% during adolescence to 13% in adulthood. For the energetic score of physical activity, the explained variance on the other and decreased from 6% during adolescence to 1% in adulthood for both sexes.[58] This strongly supports the validity of the results of animal studies in human subjects.

The preventive effect of peak strain, however, has to be confirmed in youth in true experimental design, since the significant differences in BMD can still be explained by self-selection of activity levels during the growing years.[59]

The importance of physical activity in puberty

Results from Mirwald *et al.*[60] comparing active subjects (top quartile) with inactive subjects (bottom quartile) suggested that a modifiable lifestyle factor such as physical activity plays a role in the optimization of bone mineral acquisition at the LS in boys and girls during the adolescent growth spurt. This was recently confirmed by Debar *et al.*[61] who applied a health plan-based lifestyle intervention in 14- to 16-years old girls with behavioural interventions (bimonthly group meetings, quarterly coaching telephone calls, and weekly self-monitoring) designed to improve diet and physical activity. After 1 year the girls in the intervention group had significantly higher BMD in the LS and FN compared with controls and this was maintained during the second year. A cross-sectional study of female tennis and squash players[62] showed that training started in puberty is maximally beneficial for mineralization of the bone of the playing arm. This training effect on BMD remained in adulthood (age 21–30 years) after 4 years of cessation of the training[63,64] when it was also reported that good maintenance of high impact activity induced bone gain in a 8-month follow-up of a RCT.

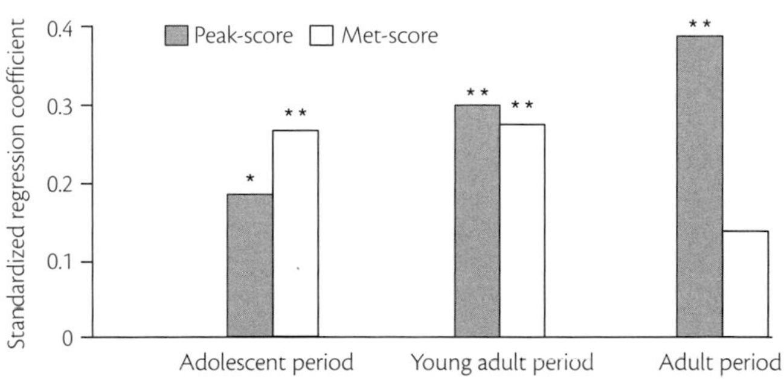

Fig. 27.6 The relationship of BMD in the lumbar spine ate age 27 years with energetic physical activity (MET) score and peak strain physical activity (peak) score during three different preceding periods in 182 males and females from the Amsterdam Growth and Health Longitudinal Study. *$p < 0.05$; **$p < 0.01$. After Groothausen *et al.*,[58] with permission.

Summary

- Bone mass increases rapidly during growth and development. The mechanism seems to be dependent on three factors: centrally regulated hormonal factors, locally determined mechanical factors, and the interaction between hormonal and mechanical factors.
- The quantitative increase of BMD during growth, measured by energy absorption methods such as DPA, SPA, and DEXA, probably gives an overestimation, because these measures do not take into consideration differences in dimensional growth of the bones in question.
- Before the age of puberty (around 12 years in girls and 13 years in boys) no significant differences in BMD between boys and girls are demonstrated.
- During the pubertal growth spurt it is now clear that the increase in BMC, on average, is 35% of total BMC increase. The clinical significance of this high percentage is that as much BMC is laid down during the four adolescent growing years, as most people will loose during all adult life.
- Investigations that measured BMD longitudinally indicate that boys and girls reach their peak BMD in their late-20s and not in their late teens. In both sexes the greatest change in BMC per year occurs 1 or 2 years after PHV.
- There are at least two exercise-related strategies to prevent osteoporosis (Fig. 27.6). One preventive strategy is to increase bone accrual during youth by increasing the amount of exercise in order to achieve a greater peak bone mass. A second strategy is to ensure that adults maintain a physically active lifestyle until old age, thus minimizing bone loss during ageing. In this way, exercise deletes the age at which the osteoporotic fracture limit is reached (Fig. 27.7).
- In young males and females, the effects of exercise intervention on BMD are scarce. Recent experimental studies show significant effects of weight-bearing activity and high impact strength training programmes on the side-specific BMD in both prepubertal and circumpubertal boys and girls. The earlier a child starts with physical activity the more bone is accumulated.

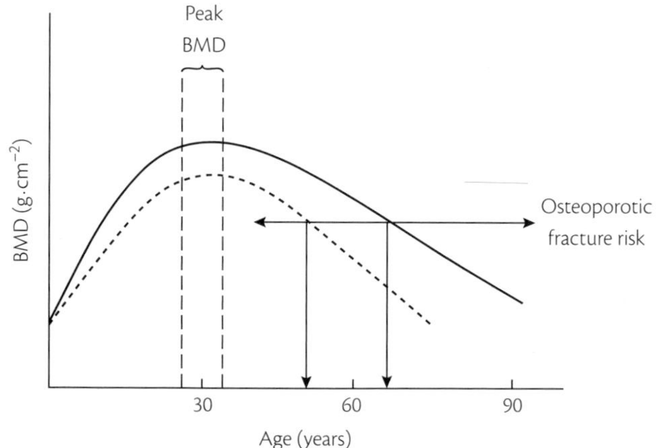

Fig. 27.7 The possible effects of lifetime exercise on the developmental curve of BMD: the average curve of inactive people (interrupted line) is shifted to the top-right (solid line) resulting in a higher BMD of any age and crossing the osteoporotic limit at a later age. After Kemper,[22] with permission.

- A preventive effect of weight-bearing activities on the PBMD is also shown in the Amsterdam Growth and Health Longitudinal study: both 27-year-old males and females, with relative high levels of peak strain weight-bearing physical activity pattern during the foregoing 15 years show significantly higher PBMD in their LS than their inactive counter parts.
- Further research is needed to establish the most effective type of exercise intervention for increasing bone mass and the most effective health-plan-based lifestyle intervention in true-experimental studies that are aimed at the possibility to increase daily physical activity patterns in both sexes in order to attain optimal maximal bone mass at young adult age.

References

1. Kemper HCG (2004). *My e-motions.* Elsevier Publishers, Maarssen.
2. Warden SJ, Fuchs RK, Castillo AB, Nelson IR, Turner CH (2007). Exercise when young provides lifelong benefits to bone structure and strength. *J Bone Miner Res* **2**, 251–9.
3. Bachrach LK (2001). Acquisition of optimal bone mass in childhood and adolescence. *Trends Endocrinol Metab* **12**, 22–8.
4. Slemenda C (1997). Prevention of hip fractures: Risk modification *Am J Med* **2A**, 65S–73S.
5. Magarey AM, Boulton TJ, Chatterton BE, Schultz C, Nordin BE, Cockington RA (1999). Bone growth from 11 to 17 years: Relationship to growth, gender and changes with pubertal stages including timing of menarche. *Acta Paediatr* **88**, 139–46.
6. Tanner JM (1955). *Growth at adolescence.* Blackwell, Oxford.
7. Tanner JM (1981). *A history of the study of human growth.* Cambridge University Press, London.
8. Weiner JS, Lourie J (1969). *Human biology, a guide to field methods IBP handbook no.9.* Blackwell, Oxford.
9. Falkner F, Tanner JM (1979). *Human growth, part 1, 2 and 3.* Plenum Press, New York.
10. Snow-Harter C, Marcus R. (1991). Exercise, bone mineral density and osteoporosis. *Exerc Sport Sci Rev* **19**, 351–88.
11. Döbeln W von (1959). Anthropometric determination of fat-free body weight. *Acta Med Scand* **165**, 37–42.
12. Roche AF, Chumlea WC, Thissen D (1988). *Assessing the skeletal maturity of the hand-wrist: Fels Method.* C.C. Thomas, Springfield, IL.
13. Roche AF, Wainer H, Thissen D (1975). *Skeletal maturity: The knee joint as a biological indicator.* Plenum, New York.
14. Tanner JM, Whitehouse RH, Marshall WA, Healy MJR, Goldstein H (1975). *Assessment of skeletal maturity and prediction of adult height (TW2 method).* Academic Press, London.
15. Sievänen H, Kannus P, Nieminen V, Heinonen A, Oja P, Vuori I (1996). Estimation of various mechanical characteristics of human bones using DEXA: Methodology and precision. *Bone* **18**, 173–5.
16. Smith EL, Raab DM (1986). Osteoporosis and physical activity. *Acta Med Scand* **711** (Suppl.), 149–56.
17. Burger EH, Klein-Nulend J (1999). Mechanotransduction in bone-role of the lacunocanalicular network. *FASEB J* **13**, S101–12.
18. Lanyon LE (1996). Using functional loading to influence bone mass and architecture: Objectives, mechanism, and relationship with estrogen of the mechanically adaptive process in bone. *Bone* 18, 37S–43S.
19. Rubin CT, Lanyon LE (1984). Regulation of bone formation by applied dynamic loads. *J Bone Joint Surg* **66A**, 397–402.
20. Umemura Y, Ishiko T, Yamauchi T, Kurono M, Mashiko S (1997). Five jumps per day increase bone mass and breaking force in rats. *J Bone Miner Res* **12**, 1480–5.
21. Turner CH (1998). Three rules for bone adaptation to mechanical stimuli. *Bone* **23**, 399–407.

22. Kemper HCG (2000). Skeletal development during childhood and adolescence and the effects of physical activity. *Pediatr Exerc Sci* **12**, 198–216.
23. Turner CH, Robling AG (2003). Designing exercise regimens to increase bone strength. *Exerc Sport Sci Rev* **31**, 45–50.
24. Gilsanz V, Gibbons DT, Roe TF, Carlson M (1988). Vertebral bone density in children: Effect of puberty. *Radiology* **166**, 847–50.
25. Glastre C, Braillon P, David L, Cochat P, Meunier PJ, Delmas PD (1990). Measurement of bone mineral content of the lumbar spine by dual energy X-ray absorptiometry in normal children: correlations with growth parameters. *J Clin Endocrinol Metab* **70**, 1330–3.
26. Gordon CL, Halton JM, Atkinson SA, Webber CE (1991). The contributions of growth and puberty to peak bone mass. *Growth Dev Aging* **55**, 257–62.
27. Southard RN, Morris JD, Hayes JR, Torch M, Sommer A (1991). Bone mass in healthy children: Measurement with quantitative DXA. *Radiology* **179**, 735–8.
28. Bonjour JF, Theintz G, Buchs B, Slosman D, Rizzoli R (1991). Critical years and stages of puberty for spinal and femoral bone mass accumulation during adolescence. *J Clin Endocrinol Metab* **73**, 555–63.
29. Geusens P, Cantatore F, Nijs J, Proesmans W, Emma F, Dequeker J (1991). Heterogeneity of growth of bone in children at the spine, radius and total skeleton. *Growth Dev Aging* **55**, 249–56.
30. Theintz G, Buchs B, Rizolli R, Slosman D, Clavien H, Sizonenko PC, Bonjour JPH. (1992). Longitudinal monitoring of bone mass accumulation in healthy adolescents: Evidence for a marked reduction after 16 years of age at the levels of lumbar spine and femoral neck in female subjects. *J Clin Endocrinol Metab* **75**, 1060–6.
31. Grimston SK, Morrison K, Harder JA, Hanley DA (1992). Bone mineral density during puberty in Western Canadian children. *J Bone Min Res* **19**, 85–96.
32. Bailey DA, Drinkwater D, Faulkner R, McKay H (1993). Proximal femur bone mineral changes in growing children: Dimensional considerations. *Pediatr Exerc Sci* **5**, 388.
33. Bailey DA, Martin AD, McKay HA (2000). Calcium accretion in girls and boys during puberty: a longitudinal analysis. *J Bone Miner Res* **15**, 2245–50.
34. Kemper HCG, Binkhorst RA (1996). Exercise and the physiological consequences of the aging process. In: Schroots JJF (ed.), *Aging, health and competence*, pp. 109–26. Elsevier, Amsterdam.
35. Buchanan JR, Meyers C, Lloyd T, Greer RB (1998). Early vertebral trabecular bone loss in normal premenopausal women. *J Bone Miner Res* **3**, 445–9.
36. Rico H, Revilla M, Hernandez ER, Villa LF, Alvarez del Buergo L (1992). Sex differences in the acquisition of total bone mineral mass peak assessed through dual energy X-ray absorptiometry. *Calcif Tissue Int* **51**, 251–4.
37. Davies KM, Recker RR, Stegman MR, Heaney RP, Kimmel DB, Leist J (1990). Third decade bone gain in women. In: Cohn DV, Glorieux FH, Martin TJ (eds.), *Calcium regulation and bone metabolism*, pp. 1497–50. Elsevier Sciences, Amsterdam.
38. Recker RR, Davies KM, Hinders SM, Heaney RP, Stegman RP, Kimmel DB (1992). Bone gain in young adult women. *JAMA* **268**, 2403–8.
39. Riggs BL, Melton J (1986). Involutional osteoporosis. *N Eng J Med* **413**, 1676–86.
40. Moen S, Sanborn C, Bonnick S, Keizer H, Gench B, DiMarco N (1992). Longitudinal lumbar bone mineral density changes in adolescent female runners. *Med Sci Sports Exerc* **38**, S12–24.
41. Slemenda CW, Miller JZ, Hui LS, Reister TK, Johnston CC (1991). Role of physical activity in the development of skeletal mass in children. *J Bone Miner Res* **6**, 1227–33.
42. Bailey DA (1997). The Saskatchewan Pediatric Bone Mineral Accrual Andy: Bone Mineral Acquisition during the growing years. *Int J Sports Med* **18**, S191–5.
43. Kahn K, McKay H, Kannus P, Bailey D, Wark J, Bennell K (2001). *Physical activity and bone health.* Human Kinetics, Champaign, IL.
44. Wolff I, Croonenberg II, Kemper HCG, Kostense PJ, Twisk JWR (1999). The effect of exercise training programs on the bone mass: A meta-analysis of published controlled trials in pre- and postmenopausal women. *Osteoporos Int* **9**, 1–12.
45. Margulies JY, Simkin A, Leichter I, Bivas A, Steinberg R, Giladi M, Stein M, Kashtan H, Milgrom C (1998). Effect of intensive physical activity on the bone mineral density content in power limbs of young adults. *J Bone Joint Surg* **68a**, 1090–3.
46. Bradney M, Pearce G, Naughton G, Sullivan C, Bass S, Beck T, Carlson J, Seeman E (1998). Moderate exercise during growth in prepubertal boys: changes in bone mass, size, volumetric density and bone strength: a controlled prospective study. *J Bone Miner Res* **13**, 1814–21.
47. Hasselstrom H, Karlsson KM, Hansen SE, Gronfeldt V, Froberg K, Andersen B (2007). Peripheral bone mineral density and different intensities of physical activity in children 6–8 years old: The Copenhagen School Child Intervention Study. *Calcif Tissue Int* **80**, 31–8.
48. Gleeson PB, Protas EJ, LeBlanc AD, Schneider VS, Evans HJ (1990). Effects of weight lifting on bone mineral density in premenopausal women. *J Bone Miner Res* **5**, 153–8.
49. Blimkie CJ, Rice S, Webber J, Martin Levy D, Parker D (1993). Bone density, physical activity, fitness, antropometry, gynaecologic, endocrine and nutrition status in adolescent girls. In: Coudert J, Praagh Ev (eds.), *Pediatric Work Physiology*, pp. 201–4. Masson, Paris.
50. Morris FL, Naughton GA, Gibbs JL, Carlson JS, Wark JD (1997). Positive effects on bone and lean mass. *J Bone Miner Res* **12**, 1453–62.
51. McKay HA, Petit MA, Schutz RW (2000) Augmented trochanteric bone mineral density after modified physical education classes: A randomized schoolbased exercise intervention in prepubertal and early pubertal children. *J Pediatr* **136**, 156–62.
52. Heinonen A, Sievanen H, Kannus P (2000). High impact exercise and bones of growing girls: A9 months controlled trial. *Osteoporos Int* **11**, 1010–17.
53. Linden C, Ahlborg HG, Besjakov J, Gardsel, P, Karlsson MK (2006). A school curriculum-based exercise program increases bone mineral accrual and bone size in prepubertal girls: Two-year data from the Pediatric Osteoporosis Prevention (POP) Study. *J Bone Miner Res* **6**, 829–35.
54. Witzke KA, Snow CM (2000). Effects of plyometric jump training on bone mass in adolescent girls. *Med Sci Sports Exerc* **32**, 1051–7.
55. Hind K, Burrows M (2007). Weight-bearing exercise and bone mineral accrual in children and adolescents: A review of controlled trials. *Bone* **40**, 14–27.
56. Welten DC, Kemper HCG, Post GB, Mechelen W van, Twisk JWR, Lips P, Teule GJ. (1994). Weight bearing activity during youth is a more important factor for peak bone mass than calcium intake. *J Bone Miner Res* **9**, 1029–96.
57. Dolan SH, Williams DP, Ainsworth BE, Shaw JM (2006). Development and reproducibility of the bone loading history questionnaire. *Med Sci Sports Exerc* **38**, 1121–31.
58. Groothausen J, Siemer H, Kemper HCG, Twisk JWR, Welten DC (1997). Influence of peak strain on lumbar bone mineral density: an analysis physical activity in young males and females. *Pediatr Exerc Sci* **9**, 159–73.
59. Kemper HCG (ed.) (2004). Amsterdam Growth and Health Longitudinal Study (AGAHLS). A 23-year follow-up from teenager to adult about lifestyle and Health. *Med Sport Sci* **47, 5–20.**
60. Mirwald RL, Bailey DA, McKay H, Crocker PE (1999). Physical activity and bone mineral acquisition at the lumbar spine during the adolescent growth spurt. Abstract at: *First International Conference on Children's Bone Health, Maastricht.* Program and Abstract Book, p. 57.

61. Debar L, Ritenbauch C, Aickin M, Orwoll E, Elliot D, Dickerson J, Vuckovic N, Stevens VJ, Moe E, Irving LM. (2006). A health plan-based lifestyle intervention increases bone mineral density in adolescent girls *Arch Pediatr Adolesc Med* **160**, 1269–76.
62. Kannus P, Haapasalo H, Sankelo M, Sievanen H, Pasanen M, Heinonen A, Oja P, Vuori I. (1995). Effect of starting age of physical activity on bone mass in the dominant arm of tennis and squash players. *Ann Intern Med* **123**, 27–31.
63. Kontulainen S, Kannus P, Haapsalo H, Heinonen A, Sievanen H, Oja P, Vuori P. (1999). Changes in bone mineral content with decreased training in competitive young adult tennis players and controls: a prospective 4-year follow-up. *Med Sci Sports Exerc* **31**, 640–52.
64. Heinonen A, Kannus P, Oja, P (1999). Good maintenance of high-impact activity-induced bone gain by voluntary, unsupervised exercises: An 8-month follow up of a randomised control trial. *J Bone Miner Res* **14**, 125–8.

CHAPTER 28

Physical activity, physical fitness, and social, psychological, and emotional health

Julie C. Garza, Nancy G. Murray, Shreela Sharma, Kelli L. Drenner, Susan R. Tortolero, and Wendell C. Taylor

Introduction

Physical activity is consistently associated with favourable physical health[1]; however, the impact of physical activity on social, psychological, and emotional health is not consistent. Given the importance of these facets of health for children and adolescents, we reviewed the literature, identified important gaps in knowledge, and recommended future research. This review includes recent literature hereby updating the earlier version of this chapter.[2]

Method of review

Published articles in English language literature from 1998 through 2007 were reviewed that included (i) subjects in the age range of 3–18 years old; (ii) measures of physical activity and/or fitness; and (iii) measures of social, psychological, emotional, and/or personality variables. The focus of our review was on the social, psychological, and emotional effects of activity and/or fitness rather than predictors and determinants of activity.

The search techniques from the earlier version of the chapter were replicated.[2] This review includes 76 articles published since 1998. Studies assessing the impact of physical activity and fitness on self-perceptions (Table 28.1), academic functioning (Table 28.2), psychological symptoms and negative affect (Table 28.3), and risk behaviours (Table 28.4) are presented in tables throughout the text. Studies included in the earlier version of this chapter have been included within the tables.[2]

Self-perceptions

The related constructs of self-perceptions have been the most extensively studied psychological outcomes of physical activity and fitness. Although many of the constructs of self-esteem, self-concept, perceived physical competence and ability, self-efficacy, and body image, are highly related, conceptually these constructs are different. The difficulty in summarizing the literature regarding these constructs is that many of these constructs are used interchangeably and terms are frequently not defined. The previous review did not identify studies that evaluated self-perception as a construct; however, this review identified six studies with self-perception as the construct of interest.[3–8] Each study reported a positive association among physical self-perceptions or health self-perceptions and physical activity.

Self-concept

Most of the studies in the previous review reported a positive association between self-concept and exercise. The most current literature is consistent with the earlier review, with five articles reporting a positive association between physical activity/fitness and global self-concept among youth (9–14 years). Only one study found no relationship between physical activity level and self-concept.[9]

The study designs used in the more recent studies were mostly cross-sectional.[9–12] A longitudinal study by Marsh *et al.*[13] examined the association between self-concept and exercise behaviour among high school students and reported a positive association between exercise and self-concept. Taylor *et al.*[14] used an experimental design to assess the effects of a physical activity intervention on self-concept and reported a positive effect of the physical activity intervention on self-concept. It is important to note that, as compared to studies in the previous review which mostly used the Piers–Harris self-concept scale to measure self-concept, the more current studies used different measures, such as the physical self-perception profile,[15] which indicates the availability of several instruments for accurate and valid measurement of self-concept.

Self-esteem

The previous review found inconsistent results regarding the relationship between physical activity and self-esteem. Three

Table 28.1 The effects of physical activity/fitness on self-perceptions

Psychosocial variable	Study design*/pop characteristics	Physical activity/fitness measure	Psychosocial well-being measure	Relationship
Aarnio[8]	LONG *n* = 5028 twins Age 16 years	Leisure time PA	Perception of current health	+
Biddle[5]	XSECT *n* = 516 girls M age 13.7 years	Physical Self-perception Profile	7-day PA questionnaire	+
Colchico[7]	EXP *n* = 30 females Age 11–14 years	Extracurricular PA intervention	Self-perceived profile for children	+
Daley[3]	EXP *n* = 90 11–16 years	Exercise therapy, attention control intervention. PA questionnaire	Physical self-perception Profile	+
Daley[4]	EXP *n* = 113 females 15–16 years	Aerobics plus PE intervention	Physical self-perception profile	+
Valois[6]	XSECT *n* = 4758 high school students Grades 9–12	CDC YRBS PA	Brief Multidimensional Student Life Satisfaction Scale	+
Self-concept				
Asci[9]	XSECT *n* = 115 M age 12.7	PA	Piers–Harris Children's Self-Concept scale (global self-concept)	0
Dishman[12]	XSECT *n* = 1250 girls Grade 12	YRBS PA and sports participation	Physical Self-Description Questionnaire (global physical self-concept)	+
Grandmontagne[10]	XSECT *n* = 740 Age 12–16 years	Physical self-concept questionnaire	Sports practice	+
Marsh[13]	LONG *n* = 2786	PA	Physical self-concept	+
Taylor[14]	EXP *n* = 92 African-American girls Age 10–12 years	PA intervention	Self-perception profile for children (physical performance self-concept)	+
Weiss[11]	XSECT *n* = 97 Age 9–43 years	Perceived Competence Scale for Special Athletes	Fitness	+
Blackman1[06]	QEXP *n* = 16 females M age 14.83	Fitness	Tennessee Self-Concept Scale (global self-concept)	0
Hatfield[107]	QEXP *n* = 14 Age 9–11 years	PA intervention	Martinek–Zaichowsky Self-Concept Scale Piers-Harris Self-Concept Scale (global self-concept)	+
MacMahon[108]	EXP CLINICAL *n* = 54 males M age 9.7 years	PA intervention	Piers–Harris Self-Concept Scale (global self-concept)	+
MacMahon[109]	QEXP CLINICAL *n* = 98 males M age 16.3 years	PA intervention	Piers–Harris Self-Concept Scale (global self-concept)	+
Overbay[110]	XSECT *n* = 61 Age 6–12 years	PA, fitness	Martinek–Zaichowsky Self-Concept Scale	+: PA 0: Fitness

continued

Table 28.1 *continued*

Psychosocial variable	Study design*/pop characteristics	Physical activity/fitness measure	Psychosocial well-being measure	Relationship
Parish–Plass[111]	QEXP CLINICAL *n* = 43 males Age 8–13.5 years	PA intervention	Tennessee Self-Concept Scale	0
Sherrill[112]	XSECT *n* = 393 Grades 4–5	Fitness	Children's Self Concept Scale	+
Young[113]	XSECT *n* = 75 females Grades 7–10th	Fitness	Tennessee Self-Concept Scale	+
Self-esteem				
Dishman [12]	XSECT *n* = 1250 females Grade 12	YRBS PA and sports participation	Physical Self-Description Questionnaire (self-esteem scale)	+
Pedersen[16]	XSECT *n* = 247 females M age 13.2 years	Team Sports Achievement and Athletic Self-evaluation	Self-perception Profile for Adolescents (self-esteem scale)	+
Strauss[17]	XSECT *n* = 92 Age 10–16 years	PA levels	Piers–Harris Children's self-concept scale (self-esteem scores)	+
Aine[114]	XSECT *n* = 90 Age 15–24 years	SR exercise	Rosenberg Self-Esteem Scale	0
Blackman[106]	QEXP *n* = 16 females M age 14.83 years	VO2 max Fitness tests	Coopersmith Self Esteem Inventory	0
Boyd[115]	QEXP *n* = 181 females Age 9–16 years	PA intervention	Self Description Questionnaire	+
Koniak–Griffin[116]	QEXP CLINICAL *n* = 58 females Age 14–20 years	PA intervention	Coopersmith Self Esteem Inventory	+
Sonstroem[40]	LONG *n* = 98 males Grades 9–12	Swim performance	Rosenberg Self-Esteem Scale	+
Body image				
Jankauskiene[30]	XSECT *n* = 405 girls M age 16.9 years	Leisure time PA	Weight related body image	+
Kelly[29]	XSECT *n* = 2357 females Grades 9–12	Peer and parent attitudes towards exercise	Body Shape Satisfaction scale	0
Kirkcaldy[28]	XSECT *n* = 1000 Age 14–18 years	Endurance sport participation	Self-image	+
Pedersen[16]	XSECT *n* = 247 females M age 13.2 years	Team Sports Achievement & Athletic Self-evaluation	Self-perception Profile for Adolescents	+
Suris[31]	XSECT *n* = 6968 14–19 years	SR PA	Catalonia Adolescent Health Survey 2001 (body image)	+

continued

Table 28.1 *continued*

Psychosocial variable	Study design*/pop characteristics	Physical activity/fitness measure	Psychosocial well-being measure	Relationship
Boyd[117]	QEXP *n* = 181 females Age 9–16 years	PA intervention	Physical Appearance Scale	+
Hatfield[107]	QEXP *n* = 11 Age 9–11 years	PA intervention	Piers–Harris Self concept Scale	0
Tuckman[118]	EXP *n* = 154 Grades 4–6	Fitness	AAHPER Youth Behaviour Rating Scale	0
Self-efficacy and perceived competence				
Paxton[34]	XSECT *n* = 63 M age 11.5 years	PA Questionnaire for Older Children	Perceived Physical Competence	+
Ryan[35]	XSECT Sample 1: *n* = 57, 25 fifth grade and 32 seventh grade. Sample 2: *n* = 49 sixth grade	PA	Self-efficacy: PA, Barriers, Asking	+
Taylor[14]	EXP *n* = 92 African-American girls Age 10–12 years	PA intervention	PA Self-Efficacy scale	+
Wang[36]	XSECT *n* = 824 Age 11–14 years	PA participation	Sports competence	+
Wu[37]	XSECT *n* = 832 M age 13.5 years	Activity log	PA Self-efficacy scale	+
Brown[38]	EXP CLINICAL M age 15.6 years	PA intervention	Self Efficacy Questionnaire	+
Holloway[39]	QEXP *n* = 59 females M age 16 years	Strength training intervention	Strength training self-efficacy	+
Sonstroem[40]	LONG *n* = 93 males Grades 9–12	Swim performance	Perceived Physical Competence	+

*XSECT is a cross-sectional study; EXP is an experimental study; QEXP is a quasi-experimental study; CASE is a case-control study; LONG is a longitudinal study; CLINICAL denotes that the study was performed in a clinical setting; M is mean age; PA is physical activity; SR is self report; + is a positive relationship, – is an inverse relationship, 0 is no association.

Table 28.2 The effects of physical activity/fitness on self-perceptions

Psychosocial variable	Study design*/pop characteristics	Physical activity/fitness measure	Psychosocial well-being measure	Relationship
Academic achievement				
Aarnio[8]	LONG (*n* = 5028) Ages 16–18 years	SR persistent inactivity (age 16)	SR of academic versus vocational school (age 18)	+
		SR persistent exercise (age 16)	SR of school grade compared with class average (age 17)	0
Ahamed[46]	EXP *n* = 288 M age 10.2 years	PA intervention	Canadian Achievement Test-3	0
Coe[47]	EXP *n* = 214 M age 11.5 years	Vigorous PA during PE ≥ HP2010 guidelines	Classroom grades	+
		PE class enrollment	Terra Nova standardized test scores	0

continued

Table 28.2 *continued*

Psychosocial variable	Study design*/pop characteristics	Physical activity/fitness measure	Psychosocial well-being measure	Relationship
Colchico[7]	QEXP *n* = 30 females M age 12.6 years	PA intervention	Self-Perception of Scholastic Competence	+
Daley[119]	XSECT *n* = 232	SR PA	Classroom grades	0
Datar[55]	LONG *n* = 11,192 Kindergarten to first grade	Parent-reported PA	Reading test scores	–: Girls 0: Boys
			Math test scores	0: Girls and Boys
Dwyer[48]	EXP *n* = 231 M age 10.3 years	PA intervention	Teacher ratings of classroom behaviour	+
			Reading and math standardized test scores	0
Dwyer[50]	XSECT *n* = 9000 Ages 9, 12, 15 years	SR lunchtime activity	School rating of academic performance	+: Boys 15 years 0: Girls and other boys
		SR weekly exercise	School rating of academic performance	+: Boys 0: Girls
Field[59]	XSECT *n* = 89 Grade 12	SR exercise level	SR grade point average	+
Grissom[58]	XSECT *n* = 888,715 Grades 5, 7, 9	Physical fitness test	Stanford 9 Reading and Math scores	+
Mahar[51]	QEXP *n* = 243 Grades 3, 4	Classroom PA intervention	Observations of on-task behavior	+
Sallis[49]	EXP *n* = 759 M age 9.5 years	Physical education intervention	Metropolitan Achievement Test-Reading, Language	+
			Metropolitan Achievement Test-Math	0
Shephard[52]	QEXP *n* = 546 Grades 1–6	PA intervention	Classroom grades	+
Sigfusdottir[56]	XSECT n = 5810 Grades 9, 10	SR PA level	SR grade average	+
		SR PA level when depressed mood, self-esteem in model	SR grade average	
Tremblay[57]	XSECT n = 6923 Grade 6	SR PA	Standardized test scores	+
Twemlow[53]	QEXP Grade 3	PE for self-regulation (1 of 4 components)	Metropolitan Achievement Test	+
Yin[54]	LONG n = 1883 Grade 8 to 10 to 12	Participation in interscholastic sports	Drop out rate	–
Bluechardt[120]	EXP CLINICAL n = 45 M age 9.4 years	PA intervention	Self Perceptions Profile for Learning Disabled Students	0
Mechanic[121]	LONG n = 1057 Grades 7–11	SR sports participation	SR academic grades	+
MacMahon[109]	QEXP CLINICAL n = 98 males Age 14–18.3 years	PA intervention	Wide Range Achievement Test	0

Table 28.3 The effects of physical activity/fitness on self-perceptions

Psychosocial variable	Study design*/pop characteristics	Physical activity/fitness measure	Psychosocial well-being measure	Relationship
Depression				
Bonhauser[67]	QEXP (*n* = 198) M age 15 years	PA intervention	Hospital Anxiety Depression Scale	0
Crews[69]	EXP *n* = 66 Grade 4	PA intervention	Beck Depression Inventory	–
Daley[68]	EXP *n* = 81 Age 11–16 years	PA intervention and behavioral counselling	Children's Depression Inventory	0
Donaldson[61]	XSECT *n* = 202 M age 12.33 years	Sports participation and sports ability teacher rating	Youth Self Report and Self-Perception Profile for Children	–
Jeong[63]	EXP *n* = 40 females M age 16 years	Dance movement therapy	Symptom Check List-90-Revision	–
			Plasma serotonin and dopamine, plasma cortisol	+
Kirkcaldy[28]	XSECT *n* = 988 M age 15.6 years	PA	Achenbach Child Behavior Checklist	–
Motl[65]	LONG *n* = 4594 M age 12.7 years	PA	Center for Epidemiological Studies Depression Scale	–
Parfitt[64]	XSECT *n* = 70 M age 10.4 years	PA	Child Depression Inventory	–
Perera[66]	XSECT *n* = 891 M age 16.4 years	PA	Center for Epidemiological Studies Depression Scale	–: Girls 0: Boys
Piko[62]	QEXP *n* = 1109 M age 16.5 years	PA	Child Depression Inventory (short version)	–
Brown[38]	EXP CLINICAL *n* = 27 M age 15.6 years	PA intervention	Beck's Depression Inventory	-: Girls 0: Boys
Brown[122]	XSECT *n* = 220 females M age 15.6 years	SR sports participation and PA	Multiple Affect Checklist-Depressed	–
Glyshaw[71]	LONG and XSECT *n* = 530	SR PA	Children's Depression Inventory	0
Koniak–Griffin[116]	QEXP CLINICAL *n* = 58 females Age 14–20 years	PA intervention	Center for Epidemiologic Studies-Depression	–: Pregnant adolescents
MacMahon[109]	QEXP CLINICAL *n* = 98 males Age 14–18.3 years	PA intervention	Beck's Depression Inventory	–
Michaud–Tomson[123]	XSECT *n* = 933	PA	Dimensions of Depression Profile	–
Milligan[124]	LONG *n* = 301 M age 18 years	SR PA	Zung Depression Scale	–: Boys 0: Girls
		Submax fitness test	Zung Depression Scale	–: Girls 0: Boys

continued

Table 28.3 *continued*

Psychosocial variable	Study design*/pop characteristics	Physical activity/fitness measure	Psychosocial well-being measure	Relationship
Norris[125]	EXP *n* = 60 M age 16.7 years	PA intervention	Multiple Affect Checklist-Depressed	0
Thorlindsson[70]	XSECT *n* = 1131 Age 15–16 years	SR sports participation	3-item depression scale	–
Anxiety				
Bonhauser[67]	QEXP *n* = 198 M age 15 years	PA intervention	Hospital Anxiety Depression Scale	–
Crews[69]	EXP *n* = 66 Grade 4	PA intervention	State-Trait Anxiety Inventory for Children (STAIC)	0
Donaldson[61]	XSECT *n* = 202 M age 12.33 years	Sports participation and sports ability teacher rating	Youth SR and Self-Perception Profile for Children	–
Jeong[63]	EXP CLINICAL *n* = 40 females M age 16 years	Dance Movement Therapy	Symptom Check List-90-Revision, plasma serotonin & dopamine , plasma cortisol	–
Kirkcaldy[28]	XSECT *n* = 988 M age 15.6 years	PA Questionnaire	Achenbach Child Behaviour Checklist	–
Parfitt[64]	XSECT *n* = 70 M age 10.4 years	PA	STAIC	–
Bahrke[126]	EXP *n* = 65 Grades 4–6	PA intervention	STAIC	0
Brown[38]	EXP CLINICAL *n* = 27 M age 15.6 years	PA intervention	Profile of Mood States	–: Girls 0: Boys
Glyshaw[71]	LONG & XSECT *n* = 530	SR physical exercise	STAIC	0
Norris[125]	EXP *n* = 60 M age 16.7 years	PA intervention	Multiple Affect Checklist-Anxiety	–
Thorlindsson[70]	XSECT *n* = 1131 Age 15–16 years	SR sports participation	3-item anxiety scale	–
Hostility				
Jeong[63]	EXP CLINICAL *n* = 40 females M age 16 years	Symptom Check List-90-Revision	Symptom Check List-90-Revision	–
Aganoff[127]	LONG *n* = 97 females Age 140–48 yeears	Menstrual Distress Questionnaire	Menstrual Distress Questionnaire	–
Brown[38]	EXP CLINICAL *n* = 27 M age 15.6 years	Profile of Mood States	Profile of Mood States	–: Girls 0: Boys
Norris[125]	EXP *n* = 60 M age 16.7 years	Menstrual Distress Questionnaire	Menstrual Distress Questionnaire	0

Table 28.4 The effects of physical activity/fitness on self-perceptions

Psychosocial variable	Study design*/pop characteristics	Physical activity/fitness measure	Psychosocial well-being measure	Relationship
Tobacco use				
Aarnio[8]	LONG *n* = 4906 Age 16 years	SR PA	SR smoking	–
Abrams[75]	XSECT *n* = 1549 Grades 6, 8, 10, and 12	SR sports participation	SR smoking	–
			SR smokeless tobacco use	+
Audrain-McGovern[74]	LONG *n* = 978 Grades 9–12	SR PA	SR smoking	–
Castrucci[76]	XSECT *n* = 16,357 Grades 9–12	SR sports participation	SR cigarette smoking	–
			SR chewing tobacco and snuff use	+
			SR lifetime cigarette use and cigar use in the past year	0
Cohen[77]	XSECT *n* = 318 Grades 9–12	SR PA	SR cigarette smoking	0
Coogan[78]	XSECT *n* = 31,861 Grades 4–12	SR PA	SR smoking	–
Easton[79]	XSECT *n* = 2410 Grades 9–12	SR vigorous PA	SR smoking	–
Ferron[80]	XSECT *n* = 9268 Age 15–20 years	SR sports participation	SR smoking	–
Frazier[81]	XSECT *n* = 12,603 Age 10–15 years	SR PA	SR cigar use	+
Garry[82]	XSECT *n* = 4346 Grades 6–8	YRBS SR sports participation	SR experimental cigarette use	+
			SR experimental chewing tobacco use and current cigarette use	0
Harrison[83]	XSECT n = 50,168 Grade 9	SR sports participation	SR smoking	–
Holmen[84]	XSECT n = 6811 Age 12–19 years	SR PA and team sports participation	SR smoking	–
Kirkcaldy[28]	XSECT n = 988 Age 14–18 years	SR PA	SR smoking	–
Kulig[85]	XSECT n = 15,349 Grades 9–12	SR PA and sports participation	SR cigarette use	–: Girls 0: Boys
Melnick[86]	XSECT n = 16,262 Grades 9–12	YRBS SR sports participation	YRBS SR smoking	–
			Smokeless tobacco use	+
			Cigar use	0

continued

Table 28.4 *continued*

Psychosocial variable	Study design*/pop characteristics	Physical activity/fitness measure	Psychosocial well-being measure	Relationship
Naylor[87]	XSECT *n* = 1515 Grades 9–12	SR sports participation	SR cigarette use	–
			SR smokeless tobacco use	0
Paavola[73]	LONG *n* = 903 Age 15 years	SR PA	SR smoking	–
Page[88]	XSECT (*n* = 12,272) Grades 9–12	YRBS SR sports participation	YRBS SR smoking	–
			Smokeless tobacco use	+: Boys 0: Girls
Papaioannou[89]	XSECT *n* = 5991 Age 11, 13, 16 years	SR sports participation	SR smoking	–
Pate[90]	XSECT *n* = 14,221 Grades 9–12	YRBS SR sports participation	YRBS SR smoking	–: White girls and Boys 0: Black and Hispanic girls
			Chewing tobacco/snuff use	–: Older girls 0: Younger girls and all boys
Rodríguez[128]	LONG *n* = 1098 Grades 9–11	SR team sport participation	SR smoking	–
Aaron[129]	LONG *n* = 1245 Age 12–16 years	SR PA	YRBS SR smoking	–: Girls 0: Boys
Baumert[23]	XSECT *n* = 6849 Grades 9–12	SR organized sports participation	YRBS SR cigarette smoking	–
			YRBS SR smokeless tobacco use	0
Coulson[130]	XSECT *n* = 932 M age 13.5 years	SR sports participation	SR smoking behaviors	–
Davis[25]	XSECT *n* = 1200 males M age 15.8 years	SR sports participation	SR smokeless tobacco use	0
		SR sports participation	SR smoking	–
Escobedo[131]	XSECT *n* = 11,248 Grade 8–12	YRBS sports team participation	YRBS SR smoking behaviour	+
Pate[26]	XSECT *n* = 11,631 Ages 12–18 years	YRBS PA	YRBS SR smoking	+
Rainey[1]	XSECT *n* = 7846 Grades 9–12			
Thorlindsson[70]	XSECT *n* = 1131 Age 15–16 years	SR sports participation	SR smoking behavior	+
Winnail[132]	XSECT *n* = 4800 Grade 9–12	YRBS number of days sweat/breathe hard	YRBS SR smoking and smokeless tobacco	–: White males 0: African-American boys/girls and White girls

continued

Table 28.4 *continued*

Psychosocial variable	Study design*/pop characteristics	Physical activity/fitness measure	Psychosocial well-being measure	Relationship
Alcohol				
Aarnio[8]	LONG n = 4906 Age 16 years	SR PA	SR alcohol use	–: Girls 0: Boys
Garry[82]	XSECT n = 4346 Grades 6–8	SR sports participation	SR current alcohol use	+
Harrison[83]	XSECT n = 50,168 Grade 9	SR sports only participation	SR binge drinking	–
			SR alcohol use	0
Kirkcaldy[28]	XSECT n = 988 Ages 14–18 years	SR PA	SR beer use	0
Kulig[85]	XSECT n = 15,349 Grades 9–12	SR PA and sports participation	SR alcohol use (binge drinking)	0
Lorente[94]	XSECT n = 816	SR sports participation	SR alcohol use	–
Nelson[93]	LONG n = 11,957 Grades 7–12	SR PA	SR being drunk in past month	–
			SR ever being drunk	0
Page[88]	XSECT n = 12,272 Grades 9–12	YRBS SR sports participation	YRBS SR alcohol use (binge drinking)	0
Pate[90]	XSECT n = 14,221 Grades 9–12	YRBS SR sports participation	YRBS SR alcohol use (binge drinking)	0
Werch[92]	QEXP n = 454 Grade 8	PA intervention	SR alcohol use	–
Aaron[129]	LONG n = 1245 Age 12–16 years	SR competitive athletics SR leisure time	YRBS SR alcohol use YRBS SR alcohol use	+: Boys 0: Girls
Baumert[23]	XSECT n = 6849 Grades 9–12	SR participation in organized sports	YRBS SR alcohol use (binge drinking)	0
Carr[21]	XSECT n = 1713 Grades 10–12	Athletic team member identification	SR alcohol use	+: Boys 0: Girls
			Abstention	–
Oler[22]	XSECT n = 823 Grades 9–12	SR competitive athletics	SR alcohol use	0
Pate[26]	XSECT n = 11,631 Age 12–18 years	YRBS PA items coded as low-high activity	YRBS SR alcohol use	+: Girls 0: Boys
Rainey[1]	XSECT n = 7846 Grades 9–12	SR athletic teams and PA	YRBS SR alcohol use & binge drinking	+

continued

Table 28.4 *continued*

Psychosocial variable	Study design*/pop characteristics	Physical activity/fitness measure	Psychosocial well-being measure	Relationship
Thorlindsson[70]	XSECT *n* = 1131 Age 15–16 years	SR sports participation	SR alcohol use (binge drinking)	+
Aggression				
Garry[82]	XSECT *n* = 4346 Grades 6–8	SR sports participation	SR physical fight	+
Harrison[83]	XSECT *n* = 50,168 Grade 9	SR sports only participation	SR physical fight and vandalism	–
Nelson[93]	LONG *n* = 11,957 Grades 7–12	SR PA	SR participation in violence	+
			SR participation in property damage	0
Pate[90]	XSECT *n* = 14,221 Grades 9–12	YRBS SR sports participation	YRBS SR physical fight injury	0
Page[88]	XSECT *n* = 12,272 Grades 9–12	YRBS SR sports participation	YRBS SR physical fight injury	0
Baumert[23]	XSECT *n* = 6849 Grades 9–12	SR sports participation	SR physical fight	0
Begg[133]	LONG *n* = 1037 Age 15–18 years	SR leisure time PA	SRed delinquency, aggressive behaviors, social competence index	+
		Sports participation	SRed delinquency, aggressive behaviors, social competence index	0
Pate[26]	XSECT *n* = 11,631 Age 12–18 years	YRBS PA	YRBS SR physical fight injury	0
Suicide				
Brosnahan[95]	XSECT *n* = 1870 Age 14–18 years	SR vigorous activity, strength and toning, and PA sessions per week	SR suicide plan	–
			Consideration of suicide	–
Ferron[80]	XSECT *n* = 9268 Age 15–20 years	SR sports participation	SR suicide attempt	–
			SR of past suicidal thoughts	0
Garry[82]	XSECT *n* = 4346 Grades 6–8	SR suicide attempt	SR sports participation	0
Harrison[83]	XSECT *n* = 50,168 Grade 9	SR sports participation	SR of suicidal thoughts and attempts	–
Page[88]	XSECT (*n* = 12,272) Grades 9–12	YRBS SR sports participation	YRBS SR suicide attempt	–

continued

Table 28.4 *continued*

Psychosocial variable	Study design*/pop characteristics	Physical activity/fitness measure	Psychosocial well-being measure	Relationship
Page[88]	XSECT (*n* = 12,272) Grades 9–12	YRBS SR sports participation	YRBS SR suicide attempt	–
Pate[90]	XSECT (*n* = 14,221) Grades 9–12	YRBS SR sports participation	YRBS SR consider suicide	–: White girls and boys +: Black boys 0: Hispanic girls and boys, Black girls
			Suicide attempt	–: White girls 0: Hispanic boys and girls, Black boys and girls, White boys
Baumert[23]	XSECT *n* = 6849 Grades 9–12	SR organized sports participation	Feelings of hopelessness	–
			Suicide ideation or attempts	0
De Wilde[134]	CASE *n* = 157	SR PA	Interviewed in year following suicide attempt	0
Oler[22]	XSECT *n* = 823 grades 9–12	SR competitive athletics	Index of potential suicide	–
			Suicide behavior questionnaire	–: Girls 0: Boys
			Children's Depression Inventory	–
Drug use				
Colingwood[96]	QEXP *n* = 329	PA intervention	SR substance use	–
Dodge[99]	LONG *n* = 15,000 Grades 7–12	SR sports participation	SR anabolic steroid use	+
Ferron[80]	XSECT *n* = 9268 Age 15–20 years	SR sports participation	SR marijuana use	–
			SR hard drug use	0
Garry[82]	XSECT *n* = 4346 Grades 6–8	SR sports participation	SR experimental cocaine and inhalant use	+
			SR experimental marijuana, steroid, and needle drug use SR current marijuana use	0
Harrison[83]	XSECT *n* = 50,168 Grade 9	SR sports only participation	SR marijuana use	–
Kirkcaldy[28]	XSECT *n* = 988 Ages 14–18 years	SR sports participation	SR marijuana use	–
Kulig[85]	XSECT *n* = 15,349 Grades 9–12	SR PA and sports participation	SR other drug use	–: Boys 0: Girls
			SR marijuana and steroid use	0
Naylor[87]	XSECT *n* = 1515 Grades 9–12	SR sports participation	SR cocaine, psychedelics, and creatine use	–
			SR marijuana, steroid, barbiturate, and amphetamine use	0

continued

Table 28.4 *continued*

Psychosocial variable	Study design*/pop characteristics	Physical activity/fitness measure	Psychosocial well-being measure	Relationship
Nelson[93]	LONG *n* = 11,957 Grades 7–12	SR PA	SR illegal drug use (except marijuana)	–
			SR marijuana use	0
Page[88]	XSECT *n* = 12,272 Grades 9–12	YRBS SR sports participation	YRBS SR cocaine, marijuana, or other illegal drug use	–
			Steroid use	+: Boys 0: Girls
Pate[90]	XSECT *n* = 14,221 Grades 9–12	YRBS SR sports participation	YRBS SR marijuana use	–: White boys/girls and Hispanic girls 0: Black boys/girls and Hispanic boys
			Cocaine use	–: White girls and all boys 0:Black and Hispanic girls
			Other illegal drug use	–: White girls and all boys +: Black girls 0: Hispanic girls
			Sniffed glue/spray cans	–: White girls/boys 0:Black boys/girls & Hispanic boys/girls
			Steroid use	–: White girls +: Hispanic girls 0: Black girls and all boys
Peretti-Watel[98]	XSECT *n* = 12,512 Age 18 years	SR formal sports practice	SR marijuana use	–
		Informal sports practice	SR marijuana use	+: Girls 0: Boys
Werch[97]	QEXP *n* = 604 Grades 9 and 11	PA intervention	SR drug use	–
Baumert[23]	XSECT *n* = 6849 Grades 9–12	SR sports participation	SR marijuana use	–
			SR use of cocaine/crack, other illicit drugs, or steroids (after controlling for age, race, and gender)	0
Collingwood[135]	QEXP CLINICAL *n* = 74 M age 16.8 years	Fitness test	SR substance use	–
Oler[22]	XSECT *n* = 823 Grades 9–12	SR competitive athletics	SR marijuana use	–
			SR cocaine use	0
Pate[26]	XSECT *n* = 11,631 Age 12–18 years	YRBS PA	YRBS self-report marijuana and cocaine use	–
Winnail[132]	XSECT *n* = 4800	YRBS number of days sweat/breathe hard	YRBS SR marijuana use	+

continued

Table 28.4 *continued*

Psychosocial variable	Study design*/pop characteristics	Physical activity/fitness measure	Psychosocial well-being measure	Relationship
Sexual activity				
Ferron[80]	XSECT *n* = 9268 Age 15–20 years	SR sports participation	SR contraception use at first intercourse and condom use at last intercourse	–
Forman[100]	XSECT *n* = 1112 Age 13–19 years	SR high school interscholastic sports	SR sexual intercourse	+
Harrison[83]	XSECT *n* = 50,168 Grade 9	SR sports only participation	SR sexual intercourse	–
Kulig[85]	XSECT *n* = 15,349 Grades 9–12	SR PA and sports participation	SR sexual activities	–: Girls 0: Boys
Miller[101]	XSECT *n* = 8979 Grades 9–12	YRBS SR sports participation	YRBS SR age at first intercourse and involvement in pregnancy	–: Girl 0: Boys
			Ever had sex, lifetime & recent sex partners	–: Girls +: Boys
			Birth control & condom use	+
			Use withdrawal method	0
Nelson[93]	LONG *n* = 11,957 Grades 7–12	SR PA	SR sexual activities	–
Page[88]	XSECT *n* = 12,272 Grades 9–12	YRBS SR sports participation	YRBS SR 4 or more sex partners; no method to prevent pregnancy	–: Boys 0: Girls
			Ever had an STD; involvement in pregnancy	–: Girls 0: Boys
			Did not use a condom	–
			Sexual intercourse ever	0
Pate[90]	XSECT *n* = 14,221 Grades 9–12		YRBS SR sexual intercourse ever	–: White girls +: Black boys 0: Black & Hispanic girls and White & Hispanic boys
			In the past 3 months	–: Girls +: Black boys 0: White & Hispanic boys
			Multiple partners in the past 3 months	–:White boys 0:All girls, Black & Hispanic boys
Sabo[102]	XSECT *n* = 699 Age 13–16 years	SR sports participation	SR frequency of sexual behavior and pregnancy risk	–: Girls 0: Boys
Forman[100]	XSECT *n* = 1112 Age 13–19 years	SR sports participation	SR sexual intercourse	+

continued

Table 28.4 *continued*

Psychosocial variable	Study design*/pop characteristics	Physical activity/fitness measure	Psychosocial well-being measure	Relationship
Miller[24]	XSECT *n* = 16,262 Grades 9–12	SR PA and sports participation	SR number of partners, lifetime sex, past year sex, early onset	–: Girls 0: Boys
Pate[26]	XSECT *n* = 11,631 Age 12–18 years	YRBS PA	No. of sex partners in past 3 months	0
Smith[20]	XSECT *n* = 1071 Grades 9–11	SR sports participation	SR sexual intercourse	+

cross-sectional studies identified for this review found a positive relationship between physical activity and self-esteem.[12,16,17] For example, a study conducted among a nationally representative sample of children/adolescents found that self-esteem scores were positively related to physical activity levels.[17] More rigorous study designs are needed to help understand the relationship between physical activity and self-esteem.

Body image

Body image or perception of physical appearance is an important construct particularly for adolescents. Both, gender and ethnic differences in perceptions of body image have been observed among adolescents.[18] Generally, females are more concerned with physical beauty and maintaining an ideal body image; whereas, boys are more concerned about body size, strength, and power.[19] Further, female adolescents generally do not match the perceived ideal body image indicated by societal expectations. In addition, it has been reported that African-American girls are more satisfied with their bodies than European American or Native American girls.[20–27]

In this review, we identified five cross-sectional studies examining the association between body image and physical activity/fitness among youth.[16,28–31] While four studies reported a positive association between exercise and body image,[16,28,30,31] one study reported no relationship.[29] Therefore, the association between physical activity/fitness and body image has not been very well studied, and the evidence that exists is inconclusive. Given the importance of body image among youth, and the reported ethnic and gender differences, further research is needed.

Self-efficacy/perceived physical competence

According to Bandura,[32] self-efficacy is the conviction that one can carry out the desired behaviour to produce the expected outcome. While self-efficacy has been shown to be predictive of a variety of health behaviours including physical activity,[33] five studies examining whether engaging in physical activity increases self-efficacy/perceived physical competence were reviewed.[13,34–37] Three additional studies were presented in the earlier review which concluded that physical activity/fitness may be positively related to self-efficacy.[38–40] Taylor *et al.*[14] employed an experimental design and concluded that a physical activity intervention was related to increased physical activity self-efficacy scale scores. The four cross-sectional studies[34–37] reported a relatively strong association between physical activity and self-efficacy or perceived self-competence. These results are consistent with the earlier review.

Summary

Overall, the conclusions are that physical activity and fitness have positive effects on self-perceptions, in particular, these effects are most evident for self-concept, self-esteem, and self-efficacy. However, data are limited about the effect of physical activity on body image because few well-designed studies have been conducted. Many studies have methodological, theoretical, and measurement problems such as inadequate study designs, absence of conceptual definitions, and theoretical models to guide the research.

Psychosocial and academic functioning

Several studies examined whether physical activity improves academic and psychosocial functioning among youth. These findings are presented in Table 28.2.

Academic functioning

In the past decade, interest in justifying physical education and physical activity opportunities in schools has fostered several review articles.[41–45] The general consensus of these reviews is that there is evidence that physical activity in children has a positive effect on cognitive functioning, that taking time out of academics for physical activity does not have a negative impact on test scores, and that additional research is needed.

Four recent studies investigating the effect of a physical activity or physical education intervention on academic performance in a school setting reported inconsistent results.[46–49] A cluster randomized-controlled trial increased physical activity 50 min per week, but did not demonstrate differences in Canadian Achievement Test scores between treatment conditions at the end of one school year.[46] While Coe *et al.*[47] did not find a significant effect of random assignment to physical education class on either standardized tests scores or classroom grades, students randomly assigned to physical education class who reported vigorous intensity physical activity scored significantly higher classroom grades than students who reported no activity. The SHAPE study demonstrated that a 14-week physical activity intervention significantly improved fitness and teacher ratings of classroom performance without any impact on academic performance despite taking an extra 1 hour and 15 min a day from the academic programme.[48,50] Project SPARK employed a randomized trial of a physical education programme that consumed twice the amount of time for physical activity compared to the comparison condition and demonstrated improvements in standardized achievement test scores for reading and language, but not for math.[49] While these rigorous studies reported inconsistent findings, they suggest that taking substantial time out of academic instruction for physical activity does not negatively impact academic performance.

Four quasi-experimental studies suggest that physical activity interventions have a positive impact on academics. A pilot project suggests that an extracurricular physical activity programme for 11- to 14-year-old girls positively impacted self-perceptions of academic performance.[7] Elementary school students who participated in classroom Energizers activities spent significantly more time in observed on-task behaviour during academic instruction time; the intervention was most effective for students who were least on-task at baseline.[51] Among Quebec students, participation in five additional hours a week of physical activity in school was associated with significantly higher classroom grades during grades 2–6 of the study (except for grade 4), especially for girls.[52] Physical education designed to teach self-regulation skills was implemented as part of a violence-reduction programme incorporating zero-tolerance for bullying, a discipline plan, and mentoring programme over 4 years.[53] The experimental school demonstrated significant improvement in standardized test scores over the comparison school; also, individual experimental students significantly improved composite and reading scores, but not math scores. These four studies are limited in sample size, research, and programme design but suggest sufficient promise to support further research.

Four longitudinal studies examine the relationship between sports participation or activity levels and academic performance. Data from the National Education Longitudinal Study in the United States found students who participated in interscholastic sports in eighth or tenth grade were less likely to drop out of school.[54] While cognitive test scores were negatively related to sports participation at baseline, there was no relationship at tenth or twelfth grade. Data from a birth cohort study of twins in Finland revealed self-reports of persistent physical inactivity at age 16 year was predictive of attendance at vocational school at age 18 year instead of academic school. However, inactivity was not predictive of self-report of school grades compared to class average at age 17 year.[8] For boys, the Early Childhood Longitudinal Study found parent-reported physical activity was negatively related to reading scores and unrelated to math scores in kindergarten (cross-sectional) and not predictive of math or reading scores in first grade.[55] For girls, there was not a cross-sectional relationship between parent-reported physical activity and math or reading scores, but a weakly significant negative longitudinal relationship for reading. These studies provide limited support for a relationship between physical activity and academic progress for adolescents, but not for very young children.

Five of six cross-sectional studies provide some support for a relationship between standardized test scores or self-reported grades and physical activity or fitness levels in adolescents. Among Icelandic children, self-report of physical activity, body mass index, and diet accounted for almost 24% of the variance in self-reported grade average (controlling for gender, parental education, family structure, and absenteeism).[56] When self-esteem and depressed mood were added to this model, the effect of physical activity on academic performance was no longer significant. Among Canadian sixth-graders, increased physical activity was weakly related to math and reading standardized test scores.[57] Among Australian high school students, self-report of lunchtime physical activity was significantly related to scholastic ratings for 15-year-old boys, but not for girls or younger boys.[50] Younger boys' (ages 9 and 12 year) scholastic ratings were related to weekly physical activity. Among California children and adolescents, the number of fitness standards achieved in the FITNESSGRAM® was significantly related to Stanford 9 reading and math scores; although, the relationship may be stronger for girls than boys, and for students of higher socio-economic status (SES).[58] In a small study of U.S. high school seniors, self-reported exercise levels were related to self-reported grade point average.[59] These cross-sectional studies provide support for a relationship between physical activity and academics but also suggest that additional constructs may mediate the relationship.

While physical activity may confer some benefit in academic functioning, the limited number of well-designed studies limits our ability to make definitive conclusions and suggests the need for further research that incorporates mediating variables.

Psychological symptoms and negative affect

A large body of literature has emerged suggesting that physical activity and fitness decrease psychological symptoms and negative affect among adults.[60] Involvement in exercise may be key to enhancing mental health. Since adolescence is characterized as a time of emotional distress, it is particularly useful to understand the benefits of physical activity in decreasing emotional distress and negative affect among youth. Table 28.3 presents the evidence for physical activity and fitness associated with depression, anxiety, negative affect, emotional distress, stress, loneliness, and hostility. It should be noted that a negative (or inverse) relationship between physical activity and/or fitness in the context of mental health is a good result. For example, as physical activity increases, negative psychological symptoms decrease.

Depression

Since 1998, 10 studies have addressed physical activity or fitness and depression among youth.[28,61–69] Cross-sectional studies account for the largest proportion of evidence for the association of physical activity and depression. With the exception of the Perera *et al.*[66] study that showed a negative association for females but not for males, all of the cross-sectional studies showed decreases in depression related to physical activity.[28,61,64,70]

Three experimental studies with physical activity interventions were reviewed.[63,68,69] Daley *et al.*[68] found no association between physical activity and depressive symptoms while two other studies[63,69] found significant reductions in depression-related symptoms for the intervention group compared to control groups. The Crews *et al.* study[69] examined the effect of aerobic exercise in 66 Hispanic 4th grade students compared to a physical activity control group. Participants in the aerobic exercise intervention group reported less depression than the control group. Jeong *et al.*[63]

reported that mildly depressed Korean middle school girls assigned to a Dance Movement Therapy (DMT) intervention group showed significant decreases in all SCL-90-R subscales in the DMT group including the depression subscale. In addition, favourable neuro-transmitter profiles in the DMT group (increased serotonin and decreased dopamine levels) suggest possible therapeutic effects of the intervention on depression.

Quasi-experimental and longitudinal studies have shown inconsistent results. One quasi-experimental study of 1109 Hungarian youth reported that self-report physical activity in boys and girls reduced depressive symptoms.[62] Bonhauser *et al.*[67] found no association between the intervention and control groups for 198 Chilean boys and girls in a 1-year, school-based physical activity intervention and scores on the Hospital Anxiety Depression Scale (HADS). A 2-year longitudinal study by Motl *et al.*[65] examined the relation between changes in self-reported physical activity and depressive symptoms in a cohort of 4594 teens. Results showed that physical activity was negatively associated with depressive symptoms in male and female youth.

In summary, physical activity appears to be associated with decreased depressive symptoms. Although much of the research on physical activity and depression has methodological flaws, the evidence indicates beneficial effects of physical activity on depressive symptoms.

Anxiety

Six studies assessed the association between physical activity/fitness and anxiety among youth.[28,61,63,64,67,69] One study found no association between self-reported anxiety and physical activity.[69,71] The evidence from the remaining five studies supports the conclusion that there is a relationship between increased physical activity and fewer symptoms of anxiety. A preliminary experimental study among girls found the DMT intervention group showed a significant decrease in anxiety symptoms compared to the control group.[63] A school-based study evaluated the effects of a 1 year physical activity programme on Chilean adolescents.[67] Compared to controls, those in the intervention schools showed a significant reduction in anxiety. Also, three cross-sectional studies found a negative relation between physical activity and measures of anxiety.[28,61,64]

The association between physical activity and anxiety is inconclusive, the research is limited, and the available studies are difficult to compare. Also, researchers used different constructs of anxiety and many of the measurement instruments were not psychometrically sound.

Hostility

Since 1998, only one study has examined the effect of physical activity on hostility levels among youth.[63] A dance movement intervention reduced hostility in a small group of mildly depressed girls.[63] Given the dearth of information in this area, future studies are needed.

Summary

Since the earlier review, more evidence has emerged indicating overall inverse relation between physical activity and emotional distress. In other words, in the presence of physical activity the symptoms of emotional distress, such as depression and anxiety, decrease. Few of the studies reviewed had an experimental design and for those with an experimental design, the results were inconsistent. To date, most of the results are cross-sectional, and inferences about causality are inappropriate. Further, it is difficult to compare the studies reviewed because a variety of methods, interventions, and measures were used. More research with randomized-controlled trials will further our understanding of the relationships between physical activity and psychological distress.

Risk behaviours

A small number of risk behaviours contribute to adverse health and social consequences for adolescents, including tobacco use, drug and alcohol use, aggression or delinquency, sexual behaviours, and suicide. We examined the effect of physical activity on those risk behaviours that are pertinent to adolescent health.

Tobacco use

The relationship between physical activity and/or sports participation and tobacco use among youth has been extensively investigated. The earlier review found that tobacco use was most often inversely related to physical activity and sports participation. However, data were limited because all but one of the studies was cross-sectional. This review identified four longitudinal studies[8,72–74] and 17 cross-sectional studies,[28,75–90] many of which used data from the Center for Disease Control and Prevention's Youth Risk Behavior Survey (YRBS).

The majority of studies assessing the relationship between physical activity and tobacco use report an inverse relationship. However, differences between genders were not as apparent in the recent literature. Of the six studies that examined smoking among boys and girls separately,[8,81,84,86,88] only one study found that cigarette smoking was inversely related to physical activity among girls but not associated with physical activity among boys.[85] When both gender and ethnicity were examined, smoking had a negative association with physical activity among White girls and all boys, but no relationship was found among Black or Hispanic girls.[90] Examination of the level of team participation between 9th and 11th grade also revealed that decreasing and erratic levels of participation from grades 9 to 11 were associated with higher levels of smoking in 9th grade and current smoking in 11th grade.[72] However, there is also an evidence suggesting the type of athletic activity (i.e. individual sport vs. team sport, high endurance vs. low endurance) may be an important factor to consider when investigating this relationship.[85,91] Three studies examined cigar use and physical activity and reported inconsistent results with two observing no association[76,86] and one observing a positive association among boys and girls.[81]

For the relationship between smokeless tobacco use and physical activity, several cross-sectional studies provide evidence of a positive relationship.[75,76,82,86,88,90] However, each of these studies examined physical activity exclusively in the context of sports participation. When examining the relationship by gender, smokeless tobacco use among males was significantly higher in athletes compared to non-athletes, even after adjusting for ethnic background and grade.[86,90] Among girls, older girls who participated in team sports were more than three times as likely to use smokeless tobacco than girls who were non-athletes.[90] These studies suggest that smokeless tobacco use may be associated with sports involvement and should be investigated further.

Alcohol use

There continues to be conflicting evidence for the relationship between physical activity, especially participation in sports teams, and alcohol use, particularly binge drinking. A quasi-experimental study found a physical activity intervention resulted in increases in physical activity and decreases in alcohol problems and consumption among eighth graders.[92] Also, two longitudinal studies found physical activity to be related to a lower likelihood of using alcohol among girls[8] and getting drunk.[93] Of seven cross-sectional studies reviewed,[28,82,83,85,88,90,94] three studies investigated males and females separately and consistently concluded that there was no association between physical activity/sports participation and alcohol use and binge drinking among either gender.[85,88,90] Studies which employed more rigorous study designs specifically assessed the relationship between physical activity and alcohol use and each reported a negative relationship; however, studies that used cross-sectional designs investigated sports participation and inconsistent results were found. Rigorous studies are needed to explore the relationship between sports participation and alcohol use and to elucidate differences between measures of physical activity and alcohol use (i.e. sports participation and alcohol use, physical activity, and alcohol use).

Aggression

The current literature has inconsistent findings for the relationship between physical activity and aggression or violence. A longitudinal study found that those who engaged in five or more sessions of moderate to vigorous intensity physical activity per week at baseline were more likely to engage in violence 1–2 years later; however, these differences were marginal.[93] In two cross-sectional studies, findings regarding sports participation and involvement in a physical fight were inconsistent, with one study reporting a positive relationship,[82] and another study reporting an inverse relationship.[83] When injuries in a physical fight and physical activity were assessed, no relationship was reported.[88,90]

Suicide

Most studies examining the relationship between physical activity/sports participation and suicidal risk have reported an inverse relationship,[80,83,88,95] however, because of the cross-sectional designs, results should be viewed cautiously given that depression is known to be associated with suicide, and that the lack of physical activity and interest in doing things is part of depressive symptomatology. Two nationally representative cross-sectional studies reported an inverse relationship between sports participation and suicidal thoughts[90] and attempts.[88,90] When gender and ethnicity were examined, only European American girls and boys who participated in sports were less likely to consider suicide than non-participants.[90] African-American boys who participated in sports were more likely to consider suicide than non-participants.[90] More conclusive studies are needed to investigate the differences by gender and ethnicity.

Drug use

Studies assessing the relationship between drug use and physical activity/sports participation continue to provide evidence of an inverse relationship for most drugs. Two quasi-experimental studies reported that participation in physical activity interventions resulted in decreases in alcohol and drug behaviours.[96,97] For marijuana use, five cross-sectional studies reported marijuana use to be inversely related to physical activity,[28,80,83,88,90] but three additional studies found no relationship.[85,87,93] A French study found that 4 or more hours in formal sports practice were related to more frequent marijuana use among both boys and girls; also, four or more hours spent in informal sports practice were related to more frequent cocaine use among girls.[98] When cocaine use was assessed among U.S. high school populations, an inverse relationship between sports participation and cocaine use was most often reported.[87,88,90] As for steroid use, two cross-sectional studies reported no relationship between physical activity/sports participation and steroid use,[82,85] but a longitudinal study reported a positive relationship.[99] Also, Page *et al.*[88] found a positive relationship between playing in three or more sports teams and steroid use among boys. Among girls, an inverse relationship was found between steroid use and team sports participation for European Americans and a positive relationship was found for Hispanics.[90] Examination of a middle school population found a positive relationship between sports participation and cocaine and inhalant use.[82]

Sexual activity

The relationship between physical activity/sports participation and sexual activity differs by gender. Overall, a nationally representative longitudinal study reported that those who participated in five or more sessions of moderate intensity physical activity per week at baseline were less likely to have sexual intercourse and to have sex without birth control 1–2 years later.[93] Eight cross-sectional studies provided further examination of the relationship between physical activity and sexual activity in adolescents.[80,83,85,88,90,100–102] In a nationally representative sample, no relationship was found between level of physical activity and number of sex partners in the past 3 months.[26] However, studies of ninth graders in Minnesota and of post-mandatory school Swedish students reported an inverse relationship for sports participation, sexual intercourse,[83] and having unprotected sex.[80] When a history of pregnancy or getting someone pregnant was assessed in relationship to athletic participation, a negative relationship was found for females but not for males.[88,101,102] The relationship between sports participation and age at initiation of sexual activity among boys remains unclear with two studies reporting a negative relationship[20,100] and four studies reporting no significant differences.[24,85,88,101] However, analysis of the YRBS found that African-American boys who participated in sports were more likely to have initiated sex and to have had sex in the past 3 months than non-participant boys.[90] While three studies reported that female athletes were less likely to have initiated sexual activity compared to female non-athletes,[24,85,101] another found this relationship to be true only among European American girls.[90] In contrast, African-American girls who participate in physical activity may be more likely to engage in sexual risk behaviours and become pregnant more often than non-participators.[85,90] More studies are needed to investigate these differences by gender and ethnicity.

Summary

The relationship between physical activity and risk behaviours is inconsistent. While children and adolescents who participate in physical activity may be less likely to smoke cigarettes and to use other drugs, they may be more likely to use alcohol and initiate sexual activity at an earlier age. Also, these relationships also differed by physical activity measure, whether it was a sports-related or non-sports-related activity. Few longitudinal studies have been conducted and many existing studies are limited and have not controlled for confounding factors. For example, there may be a risk-taking propensity among some youth that attracts them to competitive sports as well as risk-taking behaviours such as alcohol use, aggression, and sexual activity. In addition, perhaps the team environment facilitates norms for risk behaviours. Research designs that employ randomized-controlled trials to test physical activities as a preventive intervention for youth may help to answer some of the questions raised by the current research in this area.

Summary and future directions

- This chapter is an update of a review completed almost 10 years ago. In this update, we reviewed 76 articles conducted with youth from ages 3 to 18 years of age and published between 1998 and 2007.
  - (i) While several articles have been published since our last review, the evidence regarding the association between physical activity, physical fitness, sports participation, and social, psychological, and emotional health remains inconclusive.
  - (ii) Most studies (47 of 76) published in the past 10 years employ cross-sectional designs making it difficult to draw conclusions about the nature and mechanism of these associations.
  - (iii) Constructs that were consistently associated with physical activity, physical fitness, and sports participation in youth were increased self-efficacy, positive self-esteem, perceived physical competence, greater perceived psychological well-being, and decreases in anxiety and stress.
- Our findings are consistent with previous reviews among youth and psychosocial health.[40,103–105]
  - (i) A 1994 review of 20 articles, Calfas and Taylor reported that activity among youth improves self-esteem and decreases depressive symptoms, anxiety, and stress.[103]
  - (ii) A 2004 meta-analyses of 23 randomized-controlled trials in children and young people[104] and a 2005 meta-analysis of 113 studies[105] reported a positive effect of physical activity on self-esteem.
  - (iii) Reviews of the literature and meta-analyses on physical activity/fitness and academics suggest a positive effect on cognitive functioning and that taking time out of academics for physical activity does not have a negative impact on test scores and may improve them.[41–45]
- The challenges are many for future research studies on the effects of physical activity, fitness, and sports participation on the social, psychological, and emotional health of children and adolescents.
  - (i) The reliability and validity of the physical activity, sports participation, fitness, and psychosocial measures need improvement.
  - (ii) Another challenge is research design rigor; many of the findings are based on cross-sectional studies or studies without control groups. Cross-sectional designs for investigating the association between physical activity and emotional health may be problematic given that depressive signs may include symptoms of engaging in less activity and less interest in participating in activities.
  - (iii) A third challenge is generalizability. While more studies have been conducted on diverse populations (i.e. race/ethnicities, age, SES, etc.) since our last review, often the effects of physical activity, fitness, and sports participation differed by gender and racial/ethnic groups. More studies are needed with girls and a diversity of racial and ethnic groups, social classes, and health statuses (e.g. obese, hypertensive etc.). By including a broader range of youth, the confidence in the robustness of the findings will increase.
  - (iv) A fourth challenge is to conduct studies that take into account potential confounders and mediators; for example, studies on physical activity and tobacco use also should include measures of depression as a potential confounder or mediator.
- In summary, future research should strive for consistency in methods, measurement techniques, and dose effects (including intensity of physical activity). More reliable, valid, and developmentally appropriate measures, longer time periods, repeated assessments, more diverse income levels, ages, cultural settings, and ethnic backgrounds are needed. Better research will help us understand the effects of physical activity and fitness because the social, psychological, and emotional health of children and adolescents is a concern for all of society.

Acknowledgments

We gratefully acknowledge the assistance of Ms. Vaishali Shah in identifying relevant literature.

References

1. Rainey CJ, McKeown RE, Sargent RG, Valois RF (1996). Patterns of tobacco and alcohol use among sedentary, exercising, nonathletic, and athletic youth. *J School Health* **66**, 27–32.
2. Tortolero SR, Taylor WC, Murray NG (2000). Physical activity, physical fitness and social, psychological and emotional health. In: Armstrong N, Van Mechelen W (eds.), *Paediatric exercise science and medicine*, pp. 273–93. Oxford University Press, Oxford.
3. Daley AJ, Copeland RJ, Wright NP, Wales JK (2005). Protocol for: Sheffield Obesity Trial (SHOT): A randomised controlled trial of exercise therapy and mental health outcomes in obese adolescents [ISRCNT83888112]. *BMC Public Health* **5**, 113.
4. Daley AJ, Buchanan J (1999). Aerobic dance and physical self-perceptions in female adolescents: Some implications for physical education. *Res Q Exerc Sport* **70**, 196–200.
5. Biddle SJH, Wang CKJ (2003). Motivation and self-perception profiles and links with physical activity in adolescent girls. *J Adolesc* **26**, 687–701.
6. Valois RF, Zullig KJ, Huebner ES, Drane JW (2004). Physical activity behaviors and perceived life satisfaction among public high school adolescents. *J School Health* **74**, 59–65.
7. Colchico K, Zybert P, Basch CE (2000). Effects of after-school physical activity on fitness, fatness, and cognitive self-perceptions: A pilot study among urban, minority adolescent girls. *Am J Pub Health* **90**, 977–8.
8. Aarnio M, Winter T, Kujala U, Kaprio J (2002). Associations of health related behaviour, social relationships, and health status with persistent physical activity and inactivity: A study of Finnish adolescent twins. *Br J Sports Med* **36**, 360–4.

9. Aci FH, Koar SN, Iler AK (2001). The relationship of self-concept and perceived athletic competence to physical activity level and gender among Turkish early adolescents. *Adolescence* **36**, 499–507.
10. Goni Grnadmontagne A, Rodriguez Fernandez A (2004). Eating disorders, sport practice and physical self-concept in adolescents. *Actas Esp Psiquiatr* **32**, 29–36.
11. Weiss J, Diamond T, Demark J, Lovald B (2003). Involvement in Special Olympics and its relations to self-concept and actual competency in participants with developmental disabilities. *Res Dev Disabil* **24**, 281–305.
12. Dishman RK, Hales DP, Pfeiffer KA, Felton GA, Saunders R, Ward DS, Dowda M, Pate RR (2006). Physical self-concept and self-esteem mediate cross-sectional relations of physical activity and sport participation with depression symptoms among adolescent girls. *Health Psychol* **25**, 396–407.
13. Marsh HW, Papaioannou A, Theodorakis Y (2006). Causal ordering of physical self-concept and exercise behavior: Reciprocal effects model and the influence of physical education teachers. *Health Psychol* **25**, 316–28.
14. Taylor WC, Baranowski T, Klesges LM, Ey S, Pratt C, Rochon J, Zhou A (2004). Psychometric properties of optimism and pessimism: Results from the Girls' Health Enrichment Multisite Studies. *Prev Med* **38**, S69–77.
15. Harter S (1982). The Perceived Competence Scale for Children. *Child Dev* **53**, 87–97.
16. Pedersen S, Seidman E (2004). Team sports achievement and self-esteem development among urban adolescent girls. *Psychol Women Q* **28**, 412–22.
17. Strauss RS, Rodzilsky D, Burack G, Colin M (2001). Psychosocial correlates of physical activity in healthy children. *Arch Pediatr Adolesc Med* **155**, 897–902.
18. Fox KR, Corbin CC (1989). The Physical Self-Perception Profile: Development and preliminary validation. *J Sport Exerc Psych* **11**, 408–30.
19. Gill D (1995). Gender issues: A social-educational perspective. In: Murphy SM (ed.), *Sport psychology interventions,* pp. 205–34. Human Kinetics, Champaign, IL.
20. Smith EA, Caldwell LL (1994). Participation in high school sports and adolescent sexual activity. *Pediatr Exerc Sci* **6**, 69–74.
21. Carr CN, Kennedy SR, Dimick KM (1990). Alcohol use among high school athletes: A comparison of alcohol use and intoxication of male and female high school athletes and non-athletes. *J Alcohol Drug Educ* **36**, 39–43.
22. Oler MJ, Mainous AG, 3rd, Martin CA, Richardson E, Haney A, Wilson D, Adams T (1994). Depression, suicidal ideation, and substance use among adolescents: Are athletes at less risk? *Arch Fam Med* **3**, 781–5.
23. Baumert PW Jr, Henderson JM, Thompson NJ (1998). Health risk behaviors of adolescent participants in organized sports. *J Adolesc Health* **22**, 460–5.
24. Miller KE, Sabo DF, Farrell MP, Barnes GM, Melnick MJ (1998). Athletic participation and sexual behavior in adolescents: The different worlds of boys and girls. *J Health Soc Behav* **39**, 108–23.
25. Davis TC, Arnold C, Nandy I, Bocchini JA, Gottlieb A, George RB, Berkel H (1997). Tobacco use among male high school athletes. *J Adolesc Health* **21**, 97–101.
26. Pate RR, Heath GW, Dowda M, Trost SG (1996). Associations between physical activity and other health behaviors in a representative sample of US adolescents. *Am J Pub Health* **86**, 1577–81.
27. Jaffe L (1995). Adolescent girls: Factors influencing low and high body image. *Melpomen J* **14**, 14–22.
28. Kirkcaldy BD, Shephard RJ, Siefen RG (2002). The relationship between physical activity and self-image and problem behaviour among adolescents. *Soc Psych Epid* **37**, 544–50.
29. Kelly AM, Wall M, Eisenberg ME, Story M, Neumark-Sztainer D (2005). Adolescent girls with high body satisfaction: Who are they and what can they teach us? *J Adolesc Health* **37**, 391–6.
30. Jankauskiene R, Kardelis K (2005). Body image and weight reduction attempts among adolescent girls involved in physical activity. *Medicina (Kaunas)* **41**, 796–801.
31. Suris JC, Parera N (2005). Don't stop, don't stop: Physical activity and adolescence. *Int J Adolesc Med Health* **17**, 67–78.
32. Bandura A (1977). Self-efficacy: Toward a unifying theory of behavioral change. *Psychol Rev* **84**, 191–215.
33. Brawley LR, Rodgers WM (1993). Social-psychological aspects of fitness and promotion. In: Seraganian P (ed.), *Exercise psychology: The influence of physical exercise on psychological processes,* pp. 254–98. Wiley, Chichester, UK.
34. Paxton RJ, Estabrooks PA, Dzewaltowski D (2004). Attraction to physical activity mediates the relationship between perceived competence and physical activity in youth. *Res Q Exerc Sport* **75**, 107–11.
35. Ryan GJ, Dzewaltowski DA (2002) Comparing the relationships between different types of self-efficacy and physical activity in youth. *Health Educ Behav* **29**, 491–504.
36. Wang CK, Chatzisarantis NL, Spray CM, Biddle SJ (2002). Achievement goal profiles in school physical education: Differences in self-determination, sport ability beliefs, and physical activity. *Br J Educ Psychol* **72**, 433–45.
37. Wu TY, Pender N (2002). Determinants of physical activity among Taiwanese adolescents: An application of the health promotion model. *Res Nurs Health* **25**, 25–36.
38. Brown SW, Welsh MC, Labbe EE, Vitulli WF, Kulkarni P (1992). Aerobic exercise in the psychological treatment of adolescents. *Percept Mot Skills* **74**, 555–60.
39. Holloway JB, Beauter A, Duda JL (1988). Self-efficacy and training for strength in adolescent girls. *J Appl Soc Psychol* **18**, 699–719.
40. Sonstroem RJ, Harlow LL, Salisbury KS (1993). Path analysis of a self-esteem model across a competitive swim season. *Res Q Exerc Sport* **64**, 335–42.
41. Shepard RJ (1997). Curricular physical acitivity and academic performance. *Pediatr Exerc Sci* **9**, 113–26.
42. Sibley BA, Etnier JL (2003). The relationship between physical activity and cognition in children: A meta-analysis. *Pediatr Exerc Sci* **15**, 243–56.
43. Taras H (2005). Physical activity and student performance at school. *J School Health* **75**, 214–18.
44. Strong WB, Malina RM, Blimkie CJ, Daniels SR, Dishman RK, Gutin B, Hergenroeder AC, Must A, Nixon PA, Pivarnik JM, Rowland T, Trost S, Trudeau F (2005). Evidence based physical activity for school-age youth. *J Pediatr* **146**, 732–7.
45. Etnier JL, Nowell PM, Landers DM, Sibley BA (2006). A meta-regression to examine the relationship between aerobic fitness and cognitive performance. *Brain Res Rev* **52**, 119–30.
46. Ahamed Y, Macdonald H, Reed K, Naylor PJ, Liu-Ambrose T, McKay H (2007). School-based physical activity does not compromise children's academic performance. *Med Sci Sports Exerc* **39**, 371–6.
47. Coe DP, Pivarnik JM, Womack CJ, Reeves MJ, Malina RM (2006). Effect of physical education and activity levels on academic achievement in children. *Med Sci Sports Exerc* **38**, 1515–19.
48. Dwyer T, Coonan WE, Leitch DR, Hetzel BS, Baghurst RA (1983). An investigation of the effects of daily physical activity on the health of primary school students in South Australia. *Int J Epidemiol* **12**, 308–13.
49. Sallis JF, McKenzie TL, Boldan K, Lewis M, Marshall S, Rosengard P (1999). Effects of health related physical education on academic achievement: Project SPARK. *Res Q Exerc Sport* **70**, 127–34.
50. Dwyer T, Blizzard L, Dean K (1996). Physical activity and performance in children. *Nutr Rev* **54**, S27–31.
51. Mahar TM, Murphy SK, Rowe DA, Golden J, Shields AT, Raedeke TD (2006). Effect of a classroom-based program on physical activity and on-task behavior. *Med Sci Sports Exerc* **38**, 2086–94.
52. Shephard RJ, Volle M, Lavall EH, LaBarre R, Quier JC, Rajic M (1984). Required physical activity and academic grades: A controlled

longitudinal study. In: Ilmarinen J, Lim KI (eds.), *Children and sport*, pp. 58–63. Springer-Verlag, Berlin.

53. Twemlow SW, Fonagy P, Sacco FC, Gies ML, Evans R, Ewbank R (2001). Creating a peaceful school learning environment: A controlled study of an elementary school intervention to reduce violence. *Am J Psychiat* **158**, 808–10.
54. Yin Z, Moore JB (2004). Re-examining the role of interscholastic sport participation in education. *Psychol Rep* **94**, 1447–54.
55. Datar A, Sturm R, Magnabosco JL (2004). Childhood overweight and academic performance: National study of kindergartners and first-graders. *Obes Res* **12**, 58–68.
56. Sigfusdottir ID, Kristjansson AL, Allegrante JP (2007). Health behaviour and academic achievement in Icelandic school children. *Health Educ Res* **22**, 70–80.
57. Tremblay, Inman JW, Willms JD (2000). The relationship between physical activity, self-esteem, and academic achievement in 12-year-old children. *Pediatr Exerc Sci* **12**, 312–23.
58. Grissom JB (2005). Physical fitness and academic achievement. *JEP online* **8**, 11–25.
59. Field T, Diego M, Sanders CE (2001). Exercise is positively related to adolescents' relationships and academics. *Adolescence* **36**, 105–10.
60. McAuley E (1994). Physical activity and psychosocial outcomes. In: Bouchard C, Shephard RJ, Stephens T (eds.), *Physical activity, fitness and health: International proceedings and consensus statement*, pp. 551–68. Human Kinetics, Champaign, IL.
61. Donaldson SJ, Ronan KR (2006). The effects of sports participation on young adolescents' emotional well-being. *Adolescence* **41**, 369–89.
62. Piko BF, Keresztes N (2006). Physical activity, psychosocial health, and life goals among youth. *J Community Health* **31**, 136–45.
63. Jeong YJ, Hong SC, Lee MS, Park MC, Kim YK, Suh CM (2005). Dance movement therapy improves emotional responses and modulates neurohormones in adolescents with mild depression. *Int J Neurosci* **115**, 1711–20.
64. Parfitt G, Eston RG (2005). The relationship between children's habitual activity level and psychological well-being. *Acta Paediatrica* **94**, 1791–7.
65. Motl RW, Birnbaum AS, Kubik MY, Dishman RK (2004). Naturally occurring changes in physical activity are inversely related to depressive symptoms during early adolescence. *Psychosom Med* **66**, 336–42.
66. Perera B, Torabi MR, Jayawardana G, Pallethanna N (2006). Depressive symptoms among adolescents in Sri Lanka: Prevalence and behavioral correlates. *J Adolesc Health* **39**, 144–6.
67. Bonhauser M, Fernandez G, Puschel K, Yanez F, Montero J, Thompson B, Coronado G (2005). Improving physical fitness and emotional well-being in adolescents of low socioeconomic status in Chile: Results of a school-based controlled trial. *Health Promot Int* **20**, 113–22.
68. Daley AJ, Copeland RJ, Wright NP, Roalfe A, Wales JK (2006). Exercise therapy as a treatment for psychopathologic conditions in obese and morbidly obese adolescents: A randomized, controlled trial. *Pediatrics* **118**, 2126–34.
69. Crews DJ, Lochbaum MR, Landers DM (2004) Aerobic physical activity effects on psychological well-being in low-income Hispanic children. *Percept Mot Skills* **98**, 319–24.
70. Thorlindsson T, Vilhjalmsson R, Valgeirsson G (1990). Sport participation and perceived health status: A study of adolescents. *Soc Sci Med* **31**, 551–6.
71. Glyshaw K, Cohen LH, Towbes LC (1989). Coping strategies and psychological distress: Prospective analyses of early and middle adolescents. *Am J Community Psychol* **17**, 607–23.
72. Rodriguez D, Audrain-McGovern J (2004). Team sport participation and smoking: Analysis with general growth mixture modeling. *J Pediatr Psychol* **29**, 299–308.
73. Paavola M, Vartiainen E, Haukkala A (2004). Smoking, alcohol use, and physical activity: A 13-year longitudinal study ranging from adolescence into adulthood. *J Adolesc Health* **35**, 238–44.
74. Audrain-McGovern J, Rodriguez D, Moss HB (2003). Smoking progression and physical activity. *Cancer Epidem Biomar* **12**, 1121–9.
75. Abrams K, Skolnik N, Diamond JJ (1999). Patterns and correlates of tobacco use among suburban Philadelphia 6th- through 12th-grade students. *Fam Med* **31**, 128–32.
76. Castrucci BC, Gerlach KK, Kaufman NJ, Orleans CT (2004). Tobacco use and cessation behavior among adolescents participating in organized sports. *Am J Health Behav* **28**, 63–71.
77. Cohen B, Evers S, Manske S, Bercovitz K, Edward HG (2003). Smoking, physical activity and breakfast consumption among secondary school students in a southwestern Ontario community. *Can J Public Health* **94**, 41–4.
78. Coogan PF, Adams M, Geller AC, Brooks D, Miller DR, Lew RA, Koh HK (1998). Factors associated with smoking among children and adolescents in Connecticut. *Am J Prev Med* **15**, 17–24.
79. Easton A, Kiss E (2005). Covariates of current cigarette smoking among secondary school students in Budapest, Hungary, 1999. *Health Educ Res* **20**, 92–100.
80. Ferron C, Narring F, Cauderay M, Michaud PA (1999). Sport activity in adolescence: Associations with health perceptions and experimental behaviours. *Health Educ Res* **14**, 225–33.
81. Frazier AL, Fisher L, Camargo CA, Tomeo C, Colditz G (2000). Association of adolescent cigar use with other high-risk behaviors. *Pediatrics* **106**, E26.
82. Garry JP, Morrissey SL (2000). Team sports participation and risk-taking behaviors among a biracial middle school population. *Clin J Sport Med* **10**, 185–90.
83. Harrison PA, Narayan G (2003). Differences in behavior, psychological factors, and environmental factors associated with participation in school sports and other activities in adolescence. *J School Health* **73**, 113–20.
84. Holmen TL, Barrett-Connor E, Clausen J, Holmen J, Bjermer L (2002). Physical exercise, sports, and lung function in smoking versus nonsmoking adolescents. *Eur Respir J* **19**, 8–15.
85. Kulig K, Brener ND, McManus T (2003). Sexual activity and substance use among adolescents by category of physical activity plus team sports participation. *Arch Pediatr Adolesc Med* **157**, 905–12.
86. Melnick MJ, Miller KE, Sabo DF, Farrell MP, Barnes GM (2001). Tobacco use among high school athletes and nonathletes: Results of the 1997 youth risk behavior survey. *Adolescence* **36**, 727–47.
87. Naylor AH, Gardner D, Zaichkowsky L (2001). Drug use patterns among high school athletes and nonathletes. *Adolescence* **36**, 627–39.
88. Page RM, Hammermeister J, Scanlan A, Gilbert L (1998). Is school sports participation a protective factor against adolescent health risk behaviors? *J Health Educ* **29**, 186–92.
89. Papaioannou A, Karastogiannidou C, Theodorakis Y (2004). Sport involvement, sport violence and health behaviours of Greek adolescents. *Eur J Public Health* **14**, 168–72.
90. Pate RR, Trost SG, Levin S, Dowda M (2000). Sports participation and health-related behaviors among US youth. *Arch Pediatr Adolesc Med* **154**, 904–11.
91. Moore MJ, Werch CE (2005). Sport and physical activity participation and substance use among adolescents. *J Adolesc Health* **36**, 486–93.
92. Werch C, Moore M, DiClemente CC, Owen DM, Jobli E, Bledsoe R (2003). A sport-based intervention for preventing alcohol use and promoting physical activity among adolescents. *J School Health* **73**, 380–8.
93. Nelson MC, Gordon-Larsen P (2006). Physical activity and sedentary behavior patterns are associated with selected adolescent health risk behaviors. *Pediatrics* **117**, 1281–90.
94. Lorente FO, Souville M, Griffet J, Grelot L (2004). Participation in sports and alcohol consumption among French adolescents. *Addict Behav* **29**, 941–6.
95. Brosnahan J, Steffen LM, Lytle L, Patterson J, Boostrom A (2004). The relation between physical activity and mental health among Hispanic and non-Hispanic white adolescents. *Arch Pediatr Adolesc Med* **158**, 818–23.
96. Collingwood TR, Sunderlin J, Reynolds R, Kohl HW (2000). Physical training as a substance abuse prevention intervention for youth. *J Drug Educ* **30**, 435–51.

97. Werch CC, Moore MJ, DiClemente CC, Bledsoe R, Jobli E (2005). A multihealth behavior intervention integrating physical activity and substance use prevention for adolescents. *Prev Sci* **6**, 213–26.
98. Peretti-Watel P, Lorente FO (2004). Cannabis use, sport practice and other leisure activities at the end of adolescence. *Drug Alcohol Depend* **73**, 251–7.
99. Dodge TL, Jaccard JJ (2006). The effect of high school sports participation on the use of performance-enhancing substances in young adulthood. *J Adolesc Health* **39**, 367–73.
100. Forman ES, Dekker AH, Javors JR, Davison DT (1995). High-risk behaviors in teenage male athletes. *Clin J Sport Med* **5**, 36–42.
101. Miller KE, Sabo DF, Farrell MP, Barnes GM, Melnick MJ (1999). Sports, sexual behavior, contraceptive use, and pregnancy among female and male high school students: Testing cultural resource theory. *Sociol Sport J* **16**, 366–87.
102. Sabo DF, Miller KE, Farrell MP, Melnick MJ, Barnes GM (1999). High school athletic participation, sexual behavior and adolescent pregnancy: A regional study. *J Adolesc Health* **25**, 207–16.
103. Calfas KJ, Taylor WC (1994). Effects of physical activity on psychological variables of adolescents. *Pediatr Exerc Sci* **6**, 406–23.
104. Ekeland E, Heian F, Hagen KB, Abbott J, Nordheim L (2004). Exercise to improve self-esteem in children and young people. *Cochrane Database Syst Rev*, 003683.
105. Spence JC, McGannon KR, Poon P (2005). The effect of exercise on global self-esteem: A quantitative review. *J Sport Exerc Psy* **27**, 311–34.
106. Blackman L, Hunter G, Hilyer J, Harrison P (1988). The effects of dance team participation on female adolescent physical fitness and self-concept. *Adolescence* **23**, 437–48.
107. Hatfield BD, Vaccaro P, Benedict GJ (1985). Self-concept responses of children to participation in an eight-week precision jump-rope program. *Percept Mot Skills* **61**, 1275–9.
108. MacMahon JR, Gross RT (1987). Physical and psychological effects of aerobic exercise in boys with learning disabilities. *J Dev Behav Pediatr* **8**, 274–7.
109. MacMahon JR, Gross RT (1988). Physical and psychological effects of aerobic exercise in delinquent adolescent males. *Am J Dis Child* **142**, 1361–6.
110. Overbay JD, Purath J (1997). Self-concept and health status in elementary-school-aged children. *Issues Compr Pediatr Nurs* **20**, 89–101.
111. Parish-Plass J, Lufi, D (1997). Combining physical activity with a behavioral approach in the treatment of young boys with behavioral disorders. *Small Gr Res* **28**, 357–69.
112. Sherrill C, Holguin O, Caywood AJ (1989). Fitness, attitude towards physical education, and self-concept of elementary school children. *Percept Mot Skills*, **69**, 411–14.
113. Young ML (1985). Estimation of fitness and physical ability, physical performance, and self-concept among adolescent females. *J Sports Med Phys Fitness* **25**, 144–50.
114. Aine D, Lester D (1995). Exercise, depression, and self-esteem. Comment. *Percept Mot Skills* **81**, 890.
115. Boyd KR, Hrycaiko DW (1997). The effect of a physical activity intervention package on the self-esteem of pre-adolescent and adolescent females. *Adolescence* **32**, 693–708.
116. Koniak-Griffin D (1994). Aerobic exercise, psychological well-being, and physical discomforts during adolescent pregnancy. *Res Nurs Health* **17**, 253–63.
117. Boyd MP, Weinmann C, Yin Z (2002). The relationship of physical self-perceptions and goal orientations to intrinsic motivation for exercise. *J Sport Behav* **25**, 1.
118. Tuckman BW, Hinkle JS (1986). An experimental study of the physical and psychological effects of aerobic exercise on schoolchildren. *Health Psychol* **5**, 197–207.
119. Daley AJ, Ryan J (2000). Academic performance and participation in physical activity by secondary school adolescents. *Percept Mot Skills* **91**, 531–4.
120. Bluechardt MH, Wiener J, Shephard RJ (1995). Exercise programmes in the treatment of children with learning disabilities. *Sports Med* **19**, 55–72.
121. Mechanic D, Hansell S (1987). Adolescent competence, psychological well-being, and self-assessed physical health. *J Health Soc Behav* **28**, 364–74.
122. Brown JD, Lawton M (1986). Stress and well-being in adolescence: The moderating role of physical exercise. *J Human Stress* **12**, 125–31.
123. Michaud-Tomson LM (1995). *Childhood depressive symptoms, physical activity and health-related fitness.* Unpublished doctoral dissertation, Arizona State University, AZ.
124. Milligan RA, Burke V, Beilin LJ, Richards J, Dunbar D, Spencer M, Balde E, Gracey MP (1997). Health-related behaviours and psychosocial characteristics of 18 year-old Australians. *Soc Sci Med* **45**, 1549–62.
125. Norris R, Carroll D, Cochrane R (1992). The effects of physical activity and exercise training on psychological stress and well-being in an adolescent population. *J Psychosom Res* **36**, 55–65.
126. Bahrke, BG, Smith RG (1995). Alterations in anxiety of children after exercise and rest. *Am Correct Ther J* **39**, 90–4.
127. Aganoff JA, Boyle GJ (1994). Aerobic exercise, mood states and menstrual cycle symptoms. *J Psychosom Res* **38**, 183–92.
128. Rodriguez D, Audrain-McGovern J (2005). Physical activity, global physical self-concept, and adolescent smoking. *Ann Behav Med* **30**, 251–9.
129. Aaron DJ, Dearwater SR, Anderson R, Olsen T, Kriska AM, Laporte RE (1995). Physical activity and the initiation of high-risk health behaviors in adolescents. *Med Sci Sports Exerc* **27**, 1639–45.
130. Coulson NS, Eiser C, Eiser JR (1997). Diet, smoking and exercise: Interrelationships between adolescent health behaviours. *Child Care Health Dev* **23**, 207–16.
131. Escobedo LG, Marcus SE, Holtzman D, Giovino GA (1993). Sports participation, age at smoking initiation, and the risk of smoking among US high school students. *JAMA* **269**, 1391–5.
132. Winnail SD, Valois RF, McKeown RE, Saunders RP, Pate RR (1995). Relationship between physical activity level and cigarette, smokeless tobacco, and marijuana use among public high school adolescents. *J School Health* **65**, 438–42.
133. Begg DJ, Langley JD, Moffitt T, Marshall SW (1996). Sport and delinquency: An examination of the deterrence hypothesis in a longitudinal study. *Br J Sports Med* **30**, 335–41.
134. De Wilde EJ, Kienhorst CW, Diekstra RF, Wolters WH (1994). Social support, life events, and behavioral characteristics of psychologically distressed adolescents at high risk for attempting suicide. *Adolescence* **29**, 49–60.
135. Collingwood TR, Reynolds R, Kohl HW, Smith W, Sloan S (1991). Physical fitness effects on substance abuse risk factors and use patterns. *J Drug Educ* **21**, 73–84.

CHAPTER 29

Sport, physical activity, and other health behaviours

Stewart G. Trost

Introduction

Millions of children worldwide are involved in organized sports. In the United States alone, an estimated 38 million children are involved in agency sponsored programmes, such as U.S. Youth Soccer, Little League Baseball, and Pop Warner football.[1,2] Survey data from the U.S. Centers for Disease Control and Prevention (CDC) indicates that ~56% of U.S. high school students participate in at least one school or community-based sports team annually, with just over 38% of U.S. children between the ages of 9–13 years participating in sport or an organized physical activity of some kind.[3,4]

Sports participation has long been thought to provide children and adolescents with a pro-social environment that fosters basic values such as fair play, competitiveness, and achievement.[5] It is also widely believed that participation in organized sports offers protection against the negative social influences that can lead to problematic behaviour and experimentation with tobacco, alcohol, and illicit drugs.[5,6] Most youth sports programmes are offered during 'at-risk' times (after-school and weekends), thus limiting participants' opportunities to engage in risky health behaviours, and participation in school-sponsored sport programmes is often made contingent upon following rules and regulations that overtly discourage health risk behaviours such as experimentation with alcohol and drugs. Sports participation may also promote positive youth development and avoidance of certain health risk behaviours by improving social skills and enhancing self-esteem.[5,6]

A related issue that has received less research attention is the question of whether a health-promoting behaviour such as physical activity 'clusters' with other health-promoting behaviours in youth.[7,8] The existence of such clustering implies that favourable status or change in one behaviour (e.g. regular physical activity) is associated with favourable status or change in others (e.g. healthy eating, tobacco use, experimentation with illicit drugs).

The purpose of this chapter is to summarize the research literature pertaining to the relationships between sports participation, physical activity, and selected health risk behaviours in children and adolescents. The following health risk behaviours were examined: tobacco use (cigarettes and smokeless tobacco), alcohol consumption, illicit drug use, anabolic steroid use, dietary practices (fruit and vegetable intake, consumption of foods high in saturated fat), inappropriate weight control practices, sexual activity, and violence.

Method

Searches of the peer-reviewed scientific literature were conducted using several electronic databases, including PubMed, SPORT Discus, Science Citation Index, ERIC, and Readers' Guide to Periodical Literature. Searches were supplemented by direct examination of reference lists of recovered articles. The key words used for the computer searches were youth, adolescent, physical activity sports, physical education, health behaviours, violence, weight loss, and diet. No limitations were imposed as to publication date or country of origin, except that the article had to be published in the English language. Studies were included if they included children and/or adolescents and provided a measure of association between sports or physical activity participation and a specific health behaviour (e.g. correlation coefficient, beta coefficient, prevalence contrast, odds ratio). The majority of studies included participants aged 18 years or younger, although studies including college-aged athletes were included if they contributed to the breadth of the topic.

Health behaviours

Cigarette smoking

A significant number of studies have examined the association between sports participation and cigarette smoking using data collected by the CDC Youth Risk Behavior Survey (YRBS), a state and national level survey that monitors the health risk behaviours that contribute to the leading causes of mortality and morbidity among youth and adults in the United States.

Escobedo *et al.*[9] examined the relationship between participation in school sports and cigarette smoking among high school students completing the 1990 YRBS. After adjustments for age, sex, race/ethnicity, and academic performance, students reporting participation in three or more sports teams in the previous 12 months were 2.5 times less likely than non-participants to be classified as regular smokers (smoked on 5–15 of the past 30 days). In an analysis of the 1991 and 1993 South Carolina YRBS data, Rainey *et al.*[10] assessed the relationship between sports participation and cigarette smoking in approximately 8000 high school students. After controlling for race/ethnicity, sex, and participation in physical education, non-sports participants were more likely to report smoking in the past 30 days than sports participants. In an independent analysis of the

1993 South Carolina YRBS data, Winnail *et al.*[11] reported sports participation to be inversely related to cigarette smoking among white males and females. However, among African-American students, sports participation increased the risk of cigarette smoking approximately two-fold.

Pate *et al.*[12] assessed the relationship between sports participation and cigarette smoking in high school students completing the 1997 YRBS. After controlling for age, race/ethnicity, and physical activity performed outside of sport, students reporting participation in one or more sports teams during the previous 12 months were 1.2–1.3 times less likely than non-participants to report smoking in the past 30 days. This trend was observed in both genders but was only significant among females. Using data from the 1997 North Carolina YRBS, Garry and Morrissey[13] examined the association between team sports participation and cigarette smoking in an ethnically diverse sample of middle school students. In conflict with the findings of Pate and colleagues, students who participated in school or community-based sports programmes were approximately 1.3 times more likely to experiment with cigarettes smoking than non-sports participants.

Analysis of data from other population-level health surveys conducted in the United States and Europe have shown sports participation to decrease the risk of cigarette smoking in adolescents. Forman *et al.*[14] compared the smoking rates of 1117 male sports participants with normative data from the 1989 National Survey of American High School Seniors. Relative to the survey participants (65.7%), sports participants (27.9%) were significantly less likely to report smoking cigarettes. Simantov *et al.*[15] examined the factors associated with cigarette smoking in a nationally representative sample of 2574 boys and 2939 girls in grades 7 through 12 from 297 public, private, and parochial schools in the United States. Participation in extracurricular activities, defined as involvement in team sports, individual or group exercise, or after-school clubs was associated with a 60–70% reduction in the risk for regular cigarette smoking.

Nelson and Gordon-Larsen[16] analyzed data from the U.S. National Longitudinal Study of Adolescent Health to examine the association between organized sport participation and cigarette smoking. Adolescents with a high frequency of sports participation were approximately 20% less likely than non-participants to report smoking five or more cigarettes in the previous month. Thorlindsson *et al.*[17,18] examined the association between sports participation and cigarette smoking in several population-representative samples of Icelandic youth. In two random samples aged 12–15 years, sports participation was inversely associated with cigarette smoking. Depending on the definition of sports participation (structured vs. non-structured), the correlation ranged from −0.21 to −0.28. Among 12–15 year olds, both the frequency (r = −0.22) and the duration of sports participation (r = −0.24) were inversely associated with cigarette smoking.

Smaller studies involving students from a single high school or school district have also found sports participation to be inversely related to cigarette smoking among adolescents. Baumert *et al.*[19] contrasted the prevalence of cigarette smoking among sports participants (n = 4036) and non-participants (n = 2813) from a single high school in the south-eastern United States. After controlling for age, race/ethnicity, and gender, sports participants were significantly less likely than non-participants to report smoking in the past 30 days. Oler *et al.*[20] compared cigarette smoking rates in school sports participants and non-participants. After controlling for sex, race/ethnicity, and academic performance, non-participants were four times more likely than sports participants to smoke cigarettes. Davis *et al.*[21] examined the relationship between sports participation and cigarette smoking in 1200 high school-aged males. Sports participants were significantly less likely to be smokers than non-participants. However, when the relationship was adjusted for race/ethnicity and academic performance, the inverse association between sports participation and smoking was no longer significant.

A common limitation of the aforementioned studies is the use of cross-sectional study designs. Importantly, because cigarette smoking and sports participation were measured simultaneously, these studies cannot determine if non-sports participation is a cause or consequence of cigarette smoking. One study directly addressed this limitation by employing a longitudinal study design to explore the relationship between change in team sports participation between the 9th and 11th grades and 11th grade smoking status. Rodriguez and Audrain-McGovern[22] followed a cohort of approximately 1500 high school students from the 9th through 11th grade. Using general growth mixture modelling, the authors identified four distinct trajectories of sports involvement—decreasing participation, erratic participation, consistently high participation, and consistently low participation. Students exhibiting a decreasing sports participation profile were 1.9 times more likely than students with consistently low sports participation, and three times more likely than students with consistently high sports participation, to be smokers in the 11th grade. Students exhibiting an erratic participation profile were almost three times more likely to be smokers in the 11th grade than students exhibiting a consistently high participation profile. There were no differences in smoking status between high school students exhibiting erratic and decreasing sports participation profiles.

A small but significant number of studies have evaluated the relationship between physical activity participation and cigarette smoking in children and adolescents. Most studies have found physical activity to be inversely related to cigarette smoking. Kelder *et al.*[23] reported an inverse association between cigarette smoking and physical activity participation among students participating in the Minnesota Class of 1989 study. The prevalence of cigarette smoking was 14% higher in low-active students compared to high-active students.

Using data from the 1990 YRBS, Pate *et al.*[24] assessed the relationship between physical activity and cigarette smoking in a population-representative sample of U.S. high school students. After controlling for age, sex, and race/ethnicity, low active youth were found to be 1.4 times more likely than active students to have smoked in the 30 days preceding the survey. Winnail *et al.*[11] assessed the relationship between physical activity and cigarette smoking among high school students completing the 1993 South Carolina YRBS. Among white males, low-active students were almost twice as likely as high-active students to report cigarette smoking in the past 30 days. No association was observed among African-American students. In the U.S. National Longitudinal Study of Adolescent Health, adolescents who reported ≥5 bouts of moderate-to-vigorous physical activity were 22% less likely than low-active adolescents to report smoking five or more cigarettes in the previous month.[16]

Although few in number, longitudinal studies have consistently found participation in physical activity to be inversely associated with cigarette smoking in adolescent youth. Raitakari *et al.*[25] prospectively examined the association between physical activity and cigarette smoking in a representative sample of Finnish youth aged 12–18 years. Participants who remained sedentary over the 6-year follow-up period were significantly more likely than their active counterparts to either begin smoking or smoke on a daily basis. Aaron *et al.*[26] prospectively examined the relationship between leisure time physical activity and cigarette smoking in high schools students in a single city in the northeastern United States. After controlling for sex, race/ethnicity, and academic performance, a significant inverse association was observed among females but not males. Aarnio and colleagues[27] longitudinally evaluated the association between smoking status and physical activity in a population representative sample of Finnish twins. Male adolescents who were classified as regular smokers were 80% less likely than non-smokers to be persistent exercisers between the ages of 16–18.5 years. Similarly, female adolescents classified as regular smokers were 48% less likely than non-smokers to be persistent exercisers between the ages of 16–18.5 years.

In studies involving young children, among whom the prevalence of cigarette smoking or experimentation with cigarettes is comparatively low, the protective effects of physical activity are less evident. Valois *et al.*[28] investigated the relationship between physical activity and cigarette smoking in 374 fifth grade students. No association was found between self-reported physical activity and experimentation with cigarette smoking. D'Elio *et al.*[29] studied the relationship between physical activity and experimentation with cigarette smoking in 303 African-American fourth grade students. Students with moderate to high levels of physical activity were more likely than low active students to try cigarette smoking. However, the number of children experimenting with cigarettes was very small and none of the reported associations were statistically significant.

Smokeless tobacco

Smokeless tobacco (chewing tobacco, dipping tobacco, snuff) is associated with several serious health conditions including periodontal disease, nicotine addiction, and cancers of the mouth, throat, and digestive system. Because smokeless tobacco use is considered socially acceptable and often encouraged in sports such as baseball and ice hockey, the relationship between sports participation and smokeless tobacco use is a serious concern for health authorities and sports officials.[30,31] In a survey of 1226 high school baseball players from California, nearly half (46%) of the players reported historic use of smokeless tobacco, with 15% reporting current use.[31] In an additional survey of collegiate athletes from 16 Californian universities, the prevalence of smokeless tobacco use among baseball players (52%) was twice that observed for football players (26%). Of concern, 41% of the current smokeless tobacco users reported initiating regular use during their high school years.[32]

The relationship between sports participation and smokeless tobacco use has been evaluated in several population-based health surveys such as the CDC YRBS. Melnick *et al.*[33] examined the association between sports participation and smokeless tobacco use in high school students completing the 1997 YRBS. Among males, sports participants were 1.4 times more likely than non-participants to report smokeless tobacco use in the past 30 days. Among females, sports participants were 1.8 times more likely than non-participants to report smokeless tobacco use. The risk of smokeless tobacco use increased with the level of involvement in sports. Compared to non-participants, the odds of smokeless tobacco use among males and females reporting participation in three or more sports teams was 1.6 and 3.2 greater, respectively.

Rainey *et al.*[10] evaluated the relationship between sports participation and smokeless tobacco use among students completing the 1991 and 1993 South Carolina YRBS. After controlling for race/ethnicity, sex, and participation in school physical education, high school sports participation was positively associated with smokeless tobacco use in the 30 days preceding the survey; however, this trend failed to reach statistical significance. In an independent analysis of the 1993 South Carolina YRBS data, Winnail and colleagues[11] reported no association between high school sports participation and smokeless tobacco use. Karvonen *et al.*[34] assessed the relationship between sports participation and smokeless tobacco use in three population-representative samples of Finnish adolescents aged 16–18 years. After controlling for socio-economic status (SES), participation in organized sports was positively associated with smokeless tobacco use, but only among boys living in urban areas. For boys living in less urbanized areas, the prevalence of smokeless tobacco use was low and unrelated to participation in sports.

Smaller studies involving smaller, less representative samples of youth have produced equivocal findings. While some studies reported a positive relationship between sports participation and smokeless tobacco use, others have found no evidence of an association. Oler *et al.*[20] contrasted smokeless tobacco use in 243 athletes and 573 non-athletes attending a suburban high school in Kentucky. The prevalence of chewing tobacco and snuff use was found to be similar in athletes and non-athletes (~10%). Davis *et al.*[21] examined the association between sports participation and smokeless tobacco use in 1200 high school males from northwest Louisiana. After controlling for race, grade point average and sports intensity, athletes were significantly more likely than non-athletes to use chewing tobacco or snuff. On average, the rate of smokeless tobacco use was approximately 1.5 times higher among athletes than non-athletes.

Sussman *et al.*[35] examined the predictors of smokeless tobacco use in two successive cohorts of seventh grade students residing in the Los Angeles metropolitan area. Cross-sectional analyses of data collected during the participants' seventh and eight grade years showed sports participation to be unrelated to experimentation with smokeless tobacco use. However, among girls in the second cohort, sports participation in the seventh grade was significantly associated with smokeless tobacco use in the eighth grade. Seventeen per cent of the girls who reported participation in four or more competitive sports reported having tried smokeless tobacco, compared with 8.5% of girls who participated in three or less competitive sports over the same period. Sport participation in the seventh grade was not associated with smokeless tobacco use in the eighth grade among boys or girls from cohort one.

Perhaps because smokeless tobacco use is more closely linked with participation in selected sports, the association between physical activity participation and smokeless tobacco use has received little research attention. In one study that evaluated this relationship, physical activity appeared to be somewhat protective against smokeless tobacco use; however, the relationships were weak and varied by sex and race/ethnicity. Winnail and co-workers[11] assessed the relationship between physical activity level and smokeless tobacco use among high school students completing the 1993 South Carolina YRBS. Among white males and African-American females, students with low and moderate levels of physical activity were significantly more likely than those with high levels of physical activity to report smokeless tobacco use in the previous 30 days. Among white females and African-American males, low and moderate levels of physical activity were associated with decreased risk of smokeless tobacco use compared to those with high levels of physical activity; however, none of these associations reached statistical significance.

Alcohol use

The association between sports participation and alcohol use in children and adolescents has been scrutinized in numerous studies and population health surveys. The results of these investigations have been far from consistent. While some studies report a protective inverse relationship between sports participation and alcohol use, others have found sports participants to be at significantly greater risk for alcohol use and alcohol-related health risk behaviours such as driving while being intoxicated.

Buhrmann[36] examined the relationship between sport participation and alcohol use in 857 high school females from rural Iowa. After controlling for parental occupation, mother's education, cumulative grade point average, membership in out-of-school organizations, and social status, a significant inverse correlation of –0.40 was observed between sports participation and alcohol use. Thorlindsson *et al.*[17,18] examined the relationship between sports participation and alcohol consumption in a nationally representative sample of 1200 Icelandic 15–16 years old. Both the frequency of sports participation and the hours engaged in sport were inversely associated with alcohol consumption ($r = -0.19$ and –0.17, respectively). Donato *et al.*[37] compared the drinking habits of 330 elite male athletes to those of 366 male high school students residing in the same area. After controlling for social class, parental education, parental alcohol use, peer alcohol use, smoking status, and judgment of alcohol as harmful, sports participation was found to have a significant inverse relationship with total alcohol intake, frequency of wine drinking, and amount of spirits consumed. Using data from the U.S. National Longitudinal Study of Adolescent Health, Nelson and Gordon-Larsen[16] evaluated the association between sports participation and use of alcohol. Adolescents with a high frequency of sports participation were significantly less likely than sedentary adolescents to report being drunk at least once in the past year; however, no association was observed for being drunk more than once a month or driving when drunk.

In conflict with the above findings, a number of investigations have found sports participation to increase the risk of alcohol use in young people. Nativ and Puffer[38] contrasted the drinking practices of 109 intercollegiate athletes and 110 non-athletic controls. After controlling for age, sex, race, and campus living status, athletes were significantly more likely than non-athletes to report drinking three or more alcohol beverages at a sitting. Athletes and non-athletes did not differ significantly with respect to the frequency of alcohol consumption. In another survey involving university students, males and females involved in collegiate sports exhibited a significantly higher prevalence of frequent heavy drinking than students either partly involved or not involved in collegiate sports.[39] Aaron *et al.*[26] prospectively examined the relationships between participation in competitive sports and alcohol consumption in high school students from Pittsburgh. Males who reported participation in competitive sports were significantly more likely than their non-sporting counterparts to report alcohol use in the month preceding the survey. No associations were found between physical activity, sports participation, and alcohol use among female students. Garry and Morrissey[13] examined the association between team sports participation and health-risk behaviours in 3698 white and African-American middle school children completing the 1997 North Carolina YRBS. After controlling for race and gender, students reporting participation in team sports were 1.2 times more likely than non-participants to report experimenting with alcohol during past 30 days.

Inconsistent findings have also emerged from studies investigating the relationship between physical activity participation and alcohol use in children and adolescents. At least three population-based health surveys have found physically active adolescents to be less likely to consume alcohol than their low-active counterparts. Aarnio *et al.*[40] examined the association between leisure time physical activity and alcohol consumption among 1097 boys and 1014 girls from Finland. Participants were categorized into one of five physical activity levels ranging from sedentary (no leisure time physical in the previous month) to very active (vigorous physical activity 4–5 times per week). An inverse relationship was observed between physical activity level and frequency of alcohol use; however, this association was only significant among girls. Pate *et al.*[24] examined the association between physical activity and alcohol consumption in high school students completing the 1990 YRBS. After controlling for age group, gender, and race/ethnicity, females classified as physically active were significantly less likely than their low active counterparts to report alcohol use in the 30 days preceding the survey. No association was found between physical activity and alcohol use among male high school students. In the U.S. National Longitudinal Study of Adolescent Health, adolescents reporting five or more moderate to vigorous bouts of physical activity per week were 16–28% less likely than low active adolescents to report being drunk more than once per month or drive while drunk in the previous year.[16]

Opposing these findings are the results of three studies which observed a positive association between physical activity participation and alcohol use. Faulkner and Slattery[41] investigated the relationship between physical activity and alcohol use among 257 Canadian high school students. After placing students into gender specific activity tertiles, a significant positive association between physical activity level and alcohol consumption was observed in males but not females. Rainey and colleagues[10] studied the relationship between physical activity level and alcohol use in high school students completing the 1993 South Carolina YRBS. After controlling for race/ethnicity, gender, and physical education status, students with moderate and high levels of physical activity were found to be significantly more likely to report drinking on 6–19 of the 30 days preceding the survey. Physically active students also reported drinking more frequently than non-active students and were more likely than sedentary students to have engaged in episodes of binge drinking in the previous month. D'Elio *et al.*[29] evaluated the association between exercise level and alcohol experimentation in African-American fourth and fifth grade students. Students reporting moderate and high levels of physical activity were more likely than their low-active counterparts to report alcohol use; however, this association was not statistically significant when adjusted for gender, SES, use of other drugs, friends use, self-esteem, and academic performance.

Illegal drug use

Illicit drugs are pharmacological or chemical agents that are considered illegal to use, possess, or sell, without appropriate authority. Well-known examples of illicit drugs include marijuana, cocaine, heroin, amphetamines, barbiturates, PCP, LSD, and the inhalation of glues/solvents. Participation in youth sports is frequently cited as a deterrent to experimentation with drugs; however, a relatively small number of empirical studies have evaluated the relationship between sports participation and illicit drug use in children or adolescents. The majority of these studies have found sports participants to be less likely to use illicit drugs than non-participants.

Baumert *et al.*[19] compared the prevalence of marijuana use among sports participants and non-participants. After controlling for age, race, and gender, participants were significantly less likely than non-athletes to report marijuana use. Oler *et al.*[20] compared illicit drug use in high school sport participants and non-participants from Kentucky. After controlling for age, sex, race, and academic performance, non-participants were found to be twice as likely as athletes to report marijuana use. No association was found between sport participation and cocaine use. Forman *et al.*[14] compared the prevalence rates of drug use of male high school sport participants from the Chicago area with those reported in the 1989 National Survey of American High School Seniors. Relative to the survey participants, athletes were less likely to report use of marijuana, cocaine, amphetamines, barbiturates, heroin, PCP, and LSD.

Several population health surveys have shown sports participants to be less likely than non-participants to use certain illegal drugs; however, the protective effects of sports participation varies by gender, race/ethnicity, and the type of drug. Using data from the 1997 CDC YRBS, Pate *et al.*[12] assessed the relationship between sports participation and illicit drug use in U.S. high school students. Among male students, participation in school or community-based sports was protective against marijuana use in whites and Hispanics, but not in African-Americans. Sports participation significantly reduced the risk of cocaine and other illicit drug use (LSD, PCP, ecstasy, mushrooms, speed, ice, heroin) in white males; but increased the risk of use of these substances in African-American and Hispanic males. Among female students, sports participation was protective against cocaine and other illicit drugs regardless of race/ethnicity. However, only white female sports participants were at significantly decreased risk for marijuana use and sniffing glue or paint cans. Winnail *et al.*[11] examined the relationship between sports participation and illicit drug use in public high school students completing the 1993 South Carolina YRBS. After adjusting for race and gender, sports participants were significantly less likely than non-participants to report using marijuana, cocaine, and other illicit drugs such as LSD, PCP, and heroin. Using data from the National Longitudinal Study of Adolescent Health, Nelson and Gordon-Larsen[16] examined the association between sports participation and illicit drug use. Adolescents, with a high frequency of sports participation with parents and adolescents with a high frequency of sport participation at neighbourhood recreation centres, were 25–48% less likely than sedentary adolescents to report using marijuana one or more times per week or illicit drugs other than marijuana in the past year. Participation in sports at school reduced the risk of illicit drug use by 10–23%; however, this association failed to reach statistical significance.

Not all health surveys, however, have found sports participation to be protective against illicit drug use. Garry and Morrissey[13] examined the association between team sports participation and health-risk behaviours in middle school children completing the 1997 North Carolina YRBS. After controlling for race and gender, students reporting participation in team sports were 1.4 times more likely than non-participants to report inhaling glue, sprays, or paints to get high.

Fewer investigations have examined the association between physical activity and illicit drug use. Similar to sports participation, most have found physical activity to be protective against illicit drug use. Winnail *et al.*[11] contrasted marijuana use in students reporting low, moderate, and high levels of physical activity. After stratifying the sample by gender and race, moderate and high levels of physical activity were found to be negatively associated with marijuana use among white males. No association was observed among African-American males and females. Robinson *et al.*[42] examined the predictors of substance use in 1447 tenth grade students. Self-reported participation in aerobic activity did not correlate significantly with the use of illegal substances. Pate *et al.*[24] examined the relationship between physical activity status and illicit drug use in high school students completing the 1990 YRBS. After controlling for grade level, sex, and race, students classified as physically active were significantly less likely to report using cocaine and marijuana in the 30 days preceding the survey. In their analysis of data from the National Longitudinal Study of Adolescent Health, Nelson and Gordan-Larson[16] found physically active adolescents to be 27% less likely than their less active counterparts to report using illegal drugs other than marijuana in the previous year. Active adolescents were also 15% less likely than their less active counterparts to report regular marijuana use; however, this association failed to reach statistical significance.

Anabolic steroid use

Population health surveys conducted in the United States suggest that the prevalence of steroid use among adolescent youth is significant and on the rise. Between 1991 and 2003, the prevalence of anabolic steroid use among U.S. high school students increased from 2.7% to 6.1% and from 1.2% to 5.3% in males and females, respectively.[4] Although illegal and associated with numerous short- and long-term health risks, anabolic steroids are used by some athletes, including those involved in high school sports, to enhance athletic performance. Thus, the association between youth sports participation and steroid use has been scrutinized in several studies. The results of these studies, however, have been inconsistent with the strength and direction of the reported associations varying by sex and race/ethnicity.

Buckley *et al.*[43] were the first to comprehensively examine the prevalence of steroid use among high school sport participants. They drew a sample of 12th grade male students from 150 high schools across the nation. Of those eligible, only 50.3% voluntarily participated. Steroid users were more likely to participate in school sports programs than non-users. However, when examined on a sports-specific basis, steroid users were more likely to participate in football and wrestling than other school sports. Of interest, 35.2% of users did not intend to participate in school-sponsored athletics.

Several authors have contrasted anabolic steroid use among high school sports participants and non-participants completing the CDC YRBS. Using data from the 1991 YRBS, DuRant *et al.*[44] assessed the relationship between steroid use and sports participation as well as steroid use and strength training. After controlling for age, sex, academic performance, other drug use, and region of the country, students who engaged in strength training were more likely to report lifetime steroid use than students who did not engage in strength training. Students who participated on a sports team were more likely than non-participants to report steroid use; however, this association did not reach statistical significance. In the Midwest states, both strength training and sports participation were significantly associated with increased likelihood of using anabolic steroids; while in the Northeastern states, only strength training was significantly associated with steroid use. In the Southern and Western states, neither strength training nor sports participation was significantly associated with steroid use.

Using the same YRBS data, Page *et al.*[45] examined the relationship between the level of sports participation and steroid use. Male students participating in three or more sports teams were nearly twice as likely as non-participants to report ever using steroids. No association was observed among female students. Using data from the 1997 YRBS, Pate and colleagues[12] found sports participation to be positively associated with steroid use, but only among African-American males. These analyses were adjusted for age and participation in regular, vigorous physical activity. Most recently, Elliot and colleagues[46] used data from the 2003 YRBS survey to evaluate the relationship between school-sponsored sports participation and anabolic steroid use in high school girls. After adjusting for grade level and race/ethnicity, team sports participants were nearly two times less likely to be steroid users than non-participants.

Several studies conducted in non-representative samples of adolescent youth have observed a positive association between sports participation and steroid use among youth. Windsor and Dumitru[47] surveyed 901 high school students from one relatively affluent school district and one relatively lower SES school district regarding steroid use. Five per cent of males and 1.4% of females reported that they had used steroids. In comparison, 6.7% of male sport participants, and 1.8% of male non-participants took steroids. The male sport participants from the higher SES schools reported significantly greater steroid use than the male sport participants from the lower SES schools (10.2% vs. 2.8%). Tanner and colleagues[48] used a confidential survey questionnaire to assess anabolic steroid use among 6930 students from 10 high schools in Denver, Colorado. The overall prevalence of anabolic steroid use was 2.7% (4.0% for boys and 1.3% for girls). Use was slightly higher among sports participants (2.9%) than non-participants (2.2%). In a study conducted in seven high schools in Georgia, Baumert *et al.*[19] reported no significant difference in steroid use (ever or current) between sports participants and non-participants after controlling for age, race, and gender (85). Scott *et al.*[49] surveyed 4722 students from 62 high schools in Nebraska. Among all high school students, the prevalence of anabolic steroid use was low (2.5%); however, male steroid users (79.8%) were significantly more likely than non-steroid users (20.2%) to be sports participants. Steroid use was not associated with sports participation in females.

van den Berg *et al.*[50] examined the predictors of anabolic steroid use in a cohort of just over 2500 U.S. middle and high school students. Steroid use and a variety of personal, socio-environmental, and behavioral predictors of steroid use, including participation in sports related to weight concerns (wrestling, gymnastics, ballet), were measured at baseline and 5 years of follow-up. Females who reported steroid use at follow-up were 2.6 times more likely than non-users to have participated in weight-related sports at baseline. Males who reported steroid use at follow-up were 2.23 times more likely than non-users to have participated in weight-related sports at baseline, but this association failed to reach statistical significance.

Dietary practices

The positive link between nutrition and sports performance is well established. Nevertheless, the question of whether participation in youth sports promotes healthy eating in children and adolescents has not been studied extensively. French *et al.*[51] surveyed students in grades seven through ten (708 males and 786 females) in a mostly white, upper-middle class school district in Minnesota. Sports participation was assessed with a 28-item checklist representing activities of light to vigorous intensity. Students were asked to check the activities that they performed for 20 min or more and indicate one of five choices as to when the activity was last performed (e.g. today, rarely, or never). Dietary constructs were assessed with a 25-item questionnaire for preference (one through five) and recent consumption (one through five) of various foods representing sweets, salty snacks, fruits and vegetables, and protein entrees. Factor analysis was used to group the activities into leisure sports, conditioning sports, and atypical sports (sports played less frequently). Factor analysis was also used to group the foods into junk food or empty calories, salty snacks, healthy foods (e.g. fruits and vegetables, yoghurt), and protein entree (e.g. hamburger). Among both males and females, participation in leisure sports and conditioning sports was found to be positively correlated with recent healthy food choices (r = 0.26–0.36) and healthy food preferences (r = 0.13–0.20). Among females, conditioning sports (r = –0.10) and atypical sports (r = –0.09) were inversely correlated with salty snack preference, while conditioning sports were inversely associated with junk food preference (r = –0.10). Among males, conditioning sports was positively associated with protein entree preference (r = 0.11).

Baumert *et al.*[19] examined the relationship between sports participation and dietary intake in high school students from a single county in the southern United States. Compared to non-participants, sport participants were significantly more likely to report consuming breakfast, fruits, and vegetables and one serving from the dairy food group on a daily basis. They were also less likely to add salt to their foods. No differences were found in reported consumption of red meats, fried foods, and snack foods. Pate *et al.*[12] evaluated the relationship between school and community sports participation and dietary behaviours in high school students completing the 1997 YRBS. After controlling for grade level, race/ethnicity, and non-sport physical activity level, male sports participants were significantly more likely to report recent consumption of fruits and vegetables than non-participants. Female sports participants were more likely to report recent consumption of salad or vegetables than non-participants. A positive association was also observed for sports-participation and consumption of fruit or fruit juice; however, this association was only significant among white females.

Compared to sports participation, the relationship between regular physical activity and healthy dietary practices in youth has been studied more extensively. The results generally show a positive correlation between the two health behaviours. Lytle *et al.*[52] examined cross-sectional data from grades 6 through 12 of the Class of 1989 Study which was part of the Minnesota Heart Health Project. Subjects from the intervention communities were examined separately from the comparison communities. Frequency and intensity of physical activity was used to create an exercise score ranging from 0 to 9. Dietary behaviour was summarized on a scale of 0 to 18 with each point on the scale representing a healthier food choice. In both the intervention and control communities, students in the highest two quintiles for healthy food choices exhibited significantly higher levels of physical activity than students in lowest two quintiles. This difference was more evident among females in the intervention communities.

Terre *et al.*[7] studied the interrelationships among health-related behaviours in 1092 children between the ages 11 and 18 years. To examine potential developmental differences in these relationships, participants were grouped into four groups: Grade 6 (age 11), Grades 7–8 (ages 12–13), Grades 9–10 (ages 14–15), and Grades 11–12 (ages 16–18). Students completed a 35-item self-reported questionnaire designed to assess five health-related behaviours including diet and exercise. Exploratory factor analyses performed within each group revealed sedentary behaviour to be related to poor eating habits in all grade level groups with the exception of students in Grades 11 and 12.

Pate *et al.*[24] analyzed data from the national 1990 YRBS to determine if physically active adolescents were more likely than their low-active counterparts to report consumption of fruit or vegetables on the previous day. After adjustment for age group, sex, and race, students who did not eat vegetables on the previous day were almost twice as likely to be low active than students who reported eating at least one serving of vegetables. Among the Hispanic and White subgroups, students who ate no fruit on the previous day were 2.3 and 3.1 times, respectively, more likely to be low active than those who ate one or more serving of fruit on the previous day.

Several studies involving population-representative cohorts of Finnish adolescents have assessed the link between regular physical activity and healthy eating. Aarnio *et al.*[40] surveyed 1097 girls and 1014 boys in Finland from 1991 to 1993. Physical activity behaviour was classified into one of five categories from very active to inactive based on reported frequency and intensity of physical activity performed outside of school. Saturated fat intake was estimated with a single item regarding use of spread on bread. Response choices included (i) usually nothing; (ii) mostly margarine; (iii) mostly butter; (iv) butter/margarine mixtures; (v) light spread; and (vi) other. Results indicated that the highest activity group was significantly more likely to use no spread on their bread than the inactive group. For example, in the very active group, 15.4% of girls and 5.2% of boys reported using no spread; whereas among the inactive, only 1.6% of girls and none of the boys reported using no spread.

Raitakari *et al.*[25] tracked the health-related behaviours of 961 Finnish adolescents, aged 12–18 years. Leisure time physical activity was assessed by questionnaire. A physical activity index, ranging from 1 to 225, was calculated from the product of intensity, duration, and frequency. Participants with a score greater than or equal to 85 in three examinations, 3 years apart (i.e. 1980, 1983, 1986) were considered constantly active. Those with an index value less than 15 over the three examinations were considered constantly sedentary. Diet was assessed by a trained nutritionist using a 48-hour recall at the baseline examination in 1980 and again in 1986. Comparing the constantly active to the constantly sedentary, it was found that the sedentary young males consumed significantly more saturated fat and had a lower polyunsaturated to saturated fat ratio than the active males.

Most recently, Aarnio *et al.*[27] evaluated the relationship between habitual physical activity and dietary practices in a representative cohort of Finnish twins. Males reporting eating breakfast only once a week were just over 60% less likely to be persistently physically active between the ages of 16–18.5 years. Among females, persistent physical activity was associated with eating breakfast regularly; however, the association was somewhat weaker than that observed among males.

Inappropriate weight control practices

There is evidence to suggest that those who participate in sports in which leanness is emphasized, such as ballet or gymnastics, are more likely to diet inappropriately or have eating disorders such as bulimia and anorexia nervosa.[53,54] Leon[54] suggests that with the increasing participation of females in sports activities, a greater number of adolescent females may be at risk for the development of eating disorders. Others have recognized that, owing to the rules of their sport, certain athletes are subject to a particular pressure to maintain a low body weight.[55]

A study of 955 competitive male and female swimmers aged 9–18 years showed that girls, irrespective of actual weight, were more likely to engage in weight loss efforts, while boys were more likely to try to gain weight.[56] Girls were more likely than boys to use unhealthy weight loss methods, such as fasting (27.0% vs. 16.4%), self-induced vomiting (12.7% vs. 2.7%), and diet pills (10.7% vs. 6.8%). Boys used laxatives and diuretics more than girls (4.1% vs. 2.5%, 2.8% vs. 1.5%, respectively). At least one unhealthy method of weight control was used by 15.4% of the girls (24.8% among postmenarcheal girls) and 3.6% of the boys.

In a sample of high school females in a Midwestern U.S. city, the eating disorder inventory (EDI) was used to assess psychological traits known to be associated with eating disorders. Female sport participants were significantly more likely than non-participants to be a perfectionist and to engage in bulimic behaviour, such as uncontrollable overeating and self-induced vomiting. Yet, no significant differences were found on current dieting practices (28% of athletes vs. 25% of non-athletes were on a diet to lose weight).[57]

Among 64 female university students, athletes involved in sports that provided an advantage to those with a slim body (e.g. gymnastics, synchronized swimming, diving, figure skating, long-distance running, and ballet) had greater weight and diet concerns, and were more emotionally liable and dissatisfied than female athletes participating in hockey, basketball, sprinting, downhill skiing, and volleyball.[58] In their analyses of the 1993 national YRBS, Middleman and colleagues[59] found no association between high school sports participation and weight loss behaviours, including use of vomiting or diet pills to lose weight. In fact, young girls (less than 16 years) involved in sports were less likely to report trying to lose weight than non-athletes.

Pate *et al.*[12] assessed the relationship between sports participation and inappropriate weight loss practices in U.S. high school students completing the 1997 YRBS. After controlling for grade level, race/ethnicity, and non-sport physical activity, female sports participants were approximately 1.3 times less likely than non-participants to report trying to lose weight. However, female sport participants were not significantly more likely than non-participants to report use of vomiting, laxatives, or pills to lose weight. Sports participation was not associated with inappropriate weight loss practices in males.

Little is known about the association between physical activity and weight loss practices. French *et al.*[51] collected data from 708 males and 786 females in grades 7 through 10 from a suburban school district in the mid-western United States. A 21-item eating disorder checklist was developed for the study, based on previous research and DSM-III-R criteria for eating disorders. The number of affirmative responses constituted a risk score for eating disorders. Physical activity was measured using a 28-item checklist of activities. Principal components analysis resulted in three categories of sport activities: leisure or outdoor sports, conditioning sports, and atypical sports. Among males, atypical sports participation (e.g. bowling, aerobics, softball) was a significant predictor of the risk score for eating disorders. Among females, all three categories of physical activity (conditioning sports, leisure sports, and atypical sports) were significant predictors of the risk score for eating disorders. In Middleman and colleagues' analysis of the YRBS data, participation in vigorous exercise, stretching, and strength promoting exercises were associated with trying to lose weight among females and trying to gain weight in males. However, there were no indications that physical activity was associated with inappropriate weight gain or weight loss behaviours.[59]

Sexual risk behaviours

There has been considerable interest in assessing whether sports participation is associated with avoidance of sexual risk behaviours in adolescents. The available evidence, although limited, suggests that sports participation is protective against sexual risk behaviours among female adolescents. However, among adolescent males, sport and physical activity participation does not appear to be related to sexual risk behaviours.

Smith and Caldwell[60] examined the prevalence of sexual activity in 1071 high school students from a large city in the southern United States. Students classified as sports participants were significantly more likely than non-participants to report having sexual intercourse on at least one occasion (60.6% vs. 41.8%). Miller *et al.*[61] examined the effects of sports participation on sexual behaviour in a sample of 611 western New York adolescents. The authors found the relationship between sports participation and sexual behaviour to be highly gender specific. Whereas male sport participants were more likely than non-participants to report sexual activity, female sport participants were significantly less likely than non-participants to report sexual activity. These findings remained intact after controlling for race, age, socio-economic status, quality of family relations, and participation in other extracurricular activities.

Sabo *et al.*[62] examined whether high school sports participation was associated with reduced risk of sexual behaviour and pregnancy in a random sample of adolescents in the north-eastern United States. After controlling for race, age, family income, and family cohesion, female sports participants reported significantly lower rates of sexual activity within the previous year than their non-sporting counterparts. Participation in sports was not associated with pregnancy. Among males, sports participation was not associated with sexual frequency or getting a girl pregnant.

Several authors have evaluated the relationship between youth sports participation and sexual risk behaviours using data from the CDC YRBS. Using data from the 1991 YRBS, Page *et al.*[45] examined the association between school and community sports participation and sexual risk behaviour. Compared to non-participants, girls reporting participation on one or two sports teams were 1.7 times less likely to have not ever had a sexually transmitted disease, and 1.5 times less likely to have not been pregnant. Among males, there was no relationship between sports participation and sexual risk behaviour. Among high school students who had reported sexual intercourse, sports participants were significantly less likely than non-participants to have had multiple partners and were more likely than non-participants to use a condom the last time they had sexual intercourse.

Using data from the 1997 YRBS, Miller and colleagues[63] examined the association between team sports participation and sexual risk behaviours. Sexual risk was measured using the Sexual Risk Scale which included six dichotomous items related to adolescent sexual risk—intercourse prior to age 15 years, failure to use birth control at the most recent sexual intercourse, use of alcohol or drugs at most recent sexual intercourse, multiple lifetime sex partners, multiple recent sex partners, and involvement in a past pregnancy. Participants were classified as at-risk if they responded affirmatively to one or more of the six items. Girls who reported participation in team sports were significantly less likely than their non-sporting counterparts to engage in sexual risk. The protective effects of sports participation were stronger among white and Hispanic girls than African-American and Asian/Pacific Islander girls. In contrast to the girls, boys reporting participation in team sports were significantly more likely than non-participants to engage in risky sexual behaviour. However, when sexual risk was examined by race/ethnicity, sports participation was associated with a significantly lower risk among white boys, significantly higher risk for African-American boys, with no association observed among Hispanic or Asian/Pacific Islander boys.

Kulig *et al.*[64] examined the association between team sports participation and sexual risk behaviours using data from the 1999 YRBS. After controlling for grade and race/ethnicity, female sports participants classified as physically active had a significantly reduced risk of ever having had intercourse, having had four or more sexual partners in their lifetime or in the three previous months, and having been pregnant than girls not active or participating in team sports. Sports participation was not associated with sexual risk behaviours in male students.

Two studies have examined the relationship between physical activity and sexual risk behaviour. Pate *et al.*[24] examined the relationship between physical activity status and sexual activity in high school students completing the 1990 YRBS. In unadjusted analyses, students classified as low active were significantly more likely than active students to report having one or more sexual partners in the previous 3 months. However, no association was observed between physical activity and sexual activity after controlling for age-group, gender, and race/ethnicity. Nelson and Gordon-Larsen[16] analyzed data for the U.S. National Longitudinal Study of Adolescent Health to examine the association between physical activity participation and sexual activity. Adolescents reporting five or more bouts of moderate-to-vigorous physical activity were significantly less likely than low active adolescents to report having sexual intercourse in the previous year and 13% less likely to report using no birth control in their most recent sexual intercourse.

Violence

The notion that participation in sports can deter delinquent behaviours in adolescent youth has motivated a number of authors to examine the association between sports participation and behaviours that contribute to violence (i.e. carrying a weapon or being in a physical fight). Levin *et al.*[65] examined the relationship between violent behaviours and sports participation in 2436 high school students from a single county in the southwestern United States. The violent behaviours examined included assault, trouble at school, stealing, trouble with police, damaging property, carrying a weapon to get something, and carrying a weapon for protection. Among males, sports participation was not significantly associated with any of the violent behaviours; however, when male athletes were divided into contact and non-contact sports, athletes in contact sports were significantly more likely than their non-contact counterparts to assault others, get into trouble at school and carry a weapon for protection. Among females, participants from any sport were significantly less likely than non-participants to exhibit negative or violent behaviour. Similar to the males, females involved in contact sports were significantly more likely than their non-contact sporting counterparts to engage in assault and carry a weapon for protection.

Nelson and Gordon-Larsen[16] analyzed data from the U.S. National Longitudinal Study of Adolescent Health to examine the association between sports participation and violent behaviour. Adolescents with a high frequency of sports participation with parents were 12% less likely than sedentary adolescents to engage in one or more violent behaviours such as being in a serious physical fight, seriously injuring another person, participating in a group fight, using a weapon, or stabbing someone in the past year. No association was observed among adolescents reporting a high frequency of sports participation at school or neighbourhood recreation centres. Garry and Morrissey[13] examined the association between team sports participation and health-risk behaviours in 3698 white and African-American middle school children in North Carolina. After controlling for race and gender, students reporting participation in team sports were 1.3 times more likely than non-participants to report carrying a weapon (gun, knife, or club) and were 1.2 times more likely to report being in a physical fight.

Two studies have examined the association between physical activity participation and violent behaviour in youth. Aaron *et al.*[25] contrasted the prevalence of weapon carrying in high school students reporting low, medium and high levels of leisure time physical activity. Boys were significantly more likely than girls to report carrying a weapon in the previous 30 days; however, within gender groups, the prevalence of weapon carrying was similar across the three physical activity groups. Pate and colleagues[24] examined physical activity participation and the relative odds of being injured in a physical fight in a nationally representative sample of U.S. high school students. After controlling for age, sex, and race/ethnicity, no association was found between physical activity level and injury from physical fighting.

Summary

This chapter summarized the scientific evidence pertaining to the relationship between sports and/or physical activity and nine health behaviours associated with significant morbidity and mortality in children and adolescents. The findings for each health behaviour are summarized in Table 29.1.

Table 29.1 Overview of the associations between specific health behaviours and participation in sport and physical activity

Health behaviour*	Sports participation	Physical activity
Cigarette smoking	– –	– –
Smokeless Tobacco	+	–
Alcohol use	–	– +
Illegal drugs	–	–
Anabolic steroids	+	?
Improper dietary practices	– –	– –
Improper weight control practices	+	?
Sexual activity	–	–
Violence	–	↔

*Note that each health behaviour is presented as a health compromising behaviour. A negative (–) association indicates that sports participants and/or physically active individuals are ***less*** likely to engage in that behaviour. A positive (+) association indicates that sports participants and/or physically active individuals are ***more*** likely to engage in that behaviour.

– –: repeatedly documented inverse association; –: weak or mixed evidence of an inverse association; ↔: evidence of no association; +: weak or mixed evidence of a positive association; + +: repeatedly documented evidence of a positive association; – +: evidence to support both a positive and negative association; ?: insufficient data available.

- The available evidence suggests that participation in sport is protective against cigarette smoking, alcohol use and illegal drug use, unhealthy dietary practices, sexual activity, and violence. However, only the evidence related to cigarette smoking and unhealthy dietary practices can be regarded as consistent.
- For alcohol, illegal drugs, sexual activity, and violence, the reported associations vary considerably by age, gender, or race/ethnicity; and a number of studies report positive associations.
- On the negative side, participation in sport appears to increase one's risk for smokeless tobacco use, anabolic steroid use, and inappropriate weight loss practices. However, the evidence related to these health behaviours is not strong and highly dependent on the type of sport, age, gender, and race/ethnicity.
- Although fewer studies have investigated the relationship between physical activity and other health behaviours, there is evidence that regular physical activity is protective against cigarette smoking, smokeless tobacco use, illegal drug use, unhealthy dietary practices, and sexual activity. Regular physical activity is not related to violent behaviour. Of note, similar to sports participation, only the evidence related to cigarette smoking and unhealthy dietary practices can be classified as consistent. Regular physical activity may protect one against smokeless tobacco use, illegal drugs, and risky sexual behaviour, but more evidence is needed before more definite conclusions can be made about these health behaviours.
- For alcohol consumption, there is evidence that regular physical activity both increases and decreases the risk of alcohol consumption or binge drinking. However, the evidence linking physical activity to increased alcohol consumption is mainly derived from studies involving university students or young adults. For children and adolescents the association between physical activity and alcohol use is inconsistent, but tends to be protective.

- At this time, no clear conclusions can be made regarding the impact of physical activity participation on anabolic steroid use and improper weight control practices in youth. Notably, with the possible exception of alcohol use, physical activity does not increase the risk of health compromising behaviours.
- In closing, considerable caution should be exercised in interpreting the evidence summarized in Table 29.1, as the literature is, at best, inconsistent, and almost entirely composed of cross-sectional studies. There is an urgent need for longitudinal studies to more fully evaluate causal relations between sport, physical activity, and other health behaviours in youth.

References

1. National Council on Youth Sports (2001). *Report on trends and participation in organized youth sports*. National Council on Youth Sports, Stuart, FL.
2. Seefeld, VD, Ewing ME (1997). Youth sports in America: An overview. *Phys Activ Fitness Res Digest* **2**, 1–2.
3. U.S. Centers for Disease Control and Prevention (2003). Physical activity levels among children aged 9–13 years – United States, 2002. *MMWR* **52**, 785–8.
4. U.S. Centers for Disease Control and Prevention (2003). Youth Risk Behavior Survey – United States, 2005. *MMWR* **55,** SS–5.
5. Poinsett A (1996). *Carnegie meeting papers: The role of sports in youth development*. Carnegie Corporation, New York.
6. Weiss MR, Smith AL (2002). Moral development in sport and physical activity: Theory, research, and intervention. In: Horn T (ed.), *Advances in sport psychology* (2nd ed.), pp. 243–80. Human Kinetics, Champaign, IL.
7. Terre L, Drabman RS, Meydrech EF (1990). Relationships among children's health-related behaviors: Multivariate, developmental perspective. *Prev Med* **19**, 134–46.
8. Burke V, Milligan RAK, Beilin LJ, Dunbar D, Spencer M, Balde E, Gracey MP (1997). Clustering of health-related behaviors among 18-year-old Australians. *Prev Med* **26**, 724–33.
9. Escobedo LG, Marcus SE, Holtzman D, Giovano GA (1993). Sports participation, age of smoking initiation, and the risk of smoking among US high school students. *JAMA* **269**, 1391–5.
10. Rainey CJ, McKeown RE, Sargent RG, Valois RF (1996). Patterns of tobacco and alcohol use among sedentary, exercising, non-athletic, and athletic youth. *J Sch Health* **66**, 27–32.
11. Winnail SD, Valois RF, McKeown RE, Saunders RP, Pate RR (1995). Relationship between physical activity level and cigarette, smokeless tobacco use, and marijuana use among public high school adolescents. *J Sch Health* **65,** 438–42.
12. Pate RR, Trost SG, Levin S, Dowda M (2000). Sports participation and health-related behaviors among US youth. *Arch Ped Adolesc Med* **154,** 904–11.
13. Garry JP, Morrissey SL (2000). Team sports participation and risk-taking behaviors among a bi-racial middle school population. *Clin J Sports Med* **10**, 185–90.
14. Forman ES, Dekker AH, Javors JR, Davison DT (1995). High-risk behaviors in teenage male athletes. *Clin J Sports Med* **5**, 36–42.
15. Simantov E, Schoen C, Klein JD (2000). Health compromising behaviors: Why do adolescents smoke or drink? Identifying underlying risk and protective factors. *Arch Ped Adolesc Med* **154**, 1025–33.
16. Nelson MC, Gordon-Larson P (2006). Physical activity and sedentary behavior patterns are associated with selected adolescent health risk behaviors. *Pediatrics* **117**, 1281–90.
17. Thorlindsson T (1989). Sports participation, smoking, and drug and alcohol use among Icelandic youth. *Society Sport J* **6**, 136–43.
18. Thorlindsson T, Vilhjalmsson R, Valgeirsson G (1990). Sports participation and perceived health status: A study of adolescence. *Soc Sci Med* **31**, 551–6.
19. Baumert PW Jr, Henderson JM, Thompson NJ (1998). Health risk behaviors of adolescent participants in organized sports. *J Adolesc Health* **22**, 460–5.
20. Oler MJ, Mainous AG, Martin CA, Richardson E, Haney A, Wilson D, Adams T (1994). Depression, suicide ideation, and substance abuse among adolescents. Are athletes at less risk? *Arch Fam Med* **3**, 781–5.
21. Davis TC, Arnold C, Nandy I, Bocchini JA, Gottlieb A, George RB, Berkel H (1997). Tobacco use among high school athletes. *J Adolesc Health* **21**, 97–101.
22. Rodriguez D, Audrain-McGovern J (2004). Team sports participation and smoking. Analysis with general growth mixture modeling. *J Pediatr Psychol* **29**, 299–308.
23. Kelder SH, Perry CL, Klepp, K-I, Lytle LL (1994). Longitudinal tracking of adolescent smoking, physical activity and food choice behaviors. *Am J Public Health* **84**, 1121–6.
24. Pate RR, Heath GW, Dowda M, Trost SG (1996). Associations between physical activity and other health behaviors in a representative sample of US adolescents. *Am J Public Health* **86**, 1577–81.
25. Raitakari OT, Porkka KVK, Taimela S, Telema R, Rasenen L,Viikari JSA (1994). Effects of persistent physical activity and inactivity on coronary risk factors in children and young adults: The Cardiovascular Risk in Young Finns Study. *Am J Epidemiol* **140**, 195–205.
26. Aaron DJ, Dearwater SR, Anderson R, Olsen T, Kriska AM, LaPorte RE (1995). Physical activity and the initiation of high-risk health behaviors in adolescents. *Med Sci Sport Exerc* **27**, 1639–45.
27. Aarnio M, Winter T, Kujala U, Kaprio J (2002). Associations of health related behavior, social relationships, and health status with persistent physical activity and inactivity: A study of Finnish adolescent twins. *Br J Sports Med* **36**, 360–4.
28. Valois R, Dowda M, Trost SG, Weinrich M, Felton G, Pate RR (1998). Cigarette smoking experimentation among rural fifth grade students. *Am J Health Behav* **22**, 101–7.
29. D'Elio MA, Mundt DJ, Bush PJ, Iannotti RJ (1993). Healthful behaviors: Do they protect African-American, urban preadolescents from abusable substance use. *Am J Public Health* **7**, 354–63.
30. Rolandsson M, Hugoson A (2001). Factors associated with snuffing habits among ice-hockey-playing boys. *Swed Dental J* **25**, 145–54.
31. Walsh MM, Ellison J, Hilton JF, Chesney M, Ernster VL (2000). Spit (smokeless) tobacco use by high school baseball athletes in California. *Tob Control* **9** (Suppl. 2), 32–9.
32. Walsh MM, Hilton JF, Ernster VL, Masouredis CM, Grady DG (1994). Prevalence, patterns, and correlates of spit tobacco use in a college athlete population. *Addict Behav* **19**, 411–27.
33. Melnick MJ, Miller KE, Sabo DF, Farrell MP, Barnes GM (2001). Tobacco use among high school athletes and nonathletes: Results of the 1997 youth risk behavior survey. *Adolescence* **36**, 727–47.
34. Karvonen JS, Rimpela AH, Rimpela M (1995). Do sports clubs promote snuff use? Trends among Finnish boys between 1981 and 1991. *Health Educ Res* **10**, 147–54.
35. Sussman S, Holt L, Dent CW, Flay BR, Graham JW, Hanson WB, Johnson CA (1989). Activity involvement, risk taking, demographic variables, and other drug us: Prediction of trying smokeless tobacco. *NCI Monogr* **8**, 57–62.
36. Buhrman HG (1977). Athletics and deviance: An examination of the relationship between athletic participation and deviant behavior of high school girls. *Rev Sport Leisure* **2**, 17–35.
37. Donato F, Assanelli D, Marconi M, Corsini C, Rosa G, Monarca S (1994). Alcohol consumption among high school students and young athletes in north Italy. *Revue Epidemiology de la Sante Publique* **42**, 198–206.
38. Nativ A, Puffer JC (1991). Lifestyle and health risk of collegiate athletes. *J Fam Pract* **33**, 585–90.

39. Wechsler H, Davenport AE (1997). Binge drinking, tobacco, and illicit drug use and involvement in college athletics. *J Am Coll Health* **45**, 195–200.
40. Aarnio M, Kujala UM, Kaprio J (1997). Associations of health-related behaviors, school type and health status to physical activity patterns in 16 year old boys and girls. *Scand J Soc Med* **25**, 156–67.
41. Faulkner RA, Slattery CM (1990). The relationship of physical activity to alcohol consumption in youth 15–16 years of age. *Can J Public Health* **81**, 168–9.
42. Robinson TN, Killen JD, Taylor CB, Telch MJ, Bryson SW, Saylor KE, Maron DJ, Maccoby N, Farquhar JW (1987). Perspectives on adolescent substance use. A defined population study. *JAMA* **258**, 2072–6.
43. Buckley WE, Yesalis CE, Friedl KE, Anderson WA, Streit AL, Wright JE (1998). Estimated prevalence of anabolic steroid use among male high school students. *JAMA* **260**, 3441–5.
44. DuRant RH, Escobedo LG, Heath GW (1995). Anabolic-steroid use, strength training and multiple drug use among adolescents in the United States. *Pediatrics* **96**, 23–8.
45. Page RM, Hammermeister J, Scanlan A, Gilbert L (1998). Is school sports participation a protective factor against adolescent health risk behaviors. *J Health Educ* **29**, 186–92.
46. Elliot DL, Cheong J, Moe EL, Goldberg L (2007). Cross-sectional study of female students reporting anabolic steroid use. *Arch Ped Adolesc Med* **161**, 572–7.
47. Windsor R, Dumitru D (1989). Prevalence of anabolic steroid use by male and female adolescents. *Med Sci Sport Exerc* **21**, 494–7.
48. Tanner SM, Miller DW, Alongi C (1995). Anabolic steroid use by adolescents: Prevalence, motives, and knowledge of risks. *Clin J Sports Med* **5**, 108–15.
49. Scott DM, Wagner JC, Barlow TW (1996). Anabolic steroid use among adolescents in Nebraska schools. *Am J Health Syst Pharmacol* **53**, 2068–72.
50. van den Berg P, Neumark-Sztainer D, Cafri G, Wall M (2007). Steroid use among adolescents: Longitudinal findings. *Pediatrics* **119**, 476–86.
51. French SA, Perry CL, Leon GR, Fulkerson JA (1994). Food preferences, eating patterns, and physical activity among adolescents: Correlates of eating disorders symptoms. *J Adolesc Health* **15**, 286–94.
52. Lytle LA, Kelder SH, Perry CL, Klepp K-I (1995). Covariance of adolescent health behaviors: The Class of 1989 study. *Health Educ Res* **10**, 133–46.
53. Leon GR (1991). Eating disorders in female athletes. *Sports Med* **12**, 219–27.
54. Ponton LE (1995). A review of eating disorders in adolescents. *Adolesc Psychiatr* **20**, 267–85.
55. Thiel A, Gottfried H, Hesse FW (1993). Subclinical eating disorders in male athletes. A study of the low weight categories in rowers and wrestlers. *Acta Psychiatrica Scand* **88**, 259–65.
56. Drummer GM, Rosen LW, Heusner WW, Roberts PJ, Counsilman JE (1987). Pathogenic weight control behaviors of young competitive swimmers. *The Physician Sports Med* **15**, 75–84.
57. Taub DE, Blinde EM (1992). Eating disorders among adolescent female athletes: Influence of athletic participation and sport team membership. *Adolescence* **27**, 833–48.
58. Davis C, Cowles M (1989). A comparison of weight and diet concerns and personality factors among female athletes and non-athletes. *J Psychosomatic Res* **33**, 527–36.
59. Middleman AB, Vazquez I, Durant RH (1998). Eating patterns, physical activity, and attempts to change weight among adolescents. *J Adolesc Health* **22**, 37–42.
60. Smith EA, Caldwell LL (1994). Participation in high school sports and adolescent sexual activity. *Pediatr Exerc Sci* **6**, 69–74.
61. Miller KE, Sabo DF, Farrell MP, Barnes GM, Melnick MJ (1998). Athletic participation and sexual behavior in adolescents: The different worlds of boys and girls. *J Health Social Behav* **39**, 108–23.
62. Sabo DF, Miller KE, Farrell MP, Melnick MJ, Barnes GM (1999). High school athletic participation, sexual behavior and adolescent pregnancy: A regional study. *J Adolesc Health* **25**, 207–16.
63. Miller KE, Barnes GM, Melnick MJ, Sabo DF, Farrell MP (2002). Gender and racial/ethnic differences in predicting adolescent sexual risk: Athletic participation versus exercise. *J Health Social Behav* **43**, 436–50.
64. Kulig K, Brener ND, McManus T (2003). Sexual activity and substance abuse among adolescents by category of physical activity plus team sports participation. *Arch Pediatr Adolesc Med* **157**, 905–12.
65. Levin DS, Smith EA, Caldwell LL, Kimbrough J (1995). Violence and high school sports participation. *Pediatr Exerc Sci* **7**, 379–88.

CHAPTER 30

Systematic promotion of physical activity

Stef P. J. Kremers, Herman Schaalma, Ree M. Meertens, Willem van Mechelen, and Gerjo J. Kok

Introduction

It is widely acknowledged that physical activity has a positive impact on the physiological and psychological health of young people. This leads us to consider the question how we can promote such a lifestyle. In this chapter, we will present a general approach for the theory- and data-based development of health promotion interventions. We will illustrate this approach with examples concerning the promotion of physical activity amongst young people.

Planned health promotion

Health promotion is defined as 'any planned combination of educational, political, regulatory, and organizational supports for actions and conditions of living conducive to the health of individuals, groups, or communities'.[1] Health promotion objectives are (i) primary prevention, (ii) early detection and treatment (secondary prevention), and (iii) patient care and support (tertiary prevention). Health promotion strategies include (i) legislation and regulations designed to enforce behaviour change, (ii) the provision of non-compulsory services, and (iii) education that focuses on encouraging and helping people to change their behaviour of their own accord. Generally, health promotion is most effective when it involves several mutually reinforcing strategies, and when it affects different levels of society.[2,3]

When developing health promotion programmes various decisions have to be made regarding programme objectives, target population, educational methods and strategies, useful media, etc. Unfortunately, these decisions cannot be made without careful analysis of the health problem, the behavioural and environmental factors affecting this problem, and the options for corrective action. Figure 30.1 depicts a planning and evaluation model for the development of health promotion interventions.[1,4]

The first phase in the planning process addresses the social and epidemiological diagnosis of the health problem. This phase should make clear whether the health problem is linked to individual and social perceptions of quality of life, whether the assumed problem has serious individual and social consequences, and whether it relates to other health problems. This phase should also reveal which people or institutions are involved.

The second planning phase includes the diagnosis of the behavioural, social, and environmental factors that are linked to the health problem of interest. This phase should reveal whether the health problem is linked to specific behaviours, and if it is, to whose behaviours. This phase should also make clear whether reduction of the health problem needs an environmental change, and if so, the decision-makers that are responsible for environmental change should be identified.

The third phase of the model examines the determinants of the behavioural and environmental conditions that are linked to health status or quality-of-life concerns. It also identifies the factors that must be changed to initiate and sustain the process of behavioural and environmental change. Regarding individual behaviour three categories of factors can be distinguished. Predisposing factors referring to cognitive antecedents that provide a rationale or motivation for behaviour (e.g. knowledge, attitudes, values, and goal priorities). Enabling factors, that is, cognitive antecedents that enable the enactment intentions (e.g. attitudes and behaviour of peers, parents, employers, as well as individual competencies). Reinforcing factors, which, following a behaviour, enhance its persistence or repetition (e.g. availability of resources, social approval, rules, or laws). In the case of laws, rules, and the availability of resources, identification of decision-makers may be required to make further progress.

The fourth phase, intervention development, addresses the analysis of the possible usefulness of (components of) health promotion and other potential interventions (resources, regulations). This phase may include (i) the assessment of the usefulness of current health promotion interventions, (ii) the development and small-scale evaluation of new interventions or intervention components, and (iii) a diagnosis of the political, regulatory, and organizational factors that may facilitate or hinder the development and widespread implementation of a health promotion intervention.

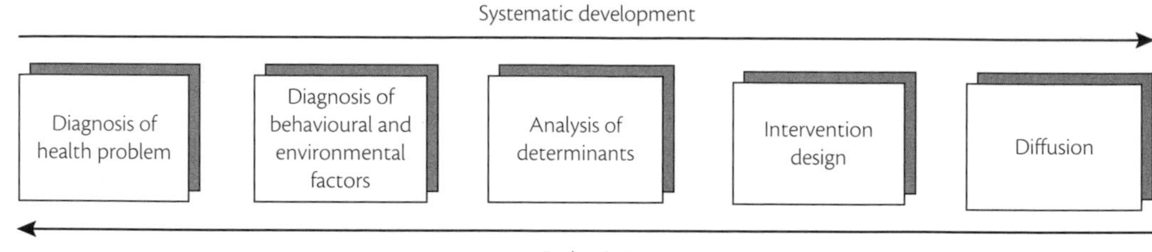

Fig. 30.1 Evidence-based development of health promotion.

The fifth planning phase addresses the diffusion of an intervention programme. This phase includes the diagnosis of the factors that are linked to the adoption, actual implementation, and institutionalization of a health promotion programme, and the launching of activities to enhance widespread programme diffusion. Awareness of the outcomes of this phase is necessary before starting the design of a practical health promotion programme.

Subsequent phases of the model all refer to the evaluation of the process, impact, and outcomes of the health promotion programme, resulting in feedback and adjustment. The core evaluation question—whether a programme results in a reduction of the health problem—often cannot be answered because of a delay between behaviour change and observable effects on the health problem. Generally, a change of behaviour is the best possible indication of the effectiveness of health promotion programmes.[5] Below, we will elaborate on each of the phases in theory- and data-based development of health promotion interventions to increase physical activity amongst children and adolescents.

Health promotion and physical activity

Problem and problem causing factors

Premature death is strongly related to chronic diseases such as heart disease, cancer, stroke, and diabetes. Lifestyle factors—such as smoking, alcohol abuse, improper diet, and physical inactivity—play an important role in the aetiology of these chronic diseases. Epidemiological studies have demonstrated that, together with smoking, physical inactivity is the most important independent risk factor for the leading causes of death in Western society.[6] Consequently, it is generally accepted that a physically active lifestyle has enormous direct and indirect health advantages for both adults and adolescents.[7–10] Not only the health of individuals, but also a nation's public health status will benefit from a physically active lifestyle. Estimates by Powell and Blair[11] showed that in the United States 35% of the coronary heart disease deaths, 32% of the colon cancer deaths, and 35% of the diabetes mellitus deaths could, theoretically, be prevented if everyone was vigorously active.

Small children seem to have a physically active lifestyle by nature. They play, jump, cycle, and run throughout the day. When they grow older, most children in Western society participate in school-based physical education (PE), organized sports, and leisure time activities in which they are physically active. For example, a nationwide survey among Dutch teenagers[12] showed that almost all participated in school-based PE with a mean of about 2 hours per week, and that about two out of three participated in organized sports for about 3 hours per week. In addition, most of them used a bicycle as a means of transportation[13] with a mean of at least 2 hours per week, and many enjoyed leisure time activities in which they are physically active for another 4 hours per week (such as street soccer, mountain biking, dancing).

Although young people seem to be fairly physically active, many young people in Western society gradually develop an inactive lifestyle during secondary school years, at least partly because of competing daily activities such as homework, watching television, playing computer games, part-time jobs, and going out.[14–17] For instance, Schaalma and colleagues[12] found a decline in physical activity with growing age for PE, organized sports, and unorganized leisure time activities, as well as for the use of a bicycle as a means of transportation. The decline in physical activity is most marked at age 13–16 years.[18] Van Mechelen and Kemper[15] found that young people who had an average of 4 hours per week of moderate physical activity at age 13 years, only had 1 hour of comparable activity at age 27 years.

Child sedentary behaviour has been assigned a specific role in the current obesity epidemic.[19] Parallel increases in the time spent on sedentary behaviours and prevalence of obesity suggest a causal relation between the two[20] and some prospective studies in children have shown a positive relationship.[21–23] 'Screen-viewing behaviour',[24] including television viewing[25–27] and computer use,[28,29] has been identified as key sedentary behaviour in this age group.[30] A systematic review by Marshall and colleagues[30] showed that most young people watch approximately 2–2.5 hours of television each day, and of those with access to computers and video games, a further 0.5 and 0.75 hours, respectively, is spent using these technologies. While the majority of young people watch television less than 2 hours per day, 28% watch more than 4 hours per day, which is double the maximum level recommended by the American Academy of Paediatrics.[31]

Children still engage in television viewing more often than in computer use, but computers have become more and more popular in recent years, even among young children. In the Netherlands, for example, the percentage of youth who use a computer more than once a week increased from 24% in 1990 to 67% in 2000.[32] In 2005, time spent on television viewing decreased for the first time in Dutch history.[33] In fact, Dutch adolescents (12–19 years) spent more time on computer use than watching television in 2005 (mean 8.6 vs. 8.4 hours per week).[33] Increased possibilities and facilities to watch television or video online may reduce time spent on television viewing even more in comparison with computer use.[34]

Determinants of physical activity

Theory

An analysis of cognitive determinants of behaviour can illustrate differences between young people's exercise behaviour. Various current social-psychological models predicting goal-oriented behaviour can be applied to health-related behaviours. Although these models include a broad range of variables, basically five general categories of core cognitive antecedents of health behaviours can be distinguished.[35]

(i) *Attitude*. This category includes beliefs and evaluations about advantages and disadvantages (e.g. health risks) of behaviour, also referred to as outcome expectations, resulting in an overall evaluation of a specific health behaviour.

(ii) *Perceived social influences*. This category includes injunctive social norms (i.e. subjective beliefs about what important others think that ought to be thought or done), descriptive social norms (i.e. perceptions of what important others generally do), and perceived direct social pressures (i.e. perceptions of direct social sanctions and rewards for behaviour).

(iii) *Self-efficacy*. This determinant category refers to perceptions of one's own capability to successfully perform a particular behaviour, also referred to as perceived behavioural control.

(iv) *Identity concerns*, that is, the extent to which a specific behaviour allows expression of, or contradicts, a valid social or personal construction of the self.

(v) *Preparation for action*, that is, the extent to which, having decided to act, people are able or are prompted to plan on how to enact their intentions amidst competing everyday priorities.

In addition to the cognitive factors as described above, actual environmental influences can be especially relevant to children and adolescents because they have less autonomy in their behavioural choices.[36] Specific recommendations for research on the determinants of physical activity in youth have emphasized the need to examine environmental influences at different levels (e.g. home, neighbourhood, school)[37,38] to better inform the development of interventions attempting to improve physical activity levels.[39,40]

Different classifications of possible environmental determinants of health behaviours have been proposed,[41–45] all of them showing great overlap and similarities. A conceptual framework that is increasingly used in the field is the ANalysis Grid for Environments Linked to Obesity (ANGELO).[46] This framework was specifically developed to conceptualize 'obesogenic' environments (i.e. those that promote excessive energy intake and low physical activity), enabling the identification of specific areas and settings to be targeted by intervention programmes. The ANGELO framework divides the variety in types of environmental determinants into four distinct types of influence: physical (what is available), economic (what are the costs), political (what are the rules), and sociocultural (what is the social and cultural background). In addition, two levels of influence are distinguished: micro-environmental settings and macro-environmental sectors. Individuals interact with the environment in multiple micro-environmental settings, including schools, workplaces, homes, and neighbourhoods, which are, in turn, influenced by broader macro-environments, including health systems, governments, and the food industry. When types and level of environment are crossed, it forms a grid that comprises four types of environment on one axis and two sizes of environment on the other.

It has been suggested that an integrated approach to the study of determinants of physical activity, in which social-psychological models are combined with ecological models of health behaviour, would improve our knowledge regarding the causal mechanisms that underlie the behaviour.[47] The EnRG framework (Environmental Research framework for weight Gain prevention; Fig. 30.2, adapted version) is an example of such an integrated framework. In this framework, environmental influences (as defined in ANGELO) are hypothesized to influence dietary intake and physical activity both indirectly and directly. The indirect causal mechanism reflects the mediating role of intrapersonal behaviour-specific cognitions and the direct influence reflects the automatic, unconscious, influence of the environment on behaviour.

EnRG hypothesizes intrapersonal factors to interact with the environment in order to determine its obesogenicity. When one wishes to gain more insight into environment–behaviour relations, it is essential to explore the more complex interactions involved in the mechanisms underlying physical activity. Distinct types of factors (e.g. demographic factors, personality, and habit strength) are postulated to moderate the causal path (i.e. inducing either the automatic or the cognitively mediated environment–behaviour relation). Especially habit strength might be an important concept in this respect. Once learned, a child's walk-

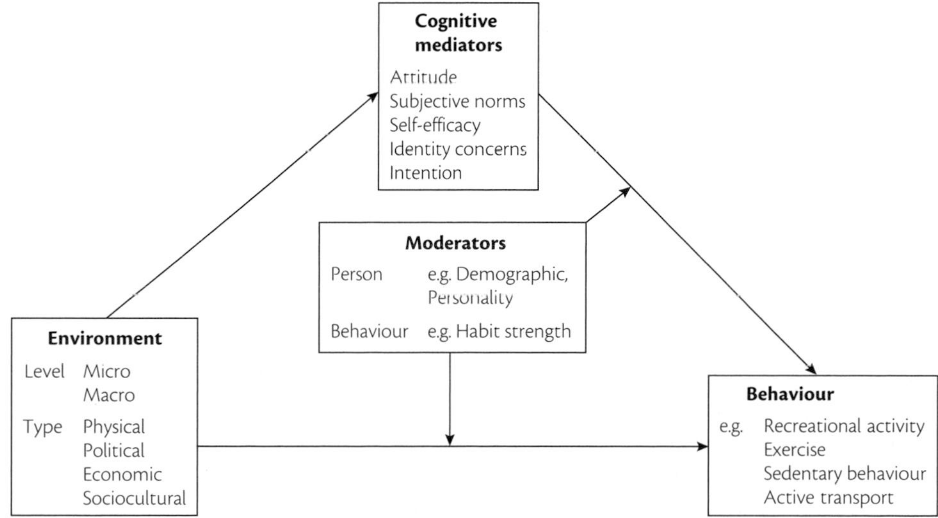

Fig. 30.2 Environmental and cognitive determinants of physical activity. Adapted from Environmental Research Framework for Weight Gain Prevention; Kremers *et al.*[47]

ing, running, and jumping would seem to be behaviours that do not require intentional efforts to be set in motion.[48] In line with this observation, Triandis[49] posited that deliberate decisions to act become irrelevant in guiding behaviour when the behaviour has been performed repeatedly in the past. Repeated behaviours may be largely determined by habit rather than by reasoned action. When habits are formed, subsequent behaviour is associated with, and automatically triggered by, specific environmental cues that normally precede the action.[48]

An example: Determinants of physical activity in young people

Many researchers have focussed on cognitive determinants of young people's exercise behaviour or their physical activity.[50–52] Multiple studies suggest that cognitive factors (attitudes, self-efficacy expectations, and perceived social influences) strongly relate to the frequency of physical activity. In the past decade, however, an increased attention to environmental determinants of physical activity in youth has been observed, which may reflect a paradigm shift from intrapersonal to determinants of physical activity.[53] A recent systematic review of the literature on environmental correlates of physical activity in children and adolescents[53] shows that factors in the home and school environments were especially associated with physical activity in young people. Most consistent positive correlates of physical activity were physical activity of the father, time spent outdoors, support from significant others, and school policies regarding physical activity. Low crime incidence (in adolescents) was a characteristic of the neighbourhood environment associated with higher physical activity. With respect to the role of habit strength in childhood physical activity, a recent study[54] investigated Triandis'[49] theoretical assumption that when strong physical (in)activity habits are formed, the behaviours are not determined by processes of reasoned action anymore. Indeed, this study indicated that a strong intention–behaviour association existed in children with weak habits, while a weak intention–behaviour association was found in the case of strong habits.[54]

Systematic development of physical activity promoting interventions

Theory

The phase following the need assessment addresses the development of a health promotion programme. In this stage, insights from theory and research have to be translated into methods and strategies. A shift must be made from *explaining* behaviour to *changing* behaviour. There is no such thing as a *magic bullet*: no intervention method is universally effective.[55] Intervention programmes have to be tailored very carefully to the behaviour, behavioural determinants, and target population. The process of intervention design includes several steps,[56] in which the Intervention Mapping (IM) protocol[57] has proven to be a helpful tool (Fig. 30.3).

IM is a systematic process that explicates a series of six steps for the development of health promotion programmes based on theory, empirical evidence, and additional research. The steps are followed in an iterative way, that is, programme planners are moving back and forth throughout the process. IM enables health promoters to create feasible and effective programmes.

In Step 1, before beginning to plan an intervention, the health problem is assessed, as well as its impact on quality of life, behavioural, and environmental causes, and determinants of behaviour and environmental causes.

Step 2 of the IM protocol focuses on desired behaviours and environments that are identified in the needs assessment. First, performance objectives (i.e. specific behaviours that the target group or key intermediaries have to adapt as a result of the programme) are specified. Then, one must specify the personal and environmental factors that are important mediators for reaching the programme objectives, that is, the predictors of healthy behaviour change need to be identified. Finally, the performance objectives are merged with these determinants, which results in matrices enabling the identification of the proximal programme objectives (i.e. statements on what must be learned by the programme participants, or what must be changed in the environment in order to enable behaviour change).

In Step 3 of IM, proximal programme objectives are linked to theory-based intervention methods and practical intervention strategies. First, theory-based methods are specified and the programme developers identify conditions under which such methods have been shown to be effective. Subsequently, these methods are translated into practical applications (strategies).

The product of Step 4 of IM is a health promotion programme. Strategies are operationalized into a programme plan, taking into account the context in which the programme will be used. Then, the programme materials are designed, pretested, and produced.

Step 5 involves the adoption and implementation plan for the health promotion programme defined in Step 4. A linkage system is developed in order to connect the developers with the users of the intervention. Next, proximal programme objectives are set with regard to the adoption and implementation of the intervention. Accordingly, an implementation programme is written.

Finally, in Step 6 of IM, a plan is prepared to evaluate the programme in order to be able to understand if and why a programme was a success or a failure.

Evidence

Although many programme developers claim that their intervention is theoretically and empirically based, descriptions of the way in which data and theories were actually applied in health promotion interventions is rare. Few programme developers have provided details regarding the underlying rationale for the intervention components, the theoretical background and behaviour change methodology (e.g. ref. 58). Consequently, we have little knowledge about the efficacy of specific teaching methods or approaches with regard to the promotion of healthy behaviours.[59] As Almond and Harris[60] concluded, 'current research does little to promote our understanding of what kind of programmes bring about health gains or outcomes that we value' (p. 145). Recent reviews do provide some insight in the effectiveness of programmes promoting physical activity, although their evaluation design could be improved in order to contribute to theory development.[61]

Studies that have focused on information provision have showed variable effects on time spent in physical activity outside the school setting.[62] Evaluations of interventions aimed at the enhancement of participation in organized exercise programmes showed that social support, commitment enhancing techniques (e.g. making a contract to complete the programme), and drop-out prevention training based on relapse prevention theory[63] can be useful in motivating young people to maintain their participation in organized sports.

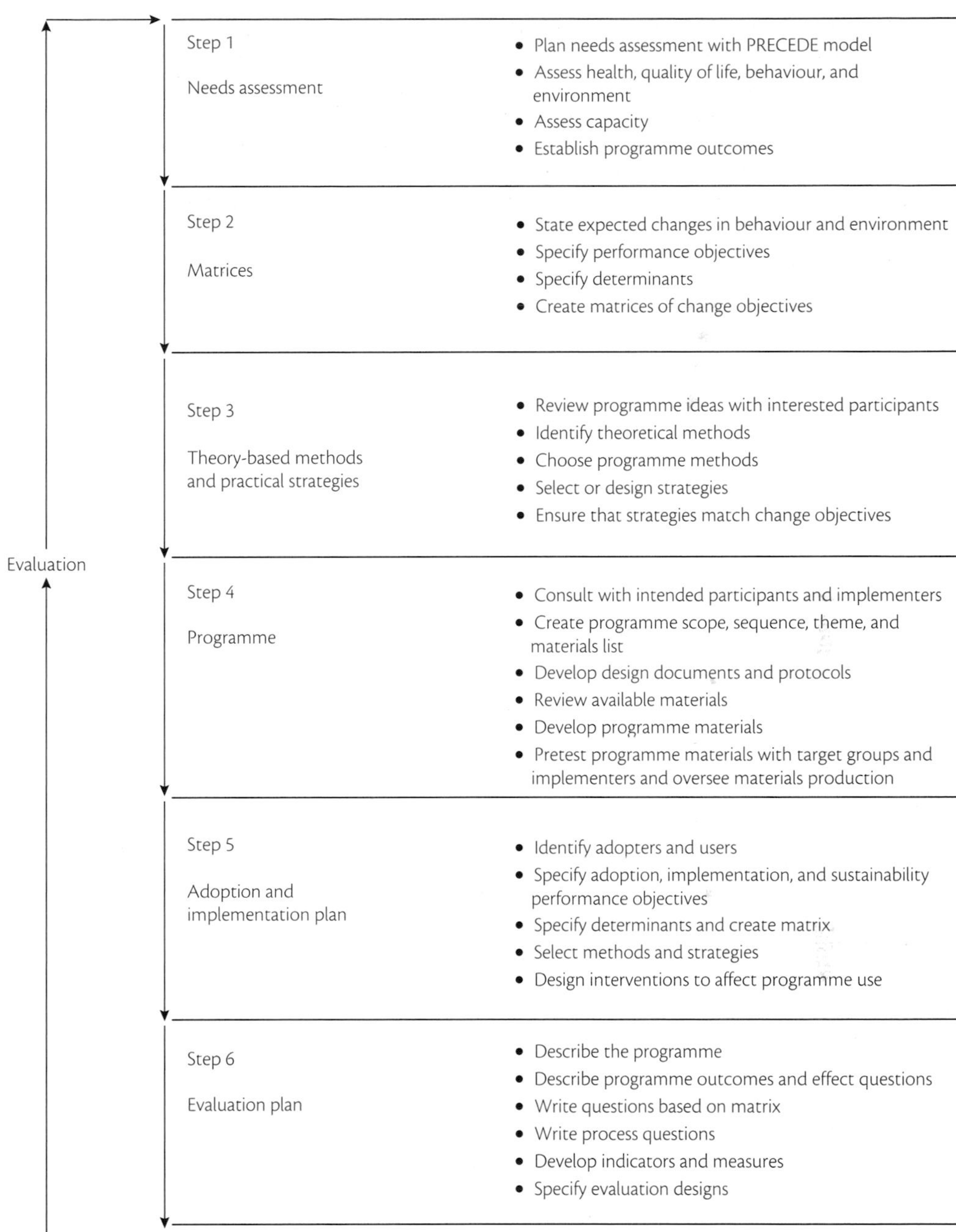

Fig. 30.3 Intervention mapping. From Bartholomew *et al.*[57]

Motivations oriented programmes, mostly based on social cognitive and social influence techniques, are least effective at this point.[64,65]

While some environmental interventions to promote physical activity in youth targeted the social environment, for instance, by teaching parents behavioural skills to influence their child's physical activity,[66] the majority of environmental interventions conducted to date are implemented in school environments through changes in PE lessons. This is usually done either by increasing length, frequency, and/or intensity of PE lessons.[62] Most of these school-based interventions have yielded positive effects on youngsters' physical activity, indicating that the school environment provides adequate possibilities to positively influence physical activity levels in youth.[62,67]

Breaking sedentary habits and promoting active habits require disrupting the environmental factors that automatically cue habit performance. Two types of potential habit change interventions have been proposed.[68] So-called downstream-plus interventions provide informational input at points when habits are vulnerable to change, such as when individuals are undergoing naturally occurring changes in environments in which many everyday physical activities are performed (e.g. moving households, changing schools). Upstream interventions are aimed at disrupting old environmental cues and establishing new ones. Typical upstream interventions involve policy changes.

One of the main problems with physical activity in young people is the maintenance of a physically active lifestyle. One of the theoretical methods that can be useful for the development of intervention components with beneficial effects on the maintenance of a physically active lifestyle is Relapse Prevention theory.[63] A study by King and Frederiksen[69] showed that drop-out prevention training that was based on Relapse Prevention theory resulted in a higher attendance to a 5-week jogging programme. This drop-out training included (i) the identification of so-called high-risk situations, that is, situations in which it would be difficult to maintain participation in the programme; and (ii) the development and practise of adequate coping responses to deal with these high-risk situations.

An example: A systematically developed intervention to promote physical activity in children

In 2002, the primary-school-based intervention programme 'JUMP-in', was started in Amsterdam.[70] JUMP-in aims to promote physical activity among primary school children. It is a systematically developed primary-school-based intervention that focuses on the use of theory, environmental changes, parental influences, and cooperation with multilevel parties (municipal authorities, local sport services, primary schools, and local sport clubs) in intervention development. The IM protocol was applied in order to systematically design the intervention, using theoretical input from the Theory of Planned Behaviour,[71] a model of physical exercise and habit formation,[48] the Precaution Adoption Process model,[72] a social ecological model of physical activity,[73] and the Service Quality Model.[74] The intervention consists of six programme components: (i) school sports activities, (ii) a pupil follow-up system, (iii) The Class Moves!®, in-class exercises, (iv) Choose your card!, lessons aimed at increasing awareness, (v) parental information services, and (vi) an Activity Week. In addition, special attention was paid to pleasure and to ethnic minorities. A pilot study in six primary schools[70] showed that JUMP-in was effective in influencing physical activity, especially among children from Grade 6. Children in the control group decreased their level of physical activity considerably, while activity levels in intervention children from Grade 6 remained stable. To embed JUMP-in in daily practice and in policy, highly structured cooperation is created between city districts, schools, youth health care, welfare organizations, school supervisory services, local municipal sport services, and local sports clubs. The wider delivery of a revised version of the JUMP-in programme incorporates 60 schools in deprived city areas of Amsterdam.

Implementation and diffusion of health promotion interventions

Theory

Implementation of a prevention programme is an essential part of the health promotion planning process. Underestimating diffusion and adoption barriers is one of the major causes of ineffectiveness in health promotion. While the need for information about the determinants of individual behaviour is commonly accepted, the need for information about the determinants of institutional 'behaviour' (such as the adoption of a prevention programme by organizations) is not widely recognized. Consequently, many expensive programmes are never adequately applied in the contexts where they are most likely to be effective.

The diffusion of a health promotion programme can be described as a process consisting of four phases: dissemination, adoption, implementation, and maintenance.[75] Dissemination concerns the transfer of information about the programme to potential users. This phase involves the selection of communication channels and systems that facilitate the diffusion of the programme to a target population. Adoption refers to potential users' intention to use the programme. This phase includes a diagnosis of the target population with regard to their needs, values, and attitudes, and their perception of programme attributes and adoption barriers, such as the relative advantage of the programme, its fit with the target population, its complexity, and the observability of programme outcomes. This phase also includes the diagnosis of the ways target adopters can be motivated to adopt the programme, and the ways to overcome barriers. Implementation refers to the actual use of the programme. The major focus in this phase is on the enhancement of adopters' self-efficacy and skills, and on encouraging trial programme implementation. Maintenance or continuation succeeds initial implementation. This phase refers to the stage in which the programme has become current practice and in which the allocation of recourses are routinely made.[76]

According to Orlandi and colleagues[77] many health promotion innovations have failed because of 'the gap that is frequently left unfilled between the point where innovation-development ends and diffusion planning begins', as if innovation-development barriers and diffusion barriers were aspects of unrelated problems. To bridge this gap, Orlandi and colleagues stressed the need for a *linkage system* between the resource system that develops and promotes the intervention (e.g. the Health Education Authority), and the user system that is supposed to adopt the intervention (e.g. sports organizations, schools). Such a liaison group should include representatives of the user system, representatives of the resource system, and a change agent facilitating the collaboration. Diffusion of the innovation may be carried out by any of the members of this liaison group. The essential point is that the innovation-development process and the diffusion planning process have been developed through co-operation, to improve the fit between innovation and user, to attune intervention innovations to practical possibilities and constraints, and to facilitate widespread implementation.

The development of a diffusion strategy can be based on a planning process that is similar to the planning of health promotion programmes. A diffusion strategy should be based on insights in the determinants of potential users' decisions regarding the adoption, implementation, and continuation of a health promoting programme. These determinants can be measured with the same kind of protocol as is used in the determinants of behaviour analyses, using the same kind of theories.[56] A diffusion strategy should further be based on useful theoretical methods and theory-based strategies.

An example: Diffusion of school-based programmes to promote physical activity

Social Cognitive Theory[78] provides a valuable framework for the development of interventions to stimulate the diffusion of school-based health promotion programmes.[79,80] A strategy for the diffusion of a school-based programme to promote physical activity may include the following objectives and methods. The objectives of a dissemination strategy could be that teachers and administrators are aware of the programme, view the programme favourably, and communicate with colleagues about the programme. Useful methods to reach these objectives are personal communication by opinion leaders, and the use of modelling showing teachers successfully using the programme, for example, through video or role-model stories in newsletters. An adoption strategy could focus on the advantages of the exercise programme in terms of outcomes, expectancies, and social reinforcements. Useful methods to reach these objectives are modelling (e.g. peer model stories in written material), incentives and social contracting, for instance, through a newsletter. An implementation strategy could focus on the reinforcement of teachers' skills and their self-efficacy to use the exercise programme with acceptable completeness, fidelity, and proficiency. Data from other implementation studies showed the importance of in-service training.[81] Methods to reach these objectives are direct modelling and guided enactment through a live workshop training, and symbolic modelling through video training. The objectives of a continuation strategy could be that teachers and administrators will have experienced positive feedback and reinforcement on the use of the exercise programme after 1 year and will continue to use it. These objectives may be accomplished by means of various kinds of incentives (social, monetary, status, and self-evaluative incentives).

Summary

From a public health perspective the promotion of physical activity has many benefits. Inactivity is a risk factor for multi-causal chronic disease, and a physically active lifestyle helps to maintain body weight. The present chapter provided an overview of relevant theoretical and empirical insights regarding the development of interventions to promote physical activity in young people.

- Physical activity promoting programmes should be based on a systematic approach combining empirical findings, theoretical insights, and practical considerations.
- Successful health promotion interventions to increase physical activity typically consist of strategies to improve intrapersonal, motivational, determinants of physical activity, as well as environmental strategies that facilitate the behaviour, break unhealthy habits, or sustain healthy ones.
- The scientific literature hardly provides any insight in the ways in which social science theory and empirical findings are applied in the design of physical activity promoting interventions, or in the effectiveness of attempts to facilitate large-scale implementation of such interventions.
- The IM protocol can be a helpful tool in the systematic development, implementation, diffusion, and evaluation of interventions aimed at the promotion of physical activity in young people.

References

1. Green LW, Kreuter MW (1991). *Health promotion planning: An educational and environmental approach*. Mountain View, Mayfield, CA.
2. De Leeuw ED (1989). *The sane revolution. Health promotion: Backgrounds, scope, prospects*. Van Gorcum, Assen, The Netherlands.
3. Milio N (1988). Strategies for health promoting policy: A study of four national case studies. *Health Promot Int* **3**, 307–11.
4. Kok GJ (1992). Quality of planning as decisive determinant of health education. *Hygie* **11**, 5–8.
5. Tones K, Tilford S, Robinson YK (1990). *Health education: Effectiveness and efficiency*. Chapman, London.
6. Pate RR, Pratt M, Blair SN, Haskell WL, Macera CA, Bouchard C, Buchner D, Ettinger W, Heath GW, King AC (1995). Physical activity and public health. A recommendation from the Centers for Disease Control and Prevention and the American College of Sports Medicine. *JAMA* **273**, 402–7.
7. Tell GS, Vellar OD (1988). Physical fitness, physical activity, and cardiovascular disease risk factors in adolescents: The Olso study. *Prev Med* **17**, 12–24.
8. World Cancer Research Fund/American Institute for Cancer Research (2007). *Food, nutrition, physical activity, and the prevention of cancer: A global perspective*. AICR, Washington, D.C.
9. NIH Consensus development panel and physical activity and cardiovascular health (1996). Physical activity and cardiovascular health. *JAMA* **276**, 241–6.
10. Suter E, Hawes MR (1993). Relationship of physical activity, body fat, diet, and blood lipid profile in youth 10–15 yr. *Med Sci Sports Exerc* **25**, 748–54.
11. Powell KE, Blair SN (1994). The public health burden of sedentary living habits: Theoretical but realistic estimates. *Med Sci Sports Exerc* **26**, 851–6.
12. Schaalma HP, Bolman C, De Nooijer J, De Vries H, Paulussen T, Aarts H, Willemse G (1997). *Prevention of cardio-vascular disease: A lifestyle and determinant analysis*. Netherlands Heart Foundation, The Hague.
13. De Bruijn GJ, Kremers SPJ, Van Mechelen W, Schaalma H, Brug J (2005). Determinants of adolescent bicycle use for transportation and snacking behavior. *Prev Med* **40**, 658–67.
14. Robinson TN, Hammer LD, Killen LD, Kraemer HC, Wilson DM, Hayward C, Taylor CB (1993). Does television viewing increase obesity and reduce physical activity in adolescents? *Prev Med* **19**, 541–51.
15. Van Mechelen W, Kemper H (1995). Habitual physical activity in longitudinal perspective In: Kemper, HCG (ed.), *The Amsterdam Growth Study: A longitudinal analysis of health, fitness, and lifestyle*, pp. 135–59. Human Kinetics, Champaign, IL.
16. Kelder SH, Perry CL, Klepp K-I (1993). Community-wide youth exercise promotion: Long term outcomes of the Minnesota Heart Health Program and the Class of 1989 study. *J School Health* **63**, 218–23.
17. Gortmaker SL, Dietz WH, Cheung LWY (1990). Inactivity, diet and the fattening of America. *J Am Diet Assoc* **90**, 1247–55.
18. Van Mechelen W, Twisk JW, Post GB, Snel J, Kemper HC (2000). Physical activity of young people: The Amsterdam Longitudinal Growth and Health Study. *Med Sci Sports Exerc* **32**, 1610–16.
19. World Health Organisation/UN Food and Agriculture Organisation (2002). *Diet, nutrition and the prevention of chronic diseases*. Report of a joint WHO/FAO expert consultation, Geneva, 28 January-1 February 2002.
20. Rennie KL, Johnson L, Jebb SA (2005). Behavioural determinants of obesity. *Best Pract Research Clin Endocrin Met* **19**, 343–58.
21. Parsons TJ, Power C, Logan S, Summerbell CD (1999). Childhood predictors of adult obesity: A systematic review. *Int J Obes* **23**, S1–107.
22. Hill JO, Wyatt HR, Melanson EL (2000). Genetic and environmental contributions to obesity. *Med Clin North Am* **84**, 333–45.
23. Hancox RJ, Milne BJ, Poulton R (2004). Association between child and adolescent television viewing and adult health: A longitudinal birth cohort study. *Lancet* **364**, 257–62.
24. He M, Irwin JD, Sangster Bouck LM, Tucker P, Pollett GL (2005). Screen-viewing behaviors among preschoolers. Parents' perceptions. *Am J Prev Med* **29**, 120–5.
25. Dietz W, Gortmaker S (1985). Do we fatten our children at the television set? *Pediatr* **75**, 807–12.
26. Gortmaker S, Sobol A, Peterson K, Colditz G, Dietz W (1996). Television viewing as a cause of increasing obesity among children in the United States, 1986–1990. *Arch Pediatr Adolesc Med* **150**, 356–62.
27. Crespo C, Smit E, Troiano R, Bartlett S, Macera C, Andersen R (2001). Television watching, energy intake, and obesity in US children: Results from the third National Health and Nutrition Examination Survey, 1988–1994. *Arch Pediatr Adolesc Med* **155**, 360–5.
28. Attewell P, Suazo-Garcia B, Battle J (2003). Computers and young children: Social benefit or social problem? *Soc Forces* **82**, 277–96.
29. Stettler N, Signer TM, Suster PM (2004). Electronic games and environmental factors associated with childhood obesity in Switzerland. *Obes Res* **12**, 896–903.

30. Marshall SJ, Gorely T, Biddle SJ (2006). A descriptive epidemiology of screen-based media use in youth: A review and critique. *J Adolesc* **29**, 333–49.
31. American Academy of Pediatrics (2001). Policy statement: Children, adolescents and television (RE0043). *Pediatr* **107**, 423–6.
32. Zeijl E (2003). *Rapportage Jeugd 2002* [in Dutch]. Sociaal en Cultureel Planbureau, Den Haag.
33. Sociaal en Cultureel Planbureau (2006). De tijd als spiegel. Hoe Nederlanders hun tijd besteden [in Dutch]. SCP, Den Haag.
34. ICM Research (2006). *Online video survey*. BBC/ICM. Available at http://www.icmresearch.co.uk/ [retrieved June 2007].
35. Abraham C, Sheeran P, Johnston M (1998). From health beliefs to self-regulation: Theoretical advances in the psychology of action control. *Psychol Health* **13**, 569–91.
36. Nutbeam D, Aar L, Catford J (1989). Understanding children's health behaviour: The implications for health promotion for young people. *Soc Sci Med* **29**, 317–25.
37. Kohl HW III, Hobbs KE (1998). Development of physical activity behaviors among children and adolescents. *Pediatr* **101**, 549–54.
38. Sallis JF, Simons-Morton BG, Stone EJ, Corbin CB, Epstein LH, Faucette N, Iannotti RJ, Killen JD, Klesges RC, Petray CK (1992). Determinants of physical activity and interventions in youth. *Med Sci Sports Exerc* **24**, S248–57.
39. Brug J, Oenema A, Ferreira I (2005). Theory, evidence and Intervention Mapping to improve behavioral nutrition and physical activity interventions. *Int J Behav Nutr Phys Act* **2**, e2.
40. Baranowski T, Cullen KW, Nicklas T, Thompson D, Baranowski J (2003). Are current health behavioral change models helpful in guiding prevention of weight gain efforts? *Obes Res* **11**, S23–43.
41. French SA, Story M, Jeffery RW (2001). Environmental influences on eating and physical activity. *Annu Rev Public Health* **22**, 309–35.
42. Story M, Neumark-Sztainer D, French S (2002). Individual and environmental influences on adolescent eating behaviors. *J Am Diet Assoc* **102**, S40–51.
43. Owen N, Leslie E, Salmon J, Fotheringham MJ (2000). Environmental determinants of physical activity and sedentary behavior. *Exerc Sport Sci Rev* **28**, 153–8.
44. Flay BR, Petraitis J (1994). The theory of triadic influence: A new theory of health behavior with implications for preventive interventions. *Adv Med Soc* **4**, 4–19.
45. Kumanyika S, Jeffery RW, Morabia A, Ritenbaugh C, Antipatis VJ (2002). Obesity prevention: The case for action. *Int J Obes* **26**, 425–36.
46. Swinburn B, Egger G, Raza F (1999). Dissecting obesogenic environments: The development and application of a framework for identifying and prioritizing environmental interventions for obesity. *Prev Med* **29**, 563–70.
47. Kremers SPJ, De Bruijn GJ, Visscher TLS, Van Mechelen W, De Vries NK, Brug J (2006). Environmental influences on energy balance-related behaviors: A dual-process view. *Int J Behav Nutr Phys Act* **3**, 9.
48. Aarts H, Paulussen T, Schaalma H (1997). Physical exercise habit: On the conceptualization and formation of habitual health behaviours. *Health Educ Res* **12**, 363–74.
49. Triandis HC (1977). *Interpersonal behavior*. Brooks/Cole, Monterey, CA.
50. De Bourdeauhuij I (1998). Behavioural factors associated with physical activity in young people. In: Biddle S, Sallis J, Cavill N (eds.), *Young and active?*, pp. 98–118. Health Education Authority, London.
51. Dishman RK, Sallis JF (1994). Determinants and interventions for physical activity and exercise. In: Bouchard C, Shepard RJ, Stephens T (eds.), *Physical activity, fitness and health: international proceedings and consensus statement 1992*. Human Kinetics, Champaign, IL.
52. Kremers SPJ, Visscher TLS, Seidell JC, Van Mechelen W, Brug J (2005). Cognitive determinants of energy balance-related behaviours: Measurement issues. *Sports Med* **35**, 923–33.
53. Ferreira I, Van der Horst K, Wendel-Vos W, Kremers S, Van Lenthe F, Brug J (2007). Environmental correlates of physical activity in youth—A review and update. *Obes Rev* **8**, 129–54.
54. Kremers SPJ, Brug J (2008). Habit strength of physical activity and sedentary behavior among children and adolescents. *Pediatr Exerc Sci* 20, 5–14.
55. Mullen PD, Green LW, Persinger G (1985). Clinical trials for patient education for chronic conditions: A comparative meta-analysis of intervention types. *Prev Med* **14**, 753–81.
56. Kok G, Schaalma H, De Vries H, Parcel G, Paulussen T (1996). Social psychology and health education. In: Stroebe W, Hewstone M (eds.), *European Review of Social Psychology*, vol. 7, pp. 210–40. John Wiley & Sons, Chichester.
57. Bartholomew LK, Parcel GS, Kok G, Gottlieb NH (2006). *Planning health promotion programs; An Intervention Mapping approach*. Jossey-Bass, San Francisco, CA.
58. Singh AS, Chin A Paw MJM, Kremers SPJ, Visscher TLS, Brug J, Van Mechelen W (2006). Design of the Dutch Obesity Intervention in Teenagers (NRG-DOiT): Systematic development, implementation and evaluation of a school-based intervention aimed at prevention of excessive weight gain in adolescents. *BMC Public Health* **6**, 304.
59. Kremers SPJ, Visscher TLS, Brug J, Chin A Paw MJM, Schouten EG, Schuit AJ, Seidell JC, Van Baak MA, Van Mechelen W, Kemper HCG, Kok FJ, Saris WHM, Kromhout D (2005). Netherlands Research programme weight Gain prevention (NHF-NRG): Rationale, objectives and strategies. *Eur J Clin Nutr* **59**, 498–507.
60. Almond L, Harris J (1998). Interventions to promote health-related physical education. In: Biddle S, Sallis J, Cavill N (eds.), *Young and active?*, pp. 133–49. Health Education Authority, London.
61. Kremers SPJ, De Bruijn GJ, Droomers M, Van Lenthe F, Brug J (2007). Moderators of environmental intervention effects on diet and activity in youth. *Am J Prev Med* **32**, 163–72.
62. Kahn EB, Ramsey LT, Brownson RC, Heath GW, Howze EH, Powell KE, Stone EJ, Rajab MW, Corso P (2002). The effectiveness of interventions to promote physical activity: A systematic review. *Am J Prev Med* **22**, S73–107.
63. Marlatt GA, Gordon J (1985). *Relapse prevention*. Guilford Press, New York.
64. Aarts H, Paulussen Th, Willemse G, Schaalma H, Bolman C, De Nooijer J (1997). *Prevention of cardiovascular disease: An analysis of international effect research on the promotion of physical exercise among young people*. Netherlands Heart Foundation, The Hague.
65. Sallis J (1998). Family and community interventions to promote physical activity in young people. In: Biddle S, Sallis J, Cavill N (eds.), *Young and active?*, pp. 150–61. Health Education Authority, London.
66. Norton DE, Froelicher ES, Waters CM, Carrieri-Kohlman V (2003). Parental influence on models of primary prevention of cardiovascular disease in children. *Eur J Cardiovasc Nurs* **2**, 311–22.
67. De Bruijn GJ, Kremers S, Wendel-Vos W, Van Lenthe F, Brug J (2005). Environmental interventions on physical activity in youth. In: Brug J, Van Lenthe F (eds.), *Environmental determinants and interventions for physical activity, nutrition and smoking: A review*, pp. 78–106. Speed-Print b.v., Zoetermeer.
68. Verplanken B, Wood W (2006). Interventions to break and create consumer habits. *J. Public Policy Market* **25**, 90–103.
69. King AC, Frederiksen LW (1984). Low-cost strategies for increasing exercise behavior. *Behav Mod* **8**, 3–21.
70. Jurg ME, Kremers SPJ, Candel MJJM, Van der Wal M, De Meij J (2006). A controlled trial of a school-based environmental intervention to improve physical activity in children: JUMP-in, kids in motion. *Health Promot Int* **21**, 320–30.
71. Ajzen I (1988). *Attitude, personality and behavior*. Open University Press, Milton Keynes, UK.

72. Weinstein ND, Sandman PM (1992). A model of the precaution adoption process: Evidence from home radon testing. *Health Psychol* **11**, 170–80.
73. Pikora T, Giles-Corti B, Bull F, Jamrozik K, Donovan R (2003). Developing a framework for assessment of environmental determinants of walking and cycling. *Soc Sci Med* **56**, 1693–703.
74. Parasuraman A, Zeithaml VA, Berry LL (1985). A conceptual model of service quality and its implications for future research. *J Market* **49**, 41–50.
75. Oldenburg B, Hardcastle D, Kok G (1997). Diffusion of innovations. In: Glanz K, Lewis FM, Rimer BK (eds.), *Health behavior and health education: Theory, research and practice* (2nd ed.), pp. 270–86. Jossey-Bass, San Francisco, CA.
76. Miles MB, Louis KS (1987). Research on institutionalization: A reflective review. In: Miles MB, Ekholm M, Vandenberghe R (eds.), *Lasting school improvement: Exploring the process of institutionalization.* ACCO, Amersfoort.
77. Orlandi MA, Landers C, Weston R, Haley N (1990). Diffusion of health promotion innovations. In: Glanz K, Lewis FM, Rimer BK (eds.), *Health behavior and health education: Theory, research and practice* (1st ed.), pp. 288–313. Jossey-Bass, San Francisco, CA.
78. Bandura A (1986). *Social foundation of thought and action: A social cognitive theory*. Prentice-Hall, NJ.
79. Parcel G, Taylor WC, Brink SG, Gottlieb NH, Enquist KE, Eriksen MP (1989). Translating theory into practice: Intervention strategies for the diffusion of a health promotion innovation. *Fam Commun Health* **12**, 1–13.
80. Parcel G, Erikson MP, Lovato CY, Gottlieb NH, Brink SG, Green LW (1989). The diffusion of school-based tobacco-use prevention programmes; project description and baseline data. *Health Educ Res* **4**, 111–24.
81. Joyce B, Showers B (1988). *Student achievement through staff development*. Longman, New York.

PART IV

Chronic Health Conditions and Physical Activity

CHAPTER 31

Exercise testing in congenital heart disease

Tony Reybrouck and Marc Gewillig

Introduction

Exercise testing in adult cardiac patients has mainly focused on ischaemic heart disease. The results of exercise testing with ECG monitoring are often helpful in diagnosing the presence of significant coronary artery disease. In children with heart disease, the type of pathology is different. Ischaemic heart disease is very rare. The majority of the patients present with congenital heart defects, which affect exercise capacity. In patients with congenital heart disease, exercise tests are frequently performed to measure exercise function or to assess abnormalities of cardiac rhythm. The risk of exercise testing is very low in the paediatric age group.[1]

To perform cardiopulmonary exercise testing in children, the same types of ergometers can be used as has been reported in adults (bicycle ergometer, treadmill).[2–6] Differences with adult exercise testing procedures[2] are adaptations of the ergometer in order to fit the size of the child, and modifications of the exercise protocols due to cooperation (motivation, anxiety).[3] Since the motivation of young children to sustain incremental exercise testing is lower than in adults, the duration of the exercise testing procedure should be shorter than in adults. Several protocols have been recommended for cycle exercise testing.[1,3] However, in children, especially in younger children, treadmill exercise testing is preferred, since younger children are more used to walking than to cycling. The most widely used protocol is the Bruce test, where the inclination and speed of the treadmill are simultaneously increased every 3 min, until exhaustion.[4] Normal values have been reported for the paediatric age group.[4,6] Other frequently used protocols are the Balke protocol[7] or variants where the speed is a function of the age of the child (4.8 km·hour^{-1} for children below 6 years of age and 5.6 km·hour^{-1} for children above that age).[8,9]

Review of commonly used parameters to assess exercise performance and aerobic exercise function in the paediatric age group

In adult exercise physiology, aerobic exercise performance is traditionally assessed by determining the maximal oxygen uptake. This reflects the highest level of oxygen ($\dot{V}O_2$ max), which does not further increase despite an increase in exercise intensity. In paediatric exercise testing, the $\dot{V}O_2$ max test is also frequently assessed. However, although the measurement of maximal oxygen uptake is useful, since it gives information about the maximal exercise tolerance, this physiological definition is not always met in children. Only about half of the children are able to reach such a plateau after repeated exercise tests (see ref. 6 and Chapter 8). Many children are not motivated to exercise till that point of exhaustion.[10] Therefore, other criteria should be used to confirm a maximal exercise test such as (i) a respiratory gas exchange ratio (VCO_2/VO_2) > 1.10; (ii) a peak heart rate, which is close to 200 beats·min^{-1}; and (iii) the subjective appearance of exhaustion. However, it should be noted that in patients with congenital heart disease the maximal heart rate cannot be used as a criterion in patients with chronotropic limitation as frequently observed in congenital heart disease.[10]

Other parameters of maximal exercise function are the measurement of the maximal work rate (kgm·min^{-1}),[5] which can be indexed by expressing it in relation to body mass and the maximal endurance time on a treadmill, while performing the Bruce protocol. Although the latter test has been shown to correlate with $\dot{V}O_2$ max (indexed per kg body weight; $r = 0.88–0.92$),[6] this measurement is strongly influenced by the motivation of the child and by the encouragement of the investigator. Maximal exercise capacity is of little relevance in daily life, while performing mild to moderate physical activity.

Because maximal exercise tests may have several drawbacks in the paediatric population, clinical investigators have tried to use submaximal exercise test procedures for application in children. In the past, the heart rate response to exercise has frequently been used to assess cardiovascular exercise performance.[11] The advantage of this measurement is its submaximal nature and minimal ergometric equipment. However, in patients with congenital heart disease several drawbacks exist, as many patients may show a relative bradycardia during exercise, which is not associated with a high value for $\dot{V}O_2$ max, as should theoretically be expected. For example, in patients after total surgical repair of tetralogy of Fallot or in patients with cardiac preload problems (Senning Mustard or Fontan operation), a reduced value for heart rate during graded exercise has been found, which was not associated with a normal value for ventilatory anaerobic threshold[12] or $\dot{V}O_2$ max.[13] Therefore, the use of heart rate response to exercise in the assessment of cardiovascular exercise performance can be misleading in patients with congenital heart disease and cannot be considered to be a valid determinant of aerobic fitness.[3]

A more sensitive assessment of aerobic exercise function can be obtained by an analysis of the gas exchange. Therefore, considerable attention has been focused on the determination of the ventilatory anaerobic threshold in children (see refs 14–17 and Chapter 6). This reflects the highest exercise intensity at which a disproportionate increase in CO_2 elimination ($\dot{V}CO_2$) is found relative to $\dot{V}O_2$.[18,19] Although in adult subjects a concomitant disproportional increase is found between the excessive CO_2 elimination and the lactate accumulation or bicarbonate decrease in the blood, a lot of experimental conditions exist, where this relationship can be disturbed [e.g. in patients with McArdle's disease who have an inability to produce lactate[20] and after glycogen depletion[21]]. However, despite this scientific debate, this exercise level has shown to be a very useful and reproducible indicator of aerobic exercise function also in the paediatric age group.[16,19] Moreover, the recent development of breath-by-breath analysis of gas exchange, with rapid responding gas analysers or mass spectrometers, allows precise and reproducible measurements of this parameter. More specifically in the paediatric age group, no ventilatory anaerobic threshold can be detected in about 10 % of the children.[16,18] Normal reference values have been reported for European[15,22] and North American children.[14,16]

More recently, newer concepts have been developed to assess dynamic changes of respiratory gas exchange during exercise, in patients with congenital heart disease. The study of the steepness of the slope of $\dot{V}CO_2$ versus $\dot{V}O_2$ above the ventilatory anaerobic threshold has been found to be a very sensitive and reproducible index for the assessment of cardiovascular exercise function in this patient group (Fig. 31.1).

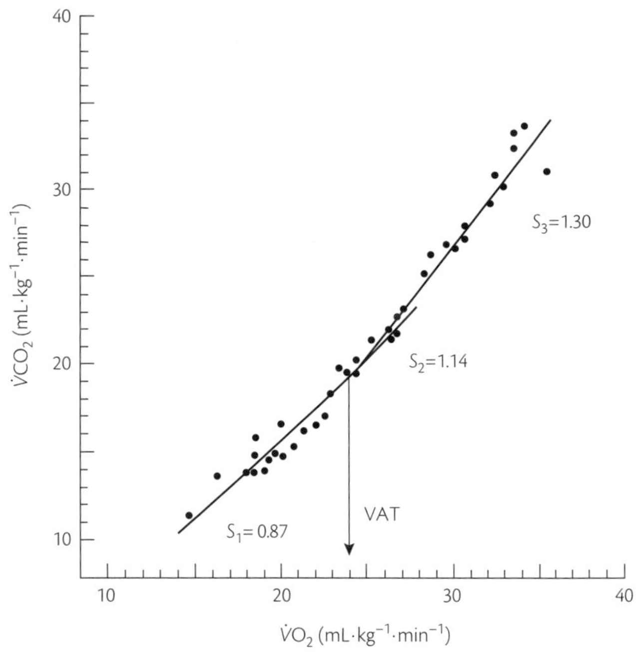

Fig. 31.1 Typical response of CO_2 output ($\dot{V}CO_2$) versus oxygen uptake ($\dot{V}O_2$) during graded treadmill exercise in an 11-year-old boy after total repair for tetralogy of Fallot.

Data represent average values for breath-by-breath measurements of $\dot{V}O_2$ and $\dot{V}CO_2$ in 10-s intervals. Exercise intensity was increased until a heart rate of 170 beats·min^{-1} was reached. S_1 is the calculated slope for increase of $\dot{V}CO_2$ versus $\dot{V}O_2$ from onset of exercise to ventilatory anaerobic threshold (VAT). S_2 is the slope between VAT and the respiratory compensation point. S_3 is the slope between VAT and exercise intensity reached at a heart rate of 170 beats·min^{-1}. Reproduced from Reybrouck *et al.*,[19] with permission.

Furthermore, the use of time constants for the assessment of the initial response of $\dot{V}O_2$ $\dot{V}CO_2$ and pulmonary ventilation ($\dot{V}_E$) during constant rate exercise, together with the recovery (half-time measurement for $\dot{V}O_2$), have been found to be sensitive indicators for the evaluation of aerobic exercise function (see refs 23–25 and Chapter 22). Also the calculation of the normalized oxygen deficit, which reflects the oxygen debt at the onset of exercise, subtracted from the steady-state value, reached after 6 min of constant work rate exercise and expressed as a percentage of the total oxygen cost of a 6-min exercise test, has been found to be a useful parameter for the assessment of cardiovascular exercise function[26] in patients with poor exercise performance and when anaerobic threshold cannot be determined (Fig. 31.2).

Parameters of aerobic exercise function, such as the steepness of the slope of $\dot{V}CO_2$, time constants, and oxygen deficit and recovery kinetics, have the advantage that they all study the dynamic change of the cardiovascular response during constant work rate exercise. The evaluation of the non-steady-state phase of the cardiorespiratory response to exercise is much more relevant to activities during daily life than maximal exercise testing. Particularly, paediatric patients and normal children perform a lot of activities during non-steady-state exercise. The speed of the response of the cardiovascular system will affect exercise tolerance and consequently the ability to perform a subsequent bout of exercise.

However, when evaluating exercise tolerance in patients with congenital heart disease, it is recommended that each laboratory determines its own normal values, because geographical differences may influence the results of aerobic exercise performance. For example, in the classical studies of Astrand[27] on Swedish children, these subjects (both adults and children) always showed superior values for maximal aerobic power, which may be related to a more active lifestyle in the Scandinavian countries.

Assessment of habitual level of physical activity in patients with congenital heart disease

Different methods for assessing the daily level of physical activity in paediatric patients have been applied. These vary from history taking, questionnaires and interviews for more direct observations, measurements of heart rate, $\dot{V}O_2$, and even long-term video recording.[28] More sophisticated methods are pedometers and actometers, which record the number of steps and vertical displacements of the body. Each of these methods has its limitations. For recall questionnaires, a low reliability and low objectivity have been experienced. When patients or parents were asked to classify themselves or their children as active or non-active, in about 30% of the cases a misclassification was found when the data were correlated with objective measurements of maximal oxygen uptake.[29,30] The same holds true for a self-keeping log. Even more sophisticated methods do not give a precise estimation of energy expenditure. For example, the measurement of $\dot{V}O_2$ is cumbersome, video recording is limited to a specific space and hard to quantify. Holter and ECG recordings are complex devices and require individual calibration. Furthermore, pedometers do not give information about vertical

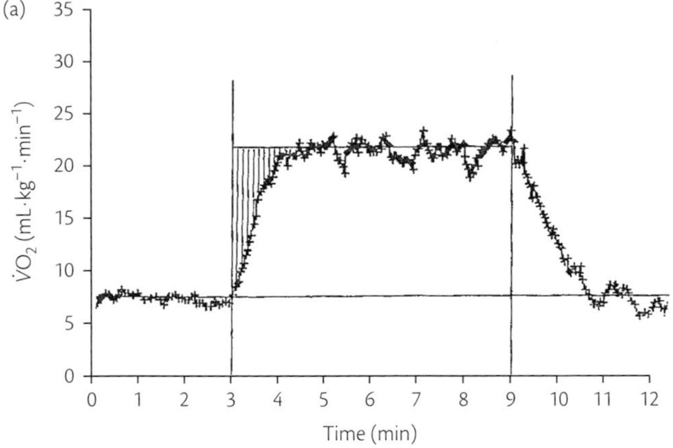

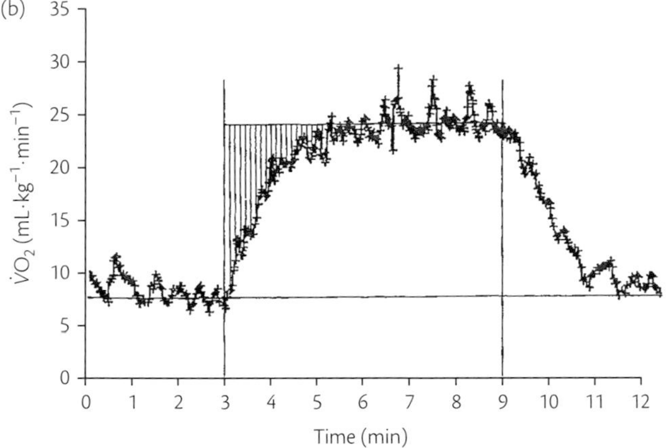

Fig. 31.2 Normalized oxygen deficit. Data for oxygen uptake were first collected during a 3-min rest period, followed by 6-min treadmill exercise at a speed of 5 km·h^{-1} and inclination of 4% and finally a recovery period for 3 min. The normalized oxygen deficit was calculated at onset of exercise as the difference between the single breath values and the steady-state value. Each point represents a five breaths moving average value for oxygen uptake, expressed as mL·kg^{-1}·min^{-1}. Data were cumulated and expressed as a percentage of the total oxygen cost for 6 min of exercise. A typical example is presented for (a) a normal child with an oxygen deficit of 8% and (b) a patient with Fontan circulation with an oxygen deficit of 14%.

displacement and do not give information about the nature of the activity (e.g. walking or running). Therefore, these devices may underestimate at high activity levels. A review of advantages and disadvantages of different systems has been published by Bar-Or[28] (see also refs 31,32 and Chapter 10).

However, despite these limitations and lack of accuracy of questionnaires, we found that the use of a standardized questionnaire, with questions about school sport, leisure time physical activity, formal sports participation during leisure time was reproducible in young children (9–13 years of age; $r = 0.98$). Furthermore, these questionnaires were able to show reduced levels of physical activity in patients with congenital heart disease and subnormal exercise tolerance.[29]

In conclusion, although the use of a standardized questionnaire to assess the daily level of physical activity is superior to the classical medical history taking, it cannot replace the objective assessment of aerobic exercise function by performing an exercise test. It should rather be considered as a complementary information which is useful in the interpretation of the exercise results.

Cardiorespiratory response to exercise in specific congenital heart defects

Left-to-right shunts

Atrial septal defect

Children with atrial septal defect (ASD) usually have a normal or near normal exercise capacity. These children can attain normal values for $\dot{V}O_2$ max or near normal values.[1,33] A number of haemodynamic abnormalities to exercise have been documented. The increase of cardiac output during exercise may be smaller than normal and maximal heart rate response has been found to be lower than normal. In those who underwent surgical closure of the ASD, the age at the time of surgery has been shown to influence exercise performance. In a consecutive series of 50 patients with ASD or ventricular septum defect, evaluated in our laboratory, the ventilatory anaerobic threshold (as an estimate of aerobic exercise performance) was at the lower limit of normal (89 ± 14.4% of normal).[9] When studying the exercise response in children who underwent surgical closure of an ASD, a normal value was found in children who underwent surgery before 5 years of age, whereas a significantly lower value was found in children operated after that age.[35]

In general, abnormalities detected in children either with unoperated or surgically closed ASD are usually minor and do not result in major limitations in exercise performance. Unless arrhythmia is a complication, these children should be encouraged to perform physical exercise and participate in all sports at all levels. Exercise testing is generally indicated if symptoms of arrhythmia or dyspnoea on exercise are reported.

Ventricular septal defect

A small ventricular septal defect (VSD) will transmit only a small amount of blood from the left to the right side of the heart. Also during exercise the shunt will remain small. Haemodynamic studies in this patient group showed that during graded exercise, patients with a VSD had a higher pulmonary circulation than systemic circulation, as could be expected. However, the relative shunt fraction decreased with increased exercise intensity.[36] Subnormal values for cardiac output were found in this patient group. Exercise performance, assessed by the measurement of maximal endurance time, maximal work rate on the cycle ergometer, and maximal heart rate were slightly reduced, when compared to normal controls (90.8 ± 1.6%).[37] Studies during submaximal exercise testing, using gas exchange measurements, showed suboptimal values for ventilatory anaerobic threshold in a consecutive series of 43 patients with an unoperated VSD, evaluated in our laboratory. This value averaged 90 ± 15.3% of normal and was below the lower limit of 95% confidence interval.[9] In this patient group, the decreased level of exercise capacity was correlated with a decreased level of habitual physical activity. In another series of patients, studied after surgical closure of a VSD, a significantly lower value was found for the ventilatory threshold (86 ± 12% of the normal value), which remains stable at re-evaluation about 3 years later on average (see Fig. 31.3 and ref 34). Finally, in a group of 18 patients who underwent surgical closure of a large VSD with pulmonary hypertension, before 1 year of life, the value for aerobic exercise performance was at the lower limit of normal (92 ± 17% of normal).[38] In a retrospective study about quality of life, Meijboom *et al.*[39] reported a normal exercise capacity in 84% of the patient group who underwent surgical closure of a VSD ($N = 109$). This shows that surgical

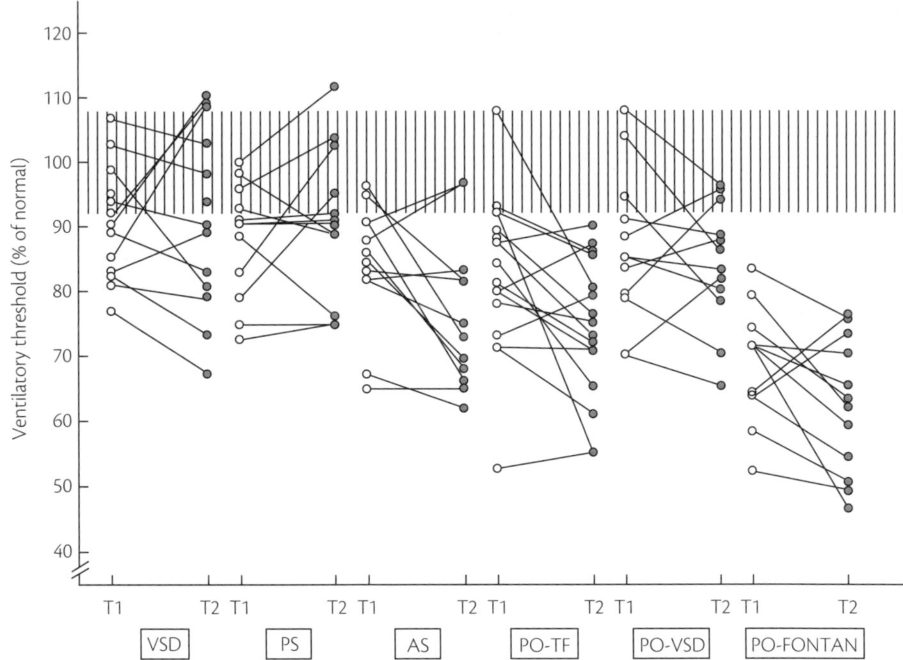

Fig. 31.3 Serial evaluation of cardiovascular exercise performance in children with congenital heart disease. Reproduced from Tuley,[25] with permission.

correction of a congenital heart defect early in life can normalize the child's exercise performance.

Patent ductus arteriosus

Similarly in this group of patients, results of exercise testing will generally be normal if the size of the shunt is moderate or small. These subjects will ordinarily be asymptomatic. In most conditions, these defects will be closed surgically or percutaneously, at an age when exercise testing is not feasible. Exercise testing will add little to the routine clinical evaluation of these patients.[1]

Valvular heart lesions

Aortic stenosis

Exercise testing in patients with aortic stenosis (AS) may show ST segment changes on the ECG, reflecting ischaemia, a drop in blood pressure or an inadequate rise in blood pressure with increasing exercise intensity, and eventually arrhythmia during exercise testing. The major haemodynamic determinant of ST segment changes during exercise is the inadequate oxygen delivery to the left ventricle. After surgical relief of the gradient, improvement of ST segment changes on the ECG during exercise has been reported.[10] A critical AS can be identified by clinical findings and confirmed by echo-Doppler examination and eventually by cardiac catheterization.

During exercise testing, most of the patients show a reduced aerobic exercise performance,[34] which may be improved after surgery. This may be related both to the inability of the cardiac output to increase adequately during exercise and further also to the effect of a medically imposed restriction of heavy physical activity and competitive sports. Sudden cardiac death during exercise has been reported and has been ascribed to malignant arrhythmias. Fortunately, this is unlikely to happen in asymptomatic patients, with mild to moderate stenosis.[33] In our experience, it has never occurred in over 200 patients in follow-up with mild to moderate AS (Doppler gradient < 60 mmHg). It allows them to perform up to moderate exercise, including recreational sports.

Pulmonary valve stenosis

Similar to AS, pulmonary valve stenosis results in a right ventricular overload. This may lead to a diminished pulmonary flow. In mild cases (PIG < 30 mmHg) normal or near normal values for ventilatory threshold have been found.[34]

During exercise, the transvalvular pressure gradient in pulmonary stenosis (PS) may increase during graded exercise testing.[1] In mild cases (gradients < 30 mmHg), values for ventilatory anaerobic threshold have been found to be at the lower limit of normal.[34] In cases with moderate to severe PS, right ventricular pressures may rise considerably during exercise, which may limit exercise capacity.[40] In patients with mild to moderate PS (Doppler > 50 mmHg), balloon valvuloplasty (or very rarely surgery) will be performed. However, exercise performance may be limited in cases with severe pulmonary incompetence.[41]

Cyanotic heart disease

Tetralogy of Fallot

Postoperative children, who are felt to have good results (no residual VSD and a pressure gradient between right ventricle and pulmonary artery below 20 mmHg), are generally asymptomatic at rest. However, a variety of abnormalities may be brought out by intensive exercise.[42] These include

- a high right ventricular pressure with values as high as 100 mmHg during maximal exercise, caused by a pressure gradient between right ventricle and pulmonary artery;
- a blunted increase in stroke volume and heart rate; and
- appearance of ventricular arrhythmia.

Despite these abnormalities, children who underwent total surgical repair for tetralogy of Fallot are usually well during daily life. However, formal exercise testing has repeatedly shown subnormal values for maximal oxygen uptake and also for ventilatory anaerobic threshold in this patient group.[13,19,43] Moreover, some individuals may reach normal values (100% normal or even higher than normal values). Furthermore after training, patients with this type of pathology can increase maximal work capacity by 25%.[44] When the adequacy of the oxygen transport during exercise in patients with tetralogy of Fallot repair was assessed by calculation of the slope of $\dot{V}O_2$ versus exercise intensity, reduced values have been found in patients after repair of tetralogy of Fallot.[45] This was associated with increased values for the physiological dead space ventilation during exercise or the slope of ventilation versus carbon dioxide output.[46,47] This is mostly attributed to significant residual haemodynamic abnormalities, such as severe pulmonary regurgitation and right ventricular dysfunction.

Postoperative tetralogy of Fallot patients may have ventricular ectopy during exercise (exercise-induced arrhythmia). Exercise-induced ventricular arrhythmias are mainly seen in patients with late repair and poor right ventricular function.[33] Patients with important residual haemodynamic abnormalities such as those mentioned above are at risk for cardiovascular events.[41,48]

Transposition of the great arteries

In simple transposition of the great arteries (TGA), the aorta arises from the right ventricle, while the pulmonary artery originates from the left ventricle. This results in severe cyanosis, as desaturated systemic venous blood is pumped into the systemic circulation, while the pulmonary venous return is pumped via left atrium and left ventricle into the lungs. Since this blood is already fully oxygenated, no more oxygen will be added to the blood.

The surgical approach to TGA from the late 1960s to the early 1980s involved baffling or rerouting the systemic venous return (from the superior and inferior vena cava) to the mitral valve and left ventricle (Mustard or Senning procedure). The desaturated blood will then be pumped through the pulmonary artery (arising from the left ventricle) to the lungs. The interatrial septum was removed and the pulmonary venous return (arterial blood) was drained to the right ventricle, and pumped into the aorta (arising from the right ventricle). In these atrial switch procedures, the right ventricle functions as the systemic ventricle. However, two major problems exist: (i) there have been extensive atrial incisions and (ii) the right ventricle is left as the systemic ventricle. Long-term problems include sinus node dysfunction, slow junctional rhythms, supraventricular tachycardias, depressed right ventricular function, right ventricular failure, and tricuspid valve insufficiency. Furthermore, because of extensive atrial surgery, the reservoir function of the atrium is seriously compromised. During ventricular filling, blood cannot 'just drop' into the ventricle, but has to come along a much longer way. Any tachycardia will shorten diastole and may critically impair ventricular filling, especially if an obstruction to the pathway is present. This may result in syncope or sudden death.[49]

Exercise testing following the atrial switch procedures has shown a variety of abnormalities even in patients who were asymptomatic at rest. Decreased endurance times, decreased $\dot{V}O_2$ max, subnormal $\dot{V}O_2$ during submaximal exercise and subnormal values for ventilatory anaerobic threshold have been reported.[10,19,50] In addition, a variety of arrhythmias have been documented during exercise testing (junctional rhythm, premature atrial contractions, and premature ventricular contractions). In addition to these abnormalities, potentially detrimental effects of vigorous training in these patients have been reported. It is unknown whether the right ventricle can dilate and hypertrophy to endurance training as does the left ventricle in highly trained young athletes.[42] For these reasons, high intensive isometric exercise or high intensive dynamic exercise and competitive sports are discouraged.

Nowadays, the arterial switch operation is the current surgical technique for TGA in the majority of the cases. Normal or near normal values for exercise performance and normal ST on ECG have been reported in this patient group.[51,52] With earlier techniques coronary problems early and late after surgery were not exceptional. Improved surgical techniques appear to have resolved these problems. However, the length of the follow-up with this procedure is still limited.[1]

Fontan circulation

In tricuspid atresia, there is a congenital absence of the tricuspid valve. In a Fontan circulation, the caval veins are currently connected directly to the pulmonary arteries, bypassing the right heart. This means that there is no effective right heart pump. Although the survival and also preoperative exercise performance of these patients improves dramatically, most of these subjects still have a limited exercise tolerance.[40–42,53–56] The circulatory output after Fontan is primordially regulated by the pulmonary vasculature, which limits ventricular preload. The ventricule usually 'will pump whatever it gets'. The heart rate response is usually blunted, but appropriate for the level of ventricular preload. A very fast heart rate with a limited preload would result in a decreased stroke volume with hypotension, syncope, and eventually death. The lower oxygen saturation in the arterial blood may be due to residual venous or atrial shunting.[56] In our series exercise performance estimated by ventilatory threshold amounted from 50% to 70%.[55]

Rhythm disturbances and conduction defects

Congenital complete atrioventricular block

In congenital complete atrioventricular block, the atrial rate increases normally, during exercise, but ventricular rate does not accelerate adequately. In some cases, these patients may develop dizziness and syncope.[57] Exercise testing in these patients shows subnormal values for $\dot{V}O_2$ max or ventilatory anaerobic threshold and even for the increase of oxygen uptake versus exercise intensity.[58] This results from the lack of acceleration of heart rate during exercise, one of the major components to increase cardiac output and consequently oxygen delivery to the exercising tissues. In some cases with severe bradycardia and syncope a pacemaker is inserted. It is obvious that these children should avoid competitive sports and physical activities with a danger of body collision in order to avoid damage to the wiring system that connects the pacemaker with the heart.

In the paediatric population, the frequency and significance of arrhythmia differs from adults.[57] As a general rule, the assessment of cardiac arrhythmia during exercise is useful in the management of these patients. If arrhythmia disappears with increased exercise intensity, the prognosis of this type of arrhythmia is usually benign.

Congenital complete atrioventricular block after surgery

The anatomic structure of the sinus node is vulnerable to damage following cardiac surgery. Damage of the sinus node has been observed after surgical procedures that require extensive manipulations and sutures in the atria. Specific defects include D-TGA, repaired by atrial baffling procedures.[59] However, fortunately surgically acquired complete atrioventricular block, despite extensive surgery in the atria as for D-TGA is relatively uncommon. In surgically acquired atrioventricular block there is usually no escape rhythm. In this case safety pacing with redundant leads is recommended. Furthermore, extra caution is warranted not to damage the pacing system with external forces. Pacemaker technology when applied in young patients has some limitations, because the upper limit of a DDD-R pacemaker (dual chamber, rate responsive: DDD-R) is often too low for these youngsters, to achieve a physiological normal value for heart rate during exercise.[59]

Natural evolution of aerobic exercise performance and daily level of physical activity in patients with congenital heart disease

To study the natural evolution of aerobic exercise performance during medium term follow-up in patients with congenital heart disease, exercise performance tests were compared in patients who underwent exercise testing at least twice with a time interval of about 3 years. Between 1980 and 1992, at our department of Paediatric Cardiology, 1982 exercise tests were performed. In 79 patients from this database,[34] exercise tests were performed at least twice in the same patient, with satisfactory respiratory gas exchange measurements on a breath-by-breath basis and a time interval of at least 2 years. These patients were divided into six subgroups. Three groups were studied for a non-operated congenital heart defect. Fourteen patients were followed for a VSD, which did not require surgical closure. Twelve patients were followed for a mild PS, with a gradient of less than 41 mmHg (average 17 ± 11 mmHg), and 12 patients with a mild AS, with a mean gradient of 36 ± 17 mmHg. Furthermore, three groups of patients who underwent surgical repair of a congenital heart defect were also studied twice. Sixteen patients who underwent total correction for tetralogy of Fallot (TF-PO) were studied, 13 patients who underwent surgical closure of a VSD (VSD-PO) and finally 12 patients with a Fontan circulation for tricuspid atresia were studied 1.9 ± 1.1 years after the Fontan operation.

The results of this study showed that at the initial evaluation all patients were in class I of the New York Heart Association. Aerobic exercise performance, assessed by the determination of the ventilatory anaerobic threshold, was at the lower limit of the normal mean value or below (Fig. 31.3). Significant differences for aerobic exercise performance were found between the different pathologies. The lowest values were found in the patients with the Fontan circulation and the highest values in patients with a VSD.

At reassessment, about 3 years later, all patients remained in NYHA class I, except for two patients with a Fontan circulation, who belonged to class II and III at re-evaluation. For patients in whom no medical restriction of physical activity was imposed (VSD, PS, and VSD-PO), no significant change was found for the value of ventilatory anaerobic threshold (expressed as a percentage of the mean value obtained in a pool of normal controls of the same age and gender) (Fig. 31.3). At variance, in patients with AS, with a medically imposed restriction of heavy physical exercise and competitive sports, a decrease was found for aerobic exercise performance, of about 8%. In patients with surgical repair of tetralogy of Fallot, a decrease in the value of ventilatory anaerobic threshold of about 9% was found over the same time interval, which was related to residual haemodynamic lesions, such as pulmonary valve incompetence.[43] Finally also in the patients with a Fontan circulation, a significant decrease in aerobic exercise performance was found over this time interval. Similarly, on reassessment the lowest values were found in this patient group. This was related to the fact that these patients were unable to perform intensive physical exercise during daily life activities and also to residual haemodynamic dysfunction.

The daily level of physical activity, assessed by a standardized questionnaire, was significantly lower both at the first and second evaluation in patients with AS, surgical repair of tetralogy of Fallot and Fontan repair. These subnormal values for the daily physical activity level were associated with a significant decrease of aerobic exercise function at reassessment. In the other patient groups (VSD, PS, VSD-PO), no significant change was found for aerobic exercise performance between the two assessments (Fig. 31.3).

These data show the combined effect of residual haemodynamic lesions and hypoactivity on the evaluation of aerobic exercise performance in these groups of patients. In children and adolescents with AS significantly lower values for aerobic exercise performance were found both at first and second assessment. Similar data have been reported by Driscoll *et al.*[37] In this group of patients heavy physical exercise and competitive sports are discouraged because of the risk of ischaemia and arrhythmia. In the other patient groups residual haemodynamic dysfunction may impede the child to perform aerobic exercise of heavy intensity, which is necessary for the normal development of the oxidative metabolism. In these patient groups (Fontan and TF-PO), subnormal values for increase in $\dot{V}O_2$ during graded exercise have also been observed.[19,47,55]

The results of these studies show that the suboptimal aerobic exercise performance in children and adolescents with congenital heart disease is to some extent attributable to residual haemodynamic lesions after corrective surgery of the defect and also to some degree of hypoactivity, which results from overprotection of the parents and the environment. However, in some patients there may also be an increase in the severity of the disease, which may impede the individual to perform the same amount of physical exercise as healthy peers. Therefore, except for some cases with the progression of the severity of the disease and medically imposed restriction of intensive dynamic or static physical exercise, children and adolescents with congenital heart disease and their parents should be strongly encouraged to be more active and to prevent the deleterious effect of physical deconditioning.

Exercise recommendations and rehabilitation of patients with congenital heart disease

Nowadays most children with congenital heart disease, both before and after surgery, are encouraged to be fully active and to participate in all recreational sport activities. These recommendations are based on clinical findings, which have shown that physical exercise in children with congenital heart disease has beneficial effects on the physical, psychological, and social levels both for the children and also for the parents. In the majority of the cases, these children do not need to participate in a formal rehabilitation programme, but they should be encouraged to participate in recreational physical activities in leisure time and at school. Even after corrective surgery, a formal rehabilitation programme is mostly restricted to the hospitalization period and consists mainly of chest physiotherapy (breathing exercises) and early mobilization. As soon as the children are discharged from the hospital, they are encouraged to resume their normal physical activities at home.

In the majority of the cases of congenital heart disease, there are only a few contraindications for physical exercise both for the non-operated cardiac defects and for the operated ones.[41] The final decision to allow the child with congenital heart disease to participate in physical exercise should always be based on a full cardiological examination.

A few controlled exercise studies in patients with congenital heart disease have shown that maximal exercise capacity can be improved following a period of physical training.[44,61] However, $\dot{V}O_2$ max was not improved in all subjects. The improvement of maximal exercise performance (expressed in Watts or kgm·min^{-1}, assessed during cycle ergometry) without an increase in $\dot{V}O_2$ max represents an improved mechanical efficiency during exercise. This may be beneficial for the patients, since the same level of exercise will be perceived as easier to perform and will induce less dyspnoea. Furthermore, especially in young children, the measurement of $\dot{V}O_2$ max is often difficult as it depends on the motivation of the child. In fact, a plateau in $\dot{V}O_2$ with increasing exercise intensity, which is a prerequisite for a true $\dot{V}O_2$ max is difficult to obtain in young children[62] (and see chapter 8).

Cumulative medical experience has shown that the potential risk of physical exercise in patients with congenital heart disease is very low.[41] In fact, only a few heart defects have been associated with sudden cardiac death, during sports participation. These include mainly hypertrophic cardiomyopathy, severe AS, congenital anomalies of the coronary arteries, Marfan's syndrome, and myocarditis. Fortunately, these anomalies represent only a small percentage of the total number of congenital heart defects.

Since children and especially children who perform competitive sports may be exposed to high levels of physiological stress a classification of sports has been made by the American College of Cardiology and American College of Sports Medicine[63] (Table 31.1). This table classifies sport activities according to the type of exercise (dynamic vs. static) and according to the intensity of exercise, which reflects the cardiovascular stress. This classification can be used for

Table 31.1 Classification of sports

	(A) Low dynamic	(B) Moderate dynamic	(C) High dynamic
(I) Low static	Bowling	Fencing	Badminton
	Cricket	Table tennis	Race walking
	Golf	Tennis (doubles)	Running (marathon)
	Riflery	Volleyball	Cross-country skiing (classic)
		Baseball*/softball*	Squash*
(II) Moderate static	Auto racing*,**	Field events (jumping)	Basketball*
	Diving**	Figure skating	Biathlon
	Equestrian*,**	Lacrosse	Ice hockey*
	Motorcycling*,**	Running (sprint)	Field hockey*
	Gymnastics*		Rugby*
	Karate/Judo*		Soccer*
	Sailing		Cross-country skiing (skating)
	Archering		Running (mid/long)
			Swimming
			Tennis (single)
			Team handball*
(III) High static	Bobsledding*,**	Body building*	Boxing*
	Field events (throwing)	Downhill skiing*,**	Canoeing, Kayaking
	Luge*,**	Wrestling*	Cycling*,**
	Rock climbing*,**	Snow boarding*,**	Decathlon
	Waterskiing*,**		Rowing
	Weight lifting*		Speed skating
	Windsurfing*,**		Thriathlon*,**

Adapted and modified after Mitchell *et al.*[64]
*Danger of bodily collision.
**Increased risk if syncope occurs.

counselling children and adolescents with congenital heart disease. An overview of the guidelines for sport participation in specific congenital heart defects, recommended by the Task Force of the European Society of Cardiology is presented in Table 31.2.

A restriction of heavy physical exercise and competitive sports is imposed in moderate to severe AS, in left-to-right shunts with pulmonary hypertension, hypertrophic cardiomyopathy, pulmonary hypertension, and arrhythmia which worsens during exercise. As a general rule, cardiopulmonary exercise testing is advised in children with congenital heart defects, before sport participation is allowed.

Summary

- As the majority of the patients with congenital heart disease belong to the paediatric age group, exercise testing equipment and exercise protocols have to be adapted for children. Functional performance should be assessed by performing exercise testing with measurement of gas exchange. Nowadays, new concepts for exercise testing in the paediatric age group are analysis of gas exchange during the non-steady state of exercise and determination of the kinetics of gas exchange during the recovery phase of exercise.
- In some groups of patients with congenital heart disease, suboptimal values have been found for aerobic exercise capacity, which can be ascribed to haemodynamic dysfunction or residual haemodynamic lesions after surgery (e.g. in TGA, tetralogy of Fallot and Fontan repair for univentricular heart). In other types of pathologies medically imposed restriction of intensive physical exercise or competitive sports may determine to some extent a subnormal value of exercise performance.
- Finally in some other types of congenital heart disease without overt haemodynamic dysfunction (e.g. VSD or ASD, with nor-

Table 31.2 Recommendations for sport participation in congenital heart diseases

Lesion	Recommendation
ASD (closed or non-significant or PFO)	No restrictions
	Scuba diving should be avoided in those with remaining shunt, due to the risk of paradoxical embolism
VSD (closed or non-significant)	No restrictions
PDA (closed or non-significant)	No restrictions
AVSD (successfully repaired)	No restrictions
Moderate MVR	Low to moderate dynamic and static sports
PAPVC/TAPVC (successfully repaired)	No restrictions
Pulmonary stenosis (mild)	No restrictions
Moderate	Low to moderate dynamic and static sports
Aortic stenosis (mild)	Low to moderate dynamic and static sports
Moderate	Low to moderate dynamic and static sports
	No competitive sport if left ventricular dysfunction of symptoms
CoA (successfully repaired)	No restrictions*
TOF (successfully repaired)	Low to moderate dynamic and static sports*
Residual disease	Low dynamic and sports*
TGA	
aso TGA (successfully repaired)	No restrictions
iar TGA, cc TGA	Low to moderate dynamic and static sports**
Ebstein anomaly	Low to moderate dynamic and static sports**
Univentricular hearts/Fontan circulation	Low to moderate dynamic and static sports**
	Low to moderate dynamic and static sports**
Eisenmenger's syndrome	Low dynamic sports**
Congenital coronary artery anomalies	No restrictions

For definitions, risk stratification, and follow-up see text. ASD = atrial septal defect; PFO = patent foramen ovale; VSD = ventricular septal defect; MVR = mitral valve regurgitation; PAPVC/TAPVC = partial or total anomalous pulmonary venous connection; CoA = coarctation of the aorta; TOF = tetralogy of Fallot; TGA = transposition of the great arteries; aso = arterial switch operation; iar = intra-atrial repair; cc = congenitally corrected.

Updated guidelines for exercise recommendation in patients with congenital heart disease (from Hirth *et al.*,[33] with permission).

*Those with conduit, interposed graft, or on anticoagulant drugs should avoid sports with the risk of bodily collision.

**No competitive sport.

mal pressures in the pulmonary circulation) a suboptimal value for aerobic exercise capacity is often related to overprotection of the parents or environment of the child. Therefore, except for some cases with medically imposed restriction of intensive physical exercise, most patients are encouraged to be fully active during leisure time and to participate at all types of physical exercise at school.

References

1. Gibbons RJ, Balady GJ, Beasley JW, Bricker JT, Duvernoy WFC, Froelicher VF, Mark DB, Marwich TH, McCallister BD, Thompson PD, Winters WL, Yanowitz FG (1997). ACC/AHA Guidelines for Exercise Testing. A Report of the American College of Cardiology/American Heart Association Task force on Practice Guidelines (Committee on Exercise Testing). *J Am Coll Cardiol* **30**, 260–315.
2. Pina IL, Balady GJ, Hanson M, Labovitz AJ, Madonna DW, Myers J (1995). Guidelines for Clinical Exercise Testing Laboratories. A Statement for Healthcare Professionals from the Committee on Exercise and Cardiac Rehabilitation, American Heart Association. *Circulation* **91**, 912–21.
3. Washington RL, Bricker JT, Alpet BS, Daniels SR, Decelbaum RJ, Fisher EA, Gidding SS, Isabel-Jones J, Kavey REW, Marx GR, Strong BW, Teske DW, Wilmore JH, Winston M (1994). Guidelines for exercise testing in the pediatric age group. *Circulation* **90**, 2166–79.
4. Cumming GR, Everatt D, Hastman L (1978). Bruce treadmill test in children: Normal values in a clinic population. *Am J Cardiol* **41**, 69–75.
5. James FW, Blomqvist CG, Freed MD, Miller WW, Moller JH, Nugent EW, Riopel DA, Strong WB, Wessel HU (1982). Standards for exercise testing in the pediatric age group. *Circulation* **66**, 1377A–97A.
6. Rowland TW (1993). Aerobic exercise testing protocols. In: Rowland TW (ed.), *Pediatric laboratory exercise testing. Clinical guidelines*, pp. 19–41. Human Kinetics, Champaign, IL.
7. Riopel DA, Taylor AB, Hohn AR (1979). Blood pressure, heart rate, pressure-rate product and electrocardiographic changes in healthy children during treadmill exercise. *Am J Cardiol* **44**, 697–704.
8. Chandramouli B, Ehmke DA, Lauer RM (1973). Exercise-induced electrocardiographic changes in children with congenital aortic stenosis. *J Pediatr* **87**, 725–30.
9. Reybrouck T, Weymans M, Stijns H, van der Hauwaert LG (1986). Ventilatory anaerobic threshold for evaluating exercise performance in children with congenital left-to-right intracardiac shunt. *Pediatr Cardiol* **7**, 19–24.
10. Pianosi PT, Driscoll DJ (2008). Exercise testing. In: Allen HE, Driscoll D, Shaddy RE, Feltes TF (eds.), *Moss' heart disease in infants, children, and adolescents*, pp. 81–94. Wolters Kluwer–Lippincott Williams and Wilkins, Philadelphia, PA.
11. Adams FH, Linde LM, Niyake H (1961). The physical working capacity of normal school children. *Pediatrics* **28**, 55–64.
12. Reybrouck T, Weymans M, Stijns H, van der Hauwaert LG (1986). Exercise testing after correction of tetralogy of Fallot: The fallacy of a reduced heart rate response. *Am Heart J* **112**, 998–1003.
13. Wessel H, Paul M (1999). Exercise studies in tetralogy of Fallot: A review. *Pediatr Cardiol* **20**, 39–48.
14. Cooper DM, Weiler-Ravell D, Whipp BJ, Wasserman K (1984). Aerobic parameters of exercise as a function of body size during growth in children. *J Appl Physiol* **56**, 628–34.
15. Reybrouck T, Weymans M, Stijns H, Van der Hauwaert LG (1985). Ventilatory anaerobic threshold in healthy children. *Eur J Appl Physiol* **54**, 278–84.
16. Washington RL, van Gundy JC, Cohen C, Sondheimer HM, Wolfe RR (1988). Normal aerobic and anaerobic exercise data for North American school-age children. *J Pediatr* **112**, 223–33.
17. Washington RL (1999). Cardiorespiratory testing: Anaerobic threshold/respiratory threshold. *Pediatr Cardiol* **20**, 12–16.
18. Wasserman K, Beaver WL, Whipp BJ (1990). Gas exchange threshold and the lactic acidosis (anaerobic) threshold. *Circulation* **81** (Suppl. 11), 14–30.
19. Reybrouck T, Mertens L, Kalis N, Weymans M, Dumoulin M, Daenen W, Gewilllig M (1996). Dynamics of respiratory gas exchange during exercise after correction of congenital heart disease. *J Appl Physiol* **80**, 458–63.
20. Hagberg JM, Coyle EF, Carroll JE, Miller JM, Martin WH, Brooke MH (1982). Exercise hyperventilation in patients with Mc Ardle's disease. *J Appl Physiol* **52**, 991–4.
21. Heigenhauser GJF, Sutton JR, Jones NL (1983). Effect of glycogen depletion on ventilatory response to exercise. *J Appl Physiol* **54**, 470–4.
22. Schulze-Neick I, Wessel HU, Lange P (1992). Heart rate and oxygen uptake response to exercise in children with low peak exercise heart rate. *Eur J Pediatr* **151**, 160–6.
23. Cooper DM, Kaplan MR, Baumgarten L, Weiler-Ravell D, Whipp BJ, Wasserman K (1987). Coupling of ventilation and CO_2 production during exercise in children. *Pediatr Res* **21**, 568–72.
24. Zanconato S, Cooper DM, Armon Y (1991). Oxygen cost and oxygen uptake dynamics and recovery with 1 min of exercise in children and adults. *J Appl Physiol* **71**, 993–8.
25. Turley KR (1997). Cardiovascular responses to exercise in children. *Sports Med* **24**, 241–57.
26. Mertens L, Reybrouck T, Eyskens B, Daenen W, Gewillig M (2003). Slow kinetics of oxygen uptake in patients with a Fontan-type circulation. *Pediatr Exerc Sci* **15**, 146–55.
27. Åstrand PO (1952). *Experimental studies of physical working capacity in relation to sex and age*. Munsgaard, Copenhagen.
28. Bar-Or O (1982). Clinical implications of pediatric exercise physiology. *Ann Clin Res* **14** (Suppl. 34), 97–106.
29. Rogers R, Reybrouck T, Weymans M, Dumoulin M, Van der Hauwaert L, Gewillig M (1994). Reliability of subjective estimates of exercise capacity after total repair of tetralogy of Fallot. *Acta Paediatr* **83**, 866–9.
30. Barber G, Heise CT (1991). Subjective estimates of exercise ability: Comparison to objective measurements. *Pediatr Exerc Sci* **3**, 327–32.
31. Saris WH, Binkhovst RA (1977). The use of pedometer and actometer in studying daily physical activity in man. Part II. Validity of pedometer and actometer in measuring the daily physical activity. *Eur J Appl Physiol* **37**, 229–35.
32. Rowland T (1996). *Developmental exercise physiology*. Human Kinetics, Champaign, IL.
33. Hirth A, Reybrouck T, Bjarnason-Wehrens B, Lawrenz W, Hoffman A (2006). Recommendations for participating in competitive and leisure sports in patients with congenital heart disease: A consensus document. *Eur J Cardiovasc Prev Rehab* **13**, 293–9.
34. Reybrouck T, Rogers R, Weymans M, Dumoulin M, Vanhove M, Daenen W, Gewillig M (1995). Serial exercise testing in patients with congenital heart disease. *Eur J Pediatr* **154**, 801–6.
35. Reybrouck T, Bisschop A, Dumoulin M, Van der Hauwaert LG (1991). Cardiorespiratory exercise capacity after surgical closure of atrial septal defect is influenced by the age at surgery. *Am Heart J* **122**, 1073–8.
36. Bendien C, Bossina KK, Buurma AE, Gerding AM, Kuipers JRG, Landsman MLJ, Mook GA, Zijlstra WG (1984). Hemodynamic effects of dynamic exercise in children and adolescents with moderate-to-small ventricular septal defects. *Circulation* **70**, 929–34.
37. Driscoll DJ, Wolfe RR, Gersony WM, Hayes CJ, Keane JF, Kidd L, O'Fallon M, Pieroni DR, Weidman WH (1993). Cardiorespiratory responses to exercise of patients with aortic stenosis, pulmonary stenosis, and ventricular septal defect. *Circulation* **87** (Suppl. 1), I-102–13.
38. Reybrouck T, Mertens L, Schulze-Neick I, Austenat I, Eyskens B, Dumoulin M, Gewillig M (1998). Ventilatory inefficiency for carbon

dioxide during exercise in patients with pulmonary hypertension. *Clin Physiol* **18**, 337–44.

39. Meijboom F, Szatmari A, Utens E, Deckers JW, Roelandt JRTC, Bos E, Hess J (1994). Long-term follow-up after surgical closure of ventricular septal defect in infancy and childhood. *J Am Coll Cardiol* **24**, 1358–64.
40. Rowland TW (1995). Congenital obstructive and valvular heart disease. In: Goldberg B (ed.), *Sports and exercise for children with chronic health conditions*, pp. 225–36. Human Kinetics, Champaign, IL.
41. Graham TW Jr, Bricker T, James FW, Strong WB (1994). Congenital heart disease. *Med Sci Sports Exerc* **26** (Suppl.), S246–53.
42. Fahey JT (1995). Congenital heart disease-shunt lesions and cyanotic heart disease. In: Goldberg B (ed.), *Sports and exercise for children with chronic health conditions*, pp. 208–24. Human Kinetics, Champaign, IL.
43. Rowe SA, Zakha KG, Manolio TA, Hornheffer PJ, Kidd L (1991). Lung function and pulmonary regurgitation limit exercise capacity in postoperative tetralogy of Fallot. *J Am Coll Cardiol* **17**, 461–6.
44. Goldberg B, Fripp RR, Lister G, Loke J, Nicholas JA, Talner NS (1981). Effect of physical training on exercise performance of children following surgical repair of congenital heart disease. *Pediatrics* **68**, 691–9.
45. Reybrouck T, Mertens L, Bruselle S (2000). Oxygen uptake versus exercise intensity: A new concept in assessing cardiovascular exercise function in patients with congenital heart disease. *Heart* **84**, 46–52.
46. Gilljam T, Eriksson BD, Six R (1998). Cardiac output and pulmonary gas exchange at maximal exercise after atrial redirection for complete transposition. *Eur Heart J* **19**, 1035–84.
47. Reybrouck T, Boshoff D, Vanhees L, Defoor J, Gewillig M (2004). Ventilatory response to exercise in patients after correction of cyanotic congenital heart disease: Relation with clinical outcome after surgery. *Heart* **90**, 215–16.
48. Roos-Hesselink JW, Perlroth MG, McGhie J, Spitaels S (1995). Atrial arrhythmias in adults after repair of tetralogy of Fallot. Correlation with clinical, exercise, and echocardiographic findings. *Circulation* **91**, 2214–19.
49. Gewillig M, Balaji S, Mertens B, Lesaffre E, Deanfield J (1991). Risk factors for arrhythmia and death after Mustard operation for simple transposition of the great arteries. *Circulation* **84**, 187–92.
50. Reybrouck T, Gewillig M, Dumoulin M, van der Hauwaert LG (1993). Cardiorespiratory exercise performance after Senning operation for transposition of the great arteries. *Br Heart J* **70**, 175–9.
51. Reybrouck T, Eyskens B, Mertens L, Defoor J, Daenen W, Gewillig M (2001). Cardiorespiratory exercise function after the atrial switch operation for transposition of the great arteries. *Eur Heart J* **22**, 1052–9.
52. Massin M, Hövels-Gürich H, Däbritz S, Messmer B, von Bernuth G (1998). Results of the Bruce treadmill test in children after arterial switch operation for simple transposition of the great arteries. *Am J Cardiol* **81**, 56–60.
53. Driscoll DJ, Danielson GK, Puga FJ, Schaff HF, Heise CT, Staats BA (1986). Exercise tolerance and cardiorespiratory response to exercise after Fontan operation for tricuspid atresia or functional single ventricle. *J Am Coll Cardiol* **7**, 1087–94.
54. Gewillig M (1994). The Fontan circulation: Late functional results. *Semin Thoracic Cardiovasc Surg* **6**, 56–63.
55. Mertens L, Rogers R, Reybrouck T, Dumoulin M, Vanhees L, Gewillig M (1996). Cardiopulmonary response to exercise after the Fontan operation—A cross sectional and longitudinal evaluation. *Cardiol Young* **6**, 136–42.
56. Gewillig M, Lündstrom R, Bull C, Wyse RKH, Deanfield JE (1990). Exercise responses in patients with congenital heart disease after Fontan repair: Patterns and determinants of performance. *J Am Coll Cardiol* **15**, 1424–32.
57. Park MK (1996). *Pediatric cardiology for practitioners* (3rd ed.). Mosby, St Louis, MO.
58. Reybrouck T, Vanden Eynde B, Dumoulin M, Van der Hauwaert LG (1989). Cardiorespiratory response to exercise in congenital complete atrioventricular block. *Am J Cardiol* **64**, 896–9.
59. Parridon SM (1997). Congenital heart disease: Cardiac performance and adaptations to exercise. *Pediatr Exerc Sci* **9**, 308–23.
60. Reybrouck T, Rogers R, Weymans M, Dumoulin M, Vanhove M, Daenen W, Van der Hauwaert L (1995). Serial cardiorespiratory exercise testing in patients with congenital heart disease. *Eur J Pediatr* **154**, 801–6.
61. Balfour IC, Drimmer AM, Nouri S, Pennington DG, Hemkens C, Harvey LL (1991). Pediatric cardiac rehabilitation. *Am J Dis Child* **145**, 627–30.
62. Armstrong N, Welsman J, Winsley R (1996). Is peak $\dot{V}O_2$ a maximal index of children's aerobic fitness ? *Int J Sports Med* **17**, 356–9.
63. American College of Sports Medicine and American College of Cardiology (1994). Recommendations for determining eligibility for competition in athletes with cardiovascular abnormalities. *Med Sci Sports Exerc* **26** (Suppl.), 223–76.
64. Mitchell JH, Haskell W, Snell P, Van Camp S (2005). Task Force 8: Classification of sports. *J Am Coll Cardiol* **45**, 1364–7.

CHAPTER 32

Exercise, physical activity, and asthma

Helge Hebestreit

Introduction

Asthma is a lung disease with the following characteristics: (i) airway obstruction that is reversible (but not completely so in some patients) either spontaneously or with treatment; (ii) airway inflammation; and (iii) increased airway responsiveness to a variety of stimuli.[1]

Information on the prevalence of asthma in children and adolescents is dependent on the diagnostic criteria used. In a study in Denmark, the prevalence of asthma in 8- to 10-year-old children, as diagnosed by their general practitioner or during a medical assessment of children who were selected based on a screening interview and monitoring of peak flow, was 6.6%.[2] In an survey on 12-year-old children,[3] a history of asthma was reported in 16.8% of children in New Zealand, while other countries showed lower prevalence (South Africa: 11.5%; Sweden: 4.0%; Wales: 12.0%). In another epidemiological study surveying 12- to 15-year-old children in Australia, England, Germany, and New Zealand, 20–27% of the participants experienced wheezing during the past 12 months, and 4–12% reported more than three episodes per year.[4] Thus, the prevalence of asthma in childhood and adolescence varies among countries and can be estimated to be somewhere between 5% and 20%. Over time, there seems to be an increasing asthma prevalence in the Western countries.[5,6]

One of the characteristics of asthma is that the bronchial system is hyper-responsive to a variety of triggers. These stimuli include airway infections, exposure to allergens or air pollutants, inhalation of dry and cold air, and, last but not least, exercise. Thus, exercise-induced asthma (EIA) is a feature of asthma and may affect any patient with asthma, provided that the exercise is of a sufficient intensity and duration.[7] Thus, knowledge about the interrelationships between asthma and exercise is of immense importance when dealing with an active paediatric population.

This chapter reviews the existing data on exercise capacity and physical activity of children with asthma. The mechanisms underlying pathologic responses to exercise in these children are summarized. Most of the information provided in this chapter is valid not only for children but also for adults.

Exercise-induced asthma

Children at risk

As stated above, EIA may possibly affect any child diagnosed to suffer from asthma. Furthermore, EIA has been described in patients with a history of bronchial pulmonary dysplasia, or with a diagnosis of hay fever or cystic fibrosis.[8,9] There are also children or adolescents suffering from EIA, who do not exhibit any of the above risk factors. It has been suggested that some 10% of adolescent athletes suffer from EIA many of them without being recognized.[10]

Symptoms of exercise-induced asthma

In most patients, EIA leads to coughing, wheezing, and shortness of breath shortly after exercise.[11] However, rather than reporting these typical respiratory symptoms, some patients complain about chest discomfort, nausea, or stomachache after exercise. In children, symptoms usually resolve within 10–90 min after the cessation of exercise although some may experience a progressive worsening of bronchoconstriction.

Pathophysiology of exercise-induced bronchial constriction

It has long been recognized that children with asthma are less likely to experience an attack when exercising in a warm and humid environment than when inhaling cold and dry air. On the basis of this observation, it was suggested that either the heat loss from the respiratory epithelium and/or the loss of water might trigger the bronchial constriction.[12] On the basis of subsequent studies, the role of airway cooling/drying during exercise and/or re-warming of the bronchi after the cessation of exertion is now generally accepted as the major mechanism responsible for EIA.[13] However, even if the respiratory heat loss is controlled for, the likelihood and severity of EIA is influenced by exercise intensity (low vs. high) and exercise mode (swimming vs. running).[14,15] Whether these latter findings indicate that airway cooling/drying/re-warming are not the exclusive pathogenic triggers responsible for EIA remains a matter of debate. It could be possible that significant local differences in respiratory heat loss occurred under the various conditions in the studies by Bar-Yishay *et al.*[14] and Noviski *et al.*[15] even though the respiratory heat loss at the level of the mouth was identical.[16]

The exact pathway linking airway cooling/re-warming/drying to bronchial obstruction is not yet completely understood.[13] The following mechanisms have been suggested:

(i) The cooling of the bronchial wall stimulates the parasympathetic system which then leads to a bronchial constriction.[17]

(ii) The cooling of the airways or the increase in bronchial surface osmolality paralleling airway drying triggers the release of neutrophil chemotactic factor of anaphylaxis, histamine, and/or leukotrienes, which then initiate a bronchial constriction.[18,19] Restitution of vagal tone after exercise and the decrease in adrenaline levels may then lead to bronchial constriction.[20]

(iii) The re-warming of the airways after exercise induces either a contraction of smooth airway muscles or a hyperaemia and swelling of the bronchial mucosa.[13,21]

Late response

Several studies have suggested that a considerable number of patients suffering from EIA experience a second fall in pulmonary function parameters several hours after the first exercise-induced airway narrowing has resolved.[22,23] These 'late responses' were reported to begin 2–4 hours after the exercise challenge, peak between 4 and 8 hours, and resolve after 12–24 hours. There are, however, some studies which could not detect a significant exercise-induced late response compared to a placebo visit.[24,25] The authors attributed the reports of late asthmatic responses after exercise to the increased spontaneous within-day variation of pulmonary mechanics in children with asthma.[24,25]

Refractory period

In patients with EIA, a second bout of exercise 1–2 hours following a first exercise task may induce less bronchial obstruction than a task of similar exercise intensity and duration which is administered without preceding exercise.[26] This reduced responsiveness is referred to as 'refractory period' and may occur even if the first challenge did not induce a significant bronchial narrowing or was performed with other muscle groups than the subsequent exercise.[27] Refractoriness can be induced not only by continuous submaximal exercise but also by intermittent sprints.[28,29]

It is important to stress that only about 40–60% of all patients with EIA show a refractory period.[30] In those patients who do exhibit this phenomenon the most effective exercise protocol seems to vary among individuals. Therefore, asthma patients who wish to utilize the refractory period to prevent EIA during training and competition should be counselled to try several exercise procedures and select the most effective routine.

The mechanisms underlying the refractory period are not yet understood. It has been suggested that mast cells might be depleted from mediators, including histamine, with the first exercise challenge and that the replenishment of the stores takes up to 2 hours.[31] Another explanation put forward is that prostaglandins, possibly type E_2, are released with the initial exercise bout and prevent a bronchial obstruction with a subsequent exercise challenge.[32] A third hypothesis is based on the assumption that a second exercise task induces less airway cooling than the first task.[33]

Diagnosing exercise-induced asthma

Exercise-induced asthma should be suspected if a patient complains about shortness of breath, wheezing, or cough during or after exercise. In children or adolescents who complain about chest pain with exercise, EIA should also be suspected.[34] In patients diagnosed to have asthma, a history of exercise-related symptoms typical for EIA justifies a medical treatment (see below) without further evaluation.[13] Only if the improvement with medication is less than expected, a further evaluation including an exercise challenge is necessary.

Children and adolescents who have no established diagnosis of asthma should be tested for impairment of resting pulmonary functions. If this test reveals bronchial obstruction which is markedly improved with the inhalation of β-adrenergic drugs, asthma as the cause for the exercise-related symptoms can be assumed. Unless required by national or international sports agencies such as the Olympic committees to allow anti-asthma medications in training and competition, no further testing is necessary to establish the diagnosis if an adequate treatment leads to satisfactory results. In all other cases, a standardized challenge to prove bronchial hyperresponsiveness is recommended.

Physical activity and exercise capacity of children and adolescents with asthma or exercise-induced asthma

Acute asthmatic attacks are often triggered by exercise.[35] It would, therefore, not be surprising, if children with asthma were less active than their peers. Astonishingly little information is available on this issue. One survey suggests that children with known asthma are physically as active as their peers,[36] another study found children with asthma to be even more active than healthy children.[37] Thus, nowadays, the average child who is known to suffer from asthma probably is as active as healthy children. This is in contrast to findings reported in the 1970s and might be the consequence of improved therapy and counselling towards physical activity. In agreement with this hypothesis, two studies have shown that children who suffer from undiagnosed or poorly controlled asthma are still at risk for hypo-activity.[38,39]

Most[40–42] but not all[43] studies have shown that children with asthma have a decreased short-term and endurance exercise capacity compared to healthy controls. The different findings between studies might reflect, in part, differences in disease severity.[41,42] Mechanisms limiting exercise capacity in asthmatic patients could be an increase in end-expiratory lung volume with exercise which results in increased work for ventilation and limitation of minute ventilation[44] and a disturbance of the ventilation–perfusion relationship in the lung.[45] However, the latter mechanisms should lead to oxygen desaturation with exercise, which is rarely seen in patients with asthma.[21]

Since there is increasing evidence that a reduced level of physical activity in children with asthma is a more important predictor of low fitness than disease severity,[43,46] a reduced fitness in a child with asthma should be primarily 'treated' with education and conditioning. An adjustment of medication might only be necessary in some cases.

Exercise-related benefits to children with asthma

Several studies have evaluated the benefits of increased physical activity in children and adolescents with asthma. In general, the effects are more pronounced in patients with severe disease compared to those with moderately severe asthma. Patients with mild asthma may not benefit from specific exercise programmes more than healthy children.

While many studies[47] showed an improvement in fitness or psychological variables in structured and supervised training programmes, some,[47] but not all,[48] observed a beneficial effect from a home-based unsupervised exercise programme. It is, therefore, advocated to refer those patients with moderate to severe asthma who might benefit from exercise rehabilitation to a structured programme. Possibly, the advantage of a structured exercise programme might be related to the effects of education[49] in addition to a more regular and intense physical training.

Improvement in fitness

Regular exercise training is effective in enhancing aerobic and anaerobic fitness and motor coordination in children with asthma.[41,50–52] The mechanisms underlying these improvements most probably act via the training effects observed also in healthy children but may also involve a more comfortable feeling of the children with asthma and their parents when the child engages in physical activities.

Psychological benefits

Children with asthma show disturbances in their psychological development, which might be tackled with an exercise programme.[53] Specifically, positive effects have been shown for ego structure, body image, social development, and concentration capacity.[53]

It should also be kept in mind that children with asthma strongly value the ability to engage in physical activities. For example, when 71 children aged 9–11 years were asked 'How do you know when you are healthy?', 46% of all responses referred to activity or other physical/functional abilities.[54] In contrast, only 9% of the responses related to the absence of asthma-specific symptoms. In other words, many children with asthma consider physical activity as an integral part of daily life. To them, being allowed to exercise means to be normal.

Reduction in asthma symptoms and exercise-induced asthma

Large randomized control trials on the effects of regular exercise on asthma morbidity are missing in children. However, some data available from relatively short exercise programmes with a duration of 2–6 months suggest that physical conditioning may reduce the frequency of asthma symptoms, hospitalizations, emergency room visits, and school absenteeism.[55,56] The effects of an exercise programme on EIA are less clear. While Fitch *et al.*[57] did not see any change in the severity of EIA after a 3-month running training programme, Svenonius *et al.*[47] and Henriksen and Nielsen[58] found a significant improvement in EIA following a combined land-based and swimming interval training programme for 3–4 months and a 6-week training programme, respectively. At least part of the improvements in hyper-responsiveness observed in the latter two studies might be attributed to the fact that the exercise challenge to determine EIA was not adjusted for the improvements in physical fitness with training. Thus, the relative intensity of the exercise was lower for the post-training tests compared to the pre-training challenge which might have been paralleled by a lower minute ventilation.

Does regular exercise reduce airway inflammation?

To the author's knowledge, no randomized control study has assessed the effects of a physical conditioning programme on airway inflammation in children with asthma. There are, however, data from a mouse model of asthma indicating that the infiltration with inflammatory cells, the number of goblet cells in airway mucosa, and the hypertrophy of airway mucosa are all decreased with regular moderate exercise following repeated exposure to inhaled ovalbumin.[59] Furthermore, the concentration of interleukin 4, one of the mediators of allergic asthma, was reduced in bronchoalveolar lavage fluid with conditioning.

Can physical training cause asthma?

Several studies on adult elite athletes have shown that the prevalence of EIA is increased in elite swimmers and endurance athletes engaging in winter sports.[60,61] Possibly, the inhalation of chemical irritants such as chlorine and/or of large amounts of cold dry air triggers airway inflammation in these athletes which results in bronchial hyper-responsiveness and EIA. When the training load is reduced the process might be reversed and symptoms cease.[62] Although allergic disease predisposes to EIA in elite athletes, it is generally assumed that the mechanism underlying EIA in many swimmers is distinct from that in allergic asthma.

Compared with the adult literature, few data are available in children. However, one study assessed the risk of children to develop asthma relative to the number of sports played and the concentration of air pollutants in their community.[63] It was shown that children playing three or more sports exposed to ozone had a higher risk of developing asthma compared with less active children or active children living in low ozone communities.

Exercise testing in children with asthma or suspected exercise-induced asthma

Indications

As pointed out above, exercise testing might be helpful to establish the diagnosis of EIA. Furthermore, once a treatment for EIA has been started, the effectiveness of that therapy can be assessed using a follow-up exercise test.

In addition, exercise testing in patients with asthma or EIA can serve several other purposes:

(i) According to the guidelines of the US National Asthma Education Program,[1] the diagnosis of asthma is based on the patient's medical history, physical examination, and, last but not least, laboratory tests. Therefore, when asthma is suspected but cannot be proven otherwise, an exercise test may help to establish the diagnosis by demonstrating a hyper-responsive airway system. The same objective can, however, be met with provocation tests using other triggers, such as hyperventilation with room air or cold air, inhalation of hypertonic saline or mannitol, or histamine/methacholine provocation. It should be kept in mind that most of these tests, including an exercise challenge, have a sensitivity to diagnose asthma of about 40–60%.[64–67] The specificity is generally somewhat higher (around 80–90%).

(ii) Exercise testing has been used as a screening tool for asthma in epidemiological research.[3] A relatively low sensitivity and a poor stability of the bronchial responses over time, however, debase its value for this purpose.[68,69]

(iii) Several studies have shown that children who are not known to have asthma but who show a pathological fall in pulmonary function parameters following an exercise challenge are at high risk to develop clinically recognizable asthma during the subsequent years.[65] Exercise testing could be, therefore, used to screen for children at risk to develop asthma. To date, however, a pathological airway response to an exercise test without any other signs of respiratory disease would not result in any treatment, so that this indication for an exercise test is hypothetical.

(iv) Many children with asthma and their parents are afraid of EIA. The patient and her/his parents might be convinced during an exercise test that exercise can be safe under certain conditions. Furthermore, the appropriate behaviour before, during, and after the exercise can be practised to prevent EIA.

(v) In children with significant asthma, a decreased fitness might be suspected. Exercise testing can provide quantitative measures of fitness and may, thereby, help to document the deficit and to follow up changes during an exercise intervention.

Who should not be tested?

Exercise testing in asthmatic patients always includes the risk of severe exercise-induced bronchial constriction. In most exercise tests, this pathological response is actually striven for. Since the decrease in pulmonary function is larger in patients with a bronchial obstruction before the test, a patient should not be subjected to an exercise test if the patient's baseline forced expiratory volume in 1 second (FEV_1) is below 60% of predicted or less than 80% of the patient's usual values.[70–72] No exercise testing should be performed during infections and in times of high seasonal allergen exposure. Furthermore, health conditions other than pulmonary impairment, such as cardiovascular or neuromuscular diseases, should also be considered.[73]

Preparation before the test and safety procedures

On the basis of the purpose of the exercise test, the child should discontinue cromoglycate sodium and short-acting β-adrenergic drugs 8 hours before testing. Four hours before the exercise test, the child should refrain from any strenuous activities and should not ingest large amounts of food. After arrival at the laboratory, the patient should be seen by a physician to obtain a recent medical history and to perform a physical examination. A test of pulmonary function at rest is mandatory to estimate the risks of an exercise test and to reconsider the indication. A resting ECG should also be written unless congenital conduction abnormalities can be excluded from an older ECG. The exercise test should then be explained in detail to the child and parents and, at least, verbal consent should be obtained.

During the exercise challenge, at least power output on the cycle ergometer or slope and speed of the belt on the treadmill, heart rate, and breath sounds should be monitored. In patients with unclear respiratory disease or severe asthma, it is recommended to further monitor ECG, blood pressure, oxygen saturation (SaO_2), minute ventilation, end tidal PCO_2, and oxygen uptake.[70] On the basis of these latter parameters, a list of situations has been compiled in which an exercise test should be terminated (Table 32.1).

Conducting the exercise challenge

Mode of exercise

Early studies indicated that the most effective exercise challenge to induce EIA was a run outdoors. However, recent research shows that treadmill running is as effective as free running in triggering EIA if climatic conditions and exercise intensity are controlled for.[74] Since there are concerns with the standardization of an exercise challenge outdoors as well as with monitoring and safety, usually a laboratory-based exercise test is used to test for EIA.

Although some studies indicate that cycling is less effective than treadmill running in triggering an EIA,[75] others suggest that the asthmatic response to various land-based exercises might be of equal magnitude, provided that the volume, temperature, and humidity of the inspired air is similar among challenges.[76,77] Both treadmill and cycle ergometer are used to test for EIA in laboratories around the world.

Duration and intensity of the exercise

It is generally agreed that an exercise of 6–10 min duration at an intensity severe enough to raise heart rate to at least 85% of predicted (about 170 beats·min^{-1} in children and adolescents) or oxygen uptake to 60–80% of maximum is best suitable to induce EIA.[13] Using a shorter duration exercise but supramaximal exercise intensities might also be effective to induce EIA.[78] However, an exercise of longer duration (and lower intensity) may result in a false-negative test because the subject may run through the temporary EIA. Although several studies suggest that a higher exercise intensity than stated here would neither affect the sensitivity of the tests to pick up EIA nor increase the severity of bronchial constriction EIA, others have shown that a heart rate of about 180 beats·min^{-1} during treadmill exercise is advantageous to a heart rate of 170 beats·min^{-1}. The required exercise intensity is usually achieved employing work rates on the cycle ergometer of 2–2.5 W·kg^{-1} body weight. Owing to the developmental changes in running economy, the optimal speed and slope during a treadmill challenge are less easy to predict.

Criteria to identify exercise-induced asthma with an exercise challenge

In order to detect an EIA, pulmonary functions are assessed before the exercise challenge, immediately afterwards and thereafter in 3–5 min intervals. Brudno *et al.*[79] suggested continuing to collect data at least until 30 min after exercise.

Table 32.1 Reasons to terminate an exercise test in children (based on Cropp[70] and Washington *et al.*[73])

◆ Patient request
◆ Diagnostic findings have been established
◆ Failure of monitoring equipment
◆ Cardiac arrhythmias precipitated or aggravated by the exercise test
◆ Myocardial ischaemia on ECG (ST segment depression or elevation > 0.3 mV)
◆ Progressive decrease in systolic blood pressure
◆ Significant respiratory distress
◆ Rise in end-tidal PCO_2 of more than 10 torr or exceeding 55 torr
◆ Drop in SaO_2 of more than 10% or below 85%

Post-exercise pulmonary function is expressed as a percentage of pre-exercise values. A fall below a certain percentage is considered indicative for EIA.

Although many different parameters derived from pulmonary function testing have been used to diagnose EIA, FEV_1 is most commonly employed. The forced expiratory flow between 25% and 75% of forced vital capacity (FEF_{25-75}) and the peak expiratory flow rate (PEFR) might also be used although sensitivity and specificity of the exercise test seems to be less with these variables compared to FEV_1.[80] Custovic *et al.*[80] suggested the use of a combination of two criteria. They felt that a fall either in FEV_1 or in FEF_{25-75} below the 95% confidence limits of normal was most sensitive to diagnose EIA. No increase in false-positive tests was observed using this approach.

Most reviews on exercise testing in asthma refer to the criteria published by Cropp[70] to diagnose EIA and to determine the severity of bronchial constriction (see Table 32.2). However, the cut-off for FEV1 and PEFR as suggested by Cropp,[70] 80% and 75%, respectively, might be too conservative. For example, on the basis of the data of Custovic *et al.*,[80] the lower borders of the 95% confidence interval for FEV1 and PEFR in 48 healthy children can be calculated to be roughly 90% and 83%. Indeed, many authors have used a fall in FEV1 of more than 10%[81] or 15%[82] as a criterion for EIA. In our laboratory, we assume EIA if the fall in FEV_1 exceeds 15%.

Reliability of bronchial responsiveness to a standardized exercise challenge

Intraclass correlation coefficients for the fall in FEV_1 with treadmill exercise while breathing dry air were reported to be 0.57.[83] The reliability, as described by the coefficient of variation, is higher in subjects with a fall in $FEV_1 > 20\%$ (CV 26%) than in subjects with a fall in $FEV_1 < 20\%$ (CV 81%).[84] This moderate reliability limits the information from repeated testing of one individual in order to assess the effectiveness of medication in preventing EIA.

Prevention of exercise-induced asthma and exercise counselling

On the basis of the reported benefits of exercise and physical activity for patients suffering from asthma or EIA (see above), every physician should try to enable a child with asthma to engage in as much physical activity as possible. The following section will summarize different approaches and principles which might be adopted to minimize exercise-related risks for the child with asthma (see also Table 32.3). The average daily doses of various drugs used to control asthma are summarized in Table 32.4.

Table 32.2 Criteria for assessing the severity of exercise-induced asthma

Parameter	Mild EIA (%)	Moderate EIA (%)	Severe EIA (%)
FVC	81–90	70–80	<70
FEV_1	66–80	50–65	<50
FEF_{25-75}	61–75	40–60	<40
PEFR	61–75	40–60	<40

Values are post-exercise pulmonary function measurements as percentage of pre-exercise determinations (based on Cropp[70]).

Control of asthma

During periods of airway inflammation, patients with asthma respond to an exercise challenge with a larger than usual fall in pulmonary function parameters. Long-term treatment of asthmatic patients with inhaled steroids such as budesonide or fluticasone propionate may decrease the hyper-responsiveness of the bronchi to a variety of stimuli, including exercise,[85,86] thereby, lowering the frequency or severity of EIA. Long-acting β_2-adrenoceptor agonists such as salmeterol or formoterol may help to reduce the risk of EIA in patients who are not symptom free with inhaled steroids alone.[87–89] Leucotriene antagonists are also effective in reducing EIA.[90]

Select the least asthmogenic activity

As pointed out above, inhaling cold and dry air while exercising increases the risk of a severe bronchial obstruction. Therefore, children with asthma are sometimes advised not to participate in winter sport activities. Using the precautions outlined in this section, such as wearing a face mask, properly administering medications, and monitoring of peak flow, exercise in cold weather can be safe for children with asthma.[91] However, if the physician is asked to provide a recommendation for appropriate activities she/he should emphasize swimming since EIA is less common during swimming

Table 32.3 Recommendations to reduce the risk of exercise-induced asthma in patients with asthma

- Control asthma (use anti-inflammatory drugs whenever bronchodilators are necessary on several days per week)
- Prefer swimming over running or cycling (note that swimming in pools with chlorinated water may lead to an asthmatic attack in some patients)
- Do not exercise during a period of severely reduced airway patency
- Be especially careful if you exercise after inhalation of allergens
- Do not exercise at high ozone levels (above 180 ppm) or in an environment with a high concentration of allergens
- Warm-up before exercise
- Inhale β_2-adrenergic agonists or cromolyn nebulizers 10–20 min before exercise
- Wear a face mask in cold weather (prevents heat/water loss from bronchial system)
- In case of exercise-induced asthma, use β_2-adrenergic agonists

Table 32.4 Recommended average daily dose for long-term nebulizer therapy in children with asthma (adapted from Reinhardt[102] and Berdel *et al.*[103])

Drug	Age 2–5 years	Age ≥6 years
Budesonide	2 × 50–200 μg	1–3 × 200–400 μg
Cromoglycate sodium	3–4 × 2–4 (–10) mg	3–4 × 2–4 mg
Fluticasone	2 × 25–100 μg	1–4 × 125–250 μg
Formoterol		2 × 6 (–12) μg
Nedocromil sodium	3–4 × 2–4 mg	3–4 × 4 mg
Salbutamol	4–6 × 100 (–400) μg	4–6 × 100–200 μg
Salmeterol		2 × 25–50 μg

than during land-based activities. However, this recommendation does not apply to those few patients who experience bronchial constriction when swimming in chlorinated water.

Select the right time to exercise

In patients with EIA, pulmonary function at rest is negatively related to the exercise-induced fall in pulmonary function.[92] Therefore, exercise should be avoided in times of bronchial obstruction. Although monitoring PEFR is not the best method to detect airway narrowing, it is recommended to measure PEFR before engaging in physical activity. If PEFR is below 80% of the child's average PEFR, short-acting β-mimetic drugs should be administered (see below) and exercise should be postponed until PEFR has improved.

The exercise-induced bronchial response is enhanced for several days after the inhalation of allergens.[93] Avoiding allergens for 1 month has been shown to reduce the risk for EIA.[94] For practical reasons, however, this recommendation can rarely be implemented. It should, however, be emphasized that exercising in an environment with a high allergen concentration may trigger EIA. Similarly, a high level of dust or ozone in the air has been linked to an increase in EIA.

Prevention of exercise-induced asthma shortly before and during exercise

As outlined above, a specific warm-up might be effective in some patients to lower the risk for EIA during the subsequent 2 hours.[28–30] However, the optimal pattern and efficacy of a warm-up protocol should be determined individually.

Several substances, such as cromoglycate sodium 20 mg, nedocromil sodium 4 mg, ipatropium bromide 80 μg, and β_2-adrenoceptor agonists such as salbutamol 0.2–0.4 mg or formoterol 6 (−12 μg), administered 10–20 min before the exercise have been shown to offer protection against EIA.[95–98] β-Adrenergic agonists seem to be more effective compared to cromoglycate or ipatropium bromide.[99] Using the same absolute dose, spacers do not improve the effect of cromoglycate or nedocromil.[100]

On the basis of the finding that an asthmatic attack with exercise most probably results from cooling and/or fluid loss of the bronchial system, the use of face masks has been recommended in cold or dry air.

Treatment of exercise-induced asthma

Once EIA has developed, it can be treated successfully with nebulized short-acting β-adrenoceptor agonists such as terbutaline sulphate or salbutamol.[101] Formoterol, one of the long-acting β_2-adrenoceptor agonists, may also be used.

Concluding remarks

Provided that the child with asthma and her or his parents are well educated and trained in the management of EIA, that the disease is treated adequately, and that the methods to prevent bronchial constriction with exercise are consequently employed, exercise can be safe. Under these conditions, nearly every patient with asthma can engage in all types of physical activities[104] and may even be successful at the very elite level of competitive athletics, for example, the Olympic games.[105]

Summary

- The incidence of asthma in children varies among countries and can be estimated to range between 5% and 20%. EIA attacks may occur in any patient with asthma and in some children without this diagnosis.
- The pathophysiology of EIA is not fully understood but airway cooling and drying with increased ventilation during exercise, and airway re-warming after exercise play an important role.
- Regular exercise may increase fitness and psychological well-being in children with asthma. Furthermore, moderate exercise may also have a beneficial effect on airway inflammation in patients with asthma.
- Typical symptoms of EIA include cough, chest tightness, and shortness of breath shortly after exercise.
- The diagnosis of EIA is based on the typical history and may be verified by an exercise challenge. Typically, a drop in FEV_1 exceeding 15% from baseline is regarded as diagnostic.
- With proper education and (pharmaco-) therapy, children with asthma can exercise safely. Even more, individuals with asthma can successfully participate in competitive sports at a very high level.

References

1. National Asthma Education Program (1991). I. Definition and diagnosis. *J Allergy Clin Immunol* **88**, 427–38.
2. Prahl P, Christiansen P, Hjuler I, Kaae HH (1997). Prevalence of asthma in Danish children aged 8–10 years. *Acta Paediatr* **86**, 1110–13.
3. Burr ML, Limb ES, Andrae S, Barry DM, Nagel F (1994). Childhood asthma in four countries: A comparative survey. *Int J Epidemiol* **23**, 341–7.
4. Pearce N, Weiland S, Keic U, Longridge P, Anderson HR, Strachow D, Baumann A, Young L, Gluyas P, Ruffin D, Crene J, Beasley R (1993). Self-reported prevalence of asthma in children in Australia, England, Germany and New Zealand: An international comparison using the JAAC protocol. *Eur Respir J* **6**, 1455–61.
5. Robertson CF, Heycock E, Bishop J, Nolan T, Olinsky A, Phelan PD (1991). Prevalence of asthma in Melbourne schoolchildren: Changes over 26 years. *BMJ* **302**,1116–18.
6. Skjonsberg OH, Clench-Aas J, Leegaard J, Skarpaas IJ, Giaever P, Bartonova A, Moseng J (1995). Prevalence of bronchial asthma in schoolchildren in Oslo, Norway. Comparison of data obtained in 1993 and 1981. *Allergy* **50**, 806–10.
7. McFadden ER (1987). Exercise induced asthma. Assessment of current etiologic concepts. *Chest* **91**, 151S–7S.
8. Badger D, Ramos AD, Lew CD, Platzker ACG, Stabile MW, Keens TG (1987). Childhood sequelae of infant lung disease: Exercise and pulmonary function abnormalities after bronchopulmonary dysplasia. *J Pediatr* **110**, 693–9.
9. Silverman M, Hobbs F, Gordon I, Carswell F (1978). Cystic fibrosis, atopy and airways lability. *Arch Dis Child* **47**, 882–9.
10. Rupp N, Guill M, Brudno D (1992). Unrecognized exercise-induced bronchospasm in adolescent athletes. *Am J Dis Child* **146**, 941–4.
11. Storms WW (1999). Exercise-induced asthma: Diagnosis and treatment for the recreational or elite athlete. *Med Sci Sports Exerc* **31** (Suppl. 1), S33–8.
12. Chen WY, Horton DJ (1977). Heat and water loss from the airways and exercise-induced asthma. *Respir* **34**, 305–10.

13. McFadden ER, Gilbert IA (1994). Exercise induced asthma. *N Engl J Med* **330**, 1362–7.
14. Bar-Yishay E, Gur I, Inbar O, Neuman I, Dlin RA, Godfrey S (1982). Differences between swimming and running as stimuli for exercise-induced asthma. *Eur J Appl Physiol* **48**, 387–97.
15. Noviski N, Bar-Yishay E, Gur I, Godfrey S (1987). Exercise intensity determines and climatic conditions modify the severity of exercise-induced asthma. *Am Rev Respir Dis* **136**, 592–4.
16. Sheppard D (1987). What does exercise have to do with 'exercise-induced' asthma? *Am Rev Respir Dis* **136**, 547–9.
17. McNally JF, Enright P, Hirsch JE, Souhrada JF (1984). The attenuation of exercise-induced bronchoconstriction by oro-pharyngeal anaesthesia. *Am Rev Respir Dis* **118**, 247–52.
18. Anderson SD (1984). Is there a unifying hypothesis for exercise induced asthma? *J Allergy Clin Immunol* **73**, 660–5.
19. Kikawa Y, Hosoi S, Inoue Y, Saito M, Nakai A, Shigematsu Y, Hirao T, Sudo M (1991). Exercise-induced urinary excretion of leukotriene E4 in children with atopic asthma. *Pediatr Res* **29**, 455–9.
20. White SW, Pitsillides KF, Parsons GH, Hayes SG, Gunther RA, Cottee DB (2001). Coronary-bronchial blood flow and airway dimensions in exercise-induced syndromes. *Clin Exp Pharmacol Physiol* **28**, 472–8.
21. Lemanske RF, Henke KG (1989). Exercise-induced asthma. In: Gisolfi CV, Lamb DR (eds.), *Youth, exercise, and sport. Perspectives in exercise science and sports medicine*, Vol. 2, pp. 465–511. Benchmark Press, Indianapolis, IN.
22. Koh YY, Lim HS, Min KU (1994). Airway responsiveness to allergen is increased 24 hours after exercise challenge. *J Allergy Clin Immunol* **94**, 507–16.
23. Speelberg B, Panis EA, Bijl D, van Herwaarden CL, Bruynzeel PL (1991). Late asthmatic responses after exercise challenge are reproducible. *J Allergy Clin Immunol* **87**, 1128–37.
24. Boner AL, Vallone G, Chiesa M, Spezia E, Fambri L, Sette L (1992). Reproducibility of late phase pulmonary response to exercise and its relationship to bronchial hyperreactivity in children with chronic asthma. *Pediatr Pulmonol* **14**, 156–9.
25. Hofstra WB, Sterk PJ, Neijens HJ, Kouwenberg JM, Mulder PG, Duiverman EJ (1996). Occurrence of a late response to exercise in asthmatic children: Multiple regression approach using time-matched baseline and histamine control days. *Eur Respir J* **9**, 1348–55.
26. Hamielec CM, Manning PJ, O'Byrne PM (1988). Exercise refractoriness after histamine inhalation in asthmatic subjects. *Am Rev Respir Dis* **138**, 794–98.
27. Wilson B, Bar-Or O, Seed L (1990). Effects of humid air breathing during arm or treadmill exercise on exercise-induced bronchoconstriction and refractoriness. *Am Rev Respir Dis* **142**, 349–52.
28. Reiff DB, Choudry NB, Pride NB, Ind PW (1989). The effect of prolonged submaximal warm-up exercise on exercise-induced asthma. *Am Rev Respir Dis* **139**, 479–84.
29. Schnall RP, Landau RI (1980). Protective effects of repeated short sprints in exercise-induced asthma. *Thorax* **35**, 828–32.
30. Lin CC, Wu JL, Huang WC, Lin CY (1991). A bronchial response comparison of exercise and methacholine in asthmatic subjects. *J Asthma* **28**, 31–40.
31. Ben-Dov I, Bar-Yishay E, Godfrey S (1982). Refractory period after exercise-induced asthma unexplained by respiratory heat loss. *Am Rev Respir Dis* **125**, 530–4.
32. Wilson B, Bar-Or O, O'Byrne PM (1994). The effects of indomethacin on refractoriness following exercise both with and without a bronchoconstrictor response. *Eur Respir J* **7**, 2174–8.
33. Gilbert IA, Fouke JM, McFadden ER (1990). The effect of repetitive exercise on airway temperatures. *Am Rev Respir Dis* **142**, 826–31.
34. Wiens L, Sabath R, Ewing L, Gowdamarajan R, Portnoy J, Scagliotti D (1992). Chest pain in otherwise healthy children and adolescents is frequently caused by exercise-induced asthma. *Pediatrics* **90**, 350–3.
35. Sarafino EP, Paterson ME, Murphy EL (1998). Age and the impacts of triggers in childhood asthma. *J Asthma* **35**, 213–17.
36. Nystad W (1997). The physical activity level in children with asthma based on a survey among 7–16 year old school children. *Scand J Med Sci Sports* **7**, 331–5.
37. Weston AR, Macfarlane DJ, Hopkins WG (1989). Physical activity of asthmatic and nonasthmatic children. *J Asthma* **26**, 279–86.
38. Hussein A, Forderer A, Abelitis M, Koch I (1988). Der Einfluss von Diagnose und Prophylaxe der anstrengungsinduzierten Bronchialobstruktion auf die sportlich Aktivitat asthmatischer Schulkinder. [Effect of the diagnosis and prevention of exercise-induced bronchial obstruction on sports participation by asthmatic school children]. *Monatsschr Kinderheilkd* **136**, 819–23.
39. Siersted HC, Boldsen J, Hansen HS, Mostgaard G, Hyldebrandt N (1998). Population based study of risk factors for underdiagnosis of asthma in adolescence: Odense schoolchild study. *BMJ* **316**, 651–5.
40. Counil FP, Varray A, Karila C, Hayot M, Voisin M, Prefaut C (1997). Wingate test performance in children with asthma: Aerobic or anaerobic limitation? *Med Sci Sports Exerc* **29**, 430–5.
41. Ludwick SK, Jones JW, Jones TK, Fukuhara JT, Strunk RC (1986). Normalization of cardiopulmonary endurance in severely asthmatic children after bicycle ergometry therapy. *J Pediatr* **109**, 446–51.
42. Strunk RC, Mrazek DA, Fukuhara JT, Masterson J, Ludwick SK, LaBreque JF (1989). Cardiovascular fitness in children with asthma correlates with psychologic functioning of the child. *Pediatrics* **84**, 460–4.
43. Santuz P, Baraldi E, Filippone M, Zacchello F (1997). Exercise performance in children with asthma: Is it different from that of healthy controls? *Eur Respir J* **10**, 1254–60.
44. Kiers A, van der Mark TW, Woldring MG, Peset R (1980). Determination of the functional residual capacity during exercise. *Ergonomics* **23**, 955–9.
45. Freyschuss UG, Hedlin G, Hedenstierna G (1984). Ventilation-perfusion relationships during exercise-induced asthma in children. *Am Rev Respir Dis* **130**, 888–94.
46. Garfinkel S, Kesten S, Chapman K, Rebuck A (1992). Physiologic and nonphysiologic determinants of aerobic fitness in mild to moderate asthma. *Am Rev Respir Dis* **145**, 741–5.
47. Svenonius E, Kautto R, Arborelius M (1983). Improvement after training of children with exercise-induced asthma. *Acta Paediatr Scand* **72**, 23–30.
48. Holzer FJ, Schnall R, Landau LI (1984). The effect of a home exercise programme in children with cystic fibrosis and asthma. *Austr Paediatr J* **20**, 297–301.
49. Perrin JM, MacLean WE, Gortmaker SL, Asher KN (1992). Improving the psychological status of children with asthma: A randomized controlled trial. *J Dev Behav Pediatr* **13**, 241–7.
50. Schmidt SM, Ballke EH, Nuske F, Leistikow G, Wiersbitzky SK (1997). Der Einfluβ einer ambulanten Sporttherapie auf das Asthma bronchiale bei Kindern. [Effect of ambulatory sports therapy on bronchial asthma in children]. *Pneumologie* **51**, 835–41.
51. Counil FP, Varray A, Matecki S, Beurey A, Marchal P, Voisin M, Prefaut C (2003). Training of aerobic and anaerobic fitness in children with asthma. *J Pediatr* **142**, 179–84.
52. Matsumoto I, Araki H, Tsuda K, Odajima H, Nishima S, Higaki Y, Tanaka H, Tanaka M, Shindo M (1999). Effects of swimming training on aerobic capacity and exercise induced bronchoconstriction in children with bronchial asthma. *Thorax* **54**, 196–201.
53. Engstrom I, Fallstrom K, Karlberg E, Sten G, Bjure J (1991). Psychological and respiratory physiological effects of a physical exercise programme on boys with severe asthma. *Acta Paediatr Scand* **80**, 1058–65.
54. Kieckhefer GM (1988). The meaning of health to 9-, 10-, and 11-year-old children with asthma. *J Asthma* **25**, 325–33.
55. Huang SW, Veiga R, Sila U, Reed E, Hines S (1989). The effect of swimming in asthmatic children—participants in a swimming program in the city of Baltimore. *J Asthma* **26**, 117–21.

56. Szentagothai K, Gyene I, Szocska M, Osvath P (1987). Physical exercise program for children with bronchial asthma. *Pediatr Pulmonol* **3**, 166–72.
57. Fitch KD, Blitvich JD, Morton AR (1986). The effect of running training on exercise-induced asthma. *Ann Allergy* **57**, 90–4.
58. Henriksen JM, Nielsen TT (1983). Effect of physical training on exercise-induced bronchoconstriction. *Acta Paediatr Scand* **72**, 31–6.
59. Pastva A, Estell K, Schoeb TR, Atkinson TP, Schwiebert LM (2004). Aerobic exercise attenuates airway inflammatory responses in a mouse model of atopic asthma. *J Immunol* **172**, 4520–6.
60. Helenius I, Haahtela T (2000). Allergy and asthma in elite summer sport athletes. *J Allergy Clin Immunol* **106**, 444–52.
61. Weiler JM, Ryan EJ 3rd (2000). Asthma in United States Olympic athletes who participated in the 1998 Olympic winter games. *J Allergy Clin Immunol* **106**, 267–71.
62. Helenius I, Rytila P, Sarna S, Lumme A, Helenius M, Remes V, Haahtela T (2002). Effect of continuing or finishing high-level sports on airway inflammation, bronchial hyperresponsiveness, and asthma: A 5-year prospective follow-up study of 42 highly trained swimmers. *J Allergy Clin Immunol* **109**, 962–8.
63. McConnell R, Barhane K, Gilliland F, London SJ, Islam T, Gaudemann JW, Avol E, Margolis HG, Peters JM (2002). Asthma in exercising children exposed to ozone: A cohort study. *Lancet* **359**, 386–91.
64. Foresi A, Corbo GM, Valente S (1988). Airway responsiveness to exercise and ultrasonically nebulized distilled water in children: Relationship to clinical and functional characteristics. *Respiration* **53**, 205–13.
65. Jones A, Bowen M (1994). Screening for childhood asthma using an exercise test. *Br J Gen Pract* **44**, 127–31.
66. Ponsonby AL, Couper D, Dwyer T, Carmichael A, Wood-Baker R (1996). Exercise-induced bronchial hyperresponsiveness and parental ISAAC questionnaire responses. *Eur Respir J* **9**, 1356–62.
67. Riedler J, Reade T, Dalton M, Holst D, Robertson C (1994). Hypertonic saline challenge in an epidemiologic survey of asthma in children. *Am J Respir Crit Care Med* **150**, 1632–9.
68. Powell CV, White RD, Primhak RA (1996). Longitudinal study of free running exercise challenge: Reproducibility. *Arch Dis Child* **74**, 108–14.
69. West JV, Robertson CF, Roberts R, Olinsky A (1996). Evaluation of bronchial responsiveness to exercise in children as an objective measure of asthma in epidemiological surveys. *Thorax* **51**, 590–5.
70. Cropp G (1979). The exercise bronchoprovocation test: Standardization of procedures and evaluation of response. *J Allergy Clin Immunol* **64**, 627–33.
71. Eggleston PA, Rosenthal RR, Anderson SA, Anderton R, Bierman CW, Bleecker ER, Chai H, Cropp GJA, Johnson JD, Konig P, Morse J, Smith LJ, Summers RJ, Trautlein JJ (1979). Guidelines for the methodology of exercise challenge testing of asthmatics. *J Allergy Clin Immunol* **64**, 642–5.
72. Russo GH, Bellia CA, Bodas AW (1986). Exercise-induced asthma (EIA): Its prevention with the combined use of ipratropium bromide and fenoterol. *Respir* **50** (Suppl. 2), 258–61.
73. Washington RL, Bricker JT, Alpert BS, Daniels SR, Deckelbaum RJ, Fisher EA, Gidding SS, Isabel-Jones J, Kavey REW, Marx GR, Strong WB, Teske DW, Wilmore JH, Winston M (1994). Guidelines for exercise testing in the pediatric age group. *Circulation* **90**, 2166–79.
74. Garcia de la Rubia S, Pajaron Fernandez MJ, Sanchez-Solis M, Martinez-Gonzalez-Moro I, Perez-Flores D, Pajaron-Ahumada M (1998). Exercise-induced asthma in children: A comparative study of free and treadmill running. *Ann Allergy Asthma Immunol* **80**, 232–6.
75. Fitch K (1975). Comparative aspects of available exercise systems. *Pediatrics* **56** (Suppl.), 904–7.
76. Bundgaard A, Ingemann-Hansen T, Schmidt A, Halkjaer-Kristensen J (1982). Exercise-induced asthma after walking, running and cycling. *Scan J Clin Lab Invest* **42**, 15–18.
77. Kilham H, Tooley M, Silverman M (1979). Running, walking, and hyperventilation causing asthma in children. *Thorax* **34**, 582–6.
78. Inbar O, Alvarez D, Lyons H (1981). Exercise-induced asthma—A comparison between two modes of exercise stress. *Eur J Respir Dis* **62**, 160–7.
79. Brudno DS, Wagner JM, Rupp NT (1994). Length of postexercise assessment in the determination of exercise-induced bronchospasm. *Ann Allergy* **73**, 227–31.
80. Custovic A, Arifhodzic N, Robinson A, Woodcock A (1994). Exercise testing revisited. The response to exercise in normal and atopic children. *Chest* **105**, 1127–32.
81. Tan RA, Spector SL (1998). Exercise-induced asthma. *Sports Med* **25**, 1–6.
82. Shapiro GG, Pierson WE, Furukawa CT, Bierman CW (1979). A comparison of the effectiveness of free-running and treadmill exercise for assessing exercise-induced bronchospasm in clinical practice. *J Allergy Clin Immunol* **64**, 609–11.
83. Hofstra WB, Sont JK, Sterk PJ, Neijens HJ, Kuethe MC, Duiverman EJ (1997). Sample size estimation in studies monitoring exercise-induced bronchoconstriction in asthmatic children. *Thorax* **52**, 739–41.
84. Eggleston PA, Guerrant JL (1976). A standardized method of evaluating exercise-induced asthma. *J Allergy Clin Immunol* **58**, 414–25.
85. Vathenen AS, Knox AJ, Wisniewski A, Tattersfield AE (1991). Effect of inhaled budesonide on bronchial reactivity to histamine, exercise, and eucapnic dry air hyperventilation in patients with asthma. *Thorax* **46**, 811–16.
86. Pedersen S, Hansen OR (1995). Budesonide treatment of moderate and severe asthma in children: A dose-response study. *J Allergy Clin Immunol* **95**, 29–33.
87. Adkins JC, McTavish D (1997). Salmeterol. A review of its pharmacological properties and clinical efficacy in the management of children with asthma. *Drugs* **54**, 331–54.
88. De Benedictis FM, Tuteri G, Pazzelli P, Niccoli A, Mezzetti D, Vaccaro R (1996). Salmeterol in exercise-induced bronchoconstriction in asthmatic children: Comparison of two doses. *Eur Respir J* **9**, 2099–103.
89. Daugbjerg P, Nielsen KG, Skov M, Bisgaard H (1996). Duration of action of formoterol and salbutamol dry-powder inhalation in prevention of exercise-induced asthma in children. *Acta Paediatr* **85**, 684–7.
90. Leff JA, Busse WW, Pearlman D, Bronsky EA, Kemp J, Hendeles L, Dockhorn R, Kundu S, Zhang J, Seidenberg BC, Reiss TF (1998). Montelukast, a leucotriene receptor antagonist, for the treatment of mild asthma and exercise induced bronchoconstriction. *N Engl J Med* **339**, 147–52.
91. Silvers W, Morrison M, Wiener M (1994). Asthma ski day: Cold air sports safe with peak flow monitoring. *Ann Allergy* **73**, 105–8.
92. Nolan P (1996). Clinical features predictive of exercise-induced asthma in children. *Respirology* **1**, 201–5.
93. Mussaffi H, Springer C, Godfrey S (1986). Increased bronchial responsiveness to exercise and histamine after allergen challenge in children with asthma. *J Allergy Clin Immunol* **77**, 48–52.
94. Benckhuijsen J, van den Bos JW, van Velzen E, de Bruijn R, Aalbers R (1996). Differences in the effect of allergen avoidance on bronchial hyperresponsiveness as measured by methacholine, adenosine 5′-monophosphate, and exercise in asthmatic children. *Pediatr Pulmonol* **22**, 147–53.
95. Ben-Dov I, Bar-Yishay E, Godfrey S (1983). Heterogeneity in the response of asthmatic patients to pre-exercise treatment with cromolyn sodium. *Am Rev Respir Dis* **127**, 113–16.
96. Boner AL, Antolini I, Andreoli A, de Stefano G, Sette L (1987). Comparison of the effects of inhaled calcium antagonist verapamil, sodium cromoglycate and ipratropium bromide on exercise-induced bronchoconstriction in children with asthma. *Eur J Pediatr* **146**, 408–11.

97. Novembre E, Frongia GF, Veneruso G, Vierucci A (1994). Inhibition of exercise-induced-asthma (EIA) by nedocromil sodium and sodium cromoglycate in children. *Pediatr Allergy Immunol* **5**, 107–10.
98. Ferrari M, Balestreri F, Baratieri S, Biasin C, Oldani V, Lo Cascio V (2000). Evidence of the rapid protective effect of formoterol dry-powder inhalation against exercise-induced bronchospasm in athletes with asthma. *Respiration* **67**, 510–13.
99. Svenonius E, Arborelius M, Wiberg R, Ekberg P (1988). Prevention of exercise-induced asthma by drugs inhaled from metered aerosols. *Allergy* **43**, 252–7.
100. Comis A, Valletta EA, Sette L, Andreoli A, Boner AL (1993). Comparison of nedocromil sodium and sodium cromoglycate administered by pressurized aerosol, with and without a spacer device in exercise-induced asthma in children. *Eur Respir J* **6**, 523–6.
101. Dos Santos JM, Costa H, Stahl E, Wiren JE (1991). Bricanyl Turbuhaler and Ventolin Rotahaler in exercise-induced asthma in children. *Allergy* **46**, 203–5.
102. Reinhardt D (1996). *Asthma bronchiale im Kindesalter.* [*Bronchial asthma in childhood*]. Springer Verlag, Berlin.
103. Berdel D, Reinhardt D, Hofmann D, Leupold W, Lindemann H (1998). *Therapie-Empfehlungen der Gesellschaft für Pädiatrische Pneumologie zur Behandlung des Asthma bronchiale bei Kindern und Jugendlichen.* [The German Society of Paediatric Pulmonology: Guidelines for asthma therapy in children] *Monatsschr Kinderheilkd* **146**, 492–7.
104. Bundgaard A (1985). Exercise and the asthmatic. *Sports Med* **2**, 254–66.
105. Voy RO (1986). The U.S. Olympic Committee experience with exercise-induced bronchospasm, 1984. *Med Sci Sports Exerc* 18, 328–30.

CHAPTER 33

Exercise, physical activity, and cystic fibrosis

Susi Kriemler

Introduction

Cystic fibrosis (CF) is the most common genetic autosomal recessive disease of the Caucasian race, generally leading to death in early adulthood.[1] The frequency of the gene carrier (heterozygote) is 1:20–25 in Caucasian populations, 1:2000 in African-Americans, and practically non-existent in Asian populations. The disease occurs in about 1 in every 2500 life births of the white population. Mean survival has risen from 8.4 years in 1969 to 32 years in 2000 due to improvements in treatment. The genetic defect causes a pathological electrolyte transport through the cell membranes by a defective chloride channel membrane transport protein [cystic fibrosis transmembrane conductance regulator (CFTR)]. With respect to the function, this affects mainly the exocrine glands of secretory cells, sinuses, lungs, pancreas, liver, and the reproductive tract of the human body leading to a highly viscous, water-depleted secretion. The secretion cannot leave the glands and in consequence causes local inflammation and destruction of various organs. The main symptoms include chronic inflammatory pulmonary disease with a progressive loss of lung function, exocrine and sometimes endocrine pancreas insufficiency, and an excessive salt loss through the sweat glands.[1] A summary of the signs and symptoms of CF will be given with a special emphasis on the effect of exercise performance and capacity.

Cystic fibrosis-related pathologies and exercise tolerance

General

Exercise tolerance in the patient with CF shows a wide variation. Some patients perform marathons or triathlons and others are hardly able to walk for a few minutes. Peak (or maximum) oxygen uptake (peak $\dot{V}O_2$ or $\dot{V}O_2$ max) is usually reduced in patients with CF even in those with mild pulmonary involvement.[2] The limitations in exercise performance increase with the progression of the disease for which several factors are responsible which have been summarized in Fig. 33.1.

In CF patients, aerobic exercise capacity correlates significantly with resting pulmonary function.[3–6] This is true, when a group of CF patients is considered, but the association is much less tight on an individual level. Nevertheless, increasing the lung function parameters, normally, results in an improved exercise capacity.[7,8] In a normal population and also in those CF patients with mild disease,[9] maximal exercise is limited by muscle fatigue when the muscles become hypoxic and accumulate lactic acid. Patients with moderate to advanced pulmonary disease are ventilatory limited in a degree which is normally correlated to the severity of the underlying lung disease. Maximal exercise performance is also influenced by other factors, such as nutrition,[3,10,11] peripheral muscle function,[12–14] and cardiac function,[15–17] as well as daily physical activity,[18–20] which we will discus in this chapter.

Respiratory system

The defect of the CFTR protein complex results in an increase of the viscosity of the bronchial secretion and its retention with the consequence of bronchial obstruction and recurrent or chronic infections in the lungs. Mechanisms include mucosal oedema secondary to chronic infection/inflammation, mechanical obstruction by abnormal viscous secretions, stimulation of autonomic nerve fibres caused by damage to the respiratory epithelium, airway smooth muscle contraction by inflammatory mediators, and dynamic collapse of airways with partly destructed walls.[21] The recurrent inflammation/infection leads to a progressive destruction of the bronchial wall with bronchiectasis and to a progressive bronchial lability with a tendency of bronchial collapse, which

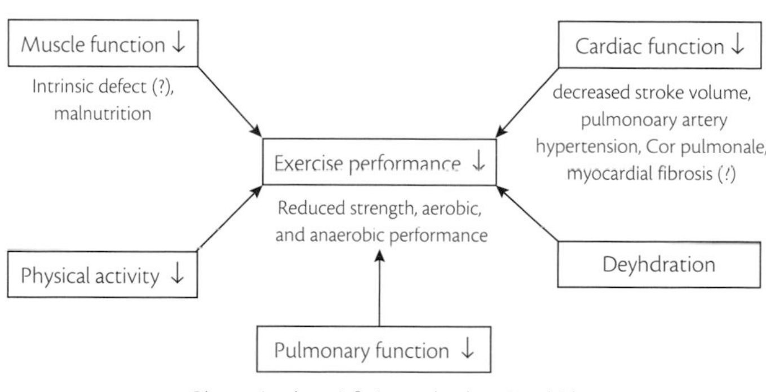

Fig. 33.1 Factors responsible für exercise limitations in patients with CF.

further provokes mucostasis and inflammation. The development of atelectatic, emphysematic, and fibrotic areas implies a progressive decline of functional lung tissue, the so-called cystic-fibrotic degeneration of the lung. The disease severity varies tremendously among patients ranging from severe obstructive pulmonary disease in the infant up to a mild cough with normal pulmonary function in a 40-year-old patient. About 10% of adolescent or adult CF patients develop a spontaneous pneumothorax mainly presenting as sharp thoracic pain and consequent tachypnoea or dyspnoea. Respiratory insufficiency with hypercapnia, chronic hypoxaemia and an exhaustion of the respiratory muscles is the cause of death in more than 95% of all CF patients.[22]

At rest, the patients normally present with an obstruction in their resting pulmonary function, including a decreased forced vital capacity (FVC), forced expiratory flow in 1 second (FEV_1), FEV between 25% and 75% of vital capacity (FEF_{25-75}), peak flow (PEF), and an increased residual volume to total lung capacity (RV/TLC).[23–25] In other words, the pulmonary function shows obstruction and hyperinflation. A first consequence is the increase of dead space ventilation (V_D). Ventilation at exercise is therefore higher for a given workload and at high work intensities peak oxygen uptake and peak work capacity will become limited.[26,27] While a healthy child uses only about 70% of his/her maximal voluntary ventilation during maximal exercise, the patient with progressed CF uses a higher percentage finally reaching 100% or even more.[28,29] Healthy people show a V_D/V_T of about 30% at rest and a lower percentage at exercise. In patients with moderate or severe CF, V_D/V_T is increased at rest and even more so at exercise due to a limited V_T and a poor matching of ventilation and perfusion of the lungs.[30] Likewise, the relative ventilation for a given workload is increased resulting in a higher oxygen cost of ventilation[31] and early fatigue of inspiratory muscle function. Oxygen cost of breathing in a healthy individual is in the range of 10% of $\dot{V}O_2$ max, but it can reach 30–40% in those patients with severe respiratory limitations.[32] If peripheral oxygen demands cannot be fulfilled, desaturation occurs which further aggravates respiratory muscle function. Furthermore, with the progression of the disease an increased arterio–alveolar oxygen gradient occurs as a manifestation of the ventilation–perfusion mismatch. In consequence oxygen desaturation occurs, first during exercise and finally also at rest.[33]

Likewise, FVC may be limited by progressive airway obstruction, which prevents a sufficient increase of tidal volume (V_T) at increasing workloads.[34] CF patients typically show lower increases in V_T, which is partially compensated by a faster respiratory rate without reaching minute ventilations of healthy controls. This adaptive strategy of rapid shallow breathing, however, has the disadvantage of increasing the cost of breathing by inefficient dead space ventilation, another factor contributing to early fatigue of the inspiratory muscles. Furthermore, time to expire a given air volume is prolonged in obstructive disease. When combined with high breathing frequencies air trapping occurs and hyperinflation is aggravated. Inspiratory muscles are shortened and the diaphragm flattened leading to a compromise of inspiratory muscle function.

High dead space ventilation can also compromise CO_2 elimination[34] and CO_2 retention occurs due to a lower increase in the minute ventilation ($\dot{V}_E$) tidal volume ratio (i.e. $\dot{V}_E/V_T$)[35–37] and changes in the chemoreceptor set point for PCO_2.[38] Carbon dioxide retention has even been described as early predictor of mortality[39] or as predictor of a faster decrement of FEV_1.[37] Whether CO_2 retention also contributes to maximal exercise limitation by increasing subjective dyspnoea sensation, is not clear.

In general, patients with a FVC or a FEV_1/FVC ratio of greater than 50% predicted are unlikely to desaturate even at high intense exercise.[9,40] In early reports, it was speculated that exercise performance in CF might be limited by oxygen availability, as indicated by a positive relationship between oxygen saturation at peak exercise and peak $\dot{V}O_2$.[41] Nixon *et al.*[42] could not induce an increase in peak workload despite oxygen supplementation in hypoxaemic CF patients which led them to conclude that maximal exercise was not oxygen limited. Another recent elegant study, however, suggests that arterial hypoxaemia is indeed responsible for the exercise limitation.[43] A group of adult CF patients with moderate to severe disease and desaturation at maximal exercise underwent maximal exercise testing with and without added dead space. The trial with added dead space was tested under normoxia as well as under hyperoxia. The addition of dead space caused reduced $\dot{V}O_2$ max with equal peak ventilation and desaturation than without added deadspace, while $\dot{V}O_2$ max increased when oxygen was added to the additional dead space. The authors concluded that oxygen supplementation might help to improve maximal exercise performance by lowering minute ventilation and as such conserving energy of the respiratory muscles. Likewise, it lowers heart rate and pulmonary artery hypertension with the consequence of an improved ventilation–perfusion time.[42] It also seems to improve aerobic metabolism in the peripheral muscles as shown in calf muscles of patients with COPD[44] or it might reduce the sensation of dyspnoea at end exercise.[43]

Some patients experience a severe cough at exercise. It is important to mention to the patient, family, and teacher that this is not dangerous. In our experience and based on scientific evidence,[45] coughing is helpful, because it facilitates the clearance of mucus from the bronchial system. Usually, a short break during exercise is sufficient to stop the spells. In some patients, however, the cough or shortness of breath is a sign of exercise-induced bronchoconstriction.[21,46,47] The diagnosis of CF asthma is problematic and it is difficult to determine which patients have a combination of CF and asthma and which have asthma-like symptoms caused by the CF lung itself. The North American and European CF databases report that 17–32% of CF patients have asthma and the higher incidences were found when patients were tested several times instead of a single test over a year.[48–50] The reported proportion of reactive airways ranges from as high as 65%[51] down to 2%,[52] but averages around 40%.[46,47,53] The therapy is the same as for exercise-induced bronchoconstriction in the non-CF population, but some CF patients do not respond to bronchodilators as well as asthmatics and should be tested repeatedly. About 10–20% of CF patients treated with bronchodilators actually demonstrate acute declines in spirometric values.[54,55] Moreover, bronchodilators do not improve maximal exercise performance in CF, despite causing significant acute bronchodilation.[54,56] This lack of benefit occurred in all patients with venilatory limitation of exercise and irrespective of a positive bronchoprovocation test.[56] Note that some authors also found bronchodilation with exercise even without treatment.[52,53,56,57] An exercise-induced increase in mucus clearance or the reopening of collapsed bronchi are thought to be the reasons for the improvement in lung function. It is also possible that bronchodilation occurs due to airway instability by loss of bronchomotor tone leading to increased dead space ventilation which could explain the lack of improvement in exercise performance.[56]

Cardiac system

Initially, the cardiovascular response to exercise appears to be relatively normal in CF and heart rates and cardiac output are adequate for a given workload.[11,27] Cardiac output is often normal due to a more rapid rise of heart rate, thus compensating for a reduced stroke volume which seems to occur even in the absence of severe lung disease.[58] With disease progression, CF patients often show a significant cor pulmonale as a consequence of the pulmonary artery hypertension. The pathophysiology of cor pulmonale and pulmonary hypertension is thought to be related to the progressive destruction of the lung parenchyma and pulmonary vasculature and to pulmonary vasoconstriction secondary to hypoxaemia. Some other authors also found right[15] and left[15,59] ventricular functional deficits during exercise while others[3,27] basically found no abnormalities. Perrault *et al.*[16] measured cardiac output response during progressive upright and supine exercise in CF patients of different severity. Cardiac output increased with exercise intensity in both positions except in those patients with severe disease (FEV_1 40%). Despite a normal cardiac output response, all CF patients irrespective of disease severity failed to increase stroke volume in response to the change from upright to the supine position. The authors concluded that this could reflect a limitation in end-diastolic ventricular filling by an alteration of ventricular diastolic function. In another study,[4] several CF patients showed a decrease in stroke volume despite a normal cardiac output. Stroke volume correlated with hypoxaemia but not with pulmonary function which is compatible with impaired left ventricular filling as a consequence of hypoxia-induced pulmonary hypertension. In contrast, another study[17] found a more striking relationship between stroke volume (% predicted) and FEV_1 than with hypoxaemia with an improvement of the stroke volume response to exercise with improvement in ventilatory mechanics in some patients who were measured twice. In summary, cardiovascular limitations in the form of decreased stroke volumes occur but are often compensated by a higher heart rate leading to a normal cardiac output. Whether the reduced stroke volume might be due to hypoxaemia causing pulmonary hypertension and in consequence an impaired left ventricular filling, or a decreased right ventricular performance as a consequence of increased pulmonary pressures and lung volumes, or due to poor nutrition or inactivity, or a combination of these factors has to be determined. A further reason could be multifocal myocardial fibrosis which has recently been described in autopsies of patients with CF.[60]

Habitual physical activity

Since exercise intervention studies have been effective in slowing down pulmonary function decline and in increasing exercise performance, habitual physical activity might have the same or even a greater long-term impact on these parameters, which are documented as predictors of mortality.[39,61,62] Indeed, in a longitudinal study[63] 7- to 17-year-old girls in the two lowest activity quartiles had a more rapid rate of decline in FEV_1 than girls in the two highest activity quartiles, while in boys physical activity was not related to FEV_1 decline. The authors concluded that an inactive lifestyle may partially explain the poorer survival of female patients with CF. Children and adults with CF have been reported to have lower[18] or similar[64] levels of daily physical activity compared to healthy children. Selvadurai *et al.*[19] documented an equal activity level in prepubertal boys and girls with CF compared to controls. After onset of puberty, physical activity was higher in boys than girls with CF. It was even higher than in controls when lung disease was mild, but lower for those with moderate to severe lung disease. The best correlates of physical activity were nutritional state, anaerobic power, aerobic capacity, and quality of life, but not lung function. So far, there are few data in the literature focusing on whether a relationship between physical activity and peak $\dot{V}O_2$ exists in CF and if so whether the relationship reflects a direct effect or is mediated by confounding factors such as pulmonary or muscle function. A cross-sectional study in 12- to 40-year-old patients with a broad range of disease severity found that physical activity beside height, sex, FEV_1, and muscle power was identified as independent predictor of $\dot{V}O_2$ max.[20]

Nutrition and muscle function

The exocrine pancreatic insufficiency with maldigestion and failure to thrive is a hallmark of CF occurring in 85–90% of the CF population. The impairment of the intraluminal digestion varies widely from the life-threatening event of a meconium ileus in the newborn to a subclinical digestive residual function in the adult patient, and the severity seems to be related to the genetic defect.[65,66] It is, nowadays, well accepted that external factors such as enzyme therapy or nutrition influence the progression and severity of the disease.[67–72] Undernutrition is often seen in patients with CF as a result of malabsorption, reduced energy intake, increased energy expenditure, and as a consequence of chronic pulmonary infection.

The chronic disease state increases energy demands, malassimilation causes energy loss, and external factors decrease energy intake. Consequently, there is a net energy deficit which is believed to impair respiratory and peripheral muscles, lead to a progressive destruction of the pulmonary parenchyma, and decrease immune regulation. This causes a worsening of the pulmonary function and increases the likeliness of pulmonary infections. Those pulmonary infections again provoke a further decrease of the lung function and on the other side may cause anorexia and vomiting which closes the vicious circle.[73]

It has to be considered that total daily energy expenditure, in a resting stage[74] as well as during exercise[75–77], is increased in persons with CF especially in the advanced stage with severe lung disease. It is therefore important that the energy intake is adjusted to the disease severity and the activity level. S. Koletzko and B. Koletzko[78] developed a simple equation to calculate the crude estimate of energy demand, on the basis of the activity level and the pulmonary function (Table 33.1).

In order to be able to calculate proper energy requirements, a first step is to assess the nutritional status and body composition. The body mass index (BMI) is widely used to assess nutritional status, but it does not inform about body composition. In patients with CF, there might be a normal BMI, although skeletal muscles might be wasted. This was indeed found in a group of young adults with CF, in whom a loss of fat-free mass (FFM) but normal fat mass measured by dual-energy X-ray absorptiometry (DXA) was found in the presence of a normal BMI.[79] The loss of FFM was related to severity of lung disease and the level of physical activity, suggesting that this pattern preferentially occurs in advanced lung disease. Whether the loss of FFM led to physical inactivity or whether the loss of FFM was rather a consequence of inappropriate use remains a matter of debate. A low FFM in adults with CF has also been

Table 33.1 Daily energy requirements, based on basal metabolic rate, activity level and lung function at rest

Daily energy requirement = BMR* × (Activity factor + Lung function factor)	
Activity factor	
Bedrest	1.3
Moderate activity	1.5
Normal activity	1.7
Lung function factor	
FEV_1 >/= 80%	0.1
FEV_1 40–79%	0.2
FEV_1 < 40%	0.3
BMR for 10- to 18-year-old children (WHO guidelines)	
12.2 × body weight + 746 (girls)	17.5 × body weight + 651 (boys)

*BMR = basal metabolic rate in kcal·d^{-1}

found in other studies[80] and was related to more severe lung disease.[81]

There are several methods that have been used in studies reporting body composition in CF, including DXA,[80–82] bioelectrical impedance[82–84], and skinfolds (see refs 82,83 and Chapter 3). DXA is the preferred method, since it has been shown to be a useful and reliable method for body composition assessment and it provides at the same time information about bone mass which is often reduced in patients with CF. Studies in children and adults with CF found that skinfold thickness and bioelectric impedance incorrectly estimate FFM in many patients compared with DXA measurements of FFM.[82,83] Although results obtained using the three methods were highly correlated for the group, values for individual subjects varied widely with limits of agreement between DXA, skinfolds, and bioelectric impedance ranging up to 19% in children and up to 7% in adults.

A better nutritional status is associated with higher aerobic[6,10] and anaerobic[85–87] exercise capacity. Likewise, a poor nutritional status is considered as a risk factor for limited exercise capacity.[3,11] An increase in body weight through an adequate nutrition has been shown to improve exercise capacity[88] and muscle strength.[89] If the increase in energy intake is combined with exercise training, an improved exercise capacity and lean tissue gain are attained in some[90] but not all studies.[89,91] In CF, chronic airway obstruction leads to a catabolic metabolism secondary to pulmonary infection and inflammation, a process which may induce protein breakdown and inhibit muscle development in patients with CF.[92,93] Yet, it is not clear, whether decreased exercise performance is caused by a decreased muscle mass or whether there is an intrinsic muscle defect. Moser *et al.*[12] tested the interaction between peak $\dot{V}O_2$ and muscle size in 7- to 18-year-old CF patients and found that the reduced peak $\dot{V}O_2$ in CF was not solely explained by a reduction in muscle size, but that the reduction in peak $\dot{V}O_2$ was observed even when normalized to muscle cross-sectional area which was only slightly lower in CF than in controls. This study is unique since it directly assessed muscle mass by magnetic resonance imaging rather than relying on indirect estimates of muscle mass. Interestingly, they found that not only peak $\dot{V}O_2$ was reduced in CF, but also $\Delta\dot{V}O_2/\Delta$workrate, decribing reduced oxygen demands of exercise in CF at any intensity level. Whether this was caused by an increased work efficiency, by slow oxygen kinetics,[94] by a higher reliance on anaerobic pathways such as in certain patients with congenital heart disease in which oxygen transport to muscle is reduced,[95] by a change in adenosine triphosphate metabolism as shown in patients with chronic disease,[96] or a altered intrinsic muscle function[14] is not clear. The latter study performed a magnetic resonance spectroscopy assessment of forearm and calf muscles of 12- to 17-year-old CF patients during isometric exercise and found higher intracellular pH with less oxidative ATP turnover than in the healthy controls suggesting an intrinsic defect in skeletal muscle function. In line with this hypothesis is the fact that although peak $\dot{V}O_2$ was lower for muscle cross-sectional area in CF subjects, the abnormality causing this did not progressively worsen in older subjects. Whether the muscle function deficit is caused by the malnutrition, by the genetic defect itself, or a combination of both, is, however, not yet clear.

Diabetes

Cystic fibrosis-related insulin-dependent diabetes mellitus (CFRDM) is an age-related complication of CF. In children less than 10 years old. CFRDM is not more prevalent than diabetes in a normal population, but 15% of patients over 35 years develop CFRDM and 43% have a pathological oral glucose tolerance test.[97] Most of the patients are treated the same way as type 1 diabetics. CFRDM can be associated with exercise intolerance, is almost always nonketotic, and has a slow, insidious onset. Physical activity should specially be promoted because it is able to smooth the glucose peaks in the blood. As in type 1 diabetes, the physically active child should be motivated to eat and drink before and during physical activity, especially when it is prolonged and intense, in order to avoid hypoglycaemia. On the basis of the better long-term prognosis in CF, it is more important than ever to provide a good management of diabetes in order to prevent microangiopathy. One way is to promote physical activity which has been described to be associated with improved glycaemic control.[98,99] This could be explained by activation of the AMP kinase system which enhances sensitivity of muscle glucose transport to insulin[100] or by the stimulation of glucose uptake by increased translocation of GLUT4 to the plasma membrane,[101] or by circumvent upstream defects in insulin signal transduction via increased mitochondrial energy metabolism.[102]

Osteopenia/osteoporosis

Children as well as adults with CF demonstrate low bone mass which may lead to osteoporosis with the potential of atraumatic bone fractures. CF patients show a reduced bone density assessed by DXA[103–105] or peripheral computer tomography (qCT).[106] Higher fracture incidences, in particular vertebral fractures, have been documented in adolescent and adult patients with CF.[103,107–110] In general, patients with advanced lung disease and those with the lowest muscle mass consistently show the least bone mass.[105,111,112] Newer data, however, show that even very small children with CF before the age of 6 years show decreased bone mineral densities comparable to older children and adolescents even in the absence of severe lung disease and normal nutritional state.[113] Pathophysiologically, there is a decrease in bone formation and sometimes,[105,114,115] but not always,[116] an increase in bone resorption. Recently, CFTR has been shown to be expressed in human osteoblasts, osteocytes, and osteoclasts,[117] and CFTR-null mice show an abnormal skeletal phenotype with striking osteopenia, reduced cortical width, and thinning of the trabeculae.[118] Although there is not yet proof, CFTR is expressed in bone cells and might have a physiological role in bone metabolism.

As in a healthy population, risk factors such as nutrition, low muscle mass, physical inactivity, delayed puberty, and steroid therapy are major causes of osteopenia. These factors often occur together in patients with CF augmenting the risk for low bone mass. There is a consistent correlation between body mass and bone density, with underweight patients showing the lowest bone mass[103,104, 106,119] compatible with the tight association between muscle and bone mass in general. There are few data on the effect of physical activity on bone mass in CF. Exercise capacity, expressed as $\dot{V}O_2$ max and BMI have been found to be significant predictors of bone mass in CF[120] and the level of physical activity was associated with bone mineral density (BMD) in children and adults with CF,[121,122] suggesting that bone mass might indeed be influenced by loading not only in the general population but also in those with CF.

Dehydration

CF patients have a low tolerance to climatic heat stress, which has been shown to increase morbidity and mortality among CF patients.[123,124] Dehydration might also decrease strength[125] and aerobic exercise performance.[126] The thermoregulatory ability among children with CF, who exercised 1.5–3 hours in a hot climate nevertheless seems to be normal. However, unlike healthy people who usually increase their extracellular osmolality as a result of sweating, CF patients had a decline in serum sodium chloride (NaCl) and osmolality during exposures to the heat.[127,128] This resulted from the much higher loss of NaCl in the sweat of exercising CF patients, compared to healthy controls. One of the triggers for thirst is an increase in extracellular osmolality which, in turn, stimulates hypothalamic osmoreceptors.[129–131] It is thus possible that patients with CF, whose sweating does not induce a normal increase in extracellular osmolality, would be deprived of this trigger for thirst. Indeed, children with CF, when allowed to drink water *ad libitum* during exposure to hot climate, drank half as much and dehydrated almost three times as much as healthy controls.[128] Children and adolescents with CF must therefore be encouraged to drink above and beyond thirst, especially when they exercise in warm or humid climates. In addition, they should be encouraged to ingest electrolyte solutions with a high-NaCl content (preferably ≥50 mmol·L^{-1}) rather than water alone which has been shown to prevent dehydration.[132] It is possible that the improvement in palatability of a high-sodium beverage would induce an even greater voluntary fluid intake.

Beneficial effects of exercise and physical activity

Many studies have been conducted over the past 30 years which suggest that exercise training can improve aerobic fitness,[133,134] maintain or lessen the decrease of pulmonary function,[135] improve health-related quality of life,[28] and possibly even prolong life. A recent Cochrane review[136] provides some limited evidence from seven randomized (see Table 33.2) or quasi-randomized controlled short- and long-term studies[8,133–135,137–139] that aerobic and anaerobic physical training has a positive effect on exercise capacity, strength, and pulmonary function. Fourteen studies were excluded as they were not randomized controlled trials or did not involve a programme of physical training or involved respiratory muscle training only.[28,90,129,140–147] They were hesitant to conclude that physical training is indeed effective due to the small sample size, short duration, and incomplete reporting of the studies. Orenstein and Higgins[148] in their recent update on the role of exercise in CF added an important reflection: on the basis of the expected decline in pulmonary function in patients with CF of 2–3% per year, an exercise intervention study shorter than 12 months may be unable to detect a difference in pulmonary function between control and intervention subjects. If we apply this statement to the existing randomized controlled studies, there are only two of the seven studies[8,135] which fulfil the criterion of a minimum of 1 year of intervention. However, both of them showed some beneficial effects including less annual decline in FVC[8,135] and exercise performance.[8]

Some authors assessed the effect of inspiratory muscle training on lung function and exercise capacity in CF.[149–152] Enright *et al.*[151] were the only ones who adjusted the workload of the inspiratory muscles to maximal inspiratory effort at each training session and thus adjusted inspiratory effort to the 80% of maximum. High-intensity inspiratory muscle training significantly improved inspiratory muscle function, aerobic work capacity, FVC and TLC, diaphragmatic thickness, and also anxiety and depression scores.

The reason why regular physical activity and exercise might be effective in decreasing the loss of pulmonary function is not well understood and still a matter of debate. It is possible that mechanical vibrations of the body and increased ventilation facilitate mechanical cleaning of the airways.[153,154] Physical activity further inhibits the Amilorid-sensitive sodium channel in respiratory epithelium.[155] As such, the inhibition of luminal sodium conductance could increase water content of the mucus in the CF lung during exercise and therefore facilitates mucus expectoration. Exercise has also been shown to stimulate anabolic mediators such as growth hormone and insulin-like growth factor I in CF[92] and might further act as in the healthy population through improvement of insulin resistance, immune function,[156] induction of tissue growth factors, or through altered neuroendocrine control of metabolism as suggested by Cooper.[157] All these factors may, at least in part, explain the beneficial effects of exercise in patients with CF.

In general, there seems to be a beneficial effect of different exercise and physical activity regimens on exercise capacity, pulmonary function, muscle strength, and quality of life in youth with CF. Many of these studies have to be interpreted with caution. Factors such as small sample sizes, the lack of an adequate control group, no follow up assessments, or short intervention periods of less than 2 months are some of the possible limitations to be considered. More studies are needed to test long-term effects, optimal training mode (aerobic vs. anaerobic vs. strength vs. inspiratory muscles) and supply (supervised vs. unsupervised, hospital vs. home based), which is most beneficial and also most attractive to patients with CF so that compliance stays high and long-term effects occur.

Harmful effects of exercise and physical activity

The risks of exercise and physical activity in patients with CF are consequences of the pathophysiological processes described above and will therefore not be discussed again but are summarized in Table 33.3.

Table 33.2 Randomized controlled exercise intervention trials in CF

Author	Training	Duration†	Age	Exercise**	Results pulmonary function	Quality of life	Weight	Follow up
Cerny[174]	AT	<1	Ch+A	ΔHR, ΔWR, ΔVE ns	ΔPF ns			
Klijn[133]	ANT	3	C	ΔVO2peak sig, ΔLac sig, ΔWR sig, ΔPP sig, ΔMP sig	ΔFVC ns	ΔQoL ns	ΔBC ns	[2]ΔPP sig, ΔMP sig, ΔQoL sig, ΔPA ns
Michel[138]	AT	<1	Ch+A					[1]ΔWt sig
Moorcroft[8]	Mixed	12	A	ΔHRleg sig, ΔVEleg ns, ΔVEarm sig, ΔLacleg sig, ΔLacarm ns, ΔBorg ns	ΔFEV1 ns, ΔFVC sig		ΔBMI ns	
Schneiderman-Walker[135]	AT	36	Ch+A	ΔVO2 ns, ΔHR ns, ΔWR ns, ΔMMV ns	ΔFEV1 ns, ΔFVC sig	ΔQoL sig	Δ%WfH ns	
Selvadurai[134]	AT, ANT	<1	Ch	AT: ΔVO2 sig, ΔSO2 sig, ΔStrength sig, ΔPA sig	AT: ΔFEV1 ns, ΔFVC ns	AT: ΔQoL sig	AT: ΔWt ns, ΔFFM ns	[1]AT: only ΔPA ns, rest idem results ANT: ΔPA ns, rest idem results
				ANT: ΔVO2 ns, ΔSO2 sig, ΔStrength sig, ΔPA sig	ANT: ΔFEV1 sig, ΔFVC ns	ANT: ΔQoL ns	ANT: ΔWt sig, ΔFFM sig	
Turchetta[139]*	AT	<1	Ch					

[1]Follow up at 1 month.

[2]Follow up at 3 months.

*Only in abstract form.

†Duration in months.

**Results at peak exercise.

AT = aerobic training, ANT = anaerobic training, mixed = AT and ANT, Ch = children, A = adults, HR = heart rate, WR = workrate, Lac = lactate, PP = peak power, MP = mean power, VE = minute ventilation, Borg = scale of perceived exertion, MMV = maximal voluntary ventilation, SO_2 = oxygen saturation, PA = physical activity, PF = pulmonary function, FVC = forced vital capacity, FEV1 = forced expiratory volume in 1 sec, QoL = quality of life, BC = body composition, BMI = body mass index, %WfH = %ideal weight for height, Wt = weight, FFM = fat-free mass.

Table 33.3 Harmful effects of exercise in patients with CF

Symptom	Comment
Hypoxaemia	Especially with FEV_1 < 50% predicted or SO_2 < 94%)
Exercise-induced bronchoconstriction	Repeated therapeutic control is recommended
Decreased body weight	When increased demands are not compensated
Dehydration	Especially with long exercise in warm environment
Hypoglycaemia	
Fractures	With osteoporosis
Pneumothorax	Contact sports, diving, weight training (?)
Trauma of liver, spleen, esophageal varices	Contact sports, bungee jumping, sky diving
Arrhythmias	

Exercise testing and recommendations

Since $\dot{V}O_2$ max has become one of the best predictors of mortality in CF[39,61] and exercise has been proven to be helpful in improving health[8,135] and quality of life in CF,[28,135] a regular exercise test is recommended for each child and adolescent. Despite the strong evidence and even recommendations in standard care guidelines for CF, exercise testing is not performed on a regular basis in most CF centres.[158,159] Beside the determination of risk factors for exercise, it might be the basis for establishing training recommendations and to document a training effect, and finally it might be a good means of motivation. If exercise testing is not done in a routine manner, it is highly recommended in all patients who

(i) experience some sort of symptoms at exercise, such as cough, dyspnoea, cyanosis, and fatigue;

(ii) are with a FEV_1 < 50% and/or FVC < 70%;

(iii) fear to have any harmful effect from any type of physical activity;

(iv) want to start a training programme;

(v) want to document training success.

We advocate a yearly exercise test in all individuals with CF in order to monitor exercise symptoms and disease progress. Most studies looking at exercise performance cross-sectionally or longitudinally have used a progressive bicycle or a treadmill test. The Godfrey protocol[160] (Table 33.4) has been used most frequently. In our experience, this is an easy protocol which is not too strenuous and takes body size and low levels of physical fitness into consideration. Alternatively, an age-adjusted ramp protocol very similar to the protocol of Godfrey, that is, 10 W·min^{-1} for age 6–9 years, 15 W·min^{-1} for age 10–13 years, and 20 W·min^{-1} for older children and adolescents has been used.[161] Likewise, 6-min walking tests[162–164] and the shuttle run test[165] have been suggested which can easily be performed. In the 6-min walking test patients walk in a hospital corridor over a distance of 8 m[163,164] and 40 m[162] back and forth while the walking distance over a 6-min period is measured. Incremental cycle ergometry,[166] the 6-min walking test,[164] and shuttle run[165] have been shown to be reliable and valid within the CF population. For those patients who are unable or unwilling to perform a maximal exercise test or to document the change in functional exercise status, submaximal testing has been proposed.[167] In order to find a level of exercise which is safe and beneficial in the patients with CF, anaerobic threshold can be determined even in the absence of a maximal exercise test. With a progressive workload increase during an incremental exercise test, a critical exercise intensity is reached above which blood lactate levels increase progressively with an abrupt rise in lactate concentration at some point, that is, at the lactate threshold. A non-invasive accurate surrogate of the lactate threshold in healthy subjects is the ventilatory threshold which is defined as the point during incremental exercise when ventilation increases out of proportion to $\dot{V}O_2$ (see ref. 168 and Chapter 6). McLoughlin *et al.*,[2] however, showed that the ventilatory threshold significantly overestimated lactate threshold in subjects with CF because of impaired CO_2 excretion. He suggested using the gas exchange threshold instead, which is the point during an incremental exercise where CO_2 increases out of proportion to $\dot{V}O_2$. This approach has been shown to correlate well with lactate threshold in chronic obstructive pulmonary disease in general[169,170] and is an easy non-invasive means of finding the anaerobic threshold. The gas exchange threshold has been shown to be reliable and valid in CF patients of all degrees of severity.[171]

Whatever test is performed, it should identify the patients whose oxygen levels fall during exercise. It is recommended that patients with CF should exercise at an intensity which allows the oxygen saturation to stay above 90%. Note that front oximetry is the preferred method, since finger oximetry has been shown to be less accurate due to motion artefacts and altered digital perfusion which can even be more altered in CF than in a healthy population.[172] The heart rate at which desaturation below 90% occurs can be noted and the patient can make sure that his exercise intensity does not exceed this level. If desaturation occurs at a very low intensity level, oxygen supplementation during exercise can be discussed. Another aim of the test is to evaluate each patient's own maximal heart rate or anaerobic threshold, to be able to prescribe an optimal training intensity. Generally, 70–80% of maximal heart rate or 85% of anaerobic threshold is considered to be beneficial for efficient aerobic training in health and disease. Retesting within 3–6 months will reassure the patient and allow the physician to evaluate the progression of the disease. We recommend performing an exercise test at least every 12 months. Always consider a change in body composition when comparing the data longitudinally. We recommend that the performance should at least be related to body weight, but better to lean body mass. Each training recommendation should include information about the frequency, intensity, and duration or time of the sport programme. Similar to healthy persons, it should be performed at least three times, better five times per week, at an intensity level of 70–80% of maximal capacity or 85% of anaerobic threshold and for the duration of 30 min. Most of the beginners are not capable of performing such a programme initially and should be allowed to reach this level within 2 or 3 months. An appropriate increase is 10% per week, either in intensity or duration. Very often, intermittent training with a lot of breaks helps to start or can be used for those not tolerating constant exercise. In this case, exercise bouts may last 2 min interspersed with 1-min breaks. The exercise intensity can be set as for the constant load exercise but might even be more intense due to the allowed recovery periods. On the basis of the information of the training programmes with CF patients, the youngsters should be informed that a clear training effect is not expected before 2–3 months. Strength training can be applied as in the healthy population.

Table 33.4 Protocol to assess aerobic exercise capacity

Rate (rpm)	Load (W)	Increment (W)	Height (cm)	Stage duration (min)
60	10	10	<120	1
60	15	15	120–150	1
60	20	20	>150	1

From Godfrey *et al.*[173]

There are several specific sports which should be prohibited for the young patient with CF, especially in an advanced stage of disease. One is scuba diving, another is sports at high altitude. In both types of activities detrimental situations can occur in which oxygen becomes limited and severe desaturation can occur over longer periods. Furthermore, contact sports can cause trauma to an enlarged liver or spleen, and bungee jumping or sky diving increase the risk for pneumothorax and variceal bleeding. For all other sports there is no contraindication.

We always recommend the young CF patient to perform various sports in combination. Team sports are extremely important for the self-esteem and social integration of any child with a chronic disease. When they are well integrated in a team, they feel healthy and 'normal' and even forget about their disease. It is helpful to inform the team and coach about the child's disease and allow him/her to take breaks or run slower whenever needed. An individual sport has the advantage that it can be performed at an individual pace without interfering with anybody else. This type of exercise is especially important, if the disease becomes advanced in order to keep the young person active but without constantly showing him/her the progression of the disease. In these progressed stages, it can be very helpful to search for sports where skills such as reactivity, coordination, and flexibility are more important than aerobic capacity or strength. Goal keeper, tennis, table tennis, rock climbing, dance, golf are some examples. In general, the child should be allowed to perform any sport beside the exceptions mentioned above. As long as the motivation and fun aspect is apparent, the best possible adherence and compliance is reached. Again, the orientation of the coach and team members about the child's health condition seems to be the best way to allow an optimal tolerance and integration of the young patient with CF into the sports world.

Summary

- Exercise capacity in CF is reduced when disease becomes moderate to severe due to a reduced function of the muscle, heart, or lungs. Whether the various functions are reduced due to the inherited genetic defect of the CF mutation itself, whether it is a consequence of progressive chronic disease, or whether it is inactivity-related which often goes hand in hand with chronic progressive disease in youth is not fully understood.
- There is evidence of positive effects of exercise training in CF on exercise performance, decline of pulmonary function, quality of life and maybe even longevity, especially when it is aerobic in nature. Possible harmful effects of exercise such as hypoxaemia, hypoglycaemia, or bleeding from altered organs have to be considered, especially with the progression of the disease.
- Different gaps in the current literature need to be filled:
  - (i) Search on pathophysiological mechanisms of exercise limitations to find out whether they can be attained (or not) by therapeutic strategies.
  - (ii) More exercise trials are needed to find the best exercise modalities to slow down disease progression, to keep the compliance of the patients high, and to reach a maximum of quality of life.

References

1. Ratjen F, Doring G (2003). Cystic fibrosis. *Lancet* **361**, 681–9.
2. McLoughlin P, McKeogh D, Byrne P, Finlay G, Hayes J, FitzGerald MX (1997). Assessment of fitness in patients with cystic fibrosis and mild lung disease. *Thorax* **52**, 425–30.
3. Marcotte JE, Canny GJ, Grisdale R (1986). Effects of nutritional status on exercise performance in advanced cystic fibrosis. *Chest* **90**, 375–9.
4. Marcotte JE, Grisdale RK, Levison H, Coates AL, Canny GJ (1986). Multiple factors limit exercise in cystic fibrosis. *Pediatr Pulmonol* **2**, 274–81.
5. Klijn PH, Terheggen-Lagro SW, Van Der Ent CK, Van Der Net J, Kimpen JL, Helders PJ (2003). Anaerobic exercise in pediatric cystic fibrosis. *Pediatr Pulmonol* **36**, 223–9.
6. Klijn PH, van der Net J, Kimpen JL, Helders PJ, van der Ent CK (2003). Longitudinal determinants of peak aerobic performance in children with cystic fibrosis. *Chest* **124**, 2215–9.
7. Cerny FJ, Pullano T, Cropp GJA (1982) Adaptation to exercise in children with cystic fibrosis. In: Nagle FJ, Montoye HJ (eds.), *Exercise in health and disease*, pp. 36–42. Thomas, Springfield, IL.
8. Moorcroft AJ, Dodd ME, Morris J, Webb AK (2004). Individualised unsupervised exercise training in adults with cystic fibrosis: A 1 year randomised controlled trial. *Thorax* **59**, 1074–80.
9. Moorcroft AJ, Dodd ME, Morris J, Webb AK (2005). Symptoms, lactate and exercise limitation at peak cycle ergometry in adults with cystic fibrosis. *Eur Respir J* **25**, 1050–6.
10. Coates AL, Boyce P, Muller D, Mearns M, Godfrey S (1980). The role of nutritional status, airway obstruction, hypoxia, and abnormalities in serum lipid composition in limiting exercise tolerance in children with cystic fibrosis. *Acta Paediatr Scand* **69**, 353–8.
11. Lands LC, Heigenhauser GJ, Jones NL (1992). Analysis of factors limiting maximal exercise performance in cystic fibrosis. *Clin Sci (Lond)* **83**, 391–7.
12. Moser C, Tirakitsoontorn P, Nussbaum E, Newcomb R, Cooper DM (2000). Muscle size and cardiorespiratory response to exercise in cystic fibrosis. *Am J Respir Crit Care Med* **162**, 1823–7.
13. Selvadurai HC, Allen J, Sachinwalla T, Macauley J, Blimkie CJ, Van Asperen PP (2003). Muscle function and resting energy expenditure in female athletes with cystic fibrosis. *Am J Respir Crit Care Med* **168**, 1476–80.
14. de Meer K, Jeneson JA, Gulmans VA, van der Laag J, Berger R (1995). Efficiency of oxidative work performance of skeletal muscle in patients with cystic fibrosis. *Thorax* **50**, 980–3.
15. Benson LN, Newth CJ, Desouza M, Lobraico R, Kartodihardjo W, Corkey C, Gilday D, Olley PM (1984). Radionuclide assessment of right and left ventricular function during bicycle exercise in young patients with cystic fibrosis. *Am Rev Respir Dis* **130**, 987–92.
16. Perrault H, Coughlan M, Marcotte JE, Drblik SP, Lamarre A (1992). Comparison of cardiac output determinants in response to upright and supine exercise in patients with cystic fibrosis. *Chest* **101**, 42–51.
17. Hortop J, Desmond KJ, Coates AL (1988). The mechanical effects of expiratory airflow limitation on cardiac performance in cystic fibrosis. *Am Rev Respir Dis* **137**, 132–7.
18. Nixon PA, Orenstein DM, Kelsey SF (2001). Habitual physical activity in children and adolescents with cystic fibrosis. *Med Sci Sports Exerc* **33**, 30–5.
19. Selvadurai HC, Blimkie CJ, Cooper PJ, Mellis CM, Van Asperen PP (2004). Gender differences in habitual activity in children with cystic fibrosis. *Arch Dis Child* **89**, 928–33.
20. Hebestreit H, Kieser S, Rudiger S, Schenk T, Junge S, Hebestreit A, Ballmann M, Posselt HG, Kriemler S (2006). Physical activity is independently related to aerobic capacity in cystic fibrosis. *Eur Respir J* **28**, 734–9.
21. Balfour-Lynn IM, Elborn JS (2002). 'CF asthma': What is it and what do we do about it? *Thorax* **57**, 742–8.
22. Davis PB (1993) *Cystic fibrosis.* Marcel Dekker Inc, New York.
23. Landau LI, Phelan PD (1973). The spectrum of cystic fibrosis. *Am Rev Respir Dis* **108**, 593–602.
24. Zapletal A, Motoyama EK, Gibson LE, Bouhuys A (1971). Pulmonary mechanics in asthma and cystic fibrosis. *Pediatrics* **48**, 64–72.
25. Corey M, McLaughlin FJ, Wiliams M, Levison H (1988). A comparison of survival, growth, and pulmonary function in patients with cystic fibrosis in Boston and Toronto. *J Clin Epidemiol* **41**, 583–91.
26. Keochkerian D, Chlif M, Delanaud S, Gauthier R, Maingourd Y, Ahmaidi S (2005). Timing and driving components of the breathing strategy in children with cystic fibrosis during exercise. *Pediatr Pulmonol* **40**, 449–56.
27. Godfrey S, Mearns M (1971). Pulmonary function and responses to exercise in cystic fibrosis. *Arch Dis Child* **46**, 144–51.
28. Orenstein DM, Franklin BA, Doershuk CF, Hellerstein HK, Germann KJ, Horowitz JG, Stern RC (1981). Exercise conditioning and cardiopulmonary fitness in cystic fibrosis. The effects of a three-month supervised running program. *Chest* **80**, 392–8.
29. Moorcroft AJ, Dodd ME, Webb AK (1997). Long-term change in exercise capacity, body mass, and pulmonary function in adults with cystic fibrosis. *Chest* **111**, 338–43.
30. Webb AK, Dodd ME, Moorcroft J (1995). Exercise in cystic fibrosis. *J Roy Soc Med* **88** (Suppl.), 30–6.
31. Mador MJ (1991). Respiratory muscle fatigue and breathing pattern. *Chest* **100**, 1430–5.
32. Levison H, Cherniack RM (1968). Ventilatory cost of exercise in chronic obstructive pulmonary disease. *J Appl Physiol* **25**, 21–7.
33. Marcus CL, Bader D, Stabile MW, Wang CI, Osher AB, Keens TG (1992). Supplemental oxygen and exercise performance in patients with cystic fibrosis with severe pulmonary disease. *Chest* **101**, 52–7.
34. Keochkerian D, Chlif M, Delanaud S, Gauthier R, Maingourd Y, Ahmaidi S (2008). Breathing pattern adopted by children with cystic fibrosis with mild to moderate pulmonary impairment during exercise. *Respiration* **75**, 170–7.

35. Coates AL, Canny G, Zinman R, Grisdale R, Desmond K, Roumeliotis D, Levision H (1988). The effects of chronic airflow limitation, increased dead space, and the pattern of ventilation on gas exchange during maximal exercise in advanced cystic fibrosis. *Am Rev Respir Dis* **138**, 1524–31.
36. Cerny FJ, Pullano T, Cropp GJA (1982). Cardiorespiratory adaptations to exercise in cystic fibrosis. *Am Rev Respir Dis* **126**, 217–20.
37. Javadpour SM, Selvadurai H, Wilkes DL, Schneiderman-Walker J, Coates AL (2005). Does carbon dioxide retention during exercise predict a more rapid decline in FEV1 in cystic fibrosis? *Arch Dis Child* **90**, 792–5.
38. Pianosi P, Wolstein R (1996). Carbon dioxide chemosensitivity and exercise ventilation in healthy children and in children with cystic fibrosis. *Pediatr Res* **40**, 508–13.
39. Nixon PA, Orenstein DM, Kelsey Sf, Doershuk CF (1992). The prognostic value of exercise testing in patients with cystic fibrosis. *N Engl J Med* **327**, 1785–8.
40. Henke KG, Orenstein DM (1984). Oxygen saturation during exercise in cystic fibrosis. *Am Rev Respir Dis* **129**, 708–11.
41. Cropp GJA, Pullano TP, Cerny FJ, Nathanson IT (1982). Exercise tolerance and cardiorespiratory adjustments at peak work capacity in cystic fibrosis. *Am Rev Respir Dis* **126**, 211–6.
42. Nixon PA, Orenstein DM, Curtis SE, Ross EA (1990). Oxygen supplementation during exercise in cystic fibrosis. *Am Rev Respir Dis* **142**, 807–11.
43. McKone EF, Barry SC, Fitzgerald MX, Gallagher CG (2005). Role of arterial hypoxemia and pulmonary mechanics in exercise limitation in adults with cystic fibrosis. *J Appl Physiol* **99**, 1012–18.
44. Payen JF, Wuyam B, Levy P (1993). Muscular metabolism during oxygen supplementation in patients with chronic hypoxemia. *Am Rev Respir Dis* **147**, 592–8.
45. King M, Brock G, Lundell C (1985). Clearance of mucus by simulated cough. *J Appl Physiol* **58**, 1776–82.
46. Holzer FJ, Olinsky A, Phelan PD (1981). Variability of airways hyperreactivity and allergy in cystic fibrosis. *Arch Dis Child* **56**, 455–9.
47. Silverman M, Hobbs FD, Gordon IR (1978). Cystic fibrosis, atopy and airways lability. *Arch Dis Child* **53**, 873–8.
48. Morgan WJ, Butler SM, Johnson CA, Colin AA, FitzSimmons SC, Geller DE, Konstan MW, Light MJ, Rabin HR, Regelmann WE, Schidlow DV, Stokes DC, Wohl ME, Kaplowitz H, Wyatt MM, Stryker S (1999). Epidemiologic study of cystic fibrosis: Design and implementation of a prospective, multicenter, observational study of patients with cystic fibrosis in the U.S. and Canada. *Pediatr Pulmonol* **28**, 231–41.
49. Koch C, McKenzie SG, Kaplowitz H, Hodson ME, Harms HK, Navarro J, Mastella G (1997). International practice patterns by age and severity of lung disease in cystic fibrosis: Data from the Epidemiologic Registry of Cystic Fibrosis (ERCF). *Pediatr Pulmonol* **24**, 147–54.
50. Konstan MW, Butler SM, Schidlow DV, Morgan WJ, Julius JR, Johnson CA (1999). Patterns of medical practice in cystic fibrosis: Part II. Use of therapies. Investigators and Coordinators of the Epidemiologic Study of Cystic Fibrosis. *Pediatr Pulmonol* **28**, 248–54.
51. Day G, Mearn HB (1973). Bronchial lability in cystic fibrosis. **48**, 355–9.
52. Skorecki K, Levison H, Crozier DN (1976). Bronchial lability in cystic fibrosis. *Acta Pediatr Scand* **65**, 39–42.
53. Price JF, Weller PH, Harper SA, Metthew DJ (1979). Response to bronchial provocation and exercise in children with cystic fibrosis. *Clin Allergy* **9**, 563–70.
54. Dodd JD, Barry SC, Daly LE, Gallagher CG (2005). Inhaled beta-agonists improve lung function but not maximal exercise capacity in cystic fibrosis. *J Cyst Fibros* **4**, 101–5.
55. Brand PL (2000). Bronchodilators in cystic fibrosis. *J R Soc Med* **93** (Suppl. 38), 37–9.
56. Serisier DJ, Coates AD, Bowler SD (2007). Effect of albuterol on maximal exercise capacity in cystic fibrosis. *Chest* **131**, 1181–7.
57. Kusenbach G, Friedrichs F, Skopnik H, Heimann G (1993). Increased physiological dead space during exercise after bronchodilation in cystic fibrosis. *Pediatr Pulmonol* **15**, 273–8.
58. Pianosi P, Pelech A (1996). Stroke volume during exercise in cystic fibrosis. *Am J Respir Crit Care Med* **153**, 1105–9.
59. Chipps BE, Alderson PO, Roland JMA, Yang AV, Martinez CR, Rosenstein BJ (1979). Non-invasive evaluation of ventricular function in cystic fibrosis. *J Pediatr* **95**, 379–84.
60. Nezelof C, Bouvier R, Dijoud F (2002). Multifocal myocardial necrosis: a distinctive cardiac lesion in cystic fibrosis, lipomatous pancreatic atrophy, and Keshan disease. *Pediatr Pathol Molec Med* **21**, 343–52.
61. Pianosi P, Leblanc J, Almudevar A (2005). Peak oxygen uptake and mortality in children with cystic fibrosis. *Thorax* **60**, 50–4.
62. Kerem E, Reisman J, Corey M, Canny GJ, Levison H (1992). Prediction of mortality in patients with cystic fibrosis. *N Engl J Med* **326**, 1187–91.
63. Schneiderman-Walker J, Wilkes DL, Strug L, Lands LC, Pollock SL, Selvadurai HC, Hay J, Coates AL, Corey M (2005). Sex differences in habitual physical activity and lung function decline in children with cystic fibrosis. *J Pediatr* **147**, 321–6.
64. Boucher GP, Lands LC, Hay JA, Hornby L (1997). Activity levels and the relationship to lung function and nutritional status in children with cystic fibrosis. *Am J Phys Med Rehab* **76**, 311–15.
65. Borgo G, Astella G, Gasparini P, Zorzanella A, Doro R, Pignatti PF (1990). Pancreatic function and gene deletion F508 in cystic fibrosis. *J Med Genet* **27**, 665–9.
66. Kerem E, Corey M, Kerem B-S, Rommens J, Markiewicz D, Levison H, Tsui L-C, Durie P (1990). The relation between genotype and phenotype in cystic fibrosis. *N Engl J Med* **323**, 1517–22.
67. Schoni MH, Casaulta-Aebischer C (2000). Nutrition and lung function in cystic fibrosis patients: Review. *Clin Nutr (Edin)* **19**, 79–85.
68. Kraemer R, Rudeberg A, Hadorn B, Rossi E (1978). Relative underweight in cystic fibrosis and its prognostic value. *Acta Paediatr Scand* **67**, 33–7.
69. Levy LD, Durie PR, Pencharz PB, Corey ML (1985). Effects of long-term nutritional rehabilitation on body composition and clinical status in malnourished children and adolescents with cystic fibrosis. *J Pediatr* **107**, 225–30.
70. Shepherd RW, Holt TL, Thomas BJ (1986). Nutritional rehabilitation in cystic fibrosis: Controlled studies of effects on nutritional growth retardation, body protein turnover, and course of pulmonary disease. *J Pediatr* **109**, 788–94.
71. Liou TG, Adler FR, Fitzsimmons SC, Cahill BC, Hibbs JR, Marshall BC (2001). Predictive 5-year survivorship model of cystic fibrosis. *Am J Epidemiol* **153**, 345–52.
72. Shale DJ (1997). Predicting survival in cystic fibrosis. *Thorax* **52**, 309.
73. Durie PR, Forstner GG (1989). Pathophysiology of sthe exocrine pancreas in cystic fibrosis. *J R Soc Med* **16**, 1–20.
74. Allen JR, McCauley JC, Selby AM, Waters DL, Gruca MA, Baur LA, Van Asperen P, Gaskin KJ (2003). Differences in resting energy expenditure between male and female children with cystic fibrosis. *J Pediatr* **142**, 15–19.
75. Vaisman N, Penchanrz PB, Corey M, Canny GJ (1987). Energy expenditure of patients with cystic fibrosis. *J Pediatr* **111**, 496–500.
76. Fried MD (1991). The cystic fibrosis gene and resting energy expenditure. *J Pediatr* **119**, 913–16.
77. Richards ML, Davies PS, Bell SC (2001). Energy cost of physical activity in cystic fibrosis. *Eur J Clin Nutr* **55**, 690–7.
78. Koletzko S, Koletzko B (1983) Zystische Fibrose—Normalernährung oder ernährungstherapien. In: Koletzko B (ed.), *Ernährung chronisch kranker kinder und jugendlicher*. Springer, Berlin, Deutschland.
79. Bolton CE, Ionescu AA, Evans WD, Pettit RJ, Shale DJ (2003). Altered tissue distribution in adults with cystic fibrosis. *Thorax* **58**, 885–9.
80. Ionescu AA, Nixon LS, Evans WD, Stone MD, Lewis-Jenkins V, Chatham K, Shale DJ (2000). Bone density, body composition, and inflammatory status in cystic fibrosis. *Am J Respir Crit Care Med* **162**, 789–94.

81. Ionescu AA, Nixon LS, Luzio S, Lewis-Jenkins V, Evans WD, Stone MD, Owens DR, Routledge PA, Shale DJ (2002). Pulmonary function, body composition, and protein catabolism in adults with cystic fibrosis. *Am J Respir Crit Care Med* **165**, 495–500.
82. Lands LC, Gordon C, Bar-Or O, Blimkie CJ, Hanning RM, Jones NL, Moss LA, Webber CE, Wilson WM, Heigenhauser GJF (1993). Comparison of three techniques for body composition analysis in cystic fibrosis. *J Appl Physiol* **75**, 162–6.
83. King S, Wilson J, Kotsimbos T, Bailey M, Nyulasi I (2005). Body composition assessment in adults with cystic fibrosis: Comparison of dual-energy X-ray absorptiometry with skinfolds and bioelectrical impedance analysis. *Nutrition* **21**, 1087–94.
84. Quirk PC, Ward LC, Thomas BJ, Holt TL, Shepherd RW, Cornish BH (1997). Evaluation of bioelectrical impedance for prospective nutritional assessment in cystic fibrosis. *Nutrition* **13**, 412–16.
85. Shah AR, Gozal D, Keens TG (1998). Determinants of aerobic and anaerobic exercise performance in cystic fibrosis. *Am J Respir Crit Care Med* **157**, 1145–50.
86. Cabrera ME, Lough MD, Doershuk CF, DeRivera GA (1993). Anaerobic performance—Assessed by the Wingate Test—In patients with cystic fibrosis. *Pediatr Exerc Sci* **5**, 78–87.
87. Boas SR, Joswiak ML, Nixon PA, Fulton JA, Orenstien DM (1996). Factors limiting anaerobic performance in adolescent males with cystic fibrosis. *Med Sci Sports Exerc* **28**, 291–8.
88. Skeie B, Askanazi J, Rothkopf MM, Rosenbaum SH, Kvetan V, Ross E (1987). Improved exercise tolerance with long-term parenteral nutrition in cystic fibrosis. *Crit Care Med* **15**, 960–2.
89. Hanning RM, Blimkie CJR, Bar-Or O, Lands LC, Moss LA, Wilson WM (1993). Relationships among nutritional status and skeletal and respiratory muscle function in cystic fibrosis: does early dietary supplementation make a difference? *Am J Clin Nutr* **57**, 580–7.
90. Heijerman HGM, Bakker W, Sterk PJ, Dijkman JH (1992). Long-term effects of exercise training and hyperalimentation in adult cystic fibrosis patients with severe pulmonary dysfunction. *Int J Rehab Res* **15**, 252–7.
91. Bertrand JM, Morin CL, Lasalle R, Ptrick J, Coates AL (1984). Short-term clinical, nutritional, and functional effects of continuous elemental enteral alimentation in children with cystic fibrosis. *J Pediatr* **104**, 41–6.
92. Tirakitsoontorn P, Nussbaum E, Moser C, Hill M, Cooper DM (2001). Fitness, acute exercise, and anabolic and catabolic mediators in cystic fibrosis. *Am J Respir Crit Care Med* **164**, 1432–7.
93. Lands LC, Grey V, Smountas AA, Kramer VG, McKenna D (1999). Lymphocyte glutathione levels in children with cystic fibrosis. *Chest* **116**, 201–5.
94. Hebestreit H, Hebestreit A, Trusen A, Hughson RL (2005). Oxygen uptake kinetics are slowed in cystic fibrosis. *Med Sci Sports Exerc* **37**, 10–7.
95. Troutman WB, Barstow TJ, Galindo AJ, Cooper DM (1998). Abnormal dynamic cardiorespiratory responses to exercise in pediatric patients after Fontan procedure. *J Am Coll Cardiol* **31**, 668–73.
96. Society AT, Society ER (1999). Skeletal muscle dysfunction in chronic obstructive pulmonary disease. *Am J Resp Crit Care Med* **159**, S1–S40.
97. Yankaskas JR, Marshall BC, Sufian B, Simon RH, Rodman D (2004). Cystic fibrosis adult care: consensus conference report. *Chest* **125**, 1S–39S.
98. Huttunen NP, Kaar ML, Knip M, Mustonen A, Puukka R, Akerblom HK (1984). Physical fitness of children and adolescents with insulin-dependent diabetes mellitus. *Ann Clin Res* **16**, 1–5.
99. Sackey AH, Jefferson IG (1996). Physical activity and glycaemic control in children with diabetes mellitus. *Diabet Med* **13**, 789–93.
100. Fisher JS, Gao J, Han DH, Holloszy JO, Nolte LA (2002). Activation of AMP kinase enhances sensitivity of muscle glucose transport to insulin. *Am J Physiol Endocrinol Metab* **282**, E18–23.
101. Towler MC, Hardie DG (2007). AMP-activated protein kinase in metabolic control and insulin signaling. *Circulation Res* **100**, 328–41.
102. Thyfault JP, Cree MG, Zheng D, Zwetsloot JJ, Tapscott EB, Koves TR, Ilkayeva O, Wolfe RR, Muoio DM, Dohm GL (2007). Contraction of insulin-resistant muscle normalizes insulin action in association with increased mitochondrial activity and fatty acid catabolism. *Am J Physiol Cell Physiol* **292**, C729–39.
103. Henderson RC, Madsen CD (1996). Bone density in children and adolescents with cystic fibrosis. *J Pediatr* **128**, 28–34.
104. Bhudhikanok GS, Lim J, Marcus R, Harkins A, Moss RB, Bachrach LK (1996). Correlates of osteopenia in patients with cystic fibrosis. *Pediatrics* **97**, 103–11.
105. Bhudhikanok GS, Wang M-C, Marcus R, Harkins A, Moss RB, Bachrach LK (1998). Bone acquisition and loss in children and adults with cystic fibrosis: a longitudinal study. *J Pediatr* **133**, 18–27.
106. Gibbens DT, Gilsanz V, Boechat MI, Dufer D, Carlson ME, Wang C-I (1988). Osteoporosis in cystic fibrosis. *J Pediatr* **113**, 295–300.
107. Elkin SL, Fairney A, Burnett S, Kemp M, Kyd P, Burgess J, Compston JE, Hodson ME (2001). Vertebral deformities and low bone mineral density in adults with cystic fibrosis: A cross-sectional study. *Osteoporos Int* **12**, 366–72.
108. Aris RM, Renner JB, Winders AD, Buell HE, Riggs DB, Lester GE, Ontjes DA (1998). Increased rate of fractures and severe kyphosis: Sequelae of living into adulthood with cystic fibrosis. *Ann Intern Med* **128**, 186–93.
109. Rossini M, Del Marco A, Dal Santo F, Gatti D, Braggion C, James G, Adami S (2004). Prevalence and correlates of vertebral fractures in adults with cystic fibrosis. *Bone* **35**, 771–6.
110. Ujhelyi R, Treszl A, Vasarhelyi B, Holics K, Toth M, Arato A, Tulassay T, Tulassay Z, Szathmari M (2004). Bone mineral density and bone acquisition in children and young adults with cystic fibrosis: A follow-up study. *J Pediatr Gastro Nutr* **38**, 401–6.
111. Haworth CS, Selby PL, Horrocks AW, Mawer EB, Adams JE, Webb AK (2002). A prospective study of change in bone mineral density over one year in adults with cystic fibrosis. *Thorax* **57**, 719–23.
112. Gronowitz E, Mellstrom D, Strandvik B (2004). Normal annual increase of bone mineral density during two years in patients with cystic fibrosis. *Pediatrics* **114**, 435–42.
113. Sermet-Gaudelus I, Souberbielle JC, Ruiz JC, Vrielynck S, Heuillon B, Azhar I, Cazenave A, Lawson-Body E, Chedevergne F, Lenoir G (2007). Low bone mineral density in young children with cystic fibrosis. *Am J Respir Crit Care Med* **175**, 951–7.
114. Baroncelli GI, De Luca F, Magazzu G, Arrigo T, Sferlazzas C, Catena C, Bertelloni S, Saggese G (1997). Bone demineralization in cystic fibrosis: evidence of imbalance between bone formation and degradation. *Pediatr Res* **41**, 397–403.
115. Greer RM, Buntain HM, Potter JM, Wainwright CE, Wong JC, O'Rourke PK, Francis PW, Bell SC, Batch JA (2003). Abnormalities of the PTH-vitamin D axis and bone turnover markers in children, adolescents and adults with cystic fibrosis: comparison with healthy controls. *Osteoporos Int* **14**, 404–11.
116. Elkin SL, Vedi S, Bord S, Garrahan NJ, Hodson ME, Compston JE (2002). Histomorphometric analysis of bone biopsies from the iliac crest of adults with cystic fibrosis. *Am J Respir Crit Care Med* **166**, 1470–4.
117. Shead EF, Haworth CS, Condliffe AM, McKeon DJ, Scott MA, Compston JE (2007). Cystic fibrosis transmembrane conductance regulator (CFTR) is expressed in human bone. *Thorax* **62**, 650–1.
118. Dif F, Marty C, Baudoin C, de Vernejoul MC, Levi G (2004). Severe osteopenia in CFTR-null mice. *Bone* **35**, 595–603.
119. Grey AB, Ames RW, Matthews RD, Reid IR (1993). Bone mineral density and body composition in adult patients with cystic fibrosis. *Thorax* **48**, 589–93.
120. Frangolias DD, Pare PD, Kendler DL, Davidson AG, Wong L, Raboud J, Wilcox PG (2003). Role of exercise and nutrition status on bone mineral density in cystic fibrosis. *J Cyst Fibros* **2**, 163–70.

121. Conway SP, Morton AM, Oldroyd B, Truscott JG, White H, Smith AH, Haigh I (2000). Osteoporosis and osteopenia in adults and adolescents with cystic fibrosis: Prevalence and associated factors. *Thorax* **55**, 798–804.
122. Buntain HM, Greer RM, Schluter PJ, Wong JC, Batch JA, Potter JM, Lewindon PJ, Powell E, Wainwright CE, Bell SC (2004). Bone mineral density in Australian children, adolescents and adults with cystic fibrosis: A controlled cross sectional study. *Thorax* **59**, 149–55.
123. Kessler WR, Andersen DH (1951). Heat prostration in fibrocystic disease of the pancreas and other conditions. *Pediatrics* **8**, 648–56.
124. Williams AJ, McKiernan J, Harris F (1976). Heat prostration in children with cystic fibrosis. *BMJ* **2**, 297.
125. Bosco JS, Terjung RL, Greenleaf JE (1968). Effects of progressive hypohydration on maximal isometric musclular strength. *J Sports Med Phys Fitness* **8**, 81–6.
126. Saltin B (1964). Aerobic and anaerobic work capacity after dehydration. *J Appl Physiol* **19**, 1114–8.
127. Orenstein DM, Henke KG, Costill DL, Doershuk CF, Lemon PJ, Stern RC (1983). Exercise and heat stress in cystic fibrosis patients. *Pediatr Res* **17**, 267–9.
128. Bar-Or O, Blimkie CJ, Hay JD, Macdougall JD, Ward DS, Wilson WM (1992). Voluntary dehydration and heat intolerance in cystic fibrosis. *Lancet* **339**, 696–9.
129. Morimoto T, Slabochova Z, Naman RK, Sargent F, 2nd (1967). Sex differences in physiological reactions to thermal stress. *J Appl Physiol* **22**, 526–32.
130. Nose H, Yawata T, Morimoto T (1985). Osmotic factors in restitution from thermal dehydration in rats. *Am J Physiol* **249**, R166–R71.
131. Nose H, Mack GW, Shi X, Nadel ER (1988). The role of plasma osmolality and plasma volume during rehydration in humans. *J Appl Physiol* **65**, 1–7.
132. Kriemler S, Wilk B, Schurer W, Wilson WM, Bar-Or O (1999). Preventing dehydration in children with cystic fibrosis who exercise in the heat. *Med Sci Sports Exerc* **31**, 774–9.
133. Klijn PH, Oudshoorn A, van der Ent CK, van der Net J, Kimpen JL, Helders PJ (2004). Effects of anaerobic training in children with cystic fibrosis: A randomized controlled study. *Chest* **125**, 1299–305.
134. Selvadurai HC, Blimkie CJ, Meyers N, Mellis CM, Cooper PJ, Van Asperen PP (2002). Randomized controlled study of in-hospital exercise training programs in children with cystic fibrosis. *Pediatr Pulmonol* **33**, 194–200.
135. Schneiderman-Walker J, Pollock SL, Corey M, Wilkes DD, Canny GJ, Pedder L, Reisman JJ (2000). A randomized controlled trial of a 3-year home exercise program in cystic fibrosis. *J Pediatr* **136**, 304–10.
136. Bradley J, Moran F (2002). Physical training for cystic fibrosis. *Cochrane database of systematic reviews (Online)*. CD002768.
137. Cerny FJ, Cropp GJA, Bye MR (1984). Hospital therapy improves exercise tolerance and lung function in cystic fibrosis. *Am J Dis Child* **138**, 261–5.
138. Michel SH, Darbee JC, Pequignot E (1989). Exercise, body composition and stregth in cystic fibrosis. *Pediatr Pulmonol* **4** (Suppl), 116.
139. Turchetta A, Bella S, Calzolari A, Castro M, Ciuffetti C, Drago F. (1991). Effect of controlled physical activity on lung function test of cystic fibrosis children. *Proceedings of the 17th European Cystic Fibrosis Conference*, p. 134. Copenhagen, Denmark.
140. Andreasson B, Jonson B, Kornfalt R, Nordmark E, Sandstrom S (1987). Long-term effects of physical exercise on working capacity and pulmonary function in cystic fibrosis. *Acta Paediatr Scand* **76**, 70–5.
141. Bilton D, Dodd ME, Abbot JV, Webb AK (1992). The benefits of exercise combined with physiotherapy in the treatment of adults with cystic fibrosis. *Respir Med* **86**, 507–11.
142. Salh W, Bilton D, Dodd M, Webb AK (1989). Effect of exercise and physiotherapy in aiding sputum expectoration in adults with cystic fibrosis. *Thorax* **44**, 1006–8.
143. de Jong W, Grevink RG, Roorda RJ, Kaptein AA, van der Schans CP (1994). Effect of a home exercise training program in patients with cystic fibrosis. *Chest* **105**, 463–8.
144. Edlund LD, French RW, Herbst JJ, Ruttenberg HD, Ruhling RO, Adams TD (1986). Effects of a swimming program on children with cystic fibrosis. *Am J Dis Child* **140**, 80–3.
145. Albinni S, Rath R, Renner S, Eichler I (2004). Additional inspiratory muscle training intensifies the beneficial effects of cycle ergometer training in patients with cystic fibrosis. *J Cyst Fibros* **3**, S63.
146. Barry SC, Dodd JD, Jensma M, Gallagher C (2001). Benefits of high intensity strength training in adults with cystic fibrosis. *Am J Resp Crit Care Med* **163 (Suppl)**, A968.
147. Kriemler S, Hebestreit A, Kieser S, Bachmann M, Hebestreit H (2001). Six months of training improves lung function and aerobic performance in CF. *J Cyst Fibrosis* **1**, P62.
148. Orenstein DM, Higgins LW (2005). Update on the role of exercise in cystic fibrosis. *Curr Opin Pulmon Med* **11**, 519–23.
149. Keens TG, Krastins IR, Wannamaker EM, Levison H, Crozier ON, Bryan C (1977). Ventilatory muscle endurance training in normal subjects and patients with cystic fibrosis. *Am Rev Respir Dis* **116**, 853–60.
150. Asher MI, Pardy RL, Coates AL, Thomas E, Macklem PT (1982). The effects of inspiratory muscle training in patients with cystic fibrosis. *Am Rev Respir Dis* **126**, 855–9.
151. Enright S, Chatham K, Ionescu AA, Unnithan VB, Shale DJ (2004). Inspiratory muscle training improves lung function and exercise capacity in adults with cystic fibrosis. *Chest* **126**, 405–11.
152. Sawyer EH, Clanton TL (1993). Improved pulmonary function and exercise tolerance with inspiratory muscle conditioning in children with cystic fibrosis. *Chest* **104**, 1490–7.
153. McIlwaine M (2007). Chest physical therapy, breathing techniques and exercise in children with CF. *Paediatr Resp Rev* **8**, 8–16.
154. Orenstein DM, Henke KG, Cerny FJ (1983). Exercise and cystic fibrosis. *Phys Sports Med* **11**, 57–63.
155. Hebestreit A, Kersting U, Basler B, Jeschke R, Hebestreit H (2001). Exercise inhibits epithelial sodium channels in patients with cystic fibrosis. *Am J Resp Crit Care* **164**, 443–6.
156. Timmons BW, Tarnopolsky MA, Snider DP, Bar-Or O (2006). Immunological changes in response to exercise: influence of age, puberty, and gender. *Med Sci Sports Exerc* **38**, 293–304.
157. Cooper DM (1998). Exercise and cystic fibrosis: The search for a therapeutic optimum. *Pediatr Pulmonol* **25**, 143–4.
158. Barker M, Hebestreit A, Gruber W, Hebestreit H (2004). Exercise testing and training in German CF centers. *Pediatr Pulmonol* **37**, 351–5.
159. Kaplan TA, ZeBranek JD, McKey RM, Jr. (1991). Use of exercise in the management of cystic fibrosis: short communication about a survey of cystic fibrosis referral centers. *Pediatr Pulmonol* **10**, 205–7.
160. Godfrey S (1974) The growth and development of the cardio-pulmonary responses to exercise. In: Davis JA, Dobbing J (eds.), *Scientific foundations of pediatrics*, pp. 271–80. W.B.Saunders, Philidelphia, PA.
161. Cooper DM, Berry C, Lamarra L, Wasserman K (1984). Aerobic parameters of exercise as a function of body size during growth in children. *J Appl Physiol* **56**, 628–34.
162. Nixon PA, Joswiak ML, Fricker FJ (1996). A six-minute walking test for assessing exercise tolerance in severely ill children. *J Pediatr* **129**, 362–6.
163. Upton CJ, Tyrrell JC, Hillser EJ (1988). Two minute walking distance in cystic fibrosis. *Arch Dis Child* **63**, 1444–8.
164. Gulmans VA, van Veldhoven NH, de Meer K, Helders PJ (1996). The six-minute walking test in children with cystic fibrosis. *Pediatr Pulmonol* **22**, 85–9.

165. Selvadurai HC, Cooper PJ, Meyers N, Blimkie CJ, Smith L, Mellis CM, Van Asperen PP (2003). Validation of shuttle tests in children with cystic fibrosis. *Pediatr Pulmonol* **35**, 133–8.
166. McKone EF, Barry SC, FitzGerald MX, Gallagher CG (1999). Reproducibility of maximal exercise ergometer testing in patients with cystic fibrosis. *Chest* **116**, 363–8.
167. Barry SC, Gallagher CG (2007). The repeatability of submaximal endurance exercise testing in cystic fibrosis. *Pediatr Pulmonol* **42**, 75–82.
168. Wasserman K (1984). The anaerobic threshold measurement to evaluate exercise performance. *Am Rev Respir Dis* **129**, S35–40.
169. Sue DY, Wasserman K, Moricca RB, Casaburi R (1988). Metabolic acidosis during exercise in patients with chronic obstructive pulmonary disease. Use of the V-slope method for anaerobic threshold determination. *Chest* **94**, 931–8.
170. Patessio A, Casaburi R, Carone M, Appendini L, Donner CF, Wasserman K (1993). Comparison of gas exchange, lactate, and lactic acidosis thresholds in patients with chronic obstructive pulmonary disease. *Am Rev Respir Dis* **148**, 622–6.
171. Thin AG, Linnane SJ, McKone EF, Freaney R, FitzGerald MX, Gallagher CG, McLoughlin P (2002). Use of the gas exchange threshold to noninvasively determine the lactate threshold in patients with cystic fibrosis. *Chest* **121**, 1761–70.
172. Yamaya Y, Bogaard HJ, Wagner PD, Niizeki K, Hopkins SR (2002). Validity of pulse oximetry during maximal exercise in normoxia, hypoxia, and hyperoxia. *J Appl Physiol* **92**, 162–8.
173. Godfrey S (1974) *Exercise testing in children: Applications in health and disease.* W.B. Saunders Co. Ltd., London.
174. Cerny FJ (1989). Relative effects of bronchial drainage and exercise for in hospital care of patients with cystic fibrosis. *Phys Ther* **69,** 633–9.

CHAPTER 34

Exercise, physical activity, and eating and weight disorders

Andrew P. Hills, Nuala M. Byrne, and Rachel E. Wood

Introduction

Obesity has been described as 'one of today's most blatantly visible—yet most neglected—public health problems' by the World Health Organization.[1,2] The escalating epidemic of overweight and obesity has been termed 'globesity' as it 'is taking over many parts of the world,'[2] including both developed and developing societies. The traditionally high prevalence of adult obesity in industrialized, mainly Western, nations is well documented; however, obesity is now also commonplace in countries undergoing economic and nutrition transition.[3,4] Recent reports suggest that approximately 20% of children and adolescents worldwide are overweight or obese, with higher rates in the Americas, Europe, and some parts of the Middle East.[5] Indeed, over the past two decades, the prevalence of excess weight in Australian children has been increasing at a rate of approximately 1% per annum.[5] As a result, the number of Australian children between the ages of 2 and 18 years who are overweight or obese rose from 12% in 1985 to 20% in 1995.[6]

Obesity is a chronic condition caused by an energy imbalance, reduced levels of energy expenditure, and/or higher than necessary energy intake which, over time, contribute to excess weight gain and unfavourable changes in body composition. However, the effects of diet and exercise are not limited to obesity. Indeed, they are contributing factors across a broad spectrum of weight disorders encompassing obesity at one extreme and the eating disorder, anorexia nervosa, as an example at the other end of this spectrum. Unfortunately, in addition to those individuals who fall at the extremes of this spectrum, many others display eating and activity behaviours which may be described as disordered.

A wide range of societal factors contribute to the spectrum of eating and weight disorders referred to above. Collectively, the wide range of determinants of the eating and weight disorders provide numerous challenges for both youngsters and adults. For example, some individuals appear to be preoccupied with body size, shape, weight, and fatness,[7,8] while others accept or appear resolved to their higher level of body fat. Diet and exercise are the primary strategies used to alter body size and shape[9,10] but what are the potential consequences if diet and/or exercise are abused, for example, in individuals whose primary motivation for physical change is for cosmetic rather than health reasons? More specifically, what constitutes an unhealthy modification to diet and/or exercise? What are the potential consequences for children and adolescents if the diet and exercise practices of their parents are inappropriate? Further, do people from different ethnic backgrounds vary in terms of diet and exercise behaviours?

A low level of body fat is considered a 'desirable' physical characteristic for most sports performances, particularly where the transfer of body weight and aesthetics is important.[11,12] Not surprisingly, many athletes train to attain a body size and shape they perceive as 'ideal' for their chosen activity area and one consistent with maximal performance. When unrealistic adjustments are made to body composition in an attempt to meet a desired size or shape, poor health outcomes may be the result.[13,14]

In parallel with the weight-related challenges facing a proportion of the athletic population, the increasing prevalence of obesity is consistent with many adults attempting to reduce body fat.[15] Unfortunately, a proportion of the adult population who are weight-conscious and desire to be slimmer may be 'normal' weight or even underweight, however, perceive themselves as being fat. To what extent are similar concerns influencing the younger population? What do we know of the eating, exercise, and weight-related behaviours of children and adolescents? Further, what is the role of medical practitioners, health professionals, and parents in this important area?

Consistent with trends in adults, the weight-control practices of children and adolescents appear to reflect a heightened concern with body image.[7,16–20] The potential long-term consequences of inappropriate weight-control practices in young people are serious and include disordered eating practices,[21–23] growth retardation, delayed menarche, amenorrhoea, osteoporosis, and psychological disturbances.[12,24–26] The commonly employed weight-control practices, dietary modification, and exercise are pervasive,[8] and not limited to the female population. As medical practitioners are widely consulted and held in high esteem by the general public, they are in a good position to identify potential problems in children and adolescents in their care.[11] The aim of this chapter is to provide an overview of the range of factors contributing to inappropriate eating and activity behaviours, particularly in children and adolescents.

A central concern: fear of fatness?

The preference for leanness in the society results in body fatness being stigmatized, which in turn places a social and psychological burden on many people.[27] Paradoxically, this preference for leanness coexists with an increased prevalence of obesity in individuals of all ages.

When physical activity and dietary restriction are taken to extremes to attain a low level of body fatness, the net result is a proliferation of poor diets, high levels of exercise, body image disturbances including weight dissatisfaction,[28] and a potential increase in eating disorders. For example, dieting can play a role in the development of eating and weight disorders, including obesity,[29–31] and is widespread in adolescent girls and to a lesser extent in boys.[32,33] However, dieting is not only restricted to overweight adolescents but is also practised by prepubertal children,[34] including those who are normal weight or underweight.[33,35] It is common for those who diet to regain weight with periods of dietary restraint followed by episodes of excessive eating.[36] If such practices are associated with adverse psychological effects this may include the contribution to clinical eating disorders.[37]

It has been suggested that for many women in society, being female is consistent with a preoccupation with weight, generally feeling too fat and wishing to weigh less.[38] The perception of fatness and the fear of being overweight in women may be more powerful determinants of eating behaviour than weight *per se*. If the fear of fatness is present in many adult women, what are the potential implications for adolescents? It is critical that youngsters are protected from extraneous pressures to lose weight[32] and this may be achieved through a sensible approach to nutrition and exercise along with an appreciation of individual differences in body size and shape. Health professionals, educators, and parents have a major responsibility to be vigilant in this area.

The 'eating and weight disorders'

Traditionally, the term 'eating disorder' has been limited to anorexia and bulimia nervosa and binge eating disorder. Each condition, along with obesity, has implications for health and well-being, including psychological health. Obesity has not been commonly described as an eating disorder, however, because of the many similarities with the eating disorders[39] in some individuals it may be described as an eating and weight disorder. For example, approximately 30% of obese adults seeking treatment for their weight disorder may also be classified as having binge eating disorder.[40] Another common feature of the eating and weight disorders in many individuals is a lack of self-esteem and a sense of effectiveness.[15]

The extent of the eating and weight disorders is difficult to quantify and there are conflicting reports in different populations.[7] Similarly, there is confusion regarding the predisposing genetic and environmental factors and the level of associated psychological ill-health,[41] potentially due to the use of different approaches to define the conditions. Beals and Houtkooper[14] have suggested that it is difficult to clearly define the boundaries between normality and abnormality regarding body weight and eating behaviour in athletic populations—perhaps the same may be true of the wider population. Despite an increased awareness of eating and weight disorders, the common perception is that a relatively small number of individuals meet the strict criteria for frank eating disorders classified according to DSM-IV. However, significantly more individuals display subclinical eating behaviours including a preoccupation with weight and food, crash diets, fasting, binge eating, and purging behaviours. In many groups, including athletes, it may be difficult to distinguish a conscientious and potentially overzealous desire to follow eating and activity guidelines from disordered eating.[14]

Contrasting scenarios: Overnutrition and physical inactivity, undernutrition and excessive physical activity

Both overnutrition and undernutrition may lead to impaired health and may predispose an individual to an increased risk of an eating or weight disorder. Overnutrition and physical inactivity characterize the most common prescription for increased body fatness and habitually low levels of physical fitness. The second scenario distinguishes individuals who combine attempts to reduce body weight (generally with the view to reducing body fatness), with heavy physical training. Consistent with this situation, concern has often been expressed for the health status of young people who participate in sport and physical activity in which size, shape, and aesthetics are paramount including gymnastics and dance. Similar concerns exist for endurance athletes, predominantly females such as swimmers and runners, who engage in heavy training over an extended period and often persist with inappropriate energy intake.[7,11]

Obesity

Obesity is a complex, multifactorial condition that commonly consists of psychosocial, anatomical, and metabolic adaptations. The numerous interrelated causes of the condition may include overnutrition, physical inactivity, genetic predisposition, psychologically determined eating disorders, and social factors.[42–44] A number of studies[39,45] have reported that the recent global increase in obesity has occurred alongside a steady level of population decrease in energy intake. Consequently, increases in body fatness are the result of a population decrease in energy expenditure including lower levels of physical activity.

There is increasing evidence for the protective effect of regular physical activity and exercise against the accumulation of excess body fat and helping in long-term weight control.[46–50] A higher prevalence of obesity is common in groups whose spontaneous habitual and occupational activity has decreased but in contrast there is a low incidence of obesity in athletic populations. Appropriate levels of body weight and adiposity are related to good health, and excess body fatness is associated with cardiorespiratory, articular, metabolic, locomotor, social, and psychological complications.[51–56] One of the most unfortunate consequences of the obesity epidemic is that the serious health consequences once limited to adults are increasingly prevalent in obese children and adolescents.[56–65]

Assessment of body fatness and criteria for obesity

A wide range of indirect and doubly indirect methods are commonly used to assess body fatness including equations derived from anthropometric measures such as skinfold thickness, bioelectrical impedance (BIA), air plethysmography (BodPod), and dual energy x-ray absorptiometry (DXA). Criteria employed to categorize overweight and obesity include simple indexes such as the body mass index [BMI = Weight (kg)/Height (m^2)], BMI *z*-scores, 120% of ideal body weight, weight-for-height, and weight-for-age percentiles (see Chapter 3).

Dwyer and Blizzard[66] suggested that the biomedical status and sum of skinfold measurements of individual children can be used to define obesity with cut-offs for obesity being 30% of total body mass as fat for girls and 20% for boys. However, Taylor *et al.* [67] have reported a large interindividual variability in per cent body fat (assessed by DXA) in children at a given BMI, which renders the use of a single cut-off problematic. Furthermore, measurements of body fat are typically not available, or practical for use in a clinical setting. Therefore, the BMI has been the most widely used indicator of overweight and obesity in epidemiological studies of adults and also in some studies of children and adolescents.[8,68,69] The major shortcoming of the BMI is its inability to distinguish weight from fatness, and the instability of the index in the growing individual.[70] Lazarus *et al.*[68] suggested that moderate obesity in youngsters was between BMI percentiles of 85 and 94 and marked obesity was over 94. Alternatively, Tell *et al.*[71] have reported age-based cut-offs for obesity using BMI: ≤14 years of age = 19–20 $kg{\cdot}m^{-2}$; 15 years of age = 25 $kg{\cdot}m^{-2}$; and ≥16 years = 28 $kg{\cdot}m^{-2}$. The most widely used international cut-offs are those developed by Cole *et al.*[72,73] In Australia, the current Clinical Practice Guidelines for the Management of Overweight and Obesity in Children and Adolescents[74] recommend that BMI-for-age percentile charts should be used to classify excess weight in children between the ages of 2 and 18 years where a child with a BMI above the 85th percentile would be classified as overweight, and a BMI above the 95th percentile as obese.

Treatment and management

Appropriate management of childhood obesity is critical, since excess body weight (fat) in childhood is associated with a greater chance of high levels of adiposity in adulthood.[75] However, the treatment and management of obesity at any age is a significant challenge, particularly in those who have been overfat for an extended period and experienced multiple failures in weight loss. To add to this, the evidence base for managing excess weight in children is limited, and even the studies that have achieved relative success have been criticised for lacking a detailed methodology.[76] It is generally agreed, however, that severe dietary restriction should be avoided, and that the key to the treatment and management of obesity, and eventually its prevention, in children and adolescents, is to modify body composition whilst promoting regular physical activity and sound nutritional practices.[77–81]

Individual assessment is strongly recommended as this can help to provide both the child and their family with an insight into both the basis of the young person's condition and be used as the basis for the necessary lifestyle changes. A thorough assessment can also help parents to modulate the guilt and blame which is commonplace with an obese child.[42,82] It is overly simplistic to attribute a child's excess weight solely to family circumstances; rather consideration should be given to the broader social context in which obesity develops.[83]

Exercise, diet, and behavioural interventions

The traditional cornerstones of obesity management are diet, exercise, and behaviour modification but many researchers suggest that the active involvement of parents and family members should be an additional element.[42,84,85] Interventions in young people based on a single component, for example, weight loss through diet alone are relatively limited—despite the potential for short-term success, weight loss is difficult to sustain for an extended period.[84] The treatment of obesity in children should aim to restore the balance between energy intake and energy expenditure,[56] and this should be done by focussing on improving health rather than emphasizing weight loss.[85] Weight loss may be both dangerous and counterproductive in the growing individual; a much better approach is to improve body composition by reducing body fat and maintaining or enhancing fat-free mass. Unfortunately, the widespread view is that the measure of success in terms of weight management is a decrease in body mass (irrespective of the consequences for body composition).[53]

In short, severe dietary restriction is contraindicated in children as growth and development may be jeopardized.[56,78] For children and adolescents who have excess body fat but are still growing, maintenance of body weight may be more important than unrealistic attempts to reduce body weight. As such individuals increase in height, the proportion of body fat will decrease. Concurrently, greater attention should be paid to increasing physical activity and exercise[53,56,86] and the development of motor skills for an active engagement in sport and physical activity. Moore and Burrows[87] contend that because exercise is active, unrestricted, and positive, whereas dieting is passive, restrictive, and negative, it is healthier to promote the benefits of a positive and rewarding activity.

Readers are referred to some of the numerous reviews of physical activity and exercise for the prevention, treatment, and management of childhood and adolescent obesity.[50,78,84,88–90] Despite the small numbers of participants in many studies, the work of Epstein[46] in family-based behavioural weight control has provided some excellent guidelines for the combined use of diet, exercise, and behaviour change. Techniques commonly used to improve obese children's eating and activity behaviours include self-monitoring, social reinforcement, modelling, and social skills.[91]

Despite the comparatively greater potential to achieve a negative energy balance through reductions in energy intake compared to increases in physical activity,[90] a combined approach is more efficacious in terms of body composition.[92,93] Most importantly, the role of physical activity in the maintenance of weight loss[84,93–95] cannot be overstated. Particular benefits are possible when individuals change from being inactive/sedentary to a regular engagement in physical activity—in children this may provide both health and motor-skill-related benefits.

The treatment and management of obesity in children and adolescents is challenging for clinicians and parents and is commonly emotionally charged. Despite the availability of general clinical guidelines for obesity management,[74] the process must be individualized and personalized, including a strong commitment and involvement of the family. Some of the key questions that may help clinicians to formalize a treatment and management plan are outlined in Table 34.1. One of the most important issues regarding interventions with overweight and obese children is that if they are driven or motivated by parents, without a commitment from the individual child, they are unlikely to succeed.

From treatment and management to prevention

The prevention and management of obesity in children should be a high priority[74,96–98] with prevention strategies including primary care, family-based, and school-based programmes.[97] High levels of physical activity are associated with greater weight loss, and

Table 34.1 Key questions that may help clinicians to formalize a treatment and management plan

◆ What is the nature of the family environment including physical characteristics of parents and siblings?
◆ How long has the individual been overweight or obese?
◆ Has the individual been relatively inactive for an extended period?
◆ Is the child or adolescent's willingness to participate in physical activity limited by low self-confidence and/or self-esteem?
◆ Has the individual been subjected to teasing and ridicule by peers?
◆ Is the individual genuinely concerned about their physical size?
◆ Is the individual self-motivated with respect to the improvement of body composition status?
◆ Does the young person have a commitment to making improvements to eating and physical activity behaviours?
◆ What is the individual's current health status and estimated risk?

the ability to maintain weight loss in overweight obese adults.[50] Similarly, for many young people, the opportunity to increase daily energy expenditure through greater participation in physical activity and exercise may be sufficient to prevent obesity.[78] If physical activity was a non-negotiable lifestyle component from birth, the prevalence of obesity in young people would be significantly less. Some[78] have proposed that a change in activity status may be simpler for non-obese youngsters than to encourage older individuals to be active once they become obese. Parents, teachers, coaches, and medical practitioners have a collective responsibility to provide every opportunity for young people to be physically active.

All children, irrespective of age, size, and shape, love to move. It is very unfortunate that an increasing number of children and adolescents are not given sufficient opportunity and encouragement to be physically active whether this is through spontaneous play and incidental activity, or more structured activity such as in school physical education and sport.

It is reasonable to suggest that quality experiences during childhood and adolescence may help to set the scene for a more active adulthood.[99] Some of the contributing factors to the maintenance of activity behaviours from childhood through to adulthood are the success, fun, and enjoyment one experiences in physical activity undertaken during the younger years.[88] Activity should not be a chore, but rather should be relevant and personally challenging for the individual. Specifically in young children, participation in a range of different activities should be encouraged, and competition should be minimized.[99] Perhaps not surprisingly, the earlier work of Epstein *et al.*[100,101] reported that activity programmes using lifestyle activities were more effective than programmed aerobic exercise.

One of the more important societal factors with the potential to impact on weight management is a greater appreciation of individual differences, including empathy for all individuals, irrespective of their size, shape, and body composition, particularly level of fatness. Despite the basic premises of the energy balance equation, we know that some individuals are both predisposed to gain weight more readily than others and also have more difficulty losing weight.[102,103] In some individuals, these processes may be more biologically determined in the same way size and shape is genetically mediated.[43,104,105] In the knowledge that they may be more predisposed than others, such individuals need to be more vigilant regarding eating and activity behaviours. It is very important that medical and other health professionals are conscious of the constellation of factors governing behaviour, including the possibility of precipitating the development of eating and weight disorders associated with a fear of fatness.[98]

While acknowledging the demands already placed on the school system,[106] the school setting could also be better utilized to foster active behaviours[42,106] with physical education programmes in infant, primary, and secondary schools and the harnessing of available professionals and equipment a high priority.[106–108] Such programmes should cater for all individuals, not just those who are physically capable.

The family environment and positive parental influences are invaluable in the management and treatment of childhood obesity.[109] However, some of the major risk factors for childhood obesity are parental obesity[42,46] and parental exercise habits.[42] Parents may facilitate and contribute to the maintenance of sedentary lifestyle behaviours[110] or parental exercise may contribute to lower levels of fatness in children, irrespective of whether the parent exercises with the child. Unfortunately, the most common scenario is that many children do not have the opportunity to walk or cycle to and from school and are not supervised by adults at home before and after school. This provides an additional opportunity for young people to make poor food choices, engage in inactive behaviours such as television viewing, and reduces the potential time for active pursuits.[91]

There is evidence that children's food choices are likely to be less healthy than their parents' choices if young people are left to their own resources.[111] Even when parents are at home, inactive pursuits such as passive television viewing may be chosen as a convenient child-minding tool. Not surprisingly, excess television viewing has been identified as one of the contributing factors to childhood obesity[112] and may also enhance the energy intake of snacks low in nutritional value.[113,114] Further, if the content of television advertising to children is not controlled, children may be exposed to less healthy food options[113,115] and the types of food that parents may wish to limit.[116]

Some research has considered the effects of reinforcing obese children for being more active and less sedentary.[101,117,118] For example, Epstein *et al.*[118] found that reducing access to preferred sedentary behaviours was superior to reinforcing active behaviour choices for weight control and fitness improvement at 1 year. Similarly, Saelens and Epstein[119] found that highly valued sedentary activities can help to reinforce physical activity participation. For example, making television viewing available to children only while they were physically active, resulted in an increase in activity time from 5 min at baseline to greater than 20 min when the contingency was in effect. Parents should be encouraged to praise and support children who participate in physical activity and also support a reduction in energy-dense foods and those low in nutritional value.

The active involvement of at least one parent in the weight management process with a child helps to improve short- and long-term weight regulation[46,120] and should be non-negotiable. All family members can benefit from the encouragement and support provided to an overweight or obese child in the adoption of new eating and exercise behaviours. Parents should take the lead and be active role models encouraging all family members to participate in physical activity, and ideally as a family unit. Numerous options exist for increased activity such as walking or cycling to and from school, taking the dog and children for a walk rather than being inactive, minimizing the use of motor vehicles, taking the stairs rather than lifts or escalators, and so on.

There is an urgent need for greater community responsibility and engagement to involve a wide range of sectors in the encouragement and promotion of exercise and physical activity.[97] Better support of obese children and adolescents would be possible if we adhered to the recommendations in Table 34.2.

In the recent past, the research community has been challenged to provide evidence-based physical activity recommendations for the health of adults. Such guidelines are now widely available; however, the same level of advice and support is not available for weight management—even less for children and adolescents. Bar-Or and Baranowski[88] summarized some of the challenges regarding exercise and weight control, including the difficulty of assessing the association between adiposity and enhanced physical activity (training) as there is a lack of standardized assessment of adiposity, physical activity, and energy expenditure. It is, therefore, difficult to recommend a dose-response or minimal dose of exercise to maintain a desirable body composition in children. However, governments and learned societies in Australia, Canada, and the United States currently recommend that children achieve at least 60–90 min of moderate to vigorous physical activity each day.[121–123] Owing to differential growth and maturation, a number of approaches to exercise prescription are required in childhood and adolescence. As such, intervention programmes for young people should account for age-related preferences in activity and changes in physical activity levels during the growing years.[78] If children are actively involved in decision-making related to physical activity and sports participation, there is likely to be greater participation rates and enjoyment.[124] Despite the lack of definitive data regarding the tracking of physical activity experiences from the growing years to adult life, there is consensus that the level of enjoyment of physical activity in early years may be a key determinant of continued participation.[125]

Table 34.2 Recommendations for better support of obese children and adolescents

◆ Educating and informing children and adolescents
◆ Actively discouraging dieting to promote weight loss
◆ Re-educating to correct poor eating and exercise habits whilst encouraging an improvement in overall health and well-being
◆ Increasing self-esteem and body image including a positive mental attitude
◆ Encouraging a positive 'can do' mentality. Everyone, irrespective of size and shape has the ability to improve their health status
◆ Encouraging an acceptance of individual variability in body size and shape
◆ Focus on health status not on weight *per se*
◆ Fostering an enjoyment in regular physical activity, commencing with low- to moderate-intensity activity and increasing as the individual improves in fitness
◆ Downplaying the 'shame and blame' mentality regarding weight and fatness
◆ Eating well and following recommended dietary guidelines

Body satisfaction during the growing years: Implications for eating and weight disorders

The physical growth and development of children, including psychosocial status, is heavily influenced by maturation and a range of external factors. However, the relationships between body size and shape and psychological health are relatively poorly understood. For example, we know there is a strong association between increased body fatness and body dissatisfaction; however, it is unclear when dissatisfaction commences and/or at what age indicators of body image such as dissatisfaction with one's body is important enough to influence the global construct of self-esteem. How are the key psychological indicators of health linked and do they track with physical growth changes? How important is the pubertal barrier in the development of particular traits in this area? Further, what is the role of physical activity participation, motor skill level, and body composition status in relation to various psychological constructs?

Despite the interest in the area, relatively few studies have considered the interrelationships between body composition *per se* and body satisfaction during childhood and adolescence.[8] We know that as for adults, preoccupation with body weight and fatness is common in childhood and adolescence; however, the strength of the association between body satisfaction and weight-related behaviours is unclear. Children as young as 3 years of age view obesity negatively,[126] and the stereotypes of thinness as attractive and desirable, and fatness as neither, are well established by 9 years of age.[127] Overweight and obese 9-year-old girls had significantly lower physical appearance and athletic competence self-esteem than their normal weight peers but body weight had no impact on girls' rated importance of self-esteem. Heavier girls were less likely to be peer nominated as pretty, but did not differ in their popularity.

One of the limiting factors in this area of research has been the nature of the methods employed. For example, in studies of body image and weight-control practices of children and adolescents, many studies have utilized instruments designed for adults.[128] We have investigated the effect of adult versus adolescent body-figure silhouette scales on ratings of body image[129] in adolescents and found significant between-scale differences. Adolescents displayed consistently lower body-image ratings when viewing adult as opposed to adolescent scales. These results confirm the need for population-specific measurement scales and the use of standardized assessment procedures.

In addition, there are differences in the measures used to assess body satisfaction, particularly with reference to the body composition of participants. Hills and Byrne[129] investigated the effect of body composition on the association among three indices of body satisfaction in a group of adolescents. For individuals with a higher weight-for-height and also greater body fat levels, Pearson correlation coefficients for body satisfaction were stronger than those for normal weight individuals. Hills and Byrne[8] also assessed appearance and weight-control attitudes and behaviours in adolescents and as for previous work with this population[129–132] found that males were significantly more satisfied than females with their physical appearance in general, and with weight-related aspects in particular. Despite both genders being less satisfied with a fatter physique, males perceived themselves as too thin and wished to be more muscular, while females felt they were too fat and desired to be thinner.

Smolak *et al.*[47] have documented an association between puberty and an increase in body dissatisfaction in females and Koff *et al.*[124] have reported a higher relationship between body image and self-concept for females at this stage of development. Earlier work by an Australian group[127] found that between 9 and 10 years of age, males and females do not differ significantly in their level of body satisfaction. Hills and Byrne[8] support the contention that the onset of puberty can influence body satisfaction, but for both sexes. In this study, a significant gender difference was found at 12 years of age, females displayed a marked level of body dissatisfaction while males were satisfied with their physical appearance. At 14 years of age, males displayed a level of dissatisfaction with their physical appearance comparable with females 2 years younger, a change which dovetailed with the average age of puberty for males. Gender differences resumed by 16 years of age, males as a group were more satisfied as they approximated their mature adult physique but females remained dissatisfied with their appearance.

It appears that current body size and fatness influences body satisfaction to some extent. A higher weight-for-height ratio and higher adiposity levels were associated with lower body satisfaction in both male and female adolescents. Those with higher adiposity thought and felt they were larger than their less obese peers. However, there were no gender differences in body and weight satisfaction in adolescent males and females with lower levels of adiposity and in addition females were no more likely than males to perceive themselves as overweight. These results confirm that body weight and level of adiposity are fundamental elements of physical attractiveness standards for both sexes.

The influence of body composition on disordered eating tendencies of adolescents

Given the higher prevalence of childhood obesity and the relationship between being above average weight and dieting in adolescence,[16] it may be hypothesized that an increasing number of adolescents will employ restrictive dietary practices. Most studies have reported that dieting is a predominantly female characteristic; however, to date more research has focused on girls than boys. In the United Kingdom, an estimated 40% of girls and 25% of boys begin dieting in adolescence.[133] Some researchers have claimed that female concerns about weight and physical appearance and associated dieting have become so pervasive that they may be considered normal behaviour.[21,22,134,135] Of particular concern is that some studies have suggested that a substantial proportion of adolescent girls have used extreme weight-loss behaviours at least occasionally. However, a major shortcoming of many studies of weight-control practices has been the failure to make any reference to the actual physical size of individuals studied.

Work by Hills and Byrne[8] assessed weight concerns and dieting practices in a group of adolescent boys and girls and consistent with previous work with a similar population[9,135,136] found that females were significantly more likely than males to diet and fast for weight control. Females also employed more pathogenic weight-control practices and counted the energy content of foods they consumed; however, it is very difficult to assess the normalcy of these results given the range of reported prevalence in adults and adolescents. The gender differences found by Hills and Byrne[8] may again relate to the greater number of females who perceived themselves as overweight. Striegel-Moore *et al.*[137] have proposed that the body weight concerns of adolescent females are due to them equating 'normal' weight with 'underweight'. Another explanation[22] may be that females are aware of appropriate weight norms, however, deliberately try to violate them, reflecting dissatisfaction with body weight.

In summary, both relative weight-for-height (BMI) and body fat levels influence body satisfaction and drive-for-thinness in males and females. Those who are bigger and fatter according to these measures are more dissatisfied with their physique, and display a greater concern with dieting, preoccupation with weight, and pursuit of thinness. These results suggest that body composition influences the prevalence of restrictive dietary practices; however, gender differences were still evident within each body composition categorization.

Exercise motivations of adolescents

In order to minimize distorted attitudes about body size and weight control one needs to determine their genesis, how they evolve over time and which individuals are most vulnerable.[128,135] Hills and Byrne[129] investigated gender differences in exercise motivations in adolescents in relation to body composition status. Males displayed significantly greater body satisfaction than females while females reported a greater concern for and preoccupation with weight and thinness. A similar proportion of males and females were overweight, however, nearly twice as many females perceived themselves as being overweight, however, more females reported exercising for weight control and to improve body tone. Those who were motivated to exercise for fitness, health, and enjoyment reported fewer disturbances in body image and body dissatisfaction compared with those motivated to exercise for weight control, tone, and attractiveness, a finding consistent with other studies.[136,138] However, once body composition was accounted for there were no significant gender differences in exercise motivation at higher body fat levels. In short, despite the evidence of gender differences being evident by adolescence, as seen in studies of adults, differences in exercise motivation may be attributed to both level of body dissatisfaction and body composition. McDonald and Thompson[136] have referenced the need to be concerned for individuals, particularly females, whose motivation for exercise is primarily cosmetic. Available evidence is particularly concerning and suggestive of an association between body composition, weight-control behaviours, and health status from an early age. All health professionals and responsible adults must help to promote exercise as a means of achieving health and wellness, rather than helping to perpetuate the restrictive approach of using exercise merely as an avenue for weight control.[125]

Anorexia nervosa, bulimia nervosa, and binge-eating disorder

Compared to anorexia, bulimia nervosa and binge-eating disorder are more commonly described as beginning in adults; however, there are large numbers of adolescents with these conditions.[139] In each condition, the individual's self-evaluation is overinfluenced by body weight and shape. Those individuals who do not meet the full DSM-IV criteria are classified as having an eating disorder not otherwise specified (EDNOS).

Both anorexia and bulimia nervosa are complex, closely related alterations in eating behaviour. Crisp[140] has suggested that both are pubertally driven disorders with the common element being an underlying 'dyslipophobia' (or distressing 'fear of fatness'). Anorexia nervosa is characterized by weight loss, poor body image, an intense fear of weight gain and obesity, particularly the 'fatness' of the normal mature female body which is instigated at puberty.[140,141] Excessive physical activity also figures prominently as a symptom.[142–144]

Mainstream bulimia nervosa, in contrast, occurs at or above normal adult body weight.[133] The condition is also characterized by an intense fear of fatness and the belief that other people consider this as a loss of control.[140] Bulimia is characterized by eating large quantities of food at one time (bingeing) which is purged from the body by vomiting, using laxatives or diuretics, fasting, and/or excessive exercise. Bulimia is also frequently related to weight reduction diets[145] and may occur in younger people who are of normal or lower than average weight where binge eating is accompanied by strict dieting, self-induced vomiting, and low body weight.[146] Obese girls who diet obsessively may be at particular risk of developing an eating disorder.

Numerous diagnostic criteria have been employed to define each condition; however, the criteria in Table 34.3 are adapted from the DSM-IV.[147]

Aetiology of anorexia and bulimia nervosa

Despite the lack of understanding of the specific aetiology of the eating disorders and the normal development of eating behaviour, there is evidence that certain critical elements may be responsible. Risk factors identified to date include familial influences and genetic predisposition,[148,149] biological mechanisms such as a serotonin deficiency[150,151] and personality and individual psychopathology.[152–154]

Table 34.3 Diagnostic criteria for anorexia nervosa, bulimia nervosa, and binge eating disorder

Diagnostic criteria for anorexia nervosa
(A) Refusal to maintain body weight at or above a minimally normal weight for age and height (e.g., weight loss leading to maintenance of body weight less than 85% of that expected; or failure to make expected weight gain during period of growth, leading to body weight less than 85% of that expected)
(B) Intense fear of gaining weight or becoming fat, even though underweight
(C) Disturbance in the way in which one's body weight or shape is experienced, undue influence of body weight or shape on self-evaluation, or denial of the seriousness of the current low body weight
(D) In post-menarcheal females, amenorrhoea, that is, the absence of at least three consecutive menstrual cycles
Diagnostic criteria for bulimia nervosa
(A) Recurrent episodes of binge eating. An episode of binge eating is characterized by both of the following: (1) Eating, in a discrete period of time (e.g. within any 2-hour period), an amount of food that is definitely larger than most people would eat during a similar period of time and under similar circumstances (2) A sense of lack of control over eating during the episode (e.g. a feeling that one cannot stop eating or control what or how much one is eating)
(B) Recurrent inappropriate compensatory behaviour in order to prevent weight gain, such as self-induced vomiting; misuse of laxatives, diuretics, enemas, or other medications; fasting; excessive exercise
(C) The binge eating and inappropriate compensatory behaviours both occur, on average, at least twice a week for 3 months
(D) Self-evaluation is unduly influenced by body shape and weight
(E) The disturbance does not occur exclusively during episodes of anorexia nervosa
Criteria for binge eating disorder
(A) Recurrent episodes of binge eating. An episode of binge eating is characterized by both of the following: (1) Eating, in a discrete period of time (e.g. within any 2-hour period), an amount of food that is definitely larger than most people would eat in a similar period of time under similar circumstances (2) A sense of lack of control over eating during the episode (e.g. a feeling that one cannot stop eating or control what or how much one is eating)
(B) The binge-eating episodes are associated with three (or more) of the following: (1) Eating much more rapidly than normal (2) Eating until feeling uncomfortably full (3) Eating large amounts of food when not feeling physically hungry (4) Eating alone because of being embarrassed by how much one is eating (5) Feeling disgusted with oneself, depressed, or very guilty after overeating
(C) Marked distress regarding binge eating is present
(D) The binge eating occurs, on average, at least 2 days a week for 6 months
(E) The binge eating is not associated with the regular use of inappropriate compensatory behaviours (e.g. purging, fasting, excessive exercise) and does not occur exclusively during the course of anorexia nervosa or bulimia nervosa

Casper[155] has outlined two categories of precipitating event in relation to the onset of anorexia nervosa—psychological or physical. Examples of psychological event include extreme disappointment in relation to an important relationship, the birth of a sibling, moving house, the loss of a friend, or a death in the family. Physical events may include early physical maturation and anxiety about puberty.

A number of researchers[7,156] have stated that participation in sport increases the risk for eating and weight problems as the biological risk for eating disorders relates to the common trend in many athletes to restrict energy intake. The dietary restraint needed to control intake may influence attitudes such as a preoccupation with eating and weight and behaviours such as binge eating.[7]

The transition from childhood to adolescence is a time of substantial biological change and in females body fat stores increase as one changes from a child to a mature young woman. As organized sport and competition in the physical activity setting are commonplace, many individuals are faced with a dilemma, a biological change in physical characteristics and a desire to control eating and weight for both appearance and performance reasons.

Crisp[140] has indicated that anorexia has physical, social, and psychological handicaps, many of which the anorectic recognizes. At the same time, the individual denies the presence of illness and weight concerns and will often be secretive and manipulative in an attempt to defend her bio-psychological avoidant stance. The individual with bulimia nervosa may also be secretive, commonly experiencing guilt, low self-esteem, and anger by his/her incapacity to control food intake.[140]

The dieting–eating disorder continuum

Numerous studies acknowledge a continuum of risks for eating disorders[14,157] ranging from normative concerns about body weight and shape, to rigid dieting, to subclinical, and subsequently, diagnosable eating disorders.[137,158–161] Similarly, Nylander[162] proposed that dieting behaviour lies on a continuum with no dieting behaviour and eating disorders at the extremes, and increasing levels of dieting severity between.

Clearly, not all individuals who diet develop eating disorders; however, dieting has been recognized as a prelude to anorexia and bulimia nervosa.[9,133,137,149,162] Smolak *et al.*[47] suggested that dieting should be viewed as a problematic behaviour as it has the potential to lead to health-threatening weight cycling and binge-eating. Dieting during adolescence is of particular concern as the highest incidence of anorexia nervosa occurs at the beginning of adolescence and bulimia nervosa at the end.[133,134,163]

Prevalence of eating disorders

A number of issues need to be addressed when discussing the prevalence of disordered eating behaviours. For example, Brownell *et al.*[7] noted that to deal only with the 'clinical' entities of anorexia and bulimia nervosa would miss many 'subclinical' problems such as preoccupation with food, obsessive thinking about weight, and disturbed body image. While the prevalence of anorexia nervosa in the general population is very low at approximately 1% and bulimia estimated to be between 1% and 3%,[164] the number of people who suffer with eating and weight problems but do not meet strict diagnostic criteria is much greater.[164–166] Despite the relatively small number of adolescent girls who suffer from clinically diagnosable eating disorders[153] (3–5%), a sizeable portion of adolescent girls (40%) and boys (25%) report dieting behaviour.[133]

As many individuals have 'unusual' eating patterns but do not meet established diagnostic criteria for an eating disorder,[167] it is important that the terminology for clinically disordered eating practices is only used where appropriate. The misuse of the term 'eating disorder', or more specifically the terms anorexia or bulimia nervosa, may be another reason for the diversity in the reported figures regarding the prevalence of eating disorders.

Binge-eating disorder

A recognized sub-population of obese individuals, estimated to approximate 25–30% of those seeking treatment for the condition[40,168] undertake periodic bouts of binge-eating. Obese binge-eaters are characterized as having experienced multiple weight loss failures followed by an abandonment of dietary restraint.[39] Interestingly, Wilson *et al.*[166] have reported that obese binge-eaters are more dissatisfied with their weight and have a higher preoccupation with their weight and food than other obese individuals.

Binge-eating is often precipitated by negative emotions and individuals report feeling out of control.[168,169] When binge eaters experience guilt, binges can be followed by increased dietary restraint which perpetuates an unbalanced relationship with food.

Prevention, treatment, and management

Treatment for each condition is largely experiential and behavioural.[140] Goals for the anorexic individual include weight gain[170] whilst weight maintenance may be more important for the bulimic or obese individual with binge-eating disorder. Robin *et al.*[167] have stressed the differential expression of anorexia and bulimia nervosa in children and adolescents compared to adults and suggested that multidisciplinary treatments should be tailored to the unique developmental, medical, nutritional, and psychological needs of young people. It is also important to acknowledge that the psychological profile in early onset (<16 years) anorexia differs from that in later onset.[171]

Recommendations for treatment and management by health professionals may include the elements of successful treatment as outlined by Comerci (1988): recognizing the disorder and restoring physiologic stability as soon as possible; establishing a trusting and therapeutic partnership with the young person; involving the family in treatment; and, using a multidisciplinary team approach.

Table 34.4 indicates some useful and practical aspects of engagement with the young eating disordered individual.

Table 34.4 Useful and practical aspects of engagement with the young eating disordered individual

1. The young person did not choose to develop an eating disorder, but they can choose to get better
2. Commonly, eating disorders reflect a means of coping with developmental issues, for example, the need to gain a sense of control, efficacy, or identity
3. The individual may become angry and frustrated with treatment requirements, including the necessity for weight gain to improve health status
4. It is pointless to assign blame or guilt for the cause of the problem
5. Professional help should focus on restoration of health (not merely weight gain)

Summary

- Youngsters often have unresolved intrapersonal (self-esteem, self-efficacy) and interpersonal (school, home, or peers) conflicts, which generally relate to the common psychosocial adjustments to adolescence.
- Weight-control practices initiated to manage these issues tend to be reinforced by feedback. Examples may include compliments regarding appearance or the perception of mastery over what is eaten (or not eaten), and attempts to manage situations of overeating through exercise, vomiting, or the taking of laxatives.
- Negative feedback may also be commonplace, usually from family members and good friends; however, this can commonly result in the opposite—further positive reinforcement.
- The use of exercise in the treatment and management of these conditions appears to have the eating and weight disorders has considerable merit. For example, anorexic adolescents who are constantly looking for opportunities to participate in aerobic-based activities may benefit from individualized resistance training sessions to help preserve and strengthen skeletal muscle tissue.
- The reader is referred to a number of other excellent sources for comprehensive details of prevention, treatment, and management.[41,172–180]

References

1. Batch JA, Baur LA (2005). Management and prevention of obesity and its complications in children and adolescents. *Med J Aust* **182**, 130–5.
2. World Health Organization. Nutrition. Controlling the global obesity epidemic. Available at: http://www.who.int/nutrition/topics/obesity/en/ (last accessed October 2007).
3. Caballero B (2005). A nutrition paradox—Underweight and obesity in developing countries. *N Engl J Med* **352**, 1514–16.
4. Asfaw A (2006). The effects of obesity on doctor-diagnosed chronic diseases in Africa: Empirical results from Senegal and South Africa. *J Pub Health Policy* **27**, 250–64.
5. Lobstein T, Baur L, Uauy R (2004). Obesity in children and young people: A crisis in public health. *Obes Rev* **5** (Suppl. 1), 4–104.
6. Magarey A, Daniels L, Boulton T (2001). Prevalence of overweight and obesity in Australian children and adolescents: Reassessment of 1985 and 1995 data against new standard international definitions. *Med J Aust* **174**, 561–4.
7. Brownell KD, Rodin J, Wilmore JH (1992). Eating, body weight and performance in athletes: An introduction. In: Brownell KD, Wilmore J (eds.), *Eating, body weight and performance*, pp. 13–14. Lea and Febiger, Philadelphia, PA.
8. Hills AP, Byrne NM (1998). Body composition, body satisfaction, eating and exercise behaviour of Australian adolescents. In: Parizkova J, Hills AP (eds.), *Physical fitness and nutrition during growth*, pp. 44–53. Karger, Basel.
9. Emmons L (1992). Dieting and purging behaviour in black and white high school students. *J Am Diet Assoc* **92**, 306–12.
10. Boutelle K, Neumark-Sztainer D, Story M, Resnick M (2002). Weight control behaviors among obese, overweight and non overweight adolescents. *J Pediatr Psychol* **27**, 531–40.
11. Committee on Sports Medicine and Fitness (2005). Promotion of healthy weight-control practices in young athletes. *Pediatrics* **116**, 1557–64.
12. Treble GF, Morton AR (1994). A recipe for success or tragedy? Selection for Australian rhythmic gymnastic representation. *Sport Health* **12**, 5–10.
13. Davis C (1992). Body image, dieting behaviours, and personality factors: A study of high-performance female athletes. *Int J Sport Psychol* **23**, 179–92.
14. Beals KA, Houtkooper L (2006). Disordered eating in athletes. In: Burke L (ed.), *Clinical sports nutrition*, pp. 201–26. McGraw-Hill, Sydney.
15. Brownell KD (1991). Dieting and the search for the perfect body: Where physiology and culture collide. *Behav Ther* **22**, 1–12.
16. Paxton SJ, Wertheim EH, Gibbons K, Szmukler GI (1991). Body image satisfaction, dieting beliefs, and weight loss behaviors in adolescent girls and boys. *J Youth Adolesc* **20**, 361–79.
17. Wertheim EH, Paxton SJ, Maude D, Szmukler GI (1992). Psychosocial predictors of weight loss behaviors and binge eating in adolescent girls and boys. *Int J Eat Disord* **12**, 151–60.
18. Maude D, Wertheim EH, Paxton S, Gibbons K (1993). Body dissatisfaction, weight loss behaviours, and bulimic tendencies in Australian adolescents with an estimate of female data representativeness. *Aust Psychol* **28**, 128–32.
19. O'Dea J (1994). Food habits, body image and self-esteem of adolescent girls from disadvantaged and non-disadvantaged backgrounds. *Aust J Nutr Diet* **51**, 74–8.
20. Nowak M, Speare R, Crawford D (1996). Gender differences in adolescent weight and shape related beliefs and behaviours. *J Paed Child Health* **32**, 148–52.
21. Mellin LM, Irwin CE, Scully S (1992). Prevalence of disordered eating in girls: A survey of middle-class children. *J Am Diet Assoc* **92**, 851–3.
22. Koff E, Rierdan J (1991). Perceptions of weight and attitudes toward eating in early adolescent girls. *J Adolesc Health* **12**, 307–12.
23. Patton GC, Selzer R, Coffey C, Carlin JB, Wolfe R (1999). Onset of adolescent eating disorders: Population based cohort study over 3 years. *BMJ* **318**, 765–8.
24. Carbon RJ (1992). Exercise, amenorrhoea and the skeleton. *Br Med Bull* **48**, 546–60.
25. Davis C, Fox J (1993). Excessive exercise and weight preoccupation in women. *Addict Behav* **18**, 201–11.
26. Greenfeld D, Quinlan D, Harding M, Glass E, Bliss A (1987). Eating behaviour in an adolescent population. *Int J Eat Disord* **6**, 99–111.
27. Spring B, Pingitore R, Bruckner E, Penava S (1994). Obesity: Idealized or stigmatized? Socio-cultural influences on the meaning and prevalence of obesity. In: Hills AP, Walqvist ML (eds.), *Exercise and obesity*, pp. 49–60. Smith-Gordon and Company, London.
28. Rosen AM, Murkofsky CA, Steckler NM, Skolnick NJ (1989). A comparison of psychological and depressive symptoms among restricting anorexic, bulimic anorexic, and normal-weight bulimic patients. *Int J Eat Disord* **8**, 657–63.
29. Polivy J, Herman P (1985). Dieting and bingeing: A causal analysis. *Am Psychol* **985**, 193–7.
30. Stice E, Presnell K, Shaw H, Rohde P (2005). Psychological and behavioral risk factors for obesity onset in adolescent girls: A prospective study. *J Consult Clin Psychol* **73**, 195–202.
31. Hill A (2007). Obesity and eating disorders. *Obes Rev* **8** (Suppl. 1), 151–5.
32. Flynn M (1997). Fear of fatness and adolescent girls: Implications for obesity prevention. *Proc Nutr Soc* **56**, 305–17.
33. Wadden T, Foster G, Stunkard A, Linowitz J (1989). Dissatisfaction with weight and figure in obese girls: Discontent but not depression. *Int J Obes Relat Metab Disord* **13**, 89–97.
34. Hill AJ, Draper E, Stack J (1994). A weight on children's minds: Body shape dissatisfactions at 9 years old. *Int J Obes Relat Metab Disord* **18**, 383–9.
35. Whitaker A, Davies M, Shaffer D, Johnson J, Abrams S, Walsh BT, Kalikow K (1989). The struggle to be thin: A survey of anorexic and bulimic symptoms in a non-referred adolescent population. *Psychol Med* **19**, 143–63.

36. Hill AJ (1993). Pre-adolescent dieting: Implications for eating disorders. *Int Rev Psychiatry* **5**, 87–99.
37. Hill AJ (1993). Causes and consequences of dieting and anorexia. *Proc Nutr Soc* **52**, 211–18.
38. Rodin J, Silberstein L, Striegel-Moore R (1985). Women and weight: A normative discontent. In: Sonderegger TB (ed.), *Psychology and gender*, pp. 267–308. University of Nebraska Press, Lincoln, NE.
39. Jebb S, Prentice A (1995). Is obesity an eating disorder? *Proc Nutr Soc* **54**, 721–8.
40. de Zwaan M (2001). Binge eating disorder and obesity. *Int J Obes Relat Metab Disord* **25** (Suppl. 1), S51–5.
41. Garfinkel P, Dorian B (1997). Factors that may influence future approaches to the eating disorders. *Eat Weight Disord* **2**, 1–16.
42. Court JM (1994). Strategies for management of obesity in children and adolescents. In: Hills AP, Wahlqvist ML (eds.), *Exercise and obesity*, pp. 181–94. Smith-Gordon and Company, London.
43. Dietz WH (1995). Childhood obesity. In: Cheung LWY, Richmond JB (eds.), *Child health, nutrition, and physical activity*, pp. 155–70, Human Kinetics, Champaign, IL.
44. Gortmaker SL, Must A, Perrin JM, Sobol AM, Dietz WH (1993). Social and economic consequences of overweight in adolescence and young adulthood. *N Engl J Med* **329**, 1008–12.
45. Parizkova J, Hainer V, Stich V, Kunesova M, Ksantini M (1994). Physiological capabilities of obese individuals and implications for exercise. In: Hills AP, Walqvist ML (eds.), *Exercise and obesity*, pp. 131–40. Smith-Gordon and Company, London.
46. Epstein L (1996). Family-based behavioural intervention for obese children. *Int J Obes Relat Metab Disord* **20** (Suppl. 1), S14–21.
47. Smolak L, Levine MP, Gralen S (1993). The impact of puberty and dating on eating problems among middle school girls. *J Youth Adolesc* **22**, 355–68.
48. Wilmore JH (1996). Increasing physical activity. *Am J Clin Nutr* **63**, 456S–60S.
49. Wadden TA, Butryn ML, Byrne KJ (2004). Efficacy of lifestyle modification for long-term weight control. *Obes Res* **12** (Suppl. 3), 151S–62.
50. Hill JO, Wyatt HR (2005). Role of physical activity in preventing and treating obesity. *J Appl Physiol* **99**, 765–70.
51. Hills AP (1994). Locomotor characteristics of obese children. In: Hills AP, Walqvist ML (eds.), *Exercise and obesity*, pp. 141–50. Smith-Gordon and Company, London.
52. Milligan R, Thompson C, Vandongen R, Beilin L, Burke V (1995). Clustering of cardiovascular risk factors in Australian adolescents: Association with dietary excesses and deficiencies. *J Cardiovasc Risk* **2**, 515–23.
53. Hills A, Byrne N (1998). Exercise prescription for weight management. *Proc Nutr Soc* **57**, 93–103.
54. Gortmaker SL, Dietz WH, Jr, Sobol AM, Wehler CA (1987). Increasing pediatric obesity in the United States. *Am J Dis Child* **141**, 535–40.
55. Labib M (2003). The investigation and management of obesity. *J Clin Pathol* **56**, 17–25.
56. Speiser PW, Rudolf MCJ, Anhalt H, Camacho-Hubner C, Chiarelli F, Eliakim A, Freemark M, Gruters A, Hershkovitz E, Iughetti L, Krude H, Latzer Y, Lustig RH, Peskovitz RH, Pinhas-Mamiel O, Rogo AD, Shalitin S, Sultan C, Stein D, Vardi P, Werther GA, Zadik Z, Zuckerman-Levin N, Hochberg Z (2005). Childhood Obesity. *J Clin Endocrinol Metab* **90**, 1871–87.
57. Haines L, Wan KC, Lynn R, Barrett TG, Shield JPH (2007). Rising incidence of type 2 diabetes in children in the UK. *Diabetes Care* **30**, 1097–101.
58. Chinn S, Rona R (1994). Trends in weight-for-height and triceps skinfold thickness for English and Scottish children, 1972–1982 and 1982–1990. *Paediatr Perinat Epidemiol* **8**, 90–106.
59. Barth N, Ziegler A, Himmelmann G, Coners H, Wabitsch M, Hennighausen K, Mayer H, Remschmidt H, Schafer H, Hebebrand J (1997). Significant weight gains in a clinical sample of obese children and adolescents between 1985 and 1995. *Int J Obes Relat Metab Disord* **21**, 122–6.
60. Himes J, Dietz W (1994). Guidelines for overweight in adolescent preventive services: Recommendations from an expert committee. The Expert Committee on clinical guidelines for overweight in adolescent preventive services. *Am J Clin Nutr* **59**, 307–16.
61. Tounian P, Aggoun Y, Dubern B, Varille V, Guy-Grand B, Sidi D, Girardet JP, Bonnet D (2001). Presence of increased stiffness of the common carotid artery and endothelial dysfunction in severely obese children: A prospective study. *Lancet* **358**, 1400–4.
62. Goran MI, Ball GDC, Cruz ML (2003). Obesity and risk of type 2 diabetes and cardiovascular disease in children and adolescents. *J Clin Endocrinol Metab* **88**, 1417–27.
63. Sorof J, Daniels S (2002). Obesity hypertension in children: A problem of epidemic proportions. *Hypertension* **40**, 441–7.
64. Groner JA, Joshi M, Bauer JA (2006). Pediatric precursors of adult cardiovascular disease: Noninvasive assessment of early vascular changes in children and adolescents. *Pediatrics* **118**, 1683–91.
65. Gielen S, Hambrecht R (2004). The childhood obesity epidemic: Impact on endothelial function. *Circulation* **109**, 1911–13.
66. Dwyer T, Blizzard C (1996). Defining obesity in children by biological endpoint rather than population distribution. *Int J Obes Relat Metab Disord* **20**, 472–80.
67. Taylor RW, Jones IE, Williams SM, Goulding A (2002). Body fat percentages measured by dual-energy X-ray absorptiometry corresponding to recently recommended body mass index cutoffs for overweight and obesity in children and adolescents aged 3–18 y. *Am J Clin Nutr* **76**, 1416–21.
68. Lazarus R, Baur L, Webb K, Blyth F, Gliksman M (1995). Recommended body mass index cut-off values for overweight screening programmes in Australian children and adolescents: Comparisons with North American values. *J Paediatr Child Health* **31**, 143–7.
69. O'Callaghan MJ, Williams GM, Andersen MJ, Bor W, Najman JM (1997). Prediction of obesity in children at 5 years: A cohort study. *J Paediatr Child Health* **33**, 311–16.
70. Wells J (2000). A Hattori chart analysis of body mass index in infants and children. *Int J Obes Relat Metab Disord* **24**, 325–9.
71. Tell GS, Tuomilehto J, Epstein FH, Strasser T (1986). Studies of atherosclerosis determinants and precursors during childhood and adolescence. *Bull World Health Organ* **64**, 595–605.
72. Cole T, Faith M, Pietrobelli A, Heo M (2005). What is the best measure of adiposity change in growing children: BMI, BMI %, BMI z-score or BMI centile? *Eur J Clin Nutr* **59**, 419–25.
73. Cole TJ, Flegal KM, Nicholls D, Jackson AA (2007). Body mass index cut offs to define thinness in children and adolescents: International survey. *BMJ* **335**, 194.
74. National Health and Medical Research Council (2003). *Obesity guidelines: Clinical practice guidelines for the management of overweight and obesity in children and adolescents*. Australian Government Publishing Service, Canberra.
75. Freedman DS, Khan LK, Serdula MK, Dietz WH, Srinivasan SR, Berenson GS (2005). The relation of childhood BMI to adult adiposity: The Bogalusa Heart Study. *Pediatrics* **115**, 22–7.
76. Collins CE, Warren J, Neve M, McCoy P, Stokes BJ (2006). Measuring effectiveness of dietetic interventions in child obesity: A systematic review of randomized trials. *Arch Pediatr Adolesc Med* **160**, 906–22.
77. Ritchie L, Welk G, Styne D, Gerstein D, Crawford P (2005). Family environment and pediatric overweight: What is a parent to do? *J Am Diet Assoc* **105** (Suppl. 1), S70–9.
78. Epstein L, Coleman K, Myers M (1996). Exercise in treating obesity in children and adolescents. *Med Sci Sports Exerc* **28**, 428–35.

79. Must A (1996). Morbidity and mortality associated with elevated body weight in children and adolescents. *Am J Clin Nutr* **63**, 445S–7S.
80. Barlow SE, Dietz WH (1998). Obesity evaluation and treatment: Expert committee recommendations. *Pediatrics* **102**, E29.
81. Council on Sports Medicine and Fitness and Council on School Health (2006). Active healthy living: Prevention of childhood obesity through increased physical activity. *Pediatrics* **117**, 1834–42.
82. Schwartz M, Puhl R (2003). Childhood obesity: A societal problem to solve. *Obes Rev* **4**, 57–71.
83. Covic T, Roufeil L, Dziurawiec S (2007). Community beliefs about childhood obesity: Its causes, consequences and potential solutions. *J Public Health Med* **29**, 123–31.
84. Foreyt JP, Goodrick GK (1997). Living without dieting: Motivating the obese to exercise and to eat prudently. *Quest* **47**, 264–73.
85. Golan M, Crow S (2004). Targeting parents exclusively in the treatment of childhood obesity: Long-term results. *Obesity Res* **12**, 357–61.
86. Schiffman S (1994). Biological and psychological benefits of exercise in obesity. In: Hills AP, Walqvist ML (eds.), *Exercise and obesity*, pp. 103–14. Smith-Gordon and Company, London.
87. Moore KA, Burrows GD (1994). Behavioural management of obesity in an exercise context. In: Hills AP, Walqvist ML (eds.), *Exercise and obesity*, pp. 207–16. Smith-Gordon and Company, London.
88. Bar-Or O, Baranowski T (1994). Physical activity, adiposity, and obesity among adolescents. *Peditar Exerc Sci* **6**, 348–60.
89. Epstein LH (1992). Exercise and obesity in children. *J Appl Sport Psychol* **4**, 120–33.
90. Epstein L (1995). Exercise in the treatment of childhood obesity. *Int J Obes Relat Metab Disord* **19** (Suppl. 4), S117–21.
91. Epstein LH, Saelens BE, O'Brien JG (1995). Effects of reinforcing increases in active behavior versus decreases in sedentary behavior for obese children. *Int J Behav Med* **2**, 41–50.
92. Stiegler P, Cunliffe A (2006). The role of diet and exercise for the maintenance of fat-free mass and resting metabolic rate during weight loss. *Sports Med* **36**, 239–62.
93. Catenacci V, Wyatt H (2007). The role of physical activity in producing and maintaining weight loss. *Nat Clin Pract Endocrinol Metab* **3**, 518–29.
94. Brownell KD, Wadden TA (1991). The heterogeneity of obesity: Fitting treatments to individuals. *Behav Ther* **22**, 153–77.
95. Saris WHM, van Baak MA (1994). Consequences of exercise on energy expenditure. In: Hills AP, Walqvist ML (eds.), *Exercise and obesity*, pp. 85–102. Smith-Gordon and Company, London.
96. Wilmore J (1997). Weight gain, weight loss, and weight control: What is the role of physical activity? *Nutrition* **13**, 820–2.
97. Gill TP (1997). Key issues in the prevention of obesity. *Br Med Bull* **53**, 359–88.
98. World Health Organization (2000). Obesity: Preventing and managing the global epidemic. World Health Organization, Geneva.
99. Allender S, Cowburn G, Foster C (2006). Understanding participation in sport and physical activity among children and adults: A review of qualitative studies. *Health Educ Res* **21**, 826–35.
100. Epstein LH (1982). A comparison of lifestyle change and programmed aerobic exercise on weight and fitness changes in obese children. *Behav Ther* **13**, 651–65.
101. Epstein LH, Wing RR, Koeske R, Valoski A (1985). A comparison of lifestyle exercise, aerobic exercise, and calisthenics on weight loss in obese children. *Behav Ther* **16**, 345–56.
102. Speakman JR (2004). Obesity: The integrated roles of environment and genetics. *J Nutr* **134**, 2090S–105S.
103. Yang W, Kelly T, He J (2007). Genetic epidemiology of obesity. *Epidemiol Rev* **29**, 49–61.
104. Bouchard C, Tremblay A, Despres J, Nadeau A, Lupien P, Theriault G, Dussault J, Moorjani S, Pinault S, Fournier G (1990). The response to long-term overfeeding in identical twins. *N Engl J Med* **322**, 1477–82.
105. Stunkard A, Harris J, Pedersen N, McClearn G (1990). The body mass index of twins who have been reared apart. *N Engl J Med* **322**, 1483–7.
106. Booth M, Okely A (2005). Promoting physical activity among children and adolescents: The strengths and limitations of school-based approaches. *Health Promot J Austr* **16**, 52–4.
107. Ward D, Bar-Or O (1986). Role of the physician and physical education teacher in the treatment of obesity at school. *Pediatrician* **13**, 44–51.
108. Sallis JF, Chen AH, Castro CM (1985). School-based interventions for childhood obesity. In: Cheung LWY, Richmond JB (eds.), *Child health, nutrition, and physical activity*, pp. 179–204. Human Kinetics, Champaign, IL.
109. Golan M (2006). Parents as agents of change in childhood obesity—From research to practice. *Int J Pediatr Obes* **1**, 66–76.
110. Dietz W (1996). The role of lifestyle in health: The epidemiology and consequences of inactivity. *Proc Nutr Soc* **55**, 829–40.
111. Klesges R, Stein R, Eck L, Isbell T, Klesges L (1991). Parental influence on food selection in young children and its relationships to childhood obesity. *Am J Clin Nutr* **53**, 859–64.
112. Gortmaker SL, Must A, Sobol AM, Peterson K, Colditz GA, Dietz WH (1996). Television viewing as a cause of increasing obesity among children in the United States, 1986–1990. *Arch Pediatr Adolesc Med* **150**, 356–62.
113. Dietz WH, Gortmaker SL (1985). Do we fatten our children at the television set? Obesity and television viewing in children and adolescents. *Pediatrics* **75**, 807–12.
114. Salmon J, Campbell K, Crawford D (2006). Television viewing habits associated with obesity risk factors: A survey of Melbourne schoolchildren. *Med J Aust* **184**, 64–7.
115. Neville L, Thomas M, Bauman A (2005). Food advertising on Australian television: The extent of children's exposure. *Health Promot Int* **20**, 105–12.
116. Wardle J (1995). Parental influences on children's diets. *Proc Nutr Soc* **54**, 747–58.
117. Epstein L, Wing R, Penner B, Kress M (1985). Effect of diet and controlled exercise on weight loss in obese children. *J Pediatr* **107**, 358–61.
118. Epstein LH, Saelens BE, Myers MD, Vito D (1997). Effects of decreasing sedentary behaviors on activity choice in obese children. *Health Psychol* **16**, 107–13.
119. Saelens B, Epstein L (1998). Behavioral engineering of activity choice in obese children. *Int J Obes Relat Metab Disord* **22**, 275–7.
120. Wrotniak BH, Epstein LH, Paluch RA, Roemmich JN (2004). Parent weight change as a predictor of child weight change in family-based behavioral obesity treatment. *Arch Pediatr Adolesc Med* **158**, 342–7.
121. Department of Health and Ageing—Commonwealth of Australia (2004). Australia's physical activity recommendations for children and young people. Available at: http://www.health.gov.au/internet/wcms/publishing.nsf/content/health-pubhlth-strateg-active-recommend.htm (last accessed October 2007).
122. Healthy Living Unit, Public Health Agency of Canada (2002). Canadian physical activity guide for children and Canadian physical activity guide for youth. Available at: http://www.phac-aspc.gc.ca/pau-uap/paguide/ (last accessed October 2007).
123. American Heart Association. AHA Scientific Position: Exercise (physical activity) and children. Available at: http://www.americanheart.org/presenter.jhtml?identifier=4596 (accessed October 2007).
124. Koff E, Rierdan J, Stubbs ML (1990). Gender, body image, and self-concept in early adolescence. *J Early Adolesc* **10**, 56–68.
125. Hills AP, Byrne NM (1994). Relationships between body dissatisfaction, disordered eating and exercise motivations. *Int J Obes Relat Metab Disord* **18** (Suppl. 2), S31.
126. Musher-Eizenman DR, Holub SC, Miller AB, Goldstein SE, Edwards-Leeper L (2004). Body size stigmatization in preschool children: The role of control attributions. *J Pediatr Psychol* **29**, 613–20.

127. Tiggerman M, Pennington B (1990). The development of gender differences in body-size satisfaction. *Aust Psychol* **41**, 246–63.
128. Byrne N, Hills AP (1996). Should body-image scales designed for adults be used with adolescents? *Percept Mot Skills* **82**, 747–53.
129. Hills AP, Byrne NM (1998). Body composition, body satisfaction, and exercise motivation of girls and boys. *Med Sci Sports Exerc* **30**, S120.
130. Hills AP, Byrne NM (1997). Body composition and body image: Implications for weight-control practices in adolescents. *Int J Obes Relat Metab Disord* **21** (Suppl. 2), S115.
131. Hill A, Silver E (1995). Fat, friendless and unhealthy: 9-year old children's perception of body shape stereotypes. *Int J Obes Relat Metab Disord* **19**, 423–30.
132. Phillips R, Hill A (1998). Fat, plain, but not friendless: Self-esteem and peer acceptance of obese pre-adolescent girls. *Int J Obes Relat Metab Disord* **22**, 287–93.
133. Nicholls D, Viner R (2005). Eating disorders and weight problems. *BMJ* **330**, 950–3.
134. Krowchuk DP, Kreiter SR, Woods CR, Sinal SH, Du Rant RH (1998). Problem dieting behaviours among young adolescents. *Arch Ped Adolesc Med* **152**, 884–8.
135. Killen JD, Taylor CB, Hammer LD, Litt I, Wilson DM, Rich T, Hayward C, Simmonds B, Kraemer H, Varady A (1993). An attempt to modify unhealthful eating attitudes and weight regulation practices of young adolescent girls. *Int J Eat Disord* **13**, 369–84.
136. McDonald K, Thompson JK (1992). Eating disturbance, body image dissatisfaction, and reasons for exercising: Gender differences and correlational findings. *Int J Eat Disord* **11**, 289–92.
137. Striegel-Moore RH, Silberstein LR, Rodin J (1986). Toward an understanding of risk factors for bulimia. *Am Psychol* **41**, 246–63.
138. Silberstein L, Striegel-Moore R, Timko C, Rodin J (1988). Behavioural and psychological implications of body dissatisfaction: Do men and women differ? *Sex Roles* **19**, 219–32.
139. Schneider M (2003). Bulimia nervosa and binge-eating disorder in adolescents. *Adolesc Med* **14**, 119–31.
140. Crisp A (1995). The dyslipophobias: A view of the psychopathologies involved and the hazards of construing anorexia nervosa and bulimia nervosa as 'eating disorders'. *Proc Nutr Soc* **54**, 701–9.
141. Herzog D, Copeland P (1985). Eating disorders. *N Engl J Med* **313**, 295–303.
142. Davis C (1997). Eating disorders and hyperactivity: A psychobiological perspective. *Can J Psychiatry* **42**, 168–75.
143. Beumont P, Arthur B, Russell J, Touyz S (1994). Excessive physical activity in dieting disorder patients: Proposals for a supervised exercise program. *Int J Eat Disord* **15**, 21–36.
144. Davis C, Blackmore E, Katzman D, Fox J (2005). Female adolescents with anorexia nervosa and their parents: A case-control study of exercise attitudes and behaviours. *Psychol Med* **35**, 377–86.
145. Westerterp KR, Saris WHM (1992). Limits of energy turnover in relation to physical performance, achievement of energy balance on a daily basis. In: Williams C, Devlin JT (ed.), *Food, nutrition and performance*, pp. 1–18. E & FN Spon, London.
146. Russell G (1979). Bulimia nervosa: An ominous variant of anorexia nervosa. *Psychol Med* **9**, 429–48.
147. American Psychiatric Association (1994). *Diagnostic and statistical manual of mental disorders—DSM-IV.* American Psychiatric Association, Washington, D.C.
148. Fichter MM, Noegel R (1990). Concordance for bulimia nervosa in twins. *Int J Eat Disord* **9**, 255–63.
149. Hsu LKG, Chesler BE, Santhouse R (1990). Bulimia nervosa in eleven sets of twins: A clinical report. *Int J Eat Disord* **9**, 275–82.
150. Goodwin GM, Fairburn CG, Cowen PJ (1987). Dieting changes serotonergic function in women, not men: Implications for the aetiology of anorexia nervosa? *Psychol Med* **17**, 839–42.
151. Kaye WH, Ballenger JC, Lydiard RB, Stuart GW, Laraia MT, O'Neil P, Fossey MD, Stevens V, Lesser S, Hsu G (1990). CSF monoamine levels in normal-weight bulimia: Evidence for abnormal noradrenergic activity. *Am J Psychiatry* **147**, 225–9.
152. Laberg JC, Wilson GT, Eldredge K, Nordby H (1991). Effects of mood on heart rate reactivity in bulimia nervosa. *Int J Eat Disord* **10**, 169–78.
153. Laessle RG, Wittchen HU, Fichter MM, Pirke KM (1989). The significance of subgroups of bulimia and anorexia nervosa: Lifetime frequency of psychiatric disorders. *Int J Eat Disord* **8**, 569–74.
154. Garner DM, Olmsted MP, Davis R, Rockert W, Goldbloom D, Eagle M (1990). The association between bulimic symptoms and reported psychopathology. *Int J Eat Disord* **9**, 1–15.
155. Casper RC (1995). Fear of fatness and anorexia nervosa in children. In: Cheung LWY (ed.), *Child health, nutrition and physical activity*, pp. 211–34. Human Kinetics, Champaign, IL.
156. Davis C, Kennedy SH, Ravelski E, Dionne M (1994). The role of physical activity in the development and maintenance of eating disorders. *Psychol Med* **24**, 957–67.
157. Garfinkel P, Kennedy SH, Kaplan A (1995). Views on classification and diagnosis of eating disorders. *Can J Psychiatry* **40**, 445–56.
158. Chamay-Weber C, Narring F, Michaud P (2005). Partial eating disorders among adolescents: A review. *J Adolesc Health* **37**, 417–27.
159. Wilson G, Eldredge I (1992). Pathology and development of eating disorders: Implications for athletes. In: Brownell K, Rodin J, Wilmore JH (eds.), *Eating, body weight, and performance in athletes*, pp. 128–45. Lea and Febiger, Philadelphia, PA.
160. Patton GC, Carlin JB, Shao Q, Hibbert ME, Rosier M, Selzer R, Bowes G (1997). Adolescent dieting: Healthy weight control or borderline eating disorder? *J Child Psychol Psychiatry* **38**, 299–306.
161. Favaro A, Ferrara S, Santonastaso P (2003). The spectrum of eating disorders in young women: A prevalence study in a general population sample. *Psychosom Med* **65**, 701–8.
162. Nylander I (1971). The feeling of being fat and dieting in a school population. Epidemiological interview investigation. *Acta Sociomed Scand* **1**, 17–26.
163. Brownell K, Fairburn C (1995). *Eating disorders and obesity.* Guilford Press, New York.
164. Bunnell DW, Shenker IR, Nussbaum MP, Jacobson MS, Cooper P (1990). Subclinical versus formal eating disorders: Differentiating psychological features. *Int J Eat Disord* **9**, 357–62.
165. Wilmore J (1991). Eating and weight disorders in the female athlete. *Int J Sport Nutr* **1**, 104–17.
166. Wilson GT, Nonas CA, Rosenblum GD (1993). Assessment of binge eating in obese patients. *Int J Eat Disord* **13**, 25–33.
167. Robin A, Gilroy M, Dennis A (1998). Treatment of eating disorders in children and adolescents. *Clin Psychol Rev* **18**, 421–46.
168. Spitzer RL, Devlin M, Walsh BT, Hasin D, Wing RR, Marcus M, Stunkard A, Wadden T, Yanovski S, Agras S, Mitchel J, Nonas C (1992). Binge eating disorder: A multisite field trial of the diagnostic criteria. *Int J Eat Disord* **11**, 191–203.
169. Stein R, Kenardy J, Wiseman C, Dounchis J, Arnow B, Wilfley D (2007). What's driving the binge in binge eating disorder? A prospective examination of precursors and consequences. *Int J Eat Disord* **40**, 195–203.
170. Patel DR, Pratt HD, Greydanus DE (2003). Treatment of adolescents with anorexia nervosa. *J Adolesc Res* **18**, 244–60.
171. Abbate-Daga G, Piero A, Rigardetto R, Gandione M, Gramaglia C, Fassino S (2007). Clinical, psychological and personality features related to age of onset of anorexia nervosa. *Psychopathology* **40**, 261–8.
172. Rome ES, Ammerman S, Rosen DS, Keller RJ, Lock J, Mammel KA, O'Toole J, Rees JM, Sanders MJ, Sawyer SM, Schneider M, Sigel E, Silber TJ (2003). Children and adolescents with eating disorders: The state of the art. *Pediatrics* **111**, e98–108.

173. Spitzer RL, Yanovski S, Wadden TA, Wing RR, Marcus MD, Stunkard A, Devlin M, Mitchell J, Hasin D, Horne L (1993). Binge eating disorder: Its further validation in a multisite study. *Int J Eat Disord* **13**, 137–53.

174. Beumont P, Russell J, Touyz S (1993). Treatment of anorexia nervosa. *Lancet* **341**, 1635–40.

175. Crisp AH, Norton K, Gowers S, Halek C (1991). A controlled study of the effect of therapies aimed at adolescent and family psychopathology in anorexia nervosa. *Br J Psychiatry* **159**, 325–33.

176. Stewart TM, Williamson DA (2004). Multidisciplinary treatment of eating disorders—Part 2: Primary goals and content of treatment. *Behav Modif* **28**, 831–53.

177. Stewart TM, Williamson DA (2004). Multidisciplinary treatment of eating disorders—Part 1: Structure and costs of treatment. *Behav Modif* **28**, 812–30.

178. Haines J, Neumark-Sztainer D (2006). Prevention of obesity and eating disorders: A consideration of shared risk factors. *Health Educ Res* **21**, 770–82.

179. Pearson J, Goldklang D, Striegel-Moore R (2002). Prevention of eating disorders: Challenges and opportunities. *Int J Eat Disord* **31**, 233–9.

180. Halmi K (1995). Prevention strategies for eating disorders. In: Cheung LWY (ed.), *Child health, nutrition and physical activity*, pp. 243–6. Human Kinetics, Champaign, IL.

CHAPTER 35

Exercise capacity and training in cerebral palsy and other neuromuscular diseases

Annet Dallmeijer and Jost Schnyder

Introduction

In children with neuromuscular diseases, exercise can be helpful not only in the assessment of physiological functions, but also as a therapeutic tool to improve functional ability and social integration. It can offer children with disabilities better self-esteem and gives a feeling of self-responsibility. Children with cerebral palsy (CP) and other neuromuscular diseases, such as progressive muscular dystrophy (PMD), were at one time restricted from physical activity and sports. Therefore, we find little information about their abilities to perform exercise, the state of their physiological parameters or their responses to exercise. In addition, little is known about the type, intensity, duration, or frequency of the physical activity they may be able to perform. This chapter intends to give an understanding of the role of exercise in the functional assessment and clinical management of children with neuromuscular diseases, especially for children with CP and PMD. Current knowledge about exercise capacity and training possibilities with respect to the different fitness components (aerobic power, anaerobic power, muscular strength) will be described as well as the level of physical activity and training recommendations. Practical advice and suggestions are given on how to build up and execute an adapted programme for physical activity, sports, and exercise. Data will be summarized to recognize the possibilities as well as the limits of exercise, and also to permit a regular evaluation and a constant adaptation of a physical activity programme.

Cerebral palsy

CP is the most common condition encountered in the large field of neuromuscular diseases in children. Its definition has recently been described by Bax *et al.*,[1] 'CP describes a group of disorders of the development of movement and posture, causing activity limitation, that are attributed to non-progressive disturbances that occurred in the developing foetal or infant brain. The motor disorders of cerebral palsy are often accompanied by disturbances of sensation, cognition, communication, perception, and/or behaviour, and/or by a seizure disorder' (p. 572). Depending on the location and the severity of the injury, symptoms may vary, ranging from severe (inability to perform movement) to very mild (only a light clumsiness) motor impairments. Apart from impairments in motor functioning (leading to activity limitations), other associated impairments may interfere with the ability to function in daily life, such as seizures, visual and auditory impairments, and cognitive and behavioural problems.[1]

In CP normal developmental processes are disturbed, resulting in different motor impairments. Abnormal muscle tone and agonist–antagonist imbalance may lead to contractures and deformities. This results in difficulty coordinating and integrating basic movement patterns. As a consequence, limitations in mobility are a prevailing aspect of CP, leading to difficulties in performing physical activities in daily life, including sports and exercise activities. A limited exercise performance and lower fitness and activity levels can be expected. In addition, associated impairments influence the acquisition and the application of new motor skills and eventually limit exercise performance.

Classification

Individuals with CP typically present a variety of observable features and consequences depending on the degree and location of brain damage. Over the years, classification has evolved that categorizes CP according to anatomical, neuromotor, and functional perspectives. The anatomic classification is based on the body segments (most limbs) involved: hemiplegia refers to unilateral involvement, diplegia refers to predominant involvement of the legs, and in quadriplegia the arms are more affected than the legs. Recently, it has been recommended to restrict the anatomical classification to uni- or bilateral involvement.[1] In the neuromotor classification, three types of CP can be distinguished: spastic, dyskinetic (dystonia or choreoathetosis), or ataxic, but mixed forms are common.[1] Spastic CP is the most common subtype.

The Gross Motor Function Classification System (GMFCS) is a five-level classification system that is based on functional abilities and limitations, with particular emphasis on sitting and walking.[2] In recent years, the GMFCS classification became the standard for classifying gross motor function in children with CP, facilitating communication among professionals and parents.[3] Distinction between the five classification levels is based on functional limitations, use of assistive mobility devices, use of wheeled mobility, and to a lesser extent, the quality of movement. GMFCS levels are described as follows: (i) Walks without restrictions; limitations in more advanced motor skills such as running and jumping. (ii) Walks without assistive devices; limitations in walking outdoors and in the community. (iii) Walks with assistive devices; limitations walking outdoors and in the community. (iv) Self-mobility with limitations; children are transported or use powered mobility outdoors and in the community. (v) Self-mobility is severely limited even with the use of assistive technology.[2]

Exercise testing

The assessment of CP patients may be difficult due to motor impairments such as spasticity, limited range of motion, impaired selective motor control, and increased level of co-activation. Nevertheless, both laboratory and field tests have been described to assess the different fitness components in children with CP, including aerobic and anaerobic capacity, and muscle strength and endurance. For all tests, one has to consider their feasibility, reproducibility, reliability, and validity (see Chapters 4, 5, and 8 for assessments of healthy children).

A number of protocols exist for assessing aerobic capacity in a laboratory setting. Protocols measuring the maximal oxygen uptake using arm[4] and leg ergometry[5] have been described, as well as a walking test on a treadmill.[6] The advantage of these laboratory tests is that test conditions can be highly standardized. Disadvantages include the need for expensive equipment and the risk of children being unable to perform the tests due to co-ordinative problems. Habituation sessions are required to establish reliable results, especially when tests are performed on a treadmill.[6] In cycle ergometry, this especially applies to children who are not used to cycling. A low maximal power output is expected in cycle ergometry, due to the reduced mechanical efficiency of children with CP (see below).

For measuring anaerobic capacity, the Wingate Anaerobic Test is used.[7] This 30-s full out cycling test on a cycle ergometer against a constant braking force showed acceptable reliability in children with CP[8] and neuromuscular disease.[9] The anaerobic tests are easier to perform in neuromuscular disease than longer lasting aerobic protocols, this being due to the muscle weakness and the resulting fatigue limiting the duration of the test.

When no equipment is available and when interest focuses on daily life circumstances field tests are indicated. Recently, a specially adapted shuttle run test was developed to measure aerobic capacity in ambulatory children with CP (GMFCS levels I and II). This highly feasible field test can be performed in any physical therapy or sport facility, and shows good validity and reliability.[10] A reliable running field test to measure anaerobic capacity has also been described by the same research group.[11] In this Muscle Power Sprint Test the children have to complete six 15-m runs at maximal speed. From time and body weight the sprint power output can be calculated.[11]

Isometric maximal muscle strength is often measured using hand-held dynamometry. It has been shown that reliability depends on standardization of the testing procedure, and experience of the tester, and that measurement error varies between muscle groups and level of impairment.[12,13] Nevertheless, taking these limitations into account, useful results regarding muscle strength (improvements) can be obtained using hand-held dynamometry. Isokinetic measurements of knee muscle strength also showed good reliability in children with CP using a dynamometer.[14]

Aerobic capacity

In children with CP, it is muscle function rather than cardiorespiratory function and, consequently, aerobic capacity that is usually affected. It is stated that in children with CP, the maximal aerobic capacity is seldom the limiting factor for the ability to perform tasks in daily life in children.[15] Nevertheless, a lower aerobic capacity has been documented by several authors in children with CP compared to healthy peers.[5,6] Physical inactivity is likely to be, at least in part, responsible for this finding. The aerobic capacity, measured as the maximal oxygen uptake in a graded exercise test on a bicycle ergometer, appeared to be up to 20% lower in children with CP.[5,16] The difference in maximal power output is even larger[8,16] due to the lower mechanical efficiency in children with CP.[16] In addition, the maximal oxygen uptake, measured in a maximal walking test on a treadmill, was considerably lower in children with CP.[6]

Training studies on aerobic capacity were until recently rare, and rather outdated.[4,17–19] Only one study was a randomized-controlled training study, reporting positive effects on aerobic power after an intensive (four times a week for 45 min) training period of 9 months in 20 school children with CP, including wheelchair bound subjects.[19,20] Training consisted predominantly of aerobic activities, such as cycling, wheelchair driving, and swimming. Aerobic power was measured as the maximal power output during arm or leg ergometry. An increase of 35% was found in the training group compared to the control group.[19,20] This considerable training effect suggests a low aerobic level of these children due to deconditioning effects, and indicates the large potential for improvements after training (see Chapters 39 and 40 for discussions of training healthy children).

Two recent randomized-controlled studies in children with CP confirmed these results, by showing improvements in aerobic capacity after a structured training programme.[21,22] Verschuren *et al.*[22] performed a well-designed training study over a period of 8 months in a large group of 65 ambulatory children with CP (GMFCS levels I and II, aged 7–20 years). A feasible group-circuit training was performed, incorporated in the school programme, with a training frequency of twice a week (45 min). The training consisted of eight standardized aerobic and anaerobic exercises. Aerobic capacity was assessed using the 10-m shuttle run test, especially adapted for children with CP.[10] Aerobic capacity increased by 38% in the training group. This effect was only partially maintained at 4 months after the end of the training, suggesting that exercise and sport opportunities are important for maintaining adequate fitness levels.[22] Another study reported on the effects of a combined strength and aerobic interval training (three times a week for 45 min) for 12 weeks in 13 children with CP (GMFCS levels II and III).[21] Both arm and leg training was included in the intervention programme. They showed an increase of approximately 20% in the training group for maximal oxygen uptake, measured using arm ergometry. In another recent study,[23] an increase in gross motor function and cycling ability after 6 weeks of adapted static bicycle training was reported in 11 non-ambulant children with CP (GMFCS levels IV and V). Although no control group was present, results also indicated that more severely impaired children do benefit from aerobic training.

Energy cost and physical activity

One of the consequences of the motor impairments of children with CP is an increased energy demand of walking compared with healthy children.[24–26] Energy cost of walking can be measured reliably by measuring oxygen uptake while children walk at self-selected speed.[27] Energy cost is defined as the energy expenditure, calculated from oxygen uptake and subsequently normalized for walking speed (i.e. expressed per metre) and body mass. Unnithan *et al.*[26] showed that the energy cost is approximately three times higher in children with CP. They assessed the contribution that co-contraction of agonist and antagonist muscles had upon the increased energy cost. Oxygen uptake and electromyographic data from the thigh (vastus lateralis and hamstrings) and lower leg (tibialis anterior and soleus) muscles were collected simultaneously. Co-contraction accounted for up to 50% of the variability in oxygen uptake for the subjects with CP, suggesting that co-contraction is a major factor responsible for the higher energy cost of walking in children with CP.[26] Johnston *et al.*[24] showed that the energy cost of walking increases with more severe functional involvement in adolescents with CP.

The increased energy cost of walking is suggested to be a cause of early fatiguability in performing activities, as seen in children with CP, which may limit their mobility and daily physical activity.[28] Maltais *et al.*[29] found a relationship between the energy cost of walking and physical activity in 11 children with mild CP, suggesting that the high-energy cost limits activity in daily life. Other studies showed that children with CP are less physically active than their healthy peers.[30–32]

Obviously, the increased energy demand, in combination with a decreased aerobic capacity, leads to high levels of relative oxygen uptake (i.e. oxygen uptake expressed as a percentage of peak value) when performing daily life activities, leaving only a small metabolic reserve. Some studies showed that the relative energy consumption of walking on a treadmill[26,29] or at a self-selected comfortable speed,[33] expressed as a percentage of peak oxygen uptake, was more than two times higher for children with CP compared with healthy children, indicating that they impose a much higher metabolic demand on their system.

As the measurement of oxygen uptake is sometimes difficult to perform, Rose *et al.*[34] proposed the energy expenditure index (EEI), on the basis of the good linear relationship between oxygen uptake and heart rate, to compare the economy of walking at various speeds between children with and without CP. Mean EEI values were significantly lower in healthy children and occurred at faster walking speeds than in children with CP.[34]

As shown in several studies[35–37] mechanical efficiency of cycling is also low in CP patients, particularly among the spastic ones. Dresen *et al.*[36] and Jones and McLaughlin[35] showed a significant reduction in mechanical efficiency at maximum stable workload, while there were no differences in resting energy expenditure between nine CP and non-disabled gender-matched children. Bar-Or *et al.*[4] also reported a low mechanical efficiency during arm crank exercise in both trained and untrained children with CP. The low efficiency of both arm and leg cycling may also be explained by motor impairments such as reduced selective motor control, increased co-contraction, and contractures and deformities.

Assessing the possibility to improve economy (i.e. reduce the energy cost) and potentially reduce fatigue through training, some studies reported an improved efficiency after training during cycling[38] and arm cranking,[21] while others found no effects.[4,18] A 10-week training programme resulted in a significant decrease of oxygen uptake at different workloads on a cycle ergometer,[38] showing that these children can perform the same amount of work after training as before, but with lower aerobic energy expenditure. This was confirmed by Unnithan *et al.*,[21] who assessed the effect of a combined strength and aerobic interval training programme on mechanical efficiency of arm cranking. They reported an increase in mechanical efficiency of arm cranking of approximately 4%. In addition, a reduction in fractional utilization (oxygen uptake expressed as a percentage of peak value) was found because of the accompanying increase in aerobic capacity.

Anaerobic capacity

Anaerobic power (or sprint power) is assumed to be a better measure of functional ability than aerobic capacity in children, because most activities of daily living of children are characterized by short bursts of exercise.[15] It is therefore suggested to be a highly relevant outcome measure for evaluating fitness or the effects of training in children with CP. Using the Wingate Anaerobic Test, Parker *et al.*[39] showed peak and mean power output values of 3–4 SD below the mean values for healthy controls in children with moderate and severe CP aged 6–14 years. Van den Berg-Emons *et al.*[8] found a 50% lower mean power output in school-aged children with CP. Possible explanations for the lower anaerobic capacity include the low functional muscle mass, an insufficient stretch in the spastic muscle caused by an exaggerated tonic reflex, and a preferential reduction in type II muscle fibres that may take place in CP. This would reduce performance in high-intensity tasks such as the anaerobic test.[15,40] The deficient synchronization between the agonist and antagonist muscle groups (co-activation) also accounts for the higher energy cost of locomotion,[26] and could therefore also explain the considerably low power outputs in an anaerobic test.

Whether anaerobic power can be trained in children with CP is equivocal. Van den Berg-Emons *et al.*[19] found no improvement in anaerobic power, measured using the Wingate test, after a 9-month aerobic training programme in 6- to 12-year-old children with spastic CP. The lack of training effect may be explained by the aerobic focus of the training. In contrast, Verschuren *et al.*[22] showed a significant increase in anaerobic power of 25% in 32 children with CP, who followed a combined aerobic and anaerobic training programme, in comparison to a non-training control group. They measured anaerobic power with the Muscle Power Sprint Test. These positive results suggest that anaerobic capacity is at least trainable in ambulant children with CP.

Muscle strength

In children with CP, muscle mass is low and muscle strength is reduced compared to healthy controls.[41,42] Strength, measured using hand-held dynamometry, showed a reduction of 37%–69% in isometric quadriceps strength, depending on knee angle. Hamstrings strength was reduced by 52%.[41] Weakness is reported to be more pronounced in the more distally located muscle groups,[42,43] and the hip extensors and ankle dorsal flexors tended to be relatively weaker than their antagonists as compared to controls.[42] Isokinetic muscle strength of the knee flexors and extensors were 53% and 48% lower in CP children.[8] Muscle weakness is therefore, apart from spasticity and decreased selective motor control, an important cause of limitation in the performance of activities of daily life and participation in children with CP. The question whether improving muscle strength will lead to improved fitness levels and functioning has been addressed by several authors.

Previously, neurological treatment methods discouraged strength training because of a hypothesized aggravating effect on spasticity. Several studies have shown that strength-training programmes can improve lower limb muscle strength in children with CP without any adverse effects such as increased spasticity.[41,44–49] Damiano *et al.*[41,45] encouraged strengthening programmes to obtain improvements in walking and crouch gait. They reported improved quadriceps strength after a 6-week muscle strengthening programme, three times weekly, at 30°, 60°, and 90° of knee flexion. The maximal voluntary contraction of the quadriceps muscle improved and was comparable to controls without CP at the end of the training period.[41] Gait analysis showed an improvement in crouch gait after a bilateral quadriceps muscle strengthening programme.[45] After an 8-week isokinetic strength-training programme, MacPhail and Kramer[48] observed a significant increase in gross motor ability and strength gains of 21–25%, similar to those reported previously for healthy individuals.

In 2002, Dodd *et al.*[50] reviewed strength-training studies in children with CP, and concluded that strength training can increase muscle strength, but that the effects were likely to be overestimated because of the low methodological quality of the included studies. All studies had a single group pre–post test design without a control group. In addition, few studies focused on functional outcomes such as gross motor function and walking ability,[46,48,49] reporting significant improvements in gross motor function, but contradictory results on walking ability. Recently, a number of randomized-controlled trials evaluating the effects of strength-training programmes have been performed[47,51–54] Dodd *et al.*[47] found significant improvements in lower limb strength, but reported only a trend for increases in gross motor function and stair climbing, and found no effect on walking speed, after a home-based strength-training programme in 21 children with CP (10 controls). Unger *et al.*[54] performed a progressive resistance school-based strength-training programme in 37 children with CP (13 controls). They reported a significant improvement in crouch gait. Although clinical relevance remains to be investigated, results agree with the earlier findings of Damiano *et al.*[45] Engsberg *et al.*[55] reported improvements in gait after ankle strength training, but these conclusions are limited by a very small sample size. Liao *et al.*[51] performed a 6-week functional strengthening programme, using loaded sit-to-stand resistance exercise in 21 children with mild spastic diplegia. The experimental group ($n = 10$) showed an improvement in gross motor function and walking efficiency, compared to the control group, but—surprisingly—no effect was found on knee extensor strength and gait. In contrast to most other studies, Patikas *et al.*[52,53] reported no effect of a post-operative strength-training programme with a 9-month duration on both strength and gross motor function in 19 children, compared to 20 controls. They suggested that a lack of compliance and low training intensity explain these findings.

In summary, several studies support the view that improving muscle strength is an important feature in the treatment of children with CP. Apart from spasticity treatment and surgical procedures, reducing the muscle paresis should receive attention in the management and therapeutic treatment of CP children. A large variation in duration, intensity, frequency, and type of exercises in strength-training programmes have been reported. A training frequency of three times a week, using high exercise intensities (65%–80% of the one repetition maximum) based on progressive resistance training, lasting at least 6 weeks, is suggested to be most effective.[56] However, the optimal training intensity, frequency, and duration remain to be investigated. Notably, no adverse effects of high-intensity training programmes have been reported.

Associated conditions and exercise

Children with CP may suffer from several associated conditions that may interfere with performing exercise. The primary motor impairments, such as impaired selective voluntary muscle control, muscle paresis, and spasticity, will limit the performance of exercise tests and training exercises. In addition, wearing orthosis will complicate performance as well. Consequently, in most cases exercises should be individually adapted for children with CP, and test reference values for able-bodied children cannot be used in this population.

Limited cognitive abilities and behavioural problems, frequently encountered in children with CP, do also interfere with exercise performance. It is necessary to take any behavioural or concentration problem into consideration. These problems are, however, rarely described in relation to exercise training and testing in the literature. It is likely that a selection bias towards mildly affected children with only minor behavioural and cognitive problems is present in literature. Most studies include only ambulatory children with spastic CP, while there is a lack of research in the more severely affected groups (GMFCS levels III and below) and other types of CP, such as athetosis, ataxia, and dystonia.[57]

Many children with CP suffer from hypoactivity or inactivity,[30] resulting in some degree of overweight or obesity.[57] Stimulating an active lifestyle may prevent obesity and delay the decline in functional status of the child. This point becomes even more important as the child develops into an adolescent.

Neuromuscular dystrophy

Diseases of skeletal muscles produce two major patterns of exercise intolerance. In disorders of muscle energy metabolism, muscle bulk and resting strength are preserved, but an imbalance in muscle energy production and utilization leads to limited strength and endurance. In PMD, there is a progressive loss of muscle fibres, which results in increasing muscle weakness, due to a loss of functional muscle mass.[58]

Muscular dystrophy is considered as a group of inherited diseases. Muscle cells degenerate and are replaced by adipose and connective tissues. Patients suffer progressively from atrophy and weakness of the muscles, and experience cardiovascular and respiratory complications due to respiratory and cardiac muscle weakness. There are different types of dystrophies such as Duchenne's dystrophy, Becker's dystrophy, myotonic dystrophy, fascio-scapulo-humeral dystrophy, and limb-girdle dystrophy.

Duchenne's muscular dystrophy is the most frequent and severe form of the disease in childhood. It affects boys and usually starts between ages 2 and 6 years. A specific protein, called dystrophin, is absent. The disease shows itself in atrophy and weakness of the thigh, hip, back, shoulder girdle, and respiratory muscles. The patients present a pseudohypertrophic appearance, especially of the calves and forearms, due to an excessive accumulation of adipose and connective tissues within the interstitial spaces between degenerated muscle cells. The progression is rapid and results in walking inability within about 10 years of onset. Difficulty in rising from a recumbent position, tendency to fall down, and pain in climbing stairs are typical symptoms. As the disease progresses, patients become confined to wheelchairs.

The group of myopathies has to be distinguished from muscle dystrophies. Genetic, metabolic, or infectious origins generate the pathology of mitochondrial myopathy, neurofibromatosis, myasthenia gravis, McArdle's disease, Prader–Willi syndrome, Friedreich's ataxia, or others. The genetic origin of several diseases is known, but still remains unclear for some others. Many recent studies have shown an improvement of muscle strength in different myopathies through exercise.[59,60] As far as exercise is concerned, these diseases can be assimilated to the group of progressive neuromuscular disorders.

Obesity is an occurring problem in patients with neuromuscular disease. Muscle cells are replaced by adipose and connective tissues, and body weight increases. Immobilization is probably the worst secondary condition. Bed rest must therefore be avoided imperatively. Some patients never recover from a prolonged illness or surgery, after having been bedridden for several weeks.

Three deficient fitness components characterize the physical working capacity of a patient with neuromuscular dystrophy: muscle strength, muscle endurance, and maximal aerobic power.

Aerobic and anaerobic capacity

In muscular dystrophy patients, deficits in aerobic and anaerobic capacity are present as a result of a decreased muscle mass due to muscle necrosis and atrophy.[9,61,62] The extent of the limitation in both anaerobic and aerobic exercise performance is related to the severity of the disease.[63] Reduced values for muscle endurance and peak anaerobic power on the Wingate test are reported for children with PMD.[9] A limited aerobic exercise performance was reported in children with PMD compared to healthy controls, owing to a lower cardiorespiratory capacity.[62] Children with PMD progressively undergo a reduction of functional motor units in the muscles and, to a lesser extent, present lower respiratory functions. This explains the observed low maximal power output and maximal oxygen uptake.[61,62] PMD patients cannot reach a very high peak heart rate and therefore have to terminate an aerobic test whereas the cardiovascular system is not fully in demand. One can assume that the main limiting factor in these children is not the oxygen transport system but rather their reduced muscle strength, endurance, and anaerobic power.

Muscle strength

Muscle strength is essential to the child's ability to accomplish daily activities such as standing, rising, or walking. Many authors have assessed muscle strength in neuromuscular dystrophy. They showed that muscle strength is markedly reduced in children with PMD, showing variable rates of deterioration across muscle groups.[15,58,63–65] Lewis and Haller[63] reviewed skeletal muscle disorders and associated factors that limit exercise performance, and noted a low muscle strength in all types of muscle dystrophy, such as Duchenne's and Becker's dystrophy. Exercise is severely impaired due to muscle wasting and weakness. McDonald *et al.*[64] studied 162 patients with Duchenne's dystrophy to provide a profile of impairment and disability. Manual muscle test (MMT) measurements showed a linear loss of strength of 0.25 MMT units per year, in boys aged 5–13 years. Legs were more affected than arms, and proximal muscle groups and extensor muscles were weaker than distal muscle groups and flexor muscles. Isometrically measured strength was 40–50% below values in healthy children. While healthy children have a constant increase in muscle strength, either measurement approach shows a continuous decline in muscle strength in Duchenne's dystrophy. Such a lack of increase in absolute muscle strength during growth corresponds with a reduction in function.[15]

Trainability

Concerning the question of trainability of muscle strength in neuromuscular dystrophy, studies in adults reported positive effects on muscle performance after a weight and strength-training programme.[66,67] A dynamic 9-week weight training programme, three times a week, in a group of five adults with different types of dystrophy[66] resulted in a strength gain from 19% to 50% in the trained limb. Results showed that the gains in strength were apparently due to a neural adaptation, rather than muscle hypertrophy. Milner-Brown and Miller[67] quantified muscle performance in 16 patients with gradually progressive neuromuscular disorders. They concluded that a high resistance weight training programme can significantly increase muscle performance, if the disease progression is slow and initial muscle strength is greater than 15% of normal. A 12-week moderate resistance exercise programme in 27 patients (and 14 controls) with slow PMD noted moderate improvement in strength measures.[68] The same research group also reported on the effects of a high resistance exercise programme in patients with slow PMD.[69] They concluded that high resistance exercise had no advantage over moderate exercise, while high resistance exercise may cause deleterious effects to the muscles. Another study in the same group of patients showed that a 12-week walking programme of moderate aerobic intensity is well tolerated and provided modest improvements of aerobic capacity.[70] This was in agreement with earlier findings reporting an increased aerobic capacity as a result of cardiovascular training adaptations, after a 12-week training programme in patients with non-PMD and slow PMD.[71] Maximal oxygen uptake increased to the same levels as in healthy subjects.

There is, however, little evidence on trainability of muscle strength in children with neuromuscular disease. In a review on the role of exercise in children with neuromuscular disease, Bar-Or[15] described results that suggest that muscle strength is trainable in children with neuromuscular dystrophy. A review by Ansved[72] summarized the literature on the influence of physical conditioning in muscular dystrophies. It was concluded that, despite the limited number and poor methodological quality of available publications, current results suggest positive effects of exercise training. Resistance and aerobic training of low-to-moderate intensity is assumed to be beneficial for patients with myopathic diseases that are slowly progressive. This type of training can prevent disuse atrophy and deconditioning in these patients. To date, there is no evidence to support the recommendation of high resistance exercise regimens over low-moderate intensity exercise in this group. In rapidly progressive dystrophy, such as Duchenne's dystrophy, low resistance endurance exercise is recommended, consisting of concentric and dynamic contractions that avoid mechanical damage. High resistance exercise and eccentric training should be avoided in these patients.[72] These findings corroborate the fact that muscle strength, muscle endurance, anaerobic power, and aerobic power are trainable in this group of children. A progressive loss of strength may be slowed down and, at least for a while, reversed, which is one of the goals of any exercise programme. However, a recent review investigating the effects of training in patients with muscle disease in randomized or quasi-experimental designs only concluded that there is insufficient evidence to ascertain that training is effective.[73]

In summary, the scientific basis for solid recommendations of different exercise regimens in muscular dystrophies is poor, but existing data suggest beneficial effects of adopting an active lifestyle. There is also no evidence that physical training can influence the evolution of muscular dystrophies in the long term.

Exercise testing

Children respond in a different way to chronic or acute exercise stress than adults. This point is even more important for patients with neuromuscular dystrophy. As tests often represent a strong demand on physical resources and may cause excess fatigue, one has to decide whether they are necessary, useful, and safe for the patient, and which type of tests are best indicated. One has to consider their feasibility, reproducibility, and reliability. In view of the fact that expensive computer-linked equipment is not commonly available, a battery of field tests can be used. Children will anyway prefer to perform tests in a group and under familiar conditions. When performing field tests, it is important to consider that the tests have to be carried out under the same conditions and with the same testing person, and that learning effects must be eliminated from initial measurements by repeated testing.

Recommendations for physical activity and training

As a consequence of the motor impairments, and concomitant limitations in mobility, children with neuromuscular diseases are more likely to develop an inactive lifestyle. A vicious cycle can develop whereby physical inactivity leads to deconditioning, that can lead in turn to lower fitness levels. The prevention of the occurrence of such a vicious cycle therefore has a priority in the management of neuromuscular diseases. A recent report of a research summit emphazised the need for promoting physical activity for maintaining fitness levels in children with CP, and stressed the need for lifelong intervention programmes, to improve health and quality of life, and prevent secondary conditions.[57] The report stated that more insight into barriers and facilitators of physical activity is required. The report also underlined the importance of becoming acquainted to enjoyable physical activity at a younger age, in order to continue an active lifestyle through adulthood.[57]

Developing a multidisciplinary training programme

As discussed above, children with neuromuscular disease can and should exercise. What kind of physical activity is indicated for them? As an example, some experience from a multidisciplinary programme for children with neuromuscular disease will be given. This programme is performed at the Centre de Medicine d'Exercise in Geneva. Twice a week, children take part in organized activities: one in the pool (45 min) and one in the gymnasium (90 min). They are followed by a physician, a nutritionist, and a psychologist. Medical and physiological evaluations are carried out twice a year. Before integrating children with neuromuscular disease in an adapted physical activity programme, one has to specify the physiological and psychological status of each child. A medical history and a general clinical examination are necessary to provide information about possible general health problems, which may have an influence on the disease itself. An underlying pathology independent from the neuromuscular disease should be clarified to prevent damaging interactions. Associated impairments, such as behavioural or hearing disorders, or troubles of vision must be taken into account particularly. Lifestyle, self-esteem, and integration are often problematic concerns in these children.

The multidisciplinary approach of such a programme has numerous advantages. The physical activity programme is performed by a therapist specialized in neuromuscular disease and a specially trained physical educator. Depending on the severity of the impairment, one instructor is necessary for a group of 3–6 children. Joining a group for specialized physical education can be a means of reducing medical support and physiotherapy sessions and be a help in becoming more independent. It can also be a way of stimulating someone who refuses to continue therapy when it is still considered necessary, for example, during the growth spurt of adolescents.

An inactive lifestyle may in the longer term lead to overweight or even obesity, which is even more serious in disabled children, because of its negative effect on physical functioning and health. A nutritional evaluation should therefore also be considered as part of a multidisciplinary approach when developing a training programme. Measurements of body mass, stature, and body composition can be performed, and used as a baseline for a training study. A questionnaire concerning eating habits should be considered. These measurements allow the evaluation of the child and for the adaptation of the programme to each child individually. The role of a nutritionist is to give advice and information to the children and the parents for their specific needs.

A psychological evaluation is of major importance to assess the child's motivations to adhere to the programme and to reveal negative thoughts and self-perceptions that might aggravate their condition. The evaluation thus serves as a basis to set realistic goals for each child and his/her parents, and also to provide topics on which to work, such as self-esteem, social integration, and unrealistic expectations about the programme. By encouraging the children to find activities that are suited to their actual capacities, the psychologist is able to create some sense of perceived competence and trust. This psychological aspect helps the children to cope better with their impairment and becomes the basis for self-acceptance in many of them. The improvement of self-esteem and well-being and the possibility of integration within a group are of greatest value, not only for the child, but also for his family.

Training programme characteristics

Training compliance is an important factor determining success in training studies. A training programme should therefore, in the first place, be attractive, enjoyable, and fun for children. These are the foremost important factors in stimulating effort and participation in training programmes. Good compliance may, for example, be achieved by including games and activities that are enjoyable for children, by applying a feasible frequency of training (usually twice a week), and by integrating the physical activities into the school programme. Learning to climb and to jump from a height can be encouraged if the descent is fun (slide, big mattress, etc.). Games can make the hard work that is necessary to improve endurance enjoyable. Creating a team spirit by training in (small) groups can also stimulate participation. The training may bring the children up to a sufficient standard, physically and psychologically, so that they are able to join a local club, group, or school lesson for some kind of sport.

Continuity of training or physical activity is important. Although improvements have been reported after short-duration programmes, it is unquestionable that training effects disappear after finishing the training or activity. Improving the children's activity levels in daily life can maintain their fitness level.

Type of physical activity

Physical activities for children with neuromuscular diseases should not differ too much from those for healthy children. The problem for the animators of such a course is to choose the correct degree of difficulty, intensity, frequency, and duration. One must show the child what he is able to do. Success in varied situations is the key to all functioning programmes.

Water is a fantastic medium in which a child with neuromuscular disease can move more freely. Sufficient time is spent in ensuring that there is an adaptation to water with little or no fear. Basic swimming techniques are taught in varying depths of water and different positions. Strength and endurance can be trained in various ways, such as running, walking, or hopping, depending on the level of impairment, in different levels of water, swimming in shallow water—with hands touching the bottom of the pool for non or poor swimmers—and, of course, swimming in medium to deep water for the good ones. Circuit training on, in, and under water is great fun and improves balance. Jumping in and out of hoops or air rings and over submerged ropes, climbing into floating objects, rowing rafts, and doing tasks forwards and backwards are means to train coordination in an entertaining way.

In the gymnasium, varied relay games have many advantages, such as memorizing instructions and preparing oneself for action. Speed is an important factor which provokes an increase in heart rate. Although the aim of each relay race is the same for all, the way in which it is performed can be varied according to individual possibilities. Balance, climbing, and swinging can be combined in different activities and circuits. Children and adolescents often enjoy the challenge of big apparatus and moving surfaces; all senses (tactile, vestibular, and proprioceptive) are stimulated and motor response is often maximal. Adapted team games, such as unihockey, volleyball, and netball, are activities where all members of the team can function and enjoy a group situation. Stretching should be a part of all lessons and adapted to the activity of the day and the individual needs of the participants.

Strength and endurance exercise are elements included in all training sessions in many different ways. Typically, one would start with a warm-up composed of a team game. The main part of the lesson could be a circuit using large apparatus. Strength, dexterity, balance, and possibly speed and endurance can be included depending on the aims and the instructions given. A calm game or stretching can be done at the end for cool-down and increasing flexibility.

Precautions

A certain selection of candidates must be made in order to obtain a smoothly running group. The purpose of the training should be carefully explained so that the children know that the difficulties of exercises will be adapted to their individual abilities, and that regular participation is needed in order to gain benefit from the programme. Each participant must find a level of activity within the course which corresponds to their abilities. If an exercise is too easy, boredom can set in. On the contrary, a too high level of difficulty can lead to frustration and negative feedback. Constant stimulation through fun learning situations, attainable aims, and encouraging programme leaders must result in regular effort and performance from the children. As a long-term aim is reintegration into non-specialized physical activities, the participants must not be overprotected within the group and should gain in independence.

Children with PMD must be carefully monitored to ensure that they do not go over their fatigue level, which may initiate accelerated degradation of residual muscle. Caution must be taken when asking for the speed of execution to ensure that not too much quality of movement is lost. Hand holds in climbing and swinging must be closely supervised: a spastic hand can slip during motion, and children with PMD are known to let go suddenly when their muscles fatigue. Foot and hand deformities can make running, jumping, and climbing very difficult and even contraindicated. All course leaders must ensure that the activity has the desired effect and not a detrimental one, may it be physical or psychological. During the programme, continuous information must be given, especially to those suffering from progressive diseases, so that poor results are correctly interpreted and that disappointment and unreasonable expectations are avoided.

Evaluation

In order to monitor the effect of participation in a physical activity programme, and to determine whether the aims of the programme have been attained, a series of useful tests can be chosen, as described above. Preferably, tests should be repeated in a systematic way and the parents, the child, and his/her doctor should be informed about the progress made. The tests also serve as a motivation for the children and their parents, and show the doctors the possible therapeutic utility of exercise and the necessity of its continuity.

Several interesting points have to be taken into consideration: (i) In children with progressive neuromuscular dystrophy one cannot expect extraordinary progression. In these children, the course is positive if no deterioration has occurred or if only little improvement of the physical parameters has been observed, as its initial goal is to slow down the progression of the physical deterioration, and secondarily to improve the performance. (ii) The regularity of physical activity is an important determinant of its success. Intercurrent illness or surgery immediately provoke a stop or regression of any previously achieved benefit. Continuity and the possibility of following a physical activity programme during the long period of the summer vacation is imperative to prevent a regression, as already mentioned by Berg in 1970.[17]

Summary

- Physical activity is suggested to be beneficial for most children with neuromuscular diseases.
- To support children to walk as long as possible and to maintain the ability to perform most common daily activities should encourage all persons involved in the approach of these diseases to motivate the children and their families to invest in physical activities.
- Even if the disease is progressive, similar to PMD, a delay in deterioration is a motivation for participating in exercise.
- A better knowledge of the innocuity of sports, if correctly practised, as well as a precise appreciation of the clinical and physiological parameters, should also help to decrease fear and overprotection and, eventually, to delay as long as possible the course towards wheelchair dependency.
- In general, further research of sufficient methodological quality is required to increase evidence on trainability of all fitness parameters and functional abilities in children with neuromuscular diseases. Special attention should be paid to (i) determining the optimal training volume for children with different levels of impairments and diseases, and (ii) establishing the trainability of muscle strength and endurance in children with neuromuscular dystrophy.
- Finally, the results described in this chapter emphasize the psychological and sociocultural benefits of exercise and encourage more research in this difficult field.

References

1. Bax M, Goldstein M, Rosenbaum P, Leviton A, Paneth N, Dan B, Jacobsson B, Damiano D (2005). Executive Committee for the Definition of Cerebral Palsy. Proposed definition and classification of cerebral palsy. *Dev Med Child Neurol* **47**, 571–6.
2. Palisano R, Rosenbaum P, Walter S, Russell D, Wood E, Galuppi B (1997). Development and reliability of a system to classify gross motor function in children with cerebral palsy. *Dev Med Child Neurol* **39**, 214–23.
3. Morris C, Bartlett D (2004). Gross Motor Function Classification System: Impact and utility. *Dev Med Child Neurol* **46**, 60–5.
4. Bar-Or O, Inbar O, Spira R (1976). Physiological effects of a sports rehabilitation program on cerebral palsied and post-poliomyelitic adolescents. *Med Sci Sports* **8**, 157–61.
5. Lundberg A (1978). Maximal aerobic capacity of young people with spastic cerebral palsy. *Dev Med Child Neurol* **20**, 205–10.
6. Hoofwijk M, Unnithan V, Bar-Or O (1995). Maximal treadmill performance of children with cerebral palsy. *Pediatr Exerc Sci* **7**, 305–13.
7. Bar-Or O (1987). The Wingate anaerobic test. An update on methodology, reliability and validity. *Sports Med* **4**, 381–94.
8. van den Berg-Emons RJ, van Baak MA, de Barbanson DC, Speth L, Saris WH (1996). Reliability of tests to determine peak aerobic power, anaerobic power and isokinetic muscle strength in children with spastic cerebral palsy. *Dev Med Child Neurol* **38**, 1117–25.
9. Tirosh E, Bar-Or O, Rosenbaum P (1990). New muscle power test in neuromuscular disease. Feasibility and reliability. *Am J Dis Child* **144**, 1083–7.
10. Verschuren O, Takken T, Ketelaar M, Gorter JW, Helders PJ (2006). Reliability and validity of data for 2 newly developed shuttle run tests in children with cerebral palsy. *Phys Ther* **86**, 1107–17.
11. Verschuren O, Takken T, Ketelaar M, Gorter JW, Helders PJ (2007). Reliability for running tests for measuring agility and anaerobic muscle power in children and adolescents with cerebral palsy. *Pediatr Phys Ther* **19**, 108–15.
12. Crompton J, Galea MP, Phillips B (2007). Hand-held dynamometry for muscle strength measurement in children with cerebral palsy. *Dev Med Child Neurol* **49**, 106–11.
13. Taylor NF, Dodd KJ, Graham HK (2004). Test-retest reliability of hand-held dynamometric strength testing in young people with cerebral palsy. *Arch Phys Med Rehabil* **85**, 77–80.
14. Ayalon M, Ben Sira D, Hutzler Y, Gilad T (2000). Reliability of isokinetic strength measurements of the knee in children with cerebral palsy. *Dev Med Child Neurol* **42**, 398–402.
15. Bar-Or O (1996). Role of exercise in the assessment and management of neuromuscular disease in children. *Med Sci Sports Exerc* **28**, 421–7.
16. Lundberg A (1984). Longitudinal study of physical working capacity of young people with spastic cerebral palsy. *Dev Med Child Neurol* **26**, 328–34.
17. Berg K (1970). Effect of physical training of school children with cerebral palsy. *Acta Paediatr Scand Suppl* **204** (Suppl.), 27–33.
18. Lundberg A, Ovenfors CO, Saltin B (1967). Effect of physical training on school-children with cerebral palsy. *Acta Paediatr Scand* **56**, 182–8.
19. van den Berg-Emons RJ, van Baak MA, Speth L, Saris WH (1998). Physical training of school children with spastic cerebral palsy: Effects on daily activity, fat mass and fitness. *Int J Rehabil Res* **21**, 179–94.
20. Emons HJ, Van Baak MA (1993). Effect of training on aerobic and anaerobic power and mechanical efficiency in spastic cerebral palsied children. *Pediatr Exerc Sci* **5**, 412.
21. Unnithan VB, Katsimanis G, Evangelinou C, Kosmas C, Kandrali I, Kellis E (2007). Effect of strength and aerobic training in children with cerebral palsy. *Med Sci Sports Exerc* **39**, 1902–9.
22. Verschuren O, Ketelaar M, Gorter JW, Helders PJ, Uiterwaal CS, Takken T (2007). Exercise training program in children and adolescents with cerebral palsy: A randomized controlled trial. *Arch Pediatr Adolesc Med* **161**, 1075–81.
23. Williams H, Pountney T (2007). Effects of a static bicycling programme on the functional ability of young people with cerebral palsy who are non-ambulant. *Dev Med Child Neurol* **49**, 522–7.
24. Johnston TE, Moore SE, Quinn LT, Smith BT (2004). Energy cost of walking in children with cerebral palsy: Relation to the Gross Motor Function Classification System. *Dev Med Child Neurol* **46**, 34–8.
25. Rose J, Gamble JG, Medeiros J, Burgos A, Haskell WL (1989). Energy cost of walking in normal children and in those with cerebral palsy: Comparison of heart rate and oxygen uptake. *J Pediatr Orthop* **9**, 276–9.
26. Unnithan VB, Dowling JJ, Frost G, Bar-Or O (1996). Role of cocontraction in the O_2 cost of walking in children with cerebral palsy. *Med Sci Sports Exerc* **28**, 1498–504.
27. Brehm MA, Becher J, Harlaar J (2007). Reproducibility evaluation of gross and net walking efficiency in children with cerebral palsy. *Dev Med Child Neurol* **49**, 45–8.
28. Dahlback GO, Norlin R (1985). The effect of corrective surgery on energy expenditure during ambulation in children with cerebral palsy. *Eur J Appl Physiol Occup Physiol* **54**, 67–70.
29. Maltais DB, Pierrynowski MR, Galea VA, Bar-Or O (2005). Physical activity level is associated with the O2 cost of walking in cerebral palsy. *Med Sci Sports Exerc* **37**, 347–53.
30. Bjornson KF, Belza B, Kartin D, Logsdon R, McLaughlin JF (2007). Ambulatory physical activity performance in youth with cerebral palsy and youth who are developing typically. *Phys Ther* **87**, 248–57.
31. Maher CA, Williams MT, Olds T, Lane AE (2007). Physical and sedentary activity in adolescents with cerebral palsy. *Dev Med Child Neurol* **49**, 450–7.
32. van den Berg-Emons HJ, Saris WH, de Barbanson DC, Westerterp KR, Huson A, van Baak MA (1995). Daily physical activity of

schoolchildren with spastic diplegia and of healthy control subjects. *J Pediatr* **127**, 578–84.

33. Dallmeijer AJ, Brehm MA, De Haas LMJ, Becher JG (2006). Physical strain of walking in children with cerebral palsy. *Presented at the European Academy of Childhood Disability*, Barcelona, Spain.
34. Rose J, Gamble JG, Burgos A, Medeiros J, Haskell WL (1990). Energy expenditure index of walking for normal children and for children with cerebral palsy. *Dev Med Child Neurol* **32**, 333–40.
35. Jones J, McLaughlin JF (1993). Mechanical efficiency of children with spastic cerebral palsy. *Dev Med Child Neurol* **35**, 614–20.
36. Dresen MH, de Groot G, Corstius JJ, Krediet GH, Meijer MG (1982). Physical work capacity and daily physical activities of handicapped and non-handicapped children. *Eur J Appl Physiol Occup Physiol* **48**, 241–51.
37. Lundberg A (1975). Mechanical efficiency in bicycle ergometer work of young adults with cerebral palsy. *Dev Med Child Neurol* **17**, 434–9.
38. Dresen MH, de Groot G, Mesa M Jr, Bouman LN (1985). Aerobic energy expenditure of handicapped children after training. *Arch Phys Med Rehabil* **66**, 302–6.
39. Parker DF, Carriere L, Hebestreit H, Bar-Or O (1992). Anaerobic endurance and peak muscle power in children with spastic cerebral palsy. *Am J Dis Child* **146**, 1069–73.
40. Unnithan VB, Clifford C, Bar-Or O (1998). Evaluation by exercise testing of the child with cerebral palsy. *Sports Med* **26**, 239–51.
41. Damiano DL, Vaughan CL, Abel MF (1995). Muscle response to heavy resistance exercise in children with spastic cerebral palsy. *Dev Med Child Neurol* **37**, 731–9.
42. Wiley ME, Damiano DL (1998). Lower-extremity strength profiles in spastic cerebral palsy. *Dev Med Child Neurol* **40**, 100–7.
43. Ross SA, Engsberg JR (2002). Relation between spasticity and strength in individuals with spastic diplegic cerebral palsy. *Dev Med Child Neurol* **44**, 148–57.
44. Blundell SW, Shepherd RB, Dean CM, Adams RD, Cahill BM (2003). Functional strength training in cerebral palsy: A pilot study of a group circuit training class for children aged 4–8 years. *Clin Rehabil* **17**, 48–57
45. Damiano DL, Kelly LE, Vaughn CL (1995). Effects of quadriceps femoris muscle strengthening on crouch gait in children with spastic diplegia. *Phys Ther* **75**, 658–67.
46. Damiano DL, Abel MF (1998). Functional outcomes of strength training in spastic cerebral palsy. *Arch Phys Med Rehabil* **79**, 119–25.
47. Dodd KJ, Taylor NF, Graham HK (2003). A randomized clinical trial of strength training in young people with cerebral palsy. *Dev Med Child Neurol* **45**, 652–7.
48. MacPhail HE, Kramer JF (1995). Effect of isokinetic strength-training on functional ability and walking efficiency in adolescents with cerebral palsy. *Dev Med Child Neurol* **37**, 763–75.
49. Morton JF, Brownlee M, McFadyen AK (2005). The effects of progressive resistance training for children with cerebral palsy. *Clin Rehabil* **19**, 283–9.
50. Dodd KJ, Taylor NF, Damiano DL (2002). A systematic review of the effectiveness of strength-training programs for people with cerebral palsy. *Arch Phys Med Rehabil* **83**, 1157–64.
51. Liao HF, Liu YC, Liu WY, Lin YT (2007). Effectiveness of loaded sit-to-stand resistance exercise for children with mild spastic diplegia: A randomized clinical trial. *Arch Phys Med Rehabil* **88**, 25–31.
52. Patikas D, Wolf SI, Armbrust P, Mund K, Schuster W, Dreher T, Doderlein L (2006). Effects of a postoperative resistive exercise program on the knee extension and flexion torque in children with cerebral palsy: A randomized clinical trial. *Arch Phys Med Rehabil* **87**, 1161–9
53. Patikas D, Wolf SI, Mund K, Armbrust P, Schuster W, Doderlein L (2006). Effects of a postoperative strength-training program on the walking ability of children with cerebral palsy: A randomized controlled trial. *Arch Phys Med Rehabil* **87**, 619–26.
54. Unger M, Faure M, Frieg A (2006). Strength training in adolescent learners with cerebral palsy: A randomized controlled trial. *Clin Rehabil* **20**, 469–77.
55. Engsberg JR, Ross SA, Collins DR (2006). Increasing ankle strength to improve gait and function in children with cerebral palsy: A pilot study. *Pediatr Phys Ther* **18**, 266–75.
56. Verschuren O, Ketelaar M, Takken T, Helders PJ, Gorter JW (2008). Exercise programs for children with cerebral palsy: A systematic review of the literature. *Am J Phys Med Rehabil* **87**, 404–17.
57. Fowler EG, Kolobe TH, Damiano DL, Thorpe DE, Morgan DW, Brunstrom JE, Coster WJ, Henderson RC, Pitetti KH, Rimmer JH, Rose J, Stevenson RD (2007). Promotion of physical fitness and prevention of secondary conditions for children with cerebral palsy: Section on pediatrics research summit proceedings. *Phys Ther* **87**, 1495–510.
58. Haller RG, Lewis SF (1984). Pathophysiology of exercise performance in muscle disease. *Med Sci Sports Exerc* **16**, 456–9.
59. Chaussain M, Camus F, Defoligny C, Eymard B, Fardeau M (1992). Exercise intolerance in patients with McArdle's disease or mitochondrial myopathies. *Eur J Med* **1**, 457–63.
60. Taivassalo T, Haller RG (2005). Exercise and training in mitochondrial myopathies. *Med Sci Sports Exerc* **37**, 2094–101.
61. Carroll JE, Hagberg JM, Brooke MH, Shumate JB (1979). Bicycle ergometry and gas exchange measurements in neuromuscular diseases. *Arch Neurol* **36**, 457–61.
62. Sockolov R, Irwin B, Dressendorfer RH, Bernauer EM (1977). Exercise performance in 6- to 11-year-old boys with Duchenne muscular dystrophy. *Arch Phys Med Rehabil* **58**, 195–201.
63. Lewis SF, Haller RG (1989). Skeletal muscle disorders and associated factors that limit exercise performance. *Exerc Sport Sci Rev* **17**, 67–113.
64. McDonald CM, Abresch RT, Carter GT, Fowler WM Jr, Johnson ER, Kilmer DD, Sigford BJ (1995). Profiles of neuromuscular diseases. Duchenne muscular dystrophy. *Am J Phys Med Rehabil* **74** (Suppl.), S70–92.
65. Brussock CM, Haley SM, Munsat TL, Bernhardt DB (1992). Measurement of isometric force in children with and without Duchenne's muscular dystrophy. *Phys Ther* **72**, 105–14.
66. McCartney N, Moroz D, Garner SH, McComas AJ (1988). The effects of strength training in patients with selected neuromuscular disorders. *Med Sci Sports Exerc* **20**, 362–8.
67. Milner-Brown HS, Miller RG (1988). Muscle strengthening through high-resistance weight training in patients with neuromuscular disorders. *Arch Phys Med Rehabil* **69**, 14–19.
68. Aitkens SG, McCrory MA, Kilmer DD, Bernauer EM (1993). Moderate resistance exercise program: Its effect in slowly progressive neuromuscular disease. *Arch Phys Med Rehabil* **74**, 711–15.
69. Kilmer DD, McCrory MA, Wright NC, Aitkens SG, Bernauer EM (1994). The effect of a high resistance exercise program in slowly progressive neuromuscular disease. *Arch Phys Med Rehabil* **75**, 560–3.
70. Wright NC, Kilmer DD, McCrory MA, Aitkens SG, Holcomb BJ, Bernauer EM (1996). Aerobic walking in slowly progressive neuromuscular disease: Effect of a 12-week program. *Arch Phys Med Rehabil* **77**, 64–9.
71. Florence JM, Hagberg JM (1984). Effect of training on the exercise responses of neuromuscular disease patients. *Med Sci Sports Exerc* **16**, 460–5.
72. Ansved T (2003). Muscular dystrophies: Influence of physical conditioning on the disease evolution. *Curr Opin Clin Nutr Metab Care* **6**, 435–9.
73. van der Kooi EL, Lindeman E, Riphagen I (2005). Strength training and aerobic exercise training for muscle disease. *Cochrane Database Syst Rev* **1**, CD003907.

CHAPTER 36

Exercise, sport, and diabetes mellitus

Edgar G. A. H. van Mil

Introduction

Definition of diabetes mellitus

Diabetes mellitus is a group of metabolic diseases characterized by chronic hyperglycaemia, resulting from defects in insulin secretion, insulin action, or both. The abnormalities in carbohydrate, fat, and protein metabolism that are found in diabetes are due to deficient action of insulin on target tissues (www.ispad.org).

Diagnostic criteria for diabetes in childhood and adolescence

Diagnostic criteria for diabetes are based on blood glucose measurement and the presence or absence of symptoms[1]:

- Symptoms of diabetes plus casual plasma glucose concentration $\geq$11.1 mmol·L^{-1} (200 mg·dL^{-1}). (Corresponding values $\geq$10.0 mmol·L^{-1} for venous whole blood and $\geq$11.1 mmol·L^{-1} for capillary whole blood.) Casual is defined as any time of day without regard to time since the last meal.

  Or

- Fasting plasma glucose $\geq$7.0 mmol·L^{-1} (126 mg·dL^{-1}). (Corresponding values are $\geq$6.3 mg·dL^{-1} for both venous and capillary whole blood.) Fasting is defined as no caloric intake for at least 8 hours.

  Or

- Two hour postload glucose 11.1 mmol·L^{-1} ($\geq$200 mg·dL^{-1}) during an oral glucose tolerance test (OGTT). The test should be performed as described by the World Health Organization, using a glucose load containing the equivalent of 75 g anhydrous glucose dissolved in water or 1.75 g·kg^{-1} of body weight to a maximum of 75 g.

Classification of diabetes

The aetiological classification recommended by the American Diabetes Association (ADA)[1] and the World Health Organization (WHO)[2] expert committee defines three groups:

(i) Type 1 diabetes mellitus (T1DM)

B-cell destruction, usually leading to absolute insulin deficiency.

(A) Autoimmune

(B) Idiopathic

(ii) Type 2 diabetes mellitus (T2DM)

May range from predominantly insulin resistance with relative deficiency to a predominantly secretory defect with or without insulin resistance.

(iii) Other specific types

  (a) Genetic defects of B-cell function [e.g. MODY (Maturity Onset Diabetes of the Young)]

  (b) Genetic defects in insulin action

  (c) Diseases of the exocrine pancreas

  (d) Endocrinopathies

  (e) Drug or chemical induced

  (f) Infections-related

  (g) Uncommon forms of immune-mediated diabetes

  (h) Other genetic syndromes sometimes associated with diabetes.

The differentiation between T1DM, T2DM, and monogenetic diabetes has important implications for both the therapeutic decisions and educational approaches. T1DM accounts for more than 90% of childhood and adolescent diabetes with annual incidence rates from 0.1 to 37.4 per 100,000 dependent on the country. Although with the increasing prevalence of childhood obesity, T2DM is becoming more common in youth,[3] this chapter is focused on T1DM.

The aetiology and incidence of type 1 diabetes mellitus

T1DM is associated with deficient insulin secretion. The beta cells of the pancreas are largely destroyed. Insulin secretory responses to standard glucose tolerance tests are markedly reduced or absent. C-peptide responses are used instead of insulin to check beta cell capacity when the diabetic is already receiving exogenous insulin. Type 1A diabetes mellitus refers to immune-related T-lymphocyte-mediated diabetes mellitus, which results in the destruction of the beta cells of the pancreas, and features anti-islet autoantibodies. Genetic factors are involved, however, there is no recog-

This chapter was based on the corresponding chapter in the previous edition written by K. D. Buchana who died on 22 July 2004.

nizable pattern of inheritance. The risk of diabetes to an identical twin of a patient with T1DM is about 36%, for a sibling, the risk is approximately 4% by the age of 20 years and 9.6% by the age of 60 years, compared with 0.5% for the general population. The HLA (human leukocyte antigen) region, also known as the human major histocompatibility complex (MHC), influences T1DM susceptibility, especially in Europe.

In Japan, the incidence of T1DM is extremely low at 1.5–2.0 per 100,000 and has a different and unique HLA association compared with Caucasians. Many countries have reported a rise in incidence of T1DM with a disproportionately greater increase in those younger than the age of 5 years.[4]

The clinical spectrum of type 1 diabetes mellitus

Presentation

Diabetes in children usually presents with characteristic symptoms such as polyuria, polydipsia, blurring of vision, and weight loss, in association with glycosuria and ketonuria. In its most severe form, ketoacidosis may develop and lead to cerebral oedema, and in the absence of effective treatment, death.

Treatment consists of dehydration, correction of electrolyte disturbances, and insulin.

In its most severe form, ketoacidosis may develop and lead to loss of consciousness, coma, and in the absence of effective treatment, death. Diabetes ketoacidosis remains the main cause of death in young T1DM.

Management

Aims

The main aim is to render as normal a lifestyle as possible to the diabetic, by three main targets of management; obtaining good metabolic control, preventing long-term complications, and promoting social competence and self-worth.[5] The main challenges are that the patient must receive insulin subcutaneously and there must be attention given to dietary factors.[6] The young person with diabetes also faces a number of hurdles mainly in the form of complications. Complications can be divided into acute and chronic. The acute complications include hypoglycaemia and diabetic ketoacidosis. The chronic complications are the triopathy of retinopathy, nephropathy, and neuropathy. Although the chronic complications may not affect the young person with diabetes, nevertheless the control of the diabetes during this time may have an impact on the development of such complications in later life. The Diabetes Control and Complications Trial (DCCT)[7] established criteria to be achieved which will lead to the prevention, at least in part, of the triopathy of complications. In an excellently controlled study, the research group concluded that intensive therapy effectively delays the onset and slows the progression of diabetic retinopathy, nephropathy, and neuropathy. Intensive therapy included the delivery of insulin by an external pump or three or more daily insulin injections. This resulted in maintaining blood glucose concentrations close to the normal range in addition to glycosylated haemoglobin. The major side effect was a two-fold to three-fold increase in severe hypoglycaemia. In a thoughtful article, Watkins[8] considered the advantages and disadvantages of conclusions of DCCT. The price of achieving excellent control will almost certainly result in more frequent insulin injections and a greater risk of hypoglycaemia. The choice for the patient and the physician is a difficult one, especially in the case of a child with diabetes. Such intensive regimes are even more daunting when the child is faced with exercise and sport. Many find that intensive insulin therapy helps with glucose management during exercise, because it allows for frequent changes in insulin dosages, particularly if they use an insulin pump. Intensive insulin therapy attempts to mimic the natural pattern of insulin secretion.[9] The major problem in the management of T1DM is that no matter how intensive the regime, it is impossible to mimic the physiological state and the second-to-second control of blood glucose by the normal pancreas.

The main aims in the management of a child or teenager with diabetes are as follows:

(i) The diet should have sufficient calories balanced among protein, fat, and carbohydrate to result in normal growth and body weight.

(ii) The diet has to be regimented in that the patient must eat on a regular basis including snacking between meals, in order to prevent hypoglycaemia.

The insulin regime should be such that it achieves the goals of DCCT within the tolerance of the young person and/or parents.

Practical aspects

To achieve such aims requires a considerable amount of education of the young patient and the parents. What can be achieved will be dependent on the age of the patient, and the younger the patient the more management will fall on the parents. The patient should be taught the core concepts of diabetes mellitus, the self-monitoring of blood glucose levels and their interpretation, and the practicalities of self-injection of insulin. The patient should fully understand the warning symptoms of hypoglycaemia, how to prevent this, and how to take action should symptoms occur. Hypoglycaemia will be covered more extensively when exercise and sport are considered. The patient (and parents) should also be aware of possible situations that may lead to ketoacidosis, and know what regimes to employ when the patient becomes ill for other reasons (most often an infective illness). The psychological aspects of diabetes should not to be ignored. The impact of diabetes can lead to emotional reactions including anger, grief, depression, anxiety, and denial. Many children maintain some endogenous insulin secretion for some time just after the diagnosis, which creates an extra challenge for metabolic control.

The adolescent with diabetes presents with other special problems. The secretion of sex hormones and an increased secretion of growth hormone in a pulsatile fashion leads to growth spurts and development of the secondary sex characteristics creating a temporary state of insulin resistance. The impact of new social interest will lead to changes in lifestyle and feelings of independence sometimes amounting to rebelliousness. Eating disorders may occur at this age.[10] This will result in increased dosage of insulin, but may also lead to deterioration in control due to all the quoted factors. So-called brittle diabetes is common at this age group, where the diabetic experiences wild swings in blood sugar with frequent hypoglycaemic attacks and ketoacidosis. The period of adolescence with all the physiological and psychological changes may be responsible, although behavioural disturbances are often behind the 'brittleness'.[11]

The insulin regime in childhood diabetes offers several choices. In the younger child, a two or three dose insulin regime is still common. This will usually consist of a mixture of soluble insulin and intermediate acting insulin before breakfast, and this is repeated in the evening.

This is conveniently given in cartridges by the pen system in a 'pre-mix' of insulin, where the ratio of the soluble and intermediate can be varied.

Another regime suitable for young children with a stable feeding pattern is a combination of a pre-mix insulin before breakfast, a short-acting insulin at dinner time, and a long-acting insulin before bedtime. Parents and patients will be instructed to vary the dose dependent on a number of factors including the prevailing blood glucose, and other factors such as intercurrent illness, exercise, etc. The preferable regime is the intensive therapy regime, either by pen or by insulin pump. The pen regime is to administer short-acting insulin before meals and long-acting insulin in the evening. The pump regime contains a pre-set insulin programme delivering a constant infusion of insulin in the subcutaneous compartment, completed by short insulin infusions before carbohydrate ingestion. This usually offers better control and more mimics the physiological situation. It also confers greater flexibility and is very suited to a busy adolescent especially one involved in sport.

Hypoglycaemia

As this is a significant problem in the exercising diabetic, it will be covered in more detail. It is also the most feared acute complication in the insulin-dependent diabetic creating havoc with lifestyle. As stated previously, insulin therapies, no matter how sophisticated the regime, cannot mimic the physiological state. If the blood runs high glucose to avoid hypoglycaemia, then the feared chronic complications are an ever-present worry. In the normal subject hypoglycaemia (blood glucose < 2.5 mmol·L^{-1}) is prevented by the inhibition of insulin secretion, secretion of counter-regulatory hormones, in particular adrenaline and glucagon, and by neural influences.[12]

The main symptoms of hypoglycaemia are a combination of the effects on the brain and catecholamines. Palpitations (tachycardia), sweating, hunger, and shaking are early warning symptoms. In mild hypoglycaemia, double vision, difficulty in concentration, and slurring of the speech occur. In moderate cases, there is confusion and behavioural changes. In severe cases, the patient can become unconscious with fits and neurological deficits such as hemiplegia.[13] The major precipitating factors are insufficient carbohydrate at meals, delayed meals, over dosage with insulin, and exercise, especially severe exercise.

There are other problems the diabetic has to contend with. Loss of awareness of hypoglycaemia is a worrying development, probably due to loss of neurohumoral responses to repeated hypoglycaemia in the past.[14] There is, however, evidence that hypoglycaemic awareness can be restored by scrupulous hypoglycaemic avoidance.[15] Preventative actions include frequent snacking, end reduced bedtime long-acting insulin after vigorous or sustained exercise on the evening after. Excess alcohol should he avoided. Both patient and doctor should be educated.

Exercise and the normal subject

In order to understand the problems facing the insulin-dependent diabetic, a knowledge of glucose homeostasis during exercise in the normal subject is required. During exercise, insulin falls and the counter-regulatory hormones glucagon and catecholamines rise. The glucagon:insulin molar ratio appears critical to glucose output from the liver, and a very small amount of insulin is all that is necessary to control glucose uptake.[16] Carbohydrate is stored as glycogen in muscle and liver, and fatty acids are stored, mainly as triglycerides, in adipose tissue. Protein may also be used as a fuel but to a lesser extent.[17] Exercise in the normal subject is usually accompanied by euglycaemia.[18] Therefore, in exercising men the glucose output from the liver matches the glucose uptake by muscle. Glucose utilization is a complex regulation by insulin, plasma glucose, alternate substrates, and other humoral and muscle factors.

At relatively low-energy levels, up to 50% $\dot{V}O_2$ max, fat (free fatty acids and muscle triglycerides) is the main source of fuel, completed by a mixture of muscle glycogen and blood glucose derived from liver glycogen. Similar effects have been demonstrated in trained individuals. Trained athletes have increased utilization of lipids compared to untrained individuals. However, as exercise intensity increases carbohydrate (muscle glycogen and plasma glucose derived from liver glycogen) becomes the main source of fuel. In adults, the plasma glucose concentration is tightly regulated in exercise up to 60% $\dot{V}O_2$ max, with the increment of uptake precisely matched by that of production. During heavy exercise, blood glucose utilization may be as great as 1.5 g·min^{-1}, and this fuel source must be continuously replaced at an equal rate or hypoglycaemia will ensue. During such exercise, insulin secretion is inhibited by B-cell α-adrenergic receptor activation. It is suggested that the catecholamine response is the primary regulator for up to eight-fold increase in glucose production during intense exercise (above 80% $\dot{V}O_2$ max).[19,20] This leads to hyperglycaemia with accompanying hyperinsulinaemia after brief intense exercise to exhaustion and persists up to 60 min of recovery.

Depletion of carbohydrate stores in muscle are the main causes of fatigue in athletes. The liver has only 2–3 hours of storage glycogen to meet the needs of a person exercising at high intensity.[21] Children have even less endogenous carbohydrate stores. Even a single bout of exercise can increase glucose uptake into skeletal muscle tissue for at least 16 hours post-exercise in healthy and in diabetic subjects.[22] Feeding on a high carbohydrate diet (70% of energy intake as carbohydrate) enabled runners who were training for 2 hours·day^{-1} to maintain muscle glycogen levels.[23] A dietary carbohydrate intake of 500–600 g may be necessary to ensure adequate glycogen re-synthesis.[24] The conclusion must be that in athletes who are competing in prolonged events at a high-energy level, increased dietary intake of carbohydrate is essential. The athlete who is also training frequently and for prolonged times must ensure that sufficient carbohydrate is ingested between training times to ensure adequate stores of glycogen in muscle and liver, otherwise fatigue will result.

Carbohydrate feeding during prolonged exercise has been shown to enhance performance.[25] This probably works to spare muscle glycogen thus delaying fatigue.[26] Alternatively, it may improve performance by maintaining blood glucose at a critical point in endurance exercise, when liver and glycogen levels are low and the uptake of glucose by skeletal muscle is increased.[27]

Physical training enhances insulin-stimulated glucose disposal in proportion to the improvement in physical fitness.[28] This appears to be mediated through increases in blood flow, the insulin-sensitive glucose transporter (Glut-4) expression, and glycogen synthase activity.[29] The increased insulin sensitivity is seen in aerobic events but not in subjects in anaerobic events.[30]

Exercise can influence intestinal absorption of fluids and glucose. Gastric emptying may be affected by exercise, the process being inhibited.[31] In post-absorptive humans, splanchnic blood flow decreases during supine[32] and upright exercise.[33] Hypoxia to mucosal cells affects sugar absorption, leading to the conclusion that intense exercise will also have this effect due to diminished blood flow.[34]

Exercise and the diabetic subject

The insulin-dependent diabetic must therefore face exercise with disordered or indeed absence of insulin secretion, and possibly with other problems relating to complications including disordered autonomic function.

Exercise may be divided into two categories:

(i) *Random and recreational exercise.* This will certainly be the category the young child with diabetes will inevitably be involved in. This includes the normal activity of the young child but on occasion will involve somewhat more extensive exercise, for example, an outing, a sports day, etc. According to the American Department of Health and Human Services 'Healthy People 2010' recommendations, young people should participate in at least 60 min·day^{-1} of moderate/intense activity for most of the week. Or, according to the ADA guidelines, 'all patients with diabetes should be given the opportunity to benefit from the many effects of exercise'.[35]

(ii) *Sport and training.* A child from about 8 years old begin to become involved in organized sport such as running, gymnastics, football, hockey, swimming, etc. This will include some training but usually not involving more than 2–3 hours per week. When the subject reaches 11 or 12 years, training will increase and intensify and will continue into adolescence and teenage years.

Philosophy of involvement of diabetics in sport

It may be argued that because of potential risks, children and teenagers with diabetes should not be involved in sport. Certainly life without sport and training will be a more sedate and less complicated existence.

Michael Hall, Chairman of the Board of Trustees, British Diabetic Association,[36] commented that diabetics should not be sheltered from the normal activities of humans, and should be able to undertake a full range of sporting activities. He quoted outstanding athletes in many sports who are diabetic and yet reached the highest levels. He found it regrettable that some sports bodies treat diabetics as disabled, and that they have been refused entry to some events. There is an International Diabetes Athletes' Association which caters for diabetics in sport.

Diabetic athletes should be treasured, since they function as role models for children and teenagers. An international organization pays tribute to these 'ambassadors in sports' (www.diabetes-exercise.org). Fortunately, a Belgium study using 24 hours continuous heart rate monitoring showed that the majority of their diabetic children and teenagers meet the guidelines for physical activity and compare favourably with their healthy peers[37] and it has also been suggested that most U.S. children with T1DM attain at least 30 min of daily exercise.[38]

Safety, however, must be the watchword, and a complete understanding by the parents or the patient as to how to control his/her diabetes is essential. Most sports have safety standards so that training is supervised and it is vital that a coach or attendant is informed that the athlete is a diabetic.

The effect of exercise in diabetics

Regular exercise will improve the health of the insulin-dependent diabetic in the following ways:

- increased cardiorespiratory fitness
- increased insulin sensitivity
- increased/maintained muscle mass to fat ratio with better weight control
- reduction in serum lipids
- decline in resting heart rate and blood pressure
- improved quality of life
- diminished glycaemic response to a meal, and a reduction in daily insulin needs.

A positive association between glycaemic control and aerobic fitness or reported physical activity exists in youth with T1DM suggesting that either increased aerobic capacity may improve metabolic control or glycaemic control maximizes aerobic capacity.[39–42] Adolescents with T1DM improve cardiorespiratory endurance and muscle strength at least as much as their non-diabetic peers after aerobic training.[40,43] Moreover, sports participation among high school students has been associated with multiple positive health behaviours, including fruit and vegetable consumption and reduced cigarette smoking.[44] Indeed, the goal of regular exercise should be to increase insulin sensitivity and to improve the overall cardiovascular and psychosocial profile of the child with T1DM, regardless of any putative benefits to blood glucose management.[9] However, diabetics will respond to exercise differently from normal subjects, particularly with respect to glucose homeostasis.

Several characteristics of exercise may strongly influence the development of exercise hypoglycaemia. Among them, duration and intensity of the exercise, physical training, and diet before the exercise are major determinants.[45]

The key problem is that the insulin-dependent diabetic does not have a normal insulin response to exercise. Peripheral insulin concentrations are tightly related by the injective therapy as well as to the site of injections and the time elapsed since the last administration. As stated previously insulin levels fall to low levels in normal subjects during exercise. The diabetic has a very significant problem in mimicking this, and indeed injected insulin often rises in the blood during exercise in the diabetic.[46] This is caused by more rapid absorption of the injected insulin particularly if the insulin is injected into the exercising part of the body.[47] A rise in body temperature and increased blood flow in subcutaneous tissue and skeletal muscle have been demonstrated to be causally related to the increased insulin concentrations during sports.[48] This rapid absorption is more marked when the insulin is given shortly before the exercise, than if given 60–90 min before the exercise. Exercise does not appear to alter insulin glargine absorption rate.[49]

The inappropriately elevated insulin levels during exercise will have undesirable effects by inhibiting hepatic glucose output and by enhancing peripheral glucose uptake and stimulating glucose uptake by exercising muscle usually within 20–60 min after the onset of exercise.[48,50] This process is also called over-insulinization. Finally, during exercise there is a dramatic increase in non-insulin-mediated glucose uptake that considerably reduces the need for circulating insulin levels.[3] Contradictory to what one might think, glucose oxidation during 60 min of intense exercise is lower in diabetic adolescent boys than in age- and weight-matched controls.[51] Possibly, because of a decreased insulin sensitivity.[52] Gluconeogenesis is also impaired. Counter-regulatory responses, such as glucagon, can be deficient in the diabetic. These changes inevitably lead to hypoglycaemia during exercise. Within 45 min of strenuous exercise performed 2 hours after a standard meal and their usual insulin dose, hypoglycaemia will develop. A reduction of 30–50% in bolus insulin delivery reduces the likelihood of developing hypoglycaemia in these patients.[40,42] Prolonged exercise (>90 min) requires a greater reduction of insulin, often up to 80% of normal.

Post-exercise hypoglycaemia can also be encountered up to several hours after exercise and even the following day.[53] In T1DM adolescents it was found to be biphasic: increased glucose requirements during and shortly after exercise and again 7–11 hours or even up to 24 hours after exercise.[54] This is probably due to increased glucose uptake and glycogen synthesis in the previously exercised muscle groups. In addition, severe post-exercise late-onset hypoglycaemia (i.e. up to 36 hours after exercise) may be particularly relevant in active children, possibly because proper insulin and nutritional strategies are not adopted while muscle and liver glycogen stores are being replaced. Strategies to limit the possibility of hypoglycaemia caused by exercise have been proposed by Riddell and Iscoe[3] as follows:

Before exercise

(i) Determine the timing, mode, duration, and intensity of exercise.

(ii) Eat a carbohydrate meal 1–3 hours before the exercise.

(iii) Assess metabolic control.

- If blood glucose is <5.0 mmol·L^{-1} and levels are decreasing, extra carbohydrates may be needed.
- If blood glucose is 5–13.9 mmol·L^{-1}, extra carbohydrates may not be needed, depending on the duration of exercise and the individual response to exercise.
- If blood glucose is >14 mmol·L^{-1} and urine or blood ketones are present, delay exercise until normalized with insulin administration.

(iv) If the activity is aerobic, estimate energy expenditure and determine if insulin or additional carbohydrate will be needed based on peak insulin activity.

- If insulin dose is to be adjusted for long-duration and/or moderate to high intensity, try a 50% pre-meal insulin dose reduction 1 hour before the exercise. Dosages can be altered on subsequent exercise days, based on the measured individual response. Insulin should be injected into a site distal to the exercising muscle and into subcutaneous tissue.
- If carbohydrate is to be increased, try 1 g·kg body weight^{-1}·hour^{-1} moderate- to high-intensity exercise performed during peak insulin activity and less carbohydrate as the time since insulin injection increases. The amount of carbohydrate can be altered on subsequent exercise days, based on the measured insulin responses. The total dose of carbohydrate should be divided equally and consumed at 20-min intervals.

(v) If the exercise is anaerobic or occurring during heat or accompanied by competition stress, an increase in insulin may be needed.

(vi) Consider fluid intake to maintain hydration (~250 mL 20 min before the exercise).

During exercise

(vii) Monitor blood glucose every 30 min.

(viii) Continue fluid intake (250 mL every 20–30 min).

(ix) If required, consume carbohydrate at 20–30 min intervals.

After exercise

(x) Monitor blood glucose, including overnight, if amount of exercise is not habitual.

(xi) Consider adjusting insulin therapy to decrease immediate and delayed insulin action.

(xii) Consider consuming additional slow-acting carbohydrate to protect against post-exercise late-onset hypoglycaemia.

The Diabetes Research in Children Network Study Group[55] demonstrated that 22% of T1DM teenagers developed hypoglycaemia overnight after an afternoon exercise session on the treadmill. The exercise session consisted of 15-min walking on a treadmill at a heart rate of approximately 140 beats·min^{-1}, followed by a 5-min rest period. This cycle was repeated three more times, for a total intervention time of 75 min. Besides the significant hypoglycaemias, the mean glucose level to 6 a.m. was lower on an exercise day compared to a sedentary day. Furthermore, the glucose level before the bedtime snack was a predictor of overnight hypoglycaemia. Hypoglycaemia was uncommon if the glucose level was above 7.2 mmol·L^{-1} (130 mg·dL^{-1}). Another study demonstrated that when exercising children maintained their basal insulin infusion rates during unplanned activity, they typically developed late-onset post-exercise hypoglycaemia during sleep, even though hypoglycaemia did not occur during exercise. Even when basal insulin rates were omitted during exercise, 6 out of 10 patients still had nocturnal hypoglycaemia.[56] Reductions in nocturnal basal insulin rates and proper bedtime snacks seem the most logical approach. A complex carbohydrate (e.g. uncooked corn starch) or a mixed snack containing fat and protein may help spread the gastrointestinal uptake during the night.[57]

Should exercise be undertaken during a state of severe insulin deficiency exercise-induced ketoacidosis can occur. During exercise under such circumstances, peripheral glucose utilization is impaired and hepatic glucose output enhanced as is lipolysis.[58] The type of exercise will make a difference. Low-to-moderate intensity exercise especially for longish spells increases the risk of hypoglycaemia.[59] In very high-intensity exercise (>80% $\dot{V}O_2$ max), blood glucose levels rise, as in healthy individuals, possibly by counter-acting hormones such as catecholamines, growth hormone, and cortisol.[60] In addition, after a short period of intense exercise, hyperglycaemia remains, but only as long as there are elevations in counter-regulatory hormones (i.e. 30–60 min).[61] As stated earlier, this is a physiological response and one could argue whether the insulin therapy should be adapted to it. Furthermore, since hypoglycaemia will be encountered in aerobic exercise especially if prolonged, it has been suggested to counter the exercise-mediated fall in glycaemia with a 10-s maximal sprint[62] or to favour intermittent high-intensity compared to continuous moderate exercise.[63] Compared to aerobic training, resistance training does not seem to have such a strong effect on metabolic control.[64]

The time of the day on which exercise is performed can make a difference. Exercise before insulin administration in the morning is associated with a low risk of hypoglycaemia, since circulating insulin levels are low and liver and muscle glycogen stores are full.[59] To a lesser extent, age, gender, level of metabolic control, and the level of aerobic fitness also contribute.

The insulin-dependent diabetic may also have gastrointestinal motor dysfunction. This includes gastric motor dysfunction, known as gastroparesis, with a significant delay in stomach emptying.[65] This can result in delay of emptying of meals thus enhancing the possibility of hypoglycaemia during exercise.

In addition, the blunted neurohormonal response to exercise that is known in diabetes appears to be exponentially increased by previous exercise performance or by antecedent hypoglycaemic episodes. Finally, in individuals with poor metabolic control, exercise can increase the risk of hyperglycaemia and ketoacidosis, causing dehydration and acidosis, both of which impair exercise performance.[3]

Practical considerations for the exercising diabetic

An exact prescription for the exercising young diabetic cannot be made. However, if major precautions and preparations are taken, then the acute problems of severe hypoglycaemia can be largely prevented. Probably, the child diabetic athlete who undertakes regular training and competition is more likely to be well educated in actions than the child who undertakes occasional and variable exercise, and will, therefore, be safer. There is extensive literature in this field.[35,66–70] In addition, there are publications which specifically cover the diabetic child athlete.[58,71–74] Diet and insulin therapy management remain the two main important strategies possible in patients with T1DM practising sports in order to minimize the occurrence of sports-related adverse events. Since children mostly perform spontaneous exercise, it is not always possible to anticipate the need to decrease exercise. In these instances, carbohydrate ingestion is a valuable option. The author will attempt to summarize the points made in these articles introducing discussion as required.

Pre-exercise assessment

Education of the patient and, if very young, the parents is essential. No young diabetic should embark on sport and exercise without having substantial awareness of the problems and how to overcome these problems. This can be appropriately undertaken by a doctor experienced in diabetes management, a specialist diabetic nurse, a dietician, and possibly also an exercise physiologist who can advise on the energy requirements of the type of exercise.

The patient should have the following training:

(i) self-monitoring of blood levels,

(ii) monitoring of ketone levels in urine,

(iii) knowledge of dietary factors, and

(iv) awareness of the symptoms of hypoglycaemia, methods of prevention, and how to treat it.

The patient should preferably be in intensive insulin therapy, either by pen or by pump. Although possibly not introducing better control, the flexibility afforded is a major advantage. Until now no significant advantages have been found for subjects with pump treatment.[56]

Should the child be undertaking regular physical training for a sport, the club coach, or teacher must be informed. Often a doctor may be involved in this sport.[75] The diabetic should wear identification indicating that he/she is a diabetic. Those supervising the training should be aware of the symptoms of hypoglycaemia and the treatment required.

It is generally recommended that the patient should have a full medical assessment before undertaking high-intensive exercise, in order to identify complicating factors such as vascular disease, microangiopathy, nephropathy, and neuropathy. Significant disease may preclude some sports, or require a modified approach to exercise. It is, however, unlikely that a young diabetic will have such significant disease. The so-called brittle diabetic, or someone with psychological problems should be cautious about involvement in highly demanding sports.

Before the exercise

The type of exercise should be assessed. This may be regularly recurring, for example, 1–2 hours of training in swimming, football, athletics, etc. The diabetic may, therefore, have a standard regime. Alternatively, the exercise may be unusual, for example, a sports day with several intermittent events. If the exercise is prolonged and aerobic, there is probably greater danger of hypoglycaemia than if the exercise is short and anaerobic.

The patient should already be well and repleted in carbohydrate stores. A meal should be taken 3–4 hours before the exercise. The meal should have a large carbohydrate component with mainly complex 'slowly absorbable' carbohydrates (at least 60%, if long-lasting aerobic exercise is programmed, it should reach 70%).

Short-acting insulin should preferably be used, since long-acting insulin would normally have to be taken the previous evening. The dose should be taken before a meal and a reduction in dosage is essential. This reduction varies by 30–50%, but will depend on the type of exercise, and the previous experience of the patient concerning insulin dosage. Flexible insulin dosing regimes, especially for pump users, will help reduce the risk of exercise-induced nocturnal hypoglycaemia. The insulin should not be injected into an exercising extremity, thus an abdominal site is usually preferable. This will prevent rapid absorption of insulin. Pre-meal insulin may be reduced by 30%–50%, and in more prolonged exercise the dose might be reduced by up to 90%. Because it is impossible to predict the exact insulin reduction needed, individuals should use records of previous experiences as a guideline and always have additional carbohydrates available. Importantly, a well-organized plan should be developed and conveyed to the child's coaches, teachers, friends, guardians, and siblings.[3] Metabolic control should be assessed. If the blood glucose is <5 mmol·L^{-1} extra calories before the exercise will be required. If the blood glucose is >15 mmol·L^{-1}, urinary ketones should be measured, and if positive, more insulin taken, and exercise delayed until blood glucose is satisfactory and urinary ketones are negative. Psychological stress before a match may also induce hyperglycaemia. Also warm and humid environments may elevate blood glucose levels. Therefore, it is advisable to check blood sugar 1 hour before and 30 min before any activity, in order to identify a trend in blood sugar concentration. For instance, a blood glucose level of 5.5 mmol·L^{-1} may be considered safe at one time, but potentially dangerous if the previous value was 10 mmol·L^{-1}. If low, a sugary drink of 15 g of simple chain molecules could be used.

During exercise

As a general rule, 1–1.5 g carbohydrate·kg body weight^{-1}·hour^{-1} should be consumed during exercise performed during peak insulin action. When the same exercise is performed 2.5 and 4 hours after insulin administration, then required carbohydrate intake will be 0.5 and only 0.25 g·kg^{-1}, respectively.[39]

If the exercise is prolonged, then further monitoring of blood may be required. This will obviously be awkward and will lose time in a prolonged marathon type event, but in a training situation should be possible. The convenience of continuous glucose-monitoring devices (e.g. Guardian RT, Medtronic) and insulin pump therapy may be ideal for youth. If the exercise is prolonged >30 min, supplemental rapidly absorbable carbohydrate (15–40 g) should be taken every 30 min. This can be made up in drinks, as fluid replacement is also essential. During a moderate-intensity exercise session of 55–60% of $\dot{V}O_2$ max for 60 min T1DM, adolescents were able to maintain the blood glucose concentration with 8–10% carbohydrate drinks.[76] Should the subjects experience symptoms of hypoglycaemia he/she should inform someone else, and take absorbable carbohydrate. Exercise can then be continued when the subject has recovered. Should severe hypoglycaemia occur and if oral administration is impossible (35–45 g of oral glucose), then intravenous glucose and/or intramuscular 1 mg of glucagon will be required.

However, to prevent strong fluctuation in blood glucose, frequent self-monitoring of blood sugar, information about the exercise, insulin administration, and carbohydrate intake should be recorded in an exercise-training log, which also documents the type, timeline, and duration of the exercise protocol.

After exercise

The main problem is delayed hypoglycaemia and a reduction in insulin dosage may be required, and possibly increased caloric intake for 12–14 hours after the activity. For patients experiencing post-exercise late-onset hypoglycaemia during the night, a complex carbohydrate (uncooked starch) or a mixed snack containing fat and protein may be particularly beneficial at bedtime. It is also useful having somewhat higher target glucose levels at bedtime on days of intense exercise, especially for those who receive prebreakfast doses of glargine insulin. Physical exercise may exacerbate abnormalities detected in patients with diabetic neuropathy, such as maximal cardiac capacity and output, decreased cardiovascular rate to response to physical exercise, orthostatic hypotension, impaired sweating, or impaired gastrointestinal function.[77–79]

Other points

It should be emphasized that exact prescriptions are impossible. Campaigne *et al.*[80] concluded that general recommendations on how to adjust insulin or diet before the exercise are difficult to provide. Individualized recommendations for treatment modification appear most appropriate. As in athletes without diabetes, the athlete with diabetes mellitus with hypoglycaemia will dramatically lower his/her exercise performance and increase his/her rating of perceived exertion. Hyperglycaemic athletes may already be dehydrated, thereby impairing performance.[50] Furthermore, hyperglycaemia has been associated with the reduced ability to secrete beta-endorphins during exercise.[81]

Short-acting insulin analogues

Tuominen *et al.*[82] found that a short-acting insulin analogue [Lys (B28) Pro (B29)] peaked earlier than human insulin and postprandial blood glucose was lower. Exercise-induced hypoglycaemia was also 2.2-fold greater during early exercise but less than 46% during late exercise. They concluded that as exercise is usually not performed until 2–3 hours after a meal, short-acting insulin analogues may be more feasible than soluble human insulin.

Exercise in type 2 diabetes mellitus

With regard to youth with type 2 diabetes, very little is known about the impact of exercise, however, one could presume similar effects.[83] Non-oxidative glucose utilization is impaired in T2DM patients, as well as in the children of T2DM patients by up to 25%.[84] This may result in impaired glucose utilization during sports activities compared to non-diabetic individuals. Intense exercise in type 2 diabetes requires additional study.

Summary

- Diabetes mellitus is a group of metabolic diseases characterized by chronic hyperglycaemia, resulting from defects in insulin secretion, insulin action, or both, leading to insufficient action of insulin on target tissue.
- Several forms of diabetes mellitus can be identified each with their specific clinical characterization and treatment. The general aim, especially for T1DM, is as normal a lifestyle as possible, through three main targets of management: obtaining good metabolic control, preventing long-term complications, and promoting social competence and self-worth.
- Intensive insulin therapy attempts to mimic the natural pattern of insulin secretion, effectively delays the late complications of T1DM and is the treatment of choice, especially for the child who is involved in sports or intensive exercise regimens.
- Hypoglycaemia remains a significant problem in the exercising diabetic. During exercise, there is a dramatic increase in non-insulin-mediated glucose uptake, which reduces the need for circulating insulin levels.
- Post-exercise hypoglycaemia in adolescents has a biphasic character with increased glucose requirements shortly after and 7–11 hours after exercise, although late-onset hypoglycaemia is known to occur up to 36 hours post-exercise.
- On the other hand, hyperglycaemia can occur during high-intensity exercise, but may also be related to pre-competition psychological stress.
- The exact prescription cannot be made, but diet and insulin therapy management remain the two main important strategies possible in patients with T1DM practising sports in order to minimize the occurrence of sports-related adverse events.

References

1. American Diabetes Association (2005). Diagnosis and classification of diabetes mellitus. *Diabetes Care* **28** (Suppl. 1), S37–42.
2. WHO Technical Report Series (1985). World Health Organisation Study Group. *Diabetic Mellitus* **727**, 1–104.
3. Riddell MC, Iscoe KE (2006). Physical activity, sport, and pediatric diabetes. *Pediatr Diabetes* **7**, 60–70.
4. Craig ME, Hattersley A, Donaghue K (2006). ISPAD Clinical Practice Consensus Guidelines 2006–2007. Definition, epidemiology and classification. *Pediatr Diabetes* **7**, 343–51.
5. Silverstein J, Klingensmith G, Copeland K, Plotnick L, Kaufman F, Laffel L, Deeb L, Grey M, Anderson B, Holzmeister LA, Clark N (2005). Care of children and adolescents with type 1 diabetes: A statement of the American Diabetes Association. *Diabetes Care* **28**, 186–212.
6. Swift PG (2007). Diabetes education. ISPAD clinical practice consensus guidelines 2006–2007. *Pediatr Diabetes* **8**, 103–9.
7. The Diabetes Control and Complications Trial Research Group (1993). The effect of intensive treatment of diabetes on the development and progression of long-term complications in insulin-dependent diabetes mellitus. *N Engl J Med* **329**, 977–86.
8. Watkins PJ (1994). DCCT: The ecstasy and the agony. *Q J Med* **87**, 315–16.
9. Riddell MC, Perkins BA (2008). Type 1 diabetes and vigorous exercise: Applications of exercise physiology to patient management. *Can J Diabetes* **30**, 63–71.
10. Steel JM, Young RJ, Lloyd GG, MacIntyre CC (1989). Abnormal eating attitudes in young insulin-dependent diabetics. *Br J Psychiatry* **155**, 515–21.
11. Thompson CJ, Cummings F, Chalmers J, Newton RW (1995). Abnormal insulin treatment behaviour: A major cause of ketoacidosis in the young adult. *Diabet Med* **12**, 429–32.
12. Frier BM (1986). Hypoglycaemia and diabetes. *Diabet Med* **3**, 513–25.
13. Watkins PJ (1982). ABC of diabetes. Hypoglycaemia. *Br Med J (Clin Res Ed)* **285**, 278–9.
14. Ryder RE, Owens DR, Hayes TM, Ghatei MA, Bloom SR (1990). Unawareness of hypoglycaemia and inadequate hypoglycaemic counterregulation: No causal relation with diabetic autonomic neuropathy. *BMJ* **301**, 783–7.
15. Cranston I, Lomas J, Maran A, Macdonald I, Amiel SA (1994). Restoration of hypoglycaemia awareness in patients with long-duration insulin-dependent diabetes. *Lancet* **344**, 283–7.
16. Wasserman DH, Vranic M (1986). Interaction between insulin and counterregulatory hormones in control of substrate utilization in health and diabetes during exercise. *Diabetes Metab Rev* **1**, 359–84.
17. Cahill GF Jr (1970). Starvation in man. *N Engl J Med* **282**, 668–75.
18. Dill DB, Edwards HT, Mead S (1935). Blood sugar regulation in exercise. *Am J Phys* **111**, 21–30.
19. Marliss EB, Vranic M (2002). Intense exercise has unique effects on both insulin release and its roles in glucoregulation: Implications for diabetes. *Diabetes* **51** (Suppl. 1), S271–83.
20. Sigal RJ, Fisher SJ, Halter JB, Vranic M, Marliss EB (1999). Glucoregulation during and after intense exercise: Effects of beta-adrenergic blockade in subjects with type 1 diabetes mellitus. *J Clin Endocrinol Metab* **84**, 3961–71.
21. Maughan RJ (1994). Nutritional aspects of endurance exercise in humans. *Proc Nutr Soc* **53**, 181–8.
22. Borghouts LB, Keizer HA (2000). Exercise and insulin sensitivity: A review. *Int J Sports Med* **21**, 1–12.
23. Costill DL (1988). Carbohydrates for exercise: Dietary demands for optimal performance. *Int J Sports Med* **9**, 1–18.
24. Coyle EF (1991). Timing and method of increased carbohydrate intake to cope with heavy training, competition and recovery. *J Sports Sci* **9**, 29–51.
25. Wilber RL, Moffatt RJ (1992). Influence of carbohydrate ingestion on blood glucose and performance in runners. *Int J Sport Nutr* **2**, 317–27.
26. Hargreaves M, Costill DL, Coggan A, Fink WJ, Nishibata I (1984). Effect of carbohydrate feedings on muscle glycogen utilization and exercise performance. *Med Sci Sports Exerc* **16**, 219–22.
27. Coyle EF, Hagberg JM, Hurley BF, Martin WH, Ehsani AA, Holloszy JO (1983). Carbohydrate feeding during prolonged strenuous exercise can delay fatigue. *J Appl Physiol* **55**, 230–5.
28. Soman VR, Koivisto VA, Deibert D, Felig P, DeFronzo RA (1979). Increased insulin sensitivity and insulin binding to monocytes after physical training. *N Engl J Med* **301**, 1200–4.
29. Ebeling P, Bourey R, Koranyi L, Tuominen JA, Groop LC, Henriksson J, Mueckler M, Sovijarvi A, Koivisto VA (1993). Mechanism of enhanced insulin sensitivity in athletes. Increased blood flow, muscle glucose transport protein (GLUT-4) concentration, and glycogen synthase activity. *J Clin Invest* **92**, 1623–31.
30. Yki-Jarvinen H, Koivisto VA (1983). Effects of body composition on insulin sensitivity. *Diabetes* **32**, 965–9.
31. Costill DL, Saltin B (1974). Factors limiting gastric emptying during rest and exercise. *J Appl Physiol* **37**, 679–83.
32. Bradley SE, Childs AW, Combes B, Cournand A, Wade OL, Wheeler HO (1956). Effects of exercise on the splanchnic blood flow and splanchnic blood volume in normal men. *Clin Sci (Lond)* **15**, 457–63.
33. Rowell LB, Blackmon JR, Bruce RA (1964). Indocyanine green clearance and estimated hepatic blood flow during mild to maximal exercise in upright man. *J Clin Invest* **43**, 1677–90.
34. Darlington WA, Quastel JH (1953). Absorption of sugars from isolated surviving intestine. *Arch Biochem Biophys* **43**, 194–207.
35. American College of Sports Medicine and American Diabetes Association joint position statement (1997). Diabetes mellitus and exercise. *Med Sci Sports Exerc* **29**, 1–6.
36. Hall M (1997). Sport and diabetes. *Br J Sports Med* **31**, 3.
37. Massin MM, Lebrethon MC, Rocour D, Gerard P, Bourguignon JP (2005). Patterns of physical activity determined by heart rate monitoring among diabetic children. *Arch Dis Child* **90**, 1223–6.
38. Raile K, Kapellen T, Schweiger A, Hunkert F, Nietzschmann U, Dost A, Kiess W (1999). Physical activity and competitive sports in children and adolescents with type 1 diabetes. *Diabetes Care* **22**, 1904–5.
39. Huttunen NP, Kaar ML, Knip M, Mustonen A, Puukka R, Akerblom HK (1984). Physical fitness of children and adolescents with insulin-dependent diabetes mellitus. *Ann Clin Res* **16**, 1–5.
40. Huttunen NP, Lankela SL, Knip M, Lautala P, Kaar ML, Laasonen K, Puukka R (1989). Effect of once-a-week training program on physical fitness and metabolic control in children with IDDM. *Diabetes Care* **12**, 737–40.
41. Ludvigsson J (1980). Physical exercise in relation to degree of metabolic control in juvenile diabetics. *Acta Paediatr Scand Suppl* **283**, 45–9.
42. Sackey AH, Jefferson IG (1996). Physical activity and glycaemic control in children with diabetes mellitus. *Diabet Med* **13**, 789–93.
43. Mosher PE, Nash MS, Perry AC, LaPerriere AR, Goldberg RB (1998). Aerobic circuit exercise training: Effect on adolescents with well-controlled insulin-dependent diabetes mellitus. *Arch Phys Med Rehabil* **79**, 652–7.
44. Pate RR, Trost SG, Levin S, Dowda M (2000). Sports participation and health-related behaviors among US youth. *Arch Pediatr Adolesc Med* **154**, 904–11.
45. Giannini C, de GT, Mohn A, Chiarelli F (2007). Role of physical exercise in children and adolescents with diabetes mellitus. *J Pediatr Endocrinol Metab* **20**, 173–84.
46. Berger M, Halban PA, Assal JP, Offord RE, Vranic M, Renold AE (1979). Pharmacokinetics of subcutaneously injected tritiated insulin: Effects of exercise. *Diabetes* **28** (Suppl. 1), 53–7.
47. Koivisto VA, Felig P (1978). Effects of leg exercise on insulin absorption in diabetic patients. *N Engl J Med* **298**, 79–83.
48. Zinman B, Murray FT, Vranic M, Albisser AM, Leibel BS, Mc Clean PA, Marliss EB (1977). Glucoregulation during moderate exercise in insulin treated diabetics. *J Clin Endocrinol Metab* **45**, 641–52.

49. Peter R, Luzio SD, dunseath G, Miles A, Hare B, Backx K, Pauvaday V, Owens DR (2005). Effects of exercise on the absorption of insulin glargine in patients with type 1 diabetes. *Diabetes Care* **28**, 560–5.
50. Riddell MC, Bar-Or O, Ayub BV, Calvert RE, Heigenhauser GJ (1999). Glucose ingestion matched with total carbohydrate utilization attenuates hypoglycemia during exercise in adolescents with IDDM. *Int J Sport Nutr* **9**, 24–34.
51. Riddell MC, Bar-Or O, Hollidge-Horvat M, Schwarcz HP, Heigenhauser GJ (2000). Glucose ingestion and substrate utilization during exercise in boys with IDDM. *J Appl Physiol* **88**, 1239–46.
52. Timmons BW, Bar-Or O, Riddell MC (2007). Energy substrate utilization during prolonged exercise with and without carbohydrate intake in preadolescent and adolescent girls. *J Appl Physiol* **103**, 995–1000.
53. McDonald MJ (1987). Post exercise late-onset hypoglycaemia in insulin-dependent diabetic patients. *Diabetes Care* **10**, 584–8.
54. McMahon SK, Ferreira LD, Ratnam N, Davey RJ, Youngs LM, Davis EA, Fournier PA, Jones TW (2007). Glucose requirements to maintain euglycemia after moderate-intensity afternoon exercise in adolescents with type 1 diabetes are increased in a biphasic manner. *J Clin Endocrinol Metab* **92**, 963–8.
55. Tsalikian E, Mauras N, Beck RW, Tamborlane WV, Janz KF, Chase HP, Wysocki T, Weinzimer SA, Buckingham BA, Kollman C, Xing D, Ruedy KJ (2005). Impact of exercise on overnight glycemic control in children with type 1 diabetes mellitus. *J Pediatr* **147**, 528–34.
56. Admon G, Weinstein Y, Falk B, Weintrob N, Benzaquen H, Ofan R, Fayman G, Zigel L, Constantini N, Phillip M (2005). Exercise with and without an insulin pump among children and adolescents with type 1 diabetes mellitus. *Pediatrics* **116**, e348–55.
57. Kalergis M, Schiffrin A, Gougeon R, Jones PJ, Yale JF (2003). Impact of bedtime snack composition on prevention of nocturnal hypoglycemia in adults with type 1 diabetes undergoing intensive insulin management using lispro insulin before meals: A randomized, placebo-controlled, crossover trial. *Diabetes Care* **26**, 9–15.
58. Horton ES (1980). *Exercise and diabetes in youth.* In: Lamb DR, Gisolfi CV (eds.), *Youth, exercise and sport*, pp. 539–74. Benchmark, Indianapolis, IN.
59. Ruegemer JJ, Squires RW, Marsh HM, Haymond MW, Cryer PE, Rizza RA, Miles JM (1990). Differences between prebreakfast and late afternoon glycemic responses to exercise in IDDM patients. *Diabetes Care* **13**, 104–10.
60. Purdon C, Brousson M, Nyveen SL, Miles PD, Halter JB, Vranic M, Marliss EB (1993). The roles of insulin and catecholamines in the glucoregulatory response during intense exercise and early recovery in insulin-dependent diabetic and control subjects. *J Clin Endocrinol Metab* **76**, 566–73.
61. Sigal RJ, Purdon C, Fisher SJ, Halter JB, Vranic M, Marliss EB (1994). Hyperinsulinemia prevents prolonged hyperglycemia after intense exercise in insulin-dependent diabetic subjects. *J Clin Endocrinol Metab* **79**, 1049–57.
62. Bussau VA, Ferreira LD, Jones TW, Fournier PA (2006). The 10-s maximal sprint: A novel approach to counter an exercise-mediated fall in glycemia in individuals with type 1 diabetes. *Diabetes Care* **29**, 601–6.
63. Guelfi KJ, Ratnam N, Smythe GA, Jones TW, Fournier PA (2007). Effect of intermittent high-intensity compared with continuous moderate exercise on glucose production and utilization in individuals with type 1 diabetes. *Am J Physiol Endocrinol Metab* **292**, E865–70.
64. Ramalho AC, de Lourdes LM, Nunes F, Cambui Z, Barbosa C, Andrade A, Viana A, Martins M, Abrantes V, Aragao C, Temistocles M (2006). The effect of resistance versus aerobic training on metabolic control in patients with type-1 diabetes mellitus. *Diabetes Res Clin Pract* **72**, 271–6.
65. Horowitz M, Dent J (1991). Disordered gastric emptying: Mechanical basis, assessment and treatment. *Baillieres Clin Gastroenterol* **5**, 371–407.
66. Choi KL, Chisholm DJ (1996). Exercise and insulin-dependent diabetes mellitus (IDDM): Benefits and pitfalls. *Aust N Z J Med* **26**, 827–33.
67. Fahey PJ, Stallkamp ET, Kwatra S (1996). The athlete with type 1 diabetes: Managing insulin, diet and exercise. *Am Fam Physician* **53**, 1611–24.
68. Horton ES (1988). Exercise and diabetes mellitus. *Med Clin North Am* **72**, 1301–21.
69. Landry GL, Allen DB (1992). Diabetes mellitus and exercise. *Clin Sports Med* **11**, 403–18.
70. Tsuei EYL, Zinman B (1995). Exercise and diabetes—New insights and therapeutic goals. *The Endocrinologist* **5**, 263–71.
71. Bar-Or O (1993). Effects of training on the child with a chronic disease. Beauty and the beast? (Editorial). *Clin J Sport Med* **3**, 2–5.
72. Byrne G (1993). Children, diabetes and sport—Yes, they do mix. *Aussie Sport Action (Canberra, Aust)* **4**, 10–11.
73. Dorchy H, Poortmans J (1989). Sport and the diabetic child. *Sports Med* **7**, 248–62.
74. Lording D (1991). The diabetic athlete today. *Sports Train Med Rehab* **2**, 197–201.
75. Jimenez CC (1997). Diabetes and exercise: The role of the athletic trainer. *J Athl Train* **32**, 339–43.
76. Perrone C, Laitano O, Meyer F (2005). Effect of carbohydrate ingestion on the glycemic response of type 1 diabetic adolescents during exercise. *Diabetes Care* **28**, 2537–8.
77. Colhoun HM, Francis DP, Rubens MB, Underwood SR, Fuller JH (2001). The association of heart-rate variability with cardiovascular risk factors and coronary artery calcification: A study in type 1 diabetic patients and the general population. *Diabetes Care* **24**, 1108–14.
78. Hilsted J, Galbo H, Christensen NJ (1979). Impaired cardiovascular responses to graded exercise in diabetic autonomic neuropathy. *Diabetes* **28**, 313–19.
79. Margonato A, Gerundini P, Vicedomini G, Gilardi MC, Pozza G, Fazio F (1986). Abnormal cardiovascular response to exercise in young asymptomatic diabetic patients with retinopathy. *Am Heart J* **112**, 554–60.
80. Campaigne BN, Wallberg-Henriksson H, Gunnarsson R (1987). Glucose and insulin responses in relation to insulin dose and caloric intake 12 h after acute physical exercise in men with IDDM. *Diabetes Care* **10**, 716–21.
81. Wanke T, Auinger M, Formanek D, Merkle M, Lahrmann H, Ogris E, Zwick H, Irsigler K (1996). Defective endogenous opioid response to exercise in type I diabetic patients. *Metabolism* **45**, 137–42.
82. Tuominen JA, Karonen SL, Melamies L, Bolli G, Koivisto VA (1995). Exercise-induced hypoglycaemia in IDDM patients treated with a short-acting insulin analogue. *Diabetologia* **38**, 106–11.
83. Kelly AS, Wetzsteon RJ, Kaiser DR, Steinberger J, Bank AJ, Dengel DR (2004). Inflammation, insulin, and endothelial function in overweight children and adolescents: The role of exercise. *J Pediatr* **145**, 731–6.
84. Laakso M, Edelman SV, Olefsky JM, Brechtel G, Wallace P, Baron AD (1990). Kinetics of *in vivo* muscle insulin-mediated glucose uptake in human obesity. *Diabetes* **39**, 965–74.

PART 5

The Elite Young Athlete

CHAPTER 37

The elite young athlete

Alison M. McManus and Neil Armstrong

Introduction

It is widely accepted that sport participation is beneficial for the physical, psychomotor, and social development of children.[1,2] Yet, for the many children who engage in sport, increasingly competitive sport leagues and exposure to intensive training means the benefits of participation are over-shadowed by risk.[3] Competitive programmes and training are commonly offered from 4 years of age, in spite of the fact that children do not understand the concept of competition until they are at least 6 years old, nor can they distinguish between effort and ability, or the effect of practice until they are at least 10 years old.[4–6] For those who show exceptional talent, the determination of the adults around them to make them champions often means they are involved in intensive training very early. These youngsters need to be provided with an environment that optimizes the development of their talent yet minimizes risk or harm.

It has been estimated that in the United States sports injuries account for nearly 20% of all emergency room visits by 5–24 year olds.[7] Particularly concerning is that the highest sports injury episode rate is for children aged 5–15 years (59.3 per 1000 persons). Sports injuries are nearly double for boys compared to girls,[8] but a surge in female participation in competitive sport has been accompanied by an increase in sports injuries in females, particularly non-contact anterior cruciate ligament tears.[9,10] Much higher sport injury rates may be expected in girls in the future.

Children and adolescents are particularly at risk from overuse sport injuries.[11] Apophysitis at the knee (Osgood–Schlatter disease), heel (Sever's disease), and elbow (Little League elbow) are common and occur in the young: Sever's disease and Little League elbow typically occur between the ages of 7–10 years, with Osgood–Schlatter disease most commonly occurring between 11 and 15 years of age.[12] The increasing number of chronic overuse injuries in the young has been attributed to early specialization in a single sport, intensive year-round training, and inadequate recovery.[13,14]

This chapter will focus on the development of elite young athletes. The chapter begins by identifying who becomes an elite young athlete. A broader discussion of how potential sporting expertise is best developed follows. The chapter then concludes with the consideration of key risks faced by youngsters involved in elite sport.

Who becomes the elite young athlete?

Talent is defined as having an aptitude for a specific area or areas.[15] Systematic programmes of talent identification have been in place for decades.[16] Since elite adult athletes generally have body characteristics and bioenergetic profiles that are specific to the event in which they compete,[17] the focus of talent identification has largely been on the identification of biological traits, particularly morphological characteristics, unique to the particular discipline of interest.[18]

The child with athletic potential is likely to be physiologically better endowed than their peers. Even prior to puberty, child athletes very often have peak oxygen uptake (peak $\dot{V}O_2$) values greater than their non-athletic peers.[19] Strength is also enhanced in athletic children, with elite girls being stronger than the normal population at all ages, whilst this advantage in strength in elite boys is conferred around the time of the pubertal growth spurt.[20]

The enhanced physiological and physical attributes in these youngsters are believed not to be the result of training, rather simply a reflection of their genetic make-up.[21] Empirical evidence that superior morphological attributes are not a product of training has been provided through a longitudinal study of youngsters considered 'elite' in soccer, swimming, and tennis.[22] Distinct differences in birth-date uniformity were found, with male swimmers, soccer, and tennis players predominately born in the first 3 months of the selection year.[22] Birth-date discrimination, a product of the time-of-year cut-off utilized by either the school system or sport leagues for class or competition grouping, is commonly referred to as the 'relative age effect' and creates a distinct advantage for those youngsters who are the oldest in their particular group.[23] This advantage is apparent for both school and elite sports where strength and size are important. At school, discrimination by birth date has been shown in rugby, soccer, hockey, and netball, with the older, autumn-born children over-represented in school teams compared to the younger summer born children.[24] An analogous birth date effect occurs for elite adult leagues. For example, there is an over representation of players born between September and November in the Football Association Premier League.[25] In youth elite leagues, the relative age effect can be even more pronounced. An over representation of those early born children was found for Canadian junior ice hockey players, with 78% of the boys selected for elite junior squads born in the first half of the selection year.[26] Likewise, elite male soccer juniors from the United Kingdom, Sweden, and Belgium have been found to have birthdays in the first half of the soccer year.[27,28]

The chronological age of a child relative to the selection year clearly influences the chances of being selected into elite junior teams. This persists into selection for senior teams and is perhaps best illustrated by data from the Football Association (see Fig. 37.1). Over a period of 6 years, 103 14-year-old boys were selected for the Football Association School of Excellence. Examination of birth-date distribution of the boys selected revealed that 65% were born in the first quarter of the selection year and less than 2% in the last quarter [see Fig. 37.1(a)]. Selection means these boys receive elite coaching from an early age, which undoubtedly enhances their chance of continued elite participation. Indeed, almost half of English premier league footballers are born in the first quarter of the youth selection year [see Fig. 37.1(b)]. Likewise, those born in the first third of the youth selection year are over-represented in the national team [see Fig. 37.1(c)]. For those born later in the selection year, the chance of being selected for the School of Excellence is slight and is most probably because these relatively younger boys are smaller and less mature. They do not receive the elite coaching opportunities afforded to the older selected boys and most likely fall behind in the development of sophisticated skills. Elite adult team selection is therefore far less likely for the relatively younger boys. It would appear being older with advanced physical development and maturation is almost a pre-requisite for elite selection into those sports, like soccer, for which there is a pronounced relative age effect.

Sherar *et al.*[26] have clearly demonstrated that alongside age, accelerated maturity confers selection advantage into elite junior sport in boys. The performance advantages resulting from maturation have been comprehensively reviewed in Chapter 12 and only the salient issues are summarized here.

The acquisition of secondary sexual characteristics commonly denotes puberty, the beginning of a much more marked period of progress toward adult maturity. Secondary sexual characteristics develop because of increased androgen production in boys and girls, testosterone production in boys, and oestrogen production in girls. The adolescent growth spurt is largely an outcome of an increase in growth hormone (GH) and insulin-like growth factor-1 (IGF-1) levels. Exercise has been shown to promote the release of various growth factors, such as GH.[29] GH is produced by the pituitary gland in a pulsatile manner and has both an anabolic and metabolic effect—inducing, for example, osteoblastic activity at the epiphyses as well as lipolysis. During childhood, the GH-IGF-1 axis is pivotal to normal physical growth.[30] IGF-1 stimulates GH and appears to be a major mediator of protein anabolism and glucose metabolism, having a pronounced effect upon muscle volume, bone growth, and cardiorespiratory fitness. There is evidence that IGF-1 influences myocardial contractility,[31] and the subsequent effect on cardiac function contributes to increases in oxygen consumption.[32] At the muscle, mechanical signals stimulate muscular IGF-1 and mechano-growth factor (MGF) is expressed. Muscle mass has been shown to increase by 25% after only 2 weeks of direct MGF injection in animals.[33] IGF-1 also enhances long bone growth through augmentation of chondrocyte proliferation.[34]

Sport-specific differences in maturation stage have been found in elite young athletes. Boys for instance who were involved in the Training Of Young Athletes (TOYA) longitudinal study all began training prior to puberty, yet the gymnasts were found to mature late whilst the swimmers were found to mature early.[22]

Boys who mature early are advantaged in a number of ways in sports requiring size and strength. Normally, peak height velocity (PHV) occurs between the ages of 11 and 13 years. Peak height gains of approximately 9.5 cm·year^{-1} are usually noted during the growth spurt in height; therefore, for those for whom PHV occurs early, these gains in stature are accelerated relative to their peer group.[35] There is a strong association between changes in height and GH secretion at puberty. IGF-1 up-regulation of GH stimulates bone and cartilage growth and increases in stature result.[36] Augmented GH release is also associated with increases in testosterone concentration, which promotes substantial increases in muscle mass.[37] Relative muscle mass increases from approximately 42% of body composition at 5 years of age to 54% at 17 years.[38] Much of this gain is during puberty and, as a result, boys experience marked increases in strength.[39]

In contrast to boys, a relative age effect is far less pronounced in girls. Only a marginal relative age effect was found amongst female elite youth soccer players from the United States.[40] Birth-date distribution was also examined amongst girls considered elite in gymnastics, swimming, and tennis as a part of the TOYA study. An unequal birth-season distribution was only found for female tennis players, with birth dates in female gymnasts distributed evenly throughout the year.[41] This is surprising as female gymnasts have been found to mature late, with peak height, leg length,

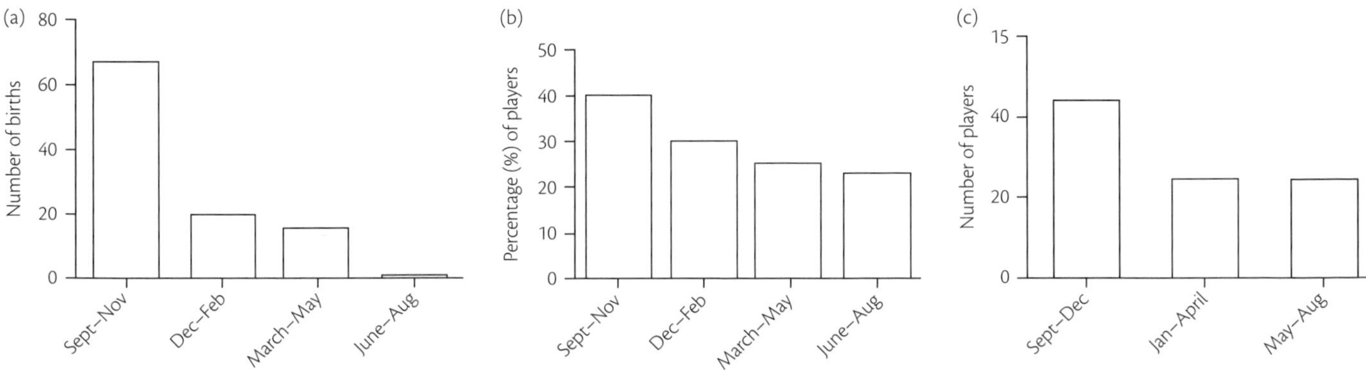

Fig. 37.1 Birthdate bias in English soccer. (a) Birthdates of boys selected for the Football Association School of Excellence. (b) English Premier League soccer players birthdate distribution. (c) Birthdates of English squad players selected for the European Championship.

and seated height velocities occurring approximately 1 year later than in non-athletic adolescent girls.[42] A number of explanations for the lack of a relative age effect in females are possible. Unlike boys, early maturation in girls may create athletic disadvantage as opposed to advantage. Although the early maturing girl is, like her male counterpart, taller and heavier than the late maturing girl, the gain in mass in girls is more a result of increased adipose tissue. Increases in muscle mass from 40% to 45% of body composition are noted in girls from 5 to 17 years of age; however, in relative terms muscle mass decreases are noted in girls after the age of 13 years due to the accumulation of body fat.[38] Girls also experience substantial changes in body shape, particularly a large adolescent spurt in hip width. As the pelvis broadens, the hips move further apart and away from the midline, causing girls to throw out their heels when they run as their thighs have to create a greater angle to bring their knees together. These changes in shape coupled with increases in adipose tissue are more likely to slow the girl down and make her less able to excel in training or in competition.[43,44] It is also possible that because girls mature earlier selection for elite teams simply occurs at a chronological point when maturational age has less impact on performance.[45] Last, there may be an interaction between maturation and socialization.[40] Sport remains a strong medium through which images of masculinity and femininity are reproduced, sustaining the same asymmetrical gender relations of the larger society.[46] The gendered identities and separate 'gendered cultures' that develop for girls are arguably at odds with the goal of achieving sporting excellence, resulting in diminished participation with increasing maturation as girls strive to conform to socially constructed gender roles.[47]

To summarize, data would imply that initial entry into many competitive sports in childhood, particularly for boys, is heavily reliant on possessing certain physical attributes such as size or maturity. This implies that those youngsters who show potential but do not confirm to the pre-requisite physical attributes may miss early selection opportunity, which clearly has an impact on later elite participation. This is less apparent for girls, but clearly maturational status exerts substantial influence on performance and the likelihood of continued participation in girls.

The development of the elite young athlete

Physiological maturation and training

Continued development and maintenance of performance in young athletes requires optimal physiological function. Children and adolescents, like adults, respond to progressive and regular training. Thorough examination of the trainability of children has been provided in Chapters 39 and 40, and only a summary of the key issues is given here.

Aerobic training has been shown to be effective when exercise at an intensity of at least 80–90% of heart rate maximum is adhered to for between 40 and 60 min, three to four times per week, for at least 12 weeks.[48] This training prescription is similar to that recommended for adults; however, the magnitude of increase in peak $\dot{V}O_2$ seems to be somewhat lower in children than that generally seen in adults,[49] with younger, prepubertal children increasing peak $\dot{V}O_2$ by approximately 7–15% following training.[50–52] The relative increase in peak $\dot{V}O_2$ following training is of a similar magnitude in both sexes, and even in the elite young athlete training results in increases in aerobic fitness.[53]

There has been much debate regarding whether a critical point in the developmental period exists when aerobic training becomes effective. Some have argued in favour of a maturational threshold or 'trigger point' before which the effects of training are negligible.[54–56] It is believed that the trigger point is influenced by the modulating effects of androgenic hormones; however, the evidence to support this hypothesis is weak. Conversely, there is evidence to support the contention that younger, prepubertal children are trainable. Using rigorous inclusion criteria, Armstrong *et al.*[48] reviewed 18 studies involving either 8–10 year olds or 11–18 year olds.[48] Of the 11 studies included for children <11 years, 6 (55%) found a training effect. Of the seven studies using participants ≥11 years, four (57%) reported significant increases in peak $\dot{V}O_2$ with training. The average increase in mass-related peak $\dot{V}O_2$ amongst participants <11 years of age was 6.5% (compared with an average control group change of −0.4%); in participants ≥11 years, an average increase of 5.5% was noted (compared with a control group average change of 0.14%). Of the eight studies included which verified the pubertal status of the participants, five (63%) showed peak $\dot{V}O_2$ increased following training. These findings are in accord with previous reviews[57,58] and suggest that the influence of age and maturation on the trainability of peak $\dot{V}O_2$ of 8–18 year olds remains to be proven.

The beneficial musculoskeletal effects of strength training have also been established in children.[59,60] Children can effectively increase strength if a training programme is introduced progressively and with appropriate supervision. Meta-analyses have shown that strength gains between 13% and 30% can be expected[61,62] and would appear to relate to quantitative and qualitative adaptations in muscle, improved motor unit activation, and neurological adaptations.[63,64]

Studies reporting the effects of training on children's anaerobic performance have found improvements, but these are varied and appear to be dependent on the mode and nature of the training. Increases in peak power between 5% and 23% have been reported following sprint running or cycle ergometer training.[50] Obert *et al.*[51] found an increase of 23% in peak power following a combined interval and continuous running training programme, whilst Rotstein *et al.*[65] reported a 13.1% increase in peak power following a continuous running programme. In contrast, Grodjinovsky *et al.*[66] found only a 5.3% increase in peak power following a sprint cycle training programme.

There is ample evidence to show that children adapt physiologically to training; however, our knowledge of the mechanisms that underpin these adaptations is scant. It is believed that increases in peak $\dot{V}O_2$ following training in children are related to changes in cardiac properties. Obert *et al.*[67] attributed increases in peak $\dot{V}O_2$ following 13 weeks of training to stroke volume, assessing stroke volume by echocardiography (ECG). The alterations in stroke volume were thought to emanate from increases in preload, decreases in afterload, and cardiac enlargement. Similar findings were reported with highly trained male child cyclists.[68] The higher peak $\dot{V}O_2$ observed in the child cyclists was again attributed to a higher stroke volume, thought to be mediated by changes in cardiac dimensions and myocardial relaxation properties. Far less is understood about the mechanisms underpinning changes in strength or anaerobic function following training in childhood.

If training practices are to be developed further so benefit can be maximized, refined quantification of training adaptations and the physiology underlying these is necessary in the elite young athlete. Recent availability of non-invasive methods, such as exercise ECG, near infra-red spectroscopy, and magnetic resonance spectroscopy, promise characterization of adaptive mechanisms during childhood, such as myocardial contractility, plasma volume, peripheral oxygen extraction, adenosine triphosphate (ATP), and phosphocreatine (PCr) activity.[69] Equally promising is the application of cellular and molecular techniques to the exercise response. Exercise training induces pleiotropic responses in skeletal muscle via complex protein signalling mechanisms. The functional consequence of the cellular and molecular response in the muscle includes improvement in metabolic profile, as well as enhanced athletic performance. Signalling mechanisms are beginning to be better understood in adults,[70] but we know far less about the signalling pathways involved in response to exercise training in the child. Is peroxisome proliferator receptor-γ co-activator-1α (PGC-1α) up-regulated in children during distance training like their adult counterparts?[71] Are increases in mitochondrial biogenesis possible during childhood, and if yes, are changes underpinned by the peroxisome proliferator activated receptors (PPARs)?[72,73] The characterization of the molecular and cellular bases and benefit of training in young athletes has yet to be achieved but promises greater insight into the muscular adaptations of current training practices, which in turn will aid the development of future training prescriptions.[70]

Attaining expertise

Whilst it is clear that those competing at a higher level possess particular inherited traits that discriminate them from more novice participants and guide entry into elite sport[74] even when optimized through physical training, these traits do not guarantee future elite performance. A myriad of factors have been shown to influence the development of expertise, and these have been extensively reviewed.[75,76] An overview of the key concepts and predominant theoretical frameworks is provided here.

Development of expert performance in any domain requires extensive periods of practice.[77] For example, by 20 years of age the most accomplished expert musicians have accumulated about 10,000 hours of deliberate practice, more than double the least accomplished expert musicians.[78] Expert performers in domains such as music or chess begin deliberate practice early and by 10 years of age have normally accumulated many more practice hours than their less accomplished peers.[78] Likewise, elite sportsmen and women spend many more hours practising in comparison to those competing at a lower level.[79] These extra hours of practice are thought to result in a wide range of benefits, many of which distinguish experts from non-experts.[80] For example, experts have an enhanced ability to interpret meaning from available information,[81] their detection and recognition of patterns of play are superior,[82] and they make more rapid and appropriate decisions.[83] In other words, the more time spent practicing appears to accelerate the ability for more complex thinking and learning structures and processes and therefore the development of more adept information processing strategies pertinent to the chosen skill.[84]

Practice is thought to follow a monotonic power function, known as the 'Power Law of Practice'.[85] This means that once the initial rapid increases in learning are achieved the rate of learning decreases and improvement levels off. It has been argued that only with years of continued 'deliberate' practice is further improvement in or maintenance of performance possible.[86] Deliberate practice is intensive and sustained, with the sole goal of increasing performance. It requires substantial effort and focus and the estimated accumulation of at least 10,000 specialized practice hours for expert development of key skills.[75]

The age at which practice is first initiated appears to be relevant. It has been suggested that deliberate practice is most effective when it commences during critical and sensitive periods of development: critical because of the quantitative and qualitative changes occurring, and sensitive because this is often a time when the system is most sensitive to manipulation.[87] The framework of 'deliberate' practice therefore advocates early specialization. Two sets of evidence have been used to support the need for early specialization. First, the highest levels of performance in sport are thought to be attained about 5 years after maturation.[88] Second, at least 10 years of preparation or 'deliberate' practice are needed to attain expertise.[89,90] If an early maturing boy is taken as an example, his performance would be predicted to peak around the age of 18–20 years, and 'deliberate' practice would need to have been initiated between 8 and 10 years of age to realize this peak.

More recent evidence provides support for the '10 year' rule in athletes; however, it also questions the need for early specialization. Baker *et al.*[91] found that expert athletes did indeed prepare for at least 10 years prior to attaining open national team selection, but the number of hours spent in deliberate, specialized practice was much less than the anticipated 10,000 hours proposed by Ericsson *et al.*[88] The negative correlation found between the number of different sporting activities experienced prior to elite adult selection and the number of hours spent in deliberate practice supports the contention that early diversification rather than specialization may be beneficial in the preparation of young athletes.

The work of Baker *et al.*[91] forms part of a growing body of evidence that questions the role of 'deliberate' practice as an optimal model for the development of young athletes[75] and proposes instead a 'developmental model' of sport participation.[92] The developmental model suggests that during early development (5–12 years) future elite youngsters, like their non-elite peers, sample a wide range of sporting activities and engage in much greater amounts of deliberate play than deliberate practice. This period ends in early adolescence and is replaced by specialization, a transition not apparent in non-elite youngsters who remain in the sampling stage.[92]

The behavioural determinants of deliberate play originate from the development of active play behaviour. Play behaviour reflects a child's physical, cognitive, social, and emotional learning,[93] and although play activity declines gradually as adulthood is attained, play activity embeds a particular pattern of behaviour. It has no specific purpose, instead it provides children with the opportunity to take in new information and develop more varied, creative, and flexible learning strategies.[94,95] There are three distinct stages of active play behaviour beginning in infancy, peaking in prepuberty, and declining thereafter.[96] Active play behaviour begins with a 'rhythmic stereotype' stage during infancy[97] and proceeds to 'exercise play' during early schooling. The salient characteristics of exercise play are spontaneity and the inclusion of gross locomotor activities such as running, chasing, and climbing.[98] As the 'exercise play' stage declines, 'rough-and-tumble' play, the final stage, increases, peaking just before the onset of puberty.[99,100]

Côté *et al.*[75] believe that the 'deliberate play' commonly engaged in by child athletes is a further extension of active play behaviour.

Deliberate play appears to combine key play behaviour attributes with unique elements of game-play associated with specific sports. Deliberate play provides exposure to relevant motor skills and game play scenarios, but in a free and unstructured environment that allows spontaneous innovation and experimentation within the context of the chosen sport. This is thought to be immensely beneficial for refining flexible and adaptive strategies that greatly augment rapid decision-making, as well as enhancing intrinsic motivation and fostering a desire for continued participation.[101] Physiological and metabolic benefits are also believed to be superior during deliberate play because the time spent being active is greater than that afforded during structured practice.

Providing children who show sporting promise with the opportunity for deliberate play and early diversified sporting experiences appears to be an important part of the development of future sporting expertise.[102,103] The ability to sample different sports and engage in deliberate play during childhood is thought to develop competence and enhance motivation.[104] The environment within which the child is reared has been shown to be highly influential for these opportunities to be realized.[105,106] Work with Canadian and American elite athletes has shown that fewer came from cities where the population was less than 10,000 or more than 500,000.[106] Cities with a population between 10,000 and 500,000 are thought to be optimal because there are more and safer open spaces for deliberate play, and youngsters are afforded access and exposure to relevant infrastructure and facilities needed to support diversified sport involvement.[105]

It would appear that one of the most pertinent benefits that emerges from early diversified participation in sport in the elite young athlete is the ability to transfer the varied skills acquired during exposure to multiple sport activities to the chosen specialization.[92] More recent theories related to knowledge transfer suggest that transfer of knowledge is most effective when varied and flexible learning opportunities have been afforded. Exposure to multiple contexts enables the learner to understand the wider application of what is being taught and be able to utilize the information flexibly in the future.[107] It is easy to see how the flexible and informal learning environment of deliberate play coupled with exposure to multiple sporting activities better facilitates transfer of key attributes, such as the identification of meaningful patterns of information.

Transfer is not confined to cognitive development, and transfer between tasks has been categorized into movement, perceptual, and conceptual.[108] Baker[80] suggests that physiological-transfer benefits are also evident and are relevant to the development of sporting expertise. Studies have shown that cross-training or physiological transfer is evident in children. Children who are trained with continuous aerobic protocols and those trained using intermittent sprint intervals both show improvement in peak $\dot{V}O_2$.[50,52,109] Intriguingly, the magnitude of change in peak $\dot{V}O_2$ has been reported to be greater in those who trained on cycle ergometers using high-intensity intermittent intervals compared to a continuous 'standard' aerobic training prescription.[109] Temporary increases in blood volume are apparent following a short burst of pedalling at a higher rather than lower exercise intensity.[110] Since a high blood volume enhances venous return and diastolic function, the peripheral response to high-intensity cycle sprints is likely mediating cardiovascular effect, in other words physiological transfer. Increases in oxygen pulse noted following cycle ergometer sprint interval training in boys suggests cardiovascular benefit transfer.[109]

Sprint training has also been reported to increase the percentage of type IIa fibres in adolescents.[111] High-intensity exercise can elevate the aerobic potential of fast-twitch motor units, which are substantially recruited above 90% of maximum $\dot{V}O_2$ in adults[112]—again, a mechanism which may contribute to high-intensity interval protocols having as much of an impact on aerobic power as anaerobic power in children. Alternatively, the apparent cardiovascular benefit following high intensity intermittent exercise in children may reflect a lower reliance on anaerobic metabolism during high intensity exercise[113] (see Chapter 16) so that a series of exercise bouts of more than 15 s will require a greater contribution from aerobic energy production in children than in adults.[114] Deliberate play has yet to be metabolically characterized, but the possibility that deliberate play creates physiological transfer opportunities in youngsters is enticing.

Exposure to risk

The child athlete is vulnerable. Vulnerable populations are characterized by having unusually high exposure to a risk, which can be modified by both innate factors, such as age or developmental stage, or acquired factors such as excessive training, influencing both the exposure and the capacity to cope with this.[115]

Exposure to excessive training during childhood unfavourably affects the very processes targeted for the enhancement of performance by slowing down or distorting them. Unfavourable effects may manifest through distortion of normal patterns of growth and maturation and/or musculoskeletal injury or cardiovascular dysfunction. Intensive involvement in competitive sport by young athletes also places them at substantial psychological risk.[116,117] Whilst it is thought that childhood activity patterns might be carried over to adult life, there is evidence to suggest the reverse with youngsters who engage in severe training, which is often accompanied by athletic 'burn-out' syndrome and a greater predisposition to injury.[118,119] Vulnerability therefore encompasses characteristics that can modify the level of risk, which in the context of elite sport may be the risk of injury, by influencing both the exposure (for instance, consideration of training practices) and the capacity to cope with it (for instance, consideration of the biological and psychological capacity to respond).

For many young athletes, the environment provided to optimize the development of their talent fails to take into account risk. Often the greatest extrinsic risk factor for the talented young athlete is the adult(s) in his/her athletic life. It has been argued that all children are at risk simply by virtue of being children because they rely on adults.[120] The child's athletic giftedness very often becomes the object of adult desire and ambition, and the environment provided to optimize their talent abuses their vulnerability and places them at considerable risk.[121] Greater success often drives the abuse, as evidenced in a recent study of former child athletes from the United Kingdom.[122] Zhang Huimin, a slight 8 year old from China, is a pertinent example. After showing an early aptitude for running, her father's development programme has recently included a 4000 km run.[123] The 55 day run required her to complete more than 60 km a day, a regime that clearly poses substantial risk to her health and development and might prevent her from attaining the elite status so desired by her father.[124]

Risk assessment has commonly been used to guide evaluation of a given risk or risks from specific exposures across a multitude of health applications.[125] Risk analysis involves identifying sources of potential harm, assesses the likelihood that harm will occur, and the consequences if harm does occur. Risk management takes this information and uses it to guide risk reduction and control. It is not possible to give a definite list of risk factors for child athletes because the level and type of risk is very individualized and depends upon the interaction of multiple factors, such as the sport, developmental age, environmental constraints, social support, etc. What this means is that some children are more vulnerable than others. Within these confines, a discussion of risk and risk management is provided for three areas that are common sources of concern for the child athlete: growth and maturation, musculoskeletal injury, and cardiac dysfunction.

Growth and maturation

A persistent anxiety has been whether intensive training and the demands of elite sport participation adversely affect the processes of growth and maturation. A certain amount of physical activity is necessary for optimal growth since activity is a known endocrine stimulant.[126] Chronic training, however, may cause less than optimal structural and functional alterations, and girls appear to be particularly at risk. A discussion of the pertinent issues related to the relationship between exercise training and growth are provided below. A thorough examination of the tempo and timing of maturation, the endocrine response to exercise, as well as the implications of differential rates of growth for physical activity is provided in Chapters 12 and 38.

Whilst there is compelling evidence that exercise provides a stimulus for growth and maturation, an equally strong case has been provided to show that excessive training may exert a negative influence on growth, particularly in girls.[127,128] Several studies have shown that female athletes in gymnastics, swimming, and ballet have delayed puberty and menarcheal age.[129] De Ridder[130] observed that, in comparison to a control group of girls matched for maturation and fatness, girls involved in competitive gymnastics exhibited delayed maturation. Theintz *et al.*[131] suggested that the delay in peak height, seated height, and leg-length velocities in girl gymnasts were evidence of an exercise-induced alteration in growth, because predicted adult height would not be attained. In contrast, others have shown that neither size nor growth are affected by elite sports participation.[132–134] Differences in stature, for example, most commonly noted in gymnastics, are believed to simply reflect the genetic predisposition in both boys and girls.[135–137] Although there is agreement that there is a delay in maturation in female gymnasts, it has been observed that later catch-up growth allows predicted adult height to be achieved and in some cases exceeded.[138] Girls who are not involved in competitive training but who mature late share similar anthropometric characteristics as their athletic peers and also display catch-up growth.[129,139]

Very delayed menarche and amenorrhea have been associated with caloric imbalance.[140] A high proportion of young female athletes suffer from disordered eating and this has been a primary risk factor for menstrual dysfunction. The intake of sufficient energy as well as vital minerals and vitamins is paramount in the young female athlete given that elite participation coincides with peak bone mineral accrual.[141] Delayed menarche places girls at risk from osteoporosis in later life because of the reduction in early bone mineralization. The inter-relationship between disordered eating, amenorrhea, and osteoporosis has been termed the 'female triad'.[142–144] Prior menstrual irregularity appears to be an important risk factor for amenorrhea in adolescent athletes,[140] and whether this is mediated by caloric restriction, excessive training, or both is not well understood. The nutritional status of some young elite gymnasts has been found to be comparable with age-matched controls.[145] By contrast, others have shown evidence of reduced energy intake in elite gymnasts.[146–148]

Many conclude that growth factors are inhibited by the combined effect of strenuous training and caloric restriction.[131,149] Nemet *et al.*[150] have attempted to tease apart the effect of intensive training and nutritional restriction on growth factors. Examining the effect of a 7 day diet alteration and strenuous exercise training programme on a group of young men, they revealed a significant decrease in IGF-1 levels in those who were underfed. Contrary to an expected increase, IGF-1 remained unchanged in those participants who were overfed. Clearly strenuous exercise is an extremely powerful mediator of IGF-1. Interestingly, these data support previous work suggesting a threshold of exercise training, beyond which the response of the GH-IGF-1 axis and related catecholamines are blunted in a manner similar to that seen in the obese.[30,151] Instead of an anabolic effect, intensive endurance training has been shown to be catabolic and related to inflammatory cytokine production. Attenuation of IGF-1 in response to intensive training mimics the GH response to trauma and has been associated with increases in the circulatory cytokines interleukin-1β and tumour necrosis factor α.[152,153] Inflammatory cytokines are critical mediators of cardiovascular dysfunction[154,155] and cause elevation of other proteins related to cardiovascular dysfunction such as high sensitive C-reactive protein (hsCRP), which itself has been linked to impaired vascular function,[156,157] an increase in insulin resistance, and metabolic disorders.[158,159] Exercise training clearly has the capacity to exert both positive anabolic as well as negative catabolic affects; however, the meaning of a blunted IGF-1 response has yet to be fully understood.

Without longitudinal studies that begin prior to the onset of both puberty and intense training, definitive conclusions on the effect of elite sport participation on growth and development are not possible. The interplay between training, GH-IGF-1, and circulating inflammatory cytokines is still not fully understood.[160] Physical activity has been shown to markedly reduce the risk of cardiovascular events;[161] attenuate the incidence of hypertension; and improve glucose tolerance, dyslipidaemia, and insulin sensitivity.[162] Yet, in children, excessive training stimulates inflammatory cytokines suggesting a boundary between healthy and unhealthy levels of exertion.[153,163]

Musculoskeletal injury

Injury is an inherent risk of participation in sport; however, many elite young athletes undergo repetitive practice extremes during training, predisposing them to increased risk.[11] For example, young divers may make up to 14,000 jumps per year, whilst a young javelin thrower may take up to 6000 throws per year.[164] Such extremes of practice can manifest in chronic overuse injuries or more permanent musculoskeletal damage.[13] Particularly concerning is the belief that overuse injuries are increasing in young athletes.[165] An overview of the literature regarding athletic injuries in the young is provided in Chapter 42 with more focused and detailed discussion of site-specific sports injuries available in Chapters 44–48.

Describing injury in a young athletic population is beset by methodological difficulties. For a start, there is no consensus on how to define an injury.[10] An injury may be defined as any trauma that occurs during practice, training, or competition *that results in* limitation, modification, or cessation of participation;[166,167] or as any trauma that occurs during practice, training, or competition *that does not result in* limitation, modification, or cessation of participation.[168] The great diversity in the definition of an injury means compiling injury rates across studies has been difficult.[169] The need to include the severity of the injury into any injury definition has been shown to be valuable for directing prevention strategies.[10,170] Time lost from participation is often used as a substitute indicator of injury severity;[169] however, these are not mutually exclusive terms, and it has been suggested that any definition of injury should include both severity and time lost.[171] This would help reduce over-estimation of injury in sports where minor injuries are common, as well as the under-estimation of more severe injuries.[10]

To facilitate the development of preventative strategies, it is important that comparison of injury rates can be made between different sports or across training practices. To do this, incidence data are necessary. Incidence rates or injuries per athlete are usually calculated by dividing the number of injuries by the total number of at-risk athletes, then multiplying with a constant k (e.g. 100), which facilitates comparisons.[172] For example, if 23 dance students sustained ankle injuries among a total of 46 participating dance students, the incidence rate would be expressed as 50 injuries per 100 participants. An injury rate per athlete exposure can also be quantified and allows injury rates to be computed that are relative to the number of hours spent in practice and/or competition.[172] Exposure can be classified in terms of practice, rehearsal, competition, 1000 hours of practice, or other risk exposure elements, such as throws, jumps, etc. For example, the incidence rate of dancers could be expressed as the number of injuries sustained divided by 1000 participation hours. Delimiting the exposure element and quantity allows for a more objective comparison of various injury rates;[173] however, use of multiple denominators on the same data would appear to provide a more thorough analysis of injury occurrence in young athletes.[10]

Up to half of all sports injuries in the young are overuse injuries.[174] The long-term implication of an overuse injury in the adolescent athlete is more severe because of the possibility of arrested growth and/or deformity of the long bones from, for example, physeal fractures.[12] Overuse injuries are most likely a result of excessive periods of specialized repetitive practice. Interestingly, a 10 year follow-up of the prospective TOYA study of elite young athletes showed that the injury rate of those youngsters who went on to become elite adults was 88% higher than those who did not attain elite adult status, suggesting the injury risk conferred by elite sports participation in the young may not be realized until a much later participation age.[175]

Cardiac dysfunction

Although the occurrence of cardiovascular disorders in the young is only a fraction of adult heart disease, of the 600 or so sudden cardiac deaths that occur per year in the United States as a result of athletic activity most occur in the young.[176,177] It is estimated that between one and three sudden cardiac deaths per 100,000 high school athletes occur per year.[178–181] A higher incidence of sudden cardiac death is noted in young male athletes than in young female athletes, probably attributable to the lower incidence of some of the more common causes of cardiac death in women and perhaps the lower rate of participation amongst girls in sport.[182] Early detection of heart disease and its proper diagnosis might prevent many of these deaths, but an effective strategy to identify those at risk continues to elude the health profession.[178,183]

There are many types of disease that are responsible for sudden cardiac death in young athletes, making detection of those at risk particularly challenging. An additional difficulty is that individual disease types often present with varying characteristics and in some cases are completely 'silent' or asymptomatic. The principal source of sudden cardiac death in young athletes is hypertrophic cardiomyopathy (HCM), which accounts for somewhere between 30% and 50% of sudden cardiac deaths.[184] HCM is essentially a myocardial disease, which is commonly inherited and characterized by one consistent feature, an unexplained hypertrophied and non-dilated left ventricle.[177] It is one of the most variable cardiac diseases in terms of symptoms, with most cases being detected during puberty.[185] This pattern of unpredictable development makes HCM one of the most difficult cardiac disorders to detect. Second to HCM as a cause of sudden cardiac death in young athletes are coronary anomalies, which account for approximately 19% of sudden cardiac deaths.[186] A myriad of other disorders such as aortic stenosis, cardiomyopathy, mitral-valve prolapse, long QT, Wolff–Parkinson–White and Marfan's Syndrome have been identified as the basis of between 0.5% and 4% of cardiac deaths in the young athletic population.[187,188]

The unexpected death of a young athlete is a uniquely poignant tragedy, representing the abrupt end of a life associated with energy and well-being. Despite recent initiatives worldwide to promote increased cardiovascular risk management in the elite young athlete, most countries, with the exception of Italy, do not endorse mandatory pre-participation screening.[189,190] There has been extensive debate over the utility of mass screening of children and adolescents before competitive sport participation.[190–195] The question of whether to screen can only be given due consideration once a range of issues are taken into account. These include the size of the population, the prevalence of the problem within that population, the specificity and sensitivity of the screening tool (i.e. how good the screening tool is and what kind of false-positive or false-negative results it produces), the costs incurred, and the legal responsibility of the activity organizer or medical support team.

The American Heart Association (AHA) recommendations are probably the most commonly used to guide the screening of young athletes.[195,196] They recommend that the basis of any screening programme should be a detailed questionnaire of medical and family history combined with a physical examination. This should be done at 2-year intervals. The questionnaire should be completed, when appropriate, by the young person or by their parents and should specifically include details of family history for known cardiovascular disorders, arrhythmia, and syncope. In the physical examination, an assessment of blood pressure, palpation of the precordium, auscultation of the heart, and measurement of pulses in the upper and lower extremities should be made. A recent study has suggested that the ability of the physical examination to detect unknown heart disorders in young people is very low. Of the 4% of children diagnosed by ECG as having heart disease, none were found to have any cardiac abnormality after physical examination by a general paediatrician. Although detection was improved when a specialist carried out the physical examination, only 54% of these cases were detected through palpation and auscultatory examination by the paediatric cardiologist.[197] The sensitivity of the AHA-recommended screening history and physical examination is not known but has been estimated to be somewhere between 3% and 6%.[198]

The ECG is a very valuable additional diagnostic tool. The less common but high-risk rhythm disorders such as long QT syndrome or Wolf–Parkinson–White syndrome can be detected with relative ease through an ECG.[199] Nearly 95% of patients with HCM also show ECG abnormalities.[200] Although varying, these can be characterized either by large Q waves in precordial leads in septal hypertrophy or by large, deeply inverted left-precordial T waves in the apical form, although in mild to moderate cases of HCM and in Marfan's syndrome the ECG might be normal. The value of the ECG can, however, be lower in an athletic population, because structural and functional changes associated with intensive training mimic those seen in certain cardiac diseases.[201] Electrocardiograph patterns common to certain disease states have often been noted in athletes under 18 years of age.[202] In a group of 1000 young athletes, 80% displayed bradycardia, 52% showed sinus arrhythmia, nearly 30% showed partial right-bundle-branch block, 45% displayed ST-segment elevation, and 22% had tall T waves.[202] Other findings included voltage criteria for left and right atrial enlargement and Romhilt–Estes score for left-ventricular hypertrophy. The latter ECG changes, however, most often occurred in isolation in the athletic group, an unusual feature for those with cardiomyopathy. Only four in this large group of young athletes had ECG findings consistent with cardiomyopathy, and subsequent ECG resulted in none being positively diagnosed. These findings indicate a 0.4% false-positive rate for the ECG. Despite the false-positive interpretation of ECG data (particularly for bradycardia and ventricular hypertrophy), as a screening tool it does offer an affordable and simple option that can substantially increase the detection ability of the screening procedure offered by the history and physical examination, with a sensitivity of about 70%.[190,203,204] The same caveat exists, however, for the ECG as for the physical examination; that is, it is probably only optimally effective when interpreted by a specialist.

ECG greatly improves the accuracy of detection of structural cardiac abnormalities in children—such as HCM and aortic dilation—and, of the available screening tools, is the only one to have 100% specificity.[198] The problem lies in the expense, the necessity for skilled specialists, and that it has a sensitivity of 80% and therefore cannot give an absolute guarantee of the absence of a cardiac disorder. ECG is unlikely to become part of a normal screening procedure given its high cost, but it does have a very important role to play for potential participants who are identified by physical examination or ECG to have unexplained cardiac abnormalities or a family history of HCM.[205]

Reducing cardiovascular risk assumes screening is a right for all young athletes, rather than simply a recommendation. Based on the success of the Italian programme of mandatory screening, a recent European consensus statement has recommended that a common European screening protocol based on 12 lead ECG should be developed and implemented across European countries.[190] Screening has, however, been described by some as searching for a needle in a haystack.[206] Even when a thorough screening system is in place, given that no tool has 100% specificity and sensitivity, no screening programme can make the claim that it can prevent all sudden cardiac death in the young.[207]

General conclusion

The elite young athlete can develop their potential within an appropriate and supportive environment; however, there are many young athletes for whom such an environment is not afforded, instead their health and well-being are regularly compromised. Those involved in the development of young athletes must have sufficient knowledge of the exercising child, physiologically and psychologically, as well as an understanding of optimal ways of developing athletic potential while minimizing risk. In 1982, Rutenfranz argued for a code of ethics to be established to protect young athletes.[164] It was suggested that such a code could apply the Declaration of Helsinki ethical guidelines for human experiments to athletic training and would serve as a code of responsibility for those involved in the development of young athletes. A little over 20 years later ministers of physical education and sport of more than 90 countries met at UNESCO headquarters for a round-table discussion that included consideration of the protection of young athletes. They concluded that a global definition of appropriate principles should be established to enable development of youngsters who show athletic potential to occur without infringement of their fundamental rights. Additionally, professions involved with the development of young athletes were encouraged to develop a 'code of good practice'.[208] Rutenfranz's belief that scientists working in paediatric exercise science and medicine have a duty to develop a 'code of good practice' to protect young athletes is as relevant today as it was in 1982.

Summary

- Entry into elite youth sport would appear to rely more upon inherited physiological attributes than specific skills. This appears to be particularly acute for boys in dynamic team sports such as soccer.
- Young athletes are generally not developmentally ready (physically, psychologically, or cognitively) for all that early sport specialization and deliberate practice entails. Intensive early involvement in a single sport is a primary antecedent for the development of overuse injuries. The deliberate practice model of talent development is more likely to predispose the young athlete to injury and drop-out than deliver future expert performance.
- Development of expertise does require many hours of concentrated practice; however, in the early developmental years, opportunity to sample many activities and engage in deliberate play appears to play a more important role in the development of future sport expertise.
- The emergence and availability of new technologies means a more detailed understanding of the mechanisms underlying the training response is possible and should be a priority for further studies in paediatric exercise physiology. Ultimately, translation of the physiological and cellular bases of training will help to refine training protocols and prescriptions for young athletes.
- Definitive conclusions on whether elite participation causes aberrations to growth are not possible; however, there is evidence

that strenuous exercise can inhibit growth factors and stimulate inflammatory cytokines. These data suggest a boundary between healthy and unhealthy levels of exertion.

- Cardiac risk is limited to a very small number of participants; however, given the potential to cause sudden death, calls for improved pre-participation screening practices continue.

References

1. Riddoch C, Boreham C (2000). Physical activity, physical fitness and children's health: Current concepts. In: Armstrong N, van Mechelen W (eds.), *Paediatric exercise science and medicine*, pp. 243–52. Oxford University Press, Oxford.
2. Trost S, Levin S, Pate R (2000). Sport, physical activity and other health behaviours in children and adolescents. In: Armstrong N, van Mechelen W (eds.), *Paediatric exercise science and medicine*, pp. 295–304. Oxford University Press, Oxford.
3. van Mechelen W, Verhagen E (2005). Injury prevention in young people—time to accept responsibility. *Lancet* **366**, 46.
4. Maffulli N (1998). At what age should a child begin regular continuous exercise at moderate or high intensity? *Br J Sports Med* **32**, 298.
5. Murphy S (1999). *The cheers and the tears. A health alternative to the dark side of youth sport today*. Jossey-Bass, San Francisco, CA.
6. Horn T, Harris A (2002). Perceived competence in young athletes: Research findings and recommendations for coaches and parents. In: Smoll F, Smith R (eds.), *Children and youth in sport: A biopsychosocial perspective*, pp. 435–64. Kendall-Hunt, Dubuque, IW.
7. Conn J, Annest J, Gilchrist J (2003). Sports and recreation related injury episodes in the US population, 1997–99. *Inj Prev* **9**, 117–23.
8. Bijur PE, Trumble A, Harel Y, Overpeck MD, Jones D, Schiedt PC (1995). Sports and recreation injuries in US children and adolescents. *Arch Pediatr Adolesc Med* **149**, 1009–16.
9. American College of Sports Medicine, American Academy of Family Physicians, American Academy of Orthopaedic Surgeons, American Medicinal Society for Sports Medicine, American Osteopathic Academy of Sports Medicine (2003). Female athlete issues for the team physician: A consensus statement. *Med Sci Sports Exerc* **35**, 1785–93.
10. Goldberg A, Moroz L, Smith A, Ganley T (2007). Injury surveillance in young athletes: A clinician's guide to sports injury literature. *Sports Med* **37**, 265–78.
11. Cassas K, Cassettari-Wayhs A (2006). Childhood and adolescent sports-related overuse injuries. *Am Fam Phys* **73**, 1014–22.
12. Adirim T, Cheng T (2003). Overview of injuries in the young athlete. *Sports Med* **33**, 75–81.
13. Emery CA (2003). Risk factors for injury in child and adolescent sport: A systematic review of the literature. *Clin J Sport Med* **13**, 256–68.
14. Benjamin H, Briner W (2005). Little league elbow. *Clin J Sport Med* **15**, 37–40.
15. Clark B (2008). *Growing up gifted*. Pearson Prentice Hall, New Jersey.
16. Durand-Bush N, Salmela J (2001). The development of talent in sport. In: Singer R, Hausenblas H, Janelle C (eds.), *Handbook of sport psychology*, pp. 269–89. John Wiley and Sons, New York.
17. Tanner JM (1964). *The physique of the Olympic athlete*. George Allen & Ungin, London.
18. Matsudo V (1996). Prediction of future athletic excellence. In: Bar-Or O (ed.), *The child and adolescent athlete*, pp. 92–112. Blackwell Science, Oxford.
19. Baxter-Jones A, Goldstein H, Helms P (1993). The development of aerobic power in young athletes. *J Appl Physiol* **75**, 1160–7.
20. Maffulli N, King J, Helms P (1994). Training in elite young athletes (the Training of Young Athletes (TOYA) Study): Injuries, flexibility and isometric strength. *Br J Sports Med* **28**, 123–36.
21. Rankinen T, Bray M, Hagberg J, Pérusse L, Roth S, Wolfarth B, Bouchard C (2006). The human gene map for performance and health-related fitness phenotypes: The 2005 update. *Med Sci Sports Exerc* **38**, 1863–88.
22. Baxter-Jones A, Helms P, Maffulli N, Baines-Preece J, Preece M (1995). Growth and development of male gymnasts, swimmers, soccer and tennis players: A longitudinal study. *Ann Hum Biol* **22**, 381–94.
23. Musch J, Grondin S (2001). Unequal competition as an impediment to personal development: A review of the relative age effect in sport. *Dev Rev* **21**, 147–67.
24. Wilson G (1999). The birthdate effect in school sports teams. *Eur J Phys Educ* **4**, 139–45.
25. Dudnik A (1994). Birth date and sporting success. *Nature* **368**, 592.
26. Sherar L, Baxter-Jones A, Faulkner R, Russell K (2007). Do physical maturity and birth date predict talent in male youth ice hockey players? *J Sports Sci* **25**, 879–86.
27. Simmons C, Paull G (2001). Season-of-birth bias in association football. *J Sports Sci* **19**, 677–86.
28. Williams A, Reilly T (2000). Talent identification and development in soccer. *J Sports Sci* **18**, 657–67.
29. Roemmich JN, Rogol AD (1997). Exercise and growth hormone: Does one affect the other? *J Pediatr* **131**, S75–80.
30. Cooper DM (1994). Evidence for and mechanisms of exercise modulation of growth—an overview. *Med Sci Sports Exerc* **26**, 733–40.
31. Donath MY, Jenni R, Brunner HP, Anrig M, Kohli S, Glatz Y, Froesch ER (1996). Cardiovascular and metabolic effects of insulin-like growth factor 1 at rest and during exercise in humans. *J Clin Endocrinol Metab* **81**, 4089–94.
32. Hütler M, Schnabel D, Staab D, Tacke A, Wahn U, Böning D, Beneke R (2002). Effect of growth hormone on exercise tolerance in children with cystic fibrosis. *Med Sci Sports Exerc* **34**, 567–72.
33. Goldspink G, Yang SY (2001). Effects of activity on growth factor expression. *Int J Sport Nutr Exerc Metab* **11**, S21–7.
34. Bonjour JP, Ammann P, Chevalley T, Rizzoli R (2001). Protein intake and bone growth. *Can J Appl Physiol* **26**, S153–66.
35. Abassi V (1998). Growth and normal puberty. *Pediatrics* **102**, S507–11.
36. Rogal A (1994). Growth at puberty: Interaction of androgens and growth hormone. *Med Sci Sports Exerc* **26**, 767–70.
37. Pomerants T, Tillmann V, Karelson K, Jürimäe J, Jürimäe T (2006). Ghrelin response to acute aerobic exercise in boys at different stages of puberty. *Horm Metab Res* **38**, 752–7.
38. Tanner J, Whitehouse R, Takaishi M (1966). Standards from birth to maturity for height, weight, height velocity and weight velocity: British children, 1965—I. *Arch Dis Child* **41**, 454–71.
39. Jones D, Round J (2000). Strength and muscle growth. In: Armstrong N, van Mechelen W (eds.), *Paediatric exercise science and medicine*, pp. 133–42. Oxford University Press, Oxford.
40. Vincent J, Glamser F (2006). Gender differences in the relative age effect among US Olympic Development Program youth soccer players. *J Sports Sci* **24**, 405–13.
41. Baxter-Jones A, Helms P (1994). Born too late to win? *Nature* **370**, 186.
42. Thomis M, Claessens A, Lefevre J, Philippaerts R, Beunen G, Malina R (2005). Adolescent growth spurts in female gymnasts. *J Pediatr* **146**, 239–44.
43. Haywood K, Getchell N (2001). *Lifespan motor development*. Human Kinetics, Champaign, IL.
44. Malina R, Bouchard C, Bar-Or O (2004). *Growth, maturation and physical activity*. Human Kinetics, Champaign, IL.
45. Sherar L, Bruner M, Munroe-Chandler K, Baxter-Jones A (2007). Relative age and fast tracking of elite major junior ice hockey players. *Percept Motor Skills* **104**, 702–6.
46. Birrell S, Cole C (1994). *Women, sport and culture*. Human Kinetics, Champaign, IL.
47. Vertinsky P, McManus A, Sit H, Liu Y (2005). The gendering of physical education in Hong Kong: East, West or global? *Int J Hist Sport* **22**, 816–39.

48. Armstrong N, Barrett N, Welsman J (2007). Cardiorespiratory training during childhood and adolescence. *J Exerc Sci Physiother* **3**, 67–75.
49. Pate RR, Ward DS (1990). Endurance exercise trainability in children and youth. In: Grana WA, Lombardo JA, Sharkey BJ, Stone JA (eds.), *Advances in sports medicine and fitness—volume 3*, pp. 37–55. Year Book Publishers, Chicago, IL.
50. McManus A, Armstrong N, Williams C (1997). Effect of training on the aerobic power and anaerobic performance of prepubertal girls. *Acta Paediatr* **86**, 456–9.
51. Obert P, Mandigout S, Vinet A, N'Guyen L, Stecken F, Courteix D (2001). Effect of aerobic training and detraining on left ventricular dimensions and diastolic function in prepubertal boys and girls. *Int J Sports Med* **22**, 90–6.
52. Baquet G, Berthoin S, Dupont G, Blondel N, Fabre C, van Praagh E (2002). Effects of high intensity intermittent training on peak VO_2 in prepubertal children. *Int J Sports Med* **23**, 439–44.
53. Baxter-Jones A, Helms P (1996). Effects if training at a young age: A review of the training of young athletes (TOYA) study. *Pediatr Exerc Sci* **8**, 310–27.
54. Katch V (1983). Physical conditioning of children. *J Adolesc Health* **3**, 241–6.
55. Mirwald R, Bailey D, Cameron N, Rasmussen R (1981). Longitudinal comparison of aerobic power in active and inactive boys age 7.0 to 17.0 Years. *Ann Hum Biol* **8**, 405–14.
56. Kobayashi K, Kitamura K, Miura M, Sodeyama H, Murase Y, Miyashita M (1978). Aerobic power as related to body growth and training in Japanese boys: A longitudinal study. *J Appl Physiol* **44**, 666–72.
57. LeMura LM, von Dullivard S, Carlonas R, Andreacci J (1999). Can exercise training improve maximal aerobic power ($\dot{V}O_2$ max) in children: A meta-analytic review. *J Exerc Physiol online* **2**, 1–22.
58. Mahon A, Vaccaro P (1989). Ventilatory threshold and $\dot{V}O_2$ max changes in children following endurance training. *Med Sci Sports Exerc* **21**, 425–31.
59. Faigenbaum A (2000). Strength training for children and adolescents. *Clin Sports Med* **19**, 593–619.
60. Malina RM (2006). Weight training in youth—growth, maturation, and safety: An evidence-based review. *Clin J Sport Med* **16**, 478–87.
61. Falk B, Tenembaum G (1996). The effectiveness of resistance training in children. *Sports Med* **22**, 176–86.
62. Payne V, Morrow J, Johnson L, Dalton S (1997). Resistance training in children and youth: Meta-analysis. *Res Q Exerc Sci* **68**, 80–8.
63. Matos N, Winsley R (2007). Trainability of young athletes and overtraining. *J Sports Sci Med* **6**, 353–67.
64. Tolfrey K (2007). Responses to training. In: Armstrong N (ed.), *Paediatric exercise science*, pp. 213–34. Churchill Livingstone, Edinburgh.
65. Rotstein A, Dotan R, Bar-Or O, Tenembaum G (1986). Effect of training on anaerobic threshold, maximal aerobic power and anaerobic performance of preadolescent boys. *Int J Sports Med* **7** 281–6.
66. Grodjinovsky A, Inbar A, Dotan R, Bar-Or O (1980). Training effect on the anaerobic performance of children as measured by the Wingate Anaerobic Test. In: Berg K, Erikkson B (eds.), *Children and exercise IX*, pp. 139–45. University Park Press, Baltimore, MD.
67. Obert P, Mandigout S, Nottin S, Vinet A, N'Guyen L, Lecoq A (2003). Cardiovascular responses to endurance training in children: Effect of gender. *Eur J Clin Invest* **33**, 199–208.
68. Nottin S, Vinet A, Stecken F, N'Guyen L, Ounissi F, Lecoq A, Obert P (2002). Central and peripheral cardiovascular adaptations to exercise in endurance-training children. *Acta Physiol Scand* **175**, 85–92.
69. Nassis G, Sidossis L (2006). Methods for assessing body composition, cardiovascular and metabolic function in children and adolescents: Implications for exercise studies. *Curr Opin Clin Nutr Metab Care* **9**, 560–7.
70. Coffey V, Hawley J (2007). The molecular bases of training adaptation. *Sports Med* **37**, 737–63.
71. Cartoni R, Léger B, Hock M, Praz M, Crettenand A, Pich S, Ziltener JL, Luthi F, Dériaz O, Zorzano A, Gobelet C, Kralli A, Russell AP (2005). Mitofusins 1/2 and ERRα expression are increase in human skeletal muscle after physical exercise. *J Physiol* **567**, 349–58.
72. Wang YX, Zhang CL, Yu RT, Cho HK, Nelson MC, Bayuga-Ocampo CR, Ham J, Kang H, Evans RM (2004). Regulation of muscle fiber type and running endurance by PPARdelta. *PLoS Biol* **2**, e294.
73. Joseph A, Pilegaard H, Litvintsev A, Leick L, Hood D (2006). Control of gene expression and mitochondrial biogenesis in the muscular adaptation to endurance exercise. *Essays Biochem* **42**, 13–29.
74. Gabbett T, Georgieff B, Domrow N (2007). The use of physiological, anthropometric, and skill data to predict selection in a talent-identified junior volleyball squad. *J Sports Sci* **25**, 1337–44.
75. Côté J, Baker J, Abernethy B (2007). Practice and play in the development of sport expertise. In: Tenenbaum G, Eklund RC (eds.), *Handbook of sport psychology*, pp. 184–202. Wiley, Hoboken, NJ.
76. Ericcson K, Nandagopal K, Roring R (in press). Toward a science of exceptional achievement: Attaining superior performance through deliberate practice. *Ann NY Acad Sci.*
77. Guest C, Regehr G, Tiberius R (2001). The life long challenge of expertise. *Med Educ* **35**, 78–81.
78. Ericsson K, Krampe R, Tesch-Romer C (1993). The role of deliberate practice in the acquisition of expert performance. *Psychol Rev* **100**, 363–406.
79. Baker J, Cote J, Abernethy B (2003). Learning from the experts: Practice activities of expert decision makers in sport. *Res Q Exerc Sport* **74**, 342–7.
80. Baker J (2003). Early specialiszation in youth sport: A requirement for adult expertise? *High Ability Stud* **14**, 85–94.
81. Abernethy B (1991). Visual search strategies and decision-making in sport. *Int J Sport Psychol* **22**, 189–210.
82. Abernethy B, Neal R, Koning P (1994). Visual-perceptual and cognitive differences between expert, intermediate and novice snooker players. *Appl Cogn Psychol* **8**, 185–211.
83. Williams A (2000). Perceptual skill in soccer: Implications for talent identification and development. *J Sports Sci* **18**, 737–50.
84. Baker J, Horton S (2004). A review of primary and secondary influences on sport expertise. *High Ability Stud* **15**, 211–28.
85. Newell A, Roesnbloom P (1981). Mechanisms of skill acquisition and the law of practice. In: Anderson J (ed.), *Cognitive skills and their acquisition*, pp. 1–55. Erlbaum, Hillsdale, NJ.
86. Krampe R, Ericsson K (1996). Maintaining excellence: Deliberate practice and elite performance in young and older pianists. *J Exp Psychol Gen* **125**, 331–59.
87. Scott JI (1988). Critical periods in organizational process. In: Falkner F, Tanner J (eds.), *Human growth volume 1: Developmental biology, prenatal growth*, pp. 181–96. Plenum Press, New York.
88. Ericsson K (1996). The acquisition of expert performance: An introduction to some of the issues. In: Ericsson K (ed.), *The road to excellence: The acquisition of expert performance in the arts, sciences, sports and games*, pp. 1–50. Lawrence Erlbaum Associates, Mahwah, NJ.
89. Simon H, Chase W (1973). Skill in chess. *Am Sci* **61**, 394–403.
90. Starkes J, Deakin J, Allard F, Hodges N, Hayes A (1996). Deliberate practice in sports: What is it anyway? In: Ericsson K (ed.), *The road to excellence: The acquisition of expert performance in the arts, sciences, sports and games*, pp. 81–106. Lawrence Erlbaum Associates, Mahwah, NJ.
91. Baker J, Côté J, Abernethy B (2003). Sport-specific practice and the development of expert decision-making in team ball sports. *J Appl Sport Psychol* **15**, 12–25.
92. Côté J (1999). The influence of the family in the development of talent in sport. *Sports Psychol* **13**, 395–417.
93. Piaget J (1962). *Play, dreams and imitation in childhood.* Norton, New York.

94. Pellegrini A, Smith P (1998). Physical activity play: The nature and function of a neglected aspect of play. *Child Dev* **69**, 577–98.
95. McCune L (1998). Immediate and ultimate functions of physical activity play. *Child Dev* **69**, 601–3.
96. Byers J (1998). The biology of human play. *Child Development* **69**, 599–600.
97. Byers J, Walker C (1995). Refining the motor training hypothesis for the evolution of play. *Am Nat* **146**, 25–40.
98. Bloch M (1989). Young boys' and girls' play in the home and in the community: A cultural ecological framework. In: Pellegrini A, Bloch M (eds.), *The ecological context of children's play*, pp. 120–54. Ablex, Norwood, NJ.
99. Humphreys A, Smith P (1987). Rough-and-tumble play, friendship and dominance in school children: Evidence for continuity and change with age. *Child Dev* **58**, 201–12.
100. Boulton M (1992). Participation in playground activities at middle school. *Educ Res* **34**, 167–82.
101. Berry J, Abernethy B, Cote J (in press). The contribution of structured practice and deliberate play to the development of expert perceptual and decision-making skill. *J Sport Exerc Psychol.*
102. Côté J, Hay J (2002). Family influences on youth sport participation and performance. In: Silva J, Stevens D (eds.), *Psychological foundations of sport*, pp. 503–19. Allyn and Bacon, Boston, MA.
103. Abernethy B, Baker J, Côté J (2005). Transfer of pattern recall skills may contribute to the development of sport expertise. *Appl Cogn Psychol* **19**, 705–18.
104. Kirk D (2005). Physical education, youth sport and lifelong participation: The importance of early learning experiences. *Eur Phys Educ Rev* **11**, 239–55.
105. Côté J, MacDonald D, Baker J, Abernethy B (2006). When "where" is more important than "when": Birthplace and birthdate effects on the achievement of sporting expertise. *J Sports Sci* **24**, 1065–73.
106. Baker J, Logan AJ (2007). Developmental contexts and sporting success: Birth date and birthplace effects in national hockey league draftees 2000–2005. *Br J Sports Med* **41**, 515–7.
107. Bransford J, Brown A, Cocking R (1999). *How people learn: Brain, mind, experience and school.* National Academy Press, Washington, DC.
108. Schmidt R, Wrisberg C (2000). *Motor learning and performance: A problem-based learning approach.* Human Kinetics, Champaign, IL.
109. McManus A, Cheng C, Leung M, Yung T, Macfarlane D (2005). Improving aerobic power in primary school boys: A comparison of continuous and interval training. *Int J Sports Med* **26**, 781–6.
110. Takaishi T, Sugiura T, Katayama K, Sato Y, Shima N, Yamamoto T, Moritani T (2002). Changes in blood volume and oxygenation level in a working muscle during a crank cycle. *Med Sci Sports Exerc* **33**, 520–8.
111. Kuno S, Takahashi H, Fujimoto K, Akima H, Miyamaru M, Nemoto I, Itai Y (1995). Muscle metabolism during exercise using phosphorus-31 nuclear magnetic resonance spectroscopy in adolescents. *Eur J Appl Physiol* **70**, 301–4.
112. Gollnick P, Piehl K, Karlsson J, Saltin B (1975). Glycogen depletion in human skeletal muscle fibres after varying types and intensities of exercise. In: Howald H, Poortmans J (eds.), *Metabolic adaptation to prolonged physical exercise: Proceedings of the 2nd International Symposium of Biochemistry and Exercise, Magglingen 1973*, pp. 416–21. Kirhauswer, Basel.
113. Zanaconata S, Buchtal S, Barstow T, Cooper D (1993). 31P-magnetic resonance spectroscopy of leg muscle metabolism during exercise in children and adults. *J Appl Physiol* **74**, 2214–18.
114. Billat V (2001). Interval training for performance: A scientific and empirical practice: Special recommendations for middle- and long-distance running. Part II: Anaerobic interval training. *Sports Med* **31**, 75–90.
115. World Health Organisation W (2004). *Health aspects of air pollution: Results from the WHO project "Systematic Review of Aspects of Air Pollution in Europe".* World Health Organisation, Copenhagen.
116. Holt N, Hoar S, Fraser S (2005). How does coping change with development? A review of childhood and adolescent sport coping research. *Eur J Sport Sci* **5**, 25–39.
117. Brustad R, Babkes M, Smith A (2001). Youth in sport: Psychological considerations. In: Singer R, Hausenblas H, Janelle C (eds.), *Handbook of sport psychology*, pp. 604–35. Wiley, New York.
118. Brenner J (2007). Council on Sports Medicine and Fitness: Overuse injuries, overtraining, and burnout in child and adolescent athletes. *Pediatrics* **119**, 1242–5.
119. Bompa T (1995). *From childhood to champion athlete.* Veritas Publishing, Toronto, Canada.
120. Finkelhor D, Dziuba-Leatherman J (1994). Victimization of children. *Am Psychol* **49**, 173–83.
121. David P (2005). *Human rights in youth sport: A critical review of children's rights in competitive sports.* Routledge, Oxford.
122. Gervis M, Dunn N (2004). The emotional abuse of elite child athletes by their coaches. *Child Abuse Rev* **13**, 215–23.
123. BBC News (2007). China girl completes 3,500 km run. Available at http://news.bbc.co.uk/2/hi/asia-pacific/6965410.stm (last accessed 27 August 2007)
124. Roberts W (2007). Can children and adolescents run marathons? *Sports Med* **37**, 299–301.
125. National Research Council (1983). *Committee of the Institutional Means for Assessment of Risks to Public Health. Risk Assessment in the Federal Government: Managing the Process.* National Academy Press, Washington, DC.
126. Gibney J, Healy M, Sonksen P (2007). The growth hormone/insulin-like growth factor-I axis in exercise and sport. *Endocrine Rev* **28**, 603–24.
127. Baxter-Jones A, Maffulli N, Mirwald R (2003). Does elite competition inhibit growth and delay maturation in some gymnasts? Probably not. *Pediatr Exerc Sci* **15**, 373–82.
128. Caine D, Bass S, Daly R (2003). Does elite competition inhibit growth and delay maturation in some gymnasts? Quite possibly. *Pediatr Exerc Sci* **15**, 360–72.
129. Malina R (1983). Menarche in athletes: A synthesis and hypothesis. *Ann Hum Biol* **10**, 1–24.
130. de Ridder C (1991). *Sexual maturation of pubertal girls: Physical and hormonal development in relation to metabolic and nutritional factors.* Unpublished PhD Thesis. University of Utrecht, the Netherlands.
131. Theintz G, Howald H, Weiss U, Sizonenko P (1993). Evidence for a reduction of growth potential in adolescent female gymnasts. *J Pediatr* **122**, 306–13.
132. Damsgaard R, Bencke J, Matthiesen G, Petersen J, Müller J (2000). Is prepubertal growth adversely affected by sport? *Med Sci Sports Exerc* **32**, 1698–703.
133. Damsgaard R, Bencke J, Matthiesen G, Petersen J, Müller J (2001). Body proportions, body composition and pubertal development of children in competitive sports. *Scand J Med Sci Sports* **11**, 54–60.
134. Malina R (1994). Physical growth and biological maturation of young athletes. *Exerc Sport Sci Rev* **22**, 389–434.
135. Daly R, Rich P, Klein R, Bass S (2000). Short stature in competitive prepubertal and early pubertal male gymnasts: The result of selection bias or intense training? *J Pediatr* **137**, 510–6.
136. Georgopoulos N, Markou K, Theodoropoulou A, Paraskevopoulou P, Varaki L, Kazantzi Z, Leglise M, Vagenakis AG (1999). Growth and pubertal development in elite female rhythmic gymnasts. *J Clin Endocrinol Metab* **84**, 4525–30.
137. Gurd B, Klentrou P (2003). Physical and pubertal development in young male gymnasts. *J Appl Physiol* **95**, 1011–5.
138. Georgopoulos NA, Markou KB, Theodoropoulou A, Vagenakis GA, Benardot D, Leglise M, Dimopoulos JC, Vagenakis AG. (2001). Height

velocity and skeletal maturation in elite female rhythmic gymnasts. *J Clin Endocrinol Metab* **86**, 5159–64.

139. de Ridder C, Thijssen J, Bruning P, Van den Brande J, Zonderland M, Erich W (1992). Body fat mass, body fat distribution, and pubertal development: A longitudinal study of physical and hormonal sexual maturation of girls. *J Clin Endocrinol Metab* **75**, 442–6.
140. Rogol A, Clark P, Roemmich J (2000). Growth and pubertal development in children and adolescents: Effects of diet and physical activity. *Am J Clin Nutr* **72**, S521–8.
141. Louis O, Demeirleir K, Kalender W, Keizer HA, Platen P, Hollmann W, Osteaux M (1991). Low vertebral bone density values in young non-elite female runners. *Int J Sports Med* **12**, 214–7.
142. Loucks A, Nattiv A (2005). Essay: The female athlete triad. *Lancet* **366**, 549–50.
143. Yeager K, Agostini R, Nativ A, Drinkwater B (1993). The female athlete triad: Disordered eating, amenorrhea, osteoporosis. *Med Sci Sports Exerc* **25**, 775–7.
144. Otis C, Drinkwater B, Johnson M, Loucks A, Wilmore J (1997). American College of Sports Medicine Position Stand: The female athlete triad. *Med Sci Sports Exerc* **29**, i–ix.
145. Filaire E, G L (2002). Nutritional status and body composition of juvenile elite female gymnasts. *J Sports Med Phys Fitness* **42**, 65–70.
146. Weimann E, Blum W, Witzel C, Schwidergall S, Bohles H (1999). Hypoleptinemia in female and male elite gymnasts. *Eur J Clin Invest* **29**, 853–60.
147. Weimann E, Witzel C, Schwidergall S, Bohles H (2000). Peripubertal perturbations in elite gymnasts caused by sport specific training regimes and inadequate nutritional intake. *Int J Sports Med* **21**, 210–5.
148. Fogelholm G, Kukkonen-Harjula T, Taipale S, Sievanen H, Oja P, Vuori I (1995). Resting metabolic rate and energy intake in female gymnasts, figure-skaters and soccer players. *Int J Sports Med* **16**, 551–6.
149. Daly R, Rich P, Klein R (1998). Hormonal responses to physical training in high-level peripubertal male gymnasts. *Eur J Appl Physiol* **79**, 74–81.
150. Nemet D, Connolly P, Pontello-Pescatello A, Rose-Gottron C, Larson J, Galassetti P, Cooper D (2004). Negative energy balance plays a major role in the IGF-I response to exercise training. *J Appl Physiol* **96**, 276–82.
151. Kanaley JA, Weatherup-Dentes MM, Jaynes EB, Hartman ML (1999). Obesity attenuates the growth hormone response to exercise. *J Clin Endocrinol Metab* **84**, 3156–61.
152. Eliakim A, Scheett T, Newcomb R, Mohan S, Cooper D (2001). Fitness, training and the growth hormone/insulin-like growth factor I axis in prepubertal girls. *J Clin Endocrinol Metab* **86**, 2797–802.
153. Scheett T, Nemet D, Stoppani J, Maresh C, Newcomb R, Cooper D (2002). The effect of endurance-type exercise training on growth mediators and inflammatory cytokines in pre-pubertal and early pubertal males. *Pediatr Res* **52**, 491–7.
154. Zoccali C, Mallamaci F, Tripepi G, Benedetto F, Cutrupi S, Parlongo S, Malatino L, Bonanno G, Seminara G, Rapisarda F, Fatuzzo P, Buemi M, Nicocia G, Tanaka S, Ouchi N, Kihara S, Funahashi T, Matsuzawa Y (2002). Adiponectin, metabolic risk factors, and cardiovascular events among patients with end-stage renal disease. *J Amer Soc Nephrol* **13**, 134–41.
155. Berg A, Scherer P (2005). Adipose tissue, inflammation, and cardiovascular disease. *Circ Res* **96**, 939–49.
156. Pasceri V, Willerson J, Yeh E (2000). Direct proinflammatory effect of C-reactive protein on human endothelial cells. *Circulation* **102**, 2165–8.
157. Pasceri V, Cheng J, Willerson J, Yeh E (2001). Modulation of C-reactive protein-mediated monocyte chemoattractant protein-1 induction in human endothelial cells by anti-atherosclerosis drugs. *Circulation* **103**, 2531–4.
158. Yudkin J, Stehouwer C, Emeis J, Coppack S (1999). C-reactive protein in healthy subjects: Associations with obesity, insulin resistance, and endothelial dysfunction: A potential role for cytokines originating from adipose tissue? *Arterioscler Thromb Vasc Biol* **19**, 972–8.
159. Festa A, D'Agostino R, Howard G, Mykkanen L, Tracy R, Haffner S (2000). Chronic subclinical inflammation as part of the insulin resistance syndrome: The Insulin Resistance Atherosclerosis Study (IRAS). *Circulation* **102**, 42–7.
160. Fredrikson G, Hedblad B, Nilsson J, Alm R, Berglund G, Nilsson J (2004). Association between diet, lifestyle, metabolic cardiovascular risk factors, and plasma C-reactive protein levels. *Metabolism* **53**, 1436–42.
161. Blair S, Brodney S (1999). Effects of physical inactivity and obesity on morbidity and mortality: Current evidence and research issues. *Med Sci Sport Exerc* **31**, S646–62.
162. Monzavi R, Dreimane D, Geffner M, Braun S, Conrad B, Klier M, Kaufman F (2006). Improvement in risk factors for metabolic syndrome and insulin resistance in overweight youth who are treated with lifestyle intervention. *Pediatrics* **117**, e1111–18.
163. Nemet D, Oh Y, Kim H, Hill M, Cooper D (2002). Effect of intense exercise on inflammatory cytokines and growth mediators in adolescent boys. *Pediatrics* **110**, 681–9.
164. Rutenfranz J (1985). Long-term effects of excessive training procedures on young athletes. In: Binkhorst RA, Kemper HCG, Saris WHM (eds.), *Children and exercise XI*, pp. 354–7. Human Kinetics, Champaign, IL.
165. Best T, van Mechelen W, Verhagen E (2006). The pediatric athlete—are we doing the right thing? *Clin J Sport Med* **16**, 455–6.
166. Gomez E, DeLee J, Farney W (1996). Incidence of injury in Texas girls' high school basketball. *Am J Sports Med* **24**, 684–7.
167. Messina D, Farney W, DeLee J (1999). The incidence of injury in Texas high school basketball: A prospective study among male and female athletes. *Amer J Sports Med* **27**, 294–6.
168. Finch C (1997). An overview of some definitional issues for sports injury surveillance. *Sports Med* **24**, 157–63.
169. Caine D, Caine C, Maffulli N (2006). Incidence and distribution of pediatric sport-related injuries. *Clin J Sport Med* **16**, 500–13.
170. van Mechelen W, Hlobil H, Kemper H (1992). Incidence, severity, aetiology and prevention of sports injuries: A review of concepts. *Sports Med* **14**, 181–3.
171. Prager B, Fitton W, Cahill B, Olson G (1989). High school football injuries: A prospective study and pitfalls of data collection. *Amer J Sports Med* **17**, 681–5.
172. Caine D, Caine C, Lindner K (1996). *Epidemiology of sports injuries*. Human Kinetics, Champaign, IL.
173. Emery CA (2005). Injury prevention and future research. *Med Sport Sci* **49**, 170–91.
174. Dalton S (1992). Overuse injuries in adolescent athletes. *Sports Med* **13**, 58–70.
175. Maffulli N, Baxter-Jones A, Grieve A (2005). Long term sport involvement and sport injury rate in elite young athletes. *Arch Dis Child* **90**, 525–7.
176. Driscoll DJ (2000). Syncope, sudden death and sensible screening. In: Quan L, Franklin WH (eds.), *Ventricular fibrillation: A pediatric problem*, pp. 269–74. Futura Pub Co, Armonk, NY.
177. Maron BJ (1988). Hypertrophic cardiomyopathy: Historical perspective, nomenclature and definition. In: Toshima H, Maron BJ (eds.), *Hypertrophic cardiomyopathy*, pp. 3–11. University of Tokyo Press, Tokyo.
178. Futterman LG, Myerburg R (1998). Sudden death in athletes: An update. *Sports Med* **26**, 335–50.
179. Garson AJ, McNamara DG (1985). Sudden death in a pediatric cardiology population, 1958 to 1983: Relation to prior arrhythmias. *J Am Coll Cardiol* **5**, S134–7.
180. Driscoll DJ, Edwards WD (1985). Sudden unexpected natural death in children and adolescents. *J Am Coll Cardiol* **5**, S118–21.

181. Topaz O, Edwards JE (1985). Pathologic features of sudden death in children, adolescents and young adults. *Chest* **87**, 476–82.

182. Liberthson RR (1996). Sudden death from cardiac causes in children and young adults. *N Engl J Med* **334**, 1039–44.

183. Wingfield K, Matheson GO, Meeuwisse WH (2004). Preparticipation evaluation: An evidence-based review. *Clin J Sport Med* **14**, 109–22.

184. Glover DW, Maron BJ (1998). Profile of pre-participation cardiovascular screening for high school athletes. *JAMA* **279**, 1817–19.

185. Goodwin JF (1988). The management of hypertrophic cardiomyopathy based on symptoms, natural history and prognosis. In: Toshima H, Maron BJ (eds.), *Hypertrophic cardiomyopathy*, pp. 335–41. University of Tokyo Press, Tokyo.

186. van Camp SP, Bloor CM, Mueller FO, Cantu RC, Olson HG (1995). Nontraumatic sports deaths in high school and college athletes. *Med Sci Sports Exerc* **27**, 641–7.

187. Soni NR, Deanfield JE (1997). Assessment of cardiovascular fitness for competitive sport in high-risk groups. *Arch Dis Child* **77**, 386–9.

188. Maron BJ, Shirani J, Poliac LC, Mathenge R, Roberts WC, Mueller FO (1996). Sudden death in young competitive athletes. *JAMA* **276**, 199–204.

189. Corrado D, Basso C, Thiene G (2005). Essay: Sudden death in young athletes. *Lancet* **366,** 47–8.

190. Corrado D, Pelliccia A, Bjornstad HH, Vanhees L, Biffi A, Borjesson M, Panhugzen-Goedkoop N, Deligiannis A, Solberg E, Dugmore D, Mellwig KP, Assanelli D, Delise P, van-Buuren F, Anastasakis A, Heidbuchel H, Hoffmann E, Fagard R, Priori SG, Basso C, Arbustini E, Blomstrom-Lundqvist C, McKenna WJ, Thiene G (2005). Cardiovascular pre-participation screening of young competitive athletes for prevention of sudden death: Proposal for a common European protocol. Consensus Statement of the Study Group of Sport Cardiology of the Working Group of Cardiac Rehabilitation and Exercise Physiology and the Working Group of Myocardial and Pericardial Diseases of the European Society of Cardiology. *Eur Heart J* **26**, 516–24.

191. Myers A, Sickles T (1998). Pre-participation sports examination. *Prim Care* **25**, 225–36.

192. Kurowksi K, Chandran S (2000). The pre-participation athletic evaluation. *Amer Fam Physician* **61**, 2683–98.

193. Lyznicki JM, Nielsen NH, Schneider JF (2000). Cardiovascular screening of student athletes. *Amer Fam Physician* **62**, 765–74.

194. Metzl JD (2000). The adolescent pre-participation physical examination: Is it helpful? *Clin Sports Med* **19**, 577–92.

195. Maron B, Thompson P, Ackerman M, Balady G, Berger S, Cohen D, Dimeff R, Douglas P, Glover D, Hutter AJ, Krauss M, Maron M, Mitten M, Roberts W, Puffer J (2007). Recommendations and considerations related to preparticipation screening for cardiovascular abnormalities in competitive athletes: 2007 update: A scientific statement from the American Heart Association Council on Nutrition, Physical Activity, and Metabolism: Endorsed by the American College of Cardiology Foundation. *Circulation* **115**, 1643–55.

196. Maron BJ, Thompson PD, Puffer JC, McGrew CA, Strong WB, Douglas PS, Clark LT, Mitten MJ, Crawford MH, Atkins DL, Driscoll DJ, Epstein AE (1996). Cardiovascular preparticipation screening of competitive athletes. A statement for health professionals from the Sudden Death Committee (Clinical Cardiology) and Congenital Cardiac Defects Committee (Cardiovascular Disease in the Young), American Heart Association. *Circulation* **94**, 850–6.

197. Steinberger J, Moller JH, Berry JM, Sinaiko AR (2000). Echocardiographic diagnosis of heart disease in apparently health adolescents. *Pediatrics* **105**, 815–18.

198. Fuller C (1999). Cost effectiveness analysis of screening of high school athletes for risk of sudden cardiac death. *Med Sci Sports Exerc* **32**, 887–90.

199. Jackson WM, Friday KJ, Anderson JL, Aliot EM, Clark M, Lazzara R (1988). The long QT syndromes: A critical review, new clinical observations and a unifying hypothesis. *Prog Cardiovasc Dis* **31**, 115–72.

200. Maron BJ, Roberts WC, Epstein SE (1982). Sudden death in hypertrophic cardiomyopathy: A profile of 78 patients. *Circulation* **65**, 1388–94.

201. Atchley AJ, Douglas P (2007). Left ventricular hypertrophy in athletes: Morphologic features and clinical correlates. *Cardiol Clin* **25**, 371–82.

202. Sharma S, Whyte G, Elliot P, Padula M, Kaushal R, Mahon N, McKenna W (1999). Electrocardiographic changes in 1000 highly training junior elite athletes. *Sports Med* **33**, 319–24.

203. Pelliccia A, Maron BJ, Culasso F, Di Paolo F, Spataro A, Biffi A, Caselli G, Piovano P (2000). Clinical significance of abnormal electrocardiographic patterns in trained athletes. *Circulation* **102**, 278–84.

204. Fuller C, McNulty C, Spring D, Arger K, Bruce S, Chryssos B, Drummer E, Kelley F, Newmark M, Whipple G (1997). Prospective screening of 5,615 high school athletes for risk of sudden cardiac death. *Med Sci Sports Exerc* **29**, 1131–8.

205. Shirley KW, Aririm TA (2005). Sudden cardiac death in young athletes. *Clin Ped Emerg Med* **6**, 194–9.

206. O'Connor FG (1998). Sudden death in young athletes: Screening for the needle in a haystack. *Amer Fam Physician* **57**, 2763–70.

207. Maron B (2007). Hypertrophic cardiomyopathy and other causes of sudden death in young competitive athletes, with considerations for preparticipation screening and criteria for disqualification. *Cardiol Clin* **25**, 399–414.

208. UNESCOPRESS (2003). Final Communique of the Round Table of Ministers and Senior Officials Responsible for Physical Education and Sport. Press Release No. 2003–02.

CHAPTER 38

Hormonal responses and adaptations

Toivo Jürimäe and Jaak Jürimäe

Introduction

Growth and maturation processes in humans are genetically determined. Linear growth and sexual maturation processes are also controlled by the secretion and action of the endocrine system, including the growth hormone (GH)–insulin-like growth factor 1 (IGF-1) axis, the hypothalamic–pituitary–gonadal (HPG) axis, and thyroid hormone concentrations. While prepubertal growth is almost exclusively dependent on GH, IGF-1, and thyroid hormones, the marked acceleration in growth velocity during puberty is dependent on the interaction of the GH–IGF-1 and HPG axes with the continued permissive effect of thyroid hormone.[1] In addition, somatic growth and maturation processes are also influenced by nutritional status and level of physical activity. Growth and maturation are slowed during undernutrition, while chronic over nutrition may result in early maturation and an increased growth velocity.[1] Similarly, levels of physical activity during childhood can also influence the development of muscle, fat, and bone tissue.[2,3] For example, basal levels of IGF-1 concentrations have been found to be related to specific fitness parameters and muscle mass in prepubertal children, adolescents, and adults.[2,3]

The influence of nutritional status on linear growth and pubertal timing is also demonstrated by the fact that a critical amount of body fat is known to be essential for onset of puberty.[4] Recently, different inflammatory markers, including leptin and ghrelin, have been demonstrated to play a role during linear growth and pubertal timing.[5,6] Specifically, leptin may be a molecular signal linking nutritional status to the pubertal activation of the HPG axis.[7] In addition, it has also been proposed that the hormone ghrelin could influence growth and physical development.[8] The initiation of puberty has been linked to increased leptin[5] and decreased ghrelin[8] concentrations in blood. Different studies have also demonstrated that acute and chronic exercise can influence leptin concentration in both adults[9] and children.[10] However, data on ghrelin concentrations through childhood have not yet been elucidated. The exact mechanisms by which leptin regulates energy balance and integrates adipose tissue with other neuroendocrine axes remain also to be fully clarified. It appears that nutritional level and more specifically energy balance has a great influence on linear growth and the timing and tempo of pubertal maturation through the influence of various hormones in children. This has led to the question of how sport training can influence the rate of growth and maturation in young athletes.[1] It is well known that young athletes train sometimes with very high training loads and achieve international recognition at a very young age in some sport disciplines (e.g. gymnasts and figure skaters). This may lead to delayed puberty and slowed growth due to large exercise energy expenditure coupled with limited nutritional intake. In contrast, another question could be whether chronic exposure to high training loads in the presence of adequate nutrition accelerates the rate of somatic growth and maturation.[1] How these situations are reflected by different basal and acute exercise-related changes in different hormones during growth and maturation are not well studied. Finally, there is not enough information about the possible overtraining syndrome in young athletes. There are several examples where some talented young athletes after long periods of intensive training end their career due to overtraining, while many late maturers may have dropped out of elite sport through the lack of success by the age of 16–17 years. The possible overtraining syndrome in young athletes has not yet been described in the literature.

This chapter focuses on the available information about the effects of acute exercise and chronic training on the secretion of different growth and energy balance related hormones at different stages of linear growth and sexual maturation throughout childhood. In addition, the role of recently discovered hormones, such as leptin and ghrelin, that assist in regulating energy balance as well as somatic and pubertal growth in children are discussed.

Hormone responses to acute exercise

Most hormones involved in linear growth and sexual maturation also play major roles in controlling macronutrient metabolism during the increased metabolic demands of acute exercise.[1] Exercise stimulates increased secretion of GH and other components of the GH–IGF-1 axis and reduces secretion of insulin to allow the increase in glucose uptake and lipolysis that are essential to meet the increased energy demands during acute exercise. Male and female sex hormones also influence carbohydrate and lipid metabolism during exercise. In addition, increased testosterone, GH, thyroid hormones, insulin, and cortisol concentrations after exercise contribute to the increased rate of adaptive protein synthesis in the target cells. However, it should be taken into account that it is still not clear whether these acute hormone responses have long-term consequences on the linear growth and sexual maturation in children. The specific responses of GH–IGF-1 and HPG axes hormones and specific markers of energy homeostasis, such as ghrelin and leptin, to acute exercise in children at different maturation levels are discussed below.

Acute exercise and the growth hormone–insulin-like growth factor 1 axis

The GH–IGF-1 axis modulates growth in many tissues and is also known to play a role in the metabolic adaptation to exercise.[2,11,12] GH and other elements of the GH–IGF-1 axis are remarkably sensitive to brief bouts of physical exercise and to fitness in general.[2,13,14] Jenkins[15] has suggested that acute exercises increase plasma GH concentration with a threshold level of approximately 30% of peak oxygen consumption (peak $\dot{V}O_2$), and the response is more pronounced in pubertal than prepubertal children. In accordance with this, our recent study[16] demonstrated that GH concentration increased during 30 min acute exercise at an intensity of 95% of anaerobic threshold in prepubertal (stage 1 of the indices described by Tanner[17]), pubertal (stages 2 and 3), and postpubertal (stages 4 and 5) groups of healthy boys. The mean increment in GH concentration was highest in boys at stages 4 and 5. Similarly, Roemmich[1] found that exercise-induced GH secretion was highest during the adolescent growth spurt. The adolescent growth spurt in boys corresponds to stage 4 as described by Tanner[17] In addition, the increment in circulating GH concentration during exercise was positively related to basal testosterone concentration.[16] Roemmich[1] has suggested that increased concentrations of sex hormones play a major role in enhancing acute exercise-induced GH release during puberty. It can be concluded that acute exercise above a certain intensity level is one of the most potent stimulators of GH secretion in boys at different maturation levels. Furthermore, it could be suggested that similar to adults[18] the magnitude of the GH response to exercise in children at different maturation levels is more closely related to the peak exercise intensity than total work output.

IGF-1 plays an important role in the GH–IGF-1 pathway, which is influenced by acute exercise.[15] Data on the influence of acute exercise on the IGF-1 concentrations in blood are contradictory. Although IGF-1 is known to mediate GH action, their reaction to acute exercise has not been confirmed to be always similar due to locally produced IGF-1 in active target tissues.[1,2] Our recent investigation demonstrated that 30 min of aerobic exercise did not change either IGF-1 or IGF binding-protein-3 (IGFBP-3) in boys at any pubertal stages[16] Since negative energy balance plays a major role in the IGF-1 and related growth mediators response to exercise,[2,12] it can be proposed that the energy expenditure during this 30 min acute exercise session was not sufficient for significant changes in IGF-1 and IGFBP-3 concentrations, although the intensity was high enough to elicit significant changes in GH concentrations in boys at different levels of puberty.[16] In another study, a 30 min exercise session at an intensity above the anaerobic threshold that caused a marked increase in post-exercise GH concentration did not affect post-exercise IGF-1 and IGFBP-3 concentrations in healthy normal weight pubertal children.[14] In contrast, prolonged and intense exercise sessions (90 min) in prepubertal children[19] and adolescents[3] caused significant decreases in IGF-1 concentrations. Both these exercise sessions were associated with increases in some inflammatory cytokines, and it was suggested that the increase in the inflammatory cytokines caused the decrease in IGF-1 concentrations.[3,19] However, the influence of acute exercise on IGF-1 and IGFBP-3 appears to depend on the pubertal stage and on the initial level before exercise as both IGF-1 and IGFBP-3 concentrations were lowest in the prepubertal boys compared to more mature boys.[16] It has to be taken into account that IGF-1 can act in an endocrine as well as an autocrine/paracrine fashion and has both metabolic (insulin-like) and anabolic (growth) functions.[20]

Insulin is essential for growth as its main function is storing excess energy substrates. Exercise has been reported to decrease insulin concentration in blood as this is essential for increased lipolysis during exercise. Similar to adults, acute exercise has been reported to cause a decrease in blood insulin concentrations in prepubertal and postpubertal children of both sexes.[21] Insulin concentrations are significantly decreased after 30 min of acute aerobic exercise in boys at different maturation levels.[16] Similarly, significant decreases in insulin concentration have been observed after 20 min of aerobic exercise at an intensity of 60% of peak $\dot{V}O_2$ in girls at different stages of sexual maturation.[22] In contrast to these findings, it has been suggested that the exercise-induced decrease in insulin concentration occurs only in advanced stages of sexual maturation.[23] Similarly, another study proposed that 15 min steady-state exercise on a cycle ergometer at an intensity of 70% of peak $\dot{V}O_2$ increased insulin concentration in prepubertal children, while no changes were observed in pubertal children and insulin concentration was decreased in postpubertal children.[24] Taken together, these studies indicate that insulin concentrations typically decrease with brief bouts of heavy exercise[14] and prolonged exercise[1] to allow the mobilization of carbohydrate and lipid metabolism during exercise in children. In addition, basal insulin concentration is significantly related to peak $\dot{V}O_2$ in children with different pubertal status.[16]

Acute exercise and the hypothalamic–pituitary–gonadal axis

In addition to the development of male sex characteristics, the male sex hormone testosterone also contributes to hormonal metabolic control during acute exercise. In adult men, a single bout of exercise increases circulating testosterone levels in direct proportion to the exercise intensity.[25] However, exercise-induced increases in testosterone are short lived and return to baseline about 40 min after the cessation of exercise.[1] Very few studies have examined the testosterone response to an acute exercise session taking into account the level of sexual maturation in boys.[16,23,26] In a study by Fahey *et al.*[23], maximal aerobic exercise did not cause a significant increase in testosterone concentration in boys regardless of the stage of pubertal development. A more recent study by Di Luigi *et al.*[26] demonstrated a significant increase in circulating testosterone after a 90 min training session in young soccer players at different levels of sexual maturation. Similar to older and more mature boys, testosterone concentration was also significantly increased in 10-year-old prepubertal boys.[26] Pomerants *et al.*[16] demonstrated that a 30 min aerobic exercise session at an intensity of 95% of anaerobic threshold did not significantly influence testosterone concentration in boys at different levels of sexual maturation. In addition, a positive association between basal testosterone level and peak $\dot{V}O_2$ was observed in healthy boys at different levels of maturation (see Fig. 38.1 and ref. 16). Taken together, this suggests that the response of testosterone to an acute exercise session may depend on the previous training history of boys. In support of this notion, Kraemer *et al.*[27] demonstrated that a resistance training session

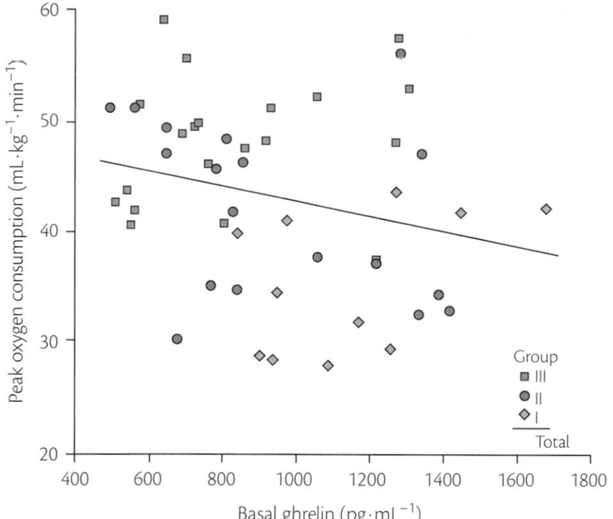

Fig. 38.1 The relationships between basal testosterone level and peak oxygen consumption ($r = 0.60$; $p < 0.001$). Reprinted from Pomerants *et al.*,[16] with permission.

significantly increased testosterone concentration in adolescent weightlifters who had trained for at least 2 or more years.

Testosterone is also important as a necessary precursor for the synthesis of oestrogens.[28] Keizer *et al.*[29] suggested that running exercise at higher intensities may increase testosterone concentration in adult females. In accordance with this, one investigation demonstrated that submaximal exercise (20 min at an intensity of 60% peak $\dot{V}O_2$) produced acute increases in testosterone concentrations in girls at stages 3–5 of the indices of sexual maturation described by Tanner[17] but not in girls at stage 2.[22] The appearance of testosterone in blood occurs in girls at sexual maturation levels 2 or 3.[22] Kraemer *et al.*[10] also demonstrated a significant post-exercise increase in testosterone concentration as a result of a graded exercise test to exhaustion in 14–16 year old adolescent female runners. Almost nothing is known about the influence of acute exercise on the reproductive hormones in girls during pubertal development. Increased oestrogen and progesterone concentrations have been found after submaximal exercise in pubertal girls.[22] The magnitude of these female sex hormone responses to acute exercise was lowest at the final period of sexual maturation (stage 4), when the basal levels of oestrogen and progesterone were significantly increased in comparison with less mature girls (stages 2 and 3).[22] These data suggest that the responses of these female sex hormones are necessary to ensure a certain level of reproductive activities in those girls who have reached puberty in conditions of negative energy balance caused by exercise.

In adults, the increases in cortisol concentration during exercise depend on the intensity threshold being close to anaerobic threshold and are significantly related to blood lactate accumulation.[30] In a recent study, Di Luigi *et al.*[26] found higher exercise-induced increases in cortisol concentrations in prepubertal boys (stage 1) compared to postpubertal boys (stage 5) and speculated that different endocrine pathways and/or different physiological and psychological characteristics may play a role in the stress reaction during the different phases of sexual maturation in boys. In another study, 20 min of cycling at 60% of peak $\dot{V}O_2$ caused an increase in post-exercise cortisol concentrations in girls at different maturation levels.[22] However, a trend towards a smaller cortisol response to the submaximal exercise was observed with advancing sexual maturation stages in girls. Two possible explanations for these findings were offered by the authors: (i) the same relative exercise intensity has a stronger influence in prepubertal children compared to pubertal and postpubertal children due to the fact that the heart rate response to submaximal exercise is reduced with advancing sexual maturation, and/or (ii) a possible new interrelationship in the production of cortisol after increased concentrations of sex hormones during the course of sexual maturation.[22]

Acute exercise and the inflammatory markers

Ghrelin, a peptide secreted by the endocrine cells in the gastrointestinal tract[31] transfers information from the stomach to the hypothalamus and influences GH release in response to changes in energy homeostasis.[32] Similarly, leptin acts directly on the hypothalamus, where it regulates a large number of molecules that are involved in energy homeostasis.[5] In adults, our recent studies have demonstrated that a single exercise session using about 400 kcal (1674.4 kJ) of energy expenditure may produce significant increases and reductions in circulating ghrelin and leptin concentrations in elite athletes, respectively.[33,34] However, there are not yet enough studies performed to draw conclusions about the effects of an acute exercise session on the ghrelin and leptin secretion in children. Clearly, further studies are warranted as the function of both ghrelin and leptin is to regulate energy homeostasis and, more importantly, energy balance is known to affect reproductive function. For example, De Souza *et al.*[35] have suggested that ghrelin is a potential discriminator between amenorrheic athletes, athletes with menstrual disturbances, and athletes with normal menstrual cycles.

In our study, we assessed the effects of 30 min acute exercise on a cycle ergometer with an intensity level slightly lower than anaerobic threshold and found that ghrelin concentration was not changed in boys with different pubertal status.[16] To our knowledge, there are no other investigations that have studied the effects of acute exercise on ghrelin concentration in children. It could be suggested that ghrelin concentrations were not changed as a result of acute exercise due to the fact that (i) less mature children have higher values of ghrelin compared to more mature children and adults and (ii) negative energy balance was not high enough to cause changes in ghrelin concentration. However, it is interesting to note that plasma ghrelin concentration before the test was negatively related to peak $\dot{V}O_2$ in boys at different maturation levels (Fig. 38.2).[16] Unfortunately, the physiological role of ghrelin in the adaptation to acute exercise has not yet been clarified, especially in children. At present, similar to adults,[36] ghrelin does not appear to regulate GH release during acute exercise in children.

Decreases in leptin concentrations have been reported to be more due to negative energy balance than to the exercise bout *per se*.[37] Probably the energy expenditure during 30 min acute exercise at an intensity of 95% of anaerobic threshold is too small for a significant reduction in plasma leptin concentration in prepubertal and pubertal boys.[16] Furthermore, surprisingly initial leptin concentration did not correlate with peak $\dot{V}O_2$ in any pubertal level of the boys studied by Pomerants *et al.*[16] It is well known that peak $\dot{V}O_2$ tends to reflect, better than total daily activity does, the type,

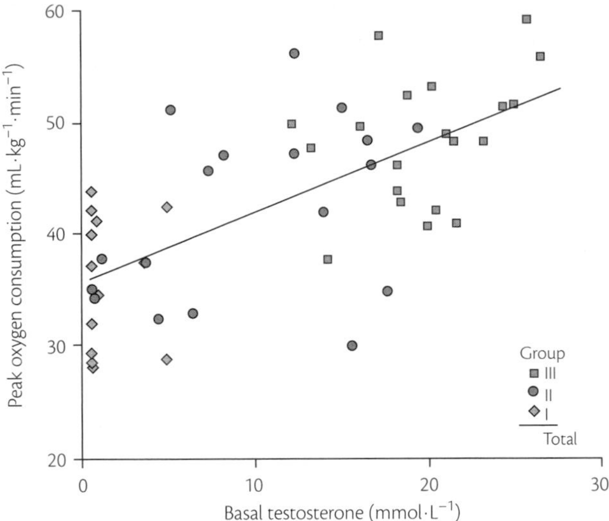

Fig. 38.2 The relationships between basal ghrelin level and peak oxygen consumption ($r = -0.35$; $p < 0.05$). Reprinted from Pomerants *et al.*,[16] with permission.

duration, and performance of exercise in a given population.[38] In support of these findings, Souza *et al.*[39] did not find any significant changes in plasma leptin concentration as a result of short treadmill exercise in prepubertal children and adolescents. The certain acute exercise conditions and the physiological condition of children under which leptin concentrations can be decreased remain to be determined. Basal leptin concentrations have been reported to increase with pubertal development and are lower in healthy children compared to adults,[5] and probably higher energy expenditure is needed to see significant changes in leptin concentrations in children at different pubertal stages.

Sport training and basal hormone concentrations

Growth and maturation processes are associated with specific modifications in numerous physical and psychological characteristics. In the world of different sport disciplines, numerous studies have evaluated different issues surrounding physical performance in children at different maturational levels. However, compared to adults, very few data are available on the role of the endocrine system that influences both athletic performance and hormone responses to frequent exercise-related stress in children.[26] In addition, it could be argued that the effects may not be similar to adults in growing children when the hormone levels could be elevated due to the process of growth rather than a reflection on a specific training environment. According to Roemmich,[1] the main adaptive changes in endocrine systems that occur during intense training periods in children include (i) altered basal and maximal exercise-induced hormone concentrations, (ii) decreased magnitude of hormonal response to acute training stimulus, and/or (iii) altered number of circulating binding proteins that bind the specific hormone. The specific effects of prolonged exercise training on the hormones of the GH–IGF-I and HPG axes and different inflammatory markers in young sportsmen at different maturation levels are discussed below.

Sport training and the growth hormone–insulin-like growth factor 1 axis

Several investigations have indicated significant relationships of aerobic fitness parameters with resting GH secretion[9,40] and resting IGF-1 concentrations,[41] while resistance training has little or no effect on resting GH secretion or resting IGF-1 concentrations[42,43] in the blood of adults. There is also evidence to suggest that aerobic fitness is related to GH secretion and resting IGF-1 concentrations in the blood of prepubertal children and adolescents.[13,44,45] Eliakim *et al.*[13] found an interesting relationship between indirect indicators of GH responsiveness [i.e. GH binding protein (GHBP)] and insulin sensitivity (i.e. IGFBP-1) with fitness and adiposity as determined by the body mass index (BMI) percentile in healthy prepubertal girls. These data suggest that there may exist a BMI percentile threshold (~70%) above which GH activity, insulin sensitivity, and aerobic fitness all begin to decrease in otherwise healthy prepubertal girls.[2] These results highlight the importance of regular physical activity on the function of the GH–IGF-1 axis in healthy prepubertal girls.

Interestingly, relatively brief periods of endurance training for 5 weeks have produced a paradoxical decrease in resting levels of IGF-1 concentrations reflecting a catabolic state in prepubertal and adolescent boys and girls.[13,44–46] Accordingly, endurance training initially causes a state of GH resistance (i.e. reduced IGF-1 and GHBP) in children,[3] which is seen under a catabolic rather than an anabolic hormonal environment.[1] Scheett *et al.*[45] suggested that this 5-week exercise programme increased specific inflammatory cytokines that can inhibit the hormones of the GH–IGF-1 axis. These catabolic alterations in the GH–IGF-1 axis may be reversed sometimes after an initial 5 weeks of training.[1] The cumulative effect of multiple exercise bouts is initially to create a metabolic state similar to the GH-resistant catabolic state in which basal IGF-1 level is reduced.[3] As training proceeds, compensatory and other yet to be determined adaptive mechanisms ensure the normalization of basal IGF-1 concentrations.[2,3] Nemet *et al.*[3] have proposed that this would explain the positive correlation that has been observed among circulating IGF-1 and different aerobic fitness parameters in several cross-sectional studies. Accordingly, Koziris *et al.*[47] reported increased concentrations in circulating IGF-1 and IGFBP-2 concentrations after 4 months of endurance training in collegiate swimmers. However, at which point of sport training a rebound in IGF-1 concentrations occurs in children has yet to be determined.[2,3] Furthermore, the effect of these exercise-associated changes in the growth factors on the overall process of growth and maturation in children has yet to be determined.[3] Eliakim *et al.*[2] have suggested that there are differences between the local and systemic GH–IGF-1 response to exercise. Specifically, skeletal muscle response is anabolic from the very early stages of sport training and results mainly from the GH-independent autocrine and paracrine IGF-1 release.[2] The systemic GH–IGF-1 response to sport training has at least two phases. The first phase is an acute catabolic-type response characterized by decreases in circulating IGF-I concentrations, and at some later and at a yet to be determined point anabolic rebound occurs and an increase in circulating IGF-1 concentrations occurs.[2]

Peak $\dot{V}O_2$ has been reported to correlate with mean overnight GH concentrations, GHBP, and IGF-1 levels in healthy prepubertal and adolescent girls.[13,44] The positive relationship between GHBP and aerobic fitness is unique.[2] GHBP is the extracellular domain of the GH receptor[48] and therefore reflects tissue GH receptor capacity.[2] In accordance with this, Eliakim *et al.*[2] have suggested that increasing levels of physical activity stimulate GH pulsatility and consequently circulating IGF-1 concentrations. The stimulation of the GH–IGF-1 axis by repetitive exercises contributes to an increase in muscle mass and also to improved peak $\dot{V}O_2$.[2] The data suggest that this mechanism works already in prepubertal and adolescent girls who are in a relatively trained or fit state even as spontaneous growth proceeds.[2]

The function of the GH–IGF-1 axis may be suppressed in child athletes during strenuous training periods showing a catabolic hormonal environment, which may be partially attributed to an imbalance between energy intake and expenditure.[1,49,50] For example, it has been demonstrated that dietary restriction during the wrestling season in adolescent wrestlers produced a partial GH resistance by late portions of the season.[50] Roemmich and Sinning[50] proposed that the partial GH resistance (increased GH concentrations) may have been caused by a reduced negative hypothalamic feedback by IGF-1 or a decrease in GHBP concentration. The growth effects of GH are enhanced by GHBP, and GH secretion would need to increase to account for the reduced GHBP concentration to ensure continuation of normal growth.[1] Accordingly, it can be suggested that the GH–IGF-1 axis is regulated by energy balance through the GH receptor, and the effects of the training season are reversible on the reduction of the training load (i.e. energy expenditure) and increase in energy intake in adolescent athletes.[50] However, Nemet *et al.*[12] demonstrated that while inadequate energy intake and negative energy balance is the major reason for the training-induced decrease in IGF-1 concentration, IGF-1 level may fall even when energy balance and weight stability are maintained. Taken together, studies on adolescent male wrestlers have demonstrated that even when incremental growth is decreased during the season, an incremental (i.e. catch-up) growth during post-season occurs.[51,52]

Sport training and the hypothalamic–pituitary–gonadal axis

The impact of sport training on testosterone concentrations in adults has been relatively well studied. Typically, circulating testosterone concentrations in blood are lowered after prolonged endurance training[9] and increased after prolonged resistance training[53] periods in adult athletes. Similarly, Rich *et al.*[54] indicated that testosterone may be lowered after 3 days of heavy training in young gymnasts, while another study reported that testosterone levels were decreased after 43 weeks of swimming training in pubertal boys.[55] In another study, adolescent wrestlers had reduced testosterone concentrations in the late season due to dietary restrictions to obtain and/or maintain the desired weight category.[50] Testosterone concentrations were returned to normal levels after the season. It was concluded that the low testosterone concentrations were caused by a reduction in testosterone production during the season as hormone binding proteins remained in the normal range.[50] There were no changes in testosterone concentration during a 2 month sport season in adolescent male runners,[54] while a 7 week competitive season caused higher resting and exercise-induced testosterone concentrations in adolescent female runners.[10] Kraemer *et al.*[10] argued that the increased testosterone response could be attributed to training and/or maturation of these adolescent female athletes. However, other studies have found no relationship between basal level of testosterone and training volume in child athletes.[56,57] It could be suggested that chronic decreases in basal testosterone concentrations are not likely to occur during the training season in maturing child athletes due to the facts that (i) it is possible that the observed lowered testosterone concentrations in children may have been a function of an increase in receptor binding, which would be a positive effect[56,57] and (ii) reductions in circulating testosterone levels have only been observed in those adult athletes who have been endurance training for several years.[58]

In children, testosterone continues to increase throughout puberty until it reaches adult levels and plays a key role in both physical and sexual maturation.[59] Studies on elite team sports players have provided some evidence that young athletes present higher values for testosterone concentrations compared to age-matched physically inactive boys.[60] As expected, the mean testosterone concentrations were significantly correlated with both chronological age and pubertal stages in young soccer players.[26] Another study in young male gymnasts found that training did not significantly change resting testosterone concentration or alter the onset of puberty.[57]

Accordingly, it can be suggested that sport training does not result in advanced onset of puberty, and taller young athletes in team sports excel because of their early maturation.[57,60] In contrast to young athletes from team sports, young gymnasts train from early age and have been found to be shorter than age-matched controls.[57,61] This has led to the question whether short stature in competitive young gymnasts is the result of selection bias or a result of delayed puberty due to altered hormonal factors during intense training.[57,61] However, no difference in basal testosterone concentrations between young gymnasts and age-matched controls has been found.[57] In another study, Daly *et al.*[49] showed no difference in resting testosterone concentrations between peripubertal gymnasts and control subjects throughout a 10 months study period. Hackney[62] found that the development of specific pubertal markers was delayed by 2 years in gymnasts and argued that this was due to selection bias and that they were likely to mature later, regardless of physical activity levels. High levels of training in young athletes appear to have no effect on pubertal development or basal testosterone concentrations in young male athletes.

Similar to testosterone concentrations, typically basal cortisol levels tend to be decreased in adult endurance-trained athletes[9] and increased in adult resistance-trained athletes.[63] In young soccer players, no differences in basal cortisol concentrations were observed between different pubertal stages.[26] In addition, there was a positive correlation between basal cortisol level and chronological age in young soccer players, while no relationship between cortisol and pubertal stages was found.[26] No difference in resting cortisol concentration at any time during a 10 month period was found in peripubertal male gymnasts and an untrained control group of boys.[49] Similarly, Kraemer *et al.*[10] reported that a 7 week high-school track season did not affect resting cortisol levels in adolescent female distance runners, while cortisol concentrations remained relatively unchanged in adolescent wrestlers and their age-matched control subjects in pre-season, late season, and post-season.[50] It is of interest to note that a relationship has been hypothesized between circulating cortisol concentration and behaviour, mood, and fitness level in children.[64,65] Shoal *et al.*[65] reported that low cortisol concentrations in pre-adolescence seem to be associated with low self-control and more aggressive behaviour. However, it is still not possible to draw conclusions about the interaction between cortisol, physical stress, and behaviour in young athletes.[26] In adult athletes, a significantly reduced cortisol value may be an indicator of chronic overtraining syndrome.[9] According to the results to date, it can be argued that basal cortisol concentrations are not affected by prolonged sport training during sexual maturation in young athletes.

Intense training has been found to delay the onset of puberty in young female athletes by altering normal hormonal development.[66] The negative impact of sport training on the female reproductive system is athletic amenorrhea.[1,67] The estimated prevalence of secondary amenorrhea among athletes is 4–20 times higher than in the general population[68] and appears to be higher mainly in younger athletes who train intensively resulting in low energy availability[67] and more specifically in those types of sport activities in which leanness may provide some competitive advantage and an aesthetic appearance (e.g. long distance runners, figure skaters, gymnasts, etc.).[1] Athletic amenorrhea is characterized by reduced oestrogen concentrations,[67] which may result in reduced bone mineral density,[67] cardiovascular risk,[69] and disordered eating.[70] In accordance with this, Loucks and Heath[71] showed that the relationship between energy expenditure and caloric intake is the major factor that alters reproductive hormone secretion in female athletes. Furthermore, it was argued that there is an energy availability threshold of about 20–25 $kcal \cdot kg^{-1}$ (83.7–104.7 $kJ \cdot kg^{-1}$) lean body mass, and menstrual disturbance occur when energy availability is below this threshold.[71] These observations together suggest that athletic amenorrhea is mainly a nutritional problem and may be reversed by dietary modifications.[67] However, nutrient deficiency is extremely concerning in young female athletes as the immature reproductive hormone axis could be less resilient to nutritional stress, which in turn may cause late menarche or primary amenorrhea[69] and perhaps even lifelong alterations in reproductive function.[1] Elite young female athletes who are training with high training volumes and limiting their dietary intake year round (e.g. gymnasts) may be at greater risk for limiting their growth and pubertal maturation.[1] For example, some studies have documented accelerated or catch-up growth after retiring from competitive gymnastics[72] suggesting reduced growth potential during training.[73] Furthermore, when the growth and maturation of female gymnasts and swimmers is compared, adolescent female gymnasts present delayed age at menarche, lower growth velocity, and lower oestradiol and IGF-1 concentrations.[73] However, in contrast, it has to be taken into account that many studies have suggested that the growth and maturation characteristics of gymnasts may be due to genetic factors since elite young gymnasts are shorter than aged-matched controls before gymnastics training and they have relatively short parents who also had later than average puberty.[74,75] At present, the separate effect of gymnastics training on the growth, maturation, and reproductive hormone system in young female gymnasts is still unclear.[1] Further longitudinal studies are needed to better understand the specific role of high training volume on sex hormones in growing and maturing young athletes.

Sport training and the inflammatory markers

Understanding the biochemical regulation of energy homeostasis in children and the effect of regular physical activity on body composition parameters at different stages of puberty will assist in the understanding and implementation of countermeasures and strategies for the prevention of obesity in children and adolescents. The discovery of different inflammatory cytokines and other peripheral markers that participate in the regulation of energy intake and energy expenditure is growing rapidly. For example, our recent study demonstrated that visfatin, a newly discovered marker of visceral adipose tissue, may have a metabolic role in adolescent male but not in female swimmers.[76] To date, the most studied inflammatory marker is leptin that is supposed to be involved in the regulation of energy intake and energy expenditure. In the light of its role as a permissive signal for the normal functioning of the HPG axis,[77] leptin appears to be the molecular link among adequate energy stores, adipose tissue, and the onset of puberty in children.[5] In addition to leptin, ghrelin is another peripheral signal, which has been associated with the appetite-regulating responses at the hypothalamic and pituitary levels.[78] Furthermore, it has also been proposed that ghrelin could influence growth and physical development.[8] The initiation of puberty has been reported to increase leptin[5] and decrease ghrelin[8] concentrations in blood. After onset of puberty, a time in which the maturation of the reproductive system is in progress,[79] a more dramatic increase in leptin concentration has been observed in girls compared with boys.[80] In contrast, there are some data to suggest that changes in plasma ghrelin concentrations are more pronounced in boys than in girls during puberty.[8] These factors together stress the importance of understanding ghrelin and leptin responses to prolonged training stress in children at different maturation levels.

Long-term chronic exercise has been reported to produce increases in ghrelin concentrations in adults.[36,81] According to Kraemer and Castracane,[36] there is a negative energy balance/weight loss threshold to increase ghrelin concentration that has not yet been determined. In addition, as ghrelin levels are higher in amenorrheic athletes than in normally ovulating exercise trainers, an association of ghrelin with reproductive function has been suggested.[36] To our knowledge, there are no longitudinal studies performed in children to monitor the ghrelin response to an exercise training programme. Our cross-sectional study found that ghrelin concentration did not change with advancing pubertal stage in adolescent swimmers and age- and BMI-matched control subjects.[82] However, significantly higher values for circulating ghrelin were observed in swimmers compared to physically inactive control subjects at different stages of puberty. This suggests that the elevated energy expenditure may have caused a significantly higher ghrelin concentration during puberty in swimmers.[82] It is well recognized that appetite and food intake increase during puberty[8] and ghrelin is known to stimulate appetite.[78] Accordingly, it could be that regular physical activity increases circulating ghrelin concentrations in order to stimulate appetite and food intake to cover the higher intake. Ghrelin may act as a hormone signalling a need for energy conservation, and ghrelin secretion is triggered to counter a further deficit of energy storage by helping to maintain body mass.[83] In our study, we also observed a negative association between basal ghrelin and leptin concentrations supporting the possibility that leptin regulates ghrelin concentration at least in normal weight healthy adolescent girls.[82] In addition, it has been previously demonstrated that ghrelin gene expression is age dependent and influenced by the level of circulating IGF-1 concentration.[84] Whatmore *et al.*[8] argued that the negative relationship of ghrelin concentration with IGF-1 level would suggest that the decrease in ghrelin facilitates growth acceleration during puberty. In our study, IGF-1 was an independent determinant of ghrelin concentration in pubertal adolescent girls.[82] It can be speculated that the increase in oestradiol levels at the onset of puberty stimulates IGF-1 secretion[85] and thus, via a negative feedback mechanism, IGF-1 may suppress ghrelin secretion during pubertal development in female swimmers.[82] Interestingly, our recent studies have demonstrated a significant negative[16] and positive[82] relationship between circulating ghrelin and peak $\dot{V}O_2$ during pubertal development in boys and girls, respectively. The results of these investigations suggest that different sex hormones may have different impacts on the possible interaction between ghrelin concentrations and peak $\dot{V}O_2$ values in boys and girls. However, since relatively little is known about the relationship between circulating oestradiol and ghrelin concentrations in girls,[86] additional studies are warranted to elucidate the physiological interaction between sex hormones and ghrelin with aerobic fitness parameters in girls throughout biological maturation. In contrast, we have shown a direct relationship between testosterone and ghrelin in boys around puberty (Fig. 38.3).[6]

Leptin concentrations have been found to be lowered after prolonged high volume training in adult athletes.[9] Intense physical training can alter the normal pattern of pubertal development in athletes,[1,87] and basal leptin levels have been reported to be lower in young athletes at different pubertal stages.[87] For example, in a study with elite female gymnasts, leptin concentrations were lower in pubertal girls compared to prepubertal girls.[87] In elite male gymnasts, leptin concentrations were also lowered in advancing maturation, but the decrease was not so pronounced compared to female gymnasts.[87] In both genders, total energy consumption and nutritional intake were insufficient, although to a lesser extent in elite young male gymnasts.[87] A long history of high-intensity (~7 years) and high volume (~22 hours per week) training during the very sensitive phases of pubertal maturation led to lowered leptin concentration in young elite female gymnasts.[87] In addition, girls also displayed low oestrogen levels, reduced body fat mass, and retarded menarche, while the pubertal development in elite male gymnasts remained almost unaltered.[87] The results of this study demonstrate

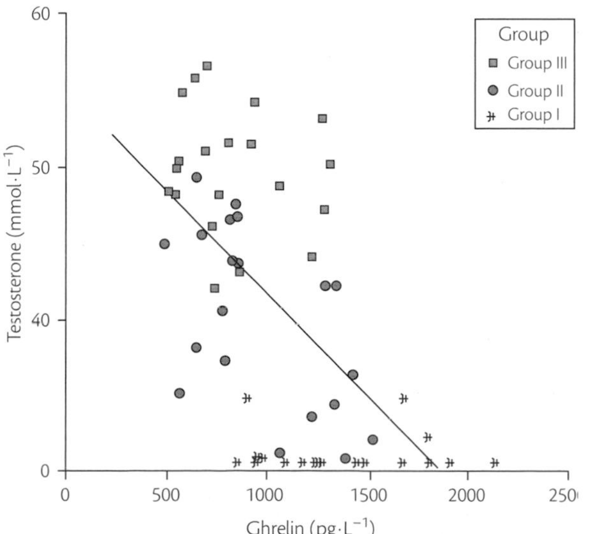

Fig. 38.3 The relationships between basal ghrelin and testosterone levels ($r = -0.59$; $p < 0.001$). Reprinted from Pomerants *et al.*,[6] with permission.

that training history has an impact on pubertal development and basal leptin concentrations in growing female athletes.[87] Similar to these results, we have also demonstrated an independent effect of training history on leptin concentration in adult male athletes.[88] Accordingly, it has to be taken into account that very intense training during pubertal development may cause a decline in leptin concentrations, which in turn exerts an overall suppressive effect on the reproductive axis especially in girls. Our recent study with sub-elite adolescent female swimmers (training for an average of 6 hours per week for at least the past 2 years) found no difference in basal leptin concentration in girls with different maturation levels after onset of puberty (stages 2 and 3 vs. stages 4 and 5 of the indices described by Tanner[82]). In addition, a 7 week high-school track season did not significantly influence resting leptin concentrations in adolescent female runners.[10] However, Kraemer *et al.*[10] argued that it is possible that a longer training season would have resulted in reduced resting leptin levels in the female adolescent runners they studied. Accordingly, it is suggested that reduced leptin concentrations could be used as a sign of increased training stress in adolescent sportsmen. For example, reduced basal and acute-exercise induced leptin levels have been suggested to be indicative of short-term overreaching state in adult male athletes.[9] Clearly, further studies are necessary to understand the exact role of leptin in conditions of high training stress and inadequate recovery in maturing young athletes.

General conclusions

Since more children worldwide practice sports, more research on the exercise-related modification of the endocrine system appears to be essential in young athletes.[26] This increased participation of children and adolescents in competitive sport in recent years, especially when associated with inadequate caloric intake, exposes young female athletes to several health risks such as menstrual irregularities and reproductive dysfunction.[67] Longitudinal studies of the relationships between hormone responses to physical stress during pubertal development in young athletes are warranted. More specifically, an effort should be made to find objective hormonal parameters to quantify the balance between actual sport training load and the tolerance of this training load by young athletes. To date, there have been no studies undertaken to find specific hormonal markers that could describe a possible overtraining syndrome in growing and maturing young athletes. It has to be taken into account that in those sport disciplines in which a thin body is required (e.g. gymnastics, figure skating) and heavy training starts at very young age there is exposure to higher risk for developing the female athletic triad.[87] The female athletic triad is characterized by late menarche, restrained eating behaviour, and increased rate of stress fractures.[87] For this reason, prepubertal and pubertal athletes should be monitored at short intervals to better understand the influence of high training load on different hormonal markers that are responsive for the overall growth and energy homeostasis in these young athletes.

Summary

- The magnitude of the GH response to acute exercise in children is closely related to peak exercise intensity rather than total work output and does not depend on the level of sexual maturation.

- The magnitude of the testosterone response to acute exercise appears not to depend on the level of sexual maturation in boys but may be more dependent on previous training history.
- The magnitude of female sex hormone responses to acute exercise is lower during the final stage of sexual maturation, when the basal levels of these hormones are higher in more mature girls compared to less mature girls.
- There appears to be a direct relationship between testosterone and ghrelin concentrations in normal healthy boys around puberty.
- Peak $\dot{V}O_2$, a marker of aerobic fitness, is positively and negatively related to basal testosterone and ghrelin concentrations, respectively, in normal healthy boys around puberty.
- Heavy training appears to have no effect on pubertal development or basal testosterone concentrations in young male athletes.
- Basal ghrelin concentrations are not different in adolescent sportsmen after onset of puberty.
- Reduced basal leptin concentrations can be used as a sign of increased training stress in adolescent sportsmen.

References

1. Roemmich JN (2005). Growth, maturation and hormonal changes during puberty: Influence of sport training. In: Kraemer WJ, Rogol AD (eds.), *The endocrine system in sports and exercise. The encyclopedia of sports medicine,* pp. 512–24. Blackwell, Oxford.
2. Eliakim A, Nemet D, Cooper DM (2005). Exercise, training and the GH-IGF-I axis. In: Kraemer WJ, Rogol AD (eds.), *The endocrine system in sports and exercise. The encyclopedia of sports medicine,* pp. 165–79. Blackwell, Oxford.
3. Nemet D, Oh Y, Kim HS, Hill M, Cooper DM (2002). Effect of intense exercise on inflammatory cytokines and growth mediators in adolescent boys. *Pediatrics* **110,** 681–9.
4. Weise M, Eisenhofer G, Merke DP (2002). Pubertal and gender-related changes in the sympathoadrenal system in healthy children. *J Clin Endoc Metab* **87,** 5038–43.
5. Clayton PE, Gill MS, Hall CM, Tillmann V, Whatmore AJ, Price DA (1997). Serum leptin through childhood and adolescence. *Clin Endocrinol* **46**, 727–33.
6. Pomerants T, Tillmann V, Jürimäe T, Jürimäe J (2006). Relationship between ghrelin and anthropometrical, body composition parameters and testosterone levels in boys at different stages of puberty. *J Endocrinol Invest* **29,** 962–7.
7. Rogol AD, Roemmich JN, Clark PA (2002). Growth at puberty. *J Adolesc Health* **31**, 192–200.
8. Whatmore AC, Hall CM, Jones J, Westwood M, Clayton PE (2003). Ghrelin concentrations in healthy children and adolescents. *Clin Endocrinol* **59**, 649–54.
9. Mäestu J, Jürimäe J, Jürimäe T (2005). Monitoring of performance and training in rowing. *Sports Med* **35**, 597–617.
10. Kraemer RR, Acevedo EO, Synovitz LB, Hebert EP, Gimpel T, Castracane VD (2001). Leptin and steroid hormone responses to exercise in adolescent female runners over a 7-week season. *Eur J Appl Physiol* **86**, 85–91.
11. Adams GR (2002). Autocrine/paracrine IGF-I and skeletal muscle adaptation. *J Appl Physiol* **93**, 1159–67.
12. Nemet D, Conolly PH, Pontello-Pescatello AM, Rose-Gottron C, Larson JK, Galassetti P, Cooper DM (2004). Negative energy balance plays a major role in the IGF-I response to exercise training. *J Appl Physiol* **96**, 276–82.
13. Eliakim A, Scheet TP, Newcomb R, Mohan S, Cooper DM (2001). Fitness, training and the growth hormone-insulin-like growth factor-I axis in prepubertal girls. *J Clin Endoc Metab* **86**, 2797–802.
14. Eliakim A, Nemet D, Zaldivar F, McMurray RG, Culler FL, Galassetti P, Cooper DM (2006). Reduced exercise-associated response of the GH-IGF-1 axis and catecholamines in obese children and adolescents. *J Appl Physiol* **100**, 1630–7.
15. Jenkins PJ (1999). Growth hormone and exercise. *Clin Endocrinol* **50**, 683–9.
16. Pomerants T, Tilmmann V, Karelson K, Jürimäe J, Jürimäe T (2006). Ghrelin response to acute aerobic exercise in boys at different stages of puberty. *Horm Metab Res* **38**, 752–7.
17. Tanner JM (1962). *Growth at adolescence* (2nd ed.). Blackwell, Oxford.
18. Ehrenborg C, Lange KH, Dall R, Christiansen JS, Lundberg PA, Baxter RC, Boroujerdi MA, Bengtsson BA, Healey ML, Petecost C, Longobardi S, Napoli R, Rosen T, GH-2000 Study Group (2003). The growth hormone/insulin-like growth factor-I axis hormones and bone markers in elite athletes in response to a maximum exercise test. *J Clin Endoc Metab* **88**, 394–401.
19. Scheett TP, Mills PJ, Ziegler MG, Stoppani J, Cooper DM (1999). Effect of exercise on cytokines and growth mediators in prepubertal children. *Pediatr Res* **46**, 429–34.
20. Jones JL, Clemmons DR (1995). Insulin-like growth factors and their binding proteins: Biological actions. *Endocr Rev* **16**, 3–34.
21. Delmarche P, Gratas-Delmarche A, Monnier M, Mavet MH, Koubi HE, Favier R (1994). Glucoregulation and hormonal changes during prolonged exercise in boys and girls. *Eur J Appl Physiol* **68**, 3–8.
22. Viru A, Laaneots L, Karelson K, Smirnova T, Viru M (1998). Exercise-induced hormone responses in girls at different stages of sexual maturation. *Eur J Appl Physiol* **77**, 401–8.
23. Fahey DT, Valle-Zuris AD, Oehlsen G, Trieb M, Seymour J (1979). Pubertal stage differences in hormonal and hematological responses to maximal exercise in males. *J Appl Physiol* **46**, 823–7.
24. Wirth A, Trager E, Scheele K, Maver D, Diehm K, Reischle K, Weicker H (1978). Cardiopulmonary adjustment and metabolic response to maximal and submaximal physical exercise of boys and girls at different stages of maturity. *Eur J Appl Physiol* **39**, 229–40.
25. Hackney AC (1996). The male reproductive system and endurance exercise. *Med Sci Sport Exerc* **28**, 180–9.
26. Di Luigi L, Baldari C, Gallotta MC, Perroni F, Romanelli F, Lenzi A, Guidetti L (2006). Salivary steroids at rest and after a training load in young male athletes: Relationship with chronological age and pubertal development. *Int J Sports Med* **27**, 709–17.
27. Kraemer WJ, Fry AC, Warren BJ, Stone MH, Fleck SJ, Kearkey JT, Conroy BP, Maresh CM, Weseman CA, Triplett NT, Gordon SE (1992). Actual hormonal responses in elite junior weightlifters. *Int J Sports Med* **13**, 103–9.
28. Kraemer RR, Heleniak RJ, Tryniecki JL, Kraemer GR, Okazaki NJ, Castracane VD (1995). Follicular and luteal phase hormonal responses to low-volume resistive exercise. *Med Sci Sport Exerc* **27**, 809–17.
29. Keizer HA, Kuipers H, de Haan J, Beckers E, Habets L (1987). Multiple hormonal responses to physical exercise in eumenorrheic trained and untrained women. *Int J Sports Med* **8**, 139–150.
30. Port K (1991). Serum and saliva cortisol responses and blood lactate accumulation during incremental exercise testing. *Int J Sports Med* **12**, 490–4.
31. Kojima M, Hosoda H, Date Y, Nakazato M, Matsuo H, Kangawa K (1999). Ghrelin is a growth-hormone-releasing acylated peptide from stomach. *Nature* **402**, 656–60.
32. Wren AM, Small CJ, Ward HJ, Murphy KG, Dakin CL, Taheri S, Kennedy AR, Roberts GH, Morgan DG, Ghatei MA, Bloom SR (2000). The novel hypothalamic peptide ghrelin stimulates food intake and growth hormone secretion. *Endocrinology* **141**, 4325–8.
33. Jürimäe J, Hofmann P, Jürimäe T, Palm R, Purge P, Sudi K, Rom K, von Duvillard SP (2007). Plasma ghrelin responses to acute sculling exercises in elite male rowers. *Eur J Appl Physiol* **99**, 467–74.

34. Jürimäe J, Jürimäe T, Purge P (2007). Plasma ghrelin is altered after maximal exercise in elite male rowers. *Exp Biol Med*, **232**, 904–9.
35. De Souza MJ, Leidy HJ, O´Donell E, Lasley B, Williams NI (2004). Fasting ghrelin levels in physically active women: Relationship with menstrual disturbances and metabolic hormones. *J Clin Endoc Metab* **89**, 3536–42.
36. Kraemer RR, Castracane VD (2007). Exercise and humoral mediators of peripheral energy balance: Ghrelin and adiponectin. *Exp Biol Med* **232**, 184–94.
37. van Aggel-Leijssen DP, van Baak MA, Tenenbaum R, Campfield LA, Saris WM (1999). Regulation of average 24 h human plasma leptin level: The influence of exercise and physiological changes in energy balance. *Int J Obesity Rel Metab Dis* **23**, 151–8.
38. Sothern MS (2001). Exercise as a modality in the treatment of childhood obesity. *Pediatr Clin N Am* **48**, 995–1015.
39. Souza MSF, Cardoso AL, Jasbek P, Faintuch J (2004). Aerobic endurance, energy expenditure, and serum leptin response in obese, sedentary, prepubertal children and adolescents participating in a short-term treadmill protocol. *Nutrition* **20**, 900–4.
40. Weltman A, Weltman JY, Shurrer R, Evans WS, Veldhuis J, Rogol AD (1992). Endurance training amplifies the pulsatile release of growth hormone: Effects of training intensity. *J Appl Physiol* **72**, 2188–96.
41. Poehlman ET, Copeland KC (1990). Influence of physical activity on insulin-like growth factor-I in healthy younger and older men. *J Clin Endoc Metab* **71**, 1468–73.
42. Häkkinen K, Pakarinen A, Kraemer WJ, Häkkinen A, Valkeinen H, Alen M (2001). Selective muscle hypertrophy, changes in EMG and force, and serum hormones during strength training in older women. *J Appl Physiol* **91**, 569–80.
43. Kramer WJ, Häkkinen K, Newton RU, Nindl BC, Volek JS, McCormick M, Gotshalk LA, Gordon SE, Fleck SJ, Campbell WW, Putukian M, Evans WJ (1999). Effect of heavy-resistance training on hormonal response patterns in younger vs. older men. *J Appl Physiol* **87**, 982–92.
44. Eliakim A, Brasel JA, Mohan S, Barstow TJ, Berman N, Cooper DM (1996). Physical fitness, endurance training, and the growth hormone-insulin-like growth factor I system in adolescent females. *J Clin Endoc Metab* **81**, 3986–92.
45. Scheett TP, Nemet D, Stoppani J, Maresh CM, Newcomb R, Cooper D (2002). The effect of endurance-type exercise training on growth mediators and inflammatory cytokines in prepubertal and early pubertal males. *Pediatr Res* **52**, 491–7.
46. Eliakim E, Brasel JA, Barstow TJ, Mohan S, Cooper DM (1998). Peak oxygen uptake, muscle volume, and the growth-hormone-insulin-like growth factor-I axis in adolescent males. *Med Sci Sport Exerc* **30**, 512–17.
47. Koziris LP, Hickson RC, Chatterton RT, Groseth RT, Christie JM, Goldflies DG, Unterman DG (1999). Serum levels of total and free IGF-I and IGFBP-3 are increased and maintained in long-term training. *J Appl Physiol* **86**, 1436–42.
48. Rosenfeld RG (1994). Circulating growth hormone binding proteins. *Horm Res* **42**, 129–32.
49. Daly RM, Rich PA, Klein R (1998). Hormonal responses to physical training in high-level peripubertal male gymnasts. *Eur J Appl Physiol* **79**, 74–81.
50. Roemmich JN, Sinning WE (1997). Weight loss and wrestling training: Effects on growth-related hormones. *J Appl Physiol* **82**, 1760–4.
51. Roemmich JN, Sinning WE (1996). Sport-seasonal changes in body composition, growth, power and strength of adolescent wrestlers. *Int J Sports Med* **17**, 92–9.
52. Roemmich JN, Sinning WE (1997). Weight loss and wrestling training: Effects on nutrition, growth, maturation, body composition, and strength. *J Appl Physiol* **82**, 1751–9.
53. Fry AC, Kraemer WJ, Ransay CT (1998). Pituitary-adrenal-gonadal responses to high-intensity resistance exercise overtraining. *J Appl Physiol* **85**, 2352–9.
54. Rich PA, Villani R, Fulton A, Ashton J, Bass S, Brinkert R, Brown P (1992). Serum cortisol concentration and testosterone to cortisol ratio in elite prepubescent male gymnasts during training. *Eur J Appl Physiol* **65**, 399–402.
55. Carli G, Martelli G, Viti A, Baldi L, Bonifazi M, Lupo di Prisco C (1983). Modulation of hormone levels in male swimmers during training. In: Hollander AP, Huijing PA, de Groot D (eds.), *Biomechanics and medicine in swimming*, pp. 33–40. Human Kinetics, Champaign, IL.
56. Rowland TW, Morris AH, Kelleher JF, Haag BL, Reiter EO (1987). Serum testosterone response to training in adolescent runners. *Am J Dis Child* **141**, 881–3.
57. Gurd B, Klentrou P (2003). Physical and pubertal development in young male gymnasts. *J Appl Physiol* **95**, 1011–15.
58. Hackney AC (2001). Endurance exercise training and reproductive endocrine dysfunction in men: Alterations in the hypothalamic-pituitary-testicular axis. *Curr Pharm Design* **7**, 261–73.
59. Rilling JK, Worthman CM, Campbell BC, Stallings JF, Mbizva M (1996). Ratios of plasma and salivary testosterone throughout puberty: Production versus bioavailability. *Steroids* **61**, 374–8.
60. Cacciari F, Mazzanti L, Tassinari D, Bergamaschi R, Magnani C, Zappulla F, Nanni G, Cobianchi C, Ghini T, Pini R (1990). Effect of sport (football) on growth: Auxological, anthropometric and hormonal aspects. *Eur J Appl Physiol* **61**, 149–58.
61. Daly RM, Rich PA, Klein R, Bass SL (2000). Short stature in competitive prepubertal and early pubertal male gymnasts: The result of selection bias or intense training? *J Pediatr* **137**, 510–16.
62. Hackney AC (1989). Endurance training and testosterone levels. *Sports Med* **8**, 117–27.
63. Fry AC, Kramer WJ, Stone MH, Warren BJ, Fleck SJ, Kearney JT, Gordon SE (1994). Endocrine responses to overreaching before and after 1 year of weightlifting. *Can J Appl Physiol* **19**, 400–10.
64. Granger DA, Shirtcliff EA, Zahn-Waxler C, Usher B, Klimes-Dougan B, Hastings P (2003). Salivary testosterone diurnal variation and psychopathology in adolescent males and females: Individual differences and developmental effects. *Dev Psychopath* **15**, 431–49.
65. Shoal GD, Giancola PR, Kirillova GP (2003). Salivary cortisol, personality, and aggressive behaviour in adolescent boys: A 5-year longitudinal study. *J Am Acad Child Psy* **42**, 1101–7.
66. Theintz GE (1994). Endocrine adaptation to intensive physical training during growth. *Clin Endocrinol* **41**, 267–72.
67. Eliakim A, Beyth Y (2003). Exercise training, menstrual irregularities and bone development in children and adolescents. *J Pediatr Adolesc Gynecol* **16**, 201–6.
68. Loucks AB, Horvath SM (1985). Athletic amenorrhea: A review. *Med Sci Sport Exerc* **17**, 56–72.
69. Constantini NW (1994). Clinical consequences of athletic amenorrhea. *Sports Med* **17**, 213–23.
70. Sabatini S (2001). The female athlete triad. *Am J Dis Child* **322**, 193–5.
71. Loucks AB, Heath EM (1994). Induction of low T_3 syndrome in exercising women occurs at a threshold of energy availability. *Am J Physiol* **266**, R817–23.
72. Caine D, Lewis R, O´Connor P, Howe W, Bass S (2001). Does gymnastics training inhibit growth of females? *Clin J Sport Med* **11**, 260–70.
73. Theintz GE, Howald H, Weiss U, Sizonenko PC (1993). Evidence for a reduction of growth potential in adolescent female gymnasts. *J Pediatr* **122**, 306–12.
74. Peltenburg AL, Erich WB, Zonderland ML, Bernick MJ, van den Brande JL, Huisveld IA (1984). A retrospective growth study of female gymnasts and girls swimmers. *Int J Sports Med* **5**, 262–7.
75. Theintz GE, Howald H, Allemann Y, Sizonenko PC (1989). Growth and pubertal development of young female gymnasts and swimmers: A correlation with parental data. *Int J Sports Med* **10**, 87–91.
76. Jürimäe J, Cicchella A, Lätt E, Haljaste K, Purge P, Zini M, Stefanelli C, Jürimäe T (2008). Plasma visfatin concentrations are related to metabolic parameters in physically active adolescent boys. In: Jürimäe T, Armstrong N, Jürimäe J (eds.), Childran and Exercise XXIV, pp. 159–62. Routledge, London.

77. Barash JA, Cheung CC, Weigle DS, Ren H, Kabigting EB, Kuijper JL, Clifton DK, Steiner RA (1996). Leptin is a metabolic signal to the reproductive system. *Endocrinology* **137**, 3144–7.
78. Nakazato M, Murukami N, Date Y, Kojima M, Matsuo H, Kangawa K, Matsukura S (2001). A role for ghrelin in the central regulation of feeding. *Nature* **409**, 194–8.
79. Sherman BM, Koreman SG (1975). Hormonal characteristics of the human menstrual cycle throughout reproductive life. *J Clin Invest* **55**, 699–706.
80. Garcia-Mayor RV, Andrade MA, Rios M, Lage M, Dieguez C, Casanueva FF (1997). Serum leptin levels in normal children: Relationship to age, gender, body mass index, pituitary-gonadal hormones, and pubertal stage. *J Clin Endoc Metab* **82**, 2849–55.
81. Leidy HJ, Gardner JK, Frye BR, Snook ML, Schuchert MK, Richard EL, Williams NI (2004). Circulating ghrelin is sensitive to changes in body weight during a diet and exercise program in normal-weight young women. *J Clin Endoc Metab* **89**, 2659–64.
82. Jürimäe J, Cicchella A, Jürimäe T, Lätt E, Haljaste K, Purge P, Hamra J, von Duvillard SP (2007). Regular physical activity influences plasma ghrelin concentration in adolescent girls. *Med Sci Sport Exerc* **39**, 1736–41.
83. St-Pierre DH, Karelis AD, Cianflone K, Conus F, Mignault D, Rabasa-Lhort R, St-Onge M, Tremblay-Lebedev A, Poelman ET (2004). Relationship between ghrelin and energy expenditure in healthy young women. *J Clin Endoc Metab* **89**, 5993–7.
84. Liu YL, Yakar S, Otero-Corchon V, Low MJ, Liu JL (2002). Ghrelin gene expression is age-dependent and influenced by gender and the level of circulating IGF-I. *Mol Cell Endocrinol* **189**, 97–103.
85. Kanber-Oksuz N, Derman O, Kinik E (2004). Correlation of sex steroids with IGF-I and IGFBP-3 during different pubertal stages. *Turkish J Pediatr* **46**, 315–21.
86. Lebenthal Y, Gat-Yablonski G, Shtaif B, Padoa A, Phillip M, Lazar R (2006). Effect of sex hormone administration on circulating ghrelin levels in peripubertal children. *J Clin Endoc Metab* **91**, 328–31.
87. Weimann E (2002). Gender-related differences in elite gymnasts: The female athlete triad. *J Appl Physiol* **92**, 2146–52.
88. Jürimäe J, Jürimäe T (2005). Leptin responses to short-term exercise in college level male rowers. *Br J Sport Med* **39**, 6–9.

CHAPTER 39

Aerobic training

Anthony D. Mahon

Introduction

Aerobic training is defined as exercise training that involves whole body endurance activity that is sustained for a sufficient length of time and at a sufficient intensity in order to improve cardiorespiratory fitness.[1] The effect of aerobic training on physiological function in children has been investigated for nearly four decades. Some of this research has focused on the health-related benefits of this type of training on children and adolescents and for good reason. With increasing rates of obesity, type 2 diabetes, metabolic syndrome, and many other physical inactivity-related disorders, there is ample reason to discern the health-related effects of aerobic training during the paediatric years.[2,3] However, there also has been a concerted effort to study the effect of aerobic training on the physiological adaptations, particularly maximal oxygen uptake ($\dot{V}O_2$ max), that are associated with endurance performance.[4] This chapter will focus on the latter consideration and will examine the effect of aerobic training in apparently healthy children and adolescents.

Knowledge of the physiological adaptations to aerobic training in children and adolescents is important for several reasons. First and foremost, establishing the aerobic trainability of the child has important implications with respect to the child's participation in this type of training.[5] Second, knowledge of the degree of the adaptation that occurs with aerobic training provides a basis for determining dose–response patterns in youths ultimately.[6] Third, identification of the training-induced adaptations that are most associated with improvement in endurance performance while minimizing the risk of injury or illness provides a starting point to implement a 'best practice' training programme during childhood.[2,5,6] Finally, physiological adaptations to aerobic training in the healthy child may provide a basis for the application of exercise training in rehabilitation programmes for children with diseases and disorders.[3,6]

General principles of training

For an exercise training stimulus to be effective in provoking a physiological adaptation, it is necessary to adhere to certain guidelines. The American College of Sports Medicine (ACSM) recommendations outline the minimal amount of aerobic training that is necessary for the development and maintenance of cardiorespiratory fitness. The latest version of these guidelines indicates that aerobic exercise should be performed 3–5 days per week, at 40–85% of $\dot{V}O_2$ reserve or heart rate (HR) reserve for 20-60 min.[1] Moreover, the activity should involve whole body aerobic exercise. Although many studies involving children and adolescents have employed training programmes consistent with the ACSM recommendations, it is important to realize that these guidelines are based on adult training responses and represent a minimal threshold of training.

In addition to this consideration, aerobic training, similar to any other form of exercise training must adhere to basic principles of exercise. Some of the principles germane to this discussion include the principle of progressive overload, the principle of hard–easy, and the principle of specificity. The progressive overload principle requires that the amount of exercise being performed in a workout must be beyond what the individual is accustomed to in order for adaptation to occur. Moreover, the application of the overload should be gradual in nature. The hard–easy principle indicates that days of intense training should be alternated with days of lighter training for the physiological adaptations to come to fruition. Finally, the specificity principle refers to the use of a training programme that will stimulate the physiological systems related to the particular exercise performance which is the focus of training.[7]

Aerobic training adaptations in adults

Maximal exercise

The benchmark measure of cardiorespiratory fitness is $\dot{V}O_2$ max. In adults, $\dot{V}O_2$ max can show significant improvement as a result of aerobic training, with typical increases averaging approximately 15–30% when a relatively sedentary individual trains.[8] However, there is marked variation in the degree of improvement in $\dot{V}O_2$ max between individuals and this variation is at least partially attributed to genetic factors.[9] The amount of training undertaken by the individual will influence the degree of improvement in a dose-dependent manner, but only up to a point, after which little or no further change occurs. Finally, the improvement in $\dot{V}O_2$ max is inversely related to the $\dot{V}O_2$ max prior to training.[8] The increase in $\dot{V}O_2$ max results in an improvement in the functional capacity of the individual to perform aerobic exercise and also makes a given submaximal level of exercise less stressful.

The physiological adaptations that lead to an increase in $\dot{V}O_2$ max can be attributed to an increase in the maximal values for cardiac output ($\dot{Q}$) and the arteriovenous oxygen difference (a-v O_2 dif). The increase in maximal $\dot{Q}$ is owing to an increase in stroke volume (SV) as maximal HR is either unchanged or decreases slightly.[10,11] The higher $\dot{Q}$, along with vascular adaptations in trained muscle, increases muscle blood flow and thus oxygen delivery.[11] Improvements in maximal a-v O_2 dif are indicated by an increase in oxygen extraction by the trained muscle. The increased capability to extract oxygen from the circulation can largely be attributed to an increase in capillary density in trained muscle that reduces the velocity of blood flow, decreases the diffusion distance, and improves the overall perfusion of the muscle.[8]

Submaximal exercise

In addition to the improvement in $\dot{V}O_2$ max, there are a number of important adaptations that occur with respect to submaximal exercise responses. From a cardiovascular perspective, HR decreases and SV increases at a given submaximal level of exercise, whereas $\dot{V}O_2$, $\dot{Q}$, and a-v O_2 dif are usually unchanged.[2,11] Ironically, there is evidence that muscle blood flow actually decreases.[11,12] Given that $\dot{Q}$ is unchanged and there is less sympathetic-mediated vasoconstriction in visceral blood flow, a higher volume of blood is directed to this region; as a result less blood flow is available to the muscle. This apparently does not compromise muscle function as muscle $\dot{V}O_2$ is unchanged, perhaps owing to the enhancement in oxygen diffusion brought about by the increase in capillary density.[11,12]

Although the extent of the cardiovascular adaptations is limited at a given submaximal level of exercise, the metabolic adaptations taking place are paramount with respect to the improvement in endurance. Specifically, there are increases in mitochondrial volume and oxidative enzyme activity.[13,14] In turn, these adaptations lead to an alteration in fuel use patterns such that the dependency on carbohydrate is reduced, whereas the use of fat as an energy source increases. Moreover, the sparing of muscle glycogen is further facilitated by an increase in glycogen storage.[14] The shift in fuel use coupled with the oxidative changes in the muscle reduces the production and accumulation of lactate,[13–15] although the accumulation of lactate is also influenced by changes in lactate clearance from the blood.[15]

Aerobic training adaptations in children

To examine aerobic training adaptations in children, researchers must decide on the experimental design that will best answer the proposed questions. In this regard, two approaches can be taken. In a cross-sectional study design, physiological assessments are made on a group of trained children and then compared to age- and sex-matched untrained (control) subjects. In other instances, a trained group might simply be profiled or described in this type of study. The main advantage in a cross-sectional study is the ability to examine children who have engaged in a high level of training; however, the drawback is the inability to establish cause and effect from aerobic training.[2,3,7] In a longitudinal research design, subjects are examined before and after participation in a training programme. It is recommended that a control group be used as growth and maturation may lead to physiological changes that are independent of the training stimulus or to simply control for a learning effect that might influence exercise test measurements and performance. Because an intervention is applied in the longitudinal approach, the ability to establish cause and effect is more certain. However, studies of this nature are more time intensive for researcher and subject and often employ relatively modest training programmes, thereby limiting the extent of the adaptations.[2,3,7]

Cross-sectional studies

There is a large body of research studies that have employed a cross-sectional design to examine $\dot{V}O_2$ max in trained children, and many of these studies are highlighted in Table 39.1. There is a paucity of data involving children under the age of 12 years, which is likely because of the limited number of young children who have been engaged in aerobic training for a sufficient amount of time to warrant examination. Many, but not all, of these studies have examined children who were training for distance running. Studies by Rowland *et al.*[16] and Mayers and Gutin[17] indicated that $\dot{V}O_2$ max per unit of mass in a group of runners (8–13 years of age) was on average 20% and 23%, respectively, higher compared to control subjects of similar age and size. Collectively, the runners in these two studies had a training history that ranged from 6 months to 4 years. van Huss *et al.*[18,19] examined a wider age range (8–15 years) and compared $\dot{V}O_2$ max in elite male and female runners to the same measurement in age- and sex-matched control groups. In one study, $\dot{V}O_2$ max averaged 63.3 and 60.2 $mL{\cdot}kg^{-1}{\cdot}min^{-1}$ in male and female runners, respectively, compared to values of 54.5 and 49.4 $mL{\cdot}kg^{-1}{\cdot}min^{-1}$ in male and female control subjects, with the difference between groups being significant.[19] In another study, van Huss *et al.*[18] also noted significantly higher $\dot{V}O_2$ max values in their male (65.9 $mL{\cdot}kg^{-1}{\cdot}min^{-1}$) and female (59.9 $mL{\cdot}kg^{-1}{\cdot}min^{-1}$) runners versus male (56.7 $mL{\cdot}kg^{-1}{\cdot}min^{-1}$) and female (47.2 $mL{\cdot}kg^{-1}{\cdot}min^{-1}$) control subjects. Unfortunately, information regarding the training programme for the runners or their level of performance was not provided.

Twelve-year-old runners in a study by Sundberg and Elovainio[20] demonstrated superior aerobic fitness compared to a control group (59.3 vs. 51.1 $mL{\cdot}kg^{-1}{\cdot}min^{-1}$); although when $\dot{V}O_2$ max was expressed in absolute terms ($L{\cdot}min^{-1}$), there was no difference between groups. Thus, the higher $\dot{V}O_2$ max per unit mass in the runners was because of their lower body mass. However, since it could be argued that the smaller runners should also have lower absolute $\dot{V}O_2$ max owing to the positive relationship between body mass and $\dot{V}O_2$ max in $L{\cdot}min^{-1}$,[21] having the same absolute $\dot{V}O_2$ max at a lower body mass could be interpreted as an adaptation to training.

A number of other studies have measured $\dot{V}O_2$ max in child and adolescent runners without the use of a control group for comparison. Despite this limitation, these studies clearly demonstrate that the average values for $\dot{V}O_2$ max are much higher than what would be expected for a given age and sex.[21] For example, in studies involving 9- to 14-year-old boys involved in distance running, the mean $\dot{V}O_2$ max values have ranged from 60 to 64 $mL{\cdot}kg^{-1}{\cdot}min^{-1}$.[20,22,23] In a group of 16 male middle-distance runners with a mean age of 13.8 years, $\dot{V}O_2$ max was 62.1 $mL{\cdot}kg^{-1}{\cdot}min^{-1}$.[24] The participants in this study were running 1 hour per day, 6 days per week for at least 1 year. In studies involving female runners 9–14 years of age average, $\dot{V}O_2$ max ranged from 51 to 58 $mL{\cdot}kg^{-1}{\cdot}min^{-1}$,[22,25–27] although one of the earliest studies that characterized $\dot{V}O_2$ max in trained females reported slightly lower values.[28] In boys and girls 15–18 years of age, a number of studies involving male runners report $\dot{V}O_2$ max values

Table 39.1 Studies examining $\dot{V}O_2$ max in trained children and adolescents using a cross-sectional research design

Citation	Group	Sex (*n*)	Age (y)	$\dot{V}O_2$ max (L·min^{-1})	$\dot{V}O_2$ max (mL·kg^{-1}·min^{-1})	Testmode	Training programme
Mayers and Gutin[17]	Run	M (8)	10.5	NR	56.6	Run	2–5 days·week^{-1}; 5–16 km·day^{-1}; 6.5–10 min·mi^{-1}; 20–55 km·week^{-1} in season with 1–2 interval sessions·week^{-1}; 5–35 km·week^{-1} out of season
	Con	M (8)	10.4	NR	45.9		
Nottin *et al.*[39]	Cyc	M (10)	11.2	NR	58.5	Cycle	Minimum of 2 years of training at 2 days·week^{-1}
	Con	M (13)	11.6	NR	45.9		
Unnithan *et al.*[23]	Run	M (13)	11.7	NR	60.5	Run	2.1 ± 0.8 year training; 11.1 ± 1.8 months·year^{-1}; 2.0 ± 0.8 days·week^{-1}; 2.7 ± 1.7 hours·week^{-1}; continuous and interval training
Rowland *et al.*[16]	Run	M (10)	12.2	NR	61.2	Run	2.2 years of training, 2–4 days·week^{-1}, 3.8 hours·week^{-1}
	Con	M (18)	11.3	NR	51.1		
Rowland *et al.*[40]	Cyc	M (7)	11.9	NR	60.0	Cycle	3.4 years of training; 4 days·week^{-1}; triathlon, run, and cycle trained
	Con	M (39)	12.2	NR	47.0		
Wolfe *et al.*[27]	Run	F (10)	10.8–13.8	NR	51.1	Run	4 days·week^{-1}; 4 × 400 m and 4.8 km·day^{-1} for 3 months
van Huss *et al.*[19]	Run	M (13)	8–15	NR	63.3	Run	Not provided
	Con	F (15)	8–15	NR	60.2		
		M (13)	8–15	NR	54.5		
		F (12)	8–15	NR	49.4		
van Huss *et al.*[18]	Run	M (20)	9–15	NR	65.9	Run	Not provided
	Con	F (22)	9–15	NR	59.9		
		M (15)	9–15	NR	56.7		
		F (11)	9–15	NR	47.2		
Maffuli *et al.*[24]	Run	M (16)	13.8	3.10	62.1	Run	6 days·week^{-1}; 1 hour·day^{-1}; 12 months
Drinkwater and Horvath[28]	Run	F (2)	12–13	2.17	48.7	Run	Not provided
		F (11)	14–15	2.53	48.5		
		F (2)	16–18	2.76	51.1		
Raven *et al.*[46]	Run	F (13)	13–18	NR	49.4	Run	Over distance and interval running
Wells *et al.*[26]	Run	F (6)	12–14	2.28	52.5	Run	Ran 4 day·week^{-1}
	XC ski	F (6)	16–18	2.66	50.2		Ran or skied > 1000 miles prior to testing
	Canoe	M (8)	15–18	3.82	57.2		Not provided
Cunningham and Eynon[42]	Swim	M (10)	11.8	2.17	52.5	Cycle	5.6 ± 2.2 days·week^{-1} (n = 9); 2471 ± 1015 yd·day^{-1} (n = 7)
		M (6)	13.5	2.65	52.9		5.1 ± 1.3 days·week^{-1} (n = 6); 2320 ± 407 yd·day^{-1} (n = 5)
		M (8)	14.9	3.37	56.6		6.8 ± 1.8 days·week^{-1} (n = 8); 3194 ± 1935 yd·day^{-1} (n = 8)
		F (8)	12.2	1.97	46.2		6.2 ± 2.7 days·week^{-1} (n = 6); 2118 ± 662 yd·day^{-1} (n = 6)
		F (6)	13.2	2.24	43.4		5.3 ± 2.0 days·week^{-1} (n = 6); 2133 ± 842 yd·day^{-1} (n = 6)
		F (5)	14.9	2.19	40.5		3.8 ± 0.8 days·week^{-1} (n = 4); 2220 ± 328 yd·d^{-1} (n = 3)
Sundberg and Elovainio[20]	Run	M (12)	12.0	2.20	59.3	Cycle	2–5 years of training; 40–100 km·week^{-1} for all run groups
	Con	M (19)	12.1	2.13	51.1		
	Run	M (10)	14.3	3.12	63.7		
	Con	M (18)	14.6	3.11	56.0		
	Run	M (12)	16.3	4.05	66.4		
	Con	M (19)	16.1	3.37	56.1		

continued

Table 39.1 *continued*

Citation	Group	Sex (*n*)	Age (y)	$\dot{V}O_2$ max (L·min^{-1})	$\dot{V}O_2$ max (mL·kg^{-1}·min^{-1})	Testmode	Training programme
Eisenmann *et al.*[22]	Run Run	M (75)† M (64)† F (66)† F (39)†	9–14 15–18 9–14 15–18	1.94–3.07 3.64–4.39 1.81–2.69 2.84–2.89	60.8–63.6 62.7–67.5 54.8–57.9 51.8–56.2	Run	For 2 subsamples (n = 48) of boys training volume prior to study was 38.9 ± 17.6 km·week^{-1} (n = 16) and 47.7 ± 22.8 km·week^{-1} For 2 subsamples (n = 22) of girls training volume prior to study was 35.8 ± 15.2 km·week^{-1} (n = 19) and 35.2 ± 13.8 km·week^{-1}
Vaccaro and Clarke[43]	Swim	M (12)	15.1	NR	56.8	Run	6 years of training; 4 days·week^{-1}; 3600–6400 m·day^{-1}
Holmer[44]	Swim	F (12)	15.3	2.96	NR	Swim Flume	2–6 years of training; 8–20 hours·week^{-1}
Butts[37]	Run	F (127)	15.6	2.58	50.8	Run	25.5 ± 12.0 mi·week^{-1} in the 2 months prior to study
Eisenmann *et al.*[25]	Run	M (48) F (22)	15.6 15.6	4.23 2.87	66.9 56.8	Run	47.7± 22.8 km·week^{-1} in the 3 months prior to study 35.2 ± 13.8 km·week^{-1} in the 3 months prior to study
Cunningham[38]	Run	F (24)	15.9	NR	61.7	Run	Not provided
Ali Almarwaey *et al.*[29]	Run	M (23) F (17)	16.1 16.0	NR NR	approximately 65.0* approximately 56.0*	Run	Not provided
Burke and Brush[36]	Run	F (13)	16.2	3.07	63.2	Run	49.5 ± 3.8 mi·week^{-1}; continuous and interval training
Fernhall *et al.*[33]	Run	M (11) F (10)	16.5 16.0	NR NR	67.7 54.6	Run	Not provided
Unnithan *et al.*[41]	Cyc Con	M (7) M (7)	16.3 15.6	4.90 3.41	71.8 55.8	Cycle	5.2 years training; 5 days·week^{-1}; 9.9 hours·week^{-1}; 205.8 km·week^{-1}
Cunningham[31]	Run	M (12) F (12)	16.6 16.2	NR NR	74.6 66.1	Run	Not provided
Kumagai *et al.*[34]	Run	M (17)	16.6	3.57	64.1	Run	Several years of intensive endurance training
Saltin *et al.*[35]	Run Con	M (20) M (6)	16.5–17.8 14.2	3.42–3.78# 2.21#	58.7–68.2# 46.4#	Run	Variety of training ranging from running to and from school to training for competition
Eisenmann *et al.*[32]	Run	M (20) F (8)	17.2 16.2	NR NR	68.0 56.1	Run	Total daily energy expenditure = 3609 ± 928 kcals·day^{-1} Total daily energy expenditure = 2467 ± 426 kcals·day^{-1}
Cole *et al.*[30]	Run	M (15)	17.3	4.66	73.4	Run	6–7 days·week^{-1}; continuous and interval training; 5 km race distance
Holmer *et al.*[45]	Swim	M (12) F (11)	18.7 17.3	5.05 3.42	NR NR	Swim flume	Not provided

Legend: Run = runners; Con = controls; Cyc = cyclists; Canoe = canoeists; XC = cross country; M = male; F = female; NR = not reported; * = $\dot{V}O_2$ max values are reported for runners in two different events (800 and 1500 m) some of whom were included in the listing of characteristics for both events; † = some subjects were tested on more than one occasion; # = $\dot{V}O_2$ max was measured at altitude (600 mmHg).

in excess of 65 mL·kg^{-1}·min^{-1}.[20,22,25,29–35] For female runners of a similar age, average $\dot{V}O_2$ max values from multiple studies range from approximately 51 to 66 mL·kg^{-1}·min^{-1}.[22,25,29,31–33,36–38] The participants in these studies were training at various levels, but all were involved in competitive distance running.

Elevated $\dot{V}O_2$ max is not restricted to children and adolescents involved with distance running. Studies by Nottin *et al.*[39] and Rowland *et al.*[40] reported that $\dot{V}O_2$ max was 58.5 and 60.0 mL·kg^{-1}·min^{-1} in trained cyclists with an average age of approximately 11.5 years. In comparison to an untrained control group of similar age, size, and sex, $\dot{V}O_2$ max was approximately 27% higher in the cyclists. In a group of seven junior members of the Great Britain cycling team (mean age 16.3 years), $\dot{V}O_2$ max was 71.8 mL·kg^{-1}·min^{-1} compared to a value of 55.8 mL·kg^{-1}·min^{-1} in control subjects.[41] Cunningham and Eynon[42] assessed $\dot{V}O_2$ max in child and adolescent club swimmers who were participating in a developmental swim training camp using a cycle ergometer. For females with mean ages of 12.2, 13.2, and 14.9 years, mean $\dot{V}O_2$ max ranged from 40.5 to 46.2 mL·kg^{-1}·min^{-1}. For males with mean ages of 11.8, 13.5, and 14.9 years, mean $\dot{V}O_2$ max ranged from 52.5 to 56.6 mL·kg^{-1}·min^{-1}. In male swimmers with a mean age of 15.1 years, $\dot{V}O_2$ max during treadmill running was 56.8 mL·kg^{-1}·min^{-1}.[43] The swimmers in this study were training an average of 6 years, 4 days per week, 3600–6400 metres per day. A comparable $\dot{V}O_2$ max value (54.3 mL·kg^{-1}·min^{-1}) was reported in female swimmers of a similar age who were training 8–20 hours per week for 2–6 years.[44] In another study conducted by Holmer,[45] $\dot{V}O_2$ max was measured in 17- and 18-year-old international calibre swimmers while swimming in a flume. The average values for $\dot{V}O_2$ max were 64.4 and 51.8 mL·kg^{-1}·min^{-1} in the male and female swimmers, respectively. Finally, average values for $\dot{V}O_2$ max in trained adolescent female (16–18 years of age) cross-country skiers and trained male canoeists (15–18 years of age) performing cycle ergometry were 50.2 and 57.2 mL·kg^{-1}·min^{-1}, respectively.[26]

The mechanisms underlying aerobic training-induced adaptations in $\dot{V}O_2$ max are fairly well established in adults; however, much less is known with regard to mechanisms that contribute to the increase in $\dot{V}O_2$ max in aerobically trained children and adolescents. In an early study involving female track athletes (sprinters and endurance runners 12–18 years of age), Raven *et al.*[46] established that SV and $\dot{Q}$ at maximal exercise were superior in the runners. More recently, SV at maximal exercise has been shown to be higher in trained versus untrained children[40,47] and $\dot{Q}$ at maximal exercise was also higher in one study,[47] but not in another study.[40] When SV and $\dot{Q}$ are indexed to body surface area (stroke index and cardiac index), there appears to be agreement that trained children have superior measurements compared to age-matched controls.[39–41,47,48] As a result, blood flow and oxygen delivery to trained muscle is likely enhanced and this, in turn, may explain the augmented $\dot{V}O_2$ max in trained children as a-v O_2 difference at maximal exercise is either similar[39,40] or lower[46] in trained versus untrained children. Thus, the augmented $\dot{V}O_2$ max observed in aerobically trained children and adolescents appears to be the result of enhanced cardiac function.

Whether increases in cardiac dimensions account for adaptations in cardiac function is less clear. Several studies found no difference in measures of left ventricular size and left ventricular mass.[16,40,49] Gutin *et al.*[50] also noted similarities in cardiac dimensions and wall thickness in three groups of boys—elite, trained, and untrained subjects of similar ages. However, when the values were adjusted statistically for age and mass, the elite runners had larger left ventricular dimensions, although wall thickness was similar to the control group. Other studies have reported larger left ventricular dimensions at rest, with and without correction for body size,[39,51] and at maximal exercise,[39] along with an increase in left ventricular mass relative to body surface area in trained versus untrained children.[51] Measures of wall thickness do not appear to be affected by training during childhood[16,40,49–51] with the exception of a study by Unnithan *et al.*[41] who noted greater posterior wall thickness in 16-year-old cyclists versus control subjects. Measures of shortening fraction and ejection fraction at rest are remarkably similar between trained and untrained children,[16,39,40,51] although Oyen *et al.*[52] indicated that trained children increased their shortening fraction to a higher level at maximal exercise compared with untrained subjects. The inconsistencies between studies is likely owing to a variety of factors including the volume (frequency, intensity, and duration) and years of training,[16,40] maturity,[16,40] the sensitivity of the measurement technique,[53] and the choice of a body size correction factor.[39]

Aerobic training-induced adaptations at a submaximal level of exercise have also been investigated, but not to the same extent that maximal exercise responses have been examined. Several studies have shown that HR at given level of submaximal exercise is lower in aerobically trained versus untrained children.[17–19,40] Reciprocating the decrease in HR is an increase in SV and stroke index in trained children.[40] At the same relative intensity (%$\dot{V}O_2$ max), Nottin *et al.*[39] noted that HR was similar between trained and untrained children; however, stroke index and cardiac index were higher in the trained boys. Gutin *et al.*[50] observed that ventilatory threshold (T_{VENT}) occurred at a higher $\dot{V}O_2$ (mL·kg^{-1}·min^{-1}) and percentage of $\dot{V}O_2$ max in elite runners with a mean age of 11.1 years, compared with less-talented runners and untrained subjects of a comparable age. In addition to these adaptations, running economy is superior[17,50] and blood lactate concentration at a given submaximal level of exercise is lower in trained versus untrained children.[18,19] This latter adaptation is consistent with a training-induced increase in muscle oxidative capacity;[13,14] although specific information on oxidative capacity in trained children and adolescents is almost non-existent. However, there is evidence that the activity of 3-hydroxylacyl-CoA dehydrogenase, a key enzyme in the beta oxidation pathway, was similar between a group of nine junior Kenyan runners (15–17 years of age) and older, more experienced adult distance runners from Kenya, and higher than in Scandinavian runners. However, the senior Kenyan runners had greater capillary density compared to the junior runners who were similar to the Scandinavian runners although citrate synthase activity was greater in both groups of adult runners compared with the younger runners.[54]

Based on this information, it appears that $\dot{V}O_2$ max in aerobically trained children and adolescents is superior to the $\dot{V}O_2$ max of untrained children of similar age and sex when direct comparisons are made. Studies not utilizing an untrained control group indicate that $\dot{V}O_2$ max in trained children exceeds the value that would be expected for a given age and sex. $\dot{V}O_2$ max appears to be higher in trained male children and adolescents compared with trained females of a similar age. This difference is likely the result of well-established sex differences in cardiovascular responses to exercise;[1,7] however, variations in the volume of training between males and females cannot be ruled out as another potential factor underlying sex differences in $\dot{V}O_2$ max in trained youth. Less certain are the underlying mechanisms of improvement, but the information to date suggests that aerobic training increases maximal SV and $\dot{Q}$; perhaps the result of left ventricular expansion. Adaptations at a submaximal level of exercise also have been examined; based on limited information, aerobic training reduces HR and increases SV. Running economy has been shown to be better in trained subjects and T_{VENT} is higher. The aerobic training-induced reduction in blood lactate concentration at a submaximal level of exercise may be due to an increase in muscle oxidative capacity.

Longitudinal studies

Examining aerobic training adaptations in children and adolescents in a longitudinal manner presents a number of methodological challenges. First and foremost, the training programme should be sufficient to provide a cardiorespiratory training effect. Although specific guidelines for children and adolescents are lacking, the recommendations of the ACSM[1] are often considered a starting point in the paediatric literature.[3,55,56] In addition, other considerations include the randomization of subjects to training or non-training groups, comparable pubertal status within and between groups, specificity of exercise training and testing, and limiting the involvement of the subjects in other physical activity regimens that might influence the training response.[57] However, in many instances some or all of these considerations are lacking in the design or not reported, thereby limiting the conclusions that can be made. Table 39.2 summarizes a selection of studies that appear to meet the following criteria for inclusion: utilization of a control group, description of the training programme that is consistent with the recommendations of the ACSM,[1] and the direct measurement of $\dot{V}O_2$ max. In some instances, studies included in Table 39.2 utilized multiple training groups and different programmes, some of which may not be in compliance with the ACSM recommendations but will be discussed for comparison purposes. In addition, a number of other studies, not included in Table 39.2 owing to their failure to meet the inclusion criteria, will be highlighted as they provide additional information on the aerobic trainability of children and adolescents.

One of the first features that might be apparent in Table 39.2 is the lack of controlled studies involving children under the age of 8 years. Although several studies have attempted to assess aerobic training adaptations in young children, methodological limitations in these studies, especially as they relate to the training programmes, confound the interpretation of the results.[58–60] For example, in the study by Yoshida *et al.*[58] 5-year-old children trained only 1 or 2 days per week and increases in absolute $\dot{V}O_2$ max, measured during over ground running, were apparent in both experimental groups and the control group but not when $\dot{V}O_2$ max was expressed relative to body mass. Studies by Yoshizawa *et al.*[59,60] reported significant increases in $\dot{V}O_2$ max (per kilogram mass) in a similar age group of children. In one study, the increase in $\dot{V}O_2$ max was apparent in both the training and control groups,[60] whereas in another study the increase in the experimental group exceeded the increase in the control group.[59] In both the studies, the children trained for 6 days per week by running 915 metres per day; however, there is no report of the intensity of training or the duration in time to run the distance.

Five studies in Table 39.2 involved boys and girls with mean ages of 8–9 years[61–65] and utilized a variety of training programmes. Of these studies, two reported a significant increase in $\dot{V}O_2$ max[63,64] and a third study[61] noted a large change (20%) that was not statistically significant in comparison to the 5% increase in $\dot{V}O_2$ max observed in the control group. McManus *et al.*[63] assessed changes in $\dot{V}O_2$ max in two groups of girls involved in different training programmes. One group performed continuous exercise on a cycle ergometer, whereas the other group performed a series of 10 and 30 s sprints. $\dot{V}O_2$ max was assessed during a graded exercise test performed on a cycle ergometer. Significant increases (8–10%) in $\dot{V}O_2$ max (L·min^{-1}) were observed in both training groups but not in the control group. Given the brief duration but high intensity of training performed by the sprint group, although the increase in $\dot{V}O_2$ max is a little surprising, it may serve to underscore the importance of intensity of training with respect to increasing $\dot{V}O_2$ max especially in short term studies. In a study by Obert *et al.*[64], young girls were examined before and after 1 year of swim training. $\dot{V}O_2$ max was assessed using a swim bench ergometer, and $\dot{V}O_2$ max increased regardless of whether it was expressed in absolute or mass relative terms. A smaller increase in absolute, but not mass relative $\dot{V}O_2$ max, was noted in a control group. Part of the increase in absolute $\dot{V}O_2$ max might have been the result of an increase in maximal HR that was noted in both groups—perhaps the result of a lack of familiarization with the unique ergometer used to assess $\dot{V}O_2$ max. Nonetheless, the increase in $\dot{V}O_2$ max in the training group far exceeded the increase in the control group. One other study, not cited in Table 39.2 because of incomplete training information reported a significant increase in $\dot{V}O_2$ max (9.5%) in 9-year-old girls who participated in 5 weeks of training that was part of a summer school programme. The girls trained using a variety of aerobic activities, 5 days per week split over two 45 min sessions each day; unfortunately the training intensity was not reported.[66] No changes were noted in a control group.

Fourteen training studies listed in Table 39.2 involved boys and girls 10–13 years of age.[67–80] Of these studies, a total of 23 experimental (trained) groups—some studies examined training adaptations separately in boys and girls, whereas other studies utilized groups engaged in different training regimens—and 18 control groups were examined. Inspection of the results presented in the table show that 14 of the 23 experimental groups experienced a significant increase in $\dot{V}O_2$ max (at least one expression and according to the authors' statistical analysis), although no significant responses were noted in the other 9 instances. A significant increase in $\dot{V}O_2$ max was noted only in 3 of the 18 control groups utilized in these studies and only for $\dot{V}O_2$ max in L·min^{-1}, but not mass relative $\dot{V}O_2$ max.[69,79]

What accounts for the discrepancy between those groups demonstrating an increase in $\dot{V}O_2$ max versus those that did not? From a sex distribution standpoint, there is a similar proportion of male and female subject groups in both categories of subjects. Furthermore, there is not a large difference in the average pre-training $\dot{V}O_2$ max between the groups demonstrating a significant change (45.0 mL·kg^{-1}·min^{-1}) versus the groups not showing a significant change (47.3 mL·kg^{-1}·min^{-1}) in $\dot{V}O_2$ max. For this calculation, two studies[76,80] did not report mass-relative $\dot{V}O_2$ max, so it was calculated based on mean values for body mass and absolute $\dot{V}O_2$ max. However, it seems unlikely that this small difference between pre-training $\dot{V}O_2$ max values (5.1%) is of sufficient

Table 39.2 Selected longitudinal studies examining aerobic training effects on $\dot{V}O_2$ max in children and adolescents

Citation	Group	Age (years)	Sex (*n*)	Training programme	Test mode	$\dot{V}O_2$ max ($L{\cdot}min^{-1}$)			$\dot{V}O_2$ max ($mL{\cdot}kg^{-1}{\cdot}min^{-1}$)		
						Pre	Post	Chg (%)	Pre	Post	Chg (%)
Children 8–9 years											
Savage *et al.*[65]	E1 E2 C	8.5 8.0 9.0	M (8) M (12) M (10)	Cont. walk/run; 3 days·week^{-1}; HR at 40% $\dot{V}O_2$ max; 1.6–4.8 km·day^{-1}; 11 weeks Cont. walk/run; 3 days·week^{-1}; HR at 75% $\dot{V}O_2$ max; 1.6–4.8 km·day^{-1}; 11 weeks	Run	NR NR NR	NR NR NR		52.2 55.9 57.0	54.6 58.5 55.7	4.6 4.7 −2.3
Gilliam and Freedson[62]	E C	8.5 8.5	M/F (11) M/F (12)	PE fitness programme; 4 days·week^{-1}; 25 min·day^{-1}; HR at approximately 165 beats·min^{-1}; 12 weeks PE classes; 2 days·week^{-1}; 25 min·day^{-1}; HR at approximately 150 beats·min^{-1}; 12 weeks	Cycle	1.29 1.34	1.34 1.40	3.9 4.5	43.4 40.5	42.9 40.9	−1.2 1.0
Becker and Vaccaro[61]	E C	9.5 10.0	M (11) M (11)	Cont. cycle; 3 day·week^{-1}; 40 min·day^{-1}; HR at 50% between T_{VENT} and $\dot{V}O_2$ max; 8 weeks	Cycle	NR NR	NR NR		39.0 41.7	47.0 44.0	20.5 5.6
Obert *et al.*[64]	E C	9.3 9.3	F (5) F (9)	Swim; 5 days·week^{-1}; 2000–4000 m·day^{-1}; HR = 170–180 beats·min^{-1}; 10 months	Swim bench	0.79 0.69	1.10 0.78	39.2* 13.0*	26.2 24.7	33.8 24.9	29.0* 0.8
McManus *et al.*[63]	E1 E2 C	9.3 9.8 9.6	F (12) F (11) F (7)	E1: Cont. cycle; 3 days·week^{-1}; 20 min·day^{-1}; HR at 160–170 beats·min^{-1}; 8 weeks E2: Int. run; 3 day·week^{-1}; 3–6 × 10 and 30 s sprints; maximal speed; 8 weeks	Run	1.30 1.54 1.49	1.43 1.67 1.46	10.0* 8.4* −2.0	NR NR NR	NR NR NR	
Children 10–13 years											
Williams *et al.*[77]	E1 E2 C	10.1 10.1 10.1	M (13) M (12) M (14)	E1: Cont. cycle; 3 days·week^{-1}; 20 min·day^{-1}; HR at 160–170 beats·min^{-1}; 8 weeks E2: Int. run; 3 days·week^{-1}; 3–6 × 10 s and 30 s sprints; maximal speed; 8 weeks	Run	1.80 1.84 1.92	1.93 1.91 1.97	7.2 3.8 2.6	54.7 54.8 56.4	57.5 53.9 56.7	5.1 −1.6 0.5
Welsman *et al.*[76]	E1 E2 C	10.2 10.1 10.2	F (17) F (18) F (16)	E1: Aerobics (2 days) and circuit exercise (1 day); 3 days·week^{-1}; 20–25 min·day^{-1}; HR at 160 beats·min^{-1}; 8 weeks E2: Cont. cycle; 3 days·week^{-1}; 20 min·day^{-1}; HR at 160–170 beats·min^{-1}; 8 weeks	Run	1.58 1.76 1.72	1.61 1.79 1.72	1.9 1.7 0.0	NR NR NR	NR NR NR	
McManus *et al.*[71]	E1 E2 C	10.4 10.4 10.5	M (10) M (10) M (15)	E1: Cont. cycle; 3 days·week^{-1}; 20 min·day^{-1}; HR at 160–170 beats·min^{-1}; 8 weeks E2: Cycle; 3 days·week^{-1}; 20 min·day^{-1} (7 × 30s with 2:45 rest); 30 s at maximal aerobic power; 8 weeks	Cycle	1.65 1.76 1.59	1.72 1.96 1.57	4.2 11.4* −1.3	47.0 45.5 44.7	50.7 50.7 45.4	7.9* 11.4* 1.6
Lussier and Buskirk[67]	E C	10.3 10.5	M/F (16) M/F (10)	Cont. run 2 days·week^{-1};10–35 min·day^{-1}; games 2 days·week^{-1} 45 min·day^{-1}; HR at 185 beats·min^{-1}; 12 weeks	Run	1.76 1.83	1.96 1.96	11.4 7.1	55.6 53.1	59.4 53.9	6.8* 1.5
Mahon and Vaccaro[68]	E C	10.6 10.2	M (13) M (13)	Cont. and int. run; 3 days·week^{-1}; 10–35 min·day^{-1} (cont.); 1.5–4.0 km·day^{-1} (int.); 70–80% (cont.) 90–100% (int.) $\dot{V}O_2$ max ;14 weeks	Run	1.47 1.51	1.71 1.49	17.0* −1.3	44.2 43.0	49.9 41.7	12.9* −3.1

continued

Table 39.2 *continued*

Citation	Group	Age (years)	Sex (*n*)	Training programme	Test mode	$\dot{V}O_2$ max (L·min^{-1})			$\dot{V}O_2$ max (mL·kg^{-1}·min^{-1})		
						Pre	Post	Chg (%)	Pre	Post	Chg (%)
Tolfrey *et al.*[75]	E C	10.6 10.6 10.3 10.5	M (12) F (14) M (10) F (9)	Cont. cycle; 3 days·week^{-1}; 30 min·day^{-1}; HR at 70.3 ± 12% max HR; 12 weeks	Cycle	1.60 1.36 1.62 1.52	1.66 1.54 1.65 1.52	3.8 13.2* 1.9 0.0	46.6 39.3 50.7 44.7 44.74 44.7	47.2 42.4 50.3 43.0	1.3 7.9 −0.8 −3.8
Mandigout *et al.*[69]	E C	10.7 10.5 10.5 10.5	M (18) F (17) M (28) F (22)	Cont. run 1 day·week^{-1}; 15–20 min·day^{-1}; HR at 75–80% max HR; Int. run;1 day·week^{-1} repeated 100–600 m runs; HR at 90% max HR; Aerobic games; 1 day·week^{-1}; 13 weeks	Cycle	1.70 1.30 1.60 1.40	1.84 1.57 1.70 1.50	8.2* 20.8* 6.4* 7.1*	47.2 38.6 46.1 39.6	49.2 41.9 45.5 39.5	4.2* 8.5* −1.3 −0.3
Obert *et al.*[72]	E C	10.5 10.4 10.7 10.7	M (9) F (10) M (9) F (7)	Cont. and int. run; 3 days·week^{-1}; 60 min·day^{-1}; Int. run HR at 90% max HR; Cont. run HR at 80% max HR; 13 weeks	Cycle	NR NR NR NR	NR NR NR NR		44.1 40.9 51.5 42.4	50.9 44.2 50.3 42.6	15.4* 8.1* −2.3 0.5
Mandigout *et al.*[70]	E1 E2 C	10–11	M (18) F (18) M (10) F (10) M (15) F (13)	E1: Cont. run 1 day·week^{-1}; 15–35 min·day^{-1}; HR at 80% max HR; Int. run; 1 day·week^{-1} repeated 100–600 m runs; HR at 90% max HR; Aerobic games; 1 day·week^{-1}; 13 weeks E2: Cont. run 1 day·week^{-1}; HR at 80% max HR; Int. run; 1 days·week^{-1} repeated 100–600 m runs; HR at 90% max HR; performed less total work during cont. and int. run than E1; 13 weeks	Cycle	1.71 1.37 1.66 1.44 1.69 1.45	1.82 1.57 1.70 1.50 1.72 1.55	18.8* 14.6* 2.4 4.2 1.8 6.9	46.9 38.2 45.5 40.1 46.6 41.1	49.3 41.5 45.2 40.6 45.6 40.1	5.1* 8.6* −0.7 1.2 −2.1 −2.4
Rowland and Boyajian[73]	E C[1]	10.9–12.8	M/F (13/24)	Aerobic activities; 3 days·week^{-1}; 20–30 min·day^{-1}; HR at 156–184 beats·min^{-1}; 12 weeks	Walk	2.02 1.96	2.24 2.02	10.9* 3.1	44.7 44.3	47.6 44.7	6.5* 0.9
Rowland *et al.*[74]	E C[1]	11.8	M/F (9/20)	Aerobic activities; 3 days·week^{-1}; 25 min·day^{-1}; HR at 153–192 beats·min^{-1}; 12 weeks	Cycle	1.92 1.86	2.07 1.92	7.8 3.2	44.3 44.2	46.7 44.3	5.4 0.2
Danis *et al.*[79]	E C	11–14#	M (9) M (9)	Cont. and int. run; 3 days·week^{-1}; 60 min·day^{-1}; 75–97% $\dot{V}O_2$ max ; 6 months	Run	2.08 2.10	2.37 2.32	13.9* 10.5*	52.1 54.0	57.5 55.4	10.4* 2.6
Mahon and Vaccaro[78]	E C	12.4 12.3	M (8) M (8)	Cont. and int. run; 4 days·week^{-1}; HR at 70–80% and 90–100% $\dot{V}O_2$ max ; 10–30 min·day^{-1} and repeated 100–800 m·day^{-1}; 8 weeks	Run	1.87 1.77	2.04 1.84	9.1* 4.0	45.9 45.4	49.4 45.9	7.6* 1.1
Stoedefalke *et al.*[80]	E C	13.6 13.7	F (20) F (18)	Aerobic activity; 3 days·week^{-1}; 20 min·day^{-1}; HR at 75–85% HRmax; 20 weeks	Run	2.25 2.39	2.32 2.45	3.1 2.5	NR NR	NR NR	
Children 14–18 years											
Burkett *et al.*[89]	E C	15.6	F (10) F (9)	Cont. and int. run; 5 days·week^{-1}; HR at 70–90% HRmax; 9.7–32 km·week^{-1}; 20 weeks	Run	NR NR	NR NR		45.1 43.2	49.4 43.2	9.5* 0.0
Rowland *et al.*[90]	E C[1]	15.7	M/F (1/14)	Cont. walking; 3 days·week^{-1}; HR at 138–169 beats·min^{-1} (3.9 mph); 27.6 min·day^{-1}; 11 weeks	Walk	2.07 2.02	2.25 2.07	8.7 2.5	30.3 30.7	33.3 30.3	9.0* −1.1

Chg = change; E = experimental group; C = control group; C[1] = experimental subjects served as their own control prior to training; M = male; F = female; Cont. = continuous; Int. = interval; HR = heart rate; T_{VENT} = ventilatory threshold;
* = significant response according to the author's statistical analysis; # = age for all subjects.

magnitude to influence the degree of improvement. Finally, the discrepancy with respect to the frequency, intensity, duration, and length of training does not appear to be large. However, there does appear to be a discrepancy with respect to the nature of the training programmes that were used. More specifically, of the 14 experimental groups in which $\dot{V}O_2$ max increased significantly, 10 of the training programmes involved a combination of interval and continuous training, whereas only continuous training or only interval training was used in 4 other instances. In contrast, six of the nine experimental groups showing no significant change in $\dot{V}O_2$ max used only continuous training, only interval training was used in one instance, and a combination of both types of training was used in two other instances. This would suggest that the combination of lower-intensity continuous training supplemented with higher-intensity interval training may be the most effective means to increase $\dot{V}O_2$ max in children in this age range, which agrees with a conclusion reached by Armstrong *et al.*[4]

There are several other studies involving children in the 10- to 13-year-old age range that employed training programmes that are either not fully described with respect to frequency, intensity, and duration of exercise or utilized programmes that fall short of the ACSM recommendations.[1] Some of the earliest studies to examine aerobic training adaptations in children were conducted by Scandinavian researchers. Ekblom[81] had six boys, 11 years of age, trained approximately 2 days per week for 6 months. Training involved a variety of activities including long- and short-interval running, continuous running, ball games, and strength training. Maximal oxygen uptake in the experimental group increased by 10.2% ($mL\cdot kg^{-1}\cdot min^{-1}$) and 15.3% ($L\cdot min^{-1}$), although no change was observed in the control group. When the training programme was extended by 26 months, the increase in $\dot{V}O_2$ max ($L\cdot min^{-1}$) was almost 50% greater (38.6% increase vs. 24.3% increase) in the training group, but when expressed relative to body mass, there was little change in either group. Studies by Eriksson and colleagues[82,83] also noted significant increases in $\dot{V}O_2$ max in 11- to 13-year-old boys, although the training programme is poorly described in both studies and a control group was not utilized for comparison purposes. Vaccaro and Clarke[84] assessed $\dot{V}O_2$ max before and after 7 months of swim training (4 days per week at 3000–10,000 yards per day) in 9- to 11-year-old boys and reported that $\dot{V}O_2$ max ($mL\cdot kg^{-1}\cdot min^{-1}$) increased by 14.6% in the swimmers and changed only by 4.5% in the control group. The increase in $\dot{V}O_2$ max in the swimmers was significant. Finally, Massicotte and MacNab[85] examined the effect of three different training intensities on changes in $\dot{V}O_2$ max in 11- to 13-year-old boys. Three groups of subjects trained 3 days per week for 12 min per day; a fourth group served as control subjects. Training intensities for the three training groups were HR of 170–180 $beats\cdot min^{-1}$, HR of 150–160 $beats\cdot min^{-1}$ and HR of 130–140 $beats\cdot min^{-1}$. A significant increase in $\dot{V}O_2$ max was noted only for the group training at the highest intensity. This might suggest that if the intensity is high and sustained, duration of exercise of less than the 20 min recommendation of ACSM may be sufficient to provoke an improvement in aerobic fitness in children.

Three other studies not cited in Table 39.2 employed short duration, high-intensity interval running as the training programme.[86–88] Two of theses studies reported a significant increase in $\dot{V}O_2$ max in boys and girls aged 8–11 years.[86,87] Rotstein *et al.*[87] used a fairly aggressive interval training programme that, after a 15–20 min warm-up period of aerobic activities, the boys ran sets of multiple repetitions over distances of 150, 400, and 600 m. Absolute $\dot{V}O_2$ max increased by 7% and mass relative $\dot{V}O_2$ max increased by 8% over the course of the training programme in the runners, but not in the control subjects. In the study by Baquet *et al.*[86], the training programme occurred 2 days per week for 7 weeks and consisted of a series of repeated sets of sprints that were 10 and 20 s in duration and performed at 110–130% of maximal aerobic speed that was calculated from maximal running speed during a shuttle run test. Maximal oxygen uptake increased significantly from 1.54 to 1.68 $L\cdot min^{-1}$ and from 43.9 to 47.5 $mL\cdot kg^{-1}\cdot min^{-1}$ in the training group although it remained unchanged in the control group. The increase in $\dot{V}O_2$ max in the trained subjects may have been facilitated by the brief nature of the recovery periods that allowed the children to maintain a high percentage of $\dot{V}O_2$ max (73–78%) during each set of intervals. This type of high-intensity training, albeit performed only 2 days per week in the study by Bacquet *et al.*, has been shown to increase $\dot{V}O_2$ max by others.[63,71] In contrast, other studies have failed to document a significant effect of this type of training on improving aerobic fitness in children.[77,88] It would seem that determining the optimal duration, repetition number, intensity, and work to rest ratio for high-intensity interval training would be fruitful.

There appears to be a void in the research literature with respect to aerobic training studies involving children over the age of 13 years when controlled studies, with respect to the use of a control group and the reporting the details of the aerobic training programme, are considered. However, the two studies cited in Table 39.2 indicate modest increases in $\dot{V}O_2$ max ($mL\cdot kg^{-1}\cdot min^{-1}$) in adolescent boys and girls engaged in aerobic training.[89,90] Interestingly, both studies report similar increases in $\dot{V}O_2$ max (~9%) despite a large difference in the pre-training $\dot{V}O_2$ max, although there is a marked difference in the training volume between these two studies.

There are several other studies that, despite incomplete information on the training programme, examined changes in $\dot{V}O_2$ max in this age group. Studies by Eliakim *et al.* examined changes in $\dot{V}O_2$ max in adolescent males[91] and females[92] who attended a 5-week summer school programme. During this programme, which occurred 5 days per week, a portion of the programme was devoted to aerobic training involving a variety of activities. Absolute $\dot{V}O_2$ max in trained girls increased significantly, but no change was observed in the untrained control group. In the study involving male subjects, there was no change in $\dot{V}O_2$ max in either the trained or control subjects. In 15-year-old female swimmers engaged in a 7-week swim training programme that took place 4 days per week and involved an average of >12,000 yards per week, $\dot{V}O_2$ max in $mL\cdot kg^{-1}\cdot min^{-1}$ increased by 14.3%. No change was noted in the control group over the same period of time.[93] Finally, Plank *et al.*[94] reported a modest increase (6%) in mass relative $\dot{V}O_2$ max in male high-school cross-country runners over the course of the competitive season. In that $\dot{V}O_2$ max averaged 61.6 $mL\cdot kg^{-1}\cdot min^{-1}$ prior to the season; the attenuated increase in $\dot{V}O_2$ max may have been partially affected by the already high value. Given that physical activity tends to decline in adolescence[95] and combined with increased opportunity for male and female children to compete in competitive endurance events, more carefully controlled exercise training studies are clearly warranted involving this age group.

As $\dot{V}O_2$ is the product of the $\dot{Q}$ and a-v O_2 dif, changes in $\dot{V}O_2$ max must be accounted for with adaptations in one or both of these factors.[8] One of the earliest studies to address this issue was carried out by Eriksson and Koch[83] who used the dye-dilution method (see Chapter 7 for a critique of methodology) to assess maximal cardiovascular function before and after training in 11- to 13-year-old boys. In their study, $\dot{V}O_2$ max in L·min^{-1} increased by approximately 19% as did $\dot{Q}$ max. The increase in $\dot{Q}$ was entirely owing to an increase in SV max that occurred despite the fact that maximal blood pressure increased. The increase in blood pressure would suggest that peripheral resistance at maximum did not decrease, as it does in adults.[11] Since the increase in $\dot{Q}$ max accounted for all the changes in $\dot{V}O_2$ max, maximal a-v O_2 dif was unchanged. Although this study provides an indication of the underlying mechanism for aerobic training-induced increase in $\dot{V}O_2$ max in children, the failure to use a control group and omission of key details with respect to the training programme that was used renders this conclusion incomplete. Obert *et al.*[72] noted significant increases in cardiac and stroke index in both boys and girls over the course of an aerobic training programme but not in the control groups. Consistent with Eriksson and Koch's observation,[83] a-v O_2 dif at maximal exercise did not change over time in any of the groups. However, contrary to these results are the findings of Weber *et al.*[96], who examined 10-, 13-, and 16-year-old boys and reported that the changes in $\dot{Q}$, SV, HR, and a-v O_2 dif did not vary significantly between trained and untrained subjects.

The limited evidence to date would suggest that most, if not all, of the training-induced increase in $\dot{V}O_2$ max can be attributed to increases in $\dot{Q}$ max and SV max. These adaptations in turn may be owing to morphological and functional changes in the myocardium. Indeed Eriksson and Koch's[83] data demonstrating an increase in SV despite a higher blood pressure would suggest that cardiac contractility was enhanced. However, other measures of cardiac contractility, such as shortening fraction and ejection fraction at rest, have been shown to be unaffected by aerobic training.[72,97–99] Increases in cardiac function can also be brought on by morphological changes in the myocardium. Ekblom[81] found no difference in the increase in heart volume over time in trained and untrained boys over 6 months, but after 26 more months of training heart volume increased more substantially in the trained subjects compared with the control subjects. Eriksson and Koch noted a small but significant increase (9.8%) in heart volume from 499 to 548 mL over the course of 4 months of training. However, without the benefit of assessing changes in an untrained group, it is not clear how much of the increase in heart volume can be attributed to training versus growth. Other studies using echocardiography techniques report mixed findings. For example, some reports indicate an increase in left ventricular end-diastolic diameter,[72,99] whereas others do not.[97,98,100] Similarly, there are inconsistent findings with respect to changes in wall thickness and left ventricular mass.[72,97–100] Given the variations between studies with respect to the nature of the training and the effectiveness in increasing $\dot{V}O_2$ max, maturation level of the subjects, the application of an appropriate size correction factor, use of control groups, and measurement technique and sensitivity to assess changes in cardiac size, definitive conclusions on the effect of aerobic training and cardiac adaptations in children and adolescents must be viewed with caution.[56] Moreover, the stimulus initiating cardiac growth in children and adolescents involved in aerobic training remains uncertain.

Researchers also have examined the effect of aerobic training on a variety of physiological responses measured during exercise at a given submaximal level. These submaximal exercise measurements provide further insight into the degree and extent of adaptability in children and adolescents involved with aerobic training. Specifically, adaptations at this level of exercise have been noted with respect to HR, SV, and $\dot{Q}$; the cardiorespiratory responses at the T_{VENT}; and metabolic responses.

A classic observation in adults who undergo aerobic training is that HR will decrease and SV will increase at a given submaximal level of exercise.[11] Likewise, there is substantial evidence that HR at given level of exercise will decrease over the course of an aerobic training programme across a wide range of children and ad olescents,[69,72,73,85,88,89,101,102] although there are some studies that have failed to observe this result.[77,86,90] Moreover, the decrease in submaximal HR occurs concomitantly with an increase in SV[72,101] while maintaining a similar value for $\dot{Q}$ and a-v O_2 dif.[72] The effects of aerobic training on the cardiovascular responses at submaximal relative exercise intensities (same % of $\dot{V}O_2$ max) have also been assessed. Mahon and Vaccaro[68] measured HR, SV, $\dot{Q}$, and a-v O_2 dif at 50% and 75% of $\dot{V}O_2$ max before and after training. HR was unchanged but SV and $\dot{Q}$ increased by about 10%, although this was not significantly different from the control group, and a-v O_2 dif increased significantly. It is interesting to note that if the findings from Mahon and Vaccaro are extrapolated to maximum—this is possible because an increase in $\dot{V}O_2$ max would result in an increase in the $\dot{V}O_2$ at any given percentage of maximum—the increased a-v O_2 dif could account for the improvement in $\dot{V}O_2$ max, a result contrary to what others have reported.[72,83,96] In contrast, Lussier and Buskirk,[67] showed HR to decline at two of four submaximal relative levels of exercise and did not observe any differences in the changes in SV, $\dot{Q}$, and a-v O_2 dif in their training and control subjects.

The decrease in submaximal HR at a given level of exercise seems to be independent of changes in $\dot{V}O_2$ max. For example, studies by Stewart and Gutin[88] and Massicotte and MacNab[85] included training groups that did not increase $\dot{V}O_2$ max, yet demonstrated a reduction in submaximal HR. Alternatively, there is evidence that fails to show significant reductions in submaximal HR, despite significant increases in $\dot{V}O_2$ max.[86,90] That changes in submaximal HR occur independently of changes in $\dot{V}O_2$ max is not surprising because an increase in $\dot{V}O_2$ max involves a number of physiological variables that are part of the oxygen transport sequence. On the other hand, HR is principally under the control of the autonomic nervous system. Thus changes in HR can probably be attributed to a training-induced alteration in balance between parasympathetic and sympathetic stimulation. In support of this, Gutin *et al.*[103], showed that exercise training reduced sympathetic to parasympathetic ratio (assessed through HR variability) at rest in obese children, although other evidence using similar techniques in healthy, non-obese children is less compelling.[104]

Studies assessing changes in T_{VENT} that occur with aerobic training have reported that the $\dot{V}O_2$ at T_{VENT} and the percentage of $\dot{V}O_2$ max at T_{VENT} will increase. Mahon and Vaccaro[78] and McManus *et al.*[71] reported significant increases in these measures of T_{VENT} in trained subjects but not in control subjects. Interestingly, the study by McManus *et al.* observed a significant increase in the T_{VENT} only in an interval-trained group but not in a continuous trained group of boys, whereas the training programme used by Mahon and Vaccaro[78] incorporated both interval and continuous training. Studies by Haffor *et al.*[105] and Becker and Vaccaro[61] also reported appreciable increases in the $\dot{V}O_2$ at T_{VENT} (~6–8 mL·kg^{-1}·min^{-1}), but in the case of Haffor *et al.* neither was the increase statistically significant nor was a control group used. In the study of Becker and Vaccaro, the difference in the increase between trained and untrained subjects was not statistically significant. It also is worth noting that in all four of these studies the percentage increase in the $\dot{V}O_2$ at T_{VENT} was markedly greater than the percentage change in $\dot{V}O_2$ max suggesting that the T_{VENT} may be more sensitive to training than $\dot{V}O_2$ max in children and adolescents.[56]

Despite the ease associated with the measurement of locomotion economy, defined as the $\dot{V}O_2$ at fixed level of submaximal exercise,[106] the effects of aerobic training on this parameter in healthy children are unclear. Studies employing comparable training and testing modes provide mixed results. Mandigout *et al.*[69] and Massicotte and MacNab[85] reported no change in submaximal cycling economy, despite significant improvements in $\dot{V}O_2$ max. Alternatively, it has been shown that cycling economy is superior in trained boys compared with control subjects at the end of training; however, there were marked differences between groups at the beginning of training in favour of the trained group that may have contributed to this difference.[101] Three studies assessing walking and running economy failed to observe improvements in economy despite significant increases in $\dot{V}O_2$ max.[73,86,90] Burkett *et al.*[89] noted a small but significant reduction in the $\dot{V}O_2$ at 9.7 km·h^{-1} in adolescent girls. A similar numerical reduction in $\dot{V}O_2$ was seen in the control group over the same time period, but that change was not statistically significant compared with the initial measurement; the difference between groups after training also was not significant. Plank *et al.*[94] showed a tendency for running economy to worsen slightly over the course of a cross-country season in adolescent boys. Two studies using different training and assessment modes also provided mixed results. Williams *et al.*[77] did not find any changes in running economy at 7 and 8 km·h^{-1} in a continuous cycle trained group, a sprint (run) interval trained group, and a control group; also there was no training effect on $\dot{V}O_2$ max in this study. Stewart and Gutin[88] used an interval running programme as the training mode and assessed economy on a cycle ergometer and a treadmill before and after training. Cycling economy was unchanged with training, however, at two of the elevations during a treadmill test, economy was significantly superior in the trained group. Given the advantages of good locomotion economy and its relationship to endurance performance[7,106–108] more research on the effect of aerobic training on this measurement is recommended.

Metabolic adaptations subsequent to aerobic training have been examined in children and adolescents but only to a small extent in comparison to the adaptations that have already been described. This may in part be attributed to challenges associated with obtaining blood samples and ethical limitations associated with other invasive procedures such as the muscle biopsy procedure.[21] Nonetheless, studies have examined changes in blood lactate concentration at a fixed submaximal level of exercise[81–83,85,94] or examined changes in the physiological responses to a fixed blood lactate concentration.[79,87] Massicotte and MacNab[85] showed a decrease in blood lactate concentration cycling at 450 kpm·min^{-1} (74 W) but only in the group training at the highest intensity. Despite the reduction in lactate, the respiratory exchange ratio was unchanged in this group and in the other groups as well. Similarly, Eriksson *et al.*[82] also reported a reduction in blood lactate concentration at one of two submaximal work rates in 11-year-old boys after 6 weeks of training. Plank *et al.*[94] reported that there was a tendency ($p < 0.06$) for blood lactate to be lower across three running speeds following training. In contrast, others have not observed a decrement in blood lactate concentration from pre- to post-training, although this may be a function of the relatively modest exercise intensities used.[81,83]

Studies by Rotstein *et al.*[87] and Danis *et al.*[79] examined the effect of aerobic training on the physiological responses at fixed blood lactate concentrations in boys between the ages of 10 and14 years. In the study by Rotstein *et al.* at the running velocity corresponding to 4 mmol·L^{-1} lactate concentration increased by approximately 0.55 km·h^{-1} in the training group, although this increase was not statistically significant. However, the velocity at the lactate threshold increased by a similar amount and was statistically significant. Paradoxically, the percentage of $\dot{V}O_2$ max corresponding to the 4 mmol·L^{-1} lactate concentration and to the lactate threshold decreased significantly in the training group. No changes were observed in the control subjects for any of these measurements. Danis *et al.* found that the running speed at the 4 mmol·L^{-1} blood lactate concentration increased significantly after 3 and 6 months of training. The $\dot{V}O_2$ at this lactate concentration was also increased but only after 6 months of training. In contrast, the percentage of $\dot{V}O_2$ max at the 4 mmol·L^{-1} lactate concentration was unchanged. All three of these measurements were unchanged over the 6-month period in the control subjects.

Favourable adaptations in the blood lactate response resulting from aerobic training generally are thought to be the result of enhanced oxidative capacity in the skeletal muscle,[13,14] although changes in lactate clearance from the blood and diffusion of lactate between muscle fibres must also be considered. As noted previously, because of ethical constraints there is very little information on these aspects in children and adolescents. One study that examined the effect of 6 weeks of aerobic training on muscle lactate concentration in 11-year-old boys did not show a decrease in muscle lactate concentration at two submaximal work rates.[82] This is surprising in light of the evidence that has shown an increase in muscle succinate dehydrogenase activity with aerobic training.[82,109] However, Eriksson *et al.*[82] also showed that muscle phosphofructokinase activity was increased and that may have served to offset the increase in oxidative capacity. It is presently unknown in children and adolescents whether changes in blood lactate concentrations brought about by aerobic training can be attributed to alterations in lactate clearance and utilization by other tissues.

In summary, longitudinal studies of aerobic training responses in children and adolescents present a number of methodological challenges to researchers. There is a paucity of aerobic training studies involving children under the age of 8 years and over the age of 13 years, as a large percentage of aerobic training studies involve children 8–13 years of age. Many, but certainly not all of these, studies indicate that $\dot{V}O_2$ max will increase with aerobic training, but there continues to be some debate regarding whether children can adapt as readily as adults (see next section for further discussion). The increase in $\dot{V}O_2$ max appears to be attributed to increases in $\dot{Q}$ max and SV max; however, the cardiac and extra-cardiac factors that account for this are not very clear. Adaptations at a submaximal level of exercise include a decrease in HR and increase in SV, an increase in T_{VENT}, improved running economy, and a reduction in blood lactate concentration and increased physiological response at a fixed lactate concentration, although these results are based on only a few studies, and results to the contrary are evident for some of these adaptations. Given the ease of measurement, it may be prudent in future studies examining the aerobic trainability of children to include submaximal exercise responses. Finally, improvements in both the muscle oxidative and glycolytic capacity have been reported, but these findings are based on very little research. In this regard, the development and availability of magnetic resonance spectroscopy serves as a promising means to study muscular adaptations to aerobic training in paediatric subjects.

Aerobic trainability

There are a number of different factors that might influence the degree in which $\dot{V}O_2$ max in children and adolescents will improve as a result of aerobic training. These factors include the volume of training, age, and maturation, $\dot{V}O_2$ max prior to training, habitual physical activity, and genetics. With respect to the volume of training, the studies listed in Table 39.2 appear to satisfy the ACSM aerobic training recommendations;[1] yet although many of these studies reported increases in $\dot{V}O_2$ max, other studies that appear to satisfy the ACSM guidelines did not observe a significant effect of training on $\dot{V}O_2$ max. Moreover, in some instances, studies utilizing training programmes that appear to be less than the ACSM recommendations report increases in $\dot{V}O_2$ max while others do not. A slightly more ambitious volume of training, particularly with respect to exercise duration and intensity, has been proposed by Armstrong *et al.*[4], but clearly there continues to be a need for additional studies to further address the optimal aerobic exercise training stimulus for children and adolescents.[56]

For some time now, there has been a notion that there is an optimal age or level of maturation in which aerobic training will be most effective in producing adaptations that increase $\dot{V}O_2$ max. Indeed, Ekblom,[81] citing earlier studies, suggested that this might be the case as early as 1969. Katch[110] proposed that there is a critical age or point during maturation when the exercise training stimulus will be most effective in provoking an adaptation. More specifically, Katch suggested that prior to puberty, the hormonal responses that initiate an anatomical or physiological adaptation to training may be blunted, a viewpoint upheld by others.[6,55,111] Furthermore, evidence from several studies that examined children and adolescents over periods of time ranging from 2 to 10 years showed increases in $\dot{V}O_2$ max in trained and/or highly active male subjects that were greatest at and after the age at peak height velocity and lends support to this concept.[112–114]

However, other evidence is contrary to the idea that there is a critical age for maximizing the degree of improvement in $\dot{V}O_2$ max.[115,116] Three other studies utilized a combined longitudinal and cross-sectional approach to study aerobic trainability in children that involved subjecting children and adults to similar aerobic training programmes and comparing changes in $\dot{V}O_2$ max between age groups. In one study, Eisenman and Golding[117] noted aerobic training increased $\dot{V}O_2$ max by a similar amount in girls (16.2%) with a mean age of 12.7 years and women (17.6%) with a mean age of 19.6 years over the course of a 14-week training programme. Likewise, Savage *et al.*[65] did not demonstrate an age by training effect with respect to $\dot{V}O_2$ max in 8- and 35-year-old males over the course of 11 weeks of training, although in comparison to Eisenman and Golding, the increase in $\dot{V}O_2$ max in both groups was quite modest. In contrast, Weber *et al.*[96] examined groups of identical twins ages 10, 13, and 16 years. Significant increases in $\dot{V}O_2$ max (mL kg^{-1}·min^{-1}) were demonstrated by the younger and older groups but not the middle age group. Moreover the youngest age group showed the largest percentage increase in $\dot{V}O_2$ max. Speculation regarding the optimal age for stimulating aerobic training adaptations in $\dot{V}O_2$ max remains intriguing, but clearly the evidence in favour of such a viewpoint is not overwhelming and the physiological factors that may be involved need to be systematically studied.

In adults there is an inverse relationship between the pre-training $\dot{V}O_2$ max and the amount that it will increase subsequent to aerobic training.[8] Whether the same relationship is apparent in children and adolescents is less certain. On one hand, a review of the literature by Pate and Ward[118] concluded that the change in $\dot{V}O_2$ max is unrelated to the initial value. This was further substantiated by data from other studies.[67,73] On the other hand, Eliakim *et al.*[92] reported a significant inverse relationship ($r = -0.68$) between pre-training $\dot{V}O_2$ max, expressed relative to the individual's predicted $\dot{V}O_2$ max, and the percentage improvement in adolescent girls. Other studies also have observed a similar inverse relationship between these variables,[69,75] although it should be noted that in the relationship reported by Tolfrey *et al.*[75], it appears that both trained and untrained subjects were included as a collective group. To further examine this issue, the relationship between pre-training $\dot{V}O_2$ max and percentage improvement was calculated using the data from the studies listed in Table 39.2. In the three studies where mass-related $\dot{V}O_2$ max was not reported,[63,76,80] a value was calculated using the mean mass and absolute $\dot{V}O_2$ max values for the trained subjects from each study. The results are shown in Fig. 39.1 and confirm that a significant inverse relationship exists between these two variables. Based on these results, it appears that approximately 52% of the variation in the amount in which $\dot{V}O_2$ max increases with training in children and adolescents can be attributed to the initial level, although it must be kept in mind that this analysis, involving studies utilizing a wide variety of training programmes, has limitations. Nonetheless, it may be prudent to account for this factor when developing subject inclusion criteria.

It has been proposed that habitual physical activity may influence the degree of aerobic training adaptations in youths.[2,3,118,119] This stems from the idea that aerobic training must provide a stimulus that is greater than the habitual physical activity of the individual—an application of the overload principle described earlier. In support of this influence, Rowland and Boyajian[73] reported a weak but significant correlation ($r = -0.35$) between the change in $\dot{V}O_2$ max and the subjects' habitual physical activity level. In contrast, Tolfrey *et al.*[75] did not document any relationship between these variables. However, Tolfrey *et al.* did observe that habitual physical activity increased in boys and girls after aerobic training but not in control subjects over the same time period. This raises a very interesting consideration with respect to the impact that aerobic training might have on promoting an increase in habitual physical activity outside of the training programme and the potential health implications.

For some time, researchers have noted that there is a large variation in the degree of adaptations resulting from aerobic training. This is apparent even when confounding factors such as age, sex, race, and pre-training $\dot{V}O_2$ max are taken into account.[120] This would imply that there is an underlying genetic predisposition with regard to the extent in which a physiological adaptation

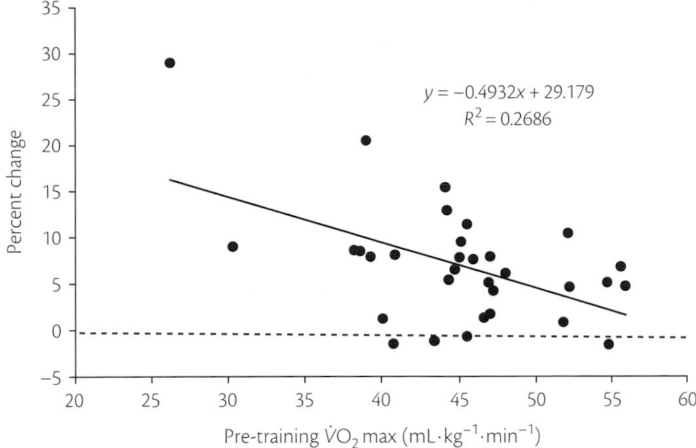

Fig. 39.1 Relationship between pre-training $\dot{V}O_2$ max and the percentage improvement with aerobic training using data from the studies listed in Table 39.2.

will manifest as a result of aerobic training.[9,120] Early evidence supporting a genetic influence on $\dot{V}O_2$ max adaptability comes from observations involving monozygous twins and showing that there is a high intraclass correlation for the within-pair change in $\dot{V}O_2$ max response as well as a much greater degree of variation between versus within pairs of twins for the aerobic training-induced increase in $\dot{V}O_2$ max.[9] More recently, it has been shown that nearly half of the change in $\dot{V}O_2$ max with aerobic training could be due to heritability,[120] and specific candidate genes have been identified that may account for individual responsiveness to aerobic training.[121–123] In children and adolescents, the genetic influence on the responsiveness of $\dot{V}O_2$ max to aerobic training is not very well understood. However, Danis *et al.*[79] recently reported a heritability estimate of 45% for the adaptation in $\dot{V}O_2$ max and 50–65% for lactate threshold (expressed several ways) over the course of 6 months in monozygous twins, where one sibling served as a training subject and the other sibling served as a control subject.

In summary, it appears that aerobic training of sufficient frequency, intensity, and duration will increase $\dot{V}O_2$ max in children and adolescents, although an exact recommendation and the interaction among these variables requires further clarification. Whether there is a critical age or level of maturation for maximizing the aerobic training adaptations in children and adolescents is unclear. The pre-training level of $\dot{V}O_2$ max may influence the amount of improvement in this variable and as such should be considered as a criterion in the subject selection process. Moreover, the degree in which the aerobic training programme exceeds the individual's habitual physical activity may be an important consideration in the design of optimal training programmes and in the interpretation of outcomes. Finally, the genetic influences on aerobic training adaptations are currently being studied in adults and evidence is accumulating with respect to specific genetic factors involved with various adaptations. The extent to which genetic factors exert the same influence on adaptability in children and adolescents is much less certain, but based on very limited evidence it appears that there is a degree of heritability with respect to some aerobic training adaptations in paediatric subjects.

Considerations for the development of aerobic training programmes

When one considers an optimal aerobic training programme for children and adolescents, a primary thought should be identifying the objective of the training programme. Consideration must also be given to the potential adverse effects of intense training during childhood.[124,125] At one end of the spectrum is aerobic training that falls into the category of fitness training that is often defined by the recommendation of the ACSM.[1] This volume of training has been utilized in the studies outlined in Table 39.2 and in most, but certainly not all, cases results in a significant increase in $\dot{V}O_2$ max. Recently, Armstrong and colleagues[4] proposed alternative recommendations, which were endorsed by the International Olympic Committee (IOC),[125] for the amount of aerobic training to increase $\dot{V}O_2$ max in children and adolescents. They suggested that training should occur three to four times per week for 40–60 min per day at 85–90% of maximal HR for 12 weeks. Moreover, Armstrong *et al.* recommend that the training programme should include both continuous and interval training.

Another consideration is the optimal mix between lower-intensity continuous training and high-intensity interval training. Since $\dot{V}O_2$ max represents 100% of maximal aerobic capacity, it makes sense that interval training performed at a high percentage of maximal ability for a sustained duration (for several minutes) and repeated multiple times would improve this parameter. This is consistent with the specificity of exercise training principle[7] as well as with recent recommendations from the adult literature.[126,127] Continuous training at a lower intensity may serve to increase endurance, more so than $\dot{V}O_2$ max and provide a reasonable training stimulus on days in between higher-intensity interval training sessions, an application of the hard easy principle. Furthermore, the collective effect of this of type of training should provide a physical activity stimulus that is over and above the child's habitual physical activity pattern and thus will provide an appropriate overload.

At the other end of the aerobic training programme spectrum is the need to better understand the physiological adaptations that result from training programmes utilized by the competitive athlete in the scholastic or club setting. These athletes usually perform more training in practice than what is recommended for improving cardiorespiratory fitness[1] and in many cases enter into a training programme in a partially trained state. Surveying the studies listed in Table 39.1 shows quite a bit of variation in the degree in which athletes were reportedly training, but it is apparent that the athletes were engaged in fairly vigorous training programmes. Although detailed information on specific aerobic training programmes utilized by child athletes is sparse, there is some information that can be highlighted. For example, Vogel[128] provided some information on the training habits in a small group of male (n = 13) and female (n = 15) age-group distance runners 7–14 years. To analyse the responses, Vogel separated the subjects into four, 2-year age groups. As might be expected, the training volume increased with age ranging from 127 km over approximately 18 weeks of training in 7- to 8-year-old boys and girls to 1453 km over approximately 38 weeks of training in 13- to 14-year-old boys and girls. When separated by sex, females ran substantially more yearly miles than the males in all age groups. Racing information was provided by Vogel and indicated that in the vast majority of instances, the runners were racing at distances ranging from just under 1 to 10 km. However, there was a very small minority of runners who reported racing distances from 10 km to the marathon. Daniels and Oldridge[115] reported that of 14 boys (10–15 years) followed over 22 months, 7 boys ran an average of 1782 km per year (range = 1200–3200 km), whereas the other 7 runners averaged 538 km per year. In a study involving nine male adolescent cross-country runners, Plank *et al.*[94] reported that pre-season training averaged approximately40 km per week, whereas in-season training (13 weeks) ranged from 45 to 80 km per week. Certainly, more studies characterizing the frequency, duration, intensity, programme length, and seasonal variations in training, along with the physiological and performance adaptations resulting from specific training programmes for competitive events are needed.

Summary

This chapter examined aerobic training-induced adaptations in children and adolescents. Based on the information presented, it appears that the following conclusions are warranted:

- Understanding aerobic training adaptations in children and adolescents has important implications with respect to health, physical fitness, the development of safe and effective training programmes, and aerobic exercise performance.
- In cross-sectional studies, $\dot{V}O_2$ max is substantially higher in aerobically trained children and adolescents compared with untrained and age-matched control subjects or in comparison to general reference values for a given age and sex. The higher $\dot{V}O_2$ max has been attributed to superior cardiac function with respect to $\dot{Q}$ max and SV max. To a much lesser extent, adaptations are also apparent at the submaximal level of exercise and include a lower HR and higher SV, a higher T_{VENT}, better running economy, and a lower blood lactate concentration at a fixed level of exercise.
- Carefully controlled longitudinal studies, albeit more difficult to conduct than cross-sectional studies; provide evidence that $\dot{V}O_2$ max is trainable in children and adolescents. However, the degree of improvement appears to be somewhat attenuated compared with adult training studies. The increase in $\dot{V}O_2$ max appears to be to the result of an increase in $\dot{Q}$ max and SV max. At a given level of submaximal exercise, adaptations include reductions in HR and blood lactate concentration, and increases in SV and T_{VENT}. In addition, the physiological responses at a fixed lactate level increase and running economy may improve.
- Although there has been a viewpoint that adaptations to aerobic training may be limited by the child's age and maturation level, the evidence to date is too varied to make a strong conclusion one way or the other. Other factors that might influence the degree in which $\dot{V}O_2$ max will increase in children and adolescents involved with aerobic training include the volume of training, $\dot{V}O_2$ max at the onset of the training programme, the relationship between the volume of training and the child's habitual physical activity level, and genetics.
- The exact amount of training necessary to increase $\dot{V}O_2$ max and other measures of aerobic function remain uncertain. Historically, the recommendations of the ACSM have been viewed as appropriate for children and adolescents, but a more recent proposal, endorsed by the IOC, suggests that the minimal level of aerobic training for children and adolescents may be greater than the guidelines proposed by ACSM. Recommendations on developmentally appropriate volumes of training for competition remain to be established, but must account for the child's unique physiological responses to exercise and the potential physical and psychological risks. Moreover, research on the effectiveness of training programmes used by scholastic and club athletes is needed.

References

1. American College of Sports Medicine (1998). The recommended quantity and quality of exercise for developing and maintaining cardiorespiratory and muscular fitness, and flexibility in healthy adults. *Med Sci Sports Exerc* **30**, 975–91.
2. Sady SP (1986). Cardiorespiratory exercise training in children. *Clin Sports Med* **5**, 493–514.
3. Vaccaro P, Mahon A (1987). Cardiorespiratory responses to endurance training in children. *Sports Med* **4**, 352–63.
4. Armstrong N, Barrett LA, Welsman JR (2007). Cardiorespiratory training during childhood and adolescence. *J Exerc Sci Physiother* **3**, 67–75.
5. Rowland TW (1997). The aerobic trainability of athletic and non-athletic children. In: Froberg K (ed.), *Exercise and fitness, benefits and risks: Children and exercise XVIII*, pp. 182–90. Odense University Press, Odense.
6. Rowland TW (1992). Trainability of the cardiorespiratory system during childhood. Can *J Sport Sci* **17**, 259–63.
7. Wilmore JH, Costil DL (2004). *Physiology of sport and exercise.* Human Kinetics, Champaign, IL.
8. Rowell L (1993). *Human cardiovascular control.* Oxford University Press, New York.
9. Bouchard C, Dionne FT, Simoneau JA, Boulay MR (1992). Genetics of aerobic and anaerobic performances. *Exerc Sports Sci Rev* **20**, 27–58.
10. Blomqvist CG, Saltin B (1983). Cardiovascular adaptations to physical training. *Ann Rev Physiol* **45**, 169–89.
11. Clausen JP (1977). Effect of physical training on cardiovascular adjustments to exercise in man. *Physiol Rev* **57**, 779–815.
12. Kiens B, Essen-Gustavsson B, Christensen NJ, Saltin B (1993). Skeletal muscle substrate utilization during submaximal exercise in man: Effect of endurance training. *J Physiol* **469**, 459–78.
13. Holloszy JO, Coyle EF (1984). Adaptations of skeletal muscle to endurance exercise and their metabolic consequences. *J Appl Physiol* **56**, 831–8.
14. Hawley JA (2002). Adaptations of skeletal muscle to prolonged, intense endurance training. *Clin Exp Pharmacol Physiol* **29**, 218–22.
15. MacRae HS, Dennis SC, Bosch AN, Noakes TD (1992). Effects of training on lactate production and removal during progressive exercise in humans. *J Appl Physiol* **72**, 1649–56.
16. Rowland TW, Unnithan VB, MacFarlane NG, Gibson NG, Paton JY (1994). Clinical manifestations of the 'athlete's heart' in prepubertal male runners. *Int J Sports Med* **15**, 515–19.
17. Mayers N, Gutin B (1979). Physiological characteristics of elite prepubertal cross-country runners. *Med Sci Sports* **11**, 172–6.
18. van Huss WD, Evans SA, Kurowski T, Anderson DJ, Allen R, Stephens K (1988). Physiological characteristics of male and female age-group runners. In: Brown EW, Branta CF (eds.), *Competitive sports for children and youth: An overview of research and issues*, pp. 143–58. Human Kinetics, Champaign, IL.
19. van Huss WD, Stephens KE, Vogel P, Anderson D, Kurowski T, Jones JA, Fitzgerald C. (1986). Physiological and perceptual responses of elite age group distance runners during progressive intermittent work to exhaustion. In: Weiss MR, Gould D (eds.), *Sport for children and youths: The 1983 Olympic scientific congress proceedings*, pp. 239–46. Human Kinetics, Champaign, IL.

20. Sundberg S, Elovainio R (1982). Cardiorespiratory function in competitive endurance runners aged 12–16 years compared with ordinary boys. *Acta Paediatr Scand* **71**, 987–92.
21. Armstrong N, Welsman JR (1994). Assessment and interpretation of aerobic fitness in children and adolescents. *Exerc Sport Sci Rev* **22**, 435–76.
22. Eisenmann JC, Pivarnik JM, Malina RM (2001). Scaling peak $\dot{V}O_2$ to body mass in young male and female distance runners. *J Appl Physiol* **90**, 2172–80.
23. Unnithan VB, Timmons JA, Paton JY, Rowland TW (1995). Physiologic correlates to running performance in pre-pubertal distance runners. *Int J Sports Med* **16**, 528–33.
24. Maffulli N, Testa V, Lancia A, Capasso G, Lombardi S (1991). Indices of sustained aerobic power in young middle distance runners. *Med Sci Sports Exercise* **23**, 1090–6.
25. Eisenmann JC, Womack CJ, Reeves MJ, Pivarnik JM, Malina RM (2001). Blood lipids of young distance runners: Distribution and inter-relationships among training volume, peak oxygen consumption, and body fatness. *Eur J Appl Physiol* **85**, 104–12.
26. Wells CL, Scrutton EW, Archibald LD, Cooke WP, De La Mothe JW (1973). Physical working capacity and maximal oxygen uptake of teenaged athletes. *Med Sci Sports* **5**, 232–8.
27. Wolfe RR, Washington R, Daberkow E, Murphy JR, Brammel HL (1986). Anaerobic threshold as a predictor of athletic performance in prepubertal female runners. *Am J Dis Child*, **140**, 922–4.
28. Drinkwater BL, Horvath SM (1972). Responses of young female track athletes to exercise. *Med Sci Sports* **3**, 56–62.
29. Ali Almarwaey O, Jones A, Tolfrey K (2003). Physiological correlates with endurance running performance in trained adolescents. *Med Sci Sports Exerc* **35**, 480–7.
30. Cole AS, Woodruff ME, Horn MP, Mahon AD (2006). Strength, power, and aerobic exercise correlates of cross-country running performance in adolescent runners. *Pediatr Exerc Sci* **18**, 374–84.
31. Cunningham LN (1990). Physiologic comparison of adolescent female and male cross-country runners. *Pediatr Exerc Sci* **2**, 313–21.
32. Eisenmann JC, Wickel EE (2007). Estimated energy expenditure and physical activity patterns of adolescent runners. *Int J Sports Nutr Exerc Metab* **17**, 178–88.
33. Fernhall B, Kohrt W, Burkett LN, Walters S (1996). Relationship between the lactate threshold and cross-country run performance in high school male and female runners *Pediatr Exerc Sci* **8**, 37–47.
34. Kumagai S, Tanaka K, Matsuura Y, Matsuzaka A, Hirakoba K, Asano K (1982). Relationships of the anaerobic threshold with the 5 km, 10 km, and 10 mile races. *Eur J Appl Physiol* **49**, 13–23.
35. Saltin B, Larsen H, Terrados N, Bangsbo J, Bak T, Kim CK, Svedenhag J, Rolf CJ (1995). Aerobic exercise capacity at sea level and at altitude in Kenyan boys, junior and senior runners compared with Scandinavian runners. *Scand J Med Sci Sports* **5**, 209–21.
36. Burke EJ, Brush FC (1979). Physiological and anthropometric assessment of successful teenage female distance runners. *Res Q* **50**, 180–7.
37. Butts NK (1982). Physiological profiles of high school female cross country runners. *Res Q Exerc Sport* **53**, 8–14.
38. Cunningham LN (1990). Relationship of running economy, ventilatory threshold, and maximal oxygen consumption to running performance in high school females. *Res Q Exerc Sport* **61**, 369–74.
39. Nottin S, Vinet A, Stecken F, N'Guyen LD, Ounissi F, Lecoq AM, Obert P (2002). Central and peripheral cardiovascular adaptations to exercise in endurance-trained children. *Acta Physiol Scand* **175**, 85–92.
40. Rowland TW, Wehnert M, Miller K (2000). Cardiac responses to exercise in competitive child cyclists. *Med Sci Sports Exerc* **32**, 747–52.
41. Unnithan VB, Rowland TW, Cable NT, Raine N (1997). Cardiac responses in elite male junior cyclists. In: Armstrong N, Kirby BJ, Welsman JR (ed.), *Children and exercise XIX: Promoting health and well being*, pp. 501–6. E & FN Spon, London.
42. Cunningham DA, Eynon RB (1973). The working capacity of young competitive simmers, 10–16 years of age. *Med Sci Sports* **5**, 227–31.
43. Vaccaro P, Clarke DH, Morris AF (1980). Physiological characteristics of young well-trained swimmers. *Eur J Appl Physiol* **44**, 61–6.
44. Holmer I (1972). Oxygen uptake during swimming in man. *J Appl Physiol* **33**, 502–9.
45. Holmer I, Lundin A, Eriksson BO (1974). Maximum oxygen uptake during swimming and running by elite swimmers. *J Appl Physiol* **36**, 711–4.
46. Raven PB, Drinkwater BL, Horvath SM (1973). Cardiovascular responses of young female track athletes during exercise. *Med Sci Sports* **4**, 205–9.
47. Rowland T, Unnithan V, Fernhall B, Baynard T, Lange C (2002). Left ventricular responses to dynamic exercise in young cyclists. *Med Sci Sports Exerc* **34**, 637–42.
48. Rowland T, Goff D, Popowski B, DeLuca P, Ferrone L (1998). Cardiac responses to exercise in child distance runners. *Int J Sports Med* **19**, 385–90.
49. Telford RD, McDonald IG, Ellis LB, Chennells MHD, Sandstrom ER, Fuller PJ (1988). Echocardiographic dimensions in trained and untrained 12-year-old boys and girls. *J Sport Sci* **6**, 49–57.
50. Gutin B, Mayers N, Levy JA, Herman MV (1988). Physiologic and echocardiographic studies of age-group runners. In: Brown EW, Branta CF (ed.), *Competitive sports for children and youth*, pp. 117–28. Human Kinetics, Champaign, IL.
51. Obert P, Stecken F, Courteix D, Lecoq AM, Guenon P (1998). Effect of long-term intensive endurance training on left ventricular structure and diastolic function in prepubertal children. *Int J Sports Med* **19**, 149–54.
52. Oyen E-M, Schuster S, Brode PE (1990). Dynamic exercise echocardiography of the left ventricle in physically trained children compared to untrained healthy children. *Int J Cardiol* **29**, 29–33.
53. Perrault H, Turcotte RA (1994). Exercise-induced cardiac hypertrophy. Fact or fallacy? *Sports Med* **17**, 288–308.
54. Saltin B, Kim CK, Terrados N, Larsen H, Svendenhag J, Rolf CJ (1995). Morphology, enzyme activities and buffer capacity in leg muscles of Kenyan and Scandinavian runners. *Scan J Med Sci Sports* **5**, 222–30.
55. Rowland TW (1985). Aerobic response to endurance training in prepubescent children: A critical analysis. *Med Sci Sports Exerc* **17**, 493–7.
56. Mahon AD (2000). Exercise training. In: Armstrong N, van Mechelen W (eds.), *Paediatric exercise science and medicine*, pp. 201–22. Oxford University Press, Oxford.
57. Baquet G, van Praagh E, Berthoin S (2003). Endurance training and aerobic fitness in young people. *Sports Med* **33**, 1127–43.
58. Yoshida T, Ishiko I, Muraoka I (1980). Effect of endurance training on cardiorespiratory functions of 5-year-old children. *Int J Sports Med* **1**, 91–4.
59. Yoshizawa S, Honda H, Nakamura N, Itoh K, Watanbe N (1997). Effects of an 18-month endurance run training program on maximal aerobic power in 4- to 6-year-old girls. *Pediatr Exerc Sci* **9**, 33–43.
60. Yoshizawa S, Honda H, Urushibara M, Nakamura N (1990). Effects of endurance run on circulorespiratory system in young children. *J Hum Ergol* **19**, 41–52.
61. Becker DM, Vaccaro P (1983). Anaerobic threshold alterations caused by endurance training in young children. *J Sports Med Phys Fitness* **23**, 445–9.
62. Gilliam TB, Freedson PS (1980). Effects of a 12-week school physical fitness program on peak $\dot{V}O_2$, body composition, and blood lipids in 7 to 9 year old children. *Int J Sports Med* **1**, 73–8.
63. McManus AM, Armstrong N, Williams CA (1997). Effect of training on the aerobic power and anaerobic performance of prepubertal girls. *Acta Paediatr* **86**, 456–9.
64. Obert P, Courteix D, Lecoq AM, Guenon P (1996). Effect of long-term intense swimming training on the upper body peak oxygen uptake of prepubertal girls. *Eur J Appl Physiol* **73**, 136–43.

65. Savage MP, Petratis MM, Thomson WH, Berg K, Smith JL, Sady SP (1986). Exercise training effects on serum lipids of prepubescent boys and adult men. *Med Sci Sports Exerc* **18**, 197–204.
66. Eliakim A, Scheett T, Allmendinger N, Brasel JA, Cooper DM (2001). Training, muscle volume, and energy expenditure in nonobese American girls. *J Appl Physiol* **90**, 35–44.
67. Lussier L, Buskirk ER (1977). Effects of an endurance training regimen on assessment of work capacity in prepubertal children. *Ann N Y Acad Sci* **301**, 734–47.
68. Mahon AD, Vaccaro P (1994). Cardiovascular adaptations in 8- to 12-year-old boys following a 14-week running program. *Can J Applied Physiol* **19**, 139–50.
69. Mandigout S, Lecoq AM, Courteix D, Guenon P, Obert P (2001). Effect of gender in response to an aerobic training programme in prepubertal children. *Acta Paediatr* **90**, 9–15.
70. Mandigout S, Melin A, Lecoq AM, Courteix D, Obert P (2002). Effect of two aerobic training regimens on the cardiorespiratory response of prepubertal boys and girls. *Acta Paediatr* **91**, 403–8.
71. McManus AM, Cheng CH, Leung MP, Yung TC, Macfarlane DJ (2005). Improving aerobic power in primary school boys: A comparison of continuous and interval training. *Int J Sports Med* **26**, 781–6.
72. Obert P, Mandigouts S, Nottin S, Vinet A, N'Guyen LD, Lecoq AM (2003). Cardiovascular responses to endurance training in children: Effect of gender. *Eur J Clin Invest* **33**, 199–208.
73. Rowland TW, Boyajian A (1995). Aerobic response to endurance exercise training in children. *Pediatrics* **96**, 654–8.
74. Rowland TW, Martel L, Vanderburgh P, Manos T, Charkoudian N (1996). The influence of short-term aerobic training on blood lipids in healthy 10–12 year old children. *Int J Sports Med* **17**, 487–92.
75. Tolfrey K, Campbell IG, Batterham AM (1998). Aerobic trainability of prepubertal boys and girls. *Pediatr Exerc Sci* **10**, 248–63.
76. Welsman JR, Armstrong N, Withers S (1997). Responses of young girls to two modes of aerobic training. *Br J Sports Med* **31**, 139–42.
77. Williams CA, Armstrong N, Powell J (2000). Aerobic responses of prepubertal boys to two modes of training. *Br J Sports Med* **34**, 168–73.
78. Mahon AD, Vaccaro P (1989). Ventilatory threshold and $\dot{V}O_2$ max changes in children following endurance training. *Med Sci Sports Exerc* **21**, 425–31.
79. Danis A, Kyriazis Y, Klissouras V (2003). The effect of training in male prepubertal and pubertal monozygotic twins. *Eur J Appl Physiol* **89**, 309–18.
80. Stoedefalke K, Armstrong N, Kirby BJ, Welsman JR (2000). Effect of training on peak oxygen uptake and blood lipids in 13 to 14-year-old girls. *Acta Paediatr* **89**, 1290–4.
81. Ekblom B (1969). Effect of physical training in adolescent boys. *J Appl Physiol* **27**, 350–5.
82. Eriksson BO, Gollnick PD, Saltin B (1973). Muscle metabolism and enzyme activities after training in boys 11–13 years old. *Acta Physiol Scand* **87**, 485–97.
83. Eriksson BO, Koch G (1973). Effect of physical training on hemodynamic response during submaximal and maximal exercise in 11–13-year old boys. *Acta Physiol Scand* **87**, 27–39.
84. Vaccaro P, Clarke DH (1978) Cardiorespiratory alterations in 9 to 11 years old children following a season of competitive swimming. *Med Sci Sports* **10**, 204–7.
85. Massicotte DR, Macnab RB (1974). Cardiorespiratory adaptations to training at specified intensities in children. *Med Sci Sports* **6**, 242–6.
86. Baquet G, Berthoin S, Dupont G, Blondel N, Fabre C, van Praagh E (2002). Effects of high intensity intermittent training on peak $\dot{V}O_2$ in prepubertal children. *Int J Sports Med* **23**, 439–44.
87. Rotstein A, Dotan R, Bar-Or O, Tenenbaum G (1986). Effect of training on anaerobic threshold, maximal aerobic power and anaerobic performance of preadolescent boys. *Int J Sports Med* **7**, 281–6.
88. Stewart KJ, Gutin B (1976). Effects of physical training on cardiorespiratory fitness in children. *Res Q* **47**, 110–20.
89. Burkett LN, Fernhall B, Walters SC (1985). Physiological effect of distance running training on teenaged females. *Res Q Exerc Sport* **56**, 215–20.
90. Rowland TW, Varzeas MR, Walsh CA (1991). Aerobic responses to walking training in sedentary adolescents. *J Adolesc Health* **12**, 30–4.
91. Eliakim A, Raisz LG, Brasel JA, Cooper DM (1997). Evidence for increased bone formation following a brief endurance-type training intervention in adolescent males. *J Bone Min Res* **12**, 1708–13.
92. Eliakim A, Barstow TJ, Brasel JA, Ajie H, Lee WN, Renslo R, Berman N, Cooper DM (1996). Effect of exercise training on energy expenditure, muscle volume, and maximal oxygen uptake in female adolescents. *J Pediatr* **129**, 537–43.
93. Stransky AW, Mickelson RJ, van Fleet C, Davis R (1979). Effects of a swimming training regimen on hematological, cardiorespiratory and body composition changes in young females. *J Sports Med Phys Fitness* **19**, 347–54.
94. Plank DM, Hipp MJ, Mahon AD (2005). Aerobic exercise adaptations in trained adolescent runners following a season of cross-country training. *Res Sports Med* **13**, 273–86.
95. Sallis JF, Simons-Morton BG, Stone EJ, Corbin CB, Epstein LH, Faucette N, Iannotti RJ, Killen JD, Klesges RC, Petray CK, Rowland TW, Taylor WC (1992). Determinants of physical activity and interventions in youth. *Med Sci Sports Exerc* **24**, S248–57.
96. Weber G, Kartodihardjo W, Klissouras V (1976). Growth and physical training with reference to heredity. *J Appl Physiol* **40**, 211–5.
97. Geenen DL, Gilliam TB, Crowley D, Moorehead-Steffens C, Rosenthal A (1982). Echocardiographic measures in 6 to 7 year old children after an 8 month exercise program. *Am J Cardiol* **49**, 1990–5.
98. George KP, Gates PE, Tolfrey K (2005). Impact of aerobic training upon left ventricular morphology and function in pre-pubescent children. *Ergonomics* **48**, 1378–89.
99. Obert P, Mandigout S, Vinet A, N'Guyen LD, Stecken F, Courteix D (2001). Effect of aerobic training and detraining on left ventricular dimensions and diastolic function in prepubertal boys and girls. *Int J Sports Med* **22**, 90–6.
100. Ricci G, Lajoie D, Petitclerc R, Peronnet F, Ferguson RJ, Fournier M, Taylor WC (1982). Left ventricular size following endurance, sprint, and strength training. *Med Sci Sports Exerc* **14**, 344–7.
101. Gatch W, Byrd AW (1979). Endurance training and cardiovascular function in 9-and 10-year-old boys. *Arch Phys Med Rehabil* **60**, 574–7.
102. Shasby GB, Hagerman FC (1975). The effects of conditioning on cardiorespiratory function in adolescent boys. *J Sports Med* **3**, 97–107.
103. Gutin B, Owens S, Slavens G, Riggs S, Treiber F (1997). Effect of physical training on heart-period variability in obese children. *J Pediatr* **130**, 938–43.
104. Mandigout S, Melin A, Fauchier L, N'Guyen LD, Courteix D, Obert P (2002). Physical training increases heart rate variability in healthy prepubertal children. *Eur J Clin Invest* **32**, 479–87.
105. Haffor AA, Kirk PA (1988). Anaerobic threshold and relation of ventilation to CO_2 output during exercise in 11 year olds. *J Sports Med Phys Fitness* **28**, 74–8.
106. Jones AM, Carter H (2000). The effect of endurance training on parameters of aerobic fitness. *Sports Med* **29**, 373–86.
107. Daniels JT (1985). A physiologist's view of running economy. *Med Sci Sports Exerc* **17**, 332–8.
108. Saunders PU, Pyne DB, Telford RD, Hawley JA (2004). Factors affecting running economy in trained distance runners. *Sports Med* **34**, 465–85.
109. Fournier M, Ricci J, Taylor AW, Ferguson RJ, Montpetit RR, Chaitman BR (1982). Skeletal muscle adaptation in adolescent boys: Sprint and endurance training and detraining. *Med Sci Sports Exerc* **14**, 453–6.
110. Katch VL (1983). Physical conditioning of children. *J Adolesc Health Care* **3**, 241–6.

111. Payne VG, Morrow JR, Jr (1993). Exercise and $\dot{V}O_2$ max in children: A meta-analysis. *Res Q Exerc Sport* **64**, 305–13.
112. Kobayashi K, Kitamura K, Miura M, Sodeyama H, Murase Y, Miyashita M, Matsui H (1978). Aerobic power as related to body growth and training in Japanese boys: A longitudinal study. *J Appl Physiol* **44**, 666–72.
113. Mercier J, Vago P, Ramonatxo M, Bauer C, Prefaut C (1987). Effect of aerobic training quantity on the $\dot{V}O_2$ max of circumpubertal swimmers. *Int J Sports Med* **8**, 26–30.
114. Mirwald RL, Bailey DA, Cameron N, Rasmussen RL (1981). Longitudinal comparison of aerobic power in active and inactive boys aged 7.0 to 17.0 years. *Ann Hum Biol* **8**, 405–14.
115. Daniels J, Oldridge N (1971). Changes in oxygen consumption of young boys during growth and running training. *Med Sci Sports* **3**, 161–5.
116. Daniels J, Oldridge N, Nagle F, White B (1978). Differences and changes in $\dot{V}O_2$ among young runners 10 to 18 years of age. *Med Sci Sports* **10**, 200–3.
117. Eisenman PA, Golding LA (1975). Comparison of effects of training on $\dot{V}O_2$ max in girls and young women. *Med Sci Sports* **7**, 136–8.
118. Pate RR, Ward DS (1990). Endurance exercise trainability in children and youth. In: Grana WA, Lombardo JA, Sharkey BJ, Stone EJ (eds.), *Advances in sports medicine and fitness*, pp. 37–55. Year Book Medical Publishers, Chicago, IL.
119. Cunningham DA, Paterson DH, Blimkie CJR (1984). The development of the cardiorespiratory system with growth and physcial activity. In: Boileau RA (ed.), *Advances in pediatric sports sciences: Volume 1 biological issues*, pp. 85–116. Human Kinetics, Champaign, IL.
120. Bouchard C, Rankinen T (2001). Individual differences in response to regular physical activity. *Med Sci Sports Exerc* **33**, S446–51.
121. Rankinen T, Bray MS, Hagberg JM, Perusse L, Roth SM, Wolfarth B, Bouchard C (2006). The human gene map for performance and health-related fitness phenotypes: The 2005 update. *Med Sci Sports Exerc* **38**, 1863–88.
122. Rivera MA, Dionne FT, Simoneau JA, Perusse L, Chagnon M, Chagnon Y, Gagnon J, Leon AS, Rao DC, Skinner JS, Wilmore JH, Bouchard C (1997). Muscle-specific creatine kinase gene polymorphism and $\dot{V}O_2$ max in the HERITAGE Family Study. *Med Sci Sports Exerc* **29**, 1311–17.
123. Rivera MA, Pérusse L, Simoneau JA, Gagnon J, Dionne FT, Leon AS, Sknneer JS, Wilmore JH, Province M, Rao DC, Bouchard C (1999). Linkage between a muscle-specific CK gene marker and $\dot{V}O_2$ max in the HERITAGE Family Study. *Med Sci Sports Exerc* **31**, 698–701.
124. American Academy of Pediatrics Committee on Sports Medicine (1990). Risks in distance running for children. *Pediatrics* **86**, 799–800.
125. Mountjoy M, Armstrong N, Bizzini L, Blimkie C, Evans J, Gerrard D, Hangen J, Knoll, K, Micheli L, Sangenis P, Van Mechelen W (2008). IOC consensus statement: Training the elite child athlete. *Br J Sports Med* **42**, 163–4.
126. Laursen PB, Jenkins DG (2002). The scientific basis for high-intensity interval training: Optimising training programmes and maximising performance in highly trained endurance athletes. *Sports Med* **32**, 53–73.
127. Midgley AW, McNaughton LR, Wilkinson M (2006). Is there an optimal training intensity for enhancing the maximal oxygen uptake of distance runners? Empirical research findings, current opinions, physiological rationale and practical recommendations. *Sports Med* **36**, 117–32.
128. Vogel PG (1986). Training and racing involvement of elite young runners. In: Weiss MR, Gould D (eds.), *Sport for children and youths: The 1983 Olympic scientific congress proceedings*, pp. 219–24. Human Kinetics, Champaign, IL.

CHAPTER 40

Maximal intensity exercise and strength training

Keith Tolfrey

Introduction

Participation in organized sports is common from a young age in the United Kingdom and other countries around the world. Sports clubs often have practice sessions that are scheduled specifically for young children. Professional clubs within some sports have recognized that it may be beneficial from both a performance and a financial standpoint to invest in what they regard as talented young players. The emergence of the Football Academy in the United Kingdom is an obvious example of this formal structure to develop young talent in the game. The role of the Football Academy has been examined elsewhere,[1] but it is important to recognize that participation in organized and competitive sport is a reality of modern society in most westernized countries. Most people are now aware that increased physical activity, through sporting or non-sporting activities, offers the potential for numerous health benefits (see Chapter 31). This chapter will focus specifically on the scientific evidence that has come from studies involving children or adolescents who have completed maximal (high-) intensity exercise training and resistance exercise training. The aim is not to explore health gains but those that might be important when considering participation in sport.

Before exploring the literature, it is worth briefly reviewing some basic research design concepts and exercise training principles that will influence our interpretation of the studies that are available currently. The main advantage of cross-sectional studies is that they can include participants who have been engaged in sport, exercise training, or physical activity for several years. The average programme length for longitudinal training studies (see Tables 40.1 and 40.2) is normally much shorter than the time that young people have been engaged in these activities in cross-sectional studies. However, it is impossible to determine cause and effect from cross-sectional research designs and the possibility of a self-selection bias cannot be discounted. Therefore, only those studies that are longitudinal in research design have been included in the present chapter. Longitudinal studies have to include several important design features in order for them to procure data that might be generalized beyond the study sample. Without a well-matched non-training control group or period (for within measures designs), it is not possible to identify changes in outcome variables that are free from the influence of growth, maturation, and development. Sample sizes are invariably relatively small in prospective training studies (Tables 40.1 and 40.2) and participants have not often been assigned randomly to groups or paired matched. Any extraneous factor that may affect the primary outcome variable, in addition to the exercise intervention, should be either controlled or at least measured so that they may be accounted for using appropriate statistical techniques. The careful standardization and quantification of exercise training programmes and measurement of physiological parameters using reliable and valid methods is critical when considering the value of research findings from the studies conducted to date. Exercise training guidelines written specifically for young people are difficult, if not impossible, to write because of the large heterogeneity within the population and the confounding influence of growth, maturation, and development. Results from the literature on adults have often been used in the design of exercise programmes with young people because the general principles are much the same. By varying the intensity, duration, frequency, and programme length it is possible to manipulate the total training volume. The relative difficulty of the exercise stress (intensity) and how long an individual is exposed to this stimulation are well recognized as the primary determinants of exercise volume. Although not as well established systematically, exercise training principles such as overload, progression, specificity, and detraining would appear to apply equally as well to young people as they do to adults.

Maximal (high-) intensity training adaptations

There is a subtle, but important difference between the assessment of maximal (high-) intensity training techniques on the one hand and the variables that reflect anaerobic energy pathways on the other. Some studies may have included measurements that are typically associated with anaerobic metabolism, directly or indirectly, but the training programme may have been neither maximal nor high in intensity. The number of studies that have systematically examined the influence of high-intensity exercise training on appropriate measures of anaerobic metabolism in young people are in short supply. Consequently, this section reviews studies that have focused on only one aspect, either outcome or appropriate training, or very rarely these in combination. There are probably two main reasons for the paucity of research in this area; (i) although many sports may benefit from an enhanced ability to utilize anaerobic

Table 40.1 Prospective high-intensity training studies with children and adolescents that included a comparison with either an untrained control or at least two different training programmes

Citation	Sample size[a]	Sex	Age (years)	Length (weeks)	Training programme	Performance change (%)[b]
Adeniran and Toriola[2]	23 and 22	F	15	8	F3[c], 4 × 4 min @ approximately 90% estimated HR_{max} (1:1 work:rest) or 4.8 km @ approximately 80–85% estimated HR_{max}	15 versus 13 versus 2[d] VJ (kg m·s^{-1})
Baquet *et al.*[3]	36	M and F	9	7	F2, 4 sets × 5–10 reps × 10–20 s @ 110–130% maximal aerobic speed (1:1 work:rest)	10 versus 3 SBJ (m)
Counil *et al.*[4]	7	M	14	6	F3, 45 min cycling @ VT with 1 min sprints @ maximal aerobic power (asthmatics)	21 versus 9 P_{max} (W·kgLBM^{-1})
Diallo *et al.*[5]	10	M	12	10	F3, plyometrics and dynamic exercises	8 versus 0 P_{max}[e] (W·kg^{-1})
Gorostiaga *et al.*[6]	8	M	17	11	F2, explosive resistance power training	median 8 versus 0 CMJ (m)
Grodjinovsky *et al.*[7]	17 and 19	M	11–13	6	F3, minimum 3 × 8 s + 3 × 30 s cycling sprints or minimum 3 × 40-m + 3 × 150-m running sprints	3 versus 4 versus –5[d] MP (W·kg^{-1}) 4 versus 3* versus –5[d] PP (W·kg^{-1})
Hetzler *et al.*[8]	10 and 10	M	13	12	F3, 3 sets × 10 reps, 50%–75%–100% 10RM (experienced or inexperienced groups)	–2 versus 3* versus 4[d,e] MP (W·kg^{-1}) –2 versus 2 versus 6[d,e] PP (W·kg^{-1})
Ingle *et al.*[9]	26	M	12	12	F3, 2–3 sets × 15–6 reps, 70–100% 10RM & low–moderate intensity plyometrics	1 versus –2 MP (W·kg^{-1}) 1 vs –1 PP (W·kg^{-1}) 4 versus 1 VJ (m) –3 vs. -1 40-m sprint (s)
McManus *et al.*[10]	10	F	9	8	F3, 3–6 × 10s + 3–6 × 30 s running sprints (1:3 work:rest)	1* versus –4 MP[e] (W·kg^{-1}) 7 versus 2 PP[e] (W·kg^{-1})
Mosher *et al.*[11]	13	M	10–11	12	F3, 6–12 reps × 4 running sprint drills lasting total 15–20 min (1:2–1:3 work:rest)	21 versus –4 AST 1* versus 0 40 yard sprint (s)
Obert *et al.*[12]	17	M and F	10–11	13	F2, running 10 × 300 m, 12 × 250 m, 4 × 600 m @ 90% HR_{max} + 15–20 min @ 75–80% HR_{max}	18 versus –2 P_{max} (W·kgLLM^{-1})
Rotstein *et al.*[13]	16	M	10–11	9	F3, 1–2 sets: 3 × 600-m + 5 × 400-m + 6 × 150-m (varied work:rest), 'high' intensity	10 versus 1 MP (W·kg^{-1}) 14 versus –1 PP (W·kg^{-1})
Sargeant *et al.*[14]	15	M	13	8	F2, mixture of short-term power, endurance, and resistance exercise (specifics not available)	5* versus 1 P_{max} (W·kg^{-1})
Siegler *et al.*[15]	17	F	16	10	15 resistance + 24 plyometric sessions, total 32 sets × approximately 10RM + variety of plyometric exercises	1* versus 0 MP (kg m·min^{-1}) 3* versus 2 PP (kg m·min^{-1}) 5* versus 7 VJ (m) –3 vs. –1 20-m sprint (s)

VJ = vertical jump; SBJ = standing broad jump; P_{max} = peak power from force–velocity protocol; CMJ = counter movement jump; MP and PP = mean power and peak power, respectively from Wingate anaerobic test; AST = anaerobic sprint test (motorized treadmill).

[a]Training group(s) sample size.

[b]Trained versus Control.

[c]F – weekly training frequency (e.g. F3 = 3 sessions per week).

[d]Three change values represent two experimental conditions and control.

[e]Power values relative to body mass (W·kg^{-1}) calculated using group data reported in these articles. Only absolute power values were reported in the original articles.

*Comparison with control group was not significant ($P > 0.05$).

Table 40.2 Prospective resistance training studies with children and adolescents that included a comparison with either an untrained control group or at least two different training programmes

Citation	Sample size[a]	Sex	Age (years)	Length (weeks)	Training programme	Strength change (%)[b]
Blanksby and Gregor[16]	20	M and F	?	?	F3[c], 2 sets, 8–12RM	18 versus −4
Blimkie *et al.*[17]	14	M	10	10	F3, 5 sets, 10–12RM (60–75% 1RM)	23 versus 3
Blimkie *et al.*[18]	16	F	16	26	F3, 4 sets, 10–12RM	22 versus 0
Christou *et al.*[19]	9	M	13	16	F2, 2–3 sets, 15–8RM (55–80% 1RM)	56 versus 10
De Konig *et al.*[20]	14	M	16	9	F3, 6 sets × 2 reps, 90% maximum isometric force	13 versus −1
DeRenne *et al.*[21]	7 and 8	M	13	12	F1 or F2, 3 sets × 10 reps, 50–75% initial 10RM (post-training maintenance programme)	2 versus 2 versus −11[d]
Faigenbaum *et al.*[22]	14	M and F	10	8	F2, 3 sets × 15–10 reps, 50–100% 10RM	78 versus 13
Faigenbaum *et al.*[23]	15	M and F	10	8	F2, 2–3 sets, 6–8RM	47 versus 8
Faigenbaum *et al.*[24]	15 and 16	M & F	8	8	F2, 1 set, 6–8RM or 13–15RM (80% or 69% 1RM)	31 versus 41 versus 14 (leg)[d,e]
Faigenbaum *et al.*[25]	15 and 16	M and F	8	8	F2, 1 set, 6–8RM & medicine ball or 13–15RM, (73% or 68% 1RM)	17 versus 16 versus 4 (chest)[d]
Faigenbaum *et al.*[26]	22 and 20	M and F	10	8	F1 or F2, 1 set, 10–15RM	9* versus 12 versus 4 (chest)[d] 14 versus 25 versus 2 (leg)[d]
Faigenbaum *et al.*[27]	12 and 19	M and F	10	8	F2, 1 set, 6–10RM or 15–20RM, (66% or 52% 1RM chest)	21 versus 23 versus 1 (chest)[d] 32* versus 42 versus 4 (leg)[d]
Gillam[28]	11–15	M	14–18	9	F1 to F5 inclusive, 18 sets, 1RM	19, 24, 32, 29 & 41[f]
Hetzler *et al.*[8]	10 and 10	M	13	12	F3, 3 sets × 10 reps, 50%–75%–100% 10RM (experienced or inexperienced groups)	25 versus 27 versus 7[d]
Ingle *et al.*[9]	26	M	12	12	F3, 2–3 sets × 15–6 reps, 70–100% 10RM & low-moderate intensity plyometrics	41 versus 1
Komi *et al.*[29]	6	M and F	14	12	F4, 5–10 maximal isometric contractions	20 versus 11 versus −2[g]
Kotzamanidis *et al.*[30]	12 and 11	M	17	9	F2, 4 sets, 8RM–6RM–3RM (3 phases)	16 versus 2
Nielsen *et al.*[31]	50	F	7–19	5	F3, 24 maximal isometric contractions	32 versus 4
Ozmun *et al.*[32]	8	M and F	10	8	F3, 3 sets, 7–10RM	23 versus 4
Pfeiffer and Francis[33]	14 and 10	M	10 and 13	9	F3, 3 sets × 10 reps, 50%–75%–100% 10RM	16 versus 9[f]
Ramsay *et al.*[34]	13	M	11	20	F3, 5 sets, 10–12RM (60–75% 1RM) then 5–7RM (60–85% 1RM) (2 × 10 week phases)	35 versus 12
Rians *et al.*[35]	18	M	8	14	F3, maximum 30 reps in 30 s, progression through resistance settings if 30+ reps	26 versus 4
Sailors and Berg[36]	5	M	12	8	F3, 3 sets × ?–7–5 reps, 65%–80%–100% 5RM	33 versus 8
Sewall and Micheli[37]	10	M and F	10–11	9	F3, 3 sets, 10–12RM	34 versus 3[h]
Weltman *et al.*[38]	16	M	8	14	F3, 30 reps in 30 s, progression through resistance settings if 30+ reps	26 versus 4

[a]Training group(s) sample size.

[b]Trained versus Control (median value of all strength measurements to reduce outlier effects). Considerable heterogeneity in the training response may exist between exercises (e.g. chest press and leg extension), muscle groups (e.g. elbow and knee), and strength tests (e.g. isotonic and isokinetic).

[c]F—weekly training frequency (e.g. F3 = 3 sessions per week).

[d]Three change values represent two experimental conditions and control.

[e]Only leg extension changes are shown—chest press changes are shown by Faigenbaum *et al.*[25]

[f]Comparison is between two or more experimental groups. An untrained control was not included in the study or change scores were not available by maturity group for the controls.

[g]Three changes represent trained leg, untrained leg (within subject), and control leg (between subject).

[h]Changes calculated from adjusted marginal means not those presented by the authors.

*Comparison with control group was not significant ($P > 0.05$).

energy pathways or from an increase in muscular power, associated health-related benefits are possibly quite limited; and (ii) it is not easy to identify exactly what constitutes anaerobic fitness or performance.

Rowland[39] suggested that it might be intuitively beneficial to approach this problem in a hierarchical manner. That is, to view measurement of anaerobic metabolism (e.g. enzyme activities and substrate availability) first as it might represent the 'purest' form of anaerobic capacity. This would be followed by power production in maximal intensity, laboratory-based standardized tests [e.g. Wingate anaerobic test (WAnT)], and finally alterations in field-based tests of speed and power (e.g. sprinting and vertical jump performance). Interestingly, it could be argued that athletes and coaches may appreciate the findings from the latter outcome measures because they may be more closely aligned to sports performance. This section of the chapter will cover all three aspects although it should be appreciated that there is very little to report and insufficient evidence is available to reach a consensus, with any confidence, regarding the trainability of this component of physical fitness. To highlight this point, a recent review that included a focus on high-intensity intermittent training and anaerobic fitness, by several leading researchers, was based on only three studies[40] (see Table 40.1 references 5,7,10). Very stringent inclusion and exclusion criteria were used before studies were retained for this review. In contrast, a more inclusive approach was adopted to construct Table 40.1 in an effort to encourage more research in this area based on the generation of research questions that should start to fill the many voids that exist currently. Furthermore, the exclusion of studies that either failed to demonstrate significant changes or had serious design faults could lead to a positive bias in the interpretation of the available literature or replication of avoidable errors in future work. Of course, those who embark upon research in this field will want to read the original studies shown in Table 40.1, but the summary should at least provide a sound foundation for further study.

Anaerobic metabolism

Measurement of metabolic factors is difficult even in adults where ethical considerations are less restrictive compared with research with more vulnerable young participants. Non-invasive techniques such as phosphorus nuclear magnetic resonance spectroscopy (^{31}P-MRS) have been used to provide some important *in vivo* insights into muscle metabolism.[41–45] However, it has not been possible to identify a study that has used this technique to assess prospective changes (pre to post) in intramuscular pH (pH_i) or the ratio of inorganic phosphate (P_i) to phosphocreatine (PCr) following chronic exercise training. A cross-sectional comparison of untrained and sprint-trained adolescent boys (12–15 years) revealed no between-group differences in pH_i or the PCr:(PCr+P_i) ratio of the rectus femoris muscle following exhaustive exercise.[42] Interestingly, although the authors did not compare the data between the four different age groups, probably because of the very small sample sizes within each cell, the graphical presentation of results suggested that the youngest trained boys (age 12 years) had both higher pH_i and PCr:(PCr+P_i) ratio than the age-matched untrained boys. The trend, if one really existed, was in the opposite direction for the other three age groups (13, 14, and 15 years). Interpretation of the results, as presented by Kuno and associates[42] or the speculation provided here, is difficult in light of the small samples and a less than clear statistical analysis provided in the original paper.

A recent reliability study of ^{31}P-MRS during exhaustive incremental exercise in children has cast doubt on the utility of this technique to detect longitudinal changes in anaerobic muscle metabolic function.[45] The coefficients of variation for subjectively estimated intracellular thresholds (IT) for P_i/PCr and pH were 10.6% and 10.3%, respectively. For end exercise (END) pH the variation was low (0.9%), but was very high for END(P_i/PCR) at 50%. The authors concluded that IT(Pi/PCR) and IT(pH) demonstrated good reliability and considered them to be stable measures for future study of developmental metabolism.[45] However, when the magnitude of training-induced change is considered in Table 40.1, it would appear that many of these gains may not be detected using the ^{31}P-MRS technique. Clearly, further work is required using this very promising but rather expensive and elusive technique and careful consideration of the stability of the measurements cannot be overlooked.

In the absence of comprehensive findings using ^{31}P-MRS, we have to rely on a handful of studies that have used the highly invasive muscle biopsy technique to further our understanding of changes in muscle metabolism with exercise training in the young. Direct measurements using the muscle biopsy technique are rare in young people for ethical reasons (see Chapter 1). In a frequently cited study, 34 training sessions were completed by 8, 11- to 13-year-old boys over a 4-month period.[46] A weakness of this study was that it was not possible to determine the specifics of the training programme characteristics from the details provided. From small samples of muscle, adenosine triphosphate (ATP), PCr, muscle glycogen, and glucose-6-phosphate (G-6-P) were quantified. Although biopsies were taken before and after the training period at rest and following submaximal and maximal exertion exercise, most of the significant training-induced adaptations occurred in the resting condition. For example, ATP increased from 4.3 to 4.8 $mmol \cdot kg^{-1}$ (wet weight of muscle, ~12%) and PCr from 14.5 to 20.2 $mmol \cdot kg^{-1}$ (~39%), but depletion patterns for both of these phosphates were not altered by exercise training. The average muscle glycogen concentration at rest increased by approximately 32% (53.9–71.0 $mmol \cdot kg^{-1}$), whereas G-6-P doubled following training (0.2–0.4 $mmol \cdot kg^{-1}$). As a consequence of these changes, both muscle and blood lactate concentrations were higher after maximal exertion exercise when comparing the post-training values with those in the untrained state (8.8–13.7 $mmol \cdot kg^{-1}$, ~56% and 4.7–5.9 $mmol \cdot L^{-1}$, ~26% respectively). In a parallel study, five different 11-year-old boys completed a 6-week training programme. Although the conventional aerobic cycling programme (3 × 20 $min \cdot week^{-1}$) employed a relatively high intensity (90% + HR_{max}), it was clearly well below the maximum intensity associated with anaerobic training. Changes in phosphofructokinase (PFK) and succinate dehydrogenase (SDH) activity were quantified from muscle biopsies taken at several time points. The SDH activity increased by approximately 30% (5.4–7.0 $\mu mol \cdot g^{-1} \cdot min^{-1}$), whereas PFK increased by approximately 83% (8.4–15.4 $\mu mol \cdot g^{-1} \cdot min^{-1}$). The combined results of these two studies led the authors to conclude that the training had increased the glycolytic capacity of skeletal muscle in the young boys that, in turn, led to the production of more lactate. Although this work appears to suggest that local adaptations may take place in the skeletal muscle of boys following training, the very small sample size does limit the extrapolation of the findings. Furthermore, changes due to normal growth could not be ascertained without a matched control group.

After analysing extracted muscle samples, Fournier *et al.*[47] did not find any changes in the relative distribution or size of different muscle fibres from six late-adolescent boys (16–17 years). However, similar to Eriksson,[46] changes in PFK activity increased by approximately 21% over the 3-month intervention period, where the boys completed interval runs varying from 50 to 250 m and some occasional stair running (4 times·week^{-1}). Of course, care must be taken when interpreting data from only six boys. With only small increases in stature and body mass, it was surmised that the increase in PFK was a direct consequence of the training rather than growth.[47] However, a substantial change in these anthropometric parameters is unlikely over just 3 months at this age, and the absence of a matched control group, though understandable, must still be viewed as a weakness. Cadefau and colleagues[48] trained 16 late-adolescent (16–18 years) athletes for 5–8 months using a combination of sprint and endurance techniques. The training programme was described as anaerobic and a high percentage of it was said to be devoted to promoting muscle strength. The majority of the training intensities for the speed and strength activities were given as 98–100%, but there was no indication of how these were measured or verified. Three distinct training groups were described in this study; however, the small discrete sample sizes means that a discussion of the pooled sample is only possible. From the 30 mg of muscle taken from the non-dominant vastus lateralis, large relative changes in muscle glycogen content (100% increase), glycogen synthase (GS, 200%), glycogen phosphorylase (GPh, 219%), PFK (43%), pyruvate kinase (PK, 111%), SDH (55%), aspartate aminotransferase (AST, 47%), and alanine aminotransferase (ALT, 56%) were reported. The changes in muscle glycogen content, associated enzymes GS and GPh, and the regulatory enzymes for glycolysis (PFK and PK) reflect some of the modifications reported in previous studies employing the invasive biopsy technique.[46,47] It is interesting that the large relative changes in these metabolites were only associated with small improvements over the intervention period in sprint running performances over 60 m (~3%) and 300 m (~4%). No correlation coefficients were provided to support the relationships, and it is difficult to gauge how meaningful the performance gains were. Large changes in performance in individuals who are already athletically trained may not be expected following brief training programmes as they may be approaching their physiologically defined upper limit. The alterations in SDH, AST, and ALT were indicative of enhancements in oxidative metabolism.[48] The training programme did include an aerobic stimulus and beneficial changes in anaerobic mechanical power have been reported elsewhere following this type of training (e.g. 12). Again, ethical restrictions precluded the inclusion of a non-training control group in this study opening up the possibility of growth and maturation changes over the 5- to 8-month period. Furthermore, strategies to control learning in the performance tasks were not described.

Power production from laboratory tests

Laboratory-based tests of mechanical power [e.g. WAnT and force–velocity test (F–V test)] are the most common for assessing changes, indirectly, of anaerobic metabolism or performance in young people (Table 40.1, and see Chapters 5 and 17 for review).

The considerable heterogeneity of the participants included in the studies measuring mechanical power coupled with the even greater variation in the training stimulus means that it is very difficult to identify meaningful trends. All of the studies in Table 40.1 have 'issues' that cloud the picture. In a study where the training programme and outcome measures were both primarily anaerobic in nature, two independent groups of primary school boys completed a 6-week programme of either maximal effort sprint cycling or sprint running.[7] The duration and intensity of the activities in the two programmes were equal in an effort to minimize the impact of differences in training volume (Table 40.1). Small gains in both body-mass-adjusted mean power (MP) and peak power (PP) were experienced by the boys completing the sprint cycling that was matched to the mode of testing (i.e. WAnT). The non-significant change in PP for the sprint running group reinforces the importance of training and testing specificity in these studies. Larger increases in MP and PP were reported by Rotstein *et al.*[13] after 16 prepubertal boys completed a 9-week training programme (Table 40.1). For children of this age, it is likely that the 600 and 400 m training distances relied, predominantly, on aerobic metabolism even if the intensity was described as suitable for each participant's physical conditioning. This was evident in the approximately 8% improvement in peak oxygen uptake (peak $\dot{V}O_2$) for the trained boys. The 10 and 14% gains in MP and PP, respectively, may be underestimations of trainability because of the lack of training and testing specificity. The only study that has focused specifically on prepubertal girls following high-intensity training suggested that absolute PP increased, whereas MP did not.[10] It is surprising that power was not scaled to account for changes in body size (e.g. body mass) to remove this as an underlying mechanism in this study. However, this estimation is available in Table 40.1, and it would appear that young girls can improve their PP after high-intensity training. The problems of specificity mentioned above also apply to this study. Furthermore, the large drop-out in the control group should not be dismissed too lightly.

Using a modification of Cunningham and Faulkner's[49] anaerobic speed test, Mosher *et al.*[11] avoided the problem of training and criterion test specificity. The 13 prepubertal male footballers who completed the assortment of sprint running drills over the 12-week programme managed to run 21% longer on the 18% inclined motorized treadmill at 11.3 km·h^{-1} (51.5–62.3 s pre-post), whereas the untrained controls fell just short of their original time when tested again (45.6–43.9 s). The reliability of measurements from this treadmill test are not available in children and the run times do not appear to have been associated with any other direct measurements of the anaerobic energy pathways. Therefore, other than showing that these boys could run for a longer period following the training, it is not possible to say what this change represents. The authors[11] implied that enhanced lactate tolerance may be a mechanism underpinning the improvement. In the absence of any blood samples, this is no more than speculation. It may be important to note that no change in 40 m sprint time was noted in this study.

Given the association between muscular force, power, and leg muscle mass,[50–52] it is not surprising that some groups (e.g. 5, 8, 9, 15) have studied the influence of resistance exercise training on power output. The changes in these studies suggest that training specificity is again a prominent issue. Aside from Diallo *et al.*[5], where maximum power (P_{max}) from the force–velocity spectrum increased by 8%, strength-induced changes have not been significant,[8,15], or they are unlikely to be meaningful from a performance standpoint.[9] It has been argued the WAnT may not provide a valid measurement of the highest attainable power and that the F–V test is more appropriate (see Chapter 5). The use of the F–V test combined with a more dynamic resistance training programme may be a factor that sets the Diallo *et al.*[5] study aside from the others. Ingle *et al.*[9], however, also used a complex training programme, but found only 1% gains in MP and PP in the trained prepubertal boys. This study also included measures to reduce the impact of learning that are more likely where children are concerned.

Obert *et al.*[12] purposely used a predominantly aerobic interval running programme that resulted in an 18% gain in P_{max} after changes in lower limb muscle mass (LLMM) had been accounted for using dual energy X-ray absorptiometry (DEXA). As no changes were noted in the optimal velocity (V_{opt}) over the 13-week training programme, the authors concluded that increases in optimal force (F_{opt}) generation must have been responsible for the improvement in P_{max}. No changes in P_{max}, V_{opt}, or F_{opt} were seen in the 16 maturity-matched control girls and boys. This study has been highlighted as it appears to be the longest available in the literature where power has been measured. The challenge of getting young people to engage in any long-term training programme is considerable, and it is possible that it might be harder to get them to commit to programmes where the exercise intensity has to be maximum (or at least close to it). This study suggests that improvements in power may be possible if the stimulus is applied for long enough (Fig. 40.1). However, the authors of this study were only able to speculate on mechanisms (qualitative skeletal muscle or neuromuscular factors) to explain such a large increase in P_{max} after an aerobic training programme.

An overview of the studies that have included laboratory-based measures of power shows that most have been short in duration, have not required the participants to train at maximal intensity, and/or have failed to match the training and criterion assessment methods. Furthermore, there does not appear to be a study where adolescents (male or female) have trained using maximal (high-) intensity exercise with power as the outcome measure. Thus, the influences of age and physical maturity on trainability are not known.

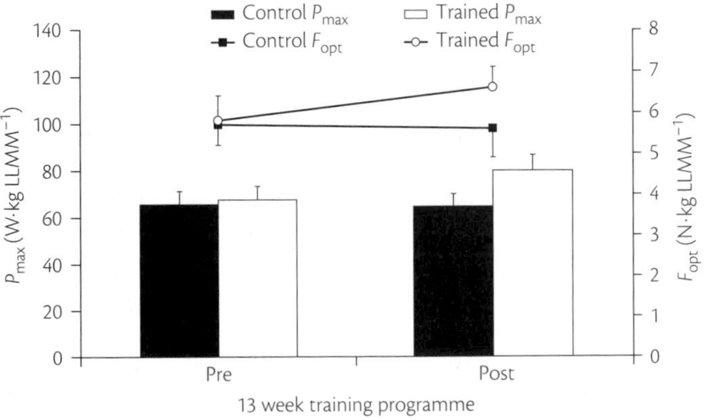

Fig. 40.1 Changes in maximal anaerobic power (P_{max}) and force at which P_{max} was attained (F_{opt}) over a 13-week intervention programme (redrawn from data in Obert *et al.*[12]). Data are mean (SD).

Field-based tests of speed and power

Whether an increased ability to generate power during cycling, to run longer on a motorized treadmill, or to increase concentrations of glycolytic enzymes translates into enhanced physical or sports performance is questionable. Of course, sports performance outcome measures are normally very complex, and it is likely that the changes reviewed above constitute an, as yet ill-defined, fraction of this outcome. Nonetheless, some studies have included physical tasks that are relatively simple to perform with a small skill component and that appear to have an implicit link with the phosphagen or glycolytic energy systems (short running sprints and vertical or horizontal jumps). In one of only two studies that have included adolescent girls, a 14.6% increase in vertical jump (VJ) performance was experienced by those who used an interval training technique with 1:1 work:rest periods.[2] The 22 girls who completed the 8-week continuous running programme also increased VJ by 13.2% compared with only 2.4% for the controls.[2] Although this study suggests that gains in short-term power may be possible through aerobic training, the efficacy of high-intensity training was not examined. The other study included 16-year-old female football players and was unable to detect any difference in VJ or 20 m sprint times between those who completed the additional training or those who simply maintained their normal football training programme [Table 40.1, (15)]. It is somewhat surprising that the combined plyometric and resistance training programme failed to increase VJ given that it included squats, leg extensions, leg curls, and calf-raises and also numerous single- and double-legged explosive exercises that replicated the VJ action.

Both Baquet *et al.*[3] and Ingle *et al.*[9] studied prepubertal boys, but the training programmes and outcomes were different. The French boys[3] completed a high-intensity interval running programme with an equal emphasis on work and rest intervals. At the end of the 7 weeks, they demonstrated an increase in standing broad jump that was approximately 7% higher than that associated with normal growth. Despite large relative increases (~50%) in muscular strength in lower body exercises (calf raise, back squat, and back squat lunges), the English boys[9] experienced modest gains in both VJ and 40 m sprint times (Table 40.1). It is possible that the low to moderate plyometric intensity was not sufficient to lead to larger improvements in the explosive VJ task. Other than completing the sprint assessment, the training did not include any running exercise. Therefore, the specificity highlighted previously is a likely factor.

At the other end of the maturity spectrum, 11 weeks of training resulted in increases in the low-force portion of the load-vertical jumping curve.[6] Improvements ranged from 5.1 to 13.9% in counter movement jump (CMJ) with external loads from 0 to 30 kg.[6] Mean group changes at the high-force portion of the curve (external loads of 40–60 kg) were similar to the low portion, but presumably a combination of larger inter-individual variation and smaller absolute changes meant that they failed to reach statistical significance. The late-adolescent boys in this study were regional footballers who had at least 5 years of experience playing the game, but none had any experience of the periodized explosive resistance training used in the experiment. The authors extended their findings to add that all increases in CMJ with external loads of 0–20 kg occurred within the first 4 weeks of training with small decrements in performance over the latter 7 weeks of the programme. The explanation posited for this decrease was a combination of pretraining status, an insufficient overload stimulus, a lack of variation in the training programme or the principle of diminishing returns.[6]

In summary, it appears as though changes in field-based tests of speed and power may increase but, as might be expected, this is largely a function of the training programme characteristics. No well-controlled studies that have used maximal intensity exercise training have included field-based measures of speed or power in young people thus precluding a direct examination of these two factors.

Resistance training

Increased muscular strength is a positive attribute for athletes to possess in most sports. It is, therefore, easy to understand why coaches, athletes, exercise trainers, and physiologists would like to identify training methods that enhance muscular strength. The extent to which a child or an adolescent increases his or her strength will be dependent upon how much effort he or she is willing, or able, to donate to the programme and the manner in which the training stimulus is structured systematically.[53] In their excellent review, Kraemer and Ratamess[53] highlighted the following components of a successful resistance training programme: (i) expert instruction, (ii) appropriate goal setting, (iii) evaluation of training progress towards predetermined goals, (iv) correct prescription of the acute programme variables, and (v) specific methods of progression targeting particular areas of muscular fitness. They indicated that these key factors to success in programme design are applicable to any level of fitness or age.

Studies with adults have been designed to identify how manipulation of specific components of the training programme might effect changes in strength. Dudley *et al.*[54] concluded that the omission of eccentric actions from a programme compromised increases in strength. It is well recognized that eccentric muscle contractions may increase the likelihood of muscle soreness in adults.[55] Although evidence linking any type of exercise to muscle soreness in young people is difficult to find, it has been suggested that they should not be deliberately exposed to exercise that might predispose them to muscle soreness.[56] When comparing total-body and upper-/lower-body split workouts in previously untrained women, it was shown that both structures resulted in similar improvements.[57] By manipulating the training load, it has been possible to demonstrate that loads in the range of 1–6RM (~100–80% of one repetition maximum; 1RM) result in the greatest improvements in maximal dynamic strength.[58] These very heavy training loads are normally only recommended for very experienced, resistance trained adults under expert supervision.[59]

Ostrowski *et al.*[60] randomly assigned men to training groups who completed either three, six, or nine sets of standard resistance exercises, four times a week for 10 weeks. Improvements in muscle size, strength, and power were found for all three groups, but there were no between-group differences. On this basis, they suggested that only three sets are necessary when designing a resistance training programme for adults. However, there is no evidence that single-set training can be superior to multiple-set training in adults.[53] The relative contribution of the three energy systems to energy expenditure during resistance exercise is influenced by the length of the rest interval between multiple sets. Therefore, longer rest intervals (i.e. 3 min) may be more effective for increasing maximum strength,[61] whereas shorter intervals (~30 s) may be preferential when muscular endurance is the primary outcome goal.[62] Keeler and colleagues[63] reported that a total (concentric/eccentric) contraction time of 6 s resulted in greater gains in maximal strength across eight different exercises compared with a super slow contraction time of 15 s (39% vs 15% increase respectively). Finally, when training frequency was manipulated, gains in maximum strength and lean body mass were different over a 12-week programme in experienced recreational resistance exercisers.[64] The improvement was approximately 1.6 times larger when spreading the same volume over three sessions per week compared with only a single session. The bites of information provided in this paragraph do not represent a critical review of resistance exercise training programme manipulations with adults. They should, however, highlight that research with adults has extended beyond just attempting to link resistance exercise training with increases in muscular strength. It is clear that more subtle attempts have been made to isolate and vary the components that characterize resistance training programmes in an effort to move closer to what might be regarded as the optimal programme. Of course, a single optimal programme cannot exist because goals vary so widely, as do the people who complete the exercise. Nevertheless, experts in the application of resistance training methods will, no doubt, combine the available scientific evidence with their own methods to design programmes that they hope will lead to optimal gains in strength.

Numerous scientific studies have examined changes in muscle strength in children and adolescents (see below). The majority of these studies were designed specifically to see whether strength *could be* increased through a systematic programme of resistance exercise. Few studies with young people appear to have advanced to the stage where the different components of resistance exercise training programmes have been isolated in an effort to examine their specific influence on muscular strength. Furthermore, given the multitude of factors that effect performance in all sports, only a very limited number of studies have extended their work to link increases in muscle strength with advances in performance directly.

Is resistance training safe?

Before a critical appraisal of the resistance training literature, it is important to review whether resistance training is considered to be safe enough to recommend for young people. Despite doubts expressed by parents, coaches, and exercise trainers who are naturally keen to protect the young people in their care, resistance exercise training can be a very safe activity for this age group. That said, it must be emphasized that children can and have sustained injuries when attempting to improve their strength through resistance training.[65–67] Closer inspection of these sources reveals that the majority of injuries have occurred when children or adolescents have attempted to use lifting techniques for which they have insufficient skill or strength to execute. The primary cause, however, appears to be the absence of appropriate supervision when using free weights. Moreover, injuries have not been reported in controlled, scientific studies that have been designed specifically to increase muscular strength using a well-designed training programme. This is not a unique feature of resistance training in the young; the likelihood of injury for adults in the same situation would also be high. One only has to look at some of the video footages that have been submitted to open-access websites for anecdotal verification of accidents (as opposed to injuries) that have happened. Although these accidents captured on film may appear light hearted, the serious nature of unsupervised resistance exercise in any age group cannot be over-emphasized.

A number of influential groups including the National Strength and Conditioning Association (NSCA),[68] the American Academy of Pediatrics,[69] the British Association of Sport and Exercise Sciences (BASES)[70] and the American College of Sports Medicine (ACSM)[71] have all published guidelines or recommendations for resistance exercise training in young people after concluding that it is a safe form of exercise provided it is closely monitored and the exercise programmes are designed appropriately. Unfortunately, many studies with young people make no reference to the number or lack of injuries sustained over the intervention period. In the absence of this information, it may be possible to conclude that nobody was injured as a direct result of completing the resistance training. However, stronger evidence is provided by studies that have indicated specifically that no injuries were sustained (e.g. 9, 22, 23, 32, 34, 37, 38, 72, 93). Two prominent studies employing retrospective survey techniques suggested lower injury rates from resistance training than in many other sports.[73,74] In the BASES Position Statement,[70] a distinction between injury owing to submaximal resistance exercise and the competitive sports of weightlifting and powerlifting was suggested. A primary goal of these two sports is to lift the maximum amount of weight possible, often using lifting techniques that require considerable expertise (e.g. clean and jerk, snatch, squat, bench press, and deadlift). It has been assumed that these activities might be associated with a higher risk of injury and should, therefore, be avoided until physical and skeletal maturity is reached.[69,75] There are some limited data that may serve to counter this stance. No training days lost to injury were reported in 70 male and female, 7- to 16- year-old weightlifters over a competitive period of 1 year.[76] As long as these young lifters could demonstrate an appropriate technique they were permitted to use maximal or near-maximal lifts in competition. More recently, no injuries were reported in eight male (12.5 years old) and three female (13.7 years old) weightlifters at the USA Weightlifting Development Centre over 28 months of training and 534 competitive clean and jerk/snatch lifts.[77] The authors indicated that medical attention was not required and there was no loss of training time. Furthermore, they emphasized the importance of proper application of scientific theory in conditioning in a conservative manner for this population.

Faigenbaum and co-workers[24–26] have tested standing and seated chest press, leg extension, and leg press strength using maximal lifts (i.e. 1RM) without incident in children ranging from 5 to 12 years. It should be recognized that the children in the aforementioned studies used child-sized resistance training equipment and those with pre-existing contraindications were excluded from the maximal testing. Nevertheless, this is still not an accepted practice universally with young people, and at least one prominent group still advises against it in immature children and adolescents.[69] Faigenbaum and colleagues[72] designed a study that included 32 girls and 64 boys to evaluate the safety and efficacy of maximal strength testing in inexperienced children less than 13 years of age. 1RM strength was assessed on either standing chest press and leg extension ($n = 41$) or on the seated chest press and leg press ($n = 55$ and 54, respectively) using plate-loaded machine exercises. A carefully planned, systematic progression of lifts was performed by each child until the 1RM was demonstrated. No injuries occurred as a direct result of participation in this study, and the participants completed all procedures without incident.[72] In addition, none of the children had to alter or stop their participation in other physical activities owing to muscle soreness. Before anyone reading this considers using the 1RM to assess muscular strength in children, especially those who are inexperienced resistance trainers, you should recognize that experienced professionals conducted the tests in the aforementioned study. Moreover, all of the children were screened for medical contraindications, they participated in an introductory training session prior to testing, and child-sized resistance exercise machines were used throughout the study. The authors did suggest that inexperienced children may require up to 11 testing sets before the 1RM is identified. They indicated that this could aid recruitment and co-ordination of the involved muscle groups. In closing, Faigenbaum *et al.*[72] stressed that unsupervised or poorly performed maximal strength tests are not recommended under any circumstances because of the potential for injury.

In contrast to most studies cited so far, Rians *et al.*[35] (also described briefly in reference 38) used a prospective design to evaluate whether a closely supervised circuit training programme was safe for 18 prepubertal boys (stage one of the secondary sexual characteristics described by Tanner[78]). The boys used eight hydraulic resistive machine stations 3 times·week^{-1} for 14 weeks. During each session, as many lifts as possible were completed within 30 s at each work station with 30 s of rest between stations—the resistance exercise lasted for 30 min. The contractions were only concentric and the load was increased progressively over the 14 weeks. Compared with 10 maturity-matched controls, the concentric work output at the end of the training programme had increased substantially in the trained group (~six-fold difference between groups). Injury surveillance, completed by a doctor, revealed one strength training injury during a shoulder press over the 14-week intervention. Although he rested the shoulder for three sessions, the boy continued to exercise his other muscle groups using the remaining machines. Numerous other musculoskeletal 'complaints' were made by the boys, but they were all resolved by improvements in technique. Biphasic scintigraphy suggested that muscle was not damaged by the training and this was confirmed when non-fractionated, creatine phosphokinase concentrations were not elevated at any stage of the study. Although the epiphyseal plates in the tibia, ulna, and radius of three boys appeared to be abnormal at various stages of the study, Rians *et al.*[35] concluded that the resistance exercise programme was unlikely to be the cause. Of course, this study cannot be used as evidence that 'any' resistance training programme is safe, but a search of the literature reveals others that support these results when a variety of programmes with different characteristics and participants have been examined (e.g. 9,22,37). A quote from the NSCA[68] is an apt way to summarize the safety aspects of resistance exercise training in young people,

'Since the goals of a resistance training program are specific to each child's needs, resistance training programs differ. Various combinations of program variables have proven safe and effective for children as long as program developers use scientific information, established training principles, and common sense. All exercises must be performed using the correct technique, and the ratio of resistance training to rest periods must be carefully monitored to ensure that each child is tolerating the prescribed regimen (p. 70).'

Strength gains

If young people complete a progressive, resistance training programme that overloads the muscle they will increase their muscular strength. This has been shown so often now that the conclusion is beyond doubt.[68,79–83] This section of the chapter will review a selection of prospective training studies that have strong research design features and may, therefore, be used as exemplars to support the efficacy of resistance exercise to increase strength in both children and adolescents. Moreover, some of the studies have been featured as most of the previous reviews pre-date their publication and they may also include sport-specific training characteristics or athletic study participants. Reference will be made to the summary of prospective resistance training studies in Table 40.2. Although other prospective training studies were located in the literature,[84–96] they have not been included in this table. This is because they have either been published in insufficient detail (e.g. missing training programme characteristics) or they include research design flaws that preclude a judgment regarding the efficacy of the intervention procedures (e.g. no control group or condition for comparison).

Training programme characteristics

The overall training volume (intensity in particular) is recognized as the most important factor when considering gains in strength following a resistance training programme.[80,97,98] This volume is made up of several different components including the resistive load, the number of times the load is moved before a rest is taken (repetitions), the number of sets (groups of repetitions), session frequency (how many per week), and total programme length (weeks). The diversity of these components within the literature precludes definitive evidence of a dose-response relationship between training volume and gains in strength in young people. However, it may be possible to tease out some trends that may be used to plan future resistance training programmes that are both safe and may lead to changes that are closer to optimal.

Programme length

The longest controlled study required the participants to train for 26 weeks,[18] whereas a less onerous commitment was required to complete the shortest that lasted only 5 weeks.[31] These extremes do not reflect the majority of training studies that range from 8 to 12 weeks in duration (Table 40.2). Studies of 2–3 months probably reflect school semester dates (i.e. when the participants are available to complete the research study) and a sense of how difficult it is to recruit and retain young volunteers to any kind of exercise intervention. This is especially pertinent if the primary purpose of the study is to examine a research-driven outcome as opposed to an intrinsically motivated goal set personally by the participants. It is interesting to note, however, that both the longest and shortest studies resulted in similar sizeable increases in strength relative to the controls. Differences in baseline strength, participant characteristics, and mode of training mean that this is an overly simplistic comparison and the discussion that follows may reveal other factors that are more important than programme length. Nevertheless, a meta-analysis indicated that programme length shared a significant positive relationship ($r = 0.22$; $p \leq 0.04$) with the 115 effect sizes for changes in muscular strength from the prospective training studies included in the analyses.[82] In contrast, Falk and Tenenbaum's meta-analysis[81] suggested that this link was still to be determined in children. The 50 girls in the Nielsen *et al.*[31] study is the largest sample identified, and they are likely to have been heterogeneous for age/maturation based on the division by stature reported in the paper. The mean change in strength was larger than the two other studies that also employed isometric training and testing modes.[20,29] This may reflect between study differences in the weekly training volume. For example, 72 maximal contractions were required each week in a study lasting only 5 weeks,[31] whereas the adolescent boys completed only 36 contractions per week at 90% of maximal force in the 9-week study of De Konig.[20]

A mid-study evaluation of strength after 13 weeks revealed that approximately 90% of the increases reported by Blimkie *et al.*[18] over the full duration of the study were present after the first half of the programme (Fig. 40.2). This might suggest that the girls' muscles had reached a point where the training volume was insufficient to stimulate any further gains in strength. However, at least half of the 16 girls in the training group were reported to have lost their enthusiasm for this modality of exercise over the latter stages of the 26 weeks; thus, a combination of submaximal effort and a lack of interest may be a factor underlying the reduced gains in strength over the final 13 weeks of the study.[18] A similar observation was made in a study of prepubertal boys when comparing changes after 10 weeks with those at the end of the 20-week intervention period[34] (Fig. 40.2). Of the 22% total gain in leg press strength (1RM), almost 17% occurred in the first half of the study. In contrast, although the 35% increase in bench press 1RM was divided equally between the two 10-week phases of the programme, both resulted in significant increases (20 and 15%). Some researchers have re-assessed strength periodically over the duration of the training programme in an effort to maintain the overload stimulus. Unfortunately, the changes in strength at these different points have not been reported precluding comparisons other than pre to post (e.g. 9,23).

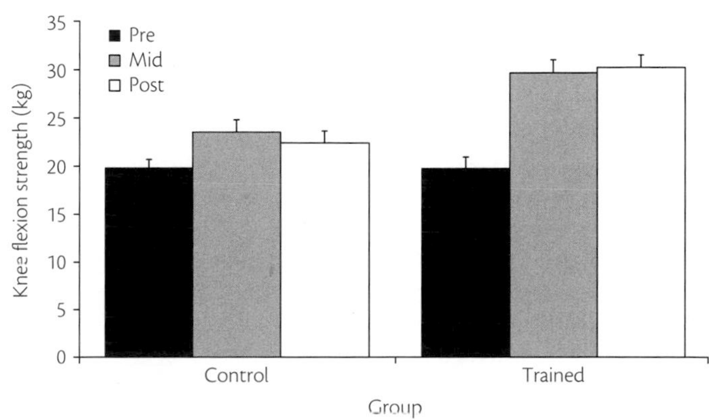

Fig. 40.2 Temporal changes in knee flexion muscular strength (kg) over a 26 week resistance training period (redrawn from data in Blimkie *et al.*[18]). Pre—before training; Mid—after 13 weeks of training; Post—after 26 weeks of training. Data are mean (SEM).

Training load

The sub-section on safety aspects provided some evidence and commentary to show that resistance training can be safe for children and adolescents. Although some of this evidence includes examples of heavy training loads[76] and even maximal testing[72] or competitive lifts,[77] most recommendations tend to adopt a cautionary tone by suggesting loads allowing at least 8–15 repetitions before momentary fatigue with a leaning towards the lighter end of this continuum. This is especially the case when considering younger children and/or those who are experiencing resistance exercise for the first time.[68,69] Of course, it is sensible for adults who are new to this mode of exercise to start gently to avoid (excessive) muscle soreness that may be felt after 48 hours of the session. However, athletes who are well accustomed to resistance exercise rarely increase maximal strength if they train with loads that permit more than 12 repetitions without failure.[58] Thus, the best combination of load and volume is probably in the 6–12RM loading range for adults[99] with only advanced levels of training using a 1–6RM range (80–85% 1RM).[100] Experts in resistance training methods suggest that focusing on just one intensity, for all sessions is very likely to lead to training plateaus or the deleterious symptoms of overtraining.[53] Thus, it is common practice for experienced resistance trainers to use various loading strategies in an effort to optimize strength, muscle size, and muscular endurance.[101] In contrast, there is insufficient evidence to determine whether any particular loading strategy results in optimal strength gains in young people while ensuring the safety of the participants.

Many of the trained participants in Table 40.2 are described explicitly as having no previous experience of resistance training. Therefore, it is not surprising that 10RM or lighter was the load of choice for a number of studies involving young people (e.g. 9, 17, 18, 21, 22, 26, 33, 35, 37, 38). However, after excluding studies that used maximal or near-maximal isometric contractions as the training load,[20,29,31] it is still clear that some researchers have encouraged the participants to exercise with loads that led to failure in less than 10 lifts.[16,19,23–25,27,28,30,32,34,36] What is particularly notable is that several of these studies with the heavier loads were also quite brief, lasting only 8 or 9 weeks and the participants were pre- or early pubescent.[23–25,27,32,36] Although the brevity of the programmes might suggest that participants must have been exposed to quite heavy lifting from the outset of the studies, closer scrutiny of the methods shows that well-established training principles and subtle research design features were used to good effect. For example, introductory training sessions[2–4] preceded the main programme to habituate the children with the lifting techniques and to reduce the impact of a learning effect on the outcome strength variable; a progressive warm-up served to ramp the load prior to the heavier exercises; child-sized machines were used in most studies by Faigenbaum;[22–27,72] elbow flexion was the only exercise performed by the participants;[32] and/or the heaviest load was only lifted in the final set of three.[36] What is remarkable about this latter study is that the boys used free weights to perform bench press and squat exercises. Both of these require more advanced technical ability than machine-based or single-joint exercises. Critically, trained professionals supervised the training sessions and spotters assisted with all lifts to eliminate any training-related injuries in this study. Faigenbaum and associates manipulated the training load in two separate studies using programmes that were designed specifically for inexperienced prepubertal boys and girls[25,27] (Fig. 40.3). In the first of these studies, greater gains than the control group in 1RM chest press strength over an 8-week intervention period were only evident in children who used either a high repetition, moderate load (13–15 repetitions; ~68% of initial 1RM) or a low repetition, heavy load (6–8 repetitions) combined with medicine ball exercises programme (complex training; ~73% of initial 1RM). A group that only trained with a heavy load (6–8 repetitions; ~79% of initial 1RM) experienced an increase in strength that was only comparable with normal growth and development (i.e. control).

The latter study examined the efficacy of using a load that would normally be associated with muscular endurance rather than strength (15–20 repetitions; ~52% of initial 1RM) and compared this with a low repetition maximum load (6–10 repetitions; ~66% of initial 1RM) (Table 40.2). Both load × repetition combinations resulted in significant increases in 1RM chest press strength (21–23%) following 8 weeks of training compared with the control (1%). However, only the high-repetition, low-load group demonstrated an increase (42%) in local muscular endurance that was significantly higher than the control group (4%). The authors emphasized that these studies were designed for practical purposes to identify the most effective programme for untrained children using only a single-set protocol (Table 40.2). Consequently, these results may not apply directly to trained children or young athletes.[25,27] It was suggested that a periodized conditioning programme may provide a yet more effective stimulus when considering training over an extended period—such a study has yet to appear in the literature. Based on these results, it was concluded that untrained children should adopt a high repetition, moderate or low load (13–15RM; ~70% 1RM or 15–20RM; ~52% 1RM), and single set approach to resistance training during the initial adaptation period.[25,27] The authors conceded that this recommendation is not necessarily based on optimizing strength gains in the long term. In order to do this, higher total training volumes using more sets and greater training frequency might be required, but at the possible expense of an enjoyable, sustainable exercise experience.[27] These results are at odds with training programmes designed to

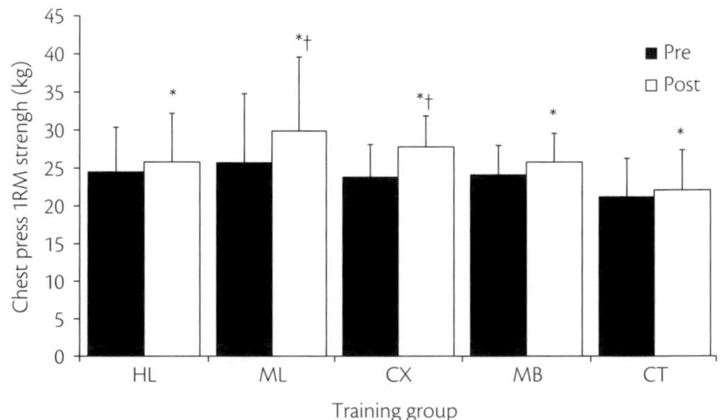

Fig. 40.3 Gains in one repetition maximum chest press strength across five groups where training load was manipulated (redrawn from data in Faigenbaum *et al.*[25]). HL = heavy load, low-repetition; ML = moderate-load, high-repetition; CX = complex training; MB = medicine ball; CT = control. Data are mean (SD). *within-group difference between pre and post ($P < 0.05$); †difference compared with CT ($P < 0.05$).

optimize strength development in adults where heavier loads are more effective where strength is the primary outcome.[102] This may be a function of differences in total training volume between programmes because this was not standardized in either study by Faigenbaum.[25,27] The long-term effects of this type of programme (beyond 8 weeks) are yet to be examined.

Frequency

Physical activity recommendations for young people suggest that they should experience resistance exercise twice a week.[103–105] Two-thirds of the studies summarized in Table 40.2 exceed this by using a frequency of three sessions per week. For young athletes to incorporate resistance training into their overall schedule, it may be prudent to identify the best combination of the main training characteristics. It is not really possible to evaluate the influence of the resistance training programme length or load without also giving due consideration to the weekly frequency that the exercise is undertaken. The combination of these factors, in conjunction with the number of sets and repetitions, determine the total training load to which the muscle is exposed during the intervention. The frequency must be viewed as an important characteristic for practical reasons because it may have a significant bearing on training compliance or the feasibility of including a resistance training component in an athlete's schedule that is already full of specific performance (skill) tasks.

In an effort to identify an optimal training frequency, Gillam[28] randomly assigned 68 mid- to late-adolescent boys to five independent groups who trained from one to five (inclusive) times a week for 9 weeks. Percentage and absolute changes in bench press 1RM tended to increase sequentially with training frequency with those training five times experiencing gains that exceeded all other groups[28] (Table 40.2, Fig. 40.4). Furthermore, there appeared to be a 'threshold' of thrice weekly training but with no discernable difference between single and twice weekly sessions. An untrained control group was not included in the study, so it is not possible to know whether the two lowest frequencies (once and twice) were any more effective than normal growth and maturation. More importantly, it is not reasonable to conclude, as Gillam did, that increased frequency is associated with greater adaptations because overall training load also varied across the five groups. Such a conclusion could only be based on a research design where total training load was equal across the groups and frequency was the only component free to vary.

In contrast, Stahle *et al.*[94] concluded that training twice per week was as effective as thrice weekly, compared with no training, over a 9-month period in a mixed maturity group of boys (7–16 years). Unfortunately, this study was published only as a conference abstract and does not include sufficient training programme details to determine whether the volume of training was equal across the two interventions described. Westcott[97] has shown in adults that the training load is more critical than frequency regardless of how it is applied. When the training volume was constant but frequency varied, upper body strength gains were similar across groups who trained one, two, three, or five times a week.[97]

Faigenbaum *et al.*[26] advanced our knowledge of training frequency by including an untrained control group but they failed to standardize the training load between groups. Thus, it is only possible to conclude from their results that one training session per week, with a single lifting set, for 8 weeks in pre- and early-pubertal children is sufficient to increase leg press 1RM strength (Table 40.2). In contrast, it was suggested that this training volume was not enough for increasing upper body strength (chest press). However, the authors did allude to low statistical power (high probability of a type II error) when considering the chest press results. Finally, increases in bench and leg press 1RM strength were induced by 12 weeks of pre-season progressive resistance training in pubescent baseball players.[21] The boys were then randomly assigned to in-season 'maintenance' resistance training groups who trained either once or twice a week. Although the training volume was double in the twice weekly group, both experimental groups were able to conserve their pre-season strength gains to the same extent when compared with an independent group who did not include resistance exercise over the same 12-week in-season period (Table 40.2). These results suggest that to maintain increases in strength may require only a single training session a week in athletic boys. It is important to note that the training load was not increased progressively over the maintenance period for fear of injuring the boys. Moreover, although the initial training programme included loads of 50 to 100% of the 10RM, the maintenance load was only 50 to 75% of

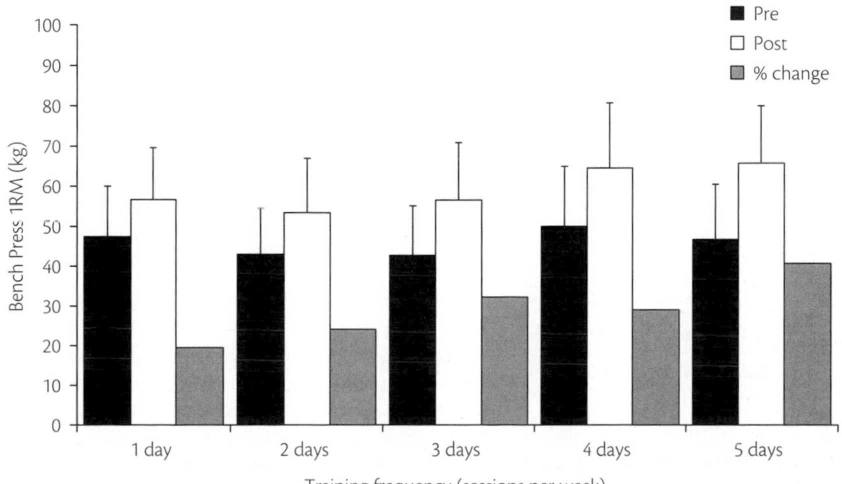

Fig. 40.4 Influence of resistance training frequency on one repetition maximum bench press strength. Training volume was not standardized across the five groups in this study. redrawn from data in Gillam[28] Data are mean (SD).

the 10RM.[21] Limitations of this study are the relatively small sample size from which to extrapolate the findings and that the boys in the independent control group appeared to experience greater pre-season gains in both absolute and relative strength than the boys in the other two groups.

Sex effect

Only a single published study has been located where the results for prepubertal girls have been analysed independently from the boys.[96] In his introduction, Westcott suggested that the number of girls and women using strength training facilities was becoming commonplace in 1979. Although it is not clear what evidence this assertion was based on, it would be hard to disagree with his sentiment that this 'fact' was long overdue and a welcome state of affairs. Sadly, a notable feature of Table 40.2 is the paucity of studies that have included just girls despite the upbeat tone from Westcott. At first glance, it would appear from Westcott's study[96] that girls (8–13 years; 23% and ~4.5 kg) may experience both larger relative and absolute increases in strength than women (19–27 years; 8% and ~2.3 kg). Furthermore, the females in this study completed just 10 training sessions spread over 3 weeks. However, a number of research design limitations mean that these results have not featured in other reviews of this topic.[39,82,83,106] Most notable is the omission of a control group although it might conceivably be argued that changes ranging from 8 to 23% across the groups are likely to be in excess of those due just to normal growth over such a short period of time. It is also not clear how many participants from each of the three age groups used the DeLorme, Berger. and Pyramid training methods that were compared in this study and, despite using pre- and post-adolescent descriptors for the two extreme groups, chronological age was used to define the groups. Finally, the conversion of changes that occurred over the 3 weeks to estimated weekly changes is based on an assumption that gains in strength are linear over time or relative to the overload. This is yet to be supported using a randomized, controlled study involving sufficient numbers of young people. Therefore, we still await stronger evidence to support these interesting, yet exploratory findings with girls of different age from almost 30 years ago.[95]

A feature of the work published by the group led by Faigenbaum is that mixed sex volunteer groups are normally included and pooled together for analyses on the grounds that the training response is 'fairly similar' prior to puberty.[26] Although there is little reason to believe that this statement is anything less than accurate, it is intriguing that supporting data do not appear to be available from a well-controlled study in which the boys and girls have been matched for potential confounding variables at the outset (e.g. physical maturation, baseline strength, training experience, muscle size, habitual physical activity) although completing an identical resistance training programme also. Although Siegel *et al.*[92] compared prepubertal boys and girls directly; they did not provide enough information to quantify the training volume, and the boys were reported to be significantly stronger at baseline. Furthermore, although the authors suggested that the training response between the sexes was similar, the elbow flexion and extension results from the cable tensiometer indicated that training resulted in reduced strength rather than the expected increase.[92] Therefore, this study does not further our understanding of potential between sex variations in resistance training adaptations. Falk and Tenenbaum's[81] meta-analysis did not unearth a distinct sex effect in prepubertal children, but the mean effect size for girls (0.81; r^2 = 0.69) in Payne *et al.*'s[82] analysis was marginally larger than that calculated from the studies involving boys (0.72; r^2 = 0.57). It is debatable whether this represents a meaningful difference between the sexes because the analysis was only based on 23 effect sizes for the girls. The authors suggested the greater effect in the girls may have reflected a more mature cohort compared with the boys, but this speculation appeared to be based primarily on chronological age data. Differences in baseline strength, with girls generally being weaker than boys of a similar age, is a more plausible explanation.[82]

Maturation effect

It is difficult to judge whether physical maturation or age influence strength trainability because of the lack of uniformity in training characteristics, strength testing methods, and participant demographics within the categories that have been compared. Direct comparisons within single studies are very rare. A study by Vrijens[95] is often cited in reviews, commentaries, and experimental research articles because it suggested that prior to the onset of puberty, at least in boys, it was not possible to increase muscular strength through resistance training. Vrijens implied that the apparent maturity effect was because of a difference in androgenic hormones. Since its original publication, this paper has gained certain notoriety because many studies with prepubertal boys (sometimes mixed with girls) have provided evidence to the contrary (Table 40.2). Furthermore, this study has been justly criticized for the omission of an untrained control group, and it has also been suggested that the mismatch between the training and testing modes of exercise, and a relatively low-training volume contributed to the null finding in the prepubertal boys.[80] In Vrijens' defense, the missing control group does not explain why leg and arm strength were not enhanced by the intervention. It is interesting to note that two separate studies that appear to have employed a lower total training volume with a similar number of prepubertal children reported large changes in strength over exactly the same training period.[24,26] Moreover, mismatches between training and testing modes have been published elsewhere (e.g. 33); in fact, Ramsay *et al.*[34] purposely adopted this strategy to eliminate a motor learning bias in the assessment of strength gains. The level of training compliance in the Vrijens' study[95] was not reported, but it might be assumed that this would have been raised in the discussion had it been a contributory factor. As expected, the prepubertal boys were weaker at baseline than their more mature counterparts; thus, a ceiling effect is also unlikely to have resulted in the depressed changes in strength experienced by this group. The beauty of this study, albeit inadvertent, is that it was the catalyst for several studies to provide the alternative prospective that is now generally accepted–prepubertal boys (and girls) are capable of increasing muscular strength via a structured, progressive resistance training programme. Whether the magnitude of this improvement is similar as children mature has yet to be unequivocally established.

Only one study to date has used a recognized method for estimating physical maturation where the experimental groups have also completed an identical resistance programme of sufficient volume to induce gains in strength.[33] However, the comparison between 9 young adults, and 14 prepubertal, and 10 pubertal boys is rather difficult to decipher despite the authors' assertion that

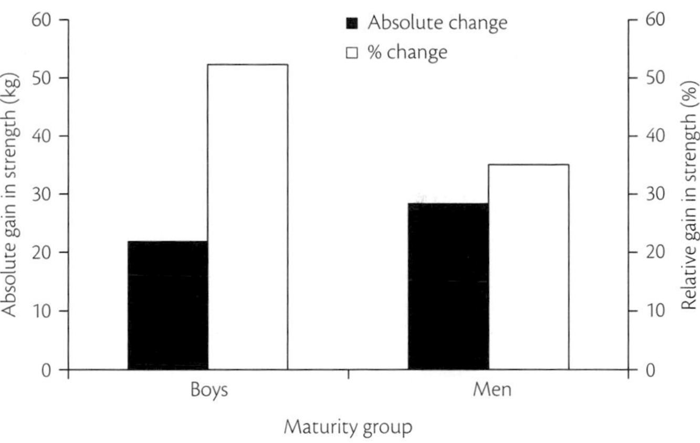

Fig. 40.5 Comparison of absolute and relative (percentage) gains in squat exercise muscular strength between pubescent boys and men (redrawn from data in Sailors and Berg,[36]).

only 3 of the 16 strength tests resulted in greater gains for the least mature group. It is not clear whether the statistical procedures were appropriate when considering the complexity of the analyses across experimental groups, left–right body side, extension–flexion contractions, and contraction speeds. Unfortunately, the authors did not provide any raw mean or standard deviation data for strength precluding an alternative interpretation.

The aforementioned meta-analysis,[81] which included 54 effect sizes (ES) from nine studies with participants who were described as children, reported that the overall weighted mean ES was 0.57. After discarding the three studies with extreme ES, the majority of studies in this analysis showed that gains in muscular strength varied between 14 and 30% above that, which would be expected from normal growth and development. Although it was not possible to determine whether age affected the strength gains identified in the meta-analysis, the authors did indicate that adolescents probably experience greater absolute increases than children following similar training programmes, but the relative improvements are larger in the youngest age groups because of the lower baseline strength. Although Sailors and Berg[36] compared small groups of pubescent boys with young men rather than preadolescents, changes in squat, bench press, and arm curl between the groups partially support these suggested patterns in relative and absolute change (Fig. 40.5). When Payne *et al.*[82] used the average age at peak height velocity (PHV) from the literature to categorize participants into 'younger' or 'older' groups it resulted in similar ES (0.75 vs 0.69). The relatively small number of ES (n = 11) for the older group means that further evidence is warranted before it can be assumed that neither age nor maturity influence strength gains following resistance training.

Longevity of strength gains

A small collection of prospective studies has reported the persistence in strength gains after the training programme had finished. Sewall and Micheli[37] did not provide any specific details of the 9-week non-training (detraining) period that followed the reported increases in strength in 10 prepubertal children (Table 40.2), and they did not track changes in an untrained control group over the same period. For knee and shoulder extension the detraining changes were very small (<–1.4%), whereas shoulder flexion strength actually increased by approximately 65.5%. Interestingly, knee flexion, which was used as a control exercise because it was not part of the initial strength training programme, decreased the maximum over the detraining period (–2.5%). Without a matched untrained comparison over the same period, it is not possible to evaluate these results with any confidence.

In another study,[85] small groups (n = 6) of prepubertal boys completed either 1 day a week maintenance training (MT) or complete detraining (DT) after demonstrating large increases in strength over a 20-week resistance training period (see Ramsay *et al.*[34] in Table 40.2). Although a matched control group was included in this study, the details have only been published in a conference abstract or in a slightly expanded form in a previous review.[80] This current interpretation is based on the figures used to illustrate the results in Blimkie's review.[80] The growth related gains in strength shown by the controls over this 8-week period were only matched by the MT group for isometric knee extension (DT regressed for this measure of strength). For bench press 1RM and isometric elbow flexion, the MT group maintained their increased level of strength relative to the controls; a similar pattern was also experienced by the DT. However, for double leg press 1RM, all three groups experienced a decline in strength, but the magnitude of change was greatest in MT and DT. It is important to note that upper body strength of the controls, prior to the 8-week experimental period, was considerably lower than that seen in both the MT and DT boys. In combination, these results suggest that although training-induced strength gains in children are not permanent, the strength advantage over untrained children is still seen after 8 weeks regardless of maintenance or complete cessation of the resistance training stimulus. However, normal growth (maturation and development) has a powerful influence on strength, but it only appears to exert this influence in children who do not express the extra advantage accrued from a 20-week resistance training programme (i.e. no additive effect). It would have been interesting to see how the three small groups of boys compared after 20 weeks.

Faigenbaum[23] advanced our understanding of the temporal changes in strength (loss) following training in children (see Table 40.2 for summary of gains) by taking measurements twice at 4-week intervals during a detraining period. Reductions in chest press were evenly distributed over the two 4-week blocks of detraining (–9% and –10%) whereas leg extension 1RM strength decreased dramatically (–21%) over the first period followed by a smaller non-significant reduction (–7%) over the latter half of detraining. A matched untrained control group did not change over this time, but their leg strength was no different to the detrained group after 8 weeks. In contrast, although the reductions in chest press were substantial, the previously trained group of children still maintained a small strength differential over the untrained controls in the upper body at the end of the study.[23] It has been suggested that decrements in strength may be related to the size of training increases, but simple measures of association did not support this in the study reviewed above (r = 0.23 and 0.33 for chest press and leg extension, respectively). The authors speculated that activities outside of the experimental manipulation may have contributed to the dramatic reductions, but there was no direct evidence to support this. Furthermore, prevailing logic might suggest that weight-bearing activities of daily living should help to maintain leg strength rather than attenuate it. Thus,

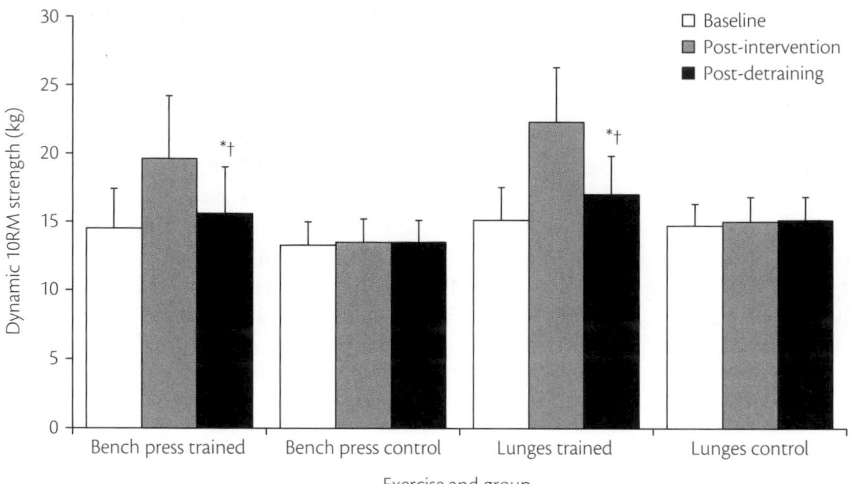

Fig. 40.6 Persistence in resistance training induced gains in muscular strength in early pubertal boys (redrawn from data in Ingle *et al.*[9]). Data are mean (SD). * difference between trained and control boys post-detraining ($P < 0.01$); †within-group difference between baseline and post-detraining ($P < 0.01$).

greater reductions might have been expected for the chest where presumably the muscles are not used to the same extent on a daily basis and rarely bear the entire body weight.

Finally, Ingle *et al.*[9] provided further supportive evidence that, regardless of the finer details of how muscular strength gains change when there is no overload stimulus, strength does regress to the untrained state given sufficient time. It was apparent in this study that both upper and lower body muscles can retain a small proportion of the hard gotten gains, but on average 75% was lost over the 12-week detraining period (Fig. 40.6).

Summary of training programmes: The variety of combinations reported in the literature does not permit the identification of an optimal resistance training programme. However, if an increase in strength is sought then it would appear that this may be achieved, in the short term, using this diversity to good effect. Most practitioners agree that resistance training needs to be enjoyable for it to be sustainable over periods longer than those seen in Table 40.2. Variety is often seen as the key to enjoyment along with measurable gains in strength and a mixture of other physical or sporting activities to accompany the resistance work. Therefore, by combining many of the features summarized in Table 40.2, it should be possible to plan a progressive programme that is fun, safe, and effective. Young athletes who have no experience of resistance training will probably benefit from an initial introductory period that provides a moderate overload stimulus and only needs to be experienced on two occasions per week. It may be prudent to start with single set exercises for a variety of muscle groups progressing to multiple sets when the total training load needs to increase to provide the necessary overload stimulus. If time is an obstacle, then athletes may wish to include only those exercises that have been shown to relate to performance in their chosen sport rather than a holistic total body programme. As resistive load shares an inverse relationship with the number of repetitions, a high repetition-moderate load regimen (13–15 repetitions; ~65–70% 1RM) should suffice in the early stages. Again, as the required overload stimulus increases, a higher load could be combined with fewer repetitions (6–12 repetitions; ~70–80% 1RM). Of course, variations around this general theme are to be encouraged if they increase the athlete's motivation to train, provided they are safe and effective in achieving planned goals.

There is not enough evidence to suggest that girls and boys should adopt different training strategies. Similarly, differences in age and/or physical maturation do not appear to be significant factors when considering programme design, although it would be wise to base decisions on previous experience of resistance training and overall body size (baseline strength) when considering the training load.

Unless young athletes (children and early adolescents) are using resistance training to compete in weight lifting events, there does not appear to be any compelling reason why they should be exposed to heavy training loads until it is evident that further gains in muscular strength may only be achieved via a carefully planned, progressive increase in this component of the programme (i.e. after increases in sets and frequency have been explored). Even then, this may only be warranted if there is unequivocal evidence that such an increase will definitely benefit their sports performance without any deleterious side effects such as overtraining or training-related injuries.

Mechanisms for increased strength

Hypertrophy

Of the eight studies summarized in Table 40.2 that included girth (circumference) measurements of various body sites as a crude estimation of changes in muscle size,[16,19,20,22,29,32,36,38] only one reported an interaction between the control and trained groups.[38] The relative increases for the trained prepubertal boys in this study ranged from 1.8% to 4.1% for chest, shoulder, and average abdomen circumference. Unfortunately, they could not be linked to the much larger increases in isokinetic strength (range 19–37%) because only torque around the knee and elbow joints were measured.[38] The characteristics (1st row Table 40.2) of this small sample of studies suggest that the training was relatively short-lived on average (~11 weeks), the participants were not previously experienced in the use of resistance training methods, and most were either prepubertal or in the early stages of puberty. Although testosterone, growth hormone (GH), insulin-like growth factor 1 (IGF-1), and insulin all influence muscle hypertrophy during normal growth and maturation,[107] their interaction with resistance training is not clear. The consensus from experts[80,108] and the empirical data suggest muscle hypertrophy is not likely to occur following a resistance training programme unless in the presence of sufficient circulating testosterone. The possibility that muscle size measurements have lacked sensitivity (precision) and the stimulus for change in muscle morphology has been lacking cannot be dismissed completely. The use of quite basic anthropometric measurements (limb girths and skinfolds) is open to considerable variation and cannot isolate the muscle tissue.

In contrast, Mersch and Stoboy[91] used the more precise technique of magnetic resonance imaging (MRI) to quantify changes in anatomical cross section area (aCSA) of the knee extensors and flexors. The two prepubertal monozygotic twin boys in this study had demonstrated a 38% increase in isometric knee strength after 10 weeks of unilateral isometric knee extensor training. Muscle hypertrophy in the trained leg varied from 4.0% to 9.2% depending on which segment of the quadriceps was measured; this is probably linked to the well-known observation that muscle tension varies over the range of movement when moving a fixed external load or it varies across the muscle length during an isometric contraction. This variation in muscle hypertrophy has been reported in other studies with adults and highlights that if the relatively small increases in muscle size that may occur in children are to be detected, then several measurements over the length of the muscle may be required.[109] Of course, it would be foolish to use the results from a single study with such a small sample to offset the weight of contrasting evidence that suggests hypertrophy is not an underlying cause of strength gains prior to puberty. However, it does provide a strong rationale for a future longer-term study where similar precise measurements of muscle size might be used to resolve this intriguing research question.

Fukunaga *et al.*[89] used ultrasonography measurements of the upper arm to conclude that it may be possible for children (skeletal age 6.2–10.7 years) to experience increases in aCSA following isometric elbow flexion training. On average, the increase in aCSA was 10.4% compared with only 5.0% in maturity-matched controls. Unfortunately, they did not give specific details of the ultrasound measurements and surprisingly the changes in elbow extensor strength and size were greater than those reported for the flexors. It was not surprising that skeletal age explained only 13% of the variance in aCSA change given all of the children in this study were probably still prepubertal. Despite the findings from these two studies procuring non-invasive *in vivo* measurements of muscle, the reported gains in strength in most studies with young people far outreach the small increases in muscle size.

If we assume that children need more testosterone to facilitate an increase in muscle size, it would make sense that adolescent boys, who experience a large increase in this androgen at the onset of puberty, should find that muscle hypertrophy parallels improvements in strength. However, a search of the literature reveals that this is not well supported by empirical data. The paucity of evidence may reflect that the majority of research in this field has been with children, that adolescents normally train only for up to 12 weeks, or that studies have simply not included an assessment of muscle size. Using soft-tissue roentgenography, Vrijens[95] measured aCSA of the thigh and upper arm before and after an 8-weeks isotonic (constant external resistance) training programme in 12 adolescent boys (16.7 years). The average increase of 25% in arm strength appeared to be due in part to a 14.3% increase in upper arm aCSA; however a similar increase in leg strength saw an increase of only 4.6% in thigh aCSA. The larger increase in arm aCSA may have been dependent on the pre-training size, or it is possible that the tissue scan was made at a point along the muscle length where the increase was at its greatest in the arm, but not the thigh. Insufficient detail is given in the paper to determine exactly where these measurements were made. The changes in aCSA are still quite small considering that boys were likely to be approaching full physical maturity; it has been suggested that the boys experienced only a relatively low volume training stimulus.[80] In the only other published study to measure both changes in size and strength in adolescent twins (14.9 years) following resistance training, Komi *et al.*[29] found that a 20% increase in maximum isometric knee extension force was not matched by a change in thigh girth (1.6%). Changes in limb girths reported in the Vrijens study[95] were much smaller than the roentgenographic scans (upper arm 3.9% and thigh 2.0%), again suggesting that this method is not sensitive enough to detect more subtle changes in the underlying muscle. Moreover, any conclusions based on data from only six participants are open to question.

The large increase in circulating hormones and growth factors at the onset of puberty stimulates a period of rapid growth and development in lean tissue in boys. It is conceivable that this stimulus might be so strong that it could override the influence of any other external factors on muscle size including resistance training. As pubertal changes in girls are different, it would be interesting to see if resistance training during a period of rapid growth in boys and girls resulted in a differential outcome. This hypothesis does not appear to have been tested in the literature, but there is some support for it when considering maximal oxygen uptake ($\dot{V}O_2$ max) measurements in twins.[110] A study with young women that assessed temporal changes in the lean mass of the trunk, legs, and arms using DEXA suggested that changes in muscle size were related to the complexity of the exercise task.[111] Those muscles that were used in more complex, multi-joint movements (e.g. bench press and leg press) experienced delays in hypertrophy relative to those used in simple movements (e.g. biceps curl). They declared that this delay reflected a prolonged neurological adaptation that needed to precede an increase in lean tissue.[111] Although this finding was not supported by the arm and leg computerized axial tomography (CAT) scans reported by Ramsay *et al.*[34], it may provide another avenue for future research where precise measurement techniques are available to quantify changes in muscle size and are used in conjunction with techniques that permit the measurement of neurological changes.

Neurological, intrinsic and motor learning

The neurological adaptations that precede and parallel muscle hypertrophy in adults completing a resistance training programme of sufficient overload are well recognized.[112] In the absence of muscle hypertrophy, the logical assumption has been that neurological mechanisms must underpin the increases in strength discussed above. However, direct evidence of this in young people is scant. In a study with adolescents, Komi *et al.*[29] used integrated electromyographic activity (iEMG) of the rectus femoris to assess whether changes in muscular strength following a 12-week resistance training programme could be ascribed to neural adaptations. In an effort to place the electrode pairs in the same place on repeat testing, each site on the skin was marked by a drop of 20% $AgNO_3$ solution. The maximum iEMG in the trained leg increased on average by 37.8%, whereas the changes in the untrained leg and the control member of the twin pair were only 0.6% and 3.3%, respectively. The authors postulated that this increase was a consequence of the training and that it suggested a reduction of inhibitory inputs to the active alpha-motor neurons resulting in a greater flow of activation reaching the muscle site. Although it did not reach statistical significance, the iEMG/tension curve shifted to the right over the 12-week training period in five of the six trained twins, which was interpreted as a more economic use of the rectus femoris. It is difficult to understand how or why the increase in iEMG was almost double the improvement reported in knee extension force; no explanation was provided in the paper.

Ozmun *et al.*[32] also used iEMG, but over the biceps brachii in eight prepubertal children who completed an 8-week elbow flexion, constant external resistance training programme. Both isokinetic (27.8% vs. 15.5%) and isotonic (22.6% vs. 3.8%) strength increased in the trained group compared with a maturity matched, randomly assigned control group. The bigger difference between the trained and control participants for the isotonic strength measurement, compared with isokinetic, was said to be a learning effect or owing to the specificity of the training. However, after initial tests revealed differences between trial one and trials two, four, and five, trial one was discarded for all subsequent ANOVA analyses to counter a potential learning effect. The 16.8% increase in iEMG amplitude for the trained group compared with a 6.0% reduction for the controls could reflect an enhancement in motor unit recruitment, improvement in the firing rate of activated motor units, or alteration of EMG firing patterns according to Ozmun and colleagues.[32] The iEMG amplitude of the trained group was approximately 21% lower than the controls prior to the intervention, whereas the post-intervention values were almost identical suggesting that the baseline values should have been included in the analyses as covariates and that changes may reflect regression to the mean. Ozmun *et al.*[32] also acknowledged that the iEMG electrode placement could have altered between the pre- and post-intervention measurements, thus introducing a source of variability to the results that could not be quantified. However, there is no reason to believe that this source of error would not be randomly distributed between the trained and control groups.

In what has, to date, become the most frequently cited resistance exercise training programme with children, Ramsay *et al.*[34] sought to identify specifically whether changes in muscular strength following resistance training were the result of hypertrophy or neurological function. The 13 boys who were randomly assigned to the 20 weeks of training increased their muscular strength above the growth experienced by the maturity-matched controls; these changes were demonstrated no matter how strength was measured (1RM, isokinetic, isometric). Mid upper-arm and thigh muscle aCSA changes assessed using CAT scans did not differ between the experimental and control boys. A rather unique feature of this study was the use of percutaneous electrical stimulation to evoke muscle contraction in the elbow flexors and knee extensors. That is, a brief electrical stimulus was applied to the muscle in order to evoke a contraction. It was possible to assess twitch torque (TT), time to peak torque (TPT), half-relaxation time (HRT)), and % motor unit activation (%MUA) using this technique. It should be recognized that these methods may be rather uncomfortable or even painful for some individuals; hence they are rarely used with young children. When the pre-intervention %MUA values for all boys were pooled, the value for elbow flexors was 89% and 78% for knee extensors. The training resulted in 13.2% and 17.4% increases, respectively, but this was not statistically significant, perhaps signalling a heterogeneous response within the group. The increases in %MUA were less than the improvements measured in isometric strength, implying that this factor may only partially explain this adaptation. The evoked TT of the elbow flexors and knee extensors both increased after training (~30%). However, no changes in TPT or HRT were reported. Evoked TT changes may be indicative of the intrinsic force-producing capacity of muscle, but the single twitch used in this study, as opposed to very painful tetanic stimulation, is unlikely to induce maximal activation of the muscle. It was suggested that the TT improvements probably meant a change in the excitation–contraction coupling. Some of the strength adaptations occurred early and others late in the 20-week study period. The temporal patterns of change were used to indirectly assess relative levels of baseline conditioning in the different muscle groups. It appears as though gains in strength in the legs may lag behind those seen in the arms because of the daily weight bearing role of the legs. Given that the TT changes were only detected beyond the mid-point of the study, it was suggested that if intrinsic muscle adaptation can be induced by training, then it is only likely to happen after at least 10 weeks of training with a specific, heavy load (refer to Table 40.2 for resistance training programme details). Finally, although modifications in motor unit co-ordination, recruitment, and firing frequency were all mentioned as possible factors, none of these was measured directly in this study.

Summary

- Well-controlled, longitudinal studies with young people that have included maximal or even high-intensity exercise as the stimulus are in short supply. Those that have also included a well-established measurement of anaerobic performance are rarer still. Consequently, it is not possible to generalize from the available research findings to the wider athletic youth population.
- Direct measurements of anaerobic metabolism using both invasive (muscle biopsy) and non-invasive (^{31}P-MRS) measurement techniques have provided some unique insights into this important aspect of paediatric exercise physiology. However, ethical considerations have limited the former studies in several ways; thus, questions still remain regarding the reliability of these findings and the ability to extrapolate beyond the small number of participants on whom they are based. Until the resolution from ^{31}P-MRS can be improved when working with the small muscles that typify children, some doubt is cast over the practical utility of this technique when considering longitudinal research designs.
- Changes in both power-production laboratory tests and field-based tests of power and speed suggest that anaerobic performance may be trainable. However, what is not known about this exercise-induced adaptation far exceeds what is understood currently. Future studies need to include outcome measures that provide a window on anaerobic metabolism but also ask the young participants to train repeatedly at maximal intensities.
- When conducted under close supervision by qualified professionals, resistance exercise training is a safe and efficacious activity that should be part of every young athlete's overall training programme. There is no doubt that children and adolescents can experience substantial gains in muscular strength if they adhere to a progressive training programme that provides

an overload stimulus that is appropriate for their immature body and mind.

- Research to move closer to the resistance training programme that might provide the 'optimal' gains in strength with young people is in its infancy compared with the adult-based scientific literature. The excellent work of Faigenbaum and colleagues has started to move us beyond just recognising that strength can improve in this segment of the population. Individual goals based on sporting needs and baseline physical attributes will dictate just how a training programme might be designed.
- As with adults, it would appear that the total training volume is critical when considering how much a young person might benefit from resistance exercise. This must be tempered with caution when considering the immature, rapidly developing and growing body. Lifting technique is more important than anything else when a person first embarks on a resistance training programme (regardless of age). Only when this is well established can a professional resistance exercise training instructor begin to consider the best training volume for their young charges.
- Data from girls are particularly sparse for both maximal (high-) intensity exercise and resistance training programmes. This ought to provide the focus for future research studies given the tenuous suggestion that young females may experience greater gains in strength than their male counterparts. Furthermore, preparation for and participation in sport by females should be just as focused and meticulously planned as it is for males.
- The mechanism for increased strength in young people is based largely on conjecture and the results from a handful of studies incorporating insightful measurements. The suggestion that muscle hypertrophy is not a significant factor prior to puberty is based on numerous studies; most of which have used imprecise estimations of actual muscle size. Although a combination of neurological, intrinsic muscular, and motor learning mechanisms appear to have received general approval, studies that have examined these systematically in children or adolescents are scarce.

References

1. Stratton G, Reilly T, Williams AM, Richardson D (2004). *Youth soccer: From science to performance*, pp. 199–211. Routledge, London.
2. Adeniran SA, Toriola AL (1988). Effects of continuous and interval running programmes on aerobic and anaerobic capacities in schoolgirls aged 13 to 17 years. *J Sports Med Phys Fitness* **28**, 260–6.
3. Baquet G, Guinhouya C, Dupont G, Nourry C, Berthoin S (2004). Effects of a short-term interval training program on physical fitness in prepubertal children. *J Strength Cond Res* **18**, 708–13.
4. Counil FP, Varray A, Matecki S, Beurey A, Marchal P, Voisin M, Prefaut C (2003). Training of aerobic and anaerobic fitness in children with asthma. *J Pediatr* **142**, 179–84.
5. Diallo O, Dore E, Duche P, Van Praagh E (2001). Effects of plyometric training followed by a reduced training programme on physical performance in prepubescent soccer players. *J Sports Med Phys Fitness* **41**, 342–8.
6. Gorostiaga EM, Izquierdo M, Ruesta M, Iribarren J, Gonzalez-Badillo JJ, Ibanez J (2004). Strength training effects on physical performance and serum hormones in young soccer players. *Eur J Appl Physiol* **91**, 698–707.
7. Grodjinovsky A, Inbar O, Dotan R, Bar-Or O (1980). Training effect on the anaerobic performance of children as measured by the Wingate anaerobic test. In: Berg K, Eriksson BO (eds.), *Children and exercise IX*, pp. 139–45. University Park Press, Baltimore, MD.
8. Hetzler RK, DeRenne C, Buxton BP, Ho KW, Chai DX, Seichi G (1997). Effects of 12 weeks of strength training on anaerobic power in prepubescent male athletes. *J Strength Cond Res* **11**, 174–81.
9. Ingle L, Sleap M, Tolfrey K (2006). The effect of a complex training and detraining programme on selected strength and power variables in early pubertal boys. *J Sports Sci* **24**, 987–97.
10. McManus AM, Armstrong N, Williams CA (1997). Effect of training on the aerobic power and anaerobic performance in prepubertal girls. *Acta Paediatr* **86**, 456–9.
11. Mosher RE, Rhodes EC, Wenger HA, Filsinger B (1985). Interval training: The effects of a 12-week programme on elite, pre-pubertal male soccer players. *J Sports Med Phys Fitness* **25**, 5–9.
12. Obert P, Mandigout M, Vinet A, Courteix D (2001). Effect of a 13-week aerobic training programme on the maximal power developed during a force-velocity test in prepubertal boys and girls. *Int J Sports Med* **22**, 442–6.
13. Rotstein A, Dotan R, Bar-Or O, Tenenbaum G (1986). Effect of training on anaerobic threshold, maximal aerobic power and anaerobic performance of preadolescent boys. *Int J Sports Med* **7**, 281–6.
14. Sargeant AJ, Dolan P, Thorne A (1985). Effects of supplementary physical activity on body composition, aerobic, and anaerobic power in 13-year-old boys. In: Binkhorst RA, Kemper HCG, Saris WH (eds.), *Children and exercise XI*, pp. 135–9. Human Kinetics, Champaign, IL.
15. Siegler J, Gaskill S, Ruby B (2003). Changes evaluated in soccer-specific power endurance either with or without a 10-week, in-season, intermittent, high-intensity training protocol. *J Strength Cond Res* **17**, 379–87.
16. Blanksby B, Gregor J (1981). Anthropometric, strength and physiological changes in male and female swimmers with progressive resistance training. *Aus J Sport Sci* **1**, 3–6.
17. Blimkie CJR, Ramsay J, Sale D, MacDougall D, Smith K, Garner S (1989). Effects of 10 weeks of resistance training on strength development in prepubertal boys. In: Oseid S, Carlsen K-H (eds.), *Children and exercise XIII*, pp. 183–97. Human Kinetics, Champaign, IL.
18. Blimkie CJR, Rice S, Webber CE, Martin J, Levy D, Gordon CL (1996). Effects of resistance training on bone mineral content and density in adolescent females. *Can J Physiol Pharmacol* **74**, 1025–33.
19. Christou M, Smilios I, Sotiropoulos K, Volaklis K, Pilianidis T, Tokmakidis SP (2006). Effects of resistance training on physical capacities of adolescent soccer players. *J Strength Cond Res* **20**, 783–91.
20. De Koning FL, Binkhorst RA, Vissers ACA, Vos JA (1982). Influence of static strength training on the force-velocity relationship of the arm flexors. *Int J Sports Med* **3**, 25–8.
21. DeRenne C, Hetzler RK, Buxton BP, Ho KW (1996). Effects of training frequency on strength maintenance in pubescent baseball players. *J Strength Cond Res* **10**, 8–14.
22. Faigenbaum AD, Zaichkowsky LD, Westcott WL, Micheli LJ, Fehlandt AF (1993). The effects of a twice-a-week strength training program on children. *Pediatr Exerc Sci* **5**, 339–46.
23. Faigenbaum AD, Westcott WL, Micheli LJ, Outerbridge AR, Long CJ, LaRosa-Loud R, Zaichkowsky LD (1996). The effects of strength training and detraining on children. *J Strength Cond Res* **10**, 109–14.
24. Faigenbaum AD, Westcott, WL, LaRosa-Loud R, Long CJ (1999). The effects of different resistance training protocols on muscular strength and endurance development in children. *Pediatrics* **104**, e5.
25. Faigenbaum AD, LaRosa-Loud R, O'Connell J, Glover S, O'Connell J, Westcott, WL (2001). Effects of different resistance training protocols on upper-body strength and endurance development in children. *J Strength Cond Res* **15**, 459–65.

26. Faigenbaum AD, Milliken LA, LaRosa-Loud R, Burak BT, Doherty CL, Westcott, WL (2002). Comparison of 1 and 2 days per week of strength training in children. *Res Q Exerc Sport* **73**, 416–24.
27. Faigenbaum AD, Milliken L, Moulton L, Westcott, WL (2005). Early muscular fitness adaptations in children in response to two different resistance training regimens. *Pediatr Exerc Sci* **17**, 237–48.
28. Gillam GM (1981). Effects of frequency of weight training on muscle strength enhancement. *J Sports Med* **21**, 432–36.
29. Komi PV, Viitasalo JT, Rauramaa R, Vihko V (1978). Effects of isometric strength training on mechanical, electrical, and metabolic aspects of muscle function. *Eur J Appl Physiol* **40**, 45–55.
30. Kotzamanidis C, Chatzopoulos D, Michailidis C, Papaiakovou G, Patikas D (2005). The effect of a combined high-intensity strength and speed training program on the running and jumping ability of soccer players. *J Strength Cond Res* **19**, 369–75.
31. Nielsen B, Nielsen M, Behrendt Hansen M, Asmussen E (1980). Training of functional muscular strength in girls 7–19 years old. In: Berg K, Eriksson BO (eds.), *Children and exercise IX*, pp. 69–78. University Park Press, Baltimore, MD.
32. Ozmun JC, Mikesky AE, Surburg PR (1994). Neuromuscular adaptations following prepubescent strength training. *Med Sci Sports Exerc* **26**, 510–14.
33. Pfeiffer RD, Francis RS (1986). Effects of strength training on muscle development in prepubescent, pubescent, and postpubescent males. *Physician Sports Med* **14**, 134–43.
34. Ramsay J, Blimkie CJR, Smith K, Garner S, MacDougall JD, Sale DG (1990). Strength training effects in prepubescent boys. *Med Sci Sports Exerc* **22**, 605–14.
35. Rians, CB, Weltman A, Cahill BR, Janney CA, Tippett SR, Katch FI (1987). Strength training for prepubescent males: Is it safe? *Am J Sports Med* **15**, 483–9.
36. Sailors M, Berg K (1987). Comparison of responses to weight training in pubescent boys and men. *J Sports Med* **27**, 30–37.
37. Sewall L, Micheli LJ (1986). Strength training for children. *J Pediatr Orthop* **6**, 143–6.
38. Weltman A, Janney C, Rians CB, Strand K, Berg B, Tippitt S, Wise J, Cahill BR, Katch FI (1986). *Med Sci Sports Exerc* **18**, 629–38.
39. Rowland TW (2005). *Children's exercise physiology* (2nd ed.). Human Kinetics, Champaign, IL.
40. Ratel S, Lazaar N, Dore E, Baquet G, Williams CA, Berthoin S, Van Praagh E, Bedu M, Duche P (2004). High-intensity intermittent activities at school: controversies and facts. *J Sports Med Phys Fitness* **44**, 272–80.
41. Zanconato S, Buchthal S, Barstow TJ, Cooper DM (1993). 31P-magnetic resonance spectroscopy of leg muscle metabolism during exercise in children and adults. *J Appl Physiol* **74**, 2214–18.
42. Kuno S, Takahashi H, Fujimoto K, Akima H, Miyamaru M, Nemoto I, Itai Y, Katsuta S (1995). Muscle metabolism during exercise using phosphorus-31 nuclear magnetic resonance spectroscopy in adolescents. *Eur J Appl Physiol* **70,** 301–4.
43. Taylor DJ, Kemp GJ, Thompson CH, Raddar GK (1997). Ageing: Effects on oxidative function of skeletal muscle in vivo. *Mol Cell Biochem* **174**, 321–4.
44. Petersen SR, Gaul CA, Stanton MM, Hanstock CC (1999). Skeletal muscle metabolism during short-term, high intensity exercise in prepubertal and pubertal girls. *J Appl Physiol* **87**, 2151–6.
45. Barker A, Welsman J, Welford D, Fulford J, Williams C, Armstrong N (2006). Reliability of 31P-magnetic resonance spectroscopy during an exhaustive incremental exercise test in children. *Eur J Appl Physiol* **98**, 556–65.
46. Eriksson BO, Gollnick PD, Saltin B. (1973). Muscle metabolism and enzyme activities after training in boys 11–13 years old. *Acta Physiol Scand* **87**, 485–97.
47. Fournier M, Ricci J, Taylor AW, Ferguson RJ, Montpetit RR, Chaitman BR (1982). Skeletal muscle adaptation in adolescent boys: Sprint and endurance training and detraining. *Med Sci Sports Exerc* **14**, 453–6.
48. Cadefau J, Casademont J, Grau JM, Fernandez J, Balaguer A, Vernet M, Cusso R, Urbano-Marquez A (1990). Biochemical and histochemical adaptation to sprint training in young athletes. *Acta Physiol Scand* **140**, 341–51.
49. Cunningham DA, Faulkner JA (1969). The effect of training on aerobic and anaerobic metabolism during a short exhaustive run. *Med Sci Sports* **1**, 65–9.
50. Hill AV (1922). The maximum work and mechanical efficiency of human muscles and their most economical speed. *J Physiol* **56**, 19–41.
51. Davies CTM, Barnes C, Godfrey S (1972). Body composition and maximal exercise performance in children. *Hum Biol* **44**, 195–214.
52. Mercier B, Mercier J, Granier P, Le Gallais D, Prefaut C (1992). Maximal anaerobic power: relationship to anthropometric characteristics during growth. *Int J Sports Med* 13, 21–6.
53. Kraemer WJ, Ratamess NA (2004). Fundamentals of resistance training: Progression and exercise prescription. *Med Sci Sports Exerc* **36**, 674–88.
54. Dudley GA, Tesch PA, Miller BJ, Buchanan MD (1991). Importance of eccentric actions in performance adaptations to resistance training. *Aviat Space Environ Med* **62**, 543–55.
55. Proske U, Allen TJ (2005). Damage to skeletal muscle from eccentric exercise. *Exerc Sport Sci Rev* **33**, 98–104.
56. Bar-Or O (1983). Pediatric sports medicine for the practitioner from physiological principles to clinical applications. Springer Verlag, New York.
57. Calder AW, Chilibeck PD, Webber CE, Sale DG (1994). Comparison of whole and split weight training routines in young women. *Can J Appl Physiol* **19**, 185–99.
58. Campos GE, Luecke TJ, Wendeln HK, Toma K, Hagerman FC, Murray TF, Ragg KE, Ratamess NA, Kraemer WJ, Staron RS. (2002). Muscular adaptations in response to three different resistance-training regimens: Specificity of repetition maximum training zones. *Eur J Appl Physiol* **88**, 50–60.
59. Fry AC, Kraemer WJ (1997). Resistance exercise overtraining and overreaching. Neuroendocrine responses. *Sports Med* **23**, 106–29.
60. Ostrowski KJ, Wilson GJ, Weatherby R, Murphy PW, Lyttle AD (1997). The effect of weight training volume on hormonal output and muscular size and function. *J Strength Cond Res* **11**, 148–54.
61. Robinson JM, Stone MH, Johnson RL, Penland CM, Warren BJ, Lewis RD (1995). Effects of different weight training exercise/rest intervals on strength, power, and high intensity exercise endurance. *J Strength Cond Res* **9**, 216–21.
62. Willardson JM (2006). A brief review: Factors affecting the length of the rest interval between resistance exercise sets. *J Strength Cond Res* **20**, 978–84.
63. Keeler LK, Finkelstein LH, Miller W, Fernhall B. (2001). Early-phase adaptations of traditional-speed vs. superslow resistance training on strength and aerobic capacity in sedentary individuals. *J Strength Cond Res* **15**, 309–14.
64. McLester JR, Bishop P, Guilliams ME (2000). Comparison of 1 day and 3 days per week of equal-volume resistance training in experienced subjects. *J Strength Cond Res* **14**, 273–81.
65. Risser WL, Risser JM, Preston D (1990). Weight-training injuries in adolescents. *Am J Dis Child* **144**, 1015–17.
66. Risser WL (1991). Weight-training injuries in children and adolescents. *Am Fam Physician* **44**, 2104–8.
67. Mazur LJ, Yetman RJ, Risser WL (1993). Weight-training injuries. Common injuries and preventative methods. *Sports Med* **16**, 57–63.
68. Faigenbaum AD, Kraemer WJ, Cahill B, Chandler J, Dziados J, Elfrink LD, Forman E, Gaudiose M, Micheli L, Nitka M, Roberts S (1996). Youth resistance training: Position statement paper and literature review. *Strength Cond* **18**, 62–75.
69. American Academy of Pediatrics Committee on Sports Medicine and Fitness: Bernhardt DT, Gomez J, Johnson MD, Martin TJ, Rowland TW, Small E, LeBlanc C, Malina R, Krein C, Young JC, Reed FE, Anderson SJ, Anderson SJ, Griesemer BA, Bar-Or O. (2001). Strength training by children and adolescents. *Pediatrics* **107**, 1470–2.

70. Stratton G, Jones M, Fox KR, Tolfrey K, Harris J, Maffulli N, Lee M, Frostick SP (2004). BASES position statement on guidelines for resistance exercise in young people. *J Sport Sci* **22**, 383–90.
71. American College of Sports Medicine (2005). *ACSM's guidelines for exercise testing and prescription* (7th ed.). Lippincott, Williams and Wilkins, Philadelphia, PA.
72. Faigenbaum AD, Milliken LA, Westcott WL (2003). Maximal strength testing in healthy children. *J Strength Cond Res* **17**, 162–6.
73. Blimkie CJ (1993). Resistance training during preadolescence. Issues and controversies. *Sports Med* **15**, 389–407.
74. Hamill BP (1994). Relative safety of weightlifting and weight training. *J Strength Cond Res* **8**, 53–7.
75. American Academy of Pediatrics: Committee on Sports Medicine. (1990). Strength training, weight and power lifting, and body building by children and adolescents. *Pediatrics* **86**, 801–3.
76. Pierce K, Byrd R, Stone M (1999). Youth weightlifting—is it safe? *Weightlifting USA* **17**, 5.
77. Byrd R, Pierce K, Reilly L, Brady J (2003). Young weightlifters' performance across time. *Sports Biomech* **2**, 133–40.
78. Tanner JM (1962). *Growth at adolescence* (2nd ed.). Blackwell, Oxford.
79. Kraemer WJ, Fry AC, Frykman PN, Conroy B, Hoffman J (1989). Resistance training and youth. *Pediatr Exerc Sci* **1**, 336–50.
80. Blimkie CJ (1992). Resistance training during pre- and early puberty: efficacy, trainability, mechanisms, and persistence. *Can J Sports Sci* **17**, 264–79.
81. Falk B, Tenenbaum G (1996). The effectiveness of resistance training in children. *Sports Med* **22**, 176–86.
82. Payne VG, Morrow JR, Johnson L, Dalton SN (1997). Resistance training in children and youth: A meta-analysis. *Res Q Exerc Sport* **68**, 80–8.
83. Mahon AD (2000) Exercise training. In: Armstrong N, Van Mechelen W (eds.), *Paediatric exercise science and medicine*, pp. 201–22. Oxford University Press, Oxford.
84. Ban-Pillarella D, Roberts SO, Robergs RA (1995). Effects of combined step aerobic and resistance training in children on cardiorespiratory endurance and strength. *Pediatr Exerc Sci* **7**, 218–19.
85. Blimkie CJR Martin J, Ramsay J, Sale D, MacDougall D (1989). The effects of detraining and maintenance weight training on strength development in prepubertal boys. *Can J Sports Sci* **14**, 102P.
86. Clarke DH, Vaccaro P, Andresen NM (1984). Physiological alterations in 7- to 9-year-old boys following a season of competitive wrestling. *Res Q Exerc Sport* **55**, 318–22.
87. Docherty D, Wenger HA, Collis ML, Quinney HA (1987). The effects of variable speed resistance training on strength development in prepubertal boys. *J Hum Mov Stud* **13**, 377–82.
88. Falk B, Mor G (1996). The effects of resistance and martial arts training in 6- to 8-year-old boys. *Pediatr Exerc Sci* **8**, *48–56.*
89. Fukunaga T, Funato K, Ikegawa, S (1992). The effects of resistance training on muscle area and strength in prepubescent age. *Ann Physiol Anthrop* **11**, 357–64.
90. Isaacs LD, Pohlman RL (1995). Specificity of strength training modes in prepubescent females. *Med Sci Sports Exerc* (Supplement) **27**, 180.
91. Mersch F, Stoboy H (1989). Strength training and muscle hypertrophy in children. In: Oseid S, Carlsen KH (eds.), *Children and exercise XIII*, pp. 165–82. Human Kinetics, Champaign, IL.
92. Siegel JA, Camaione DN, Manfredi TG (1989). The effects of upper body resistance training on prepubescent children. *Pediatr Exerc Sci* **1**, 145–54.
93. Servedio FJ, Bartels RL, Hamlin RL, Teske D, Shaffer T, Servedio A (1985). The effects of weight training, using Olympic style lifts, on various physiological variables in pre-pubescent boys. *Med Sci Sports Exerc* **17**(Suppl.), 288.
94. Stahle SD, Roberts SO, Davis B, Rybicki LA (1995). Effect of a 2 versus 3 times per week weight training program in boys aged 7 to 16. *Med Sci Sports Exerc* **27**, S114.
95. Vrijens J (1978). Muscle strength development in the pre- and post-pubescent age. *Med Sport* **11**, 152–8.
96. Westcott WL (1979). Female response to weight training. *J Phys Ed* **77**, 31–3.
97. Westcott W (1995). *Strength fitness* (4th ed.). Brown and Benchmark, Madison, WI.
98. Faigenbaum AD (2003). Youth resistance training. President's council on physical fitness and sports: research digest **4**, 1–8.
99. Kraemer WJ, Ratamess NA (2000). Physiology of resistance training: Current issues. *Orthop Phys Therapy Clin North Am Exerc Tech* **9**, 467–513.
100. Häkkinen K, Alen M, Komi PV (1985). Changes in isometric force- and relaxation-time, electromyographic and muscle fibre characteristics of human skeletal muscle during strength training and detraining. *Acta Physiol Scand* **125**, 573–85.
101. Fleck SJ (1999). Periodized strength training: A critical review. *J Strength Cond Res* **13**, 82–9.
102. Fleck S, Kraemer W (1997). *Designing resistance training programmes* (2nd ed.). Human Kinetics, Champaign, IL.
103. American College of Sports Medicine (1995). *Guidelines for exercise testing and prescription for children, the elderly, and pregnancy.* Williams and Wilkins, Philadelphia, PA.
104. Biddle S, Sallis JS, Cavill N (1998). *Young and active? Young people and health enhancing physical activity—evidence and implications.* Health Education Authority, London.
105. Department of Health (2004). *At least five a week: evidence on the impact of physical activity and its relationship to health.* A report from the Chief Medical Officer. Department of Health, London.
106. Tolfrey K (2007). Responses to training. In: Armstrong N (ed.), *Paediatric exercise physiology*, pp. 213–34. Churchill Livingstone, Edinburgh.
107. Malina RM, Bouchard C, Bar-Or O (2004). *Growth, maturation and physical activity.* Human Kinetics, Champaign, IL.
108. Sale D (1989). Strength training in children. In: Gisolfi CV, Lamb DR (eds.), *Perspectives in exercise science and sports medicine*, pp. 165–216. Benchmark Press, Indianapolis, IN.
109. Morse CI, Degens H, Jones DA (2007). The validity of estimating quadriceps volume from single MRI cross-sections in young men. *Eur J Appl Physiol* 100, 267–74.
110. Danis A, Kyriazis Y, Klissouras V (2003). The effect of training in male prepubertal and pubertal monozygotic twins. *Eur J Appl Physiol* **89**, 309–18.
111. Chilibeck PD, Calder AW, Sale DG, Webber CE (1998). A comparison of strength and muscle mass increases during resistance training in young women. *Eur J Appl Physiol* **77**, 170–5.
112. Gabriel DA, Kamen G, Frost G (2006). Neural adaptations to resistive exercise: mechanisms and recommendations for training practices. *Sports Med* **36**, 133–49.

CHAPTER 41

Young athletes with a physical or mental disability

Merrilee Zetaruk and Shareef Mustapha

Introduction

Children with disabilities, whether mental or physical, have a right to the same respect and dignity afforded to able-bodied children. Although sport participation may present more of a challenge for many with disabilities, the rewards of such activities are immeasurable. The physical and psychological benefits can have a lasting effect throughout the life of the child. Physical benefits include decreased obesity, lower lifetime risk of cardiovascular disease, improved physical skills, improved functional ability, maintenance or improvement in range of motion of joints, and increased independence.[1–7] Those with physical disabilities may have a low self-esteem[8] and children with mental disabilities often are affected more by social stigma than by their own limitations. Through sports, these children develop confidence in themselves and learn important social skills as they work together with their peers. At the same time, able-bodied children observe that despite an apparent 'handicap', children with disabilities can excel in many sports, a fact that is inspiring to both children and adults.

It was not until the Second World War that it was recognized that children and adults with visible disabilities such as amputations, spinal cord injuries, or cerebral palsy (CP) could benefit from sport participation. The first wheelchair sports began at the Stoke Mandeville Hospital in England. Since that time, national and international organizations representing a variety of athletes with disabilities have flourished and international, elite level competitions have been established. Today, spectators watch in awe as these athletes reach new heights, at times rivalling their able-bodied counterparts.

Many athletes with disabilities have demonstrated great achievements beyond the competitive field. Two athletes who deserve special mention are Terry Fox and Rick Hansen. Terry Fox lost his right leg to cancer in 1977. Three years later, with the aid of a lower-limb prosthesis, he began a run across Canada to raise money for cancer research. Although his journey was terminated early because of a recurrence of the disease, he was able to raise US$24 million for his cause. He received the prestigious Order of Canada award in 1980, 1 year before his death. Rick Hansen became paraplegic following a motor vehicle accident in 1973. In order to raise money and awareness about spinal cord injuries, this elite athlete began a world tour which took him to 34 different countries over a 2-year period. He completed over 40,000 km by wheelchair and raised millions of dollars for spinal cord research. These men have served not only as role models for young athletes with disabilities but have also become national heroes.

This chapter reviews the prevalence of some of the more common physical and mental impairments and addresses the particular challenges faced by individuals with disabilities who are participating in sports. Although the incidence of sport-significant abnormalities detected amoung able-bodied individuals on pre-participation screening is relatively low (1–3%), the rate may be as high as 40% in disabled populations.[9] As such, the injuries that athletes with disabilities are predisposed to and general strategies for prevention are reviewed in this text. In addition, the multitude of benefits that are achieved through physical activity and sport participation are discussed. Some adaptations via adjustments in rules and use of prosthetic devices that allow participation in a more diverse range of athletic activity are also reviewed. Finally, some of the opportunities that exist for athletes with disabilities who wish to participate at high levels of competition such as the Paralympic Games and Special Olympics are highlighted. Given the utility of physical activity for all and the increasing number of athletes with disabilities, it is imperative that health professionals become familiar with the unique challenges faced by these athletes. Knowledge of injuries encountered in this population as well as disability-specific modes of injury prevention is imperative.[10]

Athletes with sensory impairments

The deaf athlete

Permanent, moderate to severe bilateral sensorineural hearing loss affects 0.5–1 per 1000 live births.[11] Such hearing loss can also occur at any time during childhood resulting in a prevalence of 1.5–2 per 1000 children under 6 years of age.[11] Speech and language development can be impaired by hearing loss at a very young age as can social and emotional development, behaviour, attention, and academic achievement.[11] Sport participation for children, regardless of the status of their hearing, helps foster a healthy, active lifestyle and promotes positive attitudes toward competition and fair play.[12] There is also an opportunity for social development and increased confidence through sport participation.

Deaf athletes became involved in organized sports in the United States in the 1870s when the Ohio School for the Deaf began to offer baseball for its students.[13] Soon after, football and basketball were introduced in a number of schools for the deaf. Because there were no neuromuscular deficits in this population, deaf athletes often played against hearing athletes. Today, we see many deaf athletes who are successful in both the deaf and hearing worlds of sport.

Hearing loss does not predispose the young athlete to any specific patterns of injury. Coexisting dysfunction of the vestibular apparatus affects equilibrium; therefore, sports that require balance are more challenging. Activities that require climbing to heights, jumping on a trampoline, or diving into a pool should only be permitted if adequate safeguards are in place to prevent injury if the athlete loses balance and falls. Tumbling activities which require rotation should be attempted only if close supervision and spotting is available.[14] In the absence of concomitant vestibular dysfunction, the performance of deaf athletes compares favourably with that of able-bodied athletes since their muscle function, strength, sensation, and coordination do not differ significantly.[15,16] The greatest problem for the hard-of-hearing or deaf athlete is communication with other athletes, making participation in team sports more difficult.[17] Deaf children often participate in sports with hearing athletes but are unable to hear verbal instructions or auditory cues from coaches and other athletes. Hearing aids may be helpful for some children. Co-existing speech impairments make communication even more difficult; however, many deaf athletes facilitate communication through sign language, lip reading, and other methods of visual cueing.[18] These skills, along with maximizing powers of observation and peripheral vision, allow athletes with hearing losses to participate in almost any sport; however, individual activities which require minimal communication (e.g. running or skiing) allow for the greatest success.

The World Games for the Deaf take place every 4 years. Winter events include Alpine and Nordic skiing, ice hockey, and speed skating. Summer events include badminton, basketball, cycling, men's wrestling, shooting, soccer, swimming, table tennis, team handball, tennis, track and field, volleyball, and water polo. The rules are essentially the same as those used in hearing competitions with minor modifications such as visual cues to replace or supplement auditory cues.

The blind athlete

Visual impairment in children presents a challenge for sport participation. Approximately, three in every thousand people are blind; as a result, a number of programmes have been developed in order to allow blind athletes to participate in various sports. According to the International Blind Sports Association (IBSA), any person with less than 10% of useful vision is eligible to compete as a blind athlete. The IBSA uses the following classification of athletes based on testing of the better, corrected eye:[18]

(i) B1: No light perception or light perception with inability to recognize the shape of a hand at any distance or in any direction.

(ii) B2: Ability to recognize the shape of a hand up to a visual acuity of 2/60 and/or a field of vision less than 5 degrees.

(iii) B3: Visual acuity greater than 2/60 up to 6/60 and/or a field of vision greater than 5 degrees but less than 20 degrees.

Although visual impairment itself does not affect neuromuscular function, a fear of falling or colliding with objects results in a different pattern of movement than is observed in sighted children. Blind children have a stiffer posture, shorter stride, slower pace, and a shuffling gait. There is often hyperlordosis with a protruding abdomen.[19] Because of their restricted free movement in space, without early intervention through physical activity blind children are apt to lead a sedentary lifestyle. Sedentary children become sedentary adults; therefore, it is important to encourage physical activity in all children, especially those with visual impairments.

There are many aspects of sport participation that are of particular benefit to visually impaired children. Physical activity helps develop a sense of orientation in space and improved mobility through enhancement of sense of touch, proprioception, balance, posture, and body control.[14,19] Early physical activity enhances coordinated associated movements of the hands. Sport participation also provides psychosocial benefits such as increased self-confidence, improved social skills, and a competitive spirit.[19]

Auditory and tactile cues can be substituted for visual cues in a number of sports thereby facilitating participation of blind athletes. Through voice and touch a guide can communicate with blind athletes to teach downhill skiing. The ski bra, invented in 1974, can be used initially to help with balance. This is a rigid device that keeps the ski tips about 7.5–10 cm apart preventing crossing of the skis. Blind skiers, instructors, and guides wear a distinctive jacket or bib to allow easy identification by sighted skiers on the slopes.[20]

In addition to skiing, blind athletes compete in many different types of sports that athletes without visual impairment participate in including competitive swimming, skating, baseball, track and field, and judo. Goal ball is a game uniquely designed for blind athletes. The ball has a bell inside it allowing athletes to identify the trajectory of the ball and to prevent it from crossing their goal line or entering the net. Like hearing loss, visual impairment alone does not affect the general fitness of individuals;[19] therefore, with modifications of rules and equipment, children with visual impairment can not only become physically active but can also attain a high level of performance in many sports.

Athletes with physical impairments

Athletes who have a disability that impairs their mobility often require the use of a wheelchair for sport participation. Wheelchair sports include athletes with CP, myelomeningoceles, spinal cord injuries, or lower-extremity amputations. Not all athletes with these conditions require wheelchairs; therefore, this section will include discussion of a range of disabilities from ambulatory to wheelchair athletes.

The athlete with cerebral palsy

Cerbral palsy (CP) is a non-progressive disorder of posture and movement resulting from a defect or lesion of the developing brain. CP affects 4 per 1000 live births, with an estimated prevalence of 2 per 1000 in the general population.[21] Injuries to the cerebral cortex result in spasticity in one or more of the extremities, whereas injuries to the cerebellum or basal ganglia produce ataxia or athetosis respectively. The most common patterns of spasticity as well as physiological parameters of exercise in CP are described below:

(i) Monoplegia: one extremity involved, usually a lower extremity;

(ii) Hemiplegia: involvement of the extremities on one side of the body; associated seizure disorder in one-third of affected children and cognitive impairments in one-quarter;

(iii) Paraplegia: spasticity of both lower extremities;

(iv) Diplegia: spasticity noted in all four extremities, with the upper extremities involved to a much lesser extent; likely to have normal intellectual development with a low incidence of seizure disorders;

(v) Triplegia: three extremities involved, with sparing of one upper extremity;

(vi) Quadriplegia: involvement of all four limbs; high rate of mental retardation and seizures.

Athetoid CP is the least common form of this disorder. It is characterized by hypotonia, athetoid movements, and slurring of speech. Seizures and intellectual impairment are uncommon in this group.

There are a number of benefits to sport participation for the child with CP. A carefully designed and monitored programme of strength and flexibility training will improve flexibility, range of motion, and strength in these children.[3–5] Early physical activity helps maximize compensatory mechanisms of the central nervous system in order to decrease abnormal patterns of movement or posture.[5,22] The psychological benefits of sports are equally important to the young athlete with CP. Many forms of CP are accompanied by intellectual impairments or emotional disorders that often cause social difficulties among peers. Children with CP experience greater self-esteem and confidence through sport participation.

Although risk factors for injury are not unique to the athlete with CP, many risk factors are magnified in this population. Richter *et al.*[23] found an injury rate of 60% among athletes with CP at the 1988 Paralympic Games in South Korea. Imbalances in strength between agonist and antagonist muscle groups are risk factors for injury in children.[24,25] These imbalances are even greater in CP due to the predilection of spasticity to affect primarily agonist muscle groups. A good example of the effect of spasticity on muscle balance can be observed in the ankles. Spasticity of the gastrocnemius and soleus muscles results in tight heel cords and excessive plantar flexion of the foot.[26] Children with CP tend to be less active compared with their able-bodied peers leaving them little opportunity to stretch their muscles on a regular basis without active encouragement and assistance from caregivers.[17] Joint contractures occur frequently in this population adding to imbalances about the joints.

Patellofemoral dysfunction occurs with increased frequency as growth and spasticity lead to tightening of the quadriceps and hamstring muscles. Gait disturbances predispose children with CP to joint malalignments.[27] The result is increased stress across the patellofemoral joint, which leads to overuse injuries of the extensor mechanism. Patellofemoral syndrome, although similar to that seen in able-bodied athletes, tends to be more severe in the CP population. In addition, there is increased risk of fragmentation of the distal patellar pole such as is seen in Sinding–Larsen–Johansson syndrome. Athletes with this condition will present with pain and tenderness of the lower pole of the patella.

Spasticity not only causes an imbalance of muscles of the hip but also can result in abnormal development of the hip joint itself. These abnormalities range from acetabular dysplasia and progressive arthritis to frank dislocation of the joint. These athletes present clinically with increasing hip pain associated with physical activity such as running. Marked adductor spasticity (scissor gait) contributes to the malalignments observed in the lower extremities.[17,22]

Athletes with athetoid CP exhibit slow, writhing, involuntary movements of the extremities, head, and neck. Activities that require accuracy, such as kicking a soccer ball, may be difficult in the more severely affected children. Sports that require balance will pose the greatest challenge, and perhaps the greatest risk, to children with the ataxic or atonic forms of CP. Their unsteady gait and lack of coordination make basic skills such as running and jumping quite difficult, and may lead to injury from falls.

The diverse presentations and range of severity of CP have necessitated the development of classification systems for athletic competition. The Functional Classification System (FCS) used in the Paralympic Games assesses trunk control, gross motor control, and strength of the extremities, as well as balance and fine motor control, with or without assistive devices.[12,18,21,26] Such a classification system is designed to permit more equitable competition among CP athletes with a wide range of disabilities. Athletes with CP compete in many different sports, including cycling, powerlifting, shooting, track, archery, bowling, table-tennis, snooker, football, basketball, volleyball, and swimming. The latter is a very good sport for children with CP as swimming improves coordination and may relax spasticity.[22] Due to the high prevalence of epilepsy in CP, drowning is a real risk in this group; therefore, very close observation must be provided for all athletes with a seizure disorder. A history of a seizure disorder is not a contraindication to sports participation if the seizures are well controlled. Athletes who have had a seizure within 6 months of sport participation or have uncontrolled seizures should be carefully assessed prior to clearance.[28] Regardless of the sport, children with CP can benefit from physical activity and experience success in the competitive arena.

Athletes with myelomeningoceles

Myelomeningocele is the most common congenital anomaly of the nervous system. It results from a failure of the neural tube to close and affects approximately 1/1000 live births. Three-quarters of myelomeningoceles occur in the lumbosacral region.[21] They produce motor and sensory deficits as well as impairments in bowel and bladder function. Lesions in the lower sacral region have sparing of motor function. Eighty percent of affected children have an associated hydrocephalus that can affect cognitive function and can further impair motor function. Furthermore, there is a high incidence of obesity in children with myelomeningocele making sport participation especially important.[29]

Children with myelomeningoceles are classified according to their functional level, which corresponds to the most caudal functioning nerve root. Lower lesions may simply require bracing of the foot and ankle to permit sport participation, whereas athletes with higher lesions may perform best in a wheelchair. Swimming is a popular sport for many athletes with myelomeningoceles since the upper extremities are often unaffected (Fig. 41.1). Sport participation depends not only on the functional level, but also on the presence of mental retardation and degree of spasticity that results

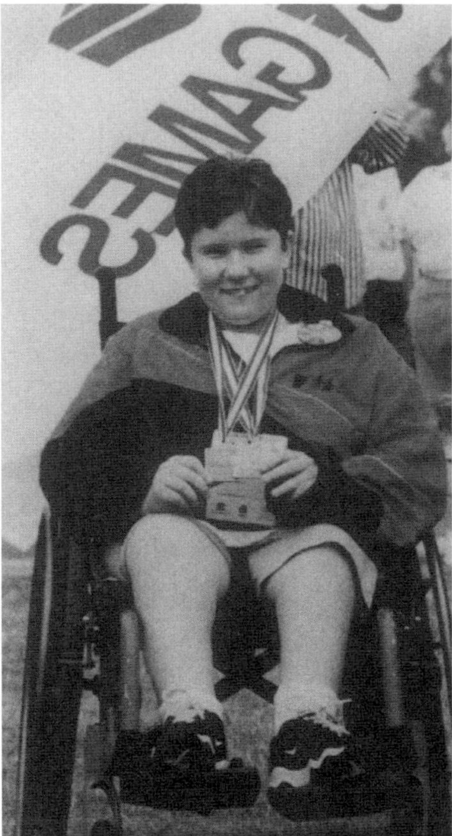

Fig. 41.1 Young competitive swimmer proudly displays medals.

from associated hydrocephalus. These factors make this group of athletes extremely heterogeneous in abilities.

Hydrocephalus, in association with a type II Chiari defect, develops in at least 80% of patients with myelomeningocele and often requires ventriculoperitoneal shunting.[30] Children with the associated Chiari malformation should be restricted from activities that have a significant risk of injury to the cervical spine such as diving, water skiing, football, and so on.[31] In general, children with shunts should wear helmets for protection when participating in physical activities.[31]

Skin, bone, and muscle–tendon units are all at increased risk of injury in athletes with myelomeningoceles. The lack of sensation below the level of the lesion leads to bruising, pressure sores, and skin breakdown from braces or wheelchair seats. Ensuring proper fit of adaptive equipment is paramount in prevention of injuries as is the use of appropriate cushioning and water absorptive clothing.[10] The risk of skin breakdown can be minimized by teaching children and their parents to inspect the skin regularly and to shift weight frequently. Lifting off the seat for 10–20 s intermittently throughout the day can be beneficial.[10] Racing wheelchair athletes may be at particularly high risk of pressure sores over the sacrum and ischium resulting from positioning of the knees higher than the hips for prolonged periods of time in these highly-specialized wheelchairs. Children who use braces should ensure that they are correctly positioned after each fall to reduce the likelihood of skin irritation from the brace.

Limited weight-bearing results in osteopaenia and increased risk of fractures. Fractures are particularly problematic in this group because of the sensory deficits that often result in delayed diagnosis. The incidence of fractures can be reduced by encouraging weight-bearing where possible and by limiting the period of immobilization following a fracture.

Soft-tissue injuries such as muscle strains occur with greater frequency in this population. This is due to muscle weaknesses just above the level of the lesion and muscle imbalances resulting from spasticity. These athletes frequently have joint contractures that can significantly limit their range of motion. Special emphasis should be placed on range of motion and flexibility in the affected limbs, particularly if joint contractures are present.

Latex allergies are another concern in individuals with myelomeningoceles. The reported prevalence of such allergies in this population ranges from 25% to 65%; therefore, it is important to ask for this pertinent past medical history and to avoid exposure in latex allergic individuals.[32]

Athletes with spinal cord injuries

Evaluation of the epidemiology of spinal cord injuries in the United States over a 30-year period (1973–2003) revealed that 3.7% of cases occurred in patients under the age of 15 and 51.6% occurred in people between the ages of 15 and 30 years.[33] Such injuries result in variable degrees of paralysis and sensory loss along with dysfunction in other areas such as thermoregulation, circulation, and bowel and bladder control. The extent of the disability depends on the level of the spinal cord lesion and whether or not it is complete. Incomplete injuries allow some communication with areas distal to the injured cord. This results in some residual motor or sensory function below the level of the injury. Classification of spinal cord injury is based upon the lowest level of motor function;[26] however, the FCS used in the Paralympic Games categorizes athletes according to their functional abilities.[18]

There are many benefits associated with participation in wheelchair sports. These include an improvement in maximal oxygen uptake by an average of 20%, reduced risk of cardiovascular disease and respiratory infection, and improved self-image. Sedentary individuals with paraplegia are at a three-fold increased risk of hospitalization compared with paraplegic athletes.[34]

The most common injuries reported in young wheelchair athletes are blisters, wheel burns, bruises, and abrasions. These injuries result from contact with the wheelchair seat back, brakes, push rims, and wheels.[34] Lacerations can occur from collisions with other wheelchairs. Due to sensory and motor deficits, spinal-cord injured athletes experience many of the same problems as athletes with myelomeningoceles. Contractures and muscle imbalances place the athletes at increased risk with the shoulder being the most common site of injury to muscle–tendon units. The anterior shoulder is prone to excessive tightness due to poor posture and wheelchair pushing.[26] The latter can also result in muscle imbalances, with the shoulder flexor muscles being stronger than the extensors. Wheelchair athletes are at increased risk of shoulder injuries such as impingement syndromes and rotator cuff tendinitis. The elbow and wrist are also frequent sites of overuse injuries with medial and lateral epicondylitis as well as de Quervain's tenosynovitis being among the more common injuries at these sites.[34] Those who present with shoulder pain often have a relative weakness of the adductor muscles. Careful attention to stretching and to achieving balanced strength can reduce the likelihood of overuse injuries in the upper extremities. Skin breakdown and osteopenia also occur in the spinal cord-injured athlete. The principles of management are the same as for athletes with myelomeningoceles.

Nerve entrapment syndromes in the upper extremities are a problem for many wheelchair athletes. The numbness and weakness associated with carpal tunnel syndrome result from repetitive pressure of the heel of the hand on the push rim. Compression of the median or ulnar nerves can occur at the elbow as well. Radial tunnel syndrome should be considered in the differential diagnosis of lateral epicondylitis.[34]

Of particular concern for the spinal cord injured athlete is the impairment of thermoregulation. Able-bodied children are less efficient than adults at compensating for changes in ambient temperature. Children with lesions above T8 cannot maintain normal body temperature in the face of extreme environmental stresses.[17] Autonomic dysfunction impedes heat production mechanisms such as shivering as well as heat dissipation mechanisms such as sweating below the level of the spinal cord injury. While this problem also occurs in athletes with myelomeningoceles, as mentioned earlier, most of these neural tube defects occur in the lumbosacral region. The higher the lesion the greater the impairment of thermoregulation; therefore, spinal-cord-injured athletes with thoracic lesions are at greatest risk. Careful observation of both groups during events that take place in either high or low ambient temperatures will prevent hyperthermia or hypothermia respectively. Physicians who provide medical coverage at wheelchair athletic events must be prepared to deal with either outcome.

Autonomic dysreflexia occurs most frequently in quadriplegics and paraplegics with lesions above T6.[26] Noxious stimuli such as a full bladder or a fracture below the lesion cause mass activation of the sympathetic nervous system. Blood pressure rises dramatically as peripheral and splanchnic blood vessels vasoconstrict.[27] Due to sympathetic activation distal to the lesion, skin will be pale, cool, and clammy below the injury. Above the lesion, parasympathetic activation from the stimulation of carotid and aortic baroreceptors leads to marked vasodilation as well as facial flushing, sweating, nasal stuffiness, and bradycardia. This condition has been considered a medical emergency for years because of the potential for stroke. It also appears to enhance performance in wheelchair racing, which has prompted athletes to intentionally induce the condition by drinking excessively prior to a race or by clamping urinary catheters. This practice is extremely dangerous and is to be condemned. In the event that a wheelchair athlete presents with signs of autonomic dysreflexia, the urinary catheter should be inspected for a clamp or kink and tight clothing or strapping of the lower extremities should be loosened. As it is difficult to place controls on the intentional induction of autonomic dysreflexia, athlete education may be the best defence against the potentially catastrophic outcome of this condition.

Amputee athletes

Amputation refers to a partial or complete loss of one or more limbs and may be either congenital or acquired. Acquired amputations may be the result of trauma, tumour, infection, or vascular insufficiency.[35] Since the number of limbs affected and the level of the amputation varies considerably among amputee athletes, classification systems based on these variables have been established. The classification systems take into account whether the amputation is confined to a single arm or leg or whether there are multiple amputations present. Athletes with amputations above the knee are distinguished from those with below-knee amputations. Similarly, athletes with above-elbow amputations compete in separate categories from those with below-elbow deficiencies. These systems provide a more equitable playing field for athletes whose disabilities vary greatly.[18]

Many amputee athletes participate in sports with the use of a prosthesis. The prosthetic device is designed to compensate for any loss of function associated with the specific amputation. In the case of acquired amputations, early use of the prosthetic device facilitates its incorporation into the child's normal body actions.[36] It is very important that the prosthesis fits the child well; any discomfort may result in posture or gait disturbances. A good prosthesis alone is not enough to replace the deficient limb. The amputee athlete must learn how to use the prosthesis with some devices requiring more extensive training. The higher the arm or leg amputation the greater the time and effort needed to master use of the prosthetic device.[36–38]

A number of highly specialized terminal prosthetic devices have been developed in order to allow children with amputations to participate in a wide variety of activities. Upper-limb prostheses have been used very successfully for swimming, baseball (Fig. 41.2), golf, basketball, skiing, and ice hockey. A device developed at the Rehabilitation Centre for Children in Winnipeg, Canada (Fig. 41.3), has allowed many young amputee athletes to participate in hockey on a level equal to their able-bodied peers up to Bantam

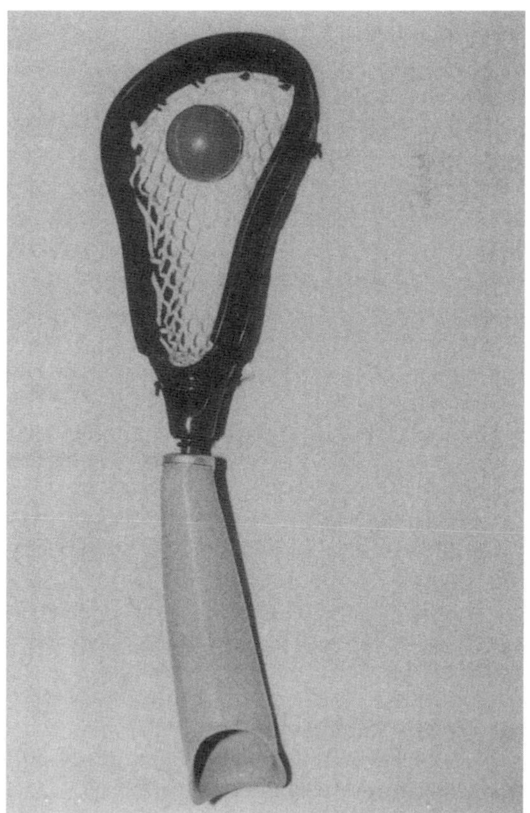

Fig. 41.2 Terminal prosthesis to facilitate participation in baseball by children with upper limb amputations.

(a)

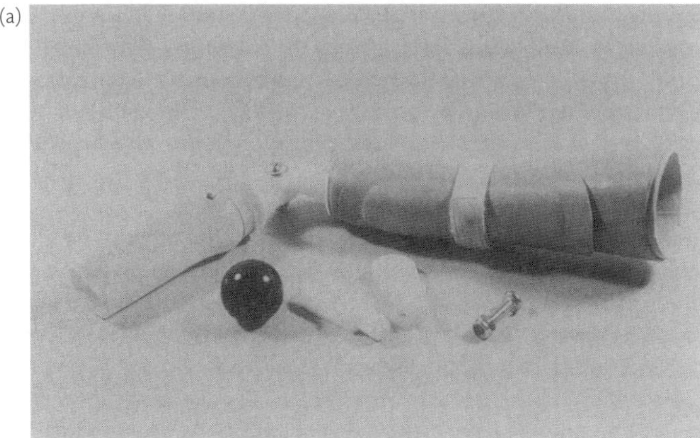

(b)

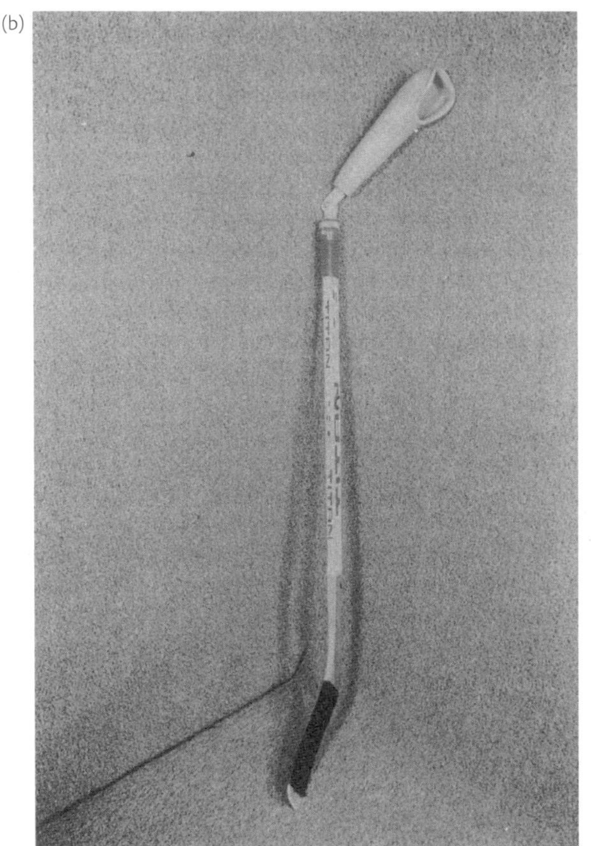

Fig. 41.3 (a) Upper limb prosthesis for participation in ice hockey. (b) Prosthesis affixed to hockey stick.

division (ages 14 and 15 years) (personal communication, Doug Paulsen, Rehabilitation Centre for Children, Winnipeg, Canada). Refinements in prosthetic design are ongoing allowing improved performance in many different sports. New lower-limb prosthetic devices provide athletes with near normal foot function. These carbon graphite prostheses store and release energy, which allows for an active push-off during running or jumping.[36] Such advances in material and design of prostheses facilitate involvement in sports such as volleyball, basketball, and track (Fig. 41.4).

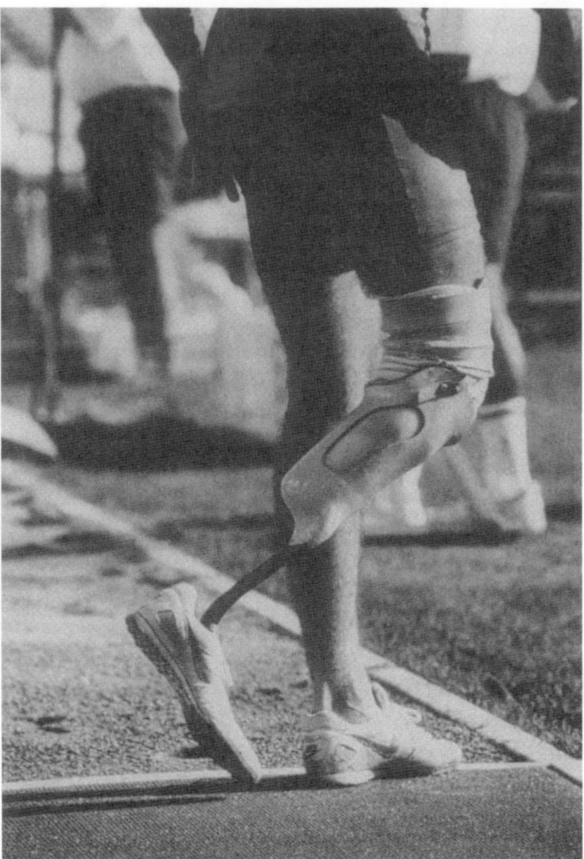

Fig. 41.4 Specialized prosthesis worn by an athlete at the Paralympic Games, Barcelona, 1992.

Special mention should be made of snow skiing for amputee athletes. In the early 1940s, Franz Wendel of Germany became the first person with a physical disability to compete as a skier after sustaining a leg injury that required amputation. Short ski tips were attached to the bottoms of crutches to aid in balance while skiing.[20] Since that time, significant improvements have been made to equipment design. Three-track skiing is used by athletes with a single leg amputation with or without one upper-extremity prosthesis. One full-length ski is attached to the sound leg while two short outrigger skis on forearm crutches are manoeuvered by the upper extremities. Children tend to ski without their lower limb prostheses for improved balance and agility, while those with below-knee amputations who begin to ski during late adolescence tend to ski with the prosthesis, primarily for cosmetic reasons. Athletes with above-knee amputations usually ski without their prosthesis.

Children and adolescents with amputations may have a decreased range of motion due to tight musculature or contractures. For example, a below-knee amputee who spends more time sitting than ambulating may develop tight hip and knee flexors. These athletes need to emphasize range of motion exercises in their training in order to reduce the risk of injuries to the muscle–tendon units. Balance is also adversely affected in athletes with amputations. For those with lower-limb amputations, this is due to the loss of proprioceptive feedback from the extremity. For those with acquired upper-limb amputations the change in weight across the shoulder girdle affects balance. This is particularly hazardous in a sport such as figure skating, where balance is critical in preventing serious injuries from falls.[37]

In children, stump overgrowth is a frequent problem.[17,39] The bone begins to grow through the soft tissue left at the end of the stump resulting in skin breakdown during physical activities. Young athletes should be instructed to inspect the stump for erythema or skin breakdown, particularly if the stump begins to lose the cushioned feeling of the soft tissues. Surgical revision of the stump will prevent severe overgrowth and will facilitate continued pain-free participation in sports.[17] For those who wear a prosthesis during skiing, padding of the stump end can help prevent pressure sores and keep the stump warm.

An additional concern is for the integrity of the prosthesis. The stresses on the prosthesis during sport participation can be quite substantial, resulting in minor or major breakdowns of the device. Amputee athletes should be instructed to inspect the prosthetic device regularly in order to detect problems before they develop into major breakdowns.

Any individual with a visible disability may be at risk for psychological and social adjustment problems. Prejudices toward cosmetic disabilities such as amputations are greater than those towards functional handicaps; therefore, children with limb deficiencies may be at particular risk. These children may be subject to bullying, marginalization, and eventual isolation by peers and society. Self-esteem can be adversely affected by these attitudes. Fortunately, sport participation and athletic competence in these individuals has been shown to correlate with higher self-esteem.[8]

Wheelchair sports

The concept of sport participation for individuals with spinal cord injuries was introduced by Sir Ludwig Guttman during the Second World War at a time when the prevailing feeling was that very little could be done for paraplegics and quadriplegics. His revolutionary approach to the spinal cord-injured patient included the introduction of the first competitive team sport for paraplegics, namely, wheelchair polo. Soon after, wheelchair basketball and badminton were added to the list of sports for patients with spinal cord injuries followed by archery and table tennis. On 28 July 1948, the Stoke Mandeville Games for the Paralysed were founded. They are held annually in Ayelsbury, England, except every fourth year when they are held in the country hosting the Olympic Games. The first city to host the International Stoke Mandeville Games outside of England was Rome in 1960 when 400 athletes from 23 countries competed in the Olympic Stadium following the Olympic Games. These Games became known as the Paraplegic Olympic Games, or Paralympics, and have grown dramatically since their inception. In 1992, more than one million spectators attended the Paralympics in Barcelona. In 2004, 3800 athletes from 136 countries participated in the Athens Paralympics (www.paralympic.org).

Popular wheelchair sports include tennis, volleyball, archery, bowling, track-and-field, marathon road racing, quad rugby, and basketball. Sport-specific modifications to wheelchairs optimize athletic performance (Fig. 41.5). Wheelchair basketball was the first organized sport for paraplegics in the United States with athletes achieving high skill levels. Modifications to rules have been made to facilitate wheelchair sports. For example, in basketball, a travelling violation occurs when an athlete performs three or more pushes of the wheelchair without bouncing the ball. Thanks to the initiative of Sir Ludwig Guttman and others around the world, spinal cord-injured individuals who were thought of as 'hopeless cripples'[2] 50 years ago now participate in sports at an elite level and achieve things unimaginable to many able-bodied athletes.

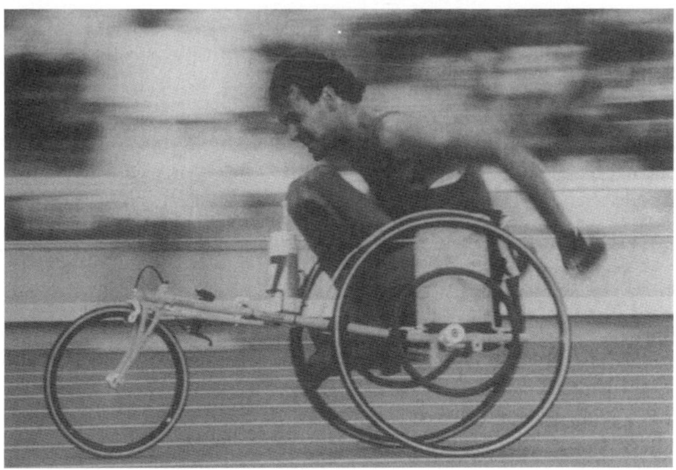

Fig. 41.5 Paralympic athlete displays speed in highly specialized wheel chair.

Athletes with mental retardation

Mental retardation (IQ < 70), which affects approximately 3% of the population, is characterized by impairments in measured intelligence and adaptive behaviour.[40] The severity of mental retardation is based upon the level of IQ. Children with borderline mental retardation (IQ = 68–83) do not all meet the criteria for mental retardation; however, they are all likely to have difficulties in school. The vast majority of children classified as mentally retarded fall into the category of mild mental retardation (IQ = 52–67). These children may require special class placement at school, but those with higher adaptive skills can become independent adults. Moderate mental retardation (IQ = 36–51) limits academic achievements to a second grade level. As adults, those who are in this category require supervision of daily activities. Children with severe mental retardation (IQ = 20–35) may learn minimal self-care skills but require extensive supervision. Profound mental retardation (IQ < 20) affects only 1% of children with cognitive impairment. These children require total supervision for all aspects of daily life.

For children with borderline or high functioning mild mental retardation, the social stigma attached to the impairment can be more handicapping than the condition itself. Sports participation can provide a means of social interaction for children with mental retardation, while improving their fitness and self-concept.[41] Exercise and activity in this population may delay the need for institutionalization as well.[42]

Adults with mild to moderate mental retardation have a higher prevalence of obesity than do their peers without mental handicaps; however, there appears to be no difference in obesity between mentally retarded children and children without cognitive impairments.[42] Physical activity reduces the likelihood of obesity in adults with mental retardation, so the trend to obesity with age in this population is most likely the result of lifestyle. Perhaps by encouraging children with mental retardation to participate in sports or other physical activities, as adults they may be more active with a lower risk of obesity and all its health implications.

Cardiovascular fitness is important in the prevention of coronary artery disease. Cardiovascular disease is the most common medical problem in adults with mental retardation.[43] Maximal oxygen uptake as a measurement of cardiovascular fitness appears to be similar among children with and without mental retardation.[42] As adolescents, those with mental retardation have a substantially lower maximal oxygen uptake than their unaffected peers.[42] This trend continues into adulthood and is particularly true for adults with Down syndrome.[42] It appears that training can improve cardiovascular fitness in all individuals with mental retardation.[42] In order to reduce the risk of premature death due to coronary artery disease, children and adults with mental retardation should be encouraged to participate in activities that improve cardiovascular fitness.

Muscular strength and endurance appear to be lower in individuals of all ages with mental retardation compared to those with normal cognitive function.[42] As in the case of obesity, this difference is thought to be primarily due to lifestyle. Through training programmes aimed at increasing muscular endurance, this problem can be largely rectified.[42] By improving muscular strength, work performance and level of independence also improve.

Down syndrome

Down syndrome, or trisomy-21, is the most frequent human chromosomal syndrome, occurring in approximately 1 in 800 live births.[44] It occurs when an extra No. 21 chromosome is present through non-disjunction or translocation. If non-disjunction occurs after the first cell division following conception, only some of the cell lines will have trisomy 21, whereas others will have a normal chromosomal complement. An individual affected by this mosaicism may have a nearly normal phenotype or may have all the characteristics of Down syndrome.[45] The craniofacial features including oblique palpebral fissures, epicanthic folds, brushfield spots, protruding tongue, prominent malformed ears, flat nasal bridge, and flat occiput make Down syndrome the best recognized of the chromosomal syndromes. Of particular interest to the sport medicine physician are the musculoskeletal and cardiovascular anomalies as well as the cognitive impairment associated with this syndrome. Through proper screening prior to sport participation, many children with Down syndrome can become active in a wide variety of sports and leisure activities.

Most of the musculoskeletal abnormalities result from a defect in collagen synthesis that leads to ligamentous laxity and contributes to generalized hypotonia. As a result, children with Down syndrome are at increased risk of problems associated with hyperflexibility including atlantoaxial instability (AAI), patellofemoral syndrome, hip joint instability, and pes planus. Slipped capital femoral epiphysis is seen with slightly increased incidence in children with Down syndrome likely due to the increased incidence of obesity and thyroid dysfunction in this population.[46,47] The development of bunions is another common complaint that is often associated with the presence of pes planus and hyperpronation of the foot and is usually managed with shoe modifications.[46]

AAI, which can lead to subsequent dislocation and spinal cord compression, is potentially the most serious musculoskeletal problem associated with Down syndrome.[48] It is also the most controversial area in the management of these athletes. The incidence of AAI in children with Down syndrome under 21 years of age is approximately 15%[49] and 1–2% of individuals with Down syndrome have symptomatic AAI.[50] The subluxation is due to laxity of the annular ligament of C1 as well as the generalized hypotonia seen in Down syndrome. Bony abnormalities such as odontoid hypoplasia, odontoid dysplasia, and the presence of os odontoideum occur in 6% of those with Down syndrome and increase the risk of atlantoaxial dislocation.

Because of the potential for permanent neurologic disability resulting from AAI, the Special Olympics issued a bulletin in 1983 restricting athletes with Down syndrome from participating in any activities that might cause injury to the neck and upper spine until they had been examined for AAI. Individuals who were found to have asymptomatic AAI were permanently restricted from participation in certain Special Olympics activities that placed them at increased risk of injury. These activities include gymnastics, diving, pentathlon, butterfly stroke in swimming, diving starts in swimming, high jump, and warm-up activities that place undue stress on the head and neck muscles.[9,51] The following year, the American Academy of Pediatrics (AAP) issued a policy statement recommending that all children with Down syndrome who wished to participate in sports that involve possible trauma to the head and neck have lateral cervical spine radiographs in neutral, flexion, and extension prior to beginning training or competition. This recommendation applied only to those who had not previously had normal radiologic findings. The AAP recommended restriction from high-risk sports when the distance between the odontoid process of the axis and the anterior arch of the atlas exceeded 4.5 mm or the odontoid was abnormal. Repeated radiographs were not indicated for those with previously normal findings. The AAP policy stated that persons with atlantoaxial subluxation or dislocation and neurologic signs or symptoms should be restricted from all strenuous activities and operative stabilization of the cervical spine be considered. The statement concluded that persons with Down syndrome who did not have evidence of AAI could participate in all sports with no further follow-up unless neurologic signs or symptoms developed.[52]

The AAP retired the 1984 policy statement following a subject review in 1995. The AAP reviewed the data on which their earlier recommendation was made and decided that there was uncertainty regarding the value of cervical spine radiographs in screening for possible catastrophic neck injury in athletes with Down syndrome. The AAP felt that radiologic screening for AAI failed to meet the criteria of Sackett *et al.*[53] stating that:

(i) Symptomatic AAI is rare in the paediatric age range.

(ii) One study has shown poor reproducibility of the radiologic tests for AAI.[54] Other studies have shown changes in radiologic status over time.[55,56]

(iii) Asymptomatic AAI, which is common, has not been proven to be a significant risk factor for symptomatic AAI, which is rare.

(iv) The AAP feels that the intervention to prevent symptomatic AAI has never been tested.

(v) Screening is expensive.

(vi) Undue anxiety may result from labelling a child as having AAI.

(vii) Many patients with symptomatic AAI have symptoms and signs of cervical spinal cord compression for weeks to years before they are recognized as having neurologic disease.

The AAP Committee on Sports Medicine and Fitness now recommends careful neurological evaluation for signs and symptoms consistent with spinal cord compromise as the best clinical predictor of AAI and that this screening should be done at least annually.[57,58] Importantly, parents of children with Down syndrome should be counselled on the early signs of AAI and to seek medical attention if present. Symptomatic children should have a magnetic resonance image (MRI) to clarify the extent of spinal cord compression and should be referred to a surgical specialist for definitive treatment if cord compression is confirmed.

Controversy still exists surrounding screening for AAI. Although not a frequent finding, symptomatic AAI may be present in as many as 5000 individuals with Down syndrome in the United States. It is argued by some experts that the associated high morbidity and mortality of symptomatic AAI should justify a screening programme.[50] O'Connor *et al.*[59] suggest that a single lateral radiograph at 1.85 m in active flexion is adequate to detect any potential AAI because flexion views are unlikely to demonstrate a lesser gap than neutral or extension views.[60] By eliminating the neutral and extension views, the cost of screening would be reduced significantly. Standardized interpretation is essential in improving reproducibility. It may also be argued that the lack of sport-related symptomatic AAI may be the result of the preventative measures in place since the 1983 bulletin by the Special Olympics restricting participation of Down syndrome athletes with AAI. Seventeen percent of Down syndrome patients with symptomatic AAI have a history of cervical spine injury which either caused or contributed to the onset of symptoms.[61] Avoiding sports which have a high risk of injury to the cervical spine could reduce the risk of symptomatic AAI in Down syndrome athletes significantly. Regarding the potential for anxiety among parents of athletes with Down syndrome and given that Special Olympics still require assessments for AAI, a screening programme would be more likely to allay fears than to create undue anxiety because the vast majority of radiographic examinations for AAI would be negative. Identification of neurologic abnormalities in Down syndrome children may be more predictive of impending progression to a more serious symptomatic AAI; however, reliance on history and physical examination alone would fail to identify any children with asymptomatic AAI who may be at risk of progression to symptomatic AAI. In addition, assessing children with Down syndrome for neurologic signs and symptoms can be extremely challenging.[62] Their ability to verbalize regarding neuromotor difficulties or neck discomfort is often limited and they may not be cooperative during physical examinations.[55]

In a more recent publication on Health supervision for children with Down syndrome by the AAP Committee on Genetics in 2001, radiographs are recommended at 3 to 5 years of age even though their utility has been called into question and state that these studies are more important in children who may participate in contact sports and are required for those who plan to participate in the Special Olympics.[63] White *et al.*[64] have found a significant relationship between neural canal width and subarachnoid space width but not with atlanto-dens interval. Narrow neural canal width appears to be a predictor of potential spinal cord compression.[64] As such, it is recommended that lateral radiographs be done with careful positioning of the neck in flexion with the chin tucked. Abnormal atlanto-dens interval should be correlated with neural canal width and any patient with narrowing of the canal or evidence of AAI should be evaluated with MRI before imposing restrictions on activities or considering surgery. White suggests that those patients with a marginally widened atlanto-dens interval but normal neural canal width may be followed up with serial radiographs; however, more research needs to be done in this area.

Cervical spine abnormalities occur in 40% of Down syndrome persons.[65] Although AAI is by far the most common, other cervical spine abnormalities exist such as abnormal vertebral bodies (especially C-2), multiple vertebral fusions, hypoplastic posterior arch of C-1, odontoid abnormalities, and spondylolysis and spondylolisthesis of the midcervical vertebrae.[66] In one series, 10 out of 12 cases of symptomatic AAI had an os odontoideum present.[48] If lateral views are performed for the purposes of screening prior to sports participation, not only should AAI be evaluated, but also other craniocervical abnormalities should be ruled out.

Instability may also occur between the atlas and the occiput increasing the risk of neurologic injury, particularly if the neck is extended. Although radiographic evaluation and normative values for Down syndrome have not been well defined for the atlantooccipital region,[17] instability may be detected on lateral radiographs.[50,51] Atlantooccipital instability (AOI) has been shown to occur in about 63% of Down syndrome patients. Neurological symptoms relating to AOI, however, are rare.[67] This suggests that radiologic screening for AOI would not be clinically helpful.

Patellofemoral instability is a concern for many Down syndrome athletes. In 32%[45] of patients with Down syndrome, the patella subluxes or dislocates resulting in significant impairment in sports and activities of daily living. This instability results from ligamentous laxity in conjunction with anatomic abnormalities such as genu valgus, patella alta, or hypoplastic medial femoral condyle. Pes planus, also due to severe, generalized ligamentous laxity, is seen frequently in Down syndrome children; therefore, use of orthotics may be necessary both in the management of patellofemoral symptoms and in the treatment of foot pain.

Excessive joint laxity may affect the hips and often presents as a loud clunking or popping sound. This condition causes gradual degeneration of the hip joint, the extent of which is not certain. These individuals have a poor gait and limited ambulation.[45] Prevention of hip damage is difficult but may be attempted using casting or abduction bracing. Even with surgical correction, hip instability may recur.

In addition to the various musculoskeletal problems that may afflict young individuals with Down syndrome, there are a myriad of medical problems that need to be followed carefully throughout infancy, childhood, and into adulthood. Children with Down syndrome have a higher prevalence of congenital heart anomalies and are at increased risk of thyroid disease, obesity, Type 2 diabetes mellitus, obstructive sleep apnoea (OSA), gastrointestinal problems (intestinal atresias, Hirschprung disease), seizures, and autoimmune conditions (celiac disease, rheumatoid arthritis, type 1 diabetes mellitus, alopecia areata, autoimmune thyroiditis).[68] In addition, there may be psychological issues such as depression, behavioural problems, and varying degrees of mental retardation that can affect sport participation.[68]

Fifty percent of children with Down syndrome have congenital heart anomalies such as atrioventricular canal defects (endocar dial cushion defects), ventricular septal defects, atrial septal defects, patent ductus arteriosus, and tetralogy of fallot. As such, a cardiology consultation and echocardiogram are recommended in the neonatal period. Valvular disease such as mitral valve prolapse, mitral regurgitation, and aortic regurgitation is found more commonly in Down syndrome than in the general population and typically presents in early adulthood;[69] therefore, prior to sport participation, children with Down syndrome should have a thorough history and physical with particular attention to the cardiovascular system.

With respect to the gastrointestinal system, intestinal atresias occur at a higher frequency in Down syndrome than in the general population and typically present in the newborn period. Hirschsprung's disease typically presents in the newborn period in Down syndrome but may present in childhood as chronic constipation.

Up to 75% of children with Down syndrome have some degree of hearing impairment; therefore, formal audiologic testing should be performed biannually until the age of 3 years and annually thereafter.[63] Opthalmologic screening should be performed yearly starting at 5 years of age because 15% of patients develop cataract and 50% of patients have severe refractive errors.[63]

It is estimated that half of all people with mental retardation are overweight.[70] With obesity comes a myriad of potential medical complications including hypertension, hypertriglyceridemia, and type 2 diabetes mellitus; therefore screening should be done at least yearly in the presence of obesity. Obesity is also associated with OSA. Symptoms of OSA such as snoring, brief periods of apnoea when sleeping, restless sleep, or excessive daytime sleepiness, should be screened for on history and patients referred to a specialist as indicated. OSA unabated can lead to sleep deprivation, symptoms of inattention, and hyperactivity and can adversely affect growth and overall development. Long term, it can have harmful affects on the cardiovascular system.[67]

Wound management in patients with Down syndrome can be a challenge. Poorly controlled diabetes is associated with delayed wound healing;[70] therefore, emphasis on good glycaemic control and prevention of skin breakdown is vital. Proper fitting footwear and orthoses are essential.

The physiologic changes that take place during regular athletic training are similar in athletes with disabilities and in non-disabled athletes. The benefits of regular physical activity should also be the similar in these two populations. In a systematic review of outcomes of cardiovascular exercise programmes for people with Down syndrome, improvement in peak oxygen consumption, peak minute ventilation and maximum work load, and increased time to exhaustion was shown.[71] Exercise fosters good physical health through improvement of strength and endurance of the musculoskeletal, nervous, cardiovascular, and endocrine systems; furthermore, it nurtures positive mental attitudes and good overall psychological health.[9] Despite proven benefits, individuals with mental or physical disabilities still tend to be less fit. Through encouragement by parents and physicians, as well as the added motivation that is provided through participation in programmes such as the Special Olympics, the overall health of individuals with disabilities will most certainly benefit.

Special Olympics

Special Olympics International began serving mentally handicapped children and adults in 1968. Participation in Special Olympics helps develop better socialization and physical skills among children and adults with mental retardation. It increases the athletes' self-confidence and independence. Today over 150 countries around the world offer this programme for children and adults with mental disabilities. Athletes, who are grouped according to age and ability, compete in summer sports such as track-and-field, swimming, powerlifting, rhythmic gymnastics, soccer, softball and bowling (Fig. 41.6). Official winter sports include Alpine and Nordic skiing, figure skating, speed skating, snowshoeing, and floor hockey. Over 30, 000 athletes participate in the programme in Canada, and many more are involved throughout the world.[72] Athletes begin with local level competitions and, like their peers without mental retardation, can progress to international competitions that are held every 4 years and are analogous to the Olympic Games.[73] The spirit of Special Olympics is encompassed in the

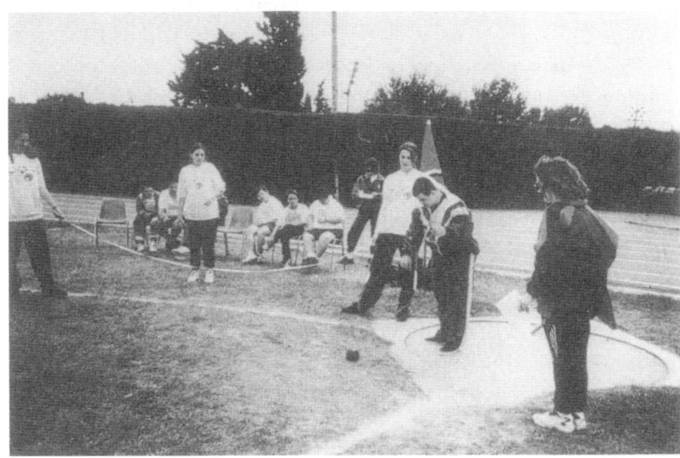

Fig. 41.6 Track and field athlete competing in the Special Olympics.

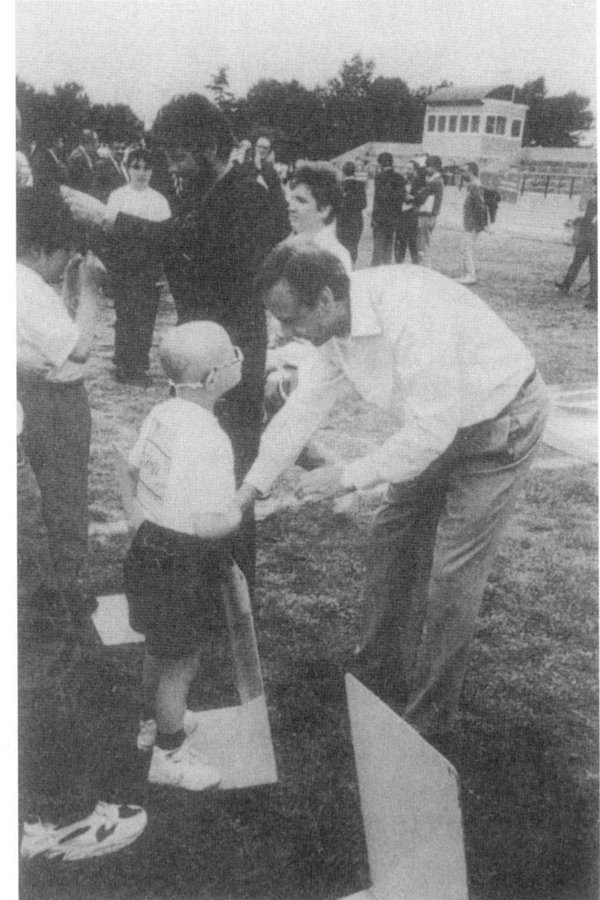

Fig. 41.7 Recognition of excellence in the Special Olympics.

Special Olympics athlete oath: 'Let me win but if I cannot win, let me be brave in the attempt' (Fig. 41.7).

Conclusion

The twentieth century witnessed a dramatic change in the public's perception of individuals with disabilities. New opportunities have allowed these young athletes to experience the many benefits of sport participation once reserved exclusively for the able-bodied child. With this new participation, the field of sport medicine has had to expand in order to allow a greater understanding of the issues unique to each athlete with a disability. From the late 1800s, when baseball was first introduced at the Ohio School for the Deaf to the world-class Paralympic Games of today, athletes with disabilities have reached heights many of us will never achieve.

> 'You are the living demonstration of the marvels of the virtue of energy. You have given a great example, which We would like to emphasize, it can be a lead to all: you have shown what an energetic soul can achieve, in spite of apparently insurmountable obstacles imposed by the body.'
>
> Pope John XXIII, at the International Stoke Mandeville Games in Rome, 1960.[74]

Summary

- Children with disabilities experience many benefits to sport participation including increased confidence and self-esteem, improved physical fitness, and opportunities for social development.
- Deaf athletes often play and compete with hearing athletes but have additional challenges related to communication with team members.
- Modifications of rules and equipment facilitate physical activity in children with visual impairment.
- Spasticity and joint contractures in children with CP increase the risks of injury.
- Lack of sensation below the lesion in myelomeningoceles or spinal cord injuries predisposes the child to pressure-related injuries; therefore, proper fit of adaptive devices and use of appropriate cushioning may prevent skin breakdown, bruising, and pressure sores.
- Osteopaenia secondary to limited weight-bearing in wheelchair athletes increases the risk of fracture, which may be masked by sensory deficits.
- Latex allergies are common in individuals with myelomeningoceles.
- Children with spinal cord lesions above T8 are particularly susceptible to heat-related illness due to impairment of heat production and dissipation mechanisms.
- Autonomic dysreflexia should be suspected in the wheelchair athlete with pale, cool, clammy skin below the lesion and facial flushing, nasal stuffiness, and sweating above the lesion. Hypertension and bradycardia are also present.
- If autonomic dysreflexia is suspected, urinary catheters should be inspected for clamps or kinks, and tight clothing or strapping of lower extremities should be loosened.
- The change in weight across the shoulder girdle in acquired upper-limb amputations affects balance and poses a greater risk for falls in some sports.
- Children with amputations should inspect their stumps regularly for skin breakdown and additional padding can help prevent pressure sores in some sports.
- Although there continues to be controversy over use of screening radiographs for AAI in Down syndrome, such investigations are still required by Special Olympics.
- A single, lateral radiograph of the cervical spine in flexion may be adequate to identify AAI although additional views may be necessary to identify other congenital anomalies of the cervical spine in Down syndrome.
- A history of associated medical conditions should be sought in any athlete with a disability.

References

1. Rimmer JH, Braddock D, Fujiura G (1993). Prevalence of obesity in adults with mental retardation: Implications for health promotion and disease prevention. *Mental Retard* **31**, 105–10.
2. Guttman L (1976). Wheelchair sports for spinal para- and tetraplegics. In: Guttman L (ed.), *Textbook of sport for the disabled*, pp. 21–46. H.M.+M. Publishers Ltd, Aylesbury.
3. Richter KJ, Gaebler-Spira D, Mushett CA (1996). Sport and the person with spasticity of cerebral origin. *Dev Med Child Neurol* **38**, 867–70.
4. Halle JW, Gabler-Halle D, Chung YB (1999). Effects of a peer-mediated aerobic conditioning program on fitness levels of youth with mental retardation: Two systematic replications. *Mental Retard* **37**, 435–48.
5. Fragala-Pinkham MA, Haley SM, Goodgold S (2000). Evaluation of a community-based group fitness program for children with disabilities. *Pediatr Phys Ther* **18**, 159–67.
6. Modan M, Peles E, Halkin H, Nitzan H, Azaria M, Gitel S, Dolfin D, Modan B (1998). Increased cardiovascular disease mortality rates in traumatic lower limb amputees. *Am J Cardiol* **82,** 1242–7.
7. Filho JA, Salvetti XM, de Mello MT, da Silva AC, Filho BL (2006). Coronary risk in a cohort of Paralympic athletes. *Br J Sports Med* **40**, 918–22.
8. Varni JW, Setoguchi Y (1991). Correlates of perceived physical appearance in children with congenital/acquired limb deficiencies. *J DevBehav Pediatr* **12**, 171–6.
9. Birrer RB (2004). The special olympics athlete: Evaluation and clearance for participation. *Clin Pediatr* **43**, 777–82.
10. Dec KL, Sparrow KJ, McKeag DB (2000). The physically-challenged athlete: Medical issues and assessment. *Sports Med* **29**, 245–58.
11. Haddad J (2004). The Ear. In: Nelson WE (ed.), *Nelson textbook of pediatrics* (17th ed.), pp. 2127–50. Saunders Company, Philadelphia, PA.
12. Hyndman JC (1998). The growing athlete. In: Harries M, Williams C, Stanish WD and Micheli LJ (eds.), *Oxford textbook of sports medicine* (2nd ed.), pp. 727–41. Oxford University Press, Oxford.
13. Winnick JP (1995). An introduction to adapted physical education and sport. In: Winnick JP (ed.), *Adapted physical education and sport*, pp. 3–16. Human Kinetics, Windsor, Ontario.
14. Craft DH (1995). Visual impairments and hearing losses. In: Winnick JP (ed.), *Adapted physical education and sport*, pp. 143–66. Human Kinetics, Windsor, Ontario.
15. Guttman L (1976). Sports for the deaf. In: Guttman L (ed.), *Textbook of sport for the disabled,* pp. 170–3. HM +M Publishers Ltd, Aylesbury.
16. Palmer T, Weber KM (2006). The deaf athlete. *Curr Sports Med Rep* **5**, 323–6.

17. Chang FM (1994). The disabled athlete. In: Stanitski CL, DeLee JC, Drez D (eds.), *Pediatric and adolescent sports medicine*—Vol. 3, pp. 48–76. W.B. Saunders Company, Philadelphia, PA.
18. Booth DW, Grogono BJ (1998). Athletes with a disability. In: Harries M, Williams C, Stanish WD, Micheli LJ (eds.), *Oxford textbook of sports medicine* (2nd ed.), pp. 815–31. Oxford University Press, Oxford.
19. Guttman L (1976). Sports for the blind and partially sighted. In: Guttman L (ed.), *Textbook of sport for the disabled*, pp. 150–61. H.M.+M. Publishers Ltd, Aylesbury.
20. Laskowski ER (1991). Snow skiing for the physically disabled. *Mayo Clinic Proc* **66**, 160–72.
21. Haslam RHA (2004). The nervous system. In: Nelson WE (ed.), *Nelson textbook of pediatrics* (17th ed.), pp. 1973–2049. W.B. Saunders Company, Philadelphia, PA.
22. Guttman L (1976). Sports for sufferers from cerebral palsy. In: Guttman L (ed.), *Textbook of sport for the disabled*, pp. 162–9. H.M.+M. Publishers Ltd, Aylesbury.
23. Richter KE, Hyman SC, Mushett-Adams CA (1991). Injuries in world-class cerebral palsy athletes at the 1988 South Korea Paralympics. *J Osteopath Sports Med* **5**, 15–8.
24. O'Neill DB, Micheli LJ (1988). Overuse injuries in the young athlete. *Clin Sports Med* **7**, 591–610.
25. Soprano JV (2005). Musculoskeletal injuries in the pediatric and adolescent athlete. *Curr Sports Med Rep* **4**, 329–34.
26. Lockette KF, Keyes AM (1994). Conditioning with spinal cord injuries, spina bifida, and poliomyelitis. In: Fowler ME (ed.), *Conditioning with physical disabilities*, pp. 91–116. Human Kinetics, Windsor, Ontario.
27. Steadward RD, Wheeler GD (1996). The young athlete with a motor disability. In: Bar-Or (ed.), *The child and adolescent athlete*, pp. 493–520. Blackwell Science Ltd., Oxford.
28. Metzl JD (2001). Preparticipation examination of the adolescent athlete: Part 1. *Pediatr Rev* **22**, 199–204.
29. van den Berg-Emons HJK, Bussmann JBJ, Meyerink HJ, Roebroeck ME, Stam HJ (2003). Body fat, fitness and level of everyday physical activity in adolescents and young adults with meningomyelocele. *J Rehab Med* **35**, 271–5.
30. Johnston MV, Kinsman S (2004). Congenital anomalies of the central nervous system. In: Nelson WE (ed.), *Nelson textbook of pediatrics* (17th ed.), pp. 1983–6. W.B. Saunders Company, Philadelphia, PA.
31. Patel DR, Greydanus DE (2002). The pediatric athlete with disabilities. *Pediatr Clin N Am* **49**, 803–27.
32. Randolph C (2001). Latex allergy in pediatrics. *Curr Prob Pediatr* **31**, 135–53.
33. Jackson AB, Dijkers M, DeVivo MJ, Poczatek RB (2004). A demographic profile of new traumatic spinal cord injuries: Change and stability over 30 years. *Arch Phys Med Rehab* **85**, 1740–8.
34. Schutz LK (1994). The wheelchair athlete. In: Buschbacher RM, Braddom RL (eds.), *Sports medicine and rehabilitation: A sport-specific approach*, pp. 267–74. Hanley & Belfus, Inc., Philadelphia, PA.
35. Lockette KF, Keyes AM (1994). Conditioning with amputations. In: Fowler ME (ed.), *Conditioning with physical disabilities*, pp. 117–34. Human Kinetics, Windsor, Ontario.
36. Poretta DL (1995). Cerebral palsy, traumatic brain injury, stroke, amputations, dwarfism, and other orthopedic impairments. In: Winnick JP (ed.), *Adapted physical education and sport*, pp. 167–91. Human Kinetics, Windsor, Ontario.
37. Guttman L (1976). Sports for amputees. In: Guttman L (ed.), *Textbook of sport for the disabled*, pp. 119–49. H.M.+M. Publishers Ltd, Aylesbury.
38. Farley R, Mitchell F, Griffiths M (2004). Custom skiing and trekking adaptations for a trans-tibial and trans-radial quadrilateral amputee. *Prosthet Orthot Int* **28**, 60–3.
39. Marquardt E, Correll J (1984). Amputations and prostheses for the lower limb. *Int Orthop (SICOT)* **8**, 139–46.
40. Shapiro BK, Bashaw ML (2004). Mental retardation. In: Nelson WE (ed.), *Nelson textbook of pediatrics* (17th ed.), pp. 138–43. W.B. Saunders Company, Philadelphia, PA.
41. Compton DM, Eisenman PA, Henderson HL (1989). Exercise and fitness for persons with disabilities. *Sports Med* **7**, 150–62.
42. Fernhall B (1993). Physical fitness and exercise training of individuals with mental retardation. *Med Sci Sports Exerc* **25**, 442–50.
43. Pitetti KH, Campbell KD (1991). Mentally retarded individuals—a population at risk? *Med Sci Sports Exerc* **23**, 586–93.
44. Hall JG (2004). Chromosomal clinical abnormalities. In: Nelson WE (ed.), *Nelson textbook of pediatrics* (17th ed.), pp. 382–91. W.B. Saunders Company, Philadelphia, PA.
45. Diamond LS, Lynne D, Sigman B (1981). Orthopedic disorders in patients with Down's syndrome. *Orthop Clin N Am* **12**, 57–71.
46. Pizzutillo PD, Herman MJ (2006). Musculoskeletal concerns in the young athlete with down syndrome. *Oper Tech Sports Med* **14**, 135–40.
47. Bosch P, Johnston CE, Karol L (2004). Slipped capital femoral epiphysis in patients with Down Syndrome. *J Pediatr Orthop* **24**, 271–7.
48. Nader-Sepahi A, Casey AT, Hayward R, Crockard HA, Thompson D (2005). Symptomatic atlantoaxial instability in Down syndrome. *J Neurosurg* **103** (Suppl. 3), 231–7.
49. American Academy of Pediatrics (1995). Atlantoaxial instability in Down syndrome: Subject review. *Pediatrics* **96**, 151–4.
50. Pueschel SM (1998). Should children with Down syndrome be screened for atlantoaxial instability? *Arch Pediatr Adolesc Med* **152**, 123–5.
51. Cohen WI (1998). Atlantoaxial instability: What's next? *Arch Pediatr Adolesc Med* **152**, 119–22.
52. Committee on Sports Medicine (1984). Atlantoaxial instability in Down syndrome. *Pediatrics* **74**, 152–4.
53. Sackett DL, Haynes RB, Guyatt GH, Tugwell P (1991). *Clinical epidemiology: A basic science for clinical medicine* (2nd ed.), pp. 153–70. Little, Brown, and Co, Boston, MA.
54. Selby KA, Newton RW, Gupta S, Hunt L (1991). Clinical predictors and radiologic reliability in atlantoaxial subluxation in Down syndrome. *Arch Dis Child* **66**, 876–8.
55. Peuschel SM, Scola FH, Pezzullo JC (1992). A longitudinal study of atlanto-dens relationships in asymptomatic individuals with Down syndrome. *Pediatrics* **89**, 1194–8.
56. Peuschel SM, Scola FH (1987). Atlantoaxial instability in individuals with Down syndrome: Epidemiologic, radiographic, and clinical studies. *Pediatrics* **80**, 555–60.
57. Committee on Sports Medicine and Fitness (1995). Atlantoaxial instability in Down syndrome: subject review. *Pediatrics* **96**, 151–4.
58. Adam HM (2003). In brief. Atlantoaxial dislocation. *Pediatr Rev* **24**, 106–7.
59. O'Connor JF, Cranley WR, McCarten KM, Feingold M (1996). Commentary: Atlantoaxial instability in Down syndrome: Reassessment by the committee on sports medicine and fitness of the American Academy of Pediatrics. *Pediatr Radiol* **26**, 748–9.
60. Ali FE, Al-Bustan MA, Al-Busairi WA, Al-Mulla FA, Esbaita EY (2006). Cervical spine abnormalities associated with Down syndrome. *Int Orthop* **30**, 284–9.
61. Pueschel SM, Herndon JH, Gelch MM, Senft KE, Scola FH, Goldberg MJ (1984). Symptomatic atlantoaxial subluxation in persons with Down syndrome. *J Pediatr Orthop* **4**, 682–8.
62. Msall ME, Reese ME, DiGaudio K, Griswold K, Granger CV, Cooke RE (1990). Symptomatic Atlantoaxial instability associated with medical and rehabilitative procedures in children with Down Syndrome. *Pediatrics* **85**, 447–9.
63. Committee on Genetics (2001). Health supervision for children with Down syndrome. *Pediatrics* **207**, 442–9.
64. White KS, Ball WS, Prenger EC, Patterson BJ, Kirks DR (1993). Evaluation of the craniocervical junction in Down syndrome:

Correlation of measurements obtained by radiography and MR imaging. *Radiology* **186**, 377–82.

65. Cope R, Olson S (1987). Abnormalities of the cervical spine in Down's syndrome: Diagnosis, risks, and review of the literature, with particular reference to the Special Olympics. *South Med J* **80**, 33–6.
66. Goldberg MJ (1993). Spine instability and the Special Olympics. *Clin Sports Med* **12**, 507–15.
67. Dincer HE, O-Neill W (2006). Deleterious effects of sleep-disordered breathing on the heart and vascular system. *Respiration* **73**, 124–30.
68. Cooley WC (2005). Down Syndrome. In: Osborn LM, DeWitt TG, First LR, Zenel JA (eds.), *Pediatrics* (1st ed.), pp. 1060–4. Mosby, Philadelphia, PA.
69. Hamada T, Gejyo F, Koshino Y, Murata T, Omori M, Nishio M, Misawa T, Isaki K (1998). Echocardiographic evaluation of cardiac valvular abnormalities in adults with Down's syndrome. *Tohoku J Exper Med* **185**, 31–5.
70. Platt LS (2001). Medical and orthopaedic conditions in Special Olympics athletes. *J Athletic Train* **36**, 74–80.
71. Dodd KJ, Shields N (2005). A systematic review of the outcomes of cardiovascular exercise programs for people with Down syndrome. *Arch Phys Med Rehab* **86**, 2051–8.
72. Special Olympics Canada (2007). Available at www.specialolympics.ca (last accessed 20 July 2007).
73. Special Olympics (2007). *World games*. Available at www.specialolympics.org (last accessed 20 July 2007).
74. Guttman L (ed.). (1976). *Textbook of sport for the disabled.* H.M.+M. Publishers Ltd, Aylesbury.

CHAPTER 42

Current concepts on the aetiology and prevention of sports injuries

Willem van Mechelen and Evert A.L.M. Verhagen

Introduction

A physically active lifestyle and active participation in sports is important, for adults as well as for children. Reasons to participate in sports and physical activity are many: pleasure and relaxation, competition, socialization, maintenance and improvement of fitness and health, etc. In general, when compared to adults, the risk for sports injury resulting from participation in sports and free play is low in children.[1] Despite this relatively low risk, sports injuries in children are a fact of life, which calls for preventive action. In order to set out effective prevention programmes, epidemiological studies need to be done on incidence, severity, and aetiology of sports injuries. Also the effect of preventive measures needs to be evaluated. In the following chapters various authors will describe these aspects of sports injuries in children, regarding specific sports. This chapter describes briefly some current concepts regarding the epidemiology and prevention of sports injuries as a means of introduction to these chapters.

The sequence of prevention

Measures to prevent sports injuries do not stand by themselves. They form part of what might be called a sequence of prevention (Fig. 42.1). First, the problem must be identified and described in terms of incidence and severity of sports injuries. Then the factors and mechanisms that play a part in the occurrence of sports injuries have to be identified. The third step is to introduce measures that are likely to reduce the future risk and/or severity of sports injuries. Such measures should be based on the aetiologic factors and the mechanisms as identified in the second step. Finally, the effect of the measures must be evaluated by repeating the first step, which will lead to so-called time-trend analysis of injury patterns. However, from an epidemiological standpoint it is preferable to evaluate the effect of preventive measures by means of a randomized controlled trial (RCT). Unfortunately, RCTs have only very rarely been conducted in sports injury prevention studies, and most of the RCTs that have been conducted so far in this area of research were carried out in adults.

Defining sports injury

When conducting (and also when interpreting the outcomes of) epidemiological sports injuries studies, one is confronted with a number of methodological issues. The first issue of importance here is the definition of sports injury. In general, sports injury is a collective name for all types of damage that can occur in relation to sporting activities. Various studies of incidence define the term sports injury in different ways. In some studies, a sports injury is defined as any injury sustained during sporting activities for which an insurance claim is submitted; in other studies, the definition is confined to injuries treated at a hospital casualty or other medical department.[2] Different definitions partly explain the differing incidences found in the literature. The results of various sports injury incidence surveys are therefore not comparable. If sports injuries are recorded through medical channels (for instance, through hospital emergency rooms), a fairly large percentage of serious, predominantly acute injuries will be observed and less serious and/or overuse injuries will not be recorded. If such a 'limited' definition is used, only part of the total sports injury problem is revealed. This 'tip-of-the-iceberg' phenomenon is commonly described in epidemiological research. This problem is to a large extent found in sports injury epidemiology in youth, where many overuse injuries are thought to be found, as well as 'minor' acute injuries.

To make sports injury surveys comparable and to avoid the 'tip-of-the-iceberg' phenomenon as far as possible, an unambiguous,

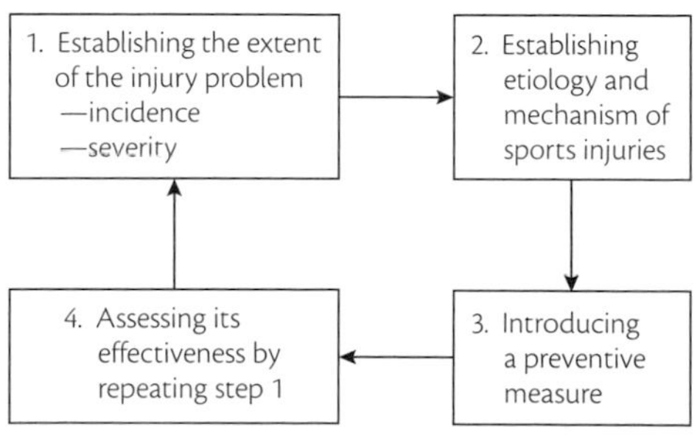

Fig. 42.1 The sequence of prevention of sports injuries.[2]

universally applicable definition of sports injury is the first prerequisite. This definition should be based on a concept of health other than that customary in standard medicine and should, for instance, take incapacitation for sports or school into account. Even if one single uniform definition of sports injury is applied, the need remains for uniform agreement on other issues. These concern, for instance, the way in which sports injury incidence is expressed and the ways in which reliable estimates are made of both the number of people engaging in sports and the number of injured sports persons.

Sports injury incidence

One way of getting an impression of the extent of the sports injury problem is by counting the absolute number of injuries. When these numbers are compared with, for instance, the number of road accidents or the number of injuries sustained during leisure time activities, the relative extent of the sports injury problem can be revealed. However, such a comparison is unable to reveal the true risk of a certain activity. One can only sustain a road accident when participating in traffic. Even so, one can only sustain a sports injury when participating in sports. While the amount of leisure time or traffic participation is usually higher than the amount of participation in sports, a comparison of absolute injury numbers are inferior from an epidemiological perspective.

The most appropriate indication of the spread of disease in the population or in a section of the population is incidence. If one substitutes 'sports injury' or 'sports accident' for 'disease', incidence can be defined as 'the number of new sports injuries or accidents sustained during a particular period, divided by the total number of sports persons at the start of the period (i.e. the population at risk)' Incidence thus defined also gives an estimate of risk. If one multiplies the obtained figure by 100, one gets the incidence percentage rate.[3] Expressed in this way, sports injury incidence figures give insight into the extent of the sports injury problem in a particular population-at-risk. It is clear from this definition of incidence that incidence can only be assessed properly if both a clear definition of sports injury as well as of the population-at-risk are present.

In many studies, the incidence rate of sports injuries is usually defined as the number of new sports injuries during a particular period (e.g. 1 year) divided by the total number of sports persons at the start of that period (population-at-risk). When interpreting and comparing the various incidence rates, to know what injury definition was used. One should also have information on the comparability of the population-at-risk. It is clear that the methods used to count injuries and to count the population-at-risk will also influence sports injury incidence figures. Finally, the length of the observation period has to be taken into account, since different lengths of observation periods will have a distinct influence on the incidences calculated.

In terms of risk assessment, another problem lies in the way incidence rates are expressed. In most cases, the number of injuries in a particular category of sports participants per season or per year is taken, or the number of injuries per player per match. In both examples no allowance is made for any differences in actual exposure (i.e. the number of hours during which the sports participant is actually at risk for being injured). This is peculiar because this factor certainly has great influence on the risk of sustaining a sports injury. Incidence figures that do not take exposure into account are therefore not a good indication of the true 'true' risk one runs, nor can the incidence rates for various sports or sporting populations be properly compared. It would be better to calculate the incidence of sports injuries in relation to exposure time (hours). The equation of Chambers,[4] adapted by De Loës and Goldi,[5] can be used to calculate injury incidence taking exposure into account:

Injury incidence = (no. of sports injuries per year) × 104 / (no. of participants) × (hours of sports participation per week) × (weeks of season/year)

Research design

The extent to which sports injury incidence can be assessed depends upon the definition of sports injury, the way in which incidence is expressed, the method used to count injuries, the method to establish population at risk, and the representativeness of the sample. Here, clearly, research design also comes into play. Injuries as well as time-at-risk can be assessed retrospectively or prospectively using questionnaires or person-to-person interviews. However, prospective studies can, by closely monitoring exposure time and injury outcome, more accurately estimate the risk and incidence of sports injury according to the level of sports participation and type of exposure of an athlete. They are therefore superior to retrospective studies. One of the main problems of retrospective studies is the inherent recall bias of the subjects participating in such a study.

A word should be said here about case studies. In sports medical journals, clinical case studies are often described. Conclusions are drawn from these case studies regarding the incidence and the risk of sustaining sports injuries. However, case studies have the drawback that no information on the population-at-risk is available. Consequently, no valid conclusions can be drawn from case studies, either with respect to sports injury incidence or with respect to injury risks.[6]

Depending upon the method of choice, the researcher will be confronted with phenomena such as recall bias, overestimation of hours of sports participation,[7] incomplete response, non-response, drop-out, invalid injury descriptions, and problems related to the duration and cost of research. These factors will clearly affect the internal validity of a study.

Special attention has to be paid to the method of assessing the population-at-risk and to the representativeness of the sample. If the population at risk is not clearly identified, it is not possible to calculate reliable incidence data. With regard to the representativeness of the study population, it has to be taken into consideration that the performance of athletes in sports, and therefore also the incidence of sports injuries, is highly determined by selection. Bol *et al.*[8] recognized four different kinds of selection:

(i) self selection (personal preferences) and/or selection by social environment (parents, friends, schools, etc.);

(ii) selection by sports environment (trainer, coach, etc.);

(iii) selection by sports organizations (organization of competitions by age and gender, the setting of participation standards, etc.); and

(iv) selection by social, medical and biological factors (socioeconomic background, mortality, age, aging, gender, etc.).

For example, within a certain sport, competing at a high level increases sports injury risk; more injuries are sustained during matches than during training; in contact sports, more injuries are sustained as compared with non-contact sports; during and shortly after the growth spurt, boys sustain more injuries than during other periods of growth; and so on.

The severity of sports injuries

A description of the severity of sports injuries is important in making a decision about whether preventive measures are needed, since the need to prevent serious injuries in a particular sport need not coincide with a high overall incidence of injuries in that sport. According to the literature, the severity of sports injuries can be described on the basis of six criteria.[9] These criteria are briefly described below.

Nature of sports injuries

The nature of sports injuries can be described in terms of medical diagnosis: sprain (of joint capsule and ligaments), strain (of muscle or tendon), contusion (bruising), dislocation, or subluxation, fracture (of bone), and so on. It is the nature of the sports injury that determines whether assistance (medical or otherwise) is sought. Recording of the nature of sports injuries enable those sports with relative serious injuries to be identified. The nature of sports injuries can also be described according to the part of the body being injured.

Duration and nature of treatment

Data on the duration and nature of treatment can be used to determine the severity of an injury more precisely, especially if it is a question of what medical bodies are involved in the treatment and what therapies used.

Sports time lost

It is important for a sports person to be able to take up his or her sport again as soon as possible after an injury. Sport and exercise play an essential part in people's free time and thus influence their mental well-being. The sporting time lost gives the most precise indication of the consequences of an injury to a sports person.

Working or school time lost

Like the cost of medical treatment, the length of working or school time lost gives an indication of the consequences of sports injuries at a societal level. Data of working or school time lost are used to compare the cost to society of sports injuries with that of other situations involving risks, such as traffic accidents.

Permanent damage

The vast majority of sports injuries heal without permanent disability. Serious injuries, such as fractures, ligament, tendon and intra-articular injuries, spinal injuries, and eye injuries, can leave permanent damage (residual symptoms). Excessive delay between the occurrence of an injury and medical assistance can aggravate the injury. If the residual symptoms are slight, they may cause the individual to modify his or her level of sporting activity. In some cases, however, the sports person may have to choose another sport or give up sport altogether. Serious physical damage can cause permanent disability or death, thus leading to reducing or eliminating the individual's capacity for work or school. When taking precautions, then, priority should be given to measures in sports where such serious injuries are common, even though the particular sport itself is characterized by a low incidence of sports injuries and/or low absolute number of participants.

Costs of sports injuries

The calculation of the costs of sports injuries essentially involves the expression of the above mentioned five categories of seriousness of sports injuries in economic terms. The economic costs can be divided into:

(i) direct costs, that is, the cost of medical treatment (diagnostic expenses such as X-rays, doctor's fee, cost of medicines, admission costs, etc.) and

(ii) indirect costs, that is, expenditure incurred in connection with the loss of productivity due to increased morbidity and mortality levels (loss of school or working time and loss of expertise due to death or handicap).

Conceptual models for the aetiology and prevention of sports injuries

Risk indicators for sports injuries can be divided into two main categories: internal risk indicators and external, environmental risk indicators.[2] This division is based on partly proven and partly supposed causal relationships between risk factors and sports injuries. However, merely to establish the cause of sports injuries, that is, the internal and external factors is not enough; the mechanism by which they occur must also be identified.[10]

As can be seen in Fig. 42.2, sports injuries result from a complex interaction of multiple risk factors, of which only a fraction have been identified. Despite this multi-causality, many epidemiological studies have concentrated on identifying single internal and external risk indicators from a medical, mono-causal point of view, rather than form a multi-causal point of view. However, studies on the aetiology of sports injuries require a dynamic model that accounts for this multi-factorial nature of sports injuries and that also takes the sequence of events eventually leading to an injury into account. One such dynamic model is the model described by Meeuwisse *et al.*[11] that describes the interplay between different factors along the path to injury. This model clearly postulates that an injury is the result of a recursive complex interaction between internal and external risk factors and is not exclusively caused by the inciting event that is generally associated with the onset of injury (see Fig. 42.3).

In studies on the aetiology of sports injuries, this model can be used to explore the inter-relationships between risk factors and their contribution to the occurrence of injury. Meeuwisse *et al.*[11] classifies the intrinsic or athlete-related factors as predisposing factors that are necessary, but seldom sufficient, to produce injury. In this theoretical model, extrinsic risk factors act on the predisposed athlete from without and are classified as enabling factors in that they facilitate the manifestation of injury. It is the presence of both intrinsic and extrinsic risk factors that render the athlete susceptible to injury, but the mere presence of these risk factors is usually not sufficient to produce injury. It is the sum of these risk factors and the interaction between them that 'prepare' the athlete for an injury to happen at a given place, in a given sports situation.

Meeuwise *et al.*[11] describe an inciting event to be the final link in the chain of causation to sports injury and state that such an inciting event is usually directly associated with the onset of injury. Such events are regarded as necessary causes. Studies on the aetiology of sports injuries tend to focus on factors proximal to the injury event (i.e. the inciting events) and tend to neglect factors more distant from the injury event (i.e. the intrinsic and extrinsic risk factors), thereby revealing only a small fraction of the factors and events that lead to sports injury. Although understandable, focusing on inciting events may lead to overweighing the importance of such events in the aetiology and prevention of sports injuries. If in aetiological studies distant factors are studied, they usually concern intrinsic, person-related risk factors. These factors are relatively easier to measure than extrinsic risk factors. Lastly, it should be noted that regarding injury aetiology there is a 'classical' linear paradigm—meaning events follow sequentially to an end-point, in this case an injury. However, an injury does not represent a finite end-point, and a linear approach does not take into account that injury occurrence or injury avoidance has an effect on future injury risk through influence on intrinsic and extrinsic risk factors. Therefore, it is a dynamic recursive model like the model of Meeuwisse *et al.*[11] that should be used to study the aetiology of sports injuries.

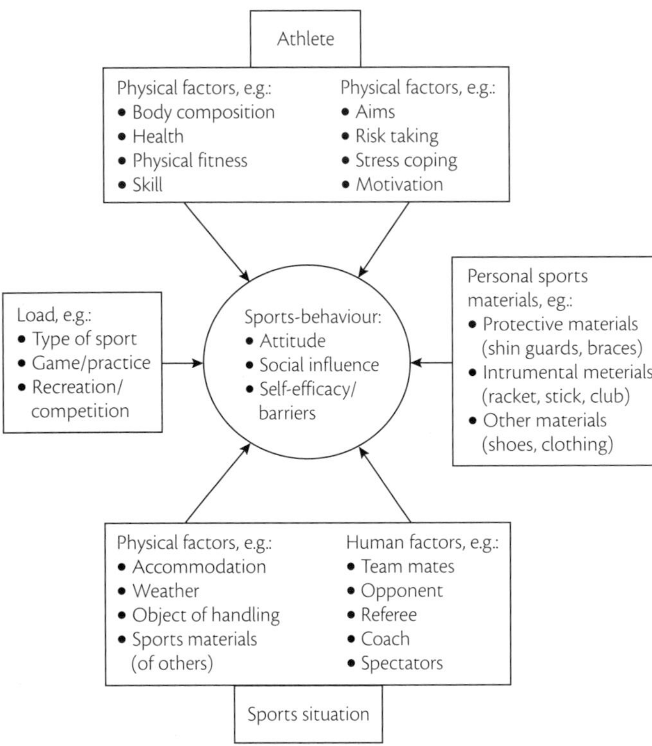

Fig. 42.2 Risk indicators for sports injuries and determinants of sports and preventive behaviour.[2]

Finally, a word should be said here about sports behaviour. Recently, debate has arisen about the true effect of proven preventive measures in a real-life sports setting.[12] In contemporary sports medicine, preventive measures are based upon risk factors and injury mechanisms, which are predominantly established through biomedical and/or biomechanical research. Bluntly put, an injury risk factor is established and one studies (preferably in a RCT) what happens to the injury risk when the risk factor is reduced or expelled from sports. Due to the controlled nature of such studies, the results of this approach can rarely be generalized to an actual sports setting and are seldom adopted by a sports population. As stated by Finch,[12] only research outcomes that will be adopted by athletes, coaches, and sporting bodies will actually prevent injuries. For this reason, Finch introduced the TRIPP model[12] as an expansion in the original sequence of prevention.[2] The TRIPP approach aims at a better understanding of the implementation context for injury prevention. Such recent advances in sports medicine lead the way to a more behavioural approach of sports injury prevention.

When trying to prevent sports injuries one should realize that participation in sports is a form of behaviour. Usually the introduction of preventive measures implies a change or modification of behaviour of the athlete and/or others involved in the athlete's care. It may very well be that the desired preventive behaviour conflicts with the actual sports behaviour, for instance, because it is believed by the athlete that the preventive behaviour will affect sports performance negatively. When introducing preventive measures and when evaluating the effect of such measures, it is therefore necessary to have knowledge of the determinants of the acting behaviours. Many models are used to explain preventive

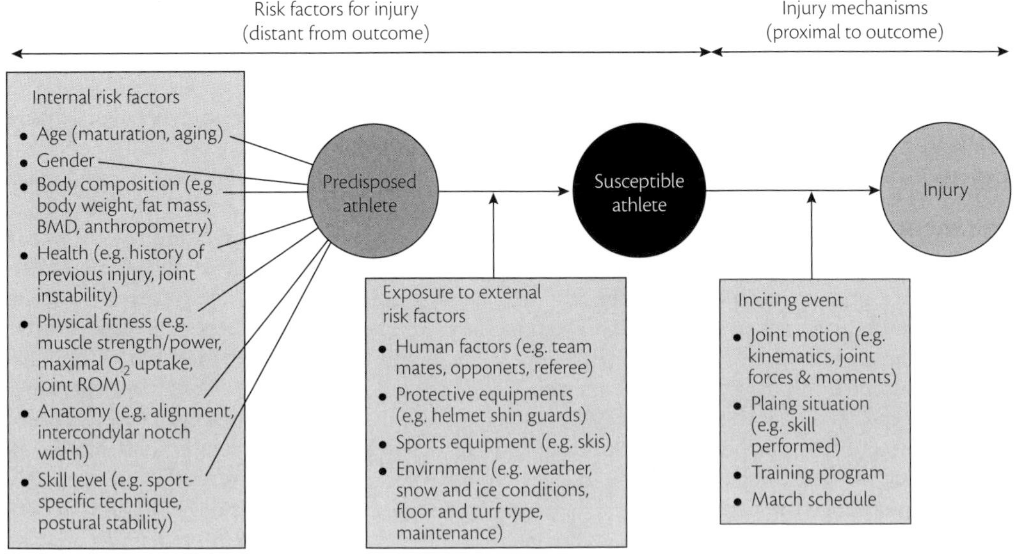

Fig. 42.3 A dynamic, multifactorial model of sports injury aetiology[10] (Reprinted with permission from British Journal of Sports Medicine).

behaviour. In general, these models include three sets of determinants: (i) knowledge and attitude, (ii) social influence and (iii) barriers and self-efficacy[13] (Fig. 42.2). These determinants are described as follows:[14]

(i) 'Attitude refers to the knowledge and beliefs of a person concerning the specific consequences of a certain form of behaviour. An attitude is the weighing of all consequences of the performance of the behaviour, as seen by the individual. Health is only seen as one of the considerations, and is often an unimportant one. When health is part of attitude one may suppose that healthy motivation is a combination of the perceived severity of the health risk, the perceived susceptibility to the health risk, and the effectiveness of preventive behaviour.

(ii) Social influence is the influence by others; directly by what others expect, indirectly by what others do (modelling). Social influence is often underestimated as a determinant of behaviour. It can lead to behaviour that conflicts with previous attitudes. Most sports situations are social situations.

(iii) Self-efficacy-cum-barriers stands for the determinant whether one is able to perform (desired) behaviour. It involves an estimation of ability, taking into account possible internal (e.g. insufficient skill, knowledge, endurance) or external barriers (e.g. resistance form others, time and money not available, etc.). Self-efficacy is the people's perception of their ability to perform the behaviour, and barriers are the real problem they face in actually performing the behaviour.

It is these determinants that should be accounted for when trying to prevent sports injuries.

Summary

- The outcome of research on the extent of the sports injury problem is highly dependant on the definitions of 'sports injury', 'sports injury incidence', and 'sports participation'.
- The outcome of sports epidemiological research also depends on the research design and methodology, the representativeness of the sample, and whether exposure time was considered when calculating incidence.
- The severity of sports injuries can be expressed by taking six indices into consideration.
- The aetiology of sports injuries is highly multi-causal and recursive. This fact, as well as the sequence of events leading to a sports injury, should be accounted for when studying the aetiology of sports injuries and when trying to prevent them.
- Finally, one should take the determinants of different behaviours (e.g. sports and preventive behaviour) into account in attempts to solve the sports injury problem.

References

1. Mechelen W van (1997). Etiology and prevention of sports injuries in youth. In: Froberg K, Pedersen P, Steen Hansen H, Blimkie CJR (eds.), *Exercise and fitness—children and exercise XVIII*, pp. 209–28. University Press, Odense.
2. Mechelen W van, Hlobil H, Kemper HCG (1992). Incidence, severity, aetiology and prevention of sports injuries. *Sports Med* **14**, 82–99.
3. Sturmans F (1984). *Epidemiologie*. Dekker and van de Vegt, Nijmegen.
4. Chambers RB (1979). Orthopedic injuries in athletes (ages 6 to 17), comparison of injuries occurring in six sports. *Am J Sports* **7**, 195–7.
5. de Loës M, Goldie MK (1988). Incidence rate of injuries during sport activity, and physical exercise in a rural Swedish municipality: Incidence rates in 17 sports. *Int J Sports Med* **9**, 461–7.
6. Walter SD, Sutton JR, McIntosh JM, Connolly C (1985). The aetiology of sports injuries. A review of methodologies. *Sports Med* **2**, 47–58.
7. Klesges RC, Eck LH, Mellon MW, Fulliton W, Somes GW, Hanson CL (1990). The accuracy of self-reports of physical activity. *Med Sci Sports Exerc* **22**, 690–7.
8. Bol E, Schmickli SL, Backx FJG, Mechelen W van (1991). *Sportblessures onder de knie*; NISGZ publication 38, Papendal.
9. Mechelen W van (1997). The severity of sports injuries. *Sports Med* **24**, 176–80.
10. Bahr R, Krosshaug T (2005). Understanding injury mechanisms; a key component of preventing injuries in sports. *Br J Sport Med* **39**, 324–9.
11. Meeuwisse WH, Tyreman H, Hagel B, Emery CA (2007). Dynamic model of etiology in sport injury: The recursive nature of risk and causation. *Clin J Sports Med* **17**, 215–9.
12. Finch C (2006). A new framework for research leading to sports injury prevention. *J Sci Med Sport* **9**, 3–9.
13. Kok GJ, Bouter LM (1990). On the importance of planned health education; prevention of ski injury as an example. *Am J Sports Med* **18**, 600–5.
14. Mechelen W van (1995). Can running injuries be effectively presented? *Sport Med* **19**, 161–5.

CHAPTER 43

Aetiology and prevention of injuries in physical education classes

Frank J.G. Backx and Dorine C.M. Collard

Introduction

In most western countries, school-aged children get 1 or 2 hours of physical education classes (PE classes) a week. Although it is questionable if this number of PE classes contribute substantially to the physical development and health of a young individual, it is presumed to be beneficial in both the short and long term.[1]

In most countries in Europe, sports activities are not explicitly incorporated into the school system as much as in the United States. On the one hand, this has resulted in PE classes being less competitive. On the other hand, club sports activities in Europe have increased. The latter has been accompanied by an increase in sports injuries.[2]

Physical education at school, in which all school-aged children participate, is aimed at all-round physical conditioning by a diversity of movements. However, the participation in PE classes diminishes as one grows older.[3] Nowadays, for instance in the Netherlands, not all secondary schools offer obligatory physical education classes at every grade level anymore.

One of the goals of PE classes should be to motivate children to practice sports over a lifetime. Negative experience like injuries during physical education will question the achievement of this objective.[4] Data concerning injuries in PE classes are mostly obtained from large epidemiological studies that do not specifically address the issue. Consequently, there are only limited specific data on this theme.

This chapter summarizes the available specific information on the epidemiology and prevention of injuries sustained in physical education.

Incidence rates

In general, sports participation and consequently the number of sports injuries in young people have increased considerably in the last three decades. Nowadays, it is evident that despite the fact that the number of school children is declining in most European countries, there still is a general increase in sports accidents.[5] Unfortunately, data concerning injuries specifically incurred in PE lessons are scarce at present. Only a few studies on sports injuries in children and adolescents have outlined the incidence and types of injuries in PE lessons. Analogous to studies performed outside the school system, these studies suffer from a lack of comparability because of:[6–8]

(i) a lack of uniform definitions of sports injury;

(ii) limited reliability of collected data;

(iii) insufficient information on the population at risk; and

(iv) insufficient information on the sports exposure time.

Furthermore, these investigations vary enormously in extent and depth. The scope of data gathered depends strongly on the methods of data acquisition, particularly on the locus of measurement.

Overall in the literature, studies on children and adolescents have rarely been population-based. Some were based on registrations in out-patient clinics or in casualty departments[9,10] and others were based on reports of PE teachers.[2,11] Probably the number of injuries that actually occur in PE classes is much higher than found in these studies because many schools do not maintain good injury records.[2,3] Another problem arises when pupils themselves have to fill in a registration form. In addition, retrospective study designs introduce recall-bias resulting in under- or over-recording.

As a result of several differences in definitions of injury, the locus of measurement, and the contents of PE classes, it is not surprising that incidence rates of injuries sustained in PE classes vary between 0.75[12] and 11.7[13] per 100 school children per year. More recently, Kelm *et al.*[4] calculated that about 5% of all school children are seriously injured during PE classes every year.

Obviously, diagnosis by medical staff or assessment by PE teachers and school-aged children themselves will affect results of studies on the incidence of injuries in PE classes considerably. It is clear that the medical system is aware of only a small and distorted segment of the total injury problem. In this context, reference is made to the well-known 'iceberg' phenomenon, discussed in Chapter 42. Therefore, the population approach to injury is preferable, as it allows considerable insight into the rate of occurrence, the causes of injury, and the identification of high-risk groups.[14] The disadvantage of this approach is the registration of a large number of less severe injuries.

The very wide variety of activities during PE classes is another point of concern. If, despite these problems, one still attempts to compare injuries sustained in physical education, because each kind of sports activity has its own characteristics, one has to deal with important differences in sports specific risk factors. This will also affect the number of injuries sustained during PE classes.

Risk of injury in physical education classes

In Germany, almost half (680,000) of all school injuries (1.34 million school accidents in total) took place during PE classes in 1994[4] which is in accord with the situation in the Netherlands.[15] Almost 12% of all the injuries sustained during PE classes (120,000) need medical treatment in the hospital. Although from all the injuries sustained during sports activities only 18.8% are sustained in PE classes (Table 43.1).[16]

A retrospective study in 11,439 junior and senior high school children in Israel, aged 12–18 years, was carried out to assess the incidence, types, and risk factors involving sports injuries among students in physical education classes. A total of 192 injuries were recorded in the survey (1.70%).[17] Sundblad *et al.*[18] studied a total of 1975 students from 48 schools (grades 3, 6, and 9) and they found an injury incidence of 2.2 injured children per 1000 PE hours.

Physical education versus (un)organized sport

Can we state that PE classes are risky? When exposure is taken into account it can be concluded that the incidence rates for PE-injuries treated in emergency departments (ED), varies between 0.5 and 2.0 (ED-consultations per 10,000 hours PE classes).[15] The overall injury incidence rates for ED-injuries in organized and non-organized sports is 1.0 (ED-consultations per 10,000 hours of sport activities). One should keep in mind that the injury incidence for ED-injuries varies for different kind of sports, for example, indoor soccer (4.6 ED-consultations per 10,000 hours) versus tennis (0.4 ED-consultations per 10,000 hours).[16]

Table 43.1 Numbers of injuries that needed medical treatment in the hospital concerning Dutch children 4–18 years old (per year)[16]

		27.700	100%	School (total)
		13.800	49.8%	School (remaining)
PE classes	18.8%	13.900	50.2%	PE classes
Sport (remaining)	81.2%	60.000		
Sport (total)	100%	73.900		

Tursz and Crost[6] stated that the frequency of accidents in out-of-school sports was higher than for those in PE classes. This is in line with other data from a population-based study in the Netherlands[2] where sports injuries were also more likely to occur during the competitive games of sports clubs rather than during PE classes or non-organized sports activities (Table 43.2; risk ratio = 1.75). Especially, the injuries sustained in organized sports matches led to more absence from physical education classes and to more medical consultation (risk ratios for both, 1.50). A comparison of year incidence rates per 1000 young athletes in organized sports and physical education is given in Table 43.3. The finding that the risk of injury in PE classes is low relative to the number of exposure hours is explained mainly by the lower intensity of the physical exertion involved. In addition, activities during PE lessons are mostly adapted to the abilities of the pupils,[5] which is in contrast to the common practice when participating in team sports.

Gender

In sports, boys have a greater risk of general injuries as they may be more aggressive, have larger body mass, experience greater physical contact, participate in vigorous exercise, and have a higher exposure time and intensity compared with girls in the same sports activities[18–20]. During PE classes, boys and girls have the same risk of injuries. In the Netherlands, both sexes are treated in the hospital due to injuries in PE classes equally.[4] Boys and girls have also fairly similar injury rates (49% girls, 51% boys) during PE classes in Israel.[16] Remarkably, Sundblad *et al.*[18] found that almost twice as many girls as boys were injured during physical education classes. Their results can be explained by the reporting factors between girls and boys and the fact that boys are less likely to report a minor injury.

Impaired vision

Twice as many children with an impaired vision reported that they had been injured during PE class.[18] Sixty seven percent of the girls and 58% of the boys reported that they did not always use their glasses or lenses while active in sports. From these findings one can

Table 43.2 Observed versus expected numbers[a] of injuries (risk ratios) according to the nature of sports participation[2]

Nature of sport	Number of school children	Risk ratio			
		All injuries	Injuries followed by non-attendence of		Injuries with medical consultations
			PE[b] classes	School	
PE	7468	0.63	0.97	1.05	0.66
Club training[c]	6458	1.04	0.99	0.76	1.05
Club match[c]	4439	1.75	1.50	1.11	1.50
Non-organized sports	4762	0.81	0.95	1.14	1.01
Total	23,127	1	1	1	1

[a]Expected numbers are based on the injury rate: that is, all injuries occurred in the total study population.
[b]Physical education.
[c]Pupils with 2, 3 memberships respectively are counted as 2, 3 persons, respectively. From Backx *et al.*[2]

Table 43.3 Incidence rates in organized sports with more than 15 participants

Type of sport	Incidence (per 1000 hours practice)	Type of sport	Incidence (per 1000 hours games)
Volleyball	6.7	Basketball	23
Handball	4.3	Handball	14
Martial arts	3.8	Korfball	12
Club Gymnastics	3.6	Soccer	8
Korfball	3.4	Field hockey	7
Baseball	3.0	Baseball	3
Horseback riding	1.7	Ballet[a]	
Soccer	1.6	Track and field[a]	
Tennis	1.5	Martial arts[a]	
Swimming	1.2	Volleyball[a]	
Field hockey	1.2	Badminton[a]	
Track and field	1.0	Tennis[a]	
Basketball[a]		Swimming[a]	
Table tennis[a]		Table tennis[a]	
Badminton[a]		Horseback riding[a]	
Ice Skating[a]		Ice Skating[a]	
Ballet[a]		Club Gymnastics[a]	
Dance[a]		Dance[a]	

[a]The incidence rate was not calculated for types of sport in which fewer than five sports injuries were registered in practice or games. From Backx *et al.*[13]

conclude that non-corrected vision impairment may possibly be a risk factor for injuries in PE classes. Further research is necessary in order to draw firm conclusions.

In conclusion, PE classes are not more risky than other sports activities, but it is interesting to focus on the type, location, and severity of the injuries in PE classes in order to develop preventive measures.

Location of injury

Comparison of medically treated home, school, and road accidents reveals that medically treated sports accidents have the highest proportion (43%) of upper limb injuries.[6] Naturally, the distribution of injuries relative to body area depends substantially on the activities programmed and instructed by the PE teachers. Figure 43.1 summarizes reported injuries by body area found in the study of Backx *et al.*[13] The distribution of injuries relative to body area and to category of sports activity revealed that PE classes gave rise to relatively more upper extremity injuries.[4,16,21] Based on the popularity of ball games in school, the ball is considered to be an important factor in sustaining a finger injury. According to Kiesslich,[22] finger injuries occur because of underdeveloped motor skills and lack of techniques while catching a ball. Finger injuries are dominant with younger children, whereas ankle joint injuries occur more in older pupils.[5,17,18]

Type of injury

PE lessons containing activities like gymnastics and ball games (soccer, basketball, volleyball, baseball) provoke most damage.[9,21] Two thirds of the injuries happen playing popular games. Most of the injuries occur while playing soccer, followed closely by basketball and gymnastic activities.[4] Vaulting block, vaulting horse, and the mini-trampoline are responsible for the most injuries during gymnastic activities.[4,9,18,21]

Rümmele[5] registered nationwide sports accidents in German schools. He found that three areas (ball games, apparatus gymnastics,

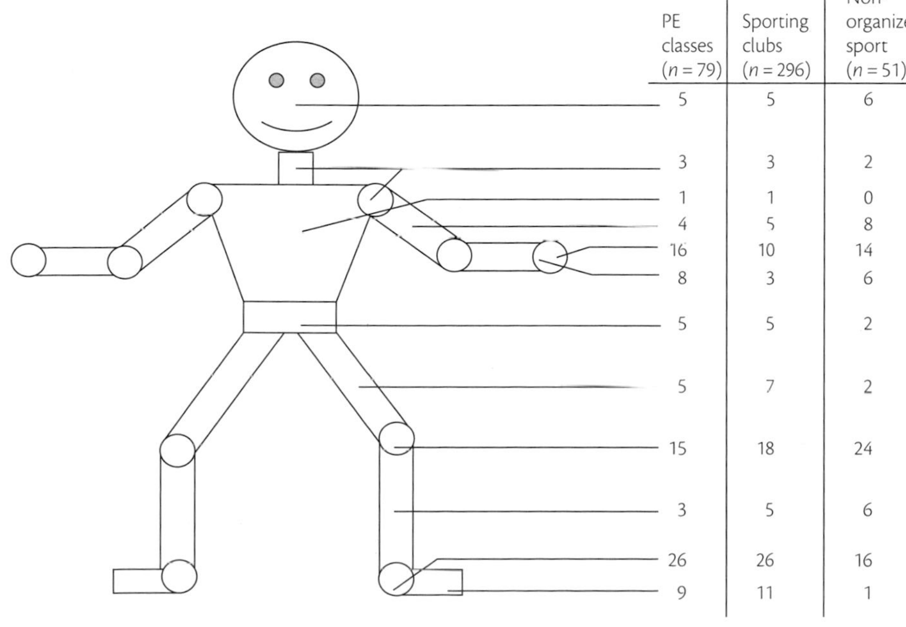

Fig. 43.1 Distribution of 399 sports injuries involving 426 body areas (%) in school children (aged 8–17) related to sports activity category. From Backx *et al.*[2]

and athletics) accounted for 88% of all sports accidents registered in schools. In comparison with the preceding two decades, accidents from ball games had increased tremendously, whereas accidents arising from gymnastics and track and field had remained relatively constant. This trend has also been seen in other countries.[13] The number of accidents due to ball games is considerable. This can be explained partially by the major role team games play in PE classes. The complexity of the game itself (sprinting, twisting, and jumping) causes a higher risk for injuries and accidents. Common sports played by individuals, like gymnastics or track-and-field, cause a smaller part of all accidents, showing that their risk has been overestimated, whereas the risk involved in ball games has been underestimated.[4]

The distribution of injury type in relation to PE classes shows no uniform pattern, which primarily is caused by the difference in injury definition, the locus of measurement, and the type of activity.

In studies using a broad injury definition, the fracture rate is low and most injuries are light contusions and sprains.[2,4,18] Measurements in hospitals have shown a different picture. Depending on the type of sport, the number of fractures varies between 15 and 60% of the total number of sports trauma.[10]

In a Dutch study,[2] significantly more fractures or dislocations occurred in PE classes in comparison with out-of-school sports. Nearly all of these fractures were located on the upper limb. Also sprains, especially involving the ankle, did often occur, although less frequently than during organized sports.[2]

Besides acute macro trauma, the importance of microtrauma and overuse injuries in children is still growing. The latter type of injury will not be described in the context of this chapter because the direct influence of PE classes on the origin of overuse injuries is unknown. Furthermore, it is important to realize that registrations of acute and chronic injuries sustained during PE classes in school will also include injuries that should primarily be attributed to biological growth. The magnitude of growth as an independent risk factor has yet to be confirmed.

Most of the injuries during PE classes are caused by the students themselves through falls or twisted movements.[4,16,18] Other common causes of injuries are collisions with another pupil and being hit by a loose object.[16,18]

Severity of injuries

It is obvious that a high incidence rate of sports injuries is no indicator of injury severity. Therefore, van Mechelen *et al.*[23] have distinguished six factors of importance to describe the severity of injuries in an efficient and practical manner. Using these factors, the following can be concluded concerning young athletes.

Nature of the sports injury

Very serious sports accidents in youth, for example, brain or spinal cord damage, or lesions of the heart or submersion, leading to permanent handicap or death, are exceptional.[6,18] This is in accord with a Swedish study[24] in which only a few such injuries were registered, ranging from life-threatening to fatal, according to the Abbreviated Injury Scale AIS severity codes 4, 5, 6. The AIS is used to classify the severity of traffic accidents. Most of the injuries sustained in PE classes have to be coded as AIS 1 and 2. Sprains are considered the most common type of injury and the ankle the most frequently injured body area.

Nature and duration of treatment

From an epidemiological point of view, one may assume that only 25% of all injuries registered call for medical attention from a general practitioner or a medical specialist.[13] Derived from a Dutch study, pupils who were injured in PE classes had to consult a medical doctor more frequently compared with those injured in other sports activities.

In the 1980s, Watson[25] observed that 13% of injured Irish school children spent one or more days in a hospital. In two other studies concerning macro trauma requiring medical care, the proportion of hospitalization was 10–11%. There is no consensus on the influence of age and gender on hospital admission.[6,21] The type and duration of treatment in the case of sports injuries in school-aged children has not been analysed as well, although there are indications that the claim on the health care system seems to be less than in adults.

The most commonly reported first aid, given immediately after the accident, was compression and thereafter ice. Most injured children were first attended by their parents or another adult member of the family, followed by the physical education teacher and physician or physical therapist.[18] Because primary care of the injured student was, with the exception of a family member, most often carried out by the PE teacher, ongoing sports medicine first aid education for this group is important.[26]

Time lost from sport

The actual number of days elapsed until the athlete returns to sports activity is often reported as a measure of injury severity. Although van Mechelen *et al.*[23] stated that the length of sports absenteeism gives the most precise indication of the consequences of a sports injury to an athlete, this is questionable with regard to school-aged children. Bias can easily be introduced, caused by factors such as an individual's tolerance to pain, type of treatment, parents, and PE-teacher/coach. A time-loss definition of a sports injury is therefore not useful in studies focusing on non-organized sports and PE classes.

Work absenteeism

In the case of youngsters, injury severity in terms of work absenteeism must be transformed into school absenteeism. Similar to days off work, defining the severity of an injury by the amount of time lost in school is highly subjective, as it is with time lost from sports. These estimates of injury severity are more practical rather than valid parameters. Work absenteeism as an outcome parameter was studied only in a Dutch study.[13] In general, most sports injuries found in this study were neither severe nor long-lasting and resulted in little loss of time from PE classes or school. Pupils who were injured in PE classes had more time loss of physical education and total school days in comparison with those whose injuries were sustained during club sports.

Permanent damage

To date there are no secure data available assessing the residual and long-term effects of injuries sustained in PE lessons. Zaricznyj *et al.*[21] recorded in school children participating in sports and physical education that 1.2% of the injured ones got a more severe injury, such as a compression fracture of the spine or a ruptured spleen, resulting in more or less permanent damage. Sundblad *et al.*[18] reported that none of their 300 students were permanently damaged. Actually, it is rather difficult to predict correctly whether or not such injuries will be permanent.

Costs

Severity in terms of costs have to include the direct costs resulting from (para)medical treatment and also the indirect social costs (i.e. sick leave) to the injured pupil, his/her family, and school.[23,24] The financial costs stemming from sports injuries in youth are not explored as a single category. Only rough calculations are known, being derived from figures concerning adults.

Aetiology

Usually the most important factors affecting sports injuries are divided in two main categories: characteristics related to the individual (intrinsic risk factors) and characteristics not related to the individual (extrinsic or environmental risk factors). Intrinsic factors are, for example, age, gender, and body composition. Examples of extrinsic risk factors are sports factors, protective equipment, and sports equipment. The inciting events are the third link in the chain that causes an injury. The description of inciting events can be grouped into four categories:[27]

(i) vital aspects of the playing (sports) situation (the situation described from a sports-specific point of view)

(ii) athlete and opponent behaviour (a qualitative description of the athlete's action and interaction with the opponent)

(iii) gross biomechanical characteristics (description of whole body biomechanics)

(iv) detailed biomechanical characteristics (description of joint/tissue biomechanics)

The dynamic model for injury causation was developed by Meeuwisse *et al.*[28] (and see Chapter 42). This model clearly shows that an injury is the result of a complex interaction between intrinsic and extrinsic risk factors and is not exclusively caused by the inciting event that is generally associated with the onset of injury.[28]

It is noticeable that specific information on the aetiology and, consequently, on the prevention of sports injuries in school-aged children is minimal. Most of the investigations according to this target group do mention causes, but this information is primarily retrieved from the subject him/herself or is reconstructed by the coach or physician. For example, retrospective data from a population-based study revealed that most reported causes of sports injuries were falling/stumbling (24%), misstep/twist (22%), and kick/push (18%) induced by the child himself instead of by other pupils.[13] In the near future, more prospective data from observational studies need to be gathered in order to provide more valid information, which can then be transferred into preventive measures.

Prevention

Injury prevention is a must, when everybody is proclaiming 'sports, a life-long activity', based on the potential benefits on health. One of the strategies in the battle against sports injuries is aimed at behaviour modification of the participants in sports.[29] Health education as a tool in realizing behavioral change can be implemented in the school's curriculum and, consequently, should be given by well-educated teachers in physical education or biology.[30]

The need for the physical educator to become involved in the field of sports injury prevention may vary from one country to another, depending on the number of other groups of professionals working in the same area. In Table 43.4, some conditions are listed which determine the need for involvement by the PE teacher.[31] The primary tasks of the physical educator must not be limited to a stimulating role in the development of skills and to applying preventive measures for safety in PE classes. The PE teacher should be, at a minimum, a message mediator, by educating school-aged children in practical and theoretical aspects of injury prevention. This kind of information will also be valuable for out-of-school sports activities. Although in this specific area the effects of health education still have to be proven, there are strong indications that in the short term it can be beneficial in reducing the number of sports injuries. The effects in the long run are only speculative.

Table 43.4 Aspects upon which the role of the teacher depends[31]

Aspects
Creating an environment for safe and fair play
Checking appropriate equipment and good condition of the playing site
Screening of physical defects
Qualification in sports medicine and injury prevention
Public awareness

In the Netherlands a controlled experimental study, focused on students of a secondary school (12–18 years old), has been performed. In this study, 24 PE lessons and 6 biology lessons were given in injury prevention.[30] The practical topics instructed in PE classes included warming up, stretching exercises, cooling down, exercises for ankle stabilization and general coordination, and techniques to fall correctly. These practical items were supported by theoretical information, taught by teachers in biology. Additional education took place concerning adequate sporting shoes, protective materials, and first aid in sports. In this study, success was achieved by clearly improving knowledge about injury prevention. This increase in knowledge led to a positive change in attitude. Although the attitude change over the 1 year period of follow-up was small, it nevertheless had a favourable influence on injury incidence, even though the explained variance was minimal. No reduction in the severity of sports injuries was seen. It can be speculated that if the intervention had been executed more frequently and for a longer period of time, the effectiveness of the educational programme would have been greater. Based on this study it was also recommended that the effects on the incidence should be monitored for a period longer than 1 year because, in health education, effects are particularly expected in the long term. Because the results of this health educational programme were very encouraging, it seems worthwhile to implement this kind of health educational intervention into the school's curriculum on a more regular basis. To do so, it is, however, necessary to compose a post-academic course for the teachers concerned, in order to optimize their role in the prevention of sports injuries.

Summary

- Injuries are more likely to occur during competitive games in sports clubs rather than during PE classes or non-organized sports activities of youngsters.
- The number of injuries occurring in PE classes might be much higher than found, because many schools do not maintain good injury records.

- Sprains are considered the most common type of injury and the ankle the most frequently injured body area. PE classes give rise to relatively more upper extremity injuries.
- The importance of microtrauma and overuse injuries in children is growing.
- PE lessons containing activities like gymnastics and ball games (soccer, basketball, volleyball, baseball) provoke most damage. The complexity of the games themselves (sprinting, twisting, and jumping) causes a higher risk for injuries and accidents.
- Most of the injuries during PE classes are caused by falls or twisted movements of the students themselves.
- Pupils injured in PE classes experienced more loss of physical education time and total school days in comparison with those whose injuries were sustained during club sports.
- The PE teacher should be a message mediator by educating school-aged children in practical and theoretical aspects of injury prevention.

References

1. Jüngst BK (1991). Schulsport; Träume und Wirklichkeit. *Dtsch Z Sportmed* **42**, 87.
2. Backx FJG, Erich WBM, Kemper ABA, Verbeek ALM (1989). Sports injuries in school-aged children: an epidemiologic study. *Am J Sports Med* **17**, 234–40.
3. Calvert R (1979). *Athletic injuries and deaths in secondary schools and colleges, 1975–76.* National Center for Education Statistics, Washington, DC.
4. Kelm J, Ahlhelm F, Pape D, Pitsch W, Engel C (2001). School sports accidents: Analysis of causes, modes and frequencies. *J Pediatr Orthop* **21**, 165–8.
5. Rümmele E (1987). Sports injuries in the Federal Republic of Germany. Part two. In: van der Togt CR, Kemper ABA, Koornneef M (eds.), *Council of Europe: Sport for all; Sports injuries and their prevention. Proceedings of the 2nd meeting*, pp. 37–49. National Institute for Sports Health Care, Oosterbeek, The Netherlands.
6. Tursz A, Crost M (1986). Sports-related injuries in children: A study of their characteristics, frequency and severity, with comparison to other types of accidental injuries. *Am J Sports Med* **14**, 294–9.
7. Emery CA, Sarah Rose M, McAllister JR, Meeuwisse WH (2007). A prevention strategy to reduce the incidence of injury in High School Basketball: A cluster randomized controlled trial. *Clin J Sport Med* **17**, 17–24.
8. Helms PJ (1997). Sports injuries in children: Should we be concerned? *Arch Dis Child* **77**, 161–3.
9. Hammer A, Schwartzbach AL, Paulev PE (1981). Children injured during physical education lessons. *J Sports Med* **21**, 423–31.
10. Sahlin Y (1990). Sport accidents in childhood. *Br J Sports Med* **24**, 40–4.
11. Medved R, Pavisic-Medved V (1973). Causes of injuries during the practical classes on physical education in schools. *J Sports Med Phys Fitness* **13**, 32–41.
12. Pospiech R (1981). Analyse von 1.000 Unfällen beim Schulsport. *Medizine Sport* **21**, 78–82.
13. Backx FJG, Beijer HJM, Bol E, Erich WBM (1991). Injuries in high-risk persons and high-risk sports. A longitudinal study of 1,818 school children. *Am J Sports Med* **19**, 124–30.
14. Walter SD, Sutton JR, McIntosh JM, Connolly C (1985). The aetiology of sports injuries: A review of methodologies. *Sports Med* **2**, 47–58.
15. Consument and Veiligheid (2005). *Monitor 'Privé- en sportongevallen 1999–2003'.* Stichting Consument en Veiligheid, the Netherlands.
16. Vriend I, Bastiaans B, Stam C (2005). *Veilig bewegingsonderwijs: van ongevallen naar preventie.* Amsterdam, Stichting Consument en Veiligheid, pp. 81. (Rapport ; 280). ISBN 9067883026 (in Dutch).
17. Carmeli E, Azencot S, Werthrim M, Coleman R (2003). Sports injuries in students aged 12–18 during physical education classes in Israel. *Biol Sport* **20**, 271–80.
18. Sundblad G, Saartok T, Engström LM, Renström P (2005). Injuries during physical activity in school children. *Scand J Med Sci Sports* **15**, 313–23.
19. Emery CA (2003). Risk factors for injury in child and adolescent sport: A systematic review of the literature. *Clin J Sport Med* **13**, 256–68.
20. Taimela S, Kujala UM, Osterman K (1990). Intrinsic risk factors and athletic injuries. *Sports Med* **9**, 205–15.
21. Zaricznyj B, Shattuck LJM, Mast TA, Robertson RV, D'Elia G (1980). Sports-related injuries in school-aged children. *Am J Sports Med* **8**, 318–24.
22. Kiesslich Th (1992). Schülerunfälle bei Sport und Spiel: Eine Auswertung des Unfallgeschehens in den Schulen. *Schulverwaltungsblatt Niedersachsen* **8**, 244–7.
23. Mechelen van W, Hlobil H, Kemper HCG (1987). *How can sports injuries be prevented?* National Institute for Sports Health Care, Oosterbeek, The Netherlands.
24. Nathorst Westfelt JAR (1982). Environmental factors in childhood accidents: A prospective study in Götenborg, Sweden. *Acta Paediatr Scand* **291(Suppl)**, 6–61.
25. Watson AWS (1986). *Sports injuries in Irish second-level schools during the school year 1984–85.* Department of Education, Dublin.
26. Abernethy L, MacAuley D, McNally O, McCann S (2003). Immediate care of school sport injury. *Inj Prev* **9**, 270–3.
27. Bahr R, Krosshaug T (2005). Understanding injury mechanisms: A key component of preventing injuries in sport. *Br J Sports Med* **39**, 324–9.
28. Meeuwisse HW, Tyreman H, Hagel B, Emery CA (2007). Dynamic model of etiology in sport injury: The recursive nature of risk and causation. *Clin J Sport Med* **17**, 215–19.
29. Kok GJ, Bouter LM (1990). On the importance of planned health education: Prevention of ski injury as an example. *Am J Sports Med* **18**, 600–5.
30. Backx FJG (1991). *Sports injuries in youth: Etiology and prevention.* University of Utrecht, Utrecht, The Netherlands.
31. Stanitski CL (1997). Pediatric and adolescent sports injuries athletes. *Clin Sports Med* **16**, 613–33.

CHAPTER 44

Aetiology and prevention of injuries in youth competitive contact sports

Evert A.L.M. Verhagen, Willem van Mechelen, Adam D.G. Baxter Jones, and Nicola Maffulli

Introduction

Other chapters in this section have covered the theoretical framework regarding the aetiology and prevention of sports injuries as well as, more specific, the aetiology and prevention of injuries in non-contact youth competition sports. This chapter will focus on sport specific injuries in contact sports. A number of sports where contact with the opponent is intentional or common have therefore been selected.

Each sport is covered in a systematic way by describing some practical information concerning the particular sport, as well as the epidemiology and aetiology of sport specific injuries, and by giving facts about the preventive strategies related to the above.

In general, sports injuries in contact sports are more frequent than in non-contact sports.[1–4] One should however keep in mind that a large proportion of sports pathology is common to both contact and non-contact sports where similar movements are involved that potentially can lead to injury, for example, running and cutting.

It should also be noted that for certain contact sports little information is available on children and that adult data have therefore been used to extrapolate where appropriate. Taking this into consideration, the present chapter summarizes certain trends that can be drawn from the literature and that give a reasonable basis on which to develop and promote prevention strategies.

American football

American football, a violent collision and contact sport, has been one of the most popular sports in the United States during the past century and has recently received support and increased participation from European nations. Given that football is a collision sport, it would be expected that most football injuries are acute, as opposed to overuse or gradual onset injuries.

To reflect the incidence and aetiology of American football injuries in youth athletes, most literature used describes high school football.

Epidemiology of American football injuries

With an increased number of athletes playing American football, an increased number of football related injuries has been documented.[5] The U.S. National Athletic Trainers Association (NATA)[6] found that 39% of varsity high school football players were injured in the 1995 season. Another study showed that at high school level, injury incidence rates range from 11.8 to 81.1 per 100 players.[7] When keeping the same definition for injury similar incidence rates are found in college football. A note of caution in interpreting such results is needed. Although rates of injuries per 100 players are frequently cited in the literature they do not take into account the varying numbers of games and practice sessions taking place. The rate of re-injury has not been extensively studied, but a study in 1995 by the NATA[6] found that 10% of high school players' injuries were re-injuries to a previously hurt area.

Different studies regarding high school football[6,8–11] found that the three most commonly occurring types of injuries are sprains (ligaments), strains (muscles), and contusions. This result was fairly consistent across all the studies.

The head is particularly susceptible to injury (~10% of all reported injuries),[12–15] with cerebral concussions (5%) as the most frequently occurring type of head injury.[12,16,17] Injuries to the upper extremities commonly occur in the game of American football (~30% of all reported injuries). Of those, the most commonly reported cases concern the shoulders (9%) and the hands/fingers (10%).[6,8–11] From the lower extremities, (~50% of all reported injuries) the knee (18%) and ankle (12%) are particularly vulnerable to injury.[6,8–11]

Aetiology of American football injuries

Concussions may occur when the skull is put into motion before the contained brain. This occurs when a moving object strikes the head in a resting state, or when the head collides with a non-moving object.[13] Injuries to the cervical spine traditionally have been attributed to hyperflexion and/or hyperextension mechanisms.[18,19]

The shoulder is often the initial contact point in tackling and blocking.[7] The hand is vulnerable to injury because it is often used in direct contact against the facemask, the opponents' body, headgear, and the shoulder pads.[7] Injuries to the fingers may occur as players grasp the opponents' pads, belts, and jerseys while blocking and tackling.[7]

Normally knee motion is limited to internal and external rotation when the leg is in extension and flexion. Therefore, injury to the knee may occur when the joint is stressed into unusual positions as the result of direct contact from other players. Non-contact injuries to the knee often involve unnatural twisting motions that prevent the natural rotation of the knee joint.

Intrinsic and extrinsic risk factors of football injuries described in the literature are listed in Table 44.1.

Leg deficiencies: There is evidence in the literature that lower extremity injuries may be the result of lower body strength imbalances and other leg deficiencies.[22] It is also believed that athletes with tight heel cords may be more susceptible to lower extremity injury.[23] Other researchers, however, have found contradicting evidence.[24,25] The role of leg deficiencies as a risk factor in injuries, therefore, is not totally clear.

Height and weight: There is a lack of statistical evidence with regard to the relationship between size, age, weight, and height and football injuries.[24,26] It is also often debated that with children of the same calendar age, the less mature player has a greater risk of sustaining an injury due to the inequality in body dimensions. Lindner *et al.*[27], however, found contradictory results, which they ascribed to more aggressive play by the more mature boys due to their advanced growth.

Previous injuries: Especially previous head injuries lead to a higher risk for future injuries to this body area.[16,28] There is also strong evidence that ankle sprains lead to chronic instability of the ankle which will result in a higher risk of sustaining ankle sprains.[29]

Players' position: Research showed that defensive and offensive line players have the highest injury incidence[32]. Possibly due to the fact that these players are involved in physical contact in every play. However, it is also stated that this high incidence in defensive and offensive line players is due to the fact that there are more line players on the field than other players.[33] When adjusting for exposure, running backs seem to be at the highest risk.[33]

Lack of well-rounded full year conditioning: Cahill and Griffith[34] found in an 8 year prospective study that pre-season conditioning of the total body decreased the incidence and severity of knee injuries throughout the season.

Cleats: Fixation of the foot through rigid cleating has been shown to be a primary factor in the production of lower extremity injuries, particularly of the knee and the ankle.[8,35,36]

Table 44.1 Intrinsic and extrinsic risk factors for football injuries, with their respective references

Intrinsic risk factors	Extrinsic risk factors
Leg deficiencies[20–25]	Players position[30–33]
Body dimensions[24,26,27]	Lack of well-rounded full year conditioning[21,34]
Previous injuries[16,28,29]	Cleats[8]
	Playing surface[37,38]
	Equipment[39–41]

Playing Surface: Grass and artificial surfaces produce similar injury rates; however, the most serious injuries occur on artificial turf.[37,38]

Equipment: Longitudinal research has shown that different helmets bring different concussion rates.[39] On the effectiveness of knee braces in the prevention of knee injuries, there is little agreement amongst researchers.[40,41] However, most of the contradiction between results stems from the variety in study designs and methodologies, which does not allow a proper comparison between study results.

Preventive strategies

Blyth and Mueller[8] found that 1.7% of all football injuries were caused by defective, broken, or ill-fitting equipment. It has also been shown that the use of improper cleats is a primary factor in lower extremity injuries.[8,35,36] The use of proven protective equipment, therefore, needs to be an integral part of all football training programmes. For instance, facial and head injuries may be prevented through the use of properly fitting helmets and padded chin straps, which eliminate helmet rotation.[39] Additional padding and/or taping for ribs, arms, ankles, and knees might help prevent some injuries. This additional protection can be individually applied depending on the athlete's position;[7] for example, defensive and offensive linemen who have continuously rough physical contact during play require additional protection compared to a wide receiver who sporadically gets extremely hard hits but needs light protection to maintain speed and agility. Which additional protection should be used for which players' position is not known from the literature. Furthermore, the use of additional protective equipment also relies on each player's individual preference.

Blyth and Mueller[7] found that 3.8% of all injuries were caused by illegal acts. This enforces the belief that stricter enforcement of rules and proper rule awareness might go a long way towards prevention of injuries in general.

Year-round mandatory football-specific conditioning and training programmes should be aimed at improving muscular and ligament imbalances and weaknesses; coordination and timing; and flexibility, mobility, and agility. Cahill and Griffith[34] showed an effect of pre-season conditioning on an incidence reduction of knee injuries. It is therefore reasonable to assume an effect of this measure on other injuries.

Furthermore, a qualified sports medicine team needs to be an integral part of all football training programmes. According to Blyth and Mueller,[7] 2.4% of all injuries could have been prevented if adequate medical supervision covered games and practices. This should lead to early and effective diagnosis, evaluation, and treatment of injuries. Proper medical supervision should also lead to better rehabilitation from an injury before returning to the game, resulting in less repeat injuries.[7]

Boxing

Unlike any other sport, boxing is associated with the intentional affliction of traumatic brain injury—that is, a concussion or knockout. Epidemiological investigations of boxing injuries have been limited both in quality and quantity. Especially on youth in boxing not much literature can be found. Therefore, it is necessary to extrapolate the limited information available about boxing injuries from adult boxers to youth boxers. When looking at boxing also a problem arises because of differences between professional and amateur boxing. Professional boxing is associated with a higher injury rate than amateur boxing. Youth boxers predominantly are amateur boxers who often do not participate in matches, but only participate in training sessions.

Epidemiology of boxing injuries

In Irish competition amateur boxing, an incidence of 0.92 injuries per man-hour of competition was reported.[42] In the literature, head injuries are described as the most common boxing injury, ranging from 27 to 93%[43–46] of all injuries. The great difference between studies is caused by the relatively flexible definition of head injury. Looking at cerebral injury, due to severe blows to the head, and facial injuries separately gives a clearer view. In Irish competition amateur boxing, an incidence of 0.47 injuries per man-hour of competition for cerebral injury was reported, followed by hand/wrist injuries (0.19 per man-hour of competition) and face/head injuries (0.19 per man-hour of competition).[42]

As mentioned, youth boxers often only participate in practice sessions. Cerebral and facial injuries are less common in training bouts where the emphasis lies on training of technique rather than on knocking down the opponent.[42] Therefore, the incidence of chronic cerebral injury might be lower and less severe in youth boxers. However, acute cerebral damage might still be a common injury in youth boxers, but unfortunately there are no data on acute cerebral damage in youth boxers.

Facial injuries most often involve facial laceration[43,45] and the nose.[44] Injuries to ears and eyes are uncommon. Injuries to lips and teeth are also rare due to the compulsory wearing of mouth guards. Injury to the spine/trunk are less frequent in boxing and comprise only 2–16% of all boxing injuries.[43–46]

Aetiology of boxing injuries

A bout finishing with a knock-out is much rarer in amateur boxing, where the emphasis is on technical superiority and not on power, than in professional boxing.[47] Furthermore, in amateur boxing the boxer is protected by strict rules which should prevent the boxer from getting serious chronic cerebral injury. Acute cerebral injuries result from intracranial bleeding, caused by a blow to the head. A blow to the head accelerates the head, but there is a delay in the brain following the head movement, which can rupture blood vessels on the surface of the brain.[48]

The incidence of hand injuries in amateur boxing is high. Most hand injuries are related to the execution of blows and/or the vulnerability of the thumb. The thumb is isolated from the other fingers in the glove, which makes it prone to forced abduction on impact.[42] The amateur boxer is only allowed to use a single encircling piece of tape and soft surgical bandages to protect the hands in competition. Shoulder injuries are the result of repetitive and forceful delivery of punches.[49]

Facial abrasions and cuts are relatively common in adult boxing, despite the use of headgear. This is because the goal of boxing is the intentional affliction of traumatic brain injury, which is achieved by giving blows to the opponent's head.

Lower extremity injuries occur more frequently during training and are likely to include overuse injuries associated with jogging and jumping rope.[49]

The intrinsic and extrinsic risk factors of boxing injuries described in the literature are listed in Table 44.2.

Table 44.2 Intrinsic and extrinsic risk factors for boxing injuries, with their respective references

Intrinsic risk factors	Extrinsic risk factors
Boxing skills[50,51]	Sparring[43,52]
	Exposure[52,53]

Boxing skills: Intuitively one would expect that more experienced boxers are able to protect themselves better against hard and repetitive blows due to better defensive skills. Research has also shown that there is a positive correlation between lost bouts and chronic brain damage.[50,51] This is only proven for professional boxers but can most likely be extrapolated to youth boxers.

Sparring (i.e. non-competitive boxing): The absolute number of injuries is higher during sparring, but the incidence is higher for competitive boxing.[44] This reflects the longer duration of time spent on sparring compared to active competition. The hypothesis that an increased exposure to head blows during sparring increases the risk for brain injury has not been confirmed in epidemiological studies.[52] Since no information on total sparring time for youth boxers was found in the literature, nothing can be said about the influence of this risk factor on injuries in youth boxing.

Exposure: This applies more to older boxers instead of youth boxers, as it seems there is a correlation between injury and longer periods of boxing—for example, 10 years or 150 fights. It is proven that the total number of boxing contests, both amateur and professional, are associated with impaired neuropsychological test performance.[52,53]

Preventive strategies

It is believed that the only way to prevent cerebral injuries, acute as well as chronic injuries, is to change the rules such that they prohibit blows to the head.[54,55] This, however, conflicts with the nature of the sport. Preventive strategies more in accordance with the sport might be a well trained ringside physician, whose duties include pre-fight medical and neurological examinations, injury surveillance during boxing competitions, and post-fight evaluations of suspected injuries.[49]

The monitoring of injuries and rehabilitation of injuries is important. A physician should allow injuries to be fully rehabilitated before the boxer re-enters the boxing ring. The length of suspensions following injury or knockout as proposed by the New York State Athletic Commission goes some way towards solving this problem. Physicians should be encouraged to apply these suspensions.[49]

It is also suggested that the floor of the ring should be sufficiently shock absorbent to reduce the risk of cerebral damage from head contact in a fall.[48] The floor should, however, not be too soft, since this hastens fatigue, which for instance results in a diminished concentration and a decreased defence.

Soccer

Soccer is considered by many as the most popular game in the world and is played by at least 40 million people. Many studies have been done to determine the injury patterns in soccer, but only a few have been taken prospectively in young players. Several factors combine to make studies of injury in young soccer players important and necessary. The first is the extent of participation in youth soccer, in 1990 it was estimated that more than 6 million youth players under 12 played on a team in the United States,[56] while soccer is even more popular in Europe. Second, there is an increased intensity of participation of youth players; some youth players nowadays play whole year round by combining outdoor and indoor soccer. These two factors combine to dramatically increase the exposure for injury risk in young soccer players.

Epidemiology of soccer injuries

As found by the NATA[7] more than 23% of high school soccer players, regardless of gender, are likely to sustain at least one time-loss injury during a season. A 4 year prospective study of youth soccer injuries has shown rates of 23.8 per 10,000 player hours.[56] A total of 4.8 injuries per 1000 hours of exposure were recorded in a 10 season study in French elite youth soccer players, injury incidences were 11.2 and 3.9 injuries per 1000 hours for matches and training, respectively[57]. In Greece, a prospective study of soccer injuries, involving 287 male youth players, from the ages of 12 to 15 years showed a total of 209 injuries sustained by 287 players.[58] The incidence of injuries was 4.0 injuries per 1000 hours of soccer time per player. Finally, a U.S. study showed that approximately 144,600 children sustained soccer-related injuries in 2000 for a rate of 2.36 injuries per 1000 children. Injury rates increased with age (0.8 for 5–9 year olds; 3.1 for 10–14 year olds; 3.2 for 15–19 year olds).[59]

The lower extremity is the most prevalent site of injury in traumatic injuries; with the thigh and hip area as the most common sites of injury (~45% of all injuries), followed by the ankle (~19% of all injuries), and knee (~16% of all injuries).[56,60] Relatively low-grade injuries such as strains and sprains (~50% of all injuries) are the most common injuries, whereas more serious injuries such as fractures (~7% of all injuries) and meniscal injuries (~4% of all injuries) are less frequent.[56,60]

Aetiology of soccer injuries

As would be expected in a contact sport, most of the injuries result from direct contact with other players.[56] Especially, hip and thigh contact is frequent during play in an attempt to push the opponent away from the ball.

The nature of the game of soccer, in which players make hard cuts, sharp turns off a planted foot, and intense contact with the ball and other players, makes players specifically vulnerable to lower extremity injury.[61] Normally, knee motion is limited to internal and external rotation when the leg is in extension and flexion. Therefore, injury to the knee may occur when the joint is stressed into unusual positions as the result of direct contact from other players. Non-contact injuries to the knee often involve unnatural twisting motions that prevent the natural rotation of the knee joint, for example, kicking the ball which forces rotation in the foot that is planted on the ground. Contact with the ground accounts for the highest number of ankle injuries, mostly ankle inversion sprains.[56] Upper extremity injuries are found more in youth players than in adult players. This may be explained by the fact that younger players are not very well coordinated when they try to keep their balance, and thus fall, trying to seek support from the upper extremity.[62]

Head injuries are usually caused when a player heads the ball, when a forcefully striked ball strikes the head, or when two players attempt to head the ball simultaneously and collide head-to-head.[61] Common soccer head injuries resulting from these mechanics include lacerations and concussions.

The higher incidence in outdoor youth female soccer players is attributed to the females' unfamiliarity and inferior technical skills when compared with males of the same age.[63,64]

The intrinsic and extrinsic risk factors of soccer injuries described in the literature are listed in Table 44.3.

Age: In younger age groups Keller *et al.*[65]documented a higher incidence of upper extremity, head, and face injuries. It is believed that this higher incidence is due to more frequent falls on outstretched hands, increased fragility of the upper extremity epiphyses, insufficient expertise in heading the ball, mechanical weaknesses of growing dental tissue, increased ball-weight to head-weight ratio, and illegal ball contact. Adolescents who lag behind in skeletal maturity are also at greater risk than their 'normal' competitors.[66]

Previous injury: Players with a history of ankle sprains are at 2.3 times greater risk for ankle injuries.[67] The same trend in ankle injuries was found by Nielsen and Yde[68] who found that 56% of all ankle injuries occurred in players with a history of ankle sprains. In general, it can be concluded that sprains of the lower extremity and overuse injuries are the most common injuries, and persistent symptoms are commonly seen after those injuries.[29]

Gender: It is believed that the females' unfamiliarity and inferior technical skills, compared with males of the same age, in youth soccer leads to the higher rate of injury found in females.[63,64,65]

Exposure: Teams with a higher practice-to-game ratio have fewer injuries, likely due to superior physical conditioning.[69] There seems to be no difference between injury occurrence and level of play.[70]

Players' position: A prospective study by Keller *et al.*[65] reported no significant differences between injury rates of players at different positions. In contrast to these results, Jörgensen[71] found in a retrospective study, a significant difference in injury incidence between players' positions. Goalkeepers and defenders sustained more injuries than attackers.

Playing surface: The rate of injury on artificial surfaces is higher than on natural surfaces[72,73]. There is also a difference in injury patterns between playing on natural surfaces and artificial surfaces.[74] More injuries affecting midfielders, injuries in tackling and sliding, and more abrasions occur on artificial surfaces.

Preventive strategies

Watson[75] found a relation between body mechanics defects and the incidence of certain kinds of sports injuries in senior Irish soccer. Teams with a higher practice-to-game ratio have fewer injuries, likely due to superior physical conditioning.[69] Youth specific conditioning and training programmes aimed at improving muscular and ligament imbalances and weaknesses; coordination and timing; flexibility, mobility, and agility, therefore are likely able to

Table 44.3 Intrinsic and extrinsic risk factors for soccer injuries, with their respective references

Intrinsic risk factors	Extrinsic risk factors
Age[65,66]	Exposure[69,70]
Previous injury[29,67,68]	Players' position[66,71]
Gender[63,64,66]	Playing surface[72–74]

reduce the incidence of injuries in youth soccer players who regularly compete at a high level.

An important role in injury prevention lies with the referee. Interviewed players in a study by Cattermole *et al.*[76] believed that their injury could have been prevented if there had been tighter refereeing control of the game. Many injuries in soccer occur during tackling and contact with an opposing player.[77] A good referee needs to keep the game under tight control and must not allow dangerous behaviour on the field.[56] An important role in reducing on-field aggressiveness also lies with the coaches. Coaching within the spirit as well as the letter of soccer laws, so that jersey pulling, deliberate 'take downs,' and tackling from behind are not condoned, should be emphasized; since these actions often lead to injuries in youth soccer.[56]

Since females seem to be at more risk of injury, adjustment in playing conditions may need to be explored.[56] Possibilities for adjustments might be ball size, closeness of refereeing, and physical conditioning. From studies on brain injury in soccer[78–80] it is suggested that the ball weight is constant and related to body weight. This implies the use of lighter balls in youth female soccer. Furthermore, it is suggested that soccer players should be advised not to head a ball that is travelling at 'high' velocity; and balls that are too hard or have become heavy with rain-water should be banned.

Proper field policing, including elimination of the holes and sharp objects and removal of bags and chairs on the perimeter of the field, should be routine. Protective padding of the goal posts has also shown to be effective in reducing injuries.[81] The use of shin guards is effective as protection against abrasions, contusions, and lacerations. It is believed that further development in shin guard technology could also prevent low impact energy injuries.[76]

Martial arts

Oriental martial sports have become increasingly popular in the west. Tournaments are not only organized for adult participants, but also for young athletes. Despite this interest in martial sports, research on the epidemiology of martial arts sports injuries is scarce and in some cases even non-existent.

In this chapter, epidemiology; aetiology; and prevention of judo, karate, and taekwondo will be discussed. These three forms of martial sports offer the majority of injury data.

In non-contact karate competitions, which is the most performed form of karate in youth, rough and uncontrolled contact with the trunk and all contacts to face, head, and neck are completely forbidden. In contrast to karate, taekwondo is mostly performed as a full contact sport by youth. At tournaments, competitors wear protective equipment including head gear, a chest and abdomen protector, a groin guard, and shin and forearm guards. As in boxing a fight can be won by knockout or on points. Judo involves no punching or kicking; judo techniques have their goal in working the opponent to the ground. This also involves physical contact but in different way than in karate and taekwondo. Competitors of all three forms of martial sports compete in divisions according to age, gender, experience, and weight.

Epidemiology of martial arts injuries

In Switzerland, an injury incidence of 2.3 injuries per 10,000 hours of exposure was found for both male and female youth judo athletes.[82] More detailed information of judo injuries is given by Kujala *et al.*[83]; unfortunately, they used an injury rate that makes the data not comparable with other studies. Overall, they found a lower injury rate for athletes under 15 years, than for athletes between the ages of 15 and 19. A higher proportion of injuries occurred in female athletes for both age groups.

A recent study showed that in the United States between 1990 and 2003 an estimated 128,400 children under the age of 17 years were treated in Emergency Departments for martial arts-related injuries from 1990 to 2003. Injured participants tended to be male 73.0% and had a mean age of 12.1 years. Most injuries were attributed to karate (79.5%).[84]

In Finland, an incidence of 0.28 injuries per bout was found in the national karate competitions.[85] Injuries were most common, however, in bouts between male adults. No exact injury incidence rates of youth karate in particular were found in the literature. Kujala *et al.*[83] found overall a lower injury rate for athletes under 15 years, than for athletes between the ages of 15 and 19 years. A higher proportion of injuries occurred in female athletes for both age groups.

For taekwondo, Pieter and Zemper[86] reported 58.34 injuries per 1000 athlete-exposures for boys and 56.57 injuries per 1000 athlete-exposures for girls. In a prospective study of youth taekwondo, Oler *et al.*[87] found a rate of 3.4 injuries per 100 athletes in one tournament; this study included both males and females.

In judo, distortions seem to have the highest injury incidence in youth male athletes (1.0 per 10,000 hours of exposure), followed by contusions (0.5 per 10,000 hours of exposure), fractures (0.4 per 10,000 hours of exposure), and luxations (0.2 per 10,000 hours of exposure).[82] The same trend was found for youth female athletes. Most injuries involve the upper extremities (45%), followed by the lower extremity (30%), and the head/spine/trunk (25%)[84] Kujala *et al.*[83] found sprains and strains to be the most occurring type of injury in judo, followed by bruises and wounds; they however did not mention youth and adult, and male and female athletes separately.

In adult male karate, contusions seem to account for 66% of all injuries, lacerations for 12%, concussions for 10%, and epistaxis for 10%.[88] No information is available on youth male and female karate, but it seems reasonable to assume that the same trend can be seen there. As in judo, Kujala *et al.*[83] found sprains and strains to be the most occurring type of injury in karate, followed by bruises and wounds.

In taekwondo, 82% of all injuries involve sprains, strains, or injuries to other soft tissue. The upper or lower leg is the most injured body part (35%), presumably due to the high number of kicks during a match. Injuries to the ankle and foot (16%), head (10%), shoulder (10%), and back (11%) are also commonly seen in taekwondo.[89]

Aetiology of martial arts injuries

Little information on the aetiology of martial arts injuries is available in the literature. Most information comes from case studies. Strangulation, a common occurrence in judo, is a major cause of brain damage; it could lead for instance to subdural haematoma[90] and reduced regional blood flow.[91] Cerebral concussions in karate are a result of blows to the head and the neck.[92] Spinning kicks are related to cervical spine injuries.[92] Punches, however, are the lead injury mechanism in karate[93] accounting for the large amount of contusions. All head and neck injuries in taekwondo are due to kicks.[94]

Fractures in the upper extremity are mostly due to improper falling techniques.[95] Being thrown on the shoulder and poorly executed breakfalls are important mechanisms of injury to the upper extremity.[96,97] In karate, detrimental change and less often loss of flexion in the dominant wrist were found.[98]

Since taekwondo has the same goal as boxing, it is believed that a majority of taekwondo injuries have the same aetiology as boxing injuries, especially when looking at head injuries.

The intrinsic and extrinsic risk factors of martial arts injuries described in the literature are listed in Table 44.4.

Physical characteristics: Age is positively related to the injury prevalence rate.[99] In young males competing in taekwondo, an increased body weight might be a risk factor for injuries but this is not the case for young females.[99]

Skill level: Skill level and flexibility have been implicated in 80% of ruptures and 76% of sprains.[100] In various studies it was found that injury prevalence increases with an increased skill level, whereas in other studies the contrary was found. Differences in study design, injury definition, and populations might account for these contrasting results.

Technique: Lack of refined technique may contribute to injury.[87] It is believed that poor fist technique leads to hand fractures in karate and taekwondo.[101,102]

Exposure: The number of bouts fought and repetitive subconcussive blows to the head could be more related to brain damage than knockouts.[103,104] No data exist however that can substantiate this.

Equipment: Although protective equipment may not reduce the chances of brain damage, it will certainly decrease the occurrence of other injuries.[105] No research has been conducted on the protective effect of the helmet and chest protector worn in taekwondo. Some evidence exists that the chest protector may do a better job in absorbing energy from rotational kicks compared to thrust kicks.[106]

Opponent: Receiving a blow is a major injury mechanism in taekwondo.[107] In judo, improper throwing techniques by the opponent are among the major injury mechanisms.[108]

Preventive strategies

Referees should have an appropriate amount of competition experience to better assess the nature of blows being exchanged in the ring and other aspects of the bout.[109] Furthermore, illegal moves should be penalized immediately and bouts interrupted if injuries are imminent.[92]

Athletes and coaches should be pointed to the potential injury risks of martial arts sports and should be taught not to enter competition prematurely.[87] Athletes should also be taught that improper attitude is a risk for injuries; the 'macho' athlete will likely receive and not less important, deliver avoidable injuries.[110]

Table 44.4 Intrinsic and extrinsic risk factors for martial arts injuries, with their respective references

Intrinsic risk factors	Extrinsic risk factors
Physical characteristics[99]	Exposure[103,104]
Skill level[100]	Equipment[105,106]
Technique[78,101,102]	Opponent[107,108]

Caution by athletes as well as coach and referee during strangulation in judo may help prevent injuries and even fatalities.[111] It is recommended that beginning karate or taekwondo athletes should not be allowed to engage in free exchange of blows.[87] Modification of the rules in karate and taekwondo, which allow blows to the head, might help to reduce serious injuries to this body part, for example, cerebral concussions.

Ice hockey

Ice hockey combines high skating speeds, individual flare for stick handling, and accurate puck shooting with team play. It enjoys an enthusiastic worldwide following and is played by all ages. The American Academy of Pediatrics classifies ice hockey as a collision sport with intentional high-energy body contact.[112] The potential for injury is always present in ice hockey and where intentional collision is allowed, injury rates have increased and the distribution of injury location and frequency has changed.

Epidemiology of ice hockey injuries

Roberts *et al.*[113] studied injury rates in American youth ice hockey tournaments for different age groups. They found incidences of 57.9 injuries per 1000 player hours for 12- to13-year-old males; 42.7 injuries per 1000 player hours for 14- to 15-year-old males; 64.8 injuries per 1000 player hours for 15- to 19-year-old males in high school; and 44.8 injuries per 1000 player hours for 15- to 19-year-old males in the junior gold competition. Lower incidence rates were found in Canadian youth ice hockey.[114] Of 986 participating players, 216 players sustained a total of 296 injuries during the 2004–2005 season. The overall injury incidence was 4.13 injuries per 1000 player hours. Almost half of all injuries occurred during body checking. In this study,[114] compared with the youngest age group (Atom), the risk of injury was 2.97 times greater in Pee Wee, 3.72 times greater in Bantam, and 5.43 times greater in the Midget league. This shows that the injury risk increases significantly with increasing age. From the literature it was impossible to provide a single approximation for the incidence rate of ice hockey injuries. This can be due to related various factors including some types of soft tissue injuries which may not be reported at all times and in all studies; various leagues have different rules regarding protective equipment that might prevent injury; and incidence rates differ between games and practices, although most studies don't stratify for this fact.[115]

Overall, contusions are the most frequent type of injury in youth ice hockey, 60% of all injuries according to Roberts *et al.*[113], followed by concussions, strains and sprains, and lacerations and fractures. In adult ice hockey, strains and sprains seem to be most common type of injury.[116] In youth ice hockey, the head and neck appear to be most frequently injured body part.[113,114] The leg and arm, however, are also body parts that frequently sustain an injury.

Aetiology of ice hockey injuries

A considerable amount of injuries are localized to the face, predominantly lacerations caused by the opponent's stick or less often by the puck.[117] The same mechanism can cause harmless facial wounds, facial fractures, or severe eye injuries resulting in blindness.[118]

The types of head injuries that may occur in ice hockey encompass the entire range, from a mild concussion to a progressive neurosurgical emergency such as an epidural trauma.[118] Most concussions occur from player collisions and rarely from the blow of the puck.

Injuries to the neck, shoulder, and arms are regularly caused by collisions with an opponent's stick, the boards, the goalposts, or other players by aggressive checking.[119,120] However, most of these injuries are classified as 'minor'.[119,120]

Injuries to the lower extremity predominantly involve soft tissues. The groin is a very common site of muscle strain because the main thrust of the skating stride involves a forceful contraction of the hip adductor muscles.[118] Contusions of the thigh are common and can occur from direct trauma when a player strikes a goalpost or an opponent's knee. Knee injuries often involve sprains of the collateral ligaments, but disruption of the anterior cruciate ligament also can occur.[118] Ankle sprains are uncommon in ice hockey, due to the stiff protective skate boot. The sharp skate blade, however, can cause tendon and vessel lacerations at the level of the ankle.

The intrinsic and extrinsic risk factors of ice hockey injuries described in the literature are listed in Table 44.5.

Physical characteristics: A relation between body weight, height, and grip strength with force of impact generated by a body check has been observed.[121,122] Other studies, in youth ice hockey, did not find this relation.[123]

Aggressive play: Over 55% of injuries are contributed to contact with an opponent,[121] these injuries include sprains, strains, contusions, ruptures, and fractures. Aggressive play, which involves large amounts of body contact, is seen by many authors as an extrinsic risk factor for ice hockey injuries.[124,125]

Equipment: It has been proven in various studies that proper use of available protective equipment can substantially reduce the incidence of injuries.[121,122,126,127]

Preventive strategies

Brust *et al.*[128] showed that only half of the 12- to 15-year-old players understood the seriousness of checking another player from behind. The coach has the power to minimize this dangerous attitude by emphasizing the magnitude of the serious injury this move can inflict. Nevertheless, body checking in youth ice hockey remains a crucial injury mechanism and prevention should have a strong focus on body checking.[114]

It is also suggested that referees are more hesitant to call penalties because referees share the same stance as players; who might have a feeling of invulnerability due to the protective equipment worn.[129] Some coaches may also share this feeling of invulnerability and may attempt to stretch the rules and instruct players to break them to gain advantage. Most concussions occur from player collisions and referees must be vigilant for checks from behind and checks after more than two strides.[130] The fact that only 8% of injuries are associated with a penalty suggests that referees may presently allow dangerous play.[117]

Table 44.5 Intrinsic and extrinsic risk factors for ice hockey injuries, with their respective references.

Intrinsic risk factors	Extrinsic risk factors
Physical characteristics[121–123]	Aggressive play[121,124,125]
	Equipment[121,122,126,127]

Mandatory use of visors is presently being introduced into Swedish youth ice hockey because it is believed to significantly reduce the incidence of facial injuries.[117]

Muscle strains involving hip flexor, adductor, and lumbar paraspinal muscles correspond to the posture and biomechanics of skating, which places these muscle groups at risk. Stretching programmes that focus on the hip flexor, adductor, and lumbar paraspinal musculature may help decrease the incidence of these strains.[131]

Basketball

Basketball has long been considered as a non-contact sport but has nowadays evolved to a game were contact is inevitable and part of the game. Modern basketball is an intense fast paced game that involves jumping, hard cuts, sharp turns off a planted foot, and intense contact with the ball and other players. Basketball continues to grow in popularity and participants at all levels of play; and as the number of players increases, so do the number of injuries. Much of the data related to basketball are found in studies comparing various sports.

Epidemiology of basketball injuries

According to the NATA injury registration system, two players on every high school basketball team in the United States, regardless of gender, are likely to be injured during a season (6). In Swiss youth athletes, an incidence rate of 3.5 injuries per 10,000 hours of exposure was found[82] for males, for females this rate was 4.9 injuries per 10,000 hours of exposure. Since most of the data related to basketball injury incidence are found in studies comparing various sports, not much can be said about the exact incidence rates of males and females. Review articles, however, have suggested that males have lower injury rates in basketball than females.[132,133]

In high school male and female basketball players, sprains and strains appear to be the most frequent types of injury, accounting for, respectively 34 and 23% of all injuries.[134] Contusions (13% of all injuries) and fracture (10% of all injuries) are also common occurring injury types. The lower extremity is the most frequently injured body part (55% of all injuries), followed by the upper extremity (20% of all injuries), and the head (10% of all injuries),[135] respectively.

From the lower extremity, the ankle is the body part most susceptible to injury (31% of all injuries).[135] Presumably this accounts for the high rate of sprains. The fingers are the most vulnerable part of the upper extremity (11% of all injuries).[135] However, injuries to knee, wrist, teeth, and back are also not uncommon in basketball.

Aetiology of basketball injuries

Ankle sprains are the most common injuries in basketball. This is due to the high jumping frequency and sharp turns needed to play the game. When jumping there is a high chance of landing on an opponent's foot and causing an ankle inversion sprain.

The fingers and wrist are the most commonly injured upper extremity body parts. The proximal interphalangeal joint is the most frequently sprained and dislocated joint in the hand.[136] These result from hyperextension and are usually associated with volar rupture and sparring of the collateral ligaments.[136] This can easily be associated with the inherent nature of the game of constant and aggressive contact with the ball. The majority of ocular injuries sustained in basketball are due to blunt trauma from fingers and elbows of other players.[137]

The intrinsic and extrinsic risk factors of basketball injuries are difficult to assess and are not well presented in the literature.[137] Identifying risk factors in basketball is an extremely complicated problem requiring a large amount of data. There are some small studies in youth that showed some insight into injury risk factors. These studies, however, presented insufficient data to provide substantial evidence that any parameter is a clear injury risk factor.

Preventive strategies

As with any sport, a pre-season conditioning programme is thought to be indicated to prevent a certain amount of injuries.[137] Throughout the season a continued condition maintenance programme should lead to less fatigue during the game and intuitively to less abnormal stresses on the lower extremity joints. Therefore, a continued conditioning programme might be able to prevent overuse syndromes and injuries.

Since the majority of ocular injuries sustained in basketball are due to blunt trauma from fingers and elbows of other players, protective eyewear is believed to help prevent ocular injury.[137]

Evidence about the effectiveness of braces, tape, and proprioceptive training on reduction of the risk for ankle injury exists.[138] The use of some of external prophylactic preventive methods (i.e. tape and brace), however, is not well tolerated by many athletes, who believe it restricts movement and therefore reduces impact on the game.

Wrestling

Wrestling is a popular sport at both the youth and high school level. Most of its popularity is ascribed to the fact that athletes of all sizes and ages can compete in the sport, although the majority of wrestlers are male. There are three different styles of wrestling and each style requires similar training techniques despite the differences in competition. The competitive season is long and practices are frequent, long, and intense. Furthermore, in wrestling there is contact 100% of the time, which increases the effective exposure period. Therefore, although wrestlers are at the same risks for injury as other contact sport athletes, the exposure for an individual wrestler is high.

Epidemiology of wrestling injuries

In wrestling, Powell[139] found an injury incidence of 9.5 injuries per 1000 athlete exposures. In high school wrestling, lower incidence rates of 7.6 injuries per 1000 athlete exposures were found.[140] Each of these studies defined injury as requiring that participation was restricted for one or more days. Athlete exposure was defined as each opportunity for an athlete to get hurt. This makes the data-from these studies comparable and makes it reasonable to assume a lower injury incidence in high school wrestling in general compared to college wrestling.

In practice, the incidence rate is lower than in competitions. In high school, incidence rates were found of 6.45 injuries per 1000 athlete exposures in practice versus 11.6 injuries per 1000 athlete exposures in competition.[140] At college, mean rates were found of 7.4 injuries per 1000 athlete exposures in practice versus 29 injuries per 1000 athlete exposures in competition.[138,139]

In general, the most commonly reported injuries in wrestling are strain and sprain injuries, accounting for approximately 15 and 28% of all injuries.[138,140] It should be noted that infections are more commonly encountered problems in wrestling. Such 'injuries' are seldom properly registered in injury registration. Infections do not seem like injuries at first sight, but they cause the athlete to have to stop wrestling for a period of time. Nevertheless, the U.S. NATA injury registration (6) found that one out of four high school wrestling teams are projected to be affected by one of numerous skin conditions during a season. The most commonly found condition is ringworm, accounting for 83.8% of all infections.

Aetiology of wrestling injuries

Injuries to the head, principally concussions, are mainly caused by head–knee or head–head collisions during takedowns; that is, working the opponent to the ground. Concussions can also be caused by contact with the mat.[141] Sprains and strains in the neck region are frequently encountered in wrestling.[142] This injury can occur when a wrestler drives the opponent with his neck and hyperextends it. Auricular haematoma or cauliflower ear, result from direct trauma to the ear. This can occur from impact with an opponent's head or knee, or by abrasive friction-causing forces.[141] Lower back injuries commonly occur during takedowns. During a match a wrestler can pull and push with the lumbar spine in mild hyperextension. This extension together with twisting results in injuries.[142] Low-back injury, however, may also result from overuse. Chest injuries can be caused in different manners, from direct trauma during takedowns or when direct pressure is applied (i.e. 'bear hug').[141]

Shoulder injuries can be caused when being thrown on the mat from a standing position. The wrestler may attempt to break his fall with an extended arm, imparting force to the shoulder girdle, if unable to extend the arm the fall is taken directly on the shoulder.[141,142] Elbow injuries are less frequent than shoulder injuries but are commonly more severe.[143]

Lower extremity injuries usually are caused by the moves used in different wrestling manoeuvres. When a move isn't executed correctly or when the opponent makes a countermove, unnatural twisting and stretching of ligaments might occur, resulting in injuries.[141] For instance, meniscus injuries occur frequently via a twisting injury to a weight bearing extremity, and a varus or valgus force to the weight-bearing extremity is commonly the cause of collateral ligament sprains. The same goes for ankle injuries. When, for instance, a wrestler attempts to throw his opponent he rises onto his toes and twists. Loss of balance will cause the wrestler to invert his ankle.

Infections and skin conditions are mainly transferred on wrestling mats or from the physical contact between competitors (6).

The intrinsic and extrinsic risk factors of wrestling injuries described in the literature are listed in Table 44.6.

Body weight: Wrestlers with higher body weights are injured more often; possibly due to the greater forces exerted by heavier wrestlers.[141] The 'weight class system' reduces the risk of injury by reducing discrepancies in weight, size, and strength between athletes. This makes it beneficial for a wrestler to lose weight prior to a match in order to fight a weaker opponent.[144,145] This rapid weight loss in itself can be a risk factor for injury, but also the weaker of the two wrestlers has a greater risk for injury.

Fatigue: The exact role of fatigue on injuries in wrestling is not totally clear, mainly due to a variety in injury definition and differences in data collection between studies. Overall, studies have shown a higher rate of injuries in the second period of wrestling

Table 44.6 Intrinsic and extrinsic risk factors for wrestling injuries, with their respective references.

Intrinsic risk factors	Extrinsic risk factors
Body weight[141,144,145]	Exposure 147,148
Fatigue[141,146,147]	Environment 141,147,149
Psychosocial characteristics[147]	Protective equipment[141,150]

matches.[146,147] The injury rates are skewed, however, due to the termination of matches after a fall, resulting in lower exposure in the second and third periods of matches. The higher rate of injury in the second period is possibly the result of an initiation of fatigue together with a relatively high exposure.[141]

Psychosocial characteristics: It has been shown for recurrence of knee injuries that compliance to medical advice by the wrestler has an effect on injury.[147] It is not known if this is also true for other injuries.

Exposure: Injury rates increase with an increase in level of wrestling. Injury rates in matches are higher than in training, due to the higher intensity of matches. Takedowns appear to be manoeuvres that account for most injuries,[147,148] and are common manoeuvres in matches.

Environment: Most injuries occur early in the season.[147,149] At this time in the season, athletes are more motivated to get starting roles and to become a member of the team.[141] Another important factor is the conditioning of the athlete, which has not reached an optimum. The environment of the wrestling room is also an important factor for injury—for example, shock absorbency of the mats, cleanliness of the mats, or obstacles near the mats.

Protective equipment: The effect of headgear on a decrease of injury has been shown[150] in wrestling. The role of other protective equipment, for example, kneepads, shoes, or mouth guards, has not been evaluated.[141] In other sports, however, these measures have been effective in preventing injuries.

Preventive strategies

Weight reduction should be limited in wrestling. There is a discrepancy in strength between two wrestlers increasing the risk of injury for the weaker athlete. Furthermore, when losing weight the wrestler loses a lot of water and tends to get dehydrated.

Strength training and conditioning might reduce the effect of fatigue on injury, especially in tournaments where there are several matches per day. Injuries are also common early in the season, suggesting a need for appropriate year-round conditioning.[147,149]

Most shoulder injuries are caused by a poor technique.[141] Training on technique will improve it and therefore reduce the risk of shoulder injuries. For other injuries the same relationship between technique and injury risk may exist, especially if the technique involves takedowns.[147,148] A proper technique is, therefore, believed to reduce the number of injuries in general.

Dermatological illnesses and bacterial infections are commonly seen in wrestling. Dermatological illnesses are transmitted by contact with the opponent,[151] and bacteria are commonly found on the mats. Proper hygiene by the wrestler, for example, daily washing of clothes after training, daily showering after training, should reduce dermatological illnesses. Proper cleaning of the mat should reduce bacterial illnesses.

The effect of headgear on a decrease of injury has been shown[150] in wrestling. The role of other protective equipment, for example, kneepads, shoes, or mouth guards, has not been evaluated.[141] In other sports, however, these measures have been effective in preventing injuries. It is reasonable to assume an effect of other protective equipment on injury reduction

Summary

- Although a large proportion of sports pathology is common to both contact and non-contact, in general sports injuries in contact sports are more frequent than in non-contact sports.
- Injuries in contact sports are generally sport specific. Nevertheless, especially in children injuries to the lower extremities and head are the most common injury locations across all sports.
- For certain contact sports little information is available on children, and adult data serve as a basis for aetiology and prevention. Although children are not miniature adults, one should question this way of thinking and focus more research specifically on children in sports.

References

1. de Loës M, Goldie I (1988). Incidence rate of injuries during sport activity and physical exercise in a rural Swedish municipality: Incidence rates in 17 sports. *Int J Sports Med* **9**, 461–7.
2. Backx FJ, Beijer HJM, Bol E, Erick WBM (1991). Injuries in high-risk persons and high-risk sports. A longitudinal study of 1818 school children. *Am J Sports Med* **19**, 124–30.
3. Kujala UM, Taimela S, Antti Poika I, Orava S, Tuominen R, Myllynen P (1995). Acute injuries in soccer, ice hockey, volleyball, basketball, judo and karate: Analysis of national registry data. *BMJ* **311**, 1465–8.
4. Mechelen W van, Twisk J, Molendijk A, Blom B, Snel J, Kemper HC (1996). Subject related risk factors for sorts-injuries: A 1-year prospective study in young adults. *Med Sci Sports Exerc* **28**, 1171–9.
5. Metzl JD (1999). Sports specific concerns in the young athlete: Football. *Pediatr Emerg Care* **15**, 363–7.
6. Powell JW, Barber-Foss KD (1999). Injury patterns in selected High School sports. *JAT* **34**, 277–84.
7. Mueller F, Zemper ED, Peters A (1996). American football. In: Caine DJ (ed.), *Epidemiology of sports injuries*, pp. 41–62. Human Kinetics, Champaign, IL.
8. Blyth C, Mueller F (1974). Where and when players get hurt. *Phys Sports Med* **2**, 45–52.
9. Culpepper M, Niemann K (1983). A comparison of game and practice injuries in high school football. *Phys Sports Med* **11**, 117–22.
10. Lackland D, Akers P, Hirata I (1982). High school football injuries in South Carolina: A computerized survey. *J S C Med Assoc* **78**, 75–8.
11. Olson O (1979). The Spokane study: High school football injuries. *Phys Sports Med* **7**, 75–82.
12. Alves W, Rimel R, Nelson W (1987). University of Virginia prospective study of football induced minor head injury: Status report. *Clin J Sports Med* **6**, 211–8.
13. Cantu R (1992). Cerebral concussions in sports. *Sports Med* **14**, 302–7.
14. Gerberich S, Priest J, Boen J, Staub C, Maxwell R (1983). Concussion incidences and severity in secondary school varsity football players. *Am J Public Health* **73**, 1370–5.
15. Kelly J, Nichols J, Filley C, Lillhei K, Rubenstein D, Kleinschmidt-DeMasters B (1991). Concussions in sports. *JAMA* **266**, 2867–9.
16. Albright J, McAuley E, Martin R, Crowley E, Foster D (1985). Head and neck injuries in college football: An eight-year analysis. *Am J Sports Med* **13**, 147–52.

17. Buckley W (1986). Concussion injury in college football: An eight-year overview. *Athletic Training* **21**(3), 207–11.
18. Carter D, Frankel V (1980). Biomechanics of hyperextension injuries to the cervical spine in football. *Am J Sports Med* **8**, 302–7.
19. Rogers B (1981). The mechanics of head and neck trauma to football players. *Athletic Training* **16**, 132–5.
20. Tamberelli A (1978). Prevention and care of the knee injury. *Athletic J* **58**, 103–5.
21. Warren R (1982). Football knee injuries. *Coaching Clinic* **20**, 16–21.
22. Darden E (1978). Prevention of knee injuries. *Audible* **40**, 30–2.
23. Walsh W, Blackburn T (1977). Prevention of ankle sprains. *Am J Sports Med* **5**, 243–5.
24. Grace T, Sweetser E, Nelson M, Ydens L, Skipper B (1984). Isokinetic muscle imbalance and knee-joint injuries. *J Bone Joint Surg* **66–A**, 734–40.
25. Kalenak A, Morehouse C (1975). Knee stability and knee ligament injuries. *JAMA* **234**, 1143–5.
26. Kaplan TA, Digel SL, Scavo SA, Arellana SB (1995). Effect of obesity on injury risk in high school football players. *Clin J Sports Med* **5**, 43–7.
27. Lindner MM., Towsend DJ, Jones JC, Balkom Il, Anthony CR (1995). Incidence of adolescent injuries in junior high school and its relation to sexual maturity. *Clin J Sports Med* **5**, 167–70.
28. Sherk A, Watters W (1981). Neck injuries in football players. *J Med Assoc NJ* **78**, 579–83.
29. Brynhildsen J, Ekstrand J, Jeppson A, Tropp H (1990). Previous injuries and persisting symptoms in female soccer players. *Int J Sports Med* **11**, 489–92.
30. Mueller F, Blyth C (1974). North Carolina high school football injury study: Equipment and prevention. *J Sports Med* **2**, 1–10.
31. Powell J (1985). Pattern of knee injuries associated with college football 1975–1982. *Athletic Training* **20**, 104–9.
32. Prager B, Fitton W, Cahill B, Olson G (1989). High school football injuries: A prospective study and pitfalls of data collection. *Am J Sports Med* **17**, 681–5.
33. Whiteside J, Fleagle S, Kalanek A, Weber H (1985). Manpower loss in football: A 12-year study at the Pennsylvania State University. *Phys Sports Med* **13**, 103–14.
34. Cahill B, Griffith E (1978). Effect of pre-season conditioning on the incidence and severity of high school football knee injuries. *Am J Sports Med* **6**, 180–4.
35. Cameron BM, Davis O (1973). The swivel football shoe: A controlled study. *J Sports Med* **1**, 16–27.
36. Torg J, Quedenfeld T, Landau S (1973). Football shoes and playing surfaces: From safe to unsafe. *Phys Sports Med* **1**, 51–4.
37. Henschen K, Heil J, Bean B, Crain S (1989). Football injuries: Is grass or astroturf the culprit? *UHPERD J* **21**, 5–7.
38. Skovron M, Levy I, Agel J (1990). Living with artificial grass: A knowledge update. *Am J Sports Med* **18**, 510–3.
39. Zemper E (1994). Analysis of cerebral concussion frequency with the most commonly used models of football helmets. *JAT*, **29**, 44–50.
40. Hansen B, Ward J, Diehl R (1985). The preventive use of the Anderson Knee Stabler in football. *Phys Sports Med* **13**, 75–7.
41. Teitz C, Hermanson B, Kronmal R, Diehr P (1987). Evaluation of the use of braces to prevent injury to the knee in collegiate football players. *J Bone Joint Surg* **69**, 1467–70.
42. Porter M, O'Brien M (1996). Incidence and severity of injuries resulting from amateur boxing in Ireland. *Clin J Sports Med* **6**, 97–101.
43. Estwanik JJ, Boitano M, Ari N (1984). Amateur boxing injuries at the 1981 and 1982 USA / ABF national championships. *Phys Sports Med* **12**, 123–8.
44. Welch MJ, Sitler M, Kroeten H (1986). Boxing injuries from an instructional program. *Phys Sports Med* **14**, 81–9.
45. Jordan BD, Campbell E (1988). Acute boxing injuries among professional boxers in New York State: A two-year survey. *Phys Sports Med* **16**, 87–91.
46. Jordan BD, Voy RO, Stone J, (1990). Amateur boxing injuries at the United States Olympic training center. *Phys Sports Med* **18**, 80–90.
47. Butler RJ (1994). Neuropsychological investigation of amateur boxers. *Br J Sports Med* **28**, 187–90.
48. Hlobil H, Mechelen W van, Kemper HCG (1987). Boxing. In: Hlobil H, Mechelen W van, Kemper HCG (eds.), *How can sports injuries be prevented*, pp. 87–93. National Institute for Sports Health Care, The Netherlands.
49. Jordan BD (1996). Boxing. In: Caine DJ (ed.), *Epidemiology of sports injuries*. pp. 113–23. Human Kinetics, Champaign, IL.
50. Drew RH, Templer DI, Schuyler BA, Newell TG, Cannon WG (1986). Neuropsychological deficits in active licensed professional boxers. *J Clin Psychol* **42**, 520–5.
51. Jordan BD, Jahre C, Hauser WA, Zimmerman RD, Zarrelli M, Lipsitz EC, Johnson V, Warren RF, Tsairis P, Folk FS (1992). CT of 338 active professional boxers. *Radiology* **185**, 509–12.
52. Stewart WF, Gordon B, Selnes O, Bandeen-Roche K, Zeger S, Tusa RJ, Celentano DD, Shechter A, Liberman J, Hall C (1994). Prospective study of central nervous system function in amateur boxers in the United States. *Am J Epidemiol* **139**, 573–88.
53. McLatchie G, Brooks N, Galbraith S, Hutchison JS, Wilson L, Melville I, Teasdale E (1987). Clinical neurological examination, neuropsychology, electroencephalography, and computed tomographic head scanning in active amateur boxers. *J Neurol Neurosurg* **50**, 96–9.
54. Unterharnscheidt F (1985). Boxing injuries In: Schneider RC (ed.), *Sports injuries*. pp. 462–95. Williams and Wilkins, Baltimore, MD.
55. Kaste M, Vilkki J, Sainio K, Kuurne T (1982). Is chronic brain damage in boxing a hazard of the past? *Lancet* **2**, 27, 1186–9.
56. Kibler BW (1993). Injuries in adolescent and preadolescent soccer players. *Med Sci Sports Exerc* **25**, 1330–2.
57. Le Gall F, Carling C, Reilly T, Vandewalle H, Church J, Rochcongar P (2006). Incidence of injuries in elite French youth soccer players: A 10-season study. Am *J Sports Med* **34**, 928–38.
58. Kakavelakis KN, Vlazakis S, Vlahakis I, Charissis G (2003). Soccer injuries in Childhood. *Scand J Med Sci Sports* **13**, 175–8.
59. Adams AL, Schiff MA (2006). Childhood soccer injuries treated in U.S. emergency departments. *Acad Emerg Med* **13**, 571–4.
60. Xethalis JL, Boiardo A (1989). Soccer injuries. In: Nicholas J (ed.), *The lower extremity in sports medicine*, pp. 1590–667. C.V. Mosby, New York.
61. Larson M, Pearl AJ, Jaffet R, Rudawsky A (1996). Soccer. In: Caine DJ (ed.), *Epidemiology of sports injuries*. pp. 387–98. Human Kinetics, Champaign, IL.
62. Schmidt-Olsen S, Jørgenson U, Kaalund S, Sørenson J (1991). Injuries among young soccer players. *Am J Sports Med* **19**, 273–5.
63. Maehlum S, Dahl E, Daljord OA (1986). Frequency of soccer injuries in a youth soccer tournament. *Phys Sports Med* **14**, 73–9.
64. Schmidt-Olsen S, Bünemann LKH, Lade V, Brassoe JOK (1985). Soccer injuries of youth. *Br J Sports Med* **19**, 161–4.
65. Keller CS, Noyes FR, Buncher CR (1987). The medical aspects of soccer injury epidemiology. *Am J Sports Med* **15**, 230–7.
66. Backous DD, Friedl KE, Schmidt NJ, Parr TJ, Carpine WD (1988). Junior Soccer injuries and their relation to physical maturity. *Sports Med* **142**, 839–42.
67. Ekstrand J, Tropp H (1990). The incidence of ankle sprains in soccer. *Foot and Ankle* **11**, 41–4.
68. Nielsen AB, Yde J (1989). Epidemiology and traumatology of injuries in soccer. *Am J Sports Med* **17**, 803–7.
69. Ekstrand J, Gillquist J, Möller M, Öberg B, Liljedahl S (1983). Incidence of soccer injuries and their relation to training and team success. *Am J Sports Med* **11**, 63–7.
70. Poulsen TD, Freund KG, Madsen F, Sandvej K (1991). Injuries in high-skilled and low-skilled soccer: A prospective study. *Br J Sports Med* **25**, 151–3.
71. Jörgensen U (1984). Epidemiology of injuries in typical Scandinavian team sports. *Br J Sports Med* **18**, 59–63.

72. Agel J, Evans TA, Dick R, Putukian M, Marshall SW (2007) Descriptive epidemiology of collegiate men's soccer injuries: National Collegiate Athletic Association Injury Surveillance System, 1988–1989 through 2002–2003. *J Ath Train* **42**, 270–7.
73. Ekstrand J, Nigg B (1989). Surface-related injuries in soccer. *Sports Med* **8**, 56–62.
74. Dick R, Putukian M, Agel J, Evans TA, Marshall SW (2007) Descriptive epidemiology of collegiate women's soccer injuries: National Collegiate Athletic Association Injury Surveillance System, 1988–89 through 2002–2003. *J Ath Train* **42**, 278–85.
75. Watson A.WS (1995). Sports injuries in footballers related to defects of posture and body mechanics. *J Sports Med Phys Fitness* **35**, 289–94.
76. Cattermole HR, Hardy JRW, Gregg PJ (1996). The footballer's fracture. *Br J Sports Med* **30**, 171–5.
77. Yde J, Nielsen AB (1990). Sports injuries in adolescents' ball games: Soccer, handball and basketball. *Br J Sports Med* **24**, 51–5.
78. Tysvaer AT, Løchen EA (1991). Soccer injuries to the brain: A neuropsychologic study of former soccer players. *Am J Sports Med* **19**, 56–69.
79. Janda DH, Bir C, Wild B, Olson S, Hensinger RN (1995). Goal posts injuries in soccer: A laboratory and field testing analysis of a preventive intervention. *Am J Sports Med* **23**, 340–4.
80. Schneider K (1984). Das risiko einer hirnverletzung beim fußball-kopfstoß. *Unfallheilkunde* **87**, 40–42.
81. Tysvaer AT, Storli OV (1989). Soccer injuries to the brain: A neurologic and electroencephalographic study of active football players. *Am J Sports Med* **17**, 573–8.
82. de Loës M (1995). Epidemiology of sports injuries in the Swiss organization "Youth and Sports" 1987–1989: Injuries, exposure and risks of main diagnosis. *Int J Sports Med* **16**, 134–8.
83. Kujala UM, Taimela S, Antti-Poika I, Orava S, Tuominen R, Myllynen P (1995). Acute injuries in soccer, ice hockey, volleyball, basketball, judo, and karate: Analysis of national registry data. *BMJ* **311**, 1465–8.
84. Yard EE, Knox CL, Smith GA, Comstock RD (2007). Pediatric martial arts injuries presenting to Emergency Departments, United States 1990–2003. *J Sci Med Sport* **10**, 219–26.
85. Tuominen R (1995). Injuries in national karate competitions in Finland. *Scand J Med Sci Sports* **5**, 44–8.
86. Pieter W, Zemper ED (1997). Injury rates in children participating in taekwondo competition. *J Trauma* **43**, 89–95.
87. Oler M, Tomson W, Pepe H, Yoon D, Branoff R, Branch J (1991). Morbidity and mortality in the martial arts: A warning. *J Trauma* **31**, 251–3.
88. Johanssen HV, Noerregaard FOH (1988). Prevention of injury in karate. *Br J Sports Med* **22**, 113–5.
89. Feehan M, Waller AE (1995). Precompetition injury and subsequent tournament performance in full-contact taekwondo. *Br J Sports Med* **29**, 258–62.
90. Nishimura K, Fujii K, Maeyama R, Saiki I, Sakata S, Kitamura K (1988). Acute subdural hematoma in judo practitioners. Report of four cases. *Neurol Med Chir* **28**, 991–3.
91. Rodriguez G, Francione S, Gardelaa M, Marenco S, Nobili F, Novellone G, Reggiani F, Rosadini G (1991). Judo and choking: EEG and regional cerebral blood flow findings. *J Sports Med Phys Fitness* **31**, 605–10.
92. McLatchie GR (1981). Injuries in combat sports In: Reilly T (ed.), *Sports fitness and sports injuries*, pp. 168–74. London, Faber and Faber.
93. Stricevic MV, Patel MR, Okazaki T, Swain BK (1993). Karate: Historical perspective and injuries sustained in national and international tournament competitions. *Am J Sports Med* **11**, 320–4.
94. Siana JE, Borum P, Kryger H (1986). Injuries in taekwondo. *Br J Sports Med* **20**, 165–6.
95. McLatchie GR, Miller JH, Morris EW (1979). Combined force injury of the elbow joint: The mechanism clarified. *Br J Sports Med* **13**, 176–9.
96. Jerosch J, Castro WHM, Geske B (1990). Damage of the long thoracic and dorsal scapular nerve after traumatic shoulder dislocation: Case report and review of the literature. *Acta Orthopedica Belgica* **56**, 625–7.
97. Russo MT, Maffulli N (1991). Dorsal dislocation of the distal end of the ulna in a judo player. *Acta Orthopedica Belgica* **57**, 442–6.
98. Danek E (1979). Martial arts: The sound of one hand chopping. *Phys Sports Med* **7**, 140–4.
99. Pieter W, Zemper ED, Heijmans J (1990). Taekwondo blessures. *Geneeskunde en Sport* **23**, 222–8.
100. Zandbergen A (no date). Taekwondo blessures en fysiotherapie. *Thesis*. Enschede, Twentse akademie voor fysiotherapie.
101. Larose JH, Kim DS (1968). Knuckle fracture. A mechanism of injury. *JAMA* **206**, 893–4.
102. Wirtz PD, Vito GR, Long DH (1988). Calcaneal apophysitis associated with taekwondo injuries. *J Am Podiatr Med Assoc* **78**, 474–5.
103. Lampert PW, Hardman JM (1984). Morphological changes in brains of boxers. *JAMA* **251**, 2676–9.
104. McCunney RJ, Russo PK (1984). Brain injuries in boxers. *Phys Sports Med* **12**, 52–67.
105. Johanssen HV, Noerregaard FOH (1988). Prevention of injury in karate. *Br J Sports Med* **22**, 113–15.
106. Chuang TY, Lieu DK (1991). A parametric study of the thoracic injury potential of basic taekwondo kicks In: Min K (ed.), *Taekwondo. USTI Instructors handbook*, pp. 118–26. United States Taekwondo Union Instructors Certification Committee, Berkeley, CA.
107. Zemper ED, Pieter W (1989). Injury rates during the 1988 US Olympic Team Trials for taekwondo. *Br J Sports Med* **23**, 161–4.
108. Koiwai EK (1965). Major accidents and injuries in judo. *J A S Med Assoc* **22**, 957–62.
109. McLatchie GR, Commandre FA, Zakarian H, Vanuxem P, Lamendin H, Barrault D, Chau PQ (1992). Injuries in the martial arts. In: Renström PAFH (ed.), *Clinical practice of sports injury prevention and care. Volume V of the encyclopaedia of sports medicine*. pp. 609–23. Blackwell Scientific, Oxford.
110. Birrer RB (1984). Martial arts injuries: Their spectrum and management. *Sports Medicine Digest* **6**, 1–3.
111. Koiwai EK (1987). Deaths allegedly caused by the use of "choke holds". *J Forensic Sci* **32**, 419–32.
112. American Academy of Pediatrics Committee on Sports Medicine and Fitness (1994). Medical conditions affecting sports participation. *Pediatrics* **94**, 757–60.
113. Roberts WO, Brust JD, Leonard B (1998). Youth ice hockey tournament injuries: Rates and patterns compared to season play. *Med Sci Sports Exerc* **31**, 46–51.
114. Emery CA, Meeuwisse WH (2006). Injury rates, risk factors, and mechanisms of injury in minor hockey. *Am J Sports Med* **34**, 1960–9.
115. Montelpare WJ, Pelletier RL, Stark RM (1996). Ice Hockey. In: Caine DJ (ed.), *Epidemiology of sports injuries*, pp. 247–67. Human Kinetics, Champaign, IL.
116. Mölsä J, Airaksinen O, Näsman O, Torstila I (1997). Ice hockey injuries in Finland: A prospective epidemiologic study. *Am J Sports Med* **25**, 495–9.
117. Tegner Y, Lorentzen R (1991). Ice hockey injuries: Incidence, nature and causes. *Br J Sports Med* **25**, 87–9.
118. Daly PJ, Sim FH, Simonet WT (1990). Ice hockey injuries: A review. *Sports Med* **10**, 122–31.
119. Fox E, Bowers R, Foss M (1993). *The physiological basis for exercise and sport, 5th edition*. Brown and Benchmark, Madison, WI.
120. Rielly M (1982). The nature and causes of hockey injuries: A five year study. *Athletic Training* **17**, 88–90.
121. Roy A, Bernard D, Roy B, Marcotte G (1989). Body checking in pee-wee hockey. *Phys Sports Med* **17**, 119–26.
122. Bernard D, Trudel P, Marcotte G, Boileau R (1993). The incidence, types and circumstances of injuries to ice hockey players at the bantam

level (14 to 15 years old). In: Castaldi C, Bishop PJ, Hoerner EF (eds.), *Safety in ice hockey: Second volume*, pp. 45–55. American Society for Testing and Materials, Philadelphia, PA.

123. Kropp D, Marchant L, Warshawski J (1975). *An analysis of head injuries in hockey and lacrosse*. Sport safety research report, fitness and amateur sport branch, Department of National Health and Welfare, USA.
124. Daly P, Foster T, Zarins B (1994). *Injuries in ice hockey*. In: Renstrom P (ed.), *Clinical practice of sports injury prevention and care*, pp. 375–91. Blackwell Scientific, London.
125. Tator C, Edmonds V, Lapczak L (1993). Spinal injuries in ice hockey: Review of 182 North American cases and analysis of etiological factors. In: Castaldi C, Bishop PJ, Hoerner EF (eds.), *Safety in ice hockey: Second volume*, pp. 95–102. American Society for Testing and Materials, Philadelphia, PA.
126. Goodwyn-Gerberich S, Finke R, Madden M, Priest J, Aamoth G, Murray K (1987). An epidemiological study of high-school ice hockey injuries. *Child's Nervous System* **3**, 59–64.
127. Dick RW (1993). Injuries in collegiate ice hockey. In: Castaldi C, Bishop PJ, Hoerner EF (eds.), *Safety in ice hockey: Second volume*, pp. 21–30. American Society for Testing and Materials, Philadelphia, PA.
128. Brust JD, Leonard BJ, Pheley A, Roberts WO (1992). Children's ice hockey injuries. *Am J Disabled Child* **146**, 741–7.
129. Tator HD, Carson JD, Edmonds VE (1996). New spinal injuries in hockey. *Clin J Sports Med* **7**, 17–21.
130. Honey CR (1997). Brain injury in ice hockey. *Clin J Sports Med* **8**, 43–6.
131. Sim FH, Chao EY (1978). Injury potential in modern ice hockey. *Am J Sports Med* **15**, 378–84.
132. Sickles RT, Lombardo JA (1993). The adolescent basketball player. *Clin Sports Med* **12**, 207–19.
133. Emerson RJ (1993). Basketball knee injuries and the anterior cruciate ligament. *Clin Sports Med* **12**(2), 317–28.
134. McClain LG, Reynolds S (1989). Sports injuries in high school. *Pediatrics* **84**, 446–50.
135. Whiteside JA, Fleagle SB, Kalenak A (1981). Fractures and refractures in intercollegiate athletes: An eleven-year experience. *Am J Sports Med* **9**, 369–77.
136. Wilson RL, McGinty LD (1993). Common hand and wrist injuries in basketball players. *Clin Sports Med* **12**, 265–91.
137. Zvijac J, Thompson W (1996). Basketball. In: Caine DJ (ed.), *Epidemiology of sports injuries*, pp. 86–97. Human Kinetics, Champaign, IL.
138. Verhagen E, Mechelen W van, De Vente W (2000). The effect of preventive measures on the incidence of ankle sprains. *Clin J Sports Med* **10**, 291–6.
139. Powell JW (1981). National athletic injuries/illness reporting system: Eye injuries in college wrestling. *Int Ophthalmol Clin* **21**, 47–58.
140. National High School Injury Registry (1988–1989). Reported in *Athletic Training*, **23**, 383–88 (1988); **24**, 360–73 (1989).
141. Wroble RR (1996). Wrestling. In: Caine DJ (ed.), *Epidemiology of sports injuries*, pp. 417–38. Human Kinetics, Champaign, IL.
142. Wroble RR, Albright JP (1986). Neck and low back injuries in wrestling. *Clin Sports Med* **5**, 295–325.
143. Estwanik JJ, Rovere GD (1983). Wrestling injuries in North Carolina high schools. *Phys Sports Med* **11**, 100–8.
144. Horswill CA (1992). Applied physiology of amateur wrestling. *Sports Med* **14**, 114–43.
145. Horswill CA (1992). When wrestler slim to win. *Phys Sports Med* **20**, 91–104.
146. Hartmann PM (1978). Injuries in preadolescent wrestlers. *Phys Sports Med* **6**, 79–82.
147. Wroble RR, Mysnyk CA, Foster DT, Albright JP (1986). Patterns of knee injuries in wrestling: A six-year study. *Am J Sports Med* **14**, 55–66.
148. Estwanik JJ, Bergfeld JA, Collins HR, Hall R (1980). Injuries in interscholastic wrestling. *Phys Sports Med* **8**, 111–21.
149. Clarke KS (1977). A survey of sports-related spinal cord injuries in schools and colleges, 1973–1975. *J Safety Research* **9**, 140–6.
150. Schuller DE, Dankle SK, Martin M, Strauss RH (1989). Auricular injury and the use of headgear in wrestlers. *Arch Otolaryngol Head Neck Surg* **115**, 714–7.
151. Belongia EA, Goodman JL, Holland EJ, Andras CW, Homann SR, Mahanti RL, Mizener MW, Erice A, Osterholm MT (1991). An outbreak of herpes gladiatorum at a high-school wrestling camp. *N Engl J Med* **325**, 906–10.

CHAPTER 45

Aetiology and prevention of injuries in youth competitive non-contact sports

Per Bo Mahler

Introduction

The global approach to aetiology and prevention of sports injuries has been covered in previous chapters, so this chapter concentrates on sports specific problems and, in particular those of non-contact sports.

A number of sports, where no intentional contact with an opponent occurs, have therefore been selected based on their world-wide popularity[1] and are discussed individually or grouped with similar sports. Certain sports that are less universally practiced or that are country specific are beyond the scope of this chapter.

Each sport is covered in a systematic way covering information about the practice of the sport, epidemiology and aetiology of sport specific injuries, risk factors (intrinsic and extrinsic), and preventive strategies related to the above.

In general, injuries in non-contact sports are less frequent than in contact sports[2–5] and more frequently fall in the overuse group. One should however keep in mind that a large proportion of sports pathology is common to both contact and non-contact sports where similar biomechanical factors are involved (running, cutting, etc.).

Unfortunately, most studies quoted in the following sections are based on case reports and case series rather than randomized prospective or intervention studies and therefore give limited significant information about risk factors and the influence of prevention on injury.[6–9] It is also noteworthy that little information is available on children in certain sports[10,11] and that adult data have therefore been used to extrapolate when appropriate. Taking this in to consideration, the present chapter underlines certain trends that can be drawn from the literature and that give a reasonable basis on which to develop and promote prevention strategies.

Bicycling

Apart from being a popular sport, cycling is an equally popular means of transport and leisure activity. It is therefore difficult to differentiate between sports-related and sports-independent injuries, a lot of the risk factors being present in both activities. Special emphasis will be placed on competitive cycling injuries when possible.

Epidemiology of cycling injuries

Two studies concerning competitive cycling in adults cite an injury incidence of about 2–3%[12,13] for punctual competitive events, with a potentially higher incidence in mountain biking.[14] In competitive mountain biking, Kronisch *et al.* found an injury rate at 0.77% for women and 0.40% for men[15] whilst Gaulrapp *et al.*[16] found an overall injury rate in mountain biking of one per 1,000 hours.

A large scale study drawn from the National Electronic Injury Surveillance System USA 1987,1989 and 1990[17] shows an age- and sex-related prevalence of injuries with females age 5–9 years (730 injuries) and males age 10–14 years (1311 injuries) having the highest injury rates per 100,000 population. When expressed per million trips, children age 5–15 years (430.7 injuries) and adults over 50 years (296.2 injuries) have the highest injury rates.

Injuries can be divided into accidents and overuse (gradual onset), the second group being more specific to competitive cycling. Injuries resulting from accidents include abrasions, lacerations (63%), fractures (16%), closed head injuries and concussions (2%).[17] In the overuse group one finds anterior and lateral knee pain,[18] neck and low back pain,[19] ischial pain and pudendal nerve palsy,[20] microtrauma to the scrotal contents,[21] ulnar nerve pain,[22] and stenotic thickening of the external iliac artery[23] but these mostly concern adults even though the foundations may be laid at a younger age.

Aetiology of cycling injuries

Falls are the most frequent source of accidental injuries followed by hitting a stationary object, hitting or being hit by a motor vehicle, hitting another cyclist, pedestrian or animal, and finally bicycle malfunction.[24] Motor vehicles are involved in the minority of accidents (10–35%) but are responsible for about 90% of fatalities. Accidents also correlate with the type of road (more fatal accidents on high speed-limit roads), damaged or slippery roads, the availability of cycle tracks, excessive speed, and poor judgement.[16] Intersections are a frequent location for accidents.[17]

The non-use of helmets has been shown to be a major risk factor for head and brain injuries and the use of helmets decreases head injuries by up to 80%.[25] Some debate however still exists as to the evidence to enforce helmet use.[26]

Overuse injuries seem to be linked to biomechanical and training factors. As in other sports, training volume and progression are important. Bicycle fit (saddle position, foot clips, frame size) should be carefully evaluated and re-evaluated in the case of injury.[19,27,28] Cycling technique (foot, hip, and arm position) should also be analyzed[29,30] (Table 45.1).

Preventive strategies

Accidents are responsible for the most serious injuries and their prevention should therefore receive special attention. The Haddon Matrix[17] that identifies modifiable risk factors and divides them into three phases (preimpact, during impact, postimpact) is a valuable model for cycle injury prevention. Important factors like helmet use, cyclist education, bicycle design, road/path design, emergency service, and rehabilitation are stressed.

As previously mentioned, certain age groups are more at risk for cycle accidents and should therefore receive special attention in prevention campaigns.

Overuse injuries are mostly due to bicycle-rider misfit or training errors, hence bicycle choice (accessories) and adjustment should when possible be carried out by a professional and adapted to growth. Other modalities like muscle stretching and strengthening as well as specific protective equipment can also be useful in preventing injury.[22,30]

Dance

Dance in its various forms (ballet, jazz, rock and roll, fitness etc.) can be compared with other sports when considering athletic qualities required, methodical training programs and injuries.[32] Dancing is a popular activity amongst youth and often requires intensive involvement in training at a young age.

Because of the paucity of information and the higher age of participants, 'aerobic' (fitness) dancing is not included.

Epidemiology of dance injuries

As for other sports, data are flawed by lack of uniformity in injury definition and severity, exposure rates, sample size, and controlled data collection. A prospective study conducted by Reid *et al.*[33] on a group of young (mean age: 13.5 years) ballet dancers, showed an injury incidence of 0.9 injuries per 1000 hours. This was lower than that found by Rovere *et al.*[34] in slightly older (15–22 years) and more advanced dancers (2.8 per 1000 hours) but higher than that found in a Swedish professional ballet company (0.6 per 1000 hours).[35] The incidence of reinjury reported in Clanin *et al.*'s study,[36] was 0.02 reinjuries per 100 hours of exposure. Few data relate to the type of activity and injury in children, Bowling's data on professional dancers gives us some insight,[37] with 15.5% of injuries occurring in class, 27.6% in rehearsal and 32.8% during performance.

Injuries mostly fall in the overuse group[36] and are two times more frequent in ballet than in modern dance and five times more frequent in ballet than in jazz. This trend was not found by Wiesler *et al.*[38] who found nearly twice the number of injuries in modern dance than in ballet. The majority (33%–60%) of injuries recorded in literature are sprains and strains, followed by tendinits and contusions.[39] Stress fractures are not uncommon and concern mainly girls with irregular or absent menses.[40] Overall, knee injuries are the most frequent (14.5%–20.1%) followed by ankle (15.4%), foot and toes (13.1%–14.8%), and the spine (10.7%–12.2%).[33,34]

A number of injuries found in ballet which have been the subject of case reports or case series are summarized in Caine and Garick.[39]

Table 45.1 Intrinsic and extrinsic risk factors for cycling injuries, with their respective references

Intrinsic risk factors	Extrinsic risk factors
Age, gender[17,15]	**Protective equipment (helmets)**[25]
Pronation[19,27,28]	**Exposure**[19,27,28]
Cycling technique[29]	Training quality (progression, programme)[19,27,28]
	Type of roads, intersections, cycle tracks[17]
	Bicycle fit[19,27,28,31]
	Mechanical malfunction[24]

Bold factors have been confirmed in prospective studies and/or are supported by a general agreement in the literature, whilst the others still lack statistical support.

Aetiology of dance injuries

Exposure, as mentioned earlier, can influence occurrence of injury. Kadel *et al.*[41] found that the risk of sustaining a stress fracture increased significantly in professional dancers who danced over 5 hours a day or who had amenohroeic intervals extending beyond 6 months. Dancers are at increased risk of bone injuries because of their extreme nutritional habits (to minimize body fat) and heavy training loads, which when combined can lead to hormonal perturbations and delayed bone growth.[42,43] It is noteworthy that dancers are at high risk for nutrient deficiency and anorexia nervosa.[44]

Malalignment of the lower extremity and subtalar pronation resulting in a lack of turnout and a shallow 'demi plie' have been shown to be related to knee injuries.[45] Reduced functional turnout has been shown to be related to an increased overall risk of injury.[46,47] Dancing 'en pointe' has been proposed as a potential mechanism for low back stress, leading to spondylolysis, because of the biomechanical loading of the pedicles and the pars interarticularis of the vertebrae.[48]

Dancing 'en pointe' and 'demi-pointe', and pronation[49] have been incriminated in various injuries of the ankle, resulting in tendinitis of the flexor hallucis longus and Achilles tendon,[50] osteochodral fractures of the talus, sprains and anterior impingement syndromes of the ankle.[51] Overstress of the forefoot has been shown to result in injuries to the hallucis longus tendon, to the metatarsophalangeal joints, to the cuboid (subluxations) and to sesamoid bones. Isolated cases of Iselin's disease of the fifth metatarsal[52] and stress fractures involving the Lisfranc joint in dancers with a hyperflexed forefoot have also been reported.[53]

Stretching (overstretching) has also been shown to be at the origin of acute hamstring injuries in student-dancers[54] (Table 45.2).

Preventive strategies

A preventive approach includes proper treatment of injuries (rest), careful monitoring of individual stretching routines, good nutritional counselling and follow up, close monitoring of any menstrual

Table 45.2 Intrinsic and extrinsic risk factors for dance injuries, with their respective references

Intrinsic risk factors	Extrinsic risk factors
Previous injury[38]	**Exposure**[41]
Low body mass index (Nutrition)[42]	Dancing surface[55]
Irregular menstrual cycles[40,41]	Type of shoe[56]
Hypermobility[57]	Stretching[54]
Restricted joint mobility[33]	'negative' stress[58]
Flaws in technique[59,60]	
Hyperflexed forefoot[53]	
Pronation[45,49]	

Bold factors have been confirmed in prospective studies and/or are supported by a general agreement in the literature, whilst the others still lack statistical support.

irregularities and the constant re-evaluation of training load. Reid[61] suggests that young dancers should be allowed at least a 6 week block of rest once a year.

Joint hyper- and hypo-mobility should be recognized and corrected when possible. Adapted shoes, technique and surface may also contribute to preventing injuries.

Preparticipation examination has been shown to be useful in reducing injuries and should include an orthopaedic examination, the rehabilitation of any previous injury and a thorough nutritional and menstrual assessment.[62,63]

Gymnastics

Gymnastics is an increasingly popular sport in certain countries and requires early involvement (6–9 years of age) in intensive training . Training volume can reach 40 hours or more a week for elite gymnasts and generates significant loads to both the upper and lower extremities which potentially result in injury.

Epidemiology of gymnastics injuries

Injury rates vary considerably between studies depending on competitive level, club or school structure, gender and data processing. Injury rates for girls vary between 3.6 per 1000 hours of exposure at club level[3] to 22.7 per 1000 hours in college gymnastics.[64] For men, no data are available per hour but injury rates of 3.5 to 5.33 injuries per 1000 athletic exposures[65,66] have been observed in college gymnastics, which is lower than that observed in girls; 9.05 per 1000 athletic exposures.[66] Re-injury rates, including previous seasons, were 0.53 and 2.19 per 1000 athletic exposures in boys and girls respectively. Injury rates are higher in training than in competition for both boys and girls. However, when computed per athletic exposure, competition results in an approximately threefold higher injury incidence than training for both sexes.[66]

The majority of injuries are of sudden onset, but the difficulty in distinguishing between an acute injury and an acute injury superimposed on a predisposing overuse injury may bias this conclusion. Injury type also tends to be limb specific, more overuse injuries being observed at the upper extremity than at the lower.[67]

Sprains (15.9–43.6%) and strains (6.4–47.1%) are consistently the most frequently observed injuries[68] in women and men,[66] other injuries like fractures, contusions, and inflammation being less consistent depending on the groups studied. The lower limb is the most frequently involved body part (54.1–70.2%), followed by the upper extremity (18.1–25%) and the spine and trunk (0–16.7%). The ankle (45.7%) is most frequently injured in the lower limb followed by the knee (26.5%),[69] the heel/Achilles tendon and the foot/toes. The wrist, followed by the elbow and hands/fingers are the most frequently involved in the upper extremity and the lower back is the most often involved in injuries to the spine.[68]

Nutritional, endocrine, and psychiatric disorders have also been observed among gymnasts.[70]

Aetiology of gymnastics injuries

The high impact loads and extreme biomechanics seen in gymnastics certainly contribute to both overuse and accidental injuries. Vault takeoffs have been shown to produce ground reaction forces of up to 5.1 times body weight to the lower limb[71] whereas forces of 8.8 to 14.4 times body weight were found on landing.[72] These forces are transmitted through the lower limbs to the spine and can result in injury.[73] Extreme biomechanics involving hyperflexion, rotation, and hyperextension of the trunk can also be considered causative factors.[74] The high incidence of spondylolysis among gymnasts (19.2% in girls, 11.5% in boys), compared to 3.3% in the general population, tends to confirm the above hypothesis.[75] The upper limb is also exposed to large loads, ranging from 1.57 times body weight in vaulting[71] to 9.2 times body weight in still rings.[76] This might explain the frequently reported stress injuries involving the distal radial growth plate (51%)[77] and to a lesser extent osteochondritis dissecans of the humeral capitellum (1.2 and 2.5/100 participant seasons in girls and boys respectively), which can lead to long term complications.[78] Some data tend to show a dose-response relation between training intensity and ulna–radial–length difference resulting from distal radial physeal arrest in elite[79] and non-elite gymnasts.[80] Femoral nerve palsy due to iliacus muscle injury or direct compression has also been observed.[81] Few catastrophic injuries have been reported in gymnastics and relate mainly to trampoline (trampette) exercises.[82]

Numerous factors have been shown to relate to gymnastics injuries and are summarized below. Anthropometric factors like size, weight, and puberty[83–85] are closely related to injury in girls confirming the advantage of small size, low body weight, and retarded puberty to be successful in gymnastics and avoid injuries. Previous injury,[66] which is consistent through most sports, and high lumbar curvature can also be considered intrinsic risk factors.

External factors such as exposure,[86] competitive level,[87] and the type of event[64,88] also correlate with injury. Floor has been observed to be the source of most of the acute traumatic injuries in both boys and girls followed by uneven bars in girls and still rings in boys. This was confirmed at the world championships in 1997 where 40% of the injuries occurred during the floor exercise.[89] The first half hour of practice and certain periods of the season (following interruptions, intensive preparation, pre-competition, during competition) have also been shown to be risk factors.[87] Safe equipment is certainly of importance but can lead to more risky behavior during training. However, due to the high injury incidence during competitions, supplementary protective equipment could prove to be beneficial during competition[90] (Table 45.3).

Preventive strategies

A recent review by Caine and Nassar[96] underscores the need to establish large-scale injury surveillance systems to analyze injury

Table 45.3 Intrinsic and extrinsic risk factors for gymnastics injuries, with their respective references

Intrinsic risk factors	Extrinsic risk factors
Large body size and weight[83–85]	**Competitive level**[87]
Early maturation (high body fat)[83–85]	**Event (floor > still rings > horizontal bar)**[64,88,90]
Rapid growth[83–85]	**Protective equipment**[89,91]
High lumbar curvature[66]	Years of competition (exposure)[86,87]
Previous injury[66]	Training errors[92]
Muscle weakness[93]	Early part of practice[87]
Muscle asymmetry[94]	Period of the sports season[87]
	Coach assisted exercise (spotting)[66]
	'achievement by proxy'[70]
	Stressful life events[95]

Bold factors have been confirmed in prospective studies and/or are supported by a general agreement in the literature, whilst the others still lack statistical support

risks and identify dependable preventive measures. However, prevention should start with education of the gymnast and the coach concerning sport specific preparation, injuries, injury prevention and treatment, nutrition, and coach–child–family interaction.[92,97] Continuing education of coaches should be mandatory[98] and alternate loading, quality training, motivation, individualization, growth, and interpersonal skills should all be covered. Equipment should be adapted to exercise level and competition.[91]

A large proportion of gymnasts (51%) seem to compete despite pain.[99] Learning to differentiate between exertional soreness and pain owing to injury might help prevent reinjury.[100]

Medical support becomes important when children reach competition. Pre-season as well as post-injury medical evaluation is important to re-evaluate risk factors (orthopaedic, schooling, and family) and guide the gymnast and his or her support 'team'.

'Achievement by proxy' (parents, coaches, physicians), can be considered to be a risk factor that can lead to health disorders and should therefore be recognized as early as possible.[70]

Running

Running is a widespread activity and is common to a multitude of both contact and non-contact sports. Most of the literature concerns the adult and results concerning injury risk, male to female injury ratios and prevention are unfortunately somewhat contradictory depending on the research design.

Epidemiology of running injuries

One prospective and two retrospective studies conducted on relatively small groups of adolescents show an annual injury incidence of 18–40%[101–103] compared with 25–75% in adults.[104] The most common running injuries observed among adolescents were overuse injuries (19.5% medial tibial stress syndrome, 18% apophyseal injuries, 14.8% nonspecific knee pain, 7.3% low back pain) the rest being mainly composed of sprains and strains (3.4% ankle sprain/strain, 2.4% foot sprain/strain).[105] A majority of injuries concerned the knee and lower leg and no clear difference could be made between males and females. Isolated cases of avulsion fractures of the anterior and posterior iliac spine[106,107] and the distal femoral epiphysis[108] have been reported in children. Stress fractures of the tibia and fibula[109] as well as epiphyseal stress fractures of the calcaneum[110] and first metatarsal[111] have also been observed in children.

Table 45.4 Represents intrinsic and extrinsic risk factors for running injuries, with their respective references

Intrinsic risk factors	Extrinsic risk factors
Foot Pronation[116,118]	**Running volume (progression)**[114,119]
Lower limb (Malalignment, muscle imbalance, restricted range of motion)[110,120]	**Previous injury**[115]
Psychological factors[115]	Shoes (adapted to the foot and biomechanics)[120]
Capacity to recognize early symptoms of injury[121]	Running surface (hardness, inclination)[120]
Stride pattern[117]	Competition[122]

Bold factors have been confirmed in prospective studies and/or are supported by a general agreement in literature, whilst the others still lack statistical support.

Taunton *et al.*[112], found younger age (<34 years) to be related to patellofemoral pain across sexes. Iliotibial band friction syndrome, patellar tendinopathy, and tibial stress syndrome were also related to age (<34 years) in men.

Aetiology of running injuries

Most authors agree that a majority of running injuries are of gradual onset and linked to repetitive mechanical loading.[113] This load is more or less well tolerated depending on individual stress tolerance which is linked to a series of intrinsic and extrinsic risk factors. The only child specific reference in the literature concerns calcaneal apophysitis which was shown to be related to genu varum, subtalar varus, and forefoot varus.[110] Certain risk factors have been shown to be related to running injuries in adults and can be considered relevant in children because of the similarities in biomechanics. Exposure[114] and previous injury[115] have both been shown to be significantly correlated with running injuries. Training errors, inadequate shoes and/or running surface, warm up and stretching, certain psychological factors, lower extremity malalignment,[116] stride pattern,[117] muscular imbalance, restricted range of motion, orthotics, time of year, and participation in other sports have also been shown to correlate with injuries[115] (Table 45.4).

Preventive strategies

Adequate information should be given to the participant with respect to injury risk, risk factors and recognizing early symptoms of injury. Lower limb malalignment and muscle imbalance (strength, flexibility) should be identified and corrected (compensated) if possible.

It would seem useful to encourage the young runner to increase running volume progressively and or run on alternate days, to practice a proper warm up, to stretch after exercise, to detect and treat any injury properly and to return to running progressively. Understanding one's body is important as well as knowing how to buy adapted equipment.

'Shock absorbing' insoles seems to protect against stress fractures and stress reacions,[123] knee braces may reduce anterior knee pain and modification of training schedules effectively reduce soft tissue running injuries.[119]

One study has shown that practicing ball sports during childhood might have a protective effect on future stress fractures in runners.[124]

Preparticipation evaluation by a doctor should be encouraged if intensive participation is considered.

Skiing and snowboarding

Skiing and especially snowboarding have become increasingly popular over the last 25 years because of the facilitated access and increased capacity of ski areas. One estimate states that there are about 200 million leisure skiers in the world today.[125] Snowboarding has also contributed to the popularity of alpine sports, adding a 'fun' dimension which has attracted numerous youngsters.

No specific data are available on competitive skiing in children, so the following data include both recreational and competitive skiers and snowboarders.

Epidemiology of skiing and snowboarding injuries

Deibert *et al.*[126], prospectively collected data over a 12 year period in a ski area and found an average injury incidence of 2.79 injuries per 1000 skier days. Children (1–10 years of age) showed the highest injury incidence: 4.27 injuries per1000 days, followed by adolescents (11–16 years of age): 2.93 injuries per 1000 days. Similar results were found by Macnab and Cadman.[127] This can also be expressed as injuries per 10 km of vertical metres skied, and Matter *et al.*[128] found rates of 4 injuries per 10 km in 1972 and 1 per 10 km in 1986 for adults. This underlines the decrease in injuries observed in other studies. Using a similar unit Ronning *et al.* found a distance-correlated injury index of 3.9 for skiing and 13.5 for snowboarding per 100,000 km.[129] Snowboarding injuries have been found to have a similar[130–132] or higher[133,134,129] incidence than skiing injuries, but injury type and location vary considerably between the two. Recent publications seem to systematically show higher injury rates for snowboarding.[129,135–137]

In skiing, injuries are principally to the lower extremity (40–70%) and the trend from 1985 to 2000 showed a decrease in tibial fractures (–89%) and ankle injuries and a clear increase in knee sprains (+280%). The most frequent injuries were knee contusions in children, ulnar collateral sprains of the thumb for adolescents and grade III anterior cruciate sprains in adults.[126] On average (including adults) 10–22% of injuries involve the head and spine.[127,138] Skull fractures seem relatively frequent among children.[138] Upper extremity injuries account for 13–36% of injuries, with ulnar collateral sprains of the thumb being the most frequent injury (10–17%) followed by shoulder fractures and dislocations (5–10%).

Snowboarding injuries vary considerably from skiing injuries in that the upper extremities (mainly hand and wrist) are most frequently involved (45.1–58%). Contrary to skiing, ankle injuries have been found to be more frequent than knee injuries.[130,132,133] The injury pattern differs somewhat in competitive snowboarding (big air, boardercross, halfpipe) where knee injuries seem to be more common than wrist injuries.[139]

Skiing injuries can on the whole be classified as relatively severe and often result in prolonged absences from sport at both the recreational and competitive level.[140]

Aetiology of skiing and snowboarding injuries

The improving trend in lower extremity injuries is partly due to improvement in equipment (safety bindings, ski stoppers, boots) and better information. However, adjustment of the bindings is paramount and Deibert *et al.*[126] showed that 71% of children presenting with a spiral fracture of the lower leg had badly adjusted bindings.

Injuries to the head and spine were often due to loss of control, collisions with other skiers or trees, incorrect landings after jumps[141] and negligible helmet use among children.[142] Five mechanisms, involving rotational and translation forces in the knee, have been described by Feagin *et al.*[143] for anterior cruciate tears. This could lead to a better prevention of this injury by, for example, avoiding to ski from packed to deep snow at high speed.

In snowboarding, injuries seem to affect mainly boys and novices. Injuries vary as a function of the activity (head, face and spine injuries in aerial maneuvers), type of boots (more severe injuries with stiff boots) and snow conditions (66% of injuries on icy, hard slopes).[131,133,142] Snowboarders have been criticized for their risk-taking behavior (speed, off piste skiing), but this was not confirmed in Berghold and Seidl's study.[131]

Serious injuries in children, requiring hospitalization, have been related to ground level falls (50%), crashes into trees (18%), falls from ski lifts (13%),[144] and collisions[145] (Table 45.5).

Preventive strategies

Injury awareness programmes assisted by video presentations on risk behaviour, dangerous situations and how to avoid them have had considerable impact on ACL injuries in Vermont[155] and can serve as a model for injury prevention in skiing and other sports. Children should receive particular attention because of their relatively high injury risk. They should be informed on risk factors and how to apply them, especially if they are beginners and/or snowboarders. Using helmets[148,149] and associated wrist guards[150–152] for snowboarders is strongly recommended.[136,156]

Some improvement can certainly be made to safety equipment (skis, bindings, pole handles, gloves) by the industry but equipment should always be checked and adjusted for weight and expertise.[156]

Table 45.5 Represents intrinsic and extrinsic risk factors for skiing and snowboarding injuries, with their respective references

Intrinsic risk factors	Extrinsic risk factors
Novice skiers and snowboarders[131,133,142,136]	**Binding adjustment**[125]
Age (child > adolescent > elder)[146,147]	**Helmets**[138,148,149]
Common sense[133]	**Snow conditions and weather (avalanches)**[130,133,138]
Conditioning	**Wrist guards** (snowboarding)[150–152]
Risky behaviour[130,141]	Fatigue (more injuries in mid-late afternoon)[153]
	Skiing fast from packed to deep snow[143]
	Slope grooming[154]

Bold factors have been confirmed in prospective studies and/or are supported by a general agreement in the literature, whilst the others still lack statistical support.

Skiers should take particular care in evaluating snow conditions and the risks in skiing off the piste. Some common sense rules as those put forward by Chisell[134] can be of use: (i) quit before 3 o'clock; (ii) go shopping (or something other than skiing) on the third day; (iii) be wary when skiing at altitudes over 3000 m.

Swimming

Swimming is among the most popular leisure and competitive sports throughout the world. Participants often begin at a young age and the swimmers who chose to compete, quickly progress to intensive training which leads to significant loads on the upper extremities and, to a lesser extent the lower extremities.

Epidemiology of swimming injuries

Few data are available on the epidemiology of swimming injuries. Swimming is mostly thought of as a 'safe' sport and the available data tend to confirm this. Maffuli *et al.*[157] found an injury incidence of 0.3 injuries per 1000 hours of swimming in a group of highly trained 10- to 16-year-old swimmers. This is similar to the injury incidence found by Schnyder (personal communication) who found an injury incidence of 0.5 injuries per 1000 hours in a group of competitive 12- to 15-year-old swimmers. The injury incidence was similar for boys and girls in both groups.

Most injuries are overuse injuries (62%) and concern mainly the shoulder and arm (35%) followed by the trunk (25%) and the lower extremity (20%).[158] The majority of injuries are benign and lead to short absences from sport. In Rowley's study,[158] 65% of injuries were sustained outside the sports activity, 25% during training and about 6% during competitions.

Aetiology of swimming injuries

Most authors agree that the repetitivity and the high training volume, leading to about 2 million strokes per year in elite swimmers, is the main source of injury.[159] Injury incidence has been shown to correlate with exposure[160,161] and performance, with medal winners showing a higher incidence of injury.[162]

Injury type varies between strokes, shoulder injuries being most common in free-style, back-stroke, and butterfly swimming[159] whilst knee and groin injuries are more common in breast stroke.[163,164] This can be explained by the varying biomechanics of the strokes, stressing different structures. Shoulder problems mainly result from a sub-acromial impingement mechanism and labral pathology[165] linked to repetitive overhead motion. This phenomenon may be aggravated by muscle imbalance between internal and external rotators, shoulder instability[166,167] and acromial shape.[168] Shoulder injuries have also been shown to be related to improper technique, premature strength training, and the use of devices such as the pull buoy and paddles.[159]

Knee problems are mainly linked to patello-femoral dysfunction during kicking or medial collateral ligament stress which is more specific to breast stroke. Lower extremity malalignment and patellar instability have been suggested as risk factors.[169]

Back pain can be linked to the repeated flexion and twisting during flip turns, torsional strain if the body is not rolled as a whole unit during the stroke or to swimming techniques that lead to lumbo-sacral hyperextension [breast stroke, butterfly][170] (Table 45.6).

Table 45.6 Represents intrinsic and extrinsic risk factors for swimming injuries, with their respective references

Intrinsic risk factors	Extrinsic risk factors
Shoulder muscle imbalance[166]	**Exposure**[160,161]
Shoulder instability[167]	Technique[159,170]
Acromial shape[168]	Using a pull buoy or paddles[159]
Lower extremity malalignment or patellar instability[169]	Premature or unadapted strength training[159]
	Type of stroke[159,163,164]

Bold factors have been confirmed in prospective studies and/or are supported by a general agreement in the literature, whilst the others still lack statistical support.

Preventive strategies

Ciullo and Stevens[159] suggest a series of factors that may contribute to preventing injuries in youth; emphasis should be placed on proper stroke mechanics, little emphasis on performance, stretching should be carried out before and after swimming, sessions should be started very progressively and terminated at the first signs of fatigue (perturbed mechanics). Strength training should begin in skeletally mature swimmers, when proper swimming mechanics have been acquired and start with high repetition low resistance exercises. Bak[171] however, suggests that resistance training in prepubescent swimmers could improve muscle balance and prevent injuries. He also suggests that coaches should be informed on preventive strategies.

Tennis and badminton

Because of similarities in injury profile and biomechanics, this chapter includes both tennis and badminton. For various reasons, these sports have become increasingly popular amongst youths, leading to early specialization and intensification of training programs. This has resulted in an increase in injuries in the younger population.[172]

Epidemiology of tennis and badminton injuries

Zaricznyj[173] studied a population of school-aged children and found that 0.3% and 0.1% of the 1576 sports related injures were sustained during tennis and badminton respectively. This gives an injury incidence of 0.01 per 1000 hours for tennis and quasi 0 for badminton. A similar injury incidence (<1%) was found by Watson[174] in Irish School children. During a 2 year prospective study on high school children, Garrick and Requa[175] found a 3% incidence of injury in girls and 7% in boys for tennis and 6% for female badminton players. However, for competitive and elite tennis, injury levels seem to be substantially higher, at about 24% for the competitive level,[176] and 60% of players at the elite level having sustained an injury in the two previous years.[172] Expressed in injuries per 1000 hours, Lanese *et al.*[177] found injury rates of 1.6 per 1000 hours for boys and 1.0 per 1000 hours for girls in intercollegiate tennis. It would also seem that girls are more often injured than boys at the elite level, contrary to what was found at high school level.[178]

The majority of injuries seem to be from overuse and mainly involve the lower extremity (hamstring, knee, ankle). Injuries to the back, neck, and groin occur at a similar frequency to the upper extremity (shoulder, elbow, wrist) but half as frequently as injuries to the lower extremity.[178] In badminton, 74% of injuries are from overuse and involve mainly the lower extremity (83%).[179] In tennis the most frequently observed injuries are rotator cuff tendonitis, epicondylitis, chronic muscle strain, and stress fractures. Maquirriain and Ghisi[180] showed a particularly high incidence (12.9%) of stress fractures (tarsal navicular > pars interarticularis > metatarsals > tibia) in young elite Argentinian tennis players. Shoulder subluxation, labral tears, 'Osgood-Schlatter disease of the shoulder', slipped capital humeral epiphysis and a stress fracture of the humeral epiphysis have been described in junior tennis and badminton players' shoulders.[181,182] Eye injuries[183] and neurological injuries involving the suprascapular nerve[184] have also been described.

Aetiology of tennis and badminton injuries

Most injuries are due to repetitive microtrauma[185] as shown by the high incidence of overuse injuries in both tennis and badminton and may be higher if acute injuries secondary to overuse are included. The overuse mechanism involves mainly the upper extremity[181] and is often due to poor technique, repetitive unnatural and dynamic movements,[186] fatigue and incoordination as well as inappropriate equipment and training programmes.[187,188] Lower extremity injuries are related to the constant pounding, accelerations and decelerations during games[189] and to the high eccentric loads which can lead to muscle tears and tendinous injuries.[190,191] In badminton however, injuries are often sustained while players stumble when trying to play a stroke.[179] Range of motion may also influence predisposition to injury, internal rotation having been shown to be limited in the dominant arm of tennis players.[192] Muscle imbalances and shortness observed in the shoulder, the forearm and the trunk may also predispose the athlete to injury.[178] A higher exposure to matches, as shown by Kibler *et al.*[172] may contribute to an increase in the number of injuries in tennis, but the inverse seems to be the case in badminton[193] (Table 45.7).

Preventive strategies

Prevention should start by informing players and coaches about the risks of injury linked to the sport, injuries themselves, injury treatment, and prevention. Even though statistical evidence is poor, a good basic fitness level, specific strengthening, regular stretching exercises[196] (internal rotation of the dominant arm) and adapted equipment[197] should be encouraged. Varying the playing surface or reducing play on hard courts may also reduce lower limb injuries.

Table 45.7 Represents intrinsic and extrinsic risk factors for tennis and badminton injuries, with their respective references

Intrinsic risk factors	Extrinsic risk factors
Sex[175]	**Exposure, Elite**[172,178]
Low fitness level	Playing surface[194]
Low flexibility[172,192]	Equipment (racket, grip, cord tension, balls)[187,188]
Insufficient shoulder strength[195]	
Muscle imbalance[178]	

Bold factors have been confirmed in prospective studies and/or are supported by a general agreement in the literature, whilst the others still lack statistical support.

Volleyball

Volleyball is progressively becoming one of the more popular sports for both boys and girls with an estimated 150 million players in the world. It has also become more attractive to children with the introduction of minivolleyball and beach volleyball.

Epidemiology of volleyball injuries

Volleyball is the third greatest source of injury in Knobloch *et al.*'s study on school sport injuries in Niedersachsen, behind basketball and soccer.[198] Two studies give volleyball as being the second greatest source of injuries for girls.[198,199] In a 6 week retrospective study of 1818 school children, Backx[3] found a surprisingly high injury incidence of 6.7 per 1000 hours, compared with the data of Zaricznyj *et al.*[173] who found an injury incidence of 0.13 per 1000 hours. In Backx's study the injuries were sustained mainly during practice and were recorded at the beginning of a season. Recent data on Dutch 2nd and 3rd division volleyball give an injury rate of 2.6 per 1000 hours.[200] Injuries during practice seem to be more frequent than competitive play.[3,4,201] The evolution from being more of a leisure activity to a highly competitive sport, with the subsequent increase in training volume, may contribute to an increase in injuries as seen over the last 10–15 years.[202]

In school volleyball, Zaricznyj *et al.*[173] found that 50% of injuries concerned the hands and fingers, 20% to the ankles and 6% to the knees. Similar results were found by Knobloch *et al.*[198] This contrasts with adult data in an amateur volleyball league where 48% of injuries were to the lower extremity, 26% to the upper extremity and 26% to the trunk and head.[203] In competitive volleyball, Verhagen[200] found that 83% of acute injuries concerned the lower limb, ankle sprains being the most frequent injury (41% of the total). In Knobloch *et al.*'s study 41% of injuries were sprains and strains, 17% fractures and 16% bruises. Case series including adolescents have shown a high frequency of patellofemoral and patellar tendon pathologies.[204] Isolated cases of long thoracic nerve entrapment[205] and a stress fracture of the ulna[206] have also been reported.

Aetiology of volleyball injuries

The jumping action (eccentric loads) during offensive and defensive play and the numerous contacts between the knee and the playing surface during defensive play are said to be responsible for the majority of injuries around the knee.[3,207] Loss of balance during landing has also been incriminated in both knee and ankle injury. Jumping and landing with the knees in a valgus position,[208] landing with a twisting motion of the knee[209] as well as one legged takeoff and landing[210] all seem to contribute to injury risk. Ankle injuries are mostly sustained during collisions between players and often with the opponent under the net.[203] Verhagen *et al.*[200] also showed that a previous ankle sprain is a major risk factor for re-injury, especially during the first year post injury. Shoulder injuries including supraspinatus tendinopathy, impingement and nerve entrapment are due to the extreme mechanics of spiking and the jump serve.[211] Fingers are mainly at risk during blocking.

Condensing data from adult literature, blocking seems to be responsible for the largest number of injuries followed by spiking and defence manoeuvers.[212] However, in Knobloch *et al.*'s study of school volleyball, collisions between opponents (60%), the landing phase (9%), and striking the ball (7%) seem to be the main sources of injury (Table 45.8).

Table 45.8 Represents intrinsic and extrinsic risk factors for volleyball injuries, with their respective references

Intrinsic risk factors	Extrinsic risk factors
Previous injury (ankle)[200]	**Exposure (frequency > duration)**[207,209]
Younger age group[213]	**Position (offensive > defensive)**[203]
Growth spurt[214]	Quality of training[215]
Poor jumping technique[208,216,210]	Playing surface[217]
Malalignment of the extensor mechanism	Collision with opponent[203]
Muscle imbalance	Match play[200]
Males > Females (Injury specific trends)	

Bold factors have been confirmed in prospective studies and/or are supported by a general agreement in the literature, whilst the others still lack statistical support.

Preventive strategies

Specific attention should be given to children and their growth phases, and adapting training loads to the individual. Malalignment and muscle imbalance should be identified and corrected where possible. Jumping and landing techniques have been shown to be important and can have a protective effect on ankle injuries.[218] Wearing protective equipment should be encouraged and the majority of play should, if possible, be done on wooden or linoleum surfaces.

Considering the frequency of ankle injuries, special attention should be given to specific preparation (technical, proprioceptive),[218] avoid premature return to sport, do a proper proprioceptive rehabilitation and wear protective braces when necessary.[219]

Summary

- It becomes clear from the above data that sports medical literature and in particular paediatric sports is plagued by numerous methodological issues[220,8] and paucity of data.
- Preventive approaches like informing coaches, athletes and health professionals about prevention and risk factors, adapting the training load to growth, doing a good warm up and cool down session, stretching after exercise, taking time for recuperation and regeneration, properly treating injuries, using protective equipment, discouraging 'achievement by proxy' and insuring adequate nutrition and hydration must be encouraged and monitored in all sports.
- The prevention model described by Emery *et al.*[98] assigning least responsibility to the child and the most to sports organizations and Government is noteworthy and stresses the need for structural prevention.
- It is the right of all children to benefit from a safe environment so that we can ensure a healthy sports practice and a proper application of the 'Children's bill of rights in Sport'.[221]

Acknowledgement

My warmest thanks go to Dr. P. Fricker and Dr. F. Mahler for their help in correcting and improving this text.

References

1. DeKnop P, Engström LM, Skirstad B, Weiss MR (1996). *World-wide trends in youth sport.* Human Kinetics, Champaign, IL.
2. DeLoes M, Goldie I (1988). Incidence rate of injuries during sport activity and physical exercise in a rural Swedish municipality: Incidence rates in 17 sports. *Int J Sports Med* **9,** 461–7.
3. Backx FJ, Beijer HJ, Bol E, Erich WB (1991). Injuries in high-risk persons and high-risk sports. A longitudinal study of 1818 school children. *Am J.Sports Med* **19**, 124–30.
4. Kujala UM, Taimela S, Antti-Poika I, Orava S, Tuominen R, Myllynen P (1995). Acute injuries in soccer, ice hockey, volleyball, basketball, judo, and karate: Analysis of national registry data. *BMJ* **311**, 1465–8.
5. van Mechelen W, Twisk J, Molendijk A, Blom B, Snel J, Kemper HC (1996). Subject-related risk factors for sports injuries: A 1-yr prospective study in young adults. *Med Sci Sports Exerc* **28**, 1171–9.
6. Brooks JH Fuller CW (2006). The influence of methodological issues on the results and conclusions from epidemiological studies of sports injuries: Illustrative examples. *Sports Med* **36**, 459–72.
7. Walter SD, Sutton JR, McIntosh JM, Connolly C (1985). The aetiology of sport injuries. A review of methodologies. *Sports Med* **2**, 47–58.
8. Shephard RJ (2005). Towards an evidence based prevention of sports injuries. *Inj Prev* **11**, 65–6.
9. Chalmers DJ (2002). Injury prevention in sport: Not yet part of the game? *Inj Prev* **8**(Suppl. 4), IV22–IV25.
10. MacKay M, Scanlan A, Olsen L, Reid D, Clark M, McKim K, Raina P (2004). Looking for the evidence: A systematic review of prevention strategies addressing sport and recreational injury among children and youth. *J Sci Med Sport* **7**, 58–73.
11. Emery CA (2005). Injury prevention and future research. *Med Sport Sci* **49**, 70–191.
12. Bohlmann JT (1981). Injuries in competitive cycling. *Phys Sportsmed* **9**, 117–24.
13. McLennan JG, McLennan JC, Ungersma J (1988). Accident prevention in competitive cycling. *Am J Sports Med* **16**, 266–8.
14. Chow TK, Bracker MD, Patrick K (1993). Acute injuries from mountain biking. *West J Med* **159**, 145–8.
15. Kronisch RL, Pfeiffer RP, Chow TK, Hummel CB (2002). Gender differences in acute mountain bike racing injuries. *Clin J Sport Med* **12**, 158–64.
16. Gaulrapp H, Weber A, Rosemeyer B (2001). Injuries in mountain biking. *Knee Surg Sports Traumatol Arthrosc* **9**, 48–53.
17. Baker SP, Li G, Fowler C, Dannenberg AL (1993). *Injuries to bicyclists: A national perspective.* Report The Johns Hopkins University Injury Prevention Centre, Baltimore, MD.
18. Holmes JC, Pruitt AL, Whalen NJ (1994). Lower extremity overuse in bicycling. *Clin Sports Med* **13**, 187–205.
19. Mellion MB (1994). Neck and back pain in bicycling. *Clin Sports Med* **13**, 137–64.
20. Weiss BD (1994). Clinical syndromes associated with bicycle seats. *Clin Sports Med* **13**, 175–86.
21. Frauscher F, Klauser A, Hobisch A, Pallwein L, Stenzl A (2000). Subclinical microtraumatisation of the scrotal contents in extreme mountain biking. *Lancet* **356**, 1414.
22. Richmond DR (1994). Handlebar problems in bicycling. *Clin Sports Med* **13**, 165–73.
23. Mosimann R, Walder J, Van Melle G (1985). Stenotic intimal thickening of the external iliac artery: Illness of the competition cyclists? *Vasc Surg* **19**, 258–63.
24. Friede AM, Azzara CV, Gallagher SS, Guyer B (1985). The epidemiology of injuries to bicycle riders. *Pediatr Clin North Am* **32**, 141–51.
25. Thompson DC, Patterson MQ (1998). Cycle helmets and the prevention of injuries. Recommendations for competitive sport. *Sports Med* **25**, 213–19.

26. Robinson DL (2006). No clear evidence from countries that have enforced the wearing of helmets. *BMJ* **332**, 722–5.
27. Burke ER (1994). Proper fit of the bicycle. *Clin Sports Med* **13**, 1–14.
28. Nichols CE (1994). Injuries in cycling In: Renstöm P (ed.), *Clinical practice of sports injury prevention and care*, pp. 514–25. Blackwell Scientific Publications, Oxford.
29. Mondenard JP (1989). *Technopathies du cyclisme*. Ciba Geigy, Paris
30. Thompson MJ, Rivara FP (2001). Bicycle-related injuries. *Am Fam Physician* **63,** 2007–14.
31. Bressel E, Larson BJ (2003). Bicycle seat designs and their effect on pelvic angle, trunk angle, and comfort. *Med Sci Sports Exerc* **35,** 327–32.
32. Bejjani FJ (1987). Occupational biomechanics of athletes and dancers: A comparative approach. *Clin Podiatr Med Surg* **4,** 671–711.
33. Reid DC, Burnham RS, Saboe LA, Kushner SF (1987). Lower extremity flexibility patterns in classical ballet dancers and their correlation to lateral hip and knee injuries. *Am J Sports Med* **15,** 347–52.
34. Rovere GD, Webb LX, Gristina AG, Vogel JM (1983). Musculoskeletal injuries in theatrical dance students. *Am J Sports Med* **11**, 195–8.
35. Nilsson C, Leanderson J, Wykman A, Strender LE (2001). The injury panorama in a Swedish professional ballet company. *Knee Surg Sports Traumatol Arthrosc* **9,** 242–6.
36. Clanin DR, Davidson DM, Plastino JG (1986). Injury patterns in university dance students In: Shell CG (ed.), *The dancer as athlete*, pp. 195–9, Human Kinetics, Champaign IL.
37. Bowling A (1989). Injuries to dancers: Prevalence, treatment, and perceptions of causes. *BMJ* **298,** 731–4.
38. Wiesler ER, Hunter DM, Martin DF, Curl WW, Hoen H (1996). Ankle flexibility and injury patterns in dancers. *Am J Sports Med* **24,** 754–57.
39. Caine CG Garrick JG (1996) Dance In: Caine DJ, Caine CG. Lindner KJ (ed.), *Epidemiology of sports injuries*, pp. 130–9. Human Kinetics, Champaign, IL.
40. Benson JE, Geiger CJ, Eiserman PA, Wardlaw GM (1989). Relationship between nutrient intake, body mass index, menstrual function, and ballet injury. *J Am Diet Assoc* **89**, 58–63.
41. Kadel NJ, Teitz CC, Kronmal RA (1992). Stress fractures in ballet dancers. *Am J Sports Med* **20**, 445–9.
42. Warren MP, Brooks-Gunn J, Hamilton LH, Warren LF, Hamilton WG (1986). Scoliosis and fractures in young ballet dancers. Relation to delayed menarche and secondary amenorrhea. *N Engl J Med* **314**, 1348–53.
43. Castelo-Branco C, Reina F, Montivero AD, Colodron M, Vanrell JA (2006). Influence of high-intensity training and of dietetic and anthropometric factors on menstrual cycle disorders in ballet dancers. *Gynecol Endocrinol* **22,** 31–5.
44. Brainsted JR, Mellin L, Gong EJ, Irwin CE Jr (1985). The adolescent ballet dancer. Nutritional practices and characteristics associated with anorexia nervosa. *J Adolesc Health Care* **6,** 365–71.
45. Clippinger-Robertson KS, Hutton RS, Miller DI, Nichols TR (1986). Mechanical and anatomical factors relating to the incidence and aetiology of patello-femoral pain in dancers In: Shell CG (ed.), *The dancer as athlete*, pp. 53–72. Human Kinetics, Champaign, IL.
46. Negus V, Hopper D, Briffa NK (2005). Associations between turnout and lower extremity injuries in classical ballet dancers. *J Orthop Sports Phys Ther* **35,** 307–18.
47. Coplan JA (2002). Ballet dancer's turnout and its relationship to self-reported injury. *J Orthop Sports Phys Ther* **32,** 579–84.
48. Ireland ML, Micheli LJ (1987). Bilateral stress fracture of the lumbar pedicles in a ballet dancer. A case report. *J Bone Joint Surg Am* **69,** 140–2.
49. Kravitz SR (1990). Pronation as a predisposing factor in overuse injuries. In: Solomon R. (ed.), *Preventing dance injuries: An interdisciplinary perspective*, pp. 15–20. National Dance Association, AAHPERD Press, Reston, VA.
50. Scheller AD, Kasser JR, Quigley TB (1983). Tendon injuries about the ankle. *Clin Sports Med* **2,** 631–41.
51. Stoller SM, Hekmat F, Kleiger B (1984). A comparative study of the frequency of anterior impingement exostoses of the ankle in dancers and nondancers. *Foot Ankle* **4,** 201–3.
52. Lehman RC, Gregg JR, Torg E (1986). Iselin's disease. *Am J Sports Med* **14,** 494–6.
53. Micheli LJ, Sohn RS, Solomon R (1985). Stress fractures of the second metatarsal involving Lisfranc's joint in ballet dancers. A new overuse injury of the foot. *J Bone Joint Surg Am* **67,** 1372–5.
54. Askling C, Lund H, Saartok T, Thorstensson A (2002). Self-reported hamstring injuries in student-dancers. *Scand J Med Sci Sports* **12,** 230–5.
55. Fernandez-Palazzi F, Rivas S, Mujica P (1990). Achilles tendinitis in ballet dancers. *Clin Orthop Rel Rehab* **257,** 257–61.
56. Skrinar M, Carlson K, Jeglosky L (1981). Effect of three brands of pointed shoe on pelvic tilt *Int J Sports Med* **2,** 283.
57. Klemp P, Chalton D (1989). Articular mobility in ballet dancers. A follow-up study after four years. *Am J Sports Med* **17,** 72–5.
58. Byhring S, Bo K (2002). Musculoskeletal injuries in the Norwegian National Ballet: A prospective cohort study. *Scand J Med Sci Sports* **12,** 365–70.
59. Gans A (1985). The relationship of heel contact in ascent and descent from jumps to the incidence of shin splints in ballet dancers. *Phys Ther* **65,** 1192–6.
60. Solomon R, Micheli L (1986). Concepts in the prevention of dance injuries: A survey and analysis. In: Shell CG (ed.), *The dancer as athlete*, pp. 201–12. Human Kinetics, Champaign, IL.
61. Reid DC (1987). Preventing injuries to the young ballet dancer. *Physiotherapy, Canada* **39**, 231–6.
62. Plastino JG (1990 Physical Screening of the Dancer: General methodologies and procedure In: Solomon R (ed.), *Preventing dance injuries: An interdisciplinary perspective*, pp. 155–75. National Dance Association, AAHPERD Press, Reston, VA.
63. Lauffenburger SK (1990). Bartenieff fundamentals: Early detection of potential dance injuries In: Solomon R (ed.), *Preventing danceIlnjuries: An interdisciplinary perspective*, pp. 177–90. National Dance Association, AAHPERD, Reston, VA.
64. Sands WA, Shultz BB, Newman AP (1993). Women's gymnastics injuries. A 5-year study. *Am J Sports Med* **21**, 271–6.
65.Clark KS, Miller SJ (1977). The national athletic injury/illness system (NAIRS) In: Morehouse CH (ed.), *Sports safety II*. pp. 49–53, American Alliance for Health, Physical Education and Recreation, Washington, DC.
66. NCAA (1994). National Collegiate Athletic Association 1993–94 men's and women's gymnastics injury surveillance system. Report NCAA Report, Kansas
67. Dixon M, Fricker P (1993). Injuries to elite gymnasts over 10 yr. *Med Sci Sports Exerc* **25,** 1322–9.
68. Caine DJ, Lindner KJ, Mandelbaum BR, Sands WA (1996). Gymnastics In: Caine DJ, Caine CG, Lindener KJ (ed.), *Epidemiology of sports injuries*, pp. 219–22. Human Kinetics, Champaign, IL.
69. Kirialanis P, Malliou P, Beneka A, Giannakopoulos K (2003). Occurrence of acute lower limb injuries in artistic gymnasts in relation to event and exercise phase. *Br J Sports Med* **37**, 137–9.
70. Tofler IR, Stryer BK, Micheli LJ, Herman LR (1996). Physical and emotional problems of elite female gymnasts. *N Engl J Med.* **335**, 281–3.
71. Takai Y. (1991). A comparaison of techniques used in performing the men's compulsory gymnastic vault at the 1988 Olympics. *Intl J Sports Biomech* **7,** 54–75.
72. Panzer VP, Wood GA, Bates BT, Mason BR (1988). *Lower extremity loads in landings of elite gymnasts.* Free University Press, Amsterdam
73. Too D, Adrain M (1987). Relationship of lumbar curvature and landing surface to ground reaction forces during gymnastic landing In: Terauds J, Gowitzke BA, Holt LE (eds.), *Biomechanics in sports III and IV*, pp. 96–102. Academic Publishers, Del Mar, CA.
74. Hall SJ (1986). Mechanical contribution to lumbar stress injuries in female gymnasts. *Med Sci Sports Exerc* **18,** 599–602.

75. Hellstrom M, Jacobsson B, Sward L, Peterson L (1990). Radiologic abnormalities of the thoraco-lumbar spine in athletes. *Acta Radiol* **31**, 127–32.
76. Sands WA, Cheltham PJ (1986). Velocity of the vault run: Junior elite female gymnasts. *Technique* **6**, 10–14.
77. DiFiori JP, Puffer JC, Aish B, Dorey F (2002). Wrist pain, distal radial physeal injury, and ulnar variance in young gymnasts: Does a relationship exist? *Am J Sports Med* **30**, 879–85.
78. Dixon M, Fricker P (1993). Injuries to elite gymnasts over 10 yr. *Med Sci Sports Exerc* **25**, 1322–9.
79. Caine D, Howe W, Ross W, Bergman G (1997). Does repetitive physical loading inhibit radial growth in female gymnasts? *Clin J Sport Med* **7**, 302–8.
80. DiFiori JP, Puffer JC, Mandelbaum BR, Dorey F (1997). Distal radial growth plate injury and positive ulnar variance in nonelite gymnasts. *Am J Sports Med* **25**, 763–8.
81. Hirasawa Y, Sakakida K (1983). Sports and peripheral nerve injury. *Am J Sports Med* **11**, 420–6.
82. Torg JS (1987). Trampoline-induced quadriplegia. *Clin Sports Med* **6**, 73–85.
83. DeSmet L, Claessens A, Lefevre J, Beunen G (1994). Gymnast wrist: An epidemiologic survey of ulnar variance and stress changes of the radial physis in elite female gymnasts. *Am J Sports Med* **22**, 846–50.
84. Meeusen R, Borms J (1992). Gymnastic injuries. *Sports Med* **13**, 337–56.
85. Caine D (1988). *An epidemiological investigation of injuries affecting young competitive female gymnasts*. Thesis/Dissertation, University of Oregon, Eugene, Oregon.
86. Dzioba RB (1984). Irreversible spinal deformity in Olympic gymnasts. *Orthop Trans* **8**, 66.
87. Caine D, Cochrane B, Caine C, Zemper E (1989). An epidemiologic investigation of injuries affecting young competitive female gymnasts. *Am J Sports Med* **17**, 811–20.
88. Lueken J, Stone J, Wallach BA (1993). Olympic training centre report men's gymnastics injuries. *Gymnastics Safety Update* **8**, 4–5.
89. Gremion G, Bielinski R, Vallotton J, Augros R, Larequi Y, Leyvraz PF (1998). [Gymnastic world championship in Lausanne: Medical staffing]. *Rev Med Suisse Romande* **118**, 709–11.
90. Goldstein JD, Berger PE, Windler GE, Jackson DW (1991). Spine injuries in gymnasts and swimmers. An epidemiologic investigation. *Am J Sports Med* **19**, 463–8.
91. Daly RM, Bass SL, Finch CF (2001). Balancing the risk of injury to gymnasts: How effective are the counter measures? *Br J Sports Med* **35**, 8–18.
92. Sands WA, Crain S, Lee KM (1990). Gymnastics coaching survey. *Technique* **10**, 22–7.
93. Micheli LJ (1979). Low back pain in the adolescent: Differential diagnosis. *Am J Sports Med* **7**, 362–4.
94. Irvin R, Major J, Sands WA (1992). Lower body and torso strength norms for elite female gymnasts. In: McNitt G (ed.), *USGF sport science congress proceedings*, pp. 5–12. USGF Publications, Indianapolis.
95. Kerr GA (1988). Psychological factors related to the occurrence of athletic injuries. *J Sport Exerc Psychol* **10**, 167–73.
96. Caine DJ, Nassar L (2005). Gymnastics injuries. *Med Sport Sci* **48**, 18–58.
97. Smith AD, Andrish JT, Micheli LJ (1993). Current comment: The prevention of sport injuries of children and adolescents. *Med Sci Sports Exerc* **25**, 1–7.
98. Emery CA, Hagel B, Morrongiello BA (2006). Injury prevention in child and adolescent sport: Whose responsibility is it? *Clin J Sport Med* **16**, 514–21.
99. Harringe ML, Lindblad S, Werner S (2004). Do team gymnasts compete in spite of symptoms from an injury? *Br J Sports Med* **38**, 398–401.
100. Nemeth RL, von Baeyer CL, Rocha EM (2005). Young gymnasts' understanding of sport-related pain: A contribution to prevention of injury. *Child Care Health Dev* **31**, 615–25.
101. Orava S, Saarela J (1978). Exertion injuries to young athletes: A follow-up research of orthopaedic problems of young track and field athletes. *Am J Sports Med* **6**, 68–74.
102. Nudel DB, Hassett I, Gurian A, Diamant S, Weinhouse E, Gootman N (1989). Young long distance runners. Physiological and psychological characteristics. *Clin.Pediatr.(Phila)* **28**, 500–5.
103. Rowland TW, Walsh CA (1985). Characteristics of child distance runners. *Phys Sportsmed* **13**, 45–53.
104. van Mechelen W (1992). Running injuries. A review of the epidemiological literature. *Sports Med* **14**, 320–35.
105. Knutzen K, Hart L (1996). Running In: Caine J, Caine CG, Linder KJ (eds.), *Epidemiology of sports injuries*, p. 364. Human Kinetics, Champaign, IL.
106. Clancy WG Jr, Foltz AS (1976). Iliac apophysitis and stress fractures in adolescent runners. *Am J Sports Med* **4**, 214–8.
107. Paluska SA (2005). An overview of hip injuries in running. *Sports Med* **35**, 991–1014.
108. Godshall RW, Hansen CA, Rising DC (1981). Stress fractures through the distal femoral epiphysis in athletes. A previously unreported entity. *Am J Sports Med* **9**, 114–6.
109. Daffner RH, Martinez S, Gehweiler JA Jr, Harrelson JM (1982). Stress fractures of the proximal tibia in runners. *Radiology* **142**, 63–5.
110. McKenzie DC, Taunton JE, Clement DB, Smart GW, McNicol KL (1981). Calcaneal epiphysitis in adolescent athletes. *Can J Appl Sport Sci* **6**, 123–5.
111. Cibulka MT (1990). Management of a patient with forefoot pain. *Physical Therapy* **70**, 41–4.
112. Taunton JE, Ryan MB, Clement DB, McKenzie DC, Lloyd-Smith DR, Zumbo BD (2002). A retrospective case-control analysis of 2002 running injuries. *Br J Sports Med* **36**, 95–101.
113. Taunton JE, Clement DB, Webber D (1981). Lower extremity fractures in athletes. *Phys Sports Med* **9**, 85–6.
114. Brunet ME, Cook SD, Brinker MR, Dickinson JA (1990). A survey of running injuries in 1505 competitive and recreational runners. *J Sports Med Phys Fitness* **30**, 307–15.
115. Marti B (1988). Benefits and risks of running among women: An epidemiologic study. *Int J Sports Med* **9**, 92–8.
116. Willems TM, De Clercq D, Delbaere K, Vanderstraeten G, De Cock A, Witvrouw E (2006). A prospective study of gait related risk factors for exercise-related lower leg pain. *Gait Posture* **23**, 91–8.
117. Hreljac A, Marshall RN, Hume PA (2000). Evaluation of lower extremity overuse injury potential in runners. *Med Sci Sports Exerc* **32**, 1635–41.
118. Bennett JE, Reinking MF, Pluemer B, Pentel A, Seaton M, Killian C (2001). Factors contributing to the development of medial tibial stress syndrome in high school runners. *J Orthop Sports Phys Ther* **31**, 504–10.
119. Yeung EW, Yeung SS (2001). A systematic review of interventions to prevent lower limb soft tissue running injuries. *Br J Sports Med* **35**, 383–9.
120. van Mechelen W (1995). Can running injuries be effectively prevented? *Sports Med* **19**, 161–5.
121. Johnston CA, Taunton JE, Lloyd-Smith DR, McKenzie DC (2003). Preventing running injuries. Practical approach for family doctors. *Can.Fam.Physician* **49**, 1101–9.
122. Zemper ED (2005). Track and field injuries. *Med Sport Sci* **48**, 138–51.
123. Gillespie WJ, Grant I (2000). Interventions for preventing and treating stress fractures and stress reactions of bone of the lower limbs in young adults. *Cochrane Database Syst Rev* **2**, CD000450.
124. Fredericson M, Ngo J, Cobb K (2005). Effects of ball sports on future risk of stress fracture in runners. *Clin J Sport Med* **15**, 136–41.
125. Burns TP, Steadman JR, Rodkey WG (1991). Alpine skiing and the mature athlete. *Clin Sports Med* **10**, 327–42.
126. Deibert MC, Aronsson DD, Johnson RJ, Ettlinger CF, Shealy JE (1998). Skiing injuries in children, adolescents, and adults. *J Bone Joint Surg Am* **80**, 25–32.

127. Macnab AJ, Cadman R (1996). Demographics of alpine skiing and snowboarding injury: Lessons for prevention programs. *Inj Prev* **2,** 286–9.
128. Matter P, Ziegler WJ, Holzach P (1987). Skiing accidents in the past 15 years. *J Sports Sci* **5,** 319–26.
129. Ronning R, Gerner T, Engebretsen L (2000). Risk of injury during alpine and telemark skiing and snowboarding. The equipment-specific distance-correlated injury index. *Am J Sports Med* **28,** 506–8.
130. Pigozzi F, Santori N, Di S, V, Parisi A, Di Luigi L (1997). Snowboard traumatology: An epidemiological study. *Orthopedics* **20,** 505–9.
131. Berghold F, Seidl AM (1991). [Snowboarding accidents in the Alps. Assessment of risk, analysis of the accidents and injury profile]. *Schweiz Z Sportmed* **39,** 13–20.
132. Bladin C, McCrory P (1995). Snowboarding injuries. An overview. *Sports Med* **19,** 358–64.
133. Chow TK, Corbett SW, Farstad DJ (1996). Spectrum of injuries from snowboarding. *J Trauma* **41,** 321–5.
134. Chissell HR, Feagin JA Jr, Warme WJ, Lambert KL, King P, Johnson L (1996). Trends in ski and snowboard injuries. *Sports Med* **22,** 141–5.
135. Hagel BE, Goulet C, Platt RW, Pless IB (2004). Injuries among skiers and snowboarders in Quebec. *Epidemiology* **15,** 279–86.
136. Made C, Elmqvist LG (2004). A 10-year study of snowboard injuries in Lapland Sweden. *Scand J Med Sci Sports* **14,** 128–33.
137. Langran M, Selvaraj S (2002). Snow sports injuries in Scotland: A case-control study. *Br J Sports Med* **36,** 135–40.
138. Lystad H.(1985). A one year study of alpine ski injuries in Hemsedal, Norway 860314-325.
139. Torjussen J, Bahr R (2006). Injuries among elite snowboarders (FIS Snowboard World Cup). *Br J Sports Med* **40,** 230–4.
140. Higgins RW, Steadman JR (1987). Anterior cruciate ligament repairs in world class skiers. *Am J Sports Med* **15,** 439–47.
141. Reid DC, Saboe L (1989). Spine fractures in winter sports. *Sports Med* **7,** 393–9.
142. Shorter NA, Jensen PE, Harmon BJ, Mooney DP (1996). Skiing injuries in children and adolescents. *J Trauma* **40,** 997–1001.
143. Feagin JA Jr, Lambert KL, Cunningham RR, Anderson LM, Riegel J, King PH, VanGenderen L (1987). Consideration of the anterior cruciate ligament injury in skiing. *Clin Orthop Relat Res* **216,** 13–8.
144. Skokan EG, Junkins EP Jr, Kadish H (2003). Serious winter sport injuries in children and adolescents requiring hospitalization. *Am J Emerg Med* **21,** 95–9.
145. Xiang H, Stallones L, Smith GA (2004). Downhill skiing injury fatalities among children. *Inj Prev* **10,** 99–102.
146. Blitzer CM, Johnson RJ, Ettlinger CF, Aggeborn K (1984). Downhill skiing injuries in children. *Am J Sports Med* **12,** 142–7.
147. Xiang H, Kelleher K, Shields BJ, Brown KJ, Smith GA (2005). Skiing- and snowboarding-related injuries treated in U.S. emergency departments, 2002. *J Trauma* **58,** 112–8.
148. Hagel BE, Pless IB, Goulet C, Platt RW, Robitaille Y (2005). Effectiveness of helmets in skiers and snowboarders: Case-control and case crossover study. *BMJ* **330,** 281.
149. Sulheim S, Holme I, Ekeland A, Bahr R (2006). Helmet use and risk of head injuries in alpine skiers and snowboarders. *JAMA* **295,** 919–24.
150. O'Neill DF (2003). Wrist injuries in guarded versus unguarded first time snowboarders. *Clin Orthop Relat Res* **409,** 91–5.
151. Ronning R, Ronning I, Gerner T, Engebretsen L (2001). The efficacy of wrist protectors in preventing snowboarding injuries. *Am J Sports Med* **29,** 581–5.
152. Machold W, Kwasny O, Gassler P, Kolonja A, Reddy B, Bauer E, Lehr S (2000). Risk of injury through snowboarding. *J Trauma* **48,** 1109–14.
153. Young LR, Oman CM, Crane H, Emerton A, Heide R (1976). The etiology of ski injuries: An eight year study of the skier and his equipment. *Orthop Clin North Am* **7,** 13–29.
154. Bergstrom KA, Ekeland A (2004). Effect of trail design and grooming on the incidence of injuries at alpine ski areas. *Br J Sports Med* **38,** 264–8.
155. Ettlinger CF, Johnson RJ, Shealy JE (1995). A method to help reduce the risk of serious knee sprains incurred in alpine skiing. *Am J Sports Med* **23,** 531–7.
156. Hagel B (2005). Skiing and snowboarding injuries. *Med Sport Sci* **48,** 74–119.
157. Maffulli N, King JB, Helms P (1994). Training in elite young athletes (the Training of Young Athletes (TOYA) Study): Injuries, flexibility and isometric strength. *Br J Sports Med* **28,** 123–36.
158. Rowley S (1992). *Training of Young Athletes Study: Project Description.* Report pp. 1–17. The Sports Council, London.
159. Ciullo JV, Stevens GG (1989). The prevention and treatment of injuries to the shoulder in swimming. *Sports Med* **7,** 182–204.
160. Ciullo JV (1986). Swimmer's shoulder. *Clin Sports Med* **5,** 115–37.
161. Stocker D, Pink M, Jobe FW (1995). Comparison of shoulder injury in collegiate- and master's-level swimmers. *Clin J Sport Med* **5,** 4–8.
162. Bak K, Bue P, Olsson G (1989). [Injury patterns in Danish competitive swimming]. *Ugeskr Laeger* **151,** 2982–4.
163. Costill DL, Maglischo EW, Richardson AB (1992). Costill DL, Maglischo EW, Richardson AB (ed.), *Swimming,* pp. 190–2. Blackwell Science, Oxford.
164. Grote K, Lincoln TL, Gamble JG (2004). Hip adductor injury in competitive swimmers. *Am J Sports Med* **32,** 104–8.
165. Brushoj C, Bak K, Johannsen HV, Fauno P (2006). Swimmers' painful shoulder arthroscopic findings and return rate to sports. *Scand J Med Sci Sports* **4,** 373–7.
166. McMaster WC (1996). Swimming injuries. An overview. *Sports Med* **22,** 332–6.
167. Bak K, Magnusson SP (1997). Shoulder strength and range of motion in symptomatic and pain-free elite swimmers. *Am J Sports Med* **25,** 454–9.
168. Fowler PJ, Webster-Bogaert MS (1991). Swimming In: Reider B. (ed.), *Sports medicine, the school-age athlete,* pp. 429–46. W.B. Saunders Company, Philadelphia.
169. Fowler PJ, Regan WD (1986). Swimming injuries of the knee, foot and ankle, elbow, and back. *Clin Sports Med* **5,** 139–48.
170. Kenal KA, Knapp LD (1996). Rehabilitation of injuries in competitive swimmers. *Sports Med* **22,** 337–47.
171. Bak K (1996). Nontraumatic glenohumeral instability and coracoacromial impingement in swimmers. *Scand J Med Sci Sports* **6,** 132–44.
172. Kibler WB, McQueen C, Uhl T (1988). Fitness evaluations and fitness findings in competitive junior tennis players. *Clin Sports Med* **7,** 403–16.
173. Zaricznyj B, Shattuck LJ, Mast TA, Robertson RV, D'Elia G (1980). Sports-related injuries in school-aged children. *Am J Sports Med* **8,** 318–24.
174. Watson AW (1984). Sports injuries during one academic year in 6799 Irish school children. *Am J Sports Me* **12,** 65–71.
175. Garrick JG, Requa RK (1978). Injuries in high school sports. *Pediatrics* **61,** 465–9.
176. Lehmann RC (1988). Shoulder pain in the competitive tennis player. *Clin Sports Med* **7,** 309–27.
177. Lanese RR, Strauss RH, Leizman DJ, Rotondi AM (1990). Injury and disability in matched men's and women's intercollegiate sports. *Am J Pub Health* **80,** 1459–62.
178. Bylak J, Hutchinson MR (1998). Common sports injuries in young tennis players. *Sports Med* **26,** 119–32.
179. Kroner K, Schmidt SA, Nielsen AB, Yde J, Jakobsen BW, Moller-Madsen B, Jensen J (1990). Badminton injuries. *Br J Sports Med* **24,** 169–72.
180. Maquirriain J, Ghisi JP (2006). The incidence and distribution of stress fractures in elite tennis players. *Br J Sports Med* **40,** 454–9.
181. Gregg JR, Torg E (1988). Upper extremity injuries in adolescent tennis players. *Clin Sports Med* **7,** 371–85.
182. Boyd KT, Batt ME (1997). Stress fracture of the proximal humeral epiphysis in an elite junior badminton player. *Br J Sports Med* **31,** 252–3.

183. Larrison WI, Hersh PS, Kunzweiler T, Shingleton BJ (1990). Sports-related ocular trauma. *Ophthalmology* **97,** 1265–9.
184. Black KP, Lombardo JA (1990). Suprascapular nerve injuries with isolated paralysis of the infraspinatus. *Am J Sports Med* **18,** 225–8.
185. Kibler WB, Safran M (2005). Tennis injuries. *Med Sport Sci* **48,** 120–37.
186. van der HH, Kibler WB (2006). Shoulder injuries in tennis players. *Br J Sports Med* **40,** 435–40.
187. Nirschl R, Sobel J (1991) Tennis In: Reider B (ed.), *Sports medicine, the school-age athlete*, pp. 664–672. W.B. Saunders Company, Philadelphia.
188. Beillot J, Parier J. (1998). Tennis: Technological factors and epicondylitis. *Journal de Traumatologie du Sport* **15,** 69.
189. Gecha SR, Torg E (1988). Knee injuries in tennis. *Clin Sports Med* **7,** 435–52.
190. Miller WA (1977). Rupture of the musculotendinous juncture of the medial head of the gastrocnemius muscle. *Am J Sports Med* **5,** 191–3.
191. Silva RT, Takahashi R, Berra B, Cohen M, Matsumoto MH (2003). Medical assistance at the Brazilian juniors tennis circuit—a one-year prospective study. *J Sci Med Sport* **6,** 14–8.
192. Ellenbecker TS, Roetert EP, Piorkowski PA, Schulz DA (1996). Glenohumeral joint internal and external rotation range of motion in elite junior tennis players. *J Orthop Sports Phys Ther* **24,** 336–41.
193. Jorgensen U, Winge S (1987). Epidemiology of badminton injuries. *Int J Sports Med* **8,** 379–82.
194. Nigg BM, Segesser B (1988). The influence of playing surfaces on the load on the locomotor system and on football and tennis injuries. *Sports Med* **5,** 375–85.
195. Ellenbecker TS, Davies GJ, Rowinski MJ (1988). Concentric versus eccentric isokinetic strengthening of the rotator cuff. Objective data versus functional test. *Am J Sports Med* **16,** 64–9.
196. Kibler WB, Chandler TJ (2003). Range of motion in junior tennis players participating in an injury risk modification program. *J Sci Med Sport* **6,** 51–62.
197. Knudson DV (1991). Factors affecting force loading on the hand in the tennis forehand. *J Sports Med Phys Fitness* **31,** 527–31.
198. Knobloch K, Rossner D, Gossling T, Richter M, Krettek C (2004). Volleyball sport school injuries. *Sportverletz.Sportschaden* **18,** 185–9.
199. Belechri M, Petridou E, Kedikoglou S, Trichopoulos D (2001). Sports injuries among children in six European union countries. *Eur J Epidemiol* **17,** 1005–12.
200. Verhagen EA, van der Beek AJ, Bouter LM, Bahr RM, van Mechelen W (2004). A one season prospective cohort study of volleyball injuries. *Br J Sports Med* **38,** 477–81.
201. Ferrari GP, Turra S, Fama G, Gigante C (1990). Traumatic injury to the hand and wrist in volleyball, and its evolution. *J Sports Traumtol Rel Res* **12,** 95–9.
202. Aagaard H, Jorgensen U (1996). Injuries in elite volleyball. *Scand J Med Sci Sports* **6,** 228–32.
203. Schafle MD, Requa RK, Patton WL, Garrick JG (1990). Injuries in the 1987 national amateur volleyball tournament. *Am J Sports Med* **18,** 624–31.
204. Ferretti A (1986). Epidemiology of jumper's knee. *Sports Med* **3,** 289–95.
205. Distefano S (1989). Neuropathy due to entrapment of the long thoracic nerve. A case report. *Ital J Orthop Traumatol.* **15,** 259–62.
206. Mutoh Y, Mori T, Suzuki Y, Sugiura Y (1982). Stress fractures of the ulna in athletes. *Am J Sports Med* **10,** 365–7.
207. Ferretti A, Puddu G, Mariani PP, Neri M (1984). Jumpers knee: An epidemiological study of volleyball players. *Phys Sportsmed* **12,** 106.
208. Sommer HM (1988). Patellar chondropathy and apicitis, and muscle imbalances of the lower extremities in competitive sports. *Sports Med* **5,** 386–94.
209. Ferretti A, Papandrea P, Conteduca F, Mariani PP (1992). Knee ligament injuries in volleyball players. *Am J Sports Med* **20,** 203–7.
210. van Soest AJ, Roebroeck ME, Bobbert MF, Huijing PA, Ingen Schenau GJ (1985). A comparison of one-legged and two-legged countermovement jumps. *Med Sci Sports Exerc* **17,** 635–9.
211. Sturbois X. SR (1990). Biomechanics and instability of the shoulder in volleyball. *Hermes (Belgium)* **21,** 423–30.
212. Lindner K.J, Ferretti A. (1996). Volleyball In: Caine DJ, Caine CJ, Linder KJ (eds.), *Epidemiology of sports injuries*. Human Kinetics, Champaign, IL.
213. DeHaven KE, Lintner DM (1986). Athletic injuries: Comparison by age, sport, and gender. *Am J Sports Med* **14,** 218–24.
214. Backx FJ, Erich WB, Kemper AB, Verbeek AL (1989). Sports injuries in school-aged children. An epidemiologic study. *Am J Sports Med* **17,** 234–40.
215. Bobbert MF (1990). Drop jumping as a training method for jumping ability. *Sports Med* **9,** 7–22.
216. Ferretti A, PPCFMPP (1992). Knee ligament injuries in volleyball players. *Am J Sports Med* **20,** 203–7.
217. Giacomelli E, Grassi W, Zampa AM (1986). Athletes diseases affecting volleyball players. *Med dello Sport* **39,** 425–34.
218. Bahr R, Lian O, Bahr IA (1997). A twofold reduction in the incidence of acute ankle sprains in volleyball after the introduction of an injury prevention program: A prospective cohort study. *Scand J Med Sci Sports* **7,** 172–7.
219. Reeser JC, Verhagen E, Briner WW, Askeland TI, Bahr R (2006). Strategies for the prevention of volleyball related injuries. *Br J Sports Med* **40,** 594–600.
220. Brooks JH, Fuller CW (2006). The influence of methodological issues on the results and conclusions from epidemiological studies of sports injuries: Illustrative examples. *Sports Med* **36,** 459–72.
221. Mahler PB, Bizzini L, Marti M, Bouvier P (2006). The bill of rights for children in sport: A tool to promote the health and protect the child in sport. *Rev Med Suisse* **2,** 1774–7.

CHAPTER 46

Upper extremity and trunk injuries

Akin Cil, Lyle J. Micheli, and Mininder S. Kocher

Introduction

Injuries to the trunk and upper extremity in child and adolescent athletes are increasingly being seen with expanded participation and higher competitive levels of youth sports. Injury patterns are unique to the growing musculoskeletal system and specific to the demands of the involved sport. Recognition of injury patterns with early activity modification and the initiation of efficacious treatment can prevent deformity/disability and return the youth athlete to sport. This chapter reviews the diagnosis and management of common upper extremity and trunk injuries in the paediatric athlete.

Upper extremity injuries

Shoulder injuries

General

The shoulder complex involves four articulations and multiple ossification centres. The secondary centre of ossification of the proximal humeral epiphysis is usually seen after 6 months of age. Additional ossification centres appear at the greater tuberosity between 7 months and 3 years of age and at the lesser tuberosity 2 years later. By age between 5 and 7 years, these centres coalesce to form the proximal humeral epiphysis. The proximal humeral physis contributes approximately 80% of the longitudinal growth of the humerus and usually fuses between 19 and 22 years of age. The proximal humeral physis is extra-articular, except medially where the capsule extends beyond the anatomic neck, inserting on the medial metaphysis. The clavicle forms by intramembranous ossification in its central portion by the sixth gestational week. The medial secondary ossification centre appears between 12 and 19 years of age and does not fuse to the shaft until between 22 and 25 years of age. The lateral epiphysis is inconstant: appearing, ossifying, and fusing over a period of a few months about age 19 years. The scapula appears as a cartilaginous anlage in the first gestational week at the C4–C5 level and gradually descends to its adult-like position overlying the first to fifth ribs. Failure to descend results in persistent elevation of the scapula and limited glenohumeral motion, Sprengel's deformity. The scapula ossifies via intramembranous ossification with multiple remaining secondary ossification centres. The ossification centre of the coracoid process appears approximately at the age of 1 year, coalescing with the ossification centre of the upper glenoid by 10 years of age. The acromion ossifies by multiple[1–4] ossification centres which usually appear about puberty and fuse by 22 years of age. Failure of fusion of one of these ossification centers may result in an os acromionale. Various other scapular malformations may occur including bipartite coracoid, acromion duplication, glenoid dysplasia, and scapular clefts.

Injury patterns to the paediatric athlete's shoulder tend to be sport specific. In American gridiron football, the shoulder ranks second only to the knee in number of overall injuries.[1,2,5] Injury patterns in rugby football are similar. These injuries tend to result from macrotrauma and include glenohumeral dislocation, acromioclavicular separation, and clavicle fractures. Bicycling is a popular recreational and sporting activity among children and adolescents. About 60% of all bicycle injuries occur in children between the ages of 5 and 14 years and 85% of injuries involve the upper extremity.[4,5] A common injury pattern during bicycling involves lateral clavicle fracture or acromioclavicular separation from landing on the point of the shoulder when thrown from the bicycle. Shoulder injuries during alpine skiing and snowboarding are being seen with increased frequency and account for approximately 40% of upper extremity injuries and 10% of all injuries.[6] In wrestling, 30% of injuries occur in the upper extremity with the shoulder being the most commonly involved location.[7] Injury to the acromioclavicular joint is frequent, resulting from a direct blow of the shoulder against the mat.[7,8]

Overuse injuries to the shoulder, resulting from repetitive overhead use, are becoming more common in the paediatric age group. In baseball, injury to the paediatric shoulder from throwing is a result of microtrauma from repetitive motions of large rotational forces.[9–11] The proximal humeral physis is particularly vulnerable to these large, repetitive forces resulting in a chronic physeal stress fracture called Little League shoulder.[10–17] The shoulder in tennis is similarly subjected to repetitive overhead motions involving large torques; impingement and depression of the shoulder called tennis shoulder, may occur.[18] Repetitive microtrauma also frequently leads to shoulder dysfunction in swimmers.[19] The risk of injury is related to the level of competition and the type of event. Injuries include impingement syndrome and glenohumeral instability. Multidirectional instability is often seen and is related to the underlying ligamentous laxity often seen in swimmers. Similarly, multidirectional instability can be seen in gymnasts who also frequently demonstrate generalized ligamentous laxity. Additional shoulder injuries unique to gymnasts include cortical hypertrophy at the pectoralis major insertion, ringman's shoulder, and supraspinatus tendonitis.[20–22]

Sternoclavicular joint injury

True sternoclavicular joint dislocations are rare in the skeletally immature. The characteristic injury involves a physeal fracture of the medial clavicle, commonly a Salter–Harris I or II injury as the medial clavicular physis does not fuse until the early twenties.[23,24] The epiphysis stays attached to the sternum via the stout sternoclavicular ligaments and the medial clavicular shaft displaces posteriorly or anteriorly (Fig. 46.1). Medial clavicular injury often results from an indirect force transmitted along the clavicle from a direct blow during contact sports to the lateral shoulder. If the shoulder is driven forward, posterior displacement of the medial clavicle occurs. Conversely, if the shoulder is driven posteriorly, anterior displacement of the medial clavicle occurs. The patient often describes a pop in the region of the sternoclavicular joint and there is tenderness to palpation of the medial clavicle. The direction of displacement may be obscured by marked swelling. Posterior displacement can be a medical emergency as the medial clavicle can impinge on vital mediastinal structures including the innominate great vessels, trachea, or oesophagus.[25,26] Venous congestion, diminished pulses, dysphagia, or dyspnea should alert the clinician to the possibility of such injury. Standard anteroposterior radiographs of the chest or sternoclavicular joint are often hard to interpret given the overlapping spinal, thoracic, and mediastinal structures. A tangential X-ray taken in a 40° cephalad directed manner, the serendipity view, may aid in visualization of the medial clavicle displacement. Images of both sides should be obtained regularly for comparison purposes. Definitive delineation of the fracture pattern and direction of displacement is provided by computed tomography (CT scan).[27]

Minimally displaced fractures heal readily. Attempted reduction of anteriorly displaced fractures can be accomplished under local anaesthesia or sedation by placing the patient supine with a bolster between the scapulae. The arm is abducted 90° and then extended with gentle posterior pressure directly over the medial clavicle followed by protraction of the shoulder. After reduction, the shoulder is immobilized in a figure-of-eight dressing or shoulder immobilizer and a gentle range of motion exercises are started as pain allows. Most fractures heal in 4–6 weeks and return to sport requires full painless range of motion and strength. Unstable fractures usually heal and remodel rapidly. Posteriorly displaced medial clavicular fractures with impingement of mediastinal structures require emergent reduction with thoracic surgery standby for the rare but potential injury of the major thoracic vessels.[28] Under general anaesthesia with the patient supine, traction is applied to the arm with the shoulder extended, and a towel clip can be used to reduce the medial clavicle. Patients with acute posterior physeal injuries, which are seen within the first 10 days, should have an attempted closed reduction.[29] However, if a patient persists beyond that time and does not show any signs of compromise of the mediastinal structures, they can be treated non-operatively with close observation.[29] There is occasionally need for open reduction and internal fixation of irreducible medial clavicular physeal fractures. Care should be taken with internal fixation and pins should be removed as catastrophic complications of pin migration from hardware about the sternoclavicular joint have been reported.[30] Open reduction with stabilization of the torn periosteum and ligamentous structures with heavy non-absorbable suture should be attempted initially.

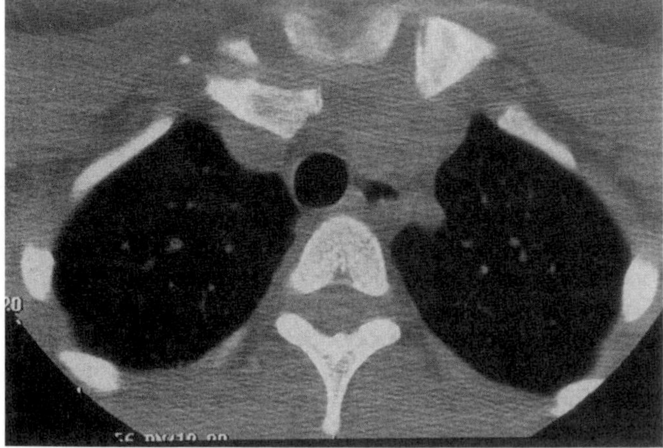

Fig. 46.1 Sternoclavicular joint injury. Axial CT scan demonstrating physeal fracture/separation of the medial clavicle with compression of the innominate vein in a 16-year-old female.

Clavicle fracture

In children, the clavicle is the most commonly fractured bone in the shoulder region, accounting for 10–15% of all children's fractures, with 90% occurring in the mid-shaft.[31,32] The clavicular shaft is vulnerable to injury from direct blows during contact sports. In addition, indirect forces on the outstretched arm may lead to clavicular fracture. The clavicular shaft is mechanically vulnerable as a strut given its S-shaped configuration and the strong ligamentous bindings at either end. With fracture, there is limited shoulder motion, tenderness over the fracture site, and the skin overlying the fracture may be tented and compromised. The proximal fragment may be elevated superiorly due to spasm of the sternocleidomastoid or trapezius muscles. Significant neurovascular injury is rare, but should be assessed clinically, given the proximity of the subclavian vessels and the brachial plexus. Plain radiographs are usually sufficient for diagnosis and management. Younger children may exhibit a greenstick fracture or plastic deformation.[33]

The prognosis of clavicular shaft fractures in children is excellent. Immobilization is accomplished by a figure-of-eight bandage or shoulder immobilizer. Slings which exert significant pressure to affect a reduction should be avoided. Even displaced fractures usually heal readily with a bump of healing callus which remodels over a period of 6–12 months. A study reported only 15 patients who had surgery for a clavicle fracture in a 21- year period.[34] Return to sport is allowed when the clavicle is non-tender; there is radiographic union and motion and strength are full. This usually occurs by 4–6 weeks in younger children and 6–10 weeks in the adolescent. Significant malunion which does not remodel and non-union of clavicular shaft fractures in the skeletally immature are rare, but they do occur.[31] Open reduction and internal fixation is indicated for open fractures, fractures with significant neurovascular compromise, threatened skin from fracture displacement, and floating shoulder injuries.[35,36]

Acromioclavicular joint injury

A fall on the point of the shoulder usually results in acromioclavicular separation in the adult and older adolescent, but often results in physeal fracture of the lateral clavicle in pre-pubescents.[37–42] With lateral clavicle fracture and true acromioclavicular separation in the paediatric patient, displacement of the proximal clavicle occurs superiorly through a tear in the thick periosteal tube surrounding the distal clavicle. The lateral clavicular epiphysis along with the acromioclavicular and coracoclavicular ligaments usually remain continuous with the periosteal tube. In the case of the paediatric athlete with lateral clavicle physeal fracture or acromioclavicular injury, the injury usually occurs after a fall or contact to the point of the shoulder. Pain and deformity are localized to the acromioclavicular joint. Plain radiographs are usually sufficient to evaluate the injury, or stress X-rays with 2.3–4.6 kg (5–10 pounds) of traction may also aid in delineating the degree of instability. An axillary lateral demonstrates anteroposterior displacement. Similar to adult acromioclavicular injuries, Rockwood[42] has classified paediatric acromioclavicular injuries based on the position of the lateral clavicle and the accompanying injury to the periosteal tube. Type I injuries involve mild sprain of the acromioclavicular ligaments without disruption of the periosteal tube. Type II injuries involve partial disruption of the dorsal periosteal tube with slight widening of the acromioclavicular joint. Type III injuries involve a large dorsal disruption of the periosteal tube with gross instability of the distal clavicle. Type IV injuries involve disruption of the periosteal tube with posterior displacement of the lateral clavicle (Fig. 46.2). Type V injuries involve periosteal tube disruption with >100% superior subcutaneous displacement of the lateral clavicle. Type VI injuries involve an inferior sub-coracoid dislocation of the lateral clavicle.

Non-operative management of acromioclavicular injuries in boys under 13 years of age is the mainstay of treatment as these injuries almost always represent a physeal fracture rather than a true acromioclavicular joint dislocation.[37–42] Thus, these injuries exhibit a great potential for healing and remodelling as the periosteal tube usually remains in continuity with the epiphyseal fragment and acromioclavicular and coracoclavicular ligaments. For type IV, V, and VI injuries with large displacement, operative stabilization may be indicated. Repair of the periosteal tube with or without internal fixation is usually performed. As with sternoclavicular injury, hardware should be removed 6 weeks after repair to avoid complications of pin migration. For late adolescent and adult-type true acromioclavicular joint separations, non-operative management results in good outcomes for type I and II injuries, while operative management is indicated for type IV, V, and VI injuries. The management of type III injuries in the athlete remains controversial, with many recommending initial non-operative management.[43–45]

Osteolysis of the distal clavicle

Osteolysis of the distal clavicle is an overuse injury resulting from repetitive microtrauma. It is seen most commonly in young adult weightlifters. It has also been described as a sequelae following traumatic injury to the distal clavicle or acromioclavicular joint. In addition, this entity is being identified in other sports as cross-training has become more popular among younger athletes who are weight training year-round for higher-level sports. Patients complain of an aching discomfort about the acromioclavicular joint after workouts, which progresses to interfere with training and eventually with activities of daily living. There is tenderness to palpation of the distal clavicle and pain with cross-chest adduction. Treatment consists of rest, particularly from weight training, and anti-inflammatory medications. For those who fail conservative treatment or who are unable to refrain from weight training, distal clavicle resection usually results in resolution of pain and return to sport.[46,47] This should be delayed to skeletal maturity, if possible, to lessen the risk of re-ossification.

(a)

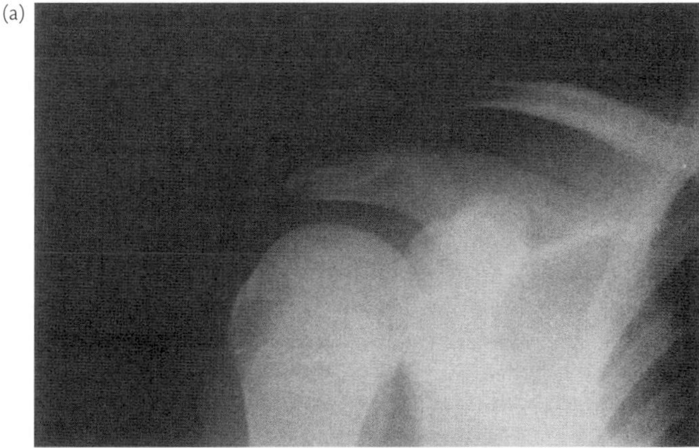

(b)

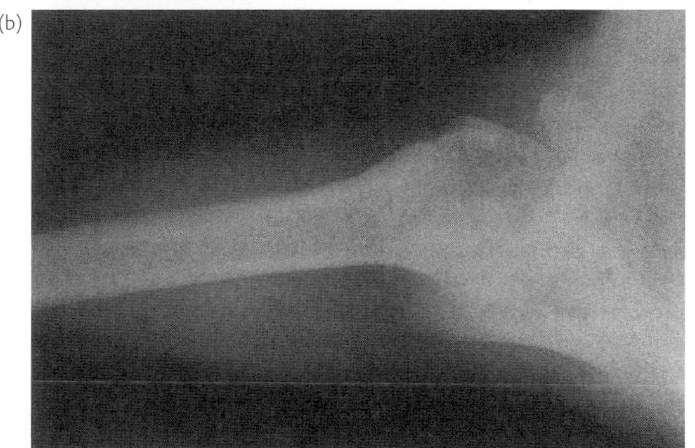

(c)

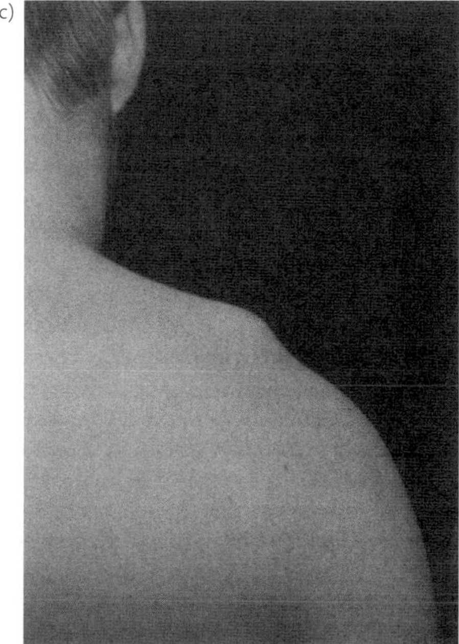

Fig. 46.2 Type IV acromioclavicular injury. (a) AP X-ray, (b) axillary lateral view demonstrating posterior displacement, and (c) photograph showing posterior prominence of lateral clavicle in a 16-year-old male.

Little League shoulder

As a result of repetitive microtrauma from the large rotational torques involved in throwing, chronic stress fracture of the proximal humeral physis can occur. This entity has been termed Little League shoulder and is most commonly seen in high-performance male pitchers between 11 and 13 years of age.[10–17,48] In addition to age and the large rotational forces of pitching, poor throwing mechanics may predispose to injury. In an extensive study of Little League pitchers, Albright[12] found that those who had poor pitching skills were more likely to be symptomatic. Patients complain of shoulder pain and there is typical widening of the proximal humeral physis on X-rays in addition to demineralization, sclerosis of the metaphysis, and fragmentation of the lateral aspect of the proximal humeral metaphysis. Often, comparative radiographs of the unaffected side are required to detect subtle physeal changes. Good results can usually be obtained by enforcing rest from pitching for the remainder of the season with a vigorous pre-season conditioning programme the subsequent year. Excessive volume of throwing is the most likely risk factor. Proper throwing mechanics should be stressed with an emphasis on control instead of speed and intensity. Despite the absence of firm evidence-based guidelines concerning throwing volume and pitch types, following guidelines from a recent study can serve as a baseline:[49] In order to minimize complaints of shoulder and elbow pain, pitchers between 9 and 14 years of age should not throw the curve ball or slider. These pitchers should use the fast ball and change-up exclusively. Baseball organizations may consider limiting pitchers in this age group to 75 pitches in a game and 600 pitches in a season. Alternatively, the number of batters faced during a game and season could be limited to 15 and 120, respectively. Furthermore, pitchers should not be allowed to circumvent pitch limits by participating in more than one league at a time. Full-effort pitching should be limited, and all organized throwing sessions should be monitored closely by a coach or parent. The recommended limits refer to full-effort, competitive game pitches and do not include warm-up pitches, practice pitches, throwing from other positions, and throwing drills, all of which are vital to a pitcher's development.[49]

Proximal humerus fracture

Approximately 20% of proximal humeral fractures in the skeletally immature occur in sporting events. The peak age is 10–14 years. Two-thirds involve the proximal humeral metaphysis and one-third involves the proximal humeral physis. Approximately one-fourth of fractures in this region occur through unicameral bone cysts.[50] Salter–Harris type I proximal humeral epiphyseal fractures occur primarily in neonates and children younger than 5 years. Metaphyseal fractures are seen mostly between 5 and 11 years of age. In older children, Salter–Harris type II fractures are predominant. With physeal fracture, the distal fragment usually displaces anteriorly and laterally through a relatively weaker area of periosteum, and the proximal fragment rotates into abduction and forward flexion due to its intact rotator cuff attachments; patients present with shoulder pain, limited motion, and tenderness to palpation. Routine roentgenograms are usually sufficient to demonstrate the fracture pattern, amount of displacement, or presence of a unicameral bone cyst.[50–56]

Non-displaced or minimally angulated metaphyseal or physeal fractures can usually be treated adequately with a shoulder immobilizer. Since most of these fractures are intrinsically stable, shoulder motion can be initiated early. There is great potential for remodelling of proximal humerus fractures since the physis is very active. Thus, many moderately displaced, angulated, or bayoneted fractures can be accepted in less-than anatomic alignment with satisfactory functional outcomes, particularly in younger children. However, in young athletes involved in overhead sports, anatomic reduction must be attained and maintained to prevent loss of abduction and external rotation. Reduction is usually achieved by bringing the distal shaft fragment into flexion, abduction, and external rotation to align it with the proximal fragment. If stable after reduction, the fracture can be immobilized next to the chest. If unstable, the reduction must be held immobilized by a shoulder spica cast or shoulder spica brace. These require experience in application and may be poorly tolerated by patients and parents. Percutaneous pinning of the anatomically reduced fracture may allow the arm to be put in a sling after reduction, but maintenance of reduction must be monitored closely with radiographs (Fig. 46.3). Open reduction is rarely indicated as a result of interposed periosteum, deltoid, capsule, or more frequently, the long head of the biceps and can result in poor outcomes.[50–56]

However, a recent study demonstrated that achieving and maintaining reduction in severely displaced proximal humeral epiphyseal fractures can be safely performed and results in excellent long-term shoulder function, especially in the older adolescent who has minimal remodelling potential.[57]

Glenohumeral instability

The glenohumeral joint is the most commonly dislocated large joint in adolescents and adults, but is less commonly involved in children before skeletal maturity. In large series of patients with glenohumeral instability, the proportion of skeletally immature patients ranges from 1%–5%.[58–63] Traumatic anterior dislocation is by far the most common type of instability seen in adolescent athletes; however, multidirectional instability, posterior subluxation, and recurrent subluxation are being recognized with increased frequency, particularly in gymnasts, swimmers, and throwers. The patient with a traumatic anterior dislocation presents with pain, limited motion, and deformity. The humeral head may be palpated anteriorly, or in the axilla, and the arm is typically held in a slightly abducted, externally rotated position. Careful examination, particularly of the axillary nerve, is essential to rule out neurovascular injury. With posterior dislocation, the coracoid process may be prominent anteriorly, and the arm is often held in internal rotation and adduction. Anteroposterior and lateral views of the glenohumeral joint demonstrate the dislocation and identify associated fractures or Hill–Sachs lesions. Posterior dislocations are frequently missed because of inadequate lateral images. Gentle reduction of an anterior dislocation is performed by one of several techniques including traction–counter traction, Stimson manoeuvre, or abduction manoeuvres. After a brief period of immobilization, a rehabilitation programme focused on rotator-cuff strengthening and avoiding the apprehension position is initiated.

Reported rates of recurrent instability after traumatic dislocation in adolescents and young adults vary between 25 and 90% in various series.[59,64–66] Rowe[61,62] reported 100% recurrence in children less than 10-years old and 94% recurrence in patients in the age group of 11 to 20 years. Rockwood[42] reported a recurrence rate of 50% in adolescent patients between 14 and 16 years of age and Marans and colleagues[60] reported a 100% recurrence rate in children between 4 and 15 years of age with open physes at the time of dislocation. Most

(a)

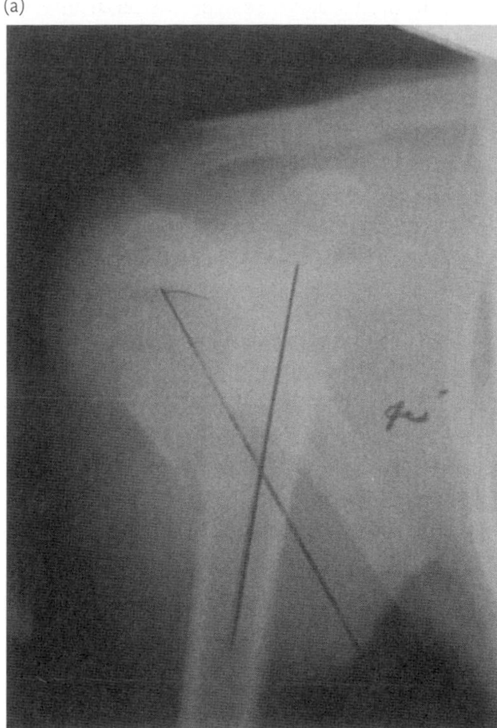

(b)

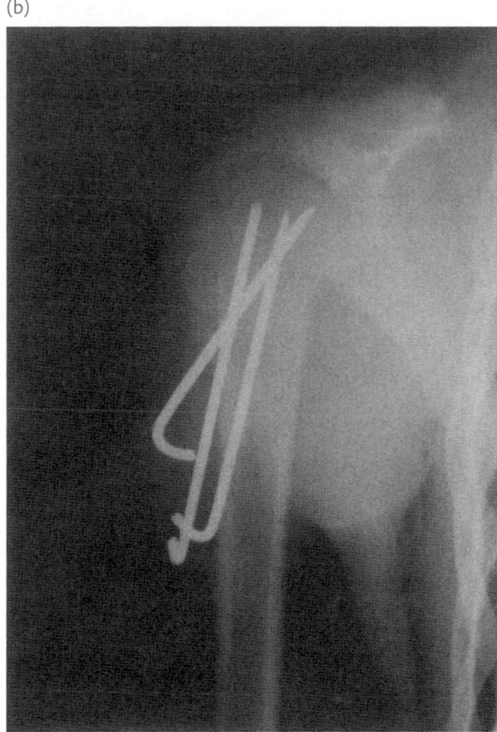

Fig. 46.3 Proximal humerus fracture. (a) Oblique view and (b) oblique view after reduction and percutaneous pinning in a 16-year-old male.

recently Deitch *et al.*[67] evaluated adolescent patients and found recurrent instability in 75% of patients which led to 50% of them requiring surgical stabilization. Management of the adolescent patient with significant recurrent instability is usually surgical involving capsulorraphy or a Bankart-type repair for capsulo-ligamentous disruption. Both arthroscopic and open techniques have been utilized with success rates of arthroscopic repair reaching the open repair in recent studies.[68]

Atraumatic instability can be seen in the paediatric athlete without a clear history of trauma and may occur with throwing, hitting, swimming, or overhead serving. There is usually a lack of pain with these episodes of subluxation with spontaneous reduction. Clinical examination often reveals signs of generalized ligamentous laxity including hyper-extensibility of the elbows, knees, and metacarpophalangeal joints.[69] Examination may also show signs of multidirectional instability, including the sulcus sign, and excessive translation with anterior and posterior drawer tests or the load and shift test. A vigorous rehabilitation programme stressing rotator-cuff strengthening is successful in most patients.[65] For patients who fail non-operative management, a capsular shift reconstruction is recommended.[70]

Rotator cuff injury

Much less common than in adults, rotator cuff tendonitis and sub-acromial impingement can occur in the paediatric overhead athlete. Repetitive microtrauma in high level overhead sports such as swimming, baseball, and tennis can lead to tendinitis, secondary muscle weakness, mechanical imbalance, and secondary instability. In the paediatric athlete with joint laxity, true extrinsic impingement with compromise of the sub-acromial space is uncommon. Rather, impingement secondary to muscle imbalance and anterior instability is seen.[17,71–74] The usual symptom is pain with overhead activities progressing to constant pain or night pain. Throwing athletes describe having pain on warm-up that does not improve. The pain tends to be worst at the top of the motion while the arm is in full external rotation or in deceleration after the ball is released. As the process continues, range of motion and strength may be diminished with loss of internal rotation, in particular. Hypermobility of the scapula with diminished periscapular strength is common. Impingement may be elicited with forward elevation or secondary to provocative instability tests. Magnetic resonance imaging (MRI) may be useful to assess the integrity of the rotator cuff; however, full-thickness tears in the paediatric or adolescent shoulder are uncommon. In competitive swimmers, a variant of impingement syndrome can be seen, which is called the swimmer's shoulder, involving anterior impingement associated with multidirectional instability and posterior subluxation.

Treatment of rotator cuff impingement consists of rest, non-steroidal anti-inflammatory medications, and a rehabilitation programme emphasizing restoration of range of motion, rotator-cuff strengthening, and scapular stabilization with the goal of restoring dynamic joint stability. For cases refractory to non-operative management, shoulder arthroscopy may be of benefit to rule out associated intra-articular pathology. Sub-acromial decompression is rarely indicated in the paediatric athlete.[17,71–74]

Elbow injuries

General

The elbow joint has three major articulations: humero-radial, humero-ulnar, and proximal radio-ulnar joints. Delineating injury patterns in children can be challenging given the cartilaginous composition of the distal humerus and the multiple ossification centres. A site-specific clinical examination and radiographs of the contralateral uninjured elbow can prove useful in identifying injury. There are six major secondary centres of ossification, which appear and unite with the epiphysis at characteristic ages (Table 46.1). Except for the medial and lateral epicondyles, the remaining ossification centres are intra-articular. The clinical carrying angle of the elbow averages 7° valgus alignment. There are several radiographic lines which are useful in assessing post-injury alignment. Bauman's angle, the angle between the capitellar physeal line and a line perpendicular to the humeral shaft, is a guide to the varus attitude of the distal humerus and should be within 5°–8° of the contralateral elbow. On the lateral X-ray, the capitellum forms an angle flexed forward 30°–40° from the humeral shaft, with the anterior humeral line bisecting the capitellum. Elbow stability is provided by congruous articular surfaces and soft-tissue constraint via capsular and ligamentous structures.

Elbow injury patterns in the paediatric athlete are dependent on the age-related stage of elbow development and the sport-specific mechanism of injury. Acute macro-traumatic injuries often result in fractures about the elbow. In younger children, supracondylar and lateral condyle fractures predominate. In adolescence and near-skeletal maturity, epicondylar and olecranon fractures are more common. In addition, elbow dislocations, ligamentous injuries, and muscular avulsions about the elbow can occur.

Repetitive microtraumatic injuries are often sport specific involving upper extremity overuse. Repetitive throwing places high demands on the vulnerable developing elbow. Tension overload of the medial-elbow restraints occurs during late cocking and can lead to medial epicondyle fragmentation, ulnar collateral ligament strain, flexor muscle strains, and traction-ulnar neuritis. Compression overload of the lateral articulation also occurs during late cocking and can lead to chondral injuries and growth disturbances of the capitellum or radial head. Posteromedial shear overload of the posterior articular surface occurs during follow-through and can lead to posterior spurs, olecranon apophysistis or avulsion, and spurs of the coronoid process.[75] In gymnastics, the elbow becomes a weight-bearing joint often subjected to repetitive large loads. Medial epicondyle traction injuries, partial tears of the flexor-origin mass, ulnar collateral ligament strains, subluxation/dislocation often with medial epicondyle avulsion, osteochondral fractures of the capitellum, and posterior elbow spurring have been described.[2,22,76] Osteochondritis dissecans of the capitellum occurs with presentation similar to throwing injuries.

Supracondylar fracture

Supracondylar humerus fractures are the most common elbow fracture in children, accounting for approximately 75% of injuries.

Table 46.1 Timing of secondary centres of ossification about the elbow

Site	Appearance	Epiphyseal Coalescence
Capitellum	18 months	14 years
Radial head	4 years	16 years
Medial epicondyle	5 years	15 years
Trochlea	8 years	14 years
Olecranon	10 years	14 years
Lateral epicondyle	12 years	16 years

The mechanism of injury is usually an acute hyperextension load on the elbow from falling on an outstretched arm. The injury typically occurs in children aged 5–10 years because of thin bony architecture in the supracondylar region and ligamentous laxity. The distal fragment displaces posteriorly in over 95% of cases and the fracture is classified according to displacement: minimally displaced (type I), posterior angulation hinged on an intact posterior cortex (type II), and completely displaced (type III) (Fig. 46.4). With complete displacement, rotational malalignment often occurs and can lead to cubitus-varus deformity if unreduced. Injury to the anterior interosseous nerve, radial nerve, median nerve, and brachial artery has been reported in 10–18% of displaced fractures.[77,78]

Type I fractures are treated in a long-arm cast for 3 weeks with the elbow flexed 90° to 100°. Type II fractures can be treated with closed reduction and casting alone; however, the elbow should be flexed beyond 90° to maintain reduction, and this position may not be tolerated secondary to vascular insufficiency and swelling. Thus, closed reduction and percutaneous pinning with two lateral pins is often the treatment of choice. Closed reduction and percutaneous pinning is the preferred method of treatment for type III fractures, obviating the problems of ischaemic contracture (compartment syndrome) and cubitus varus deformity seen with closed treatment. Reduction is accomplished by extension of the elbow, followed by correction of medial–lateral translation, followed by traction and flexion of the elbow with anterior force on the olecranon. For fractures with medial displacement, the forearm

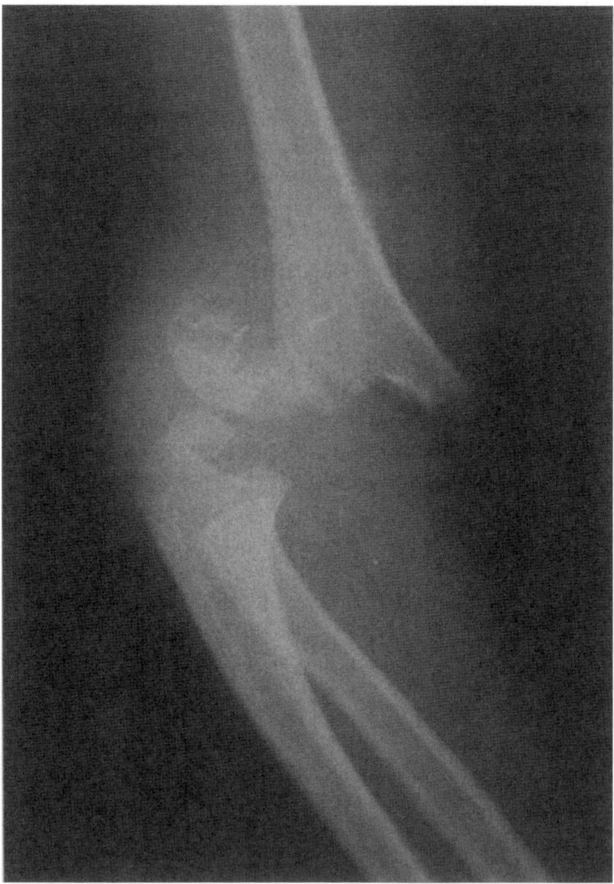

Fig. 46.4 Supracondylar humerus fracture. Oblique view of type III displaced fracture in a 6-year-old child.

is pronated which tightens the reduction against the intact medial periosteum while closing the lateral column. Systematic review of the literature suggests that the most stable pin configuration involves medial and lateral pins crossing above the fracture line.[79] However, a recent randomized clinical trial proved that both lateral-entry pin fixation and medial- and lateral-entry pin fixation are effective in the treatment of completely displaced (type III) extension supracondylar fractures of the humerus in children, without any neurological complications.[80] Motion is begun after the pins are removed at 3–4 weeks.[77,78] In cases with excessive comminution or other associated extremity injuries, skeletal traction with an olecranon pin may be beneficial.

Lateral condyle fracture

Lateral condyle fractures are the second most common elbow fractures in children and occur typically between 6 and 10 years of age. The mechanism of injury is often a valgus compressive force from the radial head or a varus tensile force on a supinated forearm from the extensor longus, brevis muscles, and collateral ligament. There is a slight increase of risk of this fracture in children with a pre-existing cubitus varus.[81] A significant portion of the fragment is unossified, leaving often only a thin lateral metaphyseal rim of bone to herald the injury. This fracture involves both the physis and the articular surface, making anatomic reduction essential. Lateral condyle fractures are classified by the Milch system as either type I or type II, depending on where the fracture line exits at the articular surface. Milch I fractures occur at the capitellotrochlear groove and correspond to classic Salter–Harris type IV fractures. These fractures also tend to leave the elbow joint more stable. Milch II fractures extend into the apex of trochlea and although resembles Salter–Harris type II, it is still an articular fracture, and hence, a Salter–Harris type IV. Displacement and rotation are common due to the lateral extensor muscle mass. Treatment depends on the degree of displacement and fragment stability. Minimally displaced fractures, <3 mm, which are demonstrated to be stable by clinical examination are treated with cast immobilization for approximately 3–4 weeks. Follow-up X-rays (particularly the oblique view) are essential 1 week after injury to rule out further displacement. Any fracture with associated elbow instability should be anatomically reduced and fixed. Fractures with initial displacement of 3–4 mm are at risk of late displacement and non-union; thus, many recommend percutaneous pinning to stabilize these fractures. Fractures with over 4 mm of displacement are often also rotated, necessitating open reduction and internal fixation to restore articular continuity. Complications of lateral condyle fractures include nonunion, progressive valgus deformity, and tardy ulnar neuritis.[78]

Radial head/neck fracture

Proximal radius injuries in the skeletally immature athlete are either physeal fractures of the radial head or fractures of the radial neck. They occur most commonly in children over the age of 9 years as the result of valgus stress with longitudinal force on an outstretched arm. Treatment depends on the degree of angulation, amount of displacement, age of child, and associated fractures (Fig. 46.5). Children less than 10-years old can tolerate up to 40°–45° of angulation of the radial neck due to expected remodelling if articular step-off is not more than 1 mm. In older children, less angulation (15°–20°) is acceptable because of less remodelling potential. For fractures with acceptable angulation, cast immobilization with early motion in 10–14 days is recommended. Closed reduction can be performed by direct pressure over the radial head with a varus stress and rotation. Alternatively, a percutaneous pin can be used to manipulate the proximal fragment. Indications for open reduction include complete displacement of the radial head, irreducible angulation over 45°, or a displaced Salter–Harris type IV fracture. Radial head fractures with significant displacement should be anatomically reduced and fixed. Radial head excision is contraindicated as proximal radial migration, radial deviation of the hand, and valgus deviation of the elbow can occur.[78,82,83] Complications of this fracture include limitations of motion and radio-ulnar synostosis.

Medial epicondyle fracture

The medial epicondyle can be avulsed from a valgus load applied to the extended elbow (Fig. 46.6). The flexor origin and the ulnar collateral ligament play a role in fracture displacement. These fractures occur typically in children 10–14 years old. Almost 50% of these injuries are thought to occur concomitantly with elbow dislocation (Fig. 46.7). For the general paediatric population, many advocate closed treatment of this injury, particularly when there is less than 5 mm of displacement. Some literature suggest they all do well without immediate or delayed sequela, regardless of the amount of displacement.[84] Although non-union may occur, it is often asymptomatic or can be treated with fragment excision when

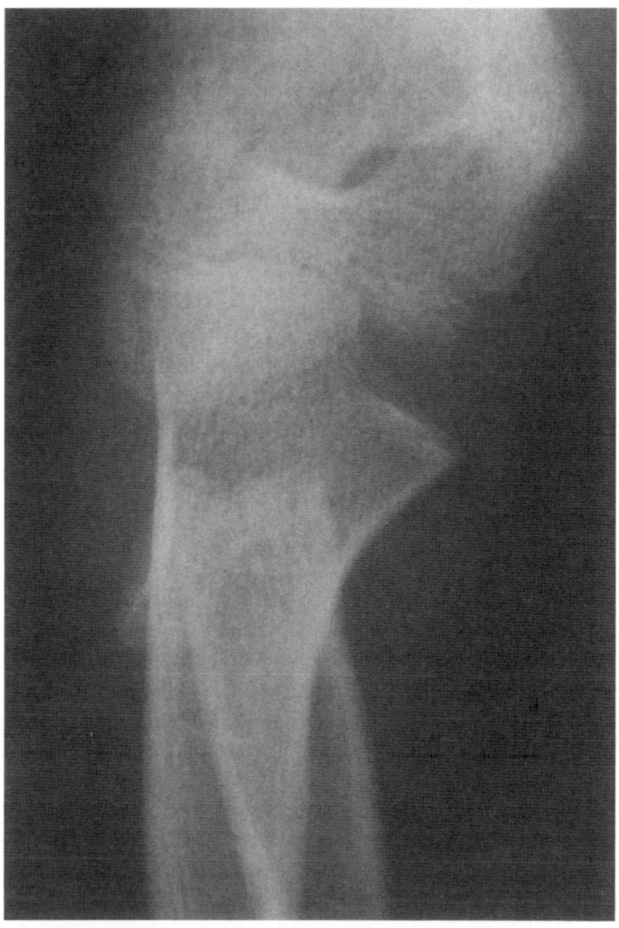

Fig. 46.5 Radial head fracture. AP view demonstrating angulation and displacement of proximal radial physeal fracture in a 12-year-old boy.

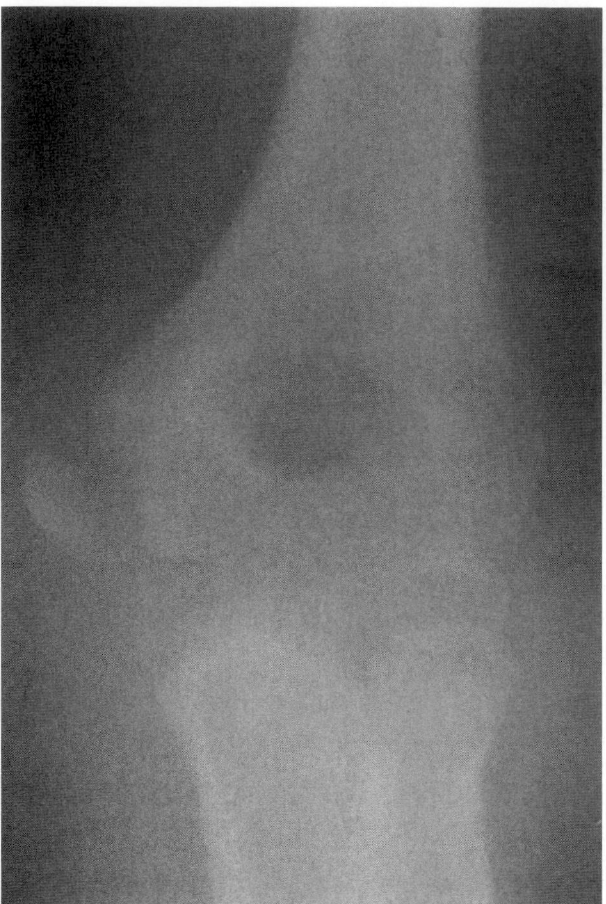

Fig. 46.6 Medial epicondyle avulsion. AP view of a displaced medial epicondyle avulsion fracture in a 14-year-old male pitcher.

symptomatic. Relative indications for open reduction and fixation include competitive athletes with >2 mm displacement or valgus instability to restore the integrity of the medial collateral ligament and retension the forearm flexors. An absolute indication for open reduction and internal fixation is medial epicondylar entrapment within the joint associated with elbow dislocation (Fig. 46.7). A common complication of medial epicondyle fracture is joint stiffness. Internal fixation allows for early post-operative range of motion at 2–3 weeks.[78,85–87]

Elbow dislocation

Elbow dislocation is relatively uncommon in the child athlete as the peak incidence is in the second decade. However, elbow dislocation may be encountered in the adolescent athlete in contact sports such as football or wrestling, or in non-contact sports such as gymnastics. The most common pattern of injury is posterolateral displacement without disruption of the proximal radio-ulnar joint. The injury may also involve disruption of the anterior capsule, tearing of the brachialis muscle, avulsion of the medial epicondyle, injury to the ulnar collateral ligament, brachial artery compromise, or nerve injury to the median or ulnar nerves. Clinical presentation is that of a grossly swollen and deformed elbow with pain on attempt at movement. Median or ulnar nerve injuries occur in up to 10% of dislocations, and a thorough neurovascular exam is crucial prior to an attempt at reduction. Prompt and gentle reduction is performed under sedation. Non-concentric reduction should alert the clinician to the possibility of interposed soft tissue or medial epicondyle (Fig. 46.7). For simple elbow dislocations, a posterior splint is used for the acute phase of pain and swelling for 10–14 days, followed by assisted range of motion and physical therapy.[78,88] Immobilization beyond 3 weeks is contraindicated due to stiffness.

Little League elbow

The term Little League elbow describes a group of pathologic entities about the elbow joint in young throwers. Originally, these findings were noted in baseball pitchers; however, the throwing motion is common to the non-pitcher's throw, the tennis serve, the javelin throw, the cricket bowl, and the football pass. The entity includes medial epicondyle fragmentation and avulsion (Fig. 46.6), growth alteration of the medial epicondyle, Panner disease or osteochondritis of the capitellum, deformation or osteochondritis of the radial head, hypertrophy of the ulna, and olecranon apophysistis. Osteochondritis of the capitellum may also be seen in high-performance female gymnasts.[89] Most cases of Little League elbow present with medial elbow complaints: medial pain and decreased throwing effectiveness/distance. Medial tension overload results from repetitive valgus stress and flexor forearm pull. Changes are age dependent. During childhood, irregular appearance of the secondary centres of ossification of the medial epicondyle may be seen. In adolescence with increasing muscle strength, avulsion fracture of the medial epicondyle may occur. After fusion of the medial epicondyle in young adulthood, injuries of the ulnar collateral ligament and flexor muscle origin become more apparent. Laterally, repetitive valgus compression may lead to damage of the radio-capitellar articulation. Panner disease is a benign form of osteochondritis dissecans of the capitellum in younger children. It is thought to be in the spectrum between normal ossification and a true osteochondritis dissecans. Osteochondritis dissecans can affect both the capitellum and the radial head. Changes include chondromalacia with softening and fissuring of the articular surface, subchondral collapse, and bony eburnation. Osteochondritis dissecans of the capitellum can present with wide variations in radiographic appearance depending on the extent of osteonecrosis and the presence of loose bodies. Availability of MRI has given opportunity for early diagnosis, prior to radiographic changes. Pain, tenderness, and contracture dominate the clinical presentation. Additional lateral injuries seen during throwing in the skeletally immature athlete include lateral apophysis avulsion from traction during follow-through and radial physeal injury from repetitive valgus overload. Posterior elbow pain in throwers is frequently due to the powerful contraction of the triceps in the early acceleration phase, coupled with the impaction of the olecranon into its humeral fossa in the late follow-through phase. Olecranon apophysistis, avulsion fracture (Fig. 46.8), posteromedial osteophytes, and loose bodies may form.[10,12,16,17,75,90–95]

Treatment of Little League elbow is directed at removing the recurrent microtrauma. Cessation of all throwing until the elbow is asymptomatic followed by reassessing throwing mechanics and number of pitches thrown is essential. More than 300 skilled throws per week may predispose to injury. Range of motion exercises and dynamic splinting may be useful for contractures. Triceps strengthening with stretching of the anterior capsule is helpful for avoidance of contracture. Arthroscopy or open surgery is useful for assessing chondral injury, removal of loose bodies, and management of osteochondritis dissecans through drilling or fragment fixation in unstable lesions.[96] Open reduction of displaced medial epicondyle fractures is indicated

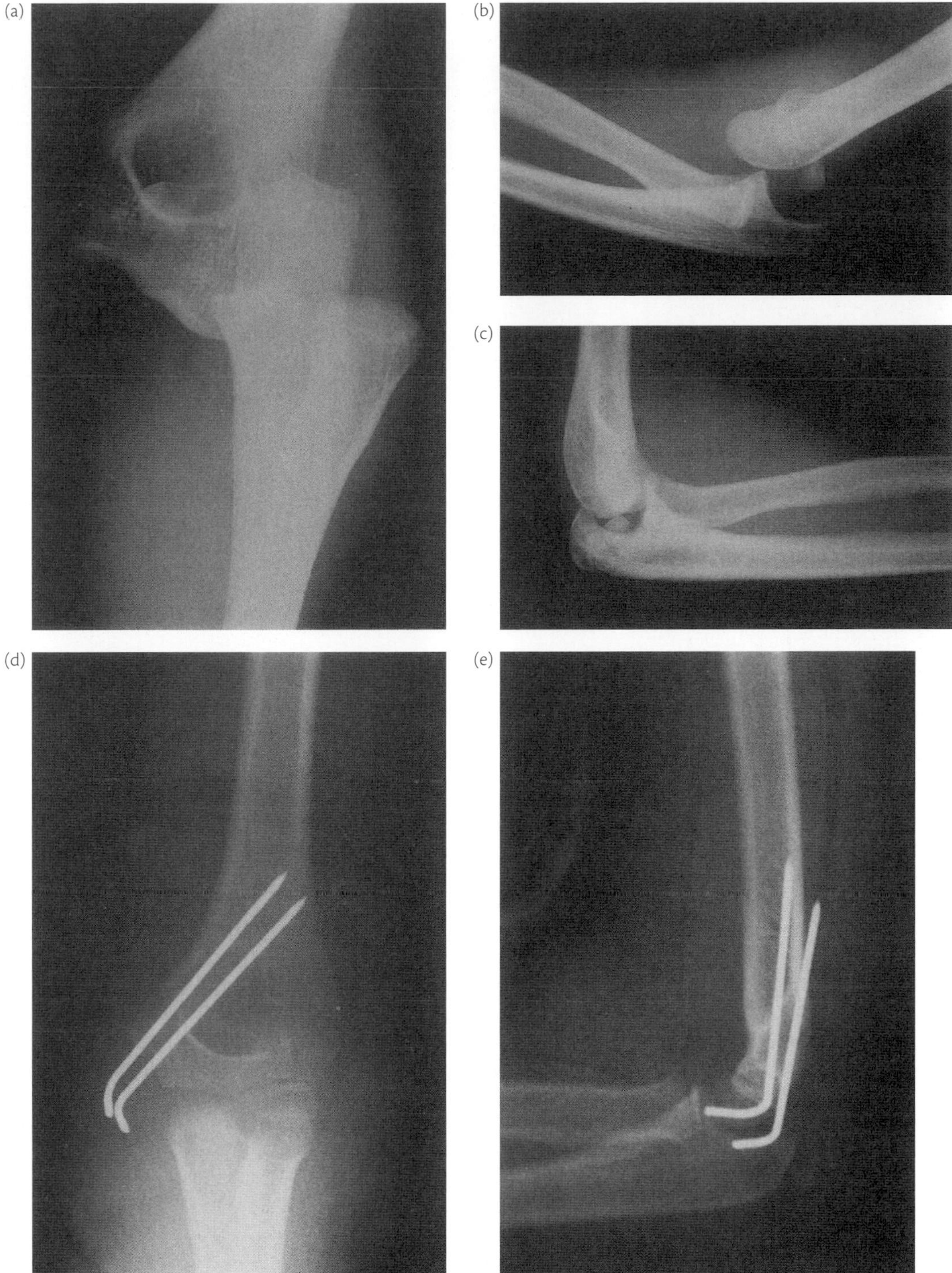

Fig. 46.7 Elbow dislocation with medial epicondyle avulsion. (a) AP and lateral (b) views demonstrating elbow dislocation with medial epicondyle avulsion in a 13-year-old female gymnast, and (c) entrapped medial epicondyle fragment, (d) AP and lateral, and (e) views after open reduction and internal fixation.

in the throwing athlete. Results of treatment of Little League elbow are generally favourable when instituted early.[10,12,16,17,75,90–95]

Wrist and hand injuries

General

In most sports, the hand and wrist are exposed, and thus are vulnerable to injury. Injury patterns are sport specific, with macrotraumatic injury or repetitive microtraumatic injury depending upon the demands placed on the upper extremity. Injuries are also age specific, related to the stage of skeletal development. In several large series of paediatric and adolescent athletic injuries, hand and wrist injury rates vary from 15 to 65% of all injuries in paediatric and adolescent athletes depending on the sport involved.[97–99] Injuries to the hand are particularly common during basketball, American football, boxing, 16-inch (41-cm) softball, skateboarding, and alpine skiing. Repetitive stress injuries, particularly of the

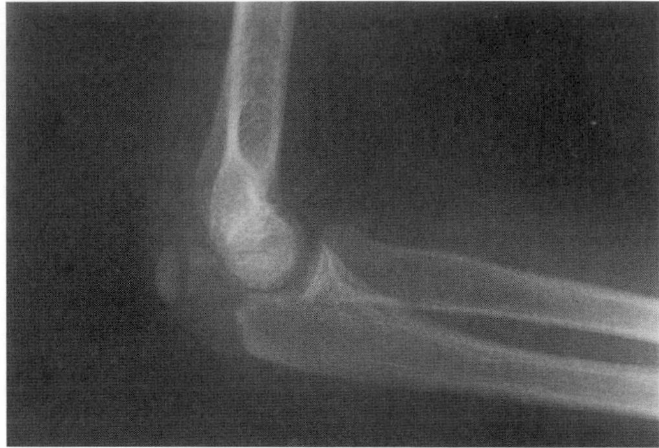

Fig. 46.8 Olecranon avulsion. Lateral view demonstrating olecranon apophysis avulsion in a 12-year-old male pitcher.

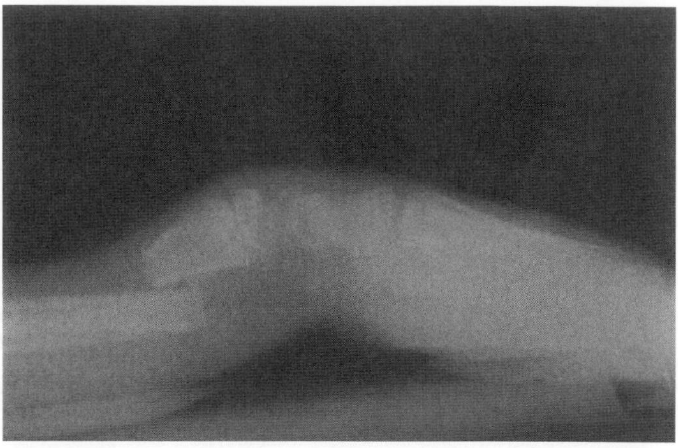

Fig. 46.9 Distal radius fracture. Lateral view in a 6-year-old boy.

wrist, are common in gymnasts. Injuries are relatively infrequent during swimming and soccer.[100–102]

Distal radius fractures

Distal radial metaphyseal fracture is the most common fracture of childhood.[103] If treated properly, these fractures usually heal without residual disability. Initial management consists of splinting and careful neurovascular evaluation of the hand. X-rays are usually sufficient to define the fracture and its angulation/displacement (Fig. 46.9). This fracture may occur in association with distal radio-ulnar joint disruption or elbow injury. Torus and greenstick fractures are often fairly stable and may be treated in a short-arm cast in older children and a long-arm cast in children under 5 years of age. The completely displaced distal radial metaphyseal fracture often requires intravenous sedation or general anaesthesia for reduction followed by long-arm casting with an appropriate mould. In the young child less than 8 years of age, bayonet apposition may be accepted. In the rare irreducible fracture, an open reduction may be necessary through a volar approach which allows for release of the carpal canal. The position of immobilization of this fracture is controversial, with advocates of pronation, neutral, and supination positioning. Approximately 10–30% of distal third radius fractures reangulate to an unacceptable position (>20°) requiring repeat closed manipulation. For the healing fracture, acceptable limits of angulation are wider. In a child aged under 8 years, up to 30° may be acceptable due to remodelling potential with an estimated correction of 1°/month.[104] In the child aged above 12 years, these fractures become increasingly unstable with less remodelling potential leading to treatment resembling that of an adult.

Galeazzi fractures are fractures of the distal radius with disruption of the radio-ulnar joint. Children may have separation of the ulnar physis instead of true disruption of the radio-ulnar joint.[105] They can be managed with closed reduction in younger children. Older children, like adults, require an open reduction.[106]

Physeal fractures of the distal radius occur most commonly in the adolescent. Salter–Harris type I and type II fracture patterns predominate. The distal fragment is usually dorsally displaced with an intact dorsal periosteum. This fracture may be associated with acute carpal tunnel syndrome or compartment syndrome. Reduction should be as atraumatic as possible to avoid further injury to the physis. The fracture should be immobilized in the position of stability as determined during reduction. Intraepiphyseal fracture extension, such as in Salter–Harris type III or IV injuries is uncommon, but should be treated with anatomical reduction of the articular surface and intraepiphyseal or transphyseal fixation.

Wrist injuries

Wrist pain has become extremely common in young, highly competitive gymnasts related to chronic, repetitive upper extremity weight bearing during growth and development. Chronic repetitive stress injury to the distal radial and ulnar physes was described by Roy and colleagues in young, highly competitive gymnasts who practised approximately 36 h·week^{-1}.[107] The presenting symptoms were stiffness and dorsiflexion pain. Radiographs showed widened physes, cystic changes, and distal metaphyseal beaking. Nearly all patients returned to competitive gymnastics without growth arrest after treatment with rest, and with or without casting. Subsequently, others have reported acquiring Madelung's deformity and increased ulnar variance in young, competitive gymnasts.[108,109] A spectrum of pathologic entities may be found on clinical examination, X-rays, MRI, and arthroscopy including stress changes of the distal radial-ulnar physes, articular cartilage changes of the wrist–carpal joints, distal radio-ulnar joint injury, triangular fibrocartilage complex (TFCC) tears, and ganglion cysts. Management is primarily non-operative with rest, immobilization, if necessary, and activity modification.

Distal radio-ulnar joint injuries in the child and adolescent athlete are rare. Acute dislocations present with pain and deformity of the joint. Acute dislocations are treated with long-arm cast immobilization with the wrist in supination for dorsal dislocations and pronation for volar dislocations. Triangular fibrocartilage injuries are increasingly being recognized in patients with repetitive wrist loading, particularly gymnasts. Patients typically present with ulnar wrist pain and injury may be demonstrated on MRI arthrogram or arthroscopy. For patients who fail non-operative management, patients with neutral or negative ulnar variance can be treated by arthroscopic debridement and patients with positive ulnar variance can be treated by ulnar shortening and/or debridement. In a child or adolescent with significant growth remaining, bony procedures should be delayed until growth ceases.[110]

The scaphoid fracture is the most common carpal fracture in children with a peak incidence between 12 and 15 years of age.

In the skeletally immature, the majority of fractures are minimally displaced. The blood supply to scaphoid enters at the distal pole, and the ossification follows the pattern of blood supply. Because of the early ossification and stout soft tissue attachments that protect its proximal pole, fractures of the scaphoid in children are often distal pole.[111] However, with increased athletic participation at increasingly intense competitive levels by children and adolescents, more adult-type displaced waist fractures are being seen. Patients present with wrist pain, limited motion, and tenderness in the anatomic snuff box. Management of minimally displaced fractures involves a short-arm thumb spica cast for 6 weeks for distal pole fractures and a long-arm thumb spica cast for 4 weeks for waist fractures, followed by short-arm casting until union occurs. Occult fractures can be diagnosed with bone scanning. Acute displaced fractures should be treated with open reduction and internal fixation. Scaphoid non-union usually requires bone grafting with or without fixation (Fig. 46.10).[112–114] Scaphoid malunion or non-union can lead to degenerative changes of the wrist in the long term. Stress fracture of the scaphoid waist can be seen particularly in competitive gymnasts.[115,116] Initial X-rays are often negative, with follow-up X-rays revealing a stress fracture.

Ligamentous injuries of the wrist are unusual in children but are being seen with increased frequency in the adolescent athlete engaged in high-level sports. The volar intercarpal ligaments, particularly the radioscapholunate and radioscaphocapitate ligaments, are important stabilizers of the wrist. Patients present with wrist pain and limited motion. X-rays may reveal widening of the scapholunate interval or alteration of the scapholunate angle (normal 30°–60°). Dorsal intercalated segment instability (DISI) can result from scaphoid fracture or scapholunate dissociation, resulting in an increased scapholunate angle. Volar intercalated segment instability (VISI) can result from disruption of the radiocarpal ligaments on the ulnar side of the wrist, resulting in a decreased scapholunate angle. Wrist arthrography, MRI, and arthroscopy can be used to further delineate the extent of ligamentous injury. Partial injuries are treated with immobilization. Acute complete ligamentous injuries are treated with ligament repair and K-wire fixation. Chronic carpal instability is usually treated with limited carpal fusions or proximal row carpectomy, often with unpredictable results.

Hand injuries

The thumb metacarpal-phalangeal joint is commonly injured, particularly during skiing. These injuries result from excessive radial deviation during a fall on the outstretched hand with the thumb in abduction. In adults and older adolescents, injury to the ulnar collateral ligament of the thumb metacarpal-phalangeal joint occurs ('gamekeeper's or skier's thumb'). In children and adolescents, physeal fracture at the base of the proximal phalanx is more common. The ulnar collateral ligament inserts onto the proximal phalangeal epiphysis, thus predisposing to a Salter–Harris type III fracture, which may involve a large portion of the articular surface (Fig. 46.11). Non-displaced fractures and partial ulnar collateral ligament injuries are treated with 4–6 weeks of immobilization in a short-arm thumb spica cast. Displaced fractures are treated with open reduction and internal fixation. Complete ligamentous injuries (>35°–40° opening in flexion without a firm end point) and Stener's lesions (interposition of the adductor aponeurosis) are treated with ligament repair.[117–121]

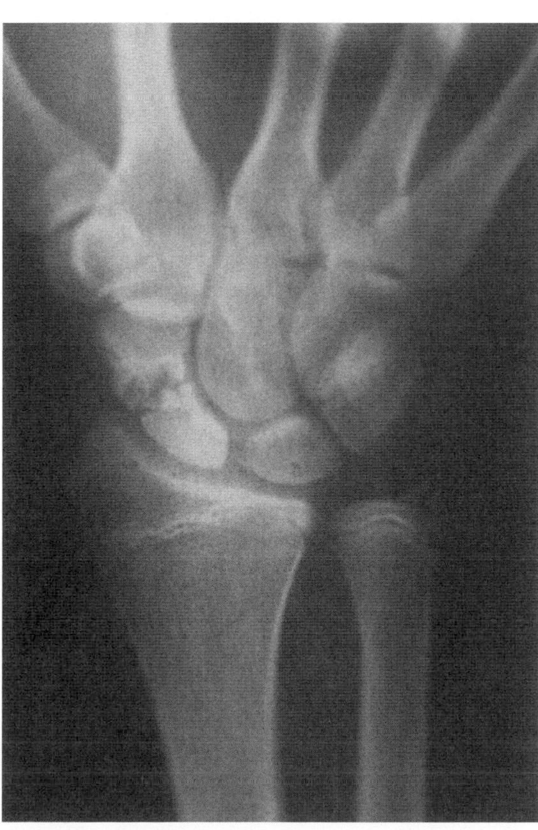

Fig. 46.10 Scaphoid nonunion.

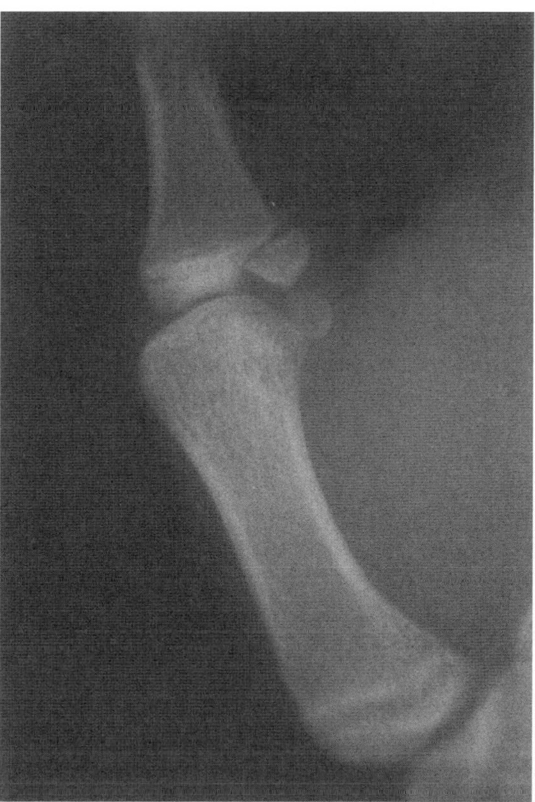

Fig. 46.11 Gamekeeper's thumb. Salter–Harris type III injury in a 10-year-old male.

The 'jammed finger' is the most common joint injury in the paediatric and adolescent athlete's hand. Axial compressive forces applied to the end of the finger can result in proximal interphalangeal joint (PIP) hyperextension with subluxation or dislocation of the joint. This injury is common in ball-catching sports such as basketball or American football. Reduction of the dislocated joint is accomplished by linear traction. Volar plate injury/avulsion or volar Salter–Harris type III fracture may be associated, but rarely requires fixation. Treatment involves a very brief period of immobilization (dorsal alumifoam splint) followed by edema control (elastoplast wrapping) and motion (buddy-taping to adjacent digit) to avoid stiffness and a fixed flexion deformity. Most athletes can return to sports (with buddy-taping) in 1–2 weeks; however, some pain and swelling may persist for months. Axial loading of the finger may also result in boutonniere deformity (PIP flexion, DIP extension) secondary to rupture of the central slip or a dorsally displaced Salter–Harris type III fracture at the base of the middle phalanx. Acute injuries should be splinted in full extension for 4–5 weeks. Chronic reconstruction results in less reliable outcomes.[117–121]

Mallet finger is the most common injury occurring at the DIP joint, resulting from hyperflexion injury producing either extensor tendon (terminal tendon) rupture or Salter–Harris type III avulsion of the distal phalangeal epiphysis (Fig. 46.12). The patient is unable to actively extend the DIP joint; however, there is full passive motion. Unless there is significant displacement of a substantial epiphyseal fragment, the DIP should be splinted with a dorsal splint in full extension for approximately 6 weeks. Terminal tendon repair may be necessary if an extensor lag persists after 10 weeks; however, this is unusual.[117–121] Hyperextension of the DIP joint may result in a dorsal DIP dislocation or avulsion of the flexor digitorum profundus (FDP). FDP avulsion most commonly involves the ring finger and occurs during American football or rugby as the finger catches on the opposing player's shirt ('jersey finger'). If identified early, the injury can be successfully treated. Missed diagnosis occurs when the patient does not recognize a significant injury or the care provider believes that the inability to flex the DIP joint is secondary to pain and swelling. Direct repair to the distal phalanx is accomplished if possible. With late diagnosis, direct repair is usually not possible as the tendon retracts and fibrosis occurs. In these cases, tendon grafts may be necessary.[122]

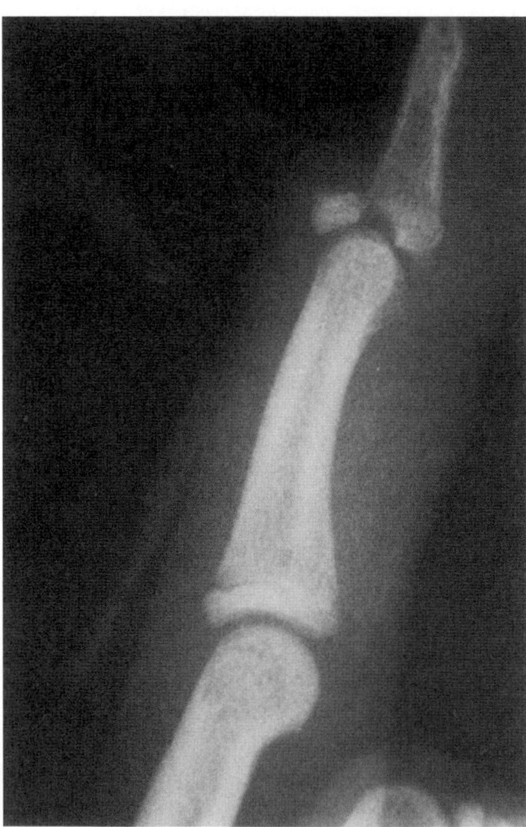

Fig. 46.12 Mallet fracture.

Hand fractures are common athletic injuries in children. Fractures involving the physis are frequent, accounting for approximately 40% of hand fractures in the skeletally immature.[101] Ossific nuclei appear in the metacarpals and phalanges by 3 years of age and fuse between 14 and 17 years of age. Remodelling potential exists for fractures near the epiphysis in the plane of motion; however, there is minimal remodelling of rotational deformity. The vast majority of hand fractures in children can be managed non-operatively with splinting of non-displaced fractures and closed reduction of angulated or displaced fractures. Fingertip crush injuries occur in tackling and collision sports. These injuries often involve a nailbed laceration and tuft fracture requiring splinting and nailbed repair. Phalangeal neck fractures typically occur between 5–10 years of age and involve the proximal phalanx. These fractures may redisplace after reduction and may have substantial rotation not appreciated on X-ray, therefore, requiring careful clinical examination. Metacarpal fractures in children are less common than adults. Little finger metacarpal neck fractures (boxer's fracture) can usually be managed by closed reduction and cast immobilization for 3 weeks. Thumb metacarpal fractures often involve a Salter–Harris type II fracture through the base of the metacarpal.[117–121]

Trunk injuries

General

Back pain and injuries to the thoracolumbar spine are not infrequent in the school-age athlete. Spine-related complaints constitute almost 10% of athletes' medical problems and approximately 75% of high-performance athletes have some sort of back pain.[27] In particular, sports that require repetitive or high-velocity twisting or bending, such as gymnastics, dancing, football, and rowing, have a predilection for back injuries.[101,123–132] With the increasing number of young athletes pursuing rigorous training and intense competition in some of these sports at an early age, the prevalence of back pain in the school-age athlete may be expected to increase.

Effective clinical management of back pain in the child and adolescent athlete requires an accurate diagnosis and a specific treatment plan. Accurate diagnosis necessitates an understanding of the differing aetiologies of back pain in the school-age athlete in contradistinction to back pain in the adult.[133] In the adult, mechanical back pain, degenerative disorders, and disc disease predominate, with symptomotology sometimes related to secondary gains, including disability and psychologic issues. In the school-age athlete with back pain, a specific diagnosis should be sought, such as spondylolysis, spondylolisthesis, apophysitis, tumor, or infection. Macrotrauma and microtrauma must be distinguished. The former involves a single-tissue overload while the latter represents cumulative trauma. Macrotrauma is typically seen in high-energy contact sports, such as rugby or football. Microtrauma is typically seen in athletes participating in sports requiring high-energy repetitive bending, twisting, or rotation, such as gymnasts, dancers, or football lineman. The growing athlete has several unique risk factors relevant to the adolescent spine. The growth cartilage of the vertebral end plates and apophyses are more susceptible to injury. Musculotendinous imbalances are quite common because of periods of rapid longitudinal growth. Eating disorders with irregular menstruation and osteoporosis are not uncommon in adolescent gymnasts and dancers. In addition, extrinsic factors such as poor technique, grouping of children by similar age despite differing abilities, and insufficient conditioning may predispose to injury.

Major anatomic differences of the spine in the skeletally immature include an increased cartilage to bone ratio and the presence of secondary centres of ossification at the vertebral end plates, which normally fuse to the vertebral bodies by maturity. Unlike adults who often have asymptomatic pre-existing degenerative changes in the fibrocartilaginous disc, intervertebral discs in the child are generally well hydrated and tightly adhered to the cartilaginous plate. The apophyseal ring is thinner in the middle than the periphery; thus, axial compression with forward flexion may force the disc through the end plates into the cancellous bone of the vertebral body as opposed to through the annulus towards the spinal canal as seen in adults. In addition, compressive and bending forces tend to fracture the weaker vertebral end plate rather than producing annulus failure and disc herniation.

A thorough history and discerning physical examination are essential in the assessment of spine injuries in child and adolescent athletes. The athlete's age, sex, pattern of complaints, location and radiation of pain, and chronology of symptoms are essential facts to obtain. Attention should be directed toward the mechanics of the sport producing the pain, such as walkovers in gymnasts, butterfly stroke in swimmers, and hyperextension and loading in linemen. A family history is implicated in scoliosis and spondylolisthesis. Night pain suggests tumor, morning stiffness associated with sacroiliac pain may be the presenting symptoms of juvenile ankylosing spondylitis, and systemic symptoms such as fever and chill suggest infection. Neurologic symptoms such as paresthesias, weakness, and bowel/bladder dysfunction require immediate attention. The physical examination should include an assessment of gait and leg lengths. The frontal and sagital contour of the spine should be examined both standing and bending to evaluate any asymmetry or deformity. Range of motion should be measured and localized areas of tenderness elicited. Provocative tests such as hyperextension or straight leg raising should be performed. Hip range of motion, muscle tightness, and generalized laxity should be assessed. Finally, a thorough neurologic examination of muscle strength, sensation, and reflexes should be performed. Radiographs and further diagnostic studies such as MRI, CT, and radionuclide scanning is individualized, depending on the differential diagnosis and symptomotology.

Spondylolysis and spondylolisthesis

Mechanical injury to the pars interarticularis is a common source of discomfort in young athletes involved in competitive sports and is probably the anatomic lesion diagnosed most frequently in young people with back pain. Spondylolysis refers to a bony defect in the pars interarticularis, and spondylolisthesis refers to translation of a vertebral body relative to an adjacent body in the sagittal plane. Fracture of the pars interarticularis occurs as a consequence of activity and is usually an overuse injury. Spondylolytic defects are rare in young children, have not been reported in newborns, are absent in other primates, and are not seen in patients who have not assumed an upright posture.[134] Nearly 50% of patients with spondylolysis relate the onset of symptoms to competitive sports training.[135] In a series of 177 male high school and college athletes, approximately 21% showed radiographic evidence of spondylolysis.[136] The incidence of spondylolysis is estimated at approximately 4% in the general adolescent population, increasing to 6% in adulthood.[137,138] Many inactive individuals are asymptomatic. The average age of diagnosis in the symptomatic school-age athletic population is between 15 and 16 years. LaFond[139] noted that 23% of spondylolysis patients in his series experienced the onset of symptoms before 20 years of age; however, only 9% of them had severe enough symptoms to seek medical attention. Approximately 85% of spondylolysis occurs at the L5 level.

It is postulated that spondylolysis and isthmic spondylolisthesis represent acquired fatigue fractures as a result of repeated microtrauma. Shear stresses of 400–600 N due to hyperextension, flexion, and torsion are concentrated across the pars interarticularis, an area calculated to be only 0.75 cm^2 at L5.[140,141] Repetitive hyperextension loading sports such as gymnastics, blocking in American football, hurdling, ballet dancing, volleyball spiking, competitive diving, tennis serving, weight lifting, and swimming turns have all been associated with spondylolysis. Pars defects occur four times more frequently in young female gymnasts than the general female population.[128] However, given the same demands within the same sport, it is difficult to determine why one athlete is predisposed to spondylolysis while another avoids injury. Genetic predisposition of spondylolytic defects has been documented.[142,143] Anatomic variations such as transitional vertebrae, spina bifida occulta, and an elongated pars may be seen. In addition, poor technique, inadequate supervision, poor conditioning, poor flexibility, and hyperlordotic posture may predispose to injury.

It is essential to make the diagnosis and initiate protective treatment as early as possible. The onset of symptoms typically coincide with the adolescent growth spurt and with the onset of strenuous, repetitive training. In athletes, symptoms are usually insidious aching low back pain without radiation. Initially, the pain is elicited by strenuous activity; however, the pain often becomes progressively more severe and becomes associated with activities of daily living. L5 radicular symptoms may arise from foraminal encroachment, fibrocartilaginous callus at the healing pars, or forward displacement of L5 on S1. Physical examination may demonstrate paraspinal tenderness, limited motion, hyperlordosis, and hamstring tightness.[144] Typically, pain can be reproduced with hyperextension and occasionally can be localized with ipsilateral hyperextension. Initial diagnostic work-up includes radiographs of the lumbosacral spine. Slippage through a pars defect may be seen on the standing lateral view, allowing for measurement of the percent slippage and slip angle (Figs. 46.13 and 46.14). A 25°–45° oblique view may demonstrate the spondylolytic defect (Fig. 46.13). Acutely, the defect appears as a narrow gap with irregular edges. Over time, the edges become rounded and smooth. Reactive sclerosis and hypertrophy of the opposite pars or lamina can be seen in unilateral spondylolysis and occasionally confused with osteoid osteoma. If spondylolysis is suspected but not demonstrated on plain films, single photon emission computed tomography (SPECT) scanning is particularly

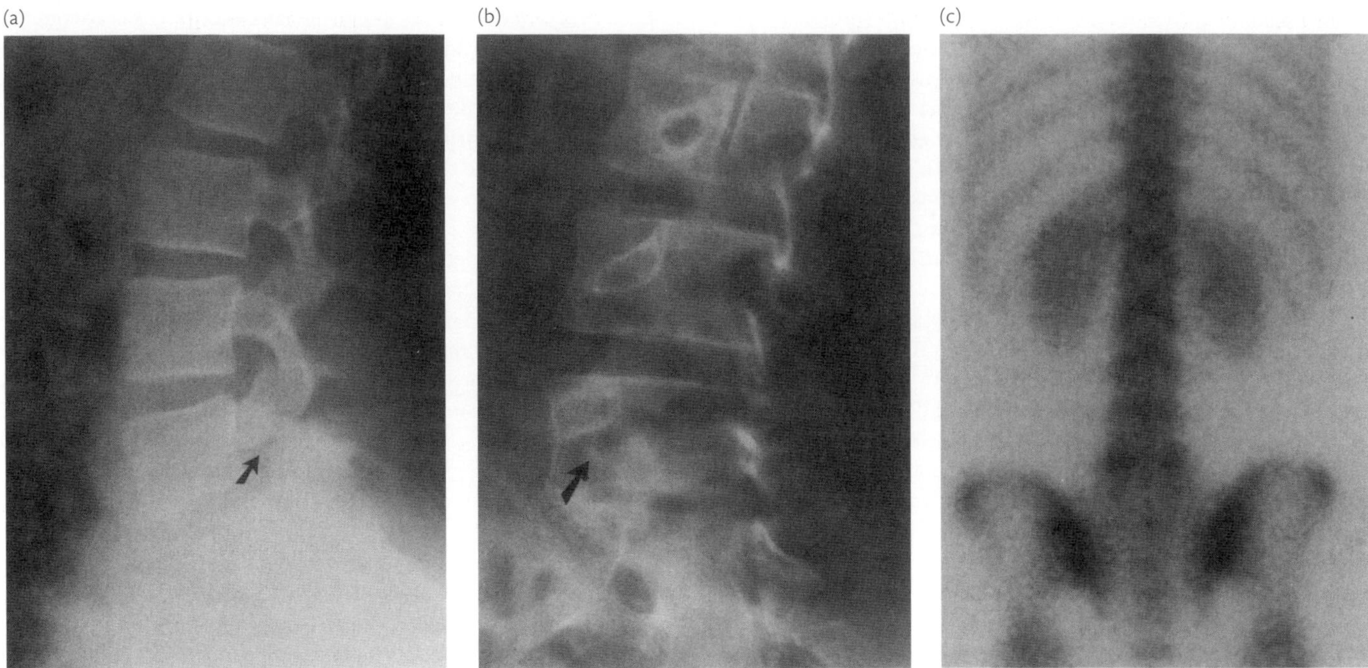

Fig. 46.13 Spondylolysis. (a) Lateral, (b) Oblique, and (c) SPECT scan in a 14-year-old female gymnast.

sensitive in detecting pars defects (Fig. 46.13).[145] More important, several studies have found that a positive bone scan or SPECT correlates with a painful pars lesion.[146] Early diagnosis with SPECT is of great practical significance as fresh pars defects may heal with early effective immobilization.[147] Computed tomography has significant limitations as a primary diagnostic tool, as an early stress reaction in pars without overt fracture results in a normal CT. However, oblique linear tomography or CT scanning may demonstrate the established pars lesion. With radicular symptoms, MRI is useful in demonstrating the aetiology of root compression. The limitations of MRI in terms of correctly grading the pars lesions are particularly apparent in patients with stress reaction in the pars without a clear fracture line.[148]

Management must consider the athlete's age, type of sport activity, severity of symptoms, and risk of progression. Risk factors for slip progression include slip percentage >50%, high slip angle, spina bifida, convex sacral contour, ligamentous laxity, and the adolescent age group.[149–153] The asymptomatic individual should be periodically followed clinically and radiographically if there are risk factors for progression. The symptomatic adolescent athlete can initially be treated with restriction of athletic activity and an abdominal- and back-strengthening program. We treat this as a stress fracture with activity modification and immobilization, using a rigid polypropylene lumbosacral brace constructed with 0° of lumbar flexion (antilordosis). The main effect of bracing appears to be restriction in gross body motion, and a brace may act as a means of restricting activity rather than stabilizing the fractures in these patients.[154] We advocate full-time brace use for approximately 3 months. Braced patients are allowed to resume limited activities several weeks after initiation of brace wear, when most have become asymptomatic. Results are promising with this treatment. In our series, 32% of 75 patients achieved bony union and 88% were able to return to previously painful sports, even if the pars defect had not healed.[155,156] A recent update from our institution revealed that a favourable clinical outcome can be achieved in 80% with bracing. However, the success of bracing depends on the type of sports participated in addition to acute onset of pain and hamstring tightness which were found to be associated with a worse outcome. With the brace treatment, the young athlete can return to sports in as little as 4–6 weeks.[157]

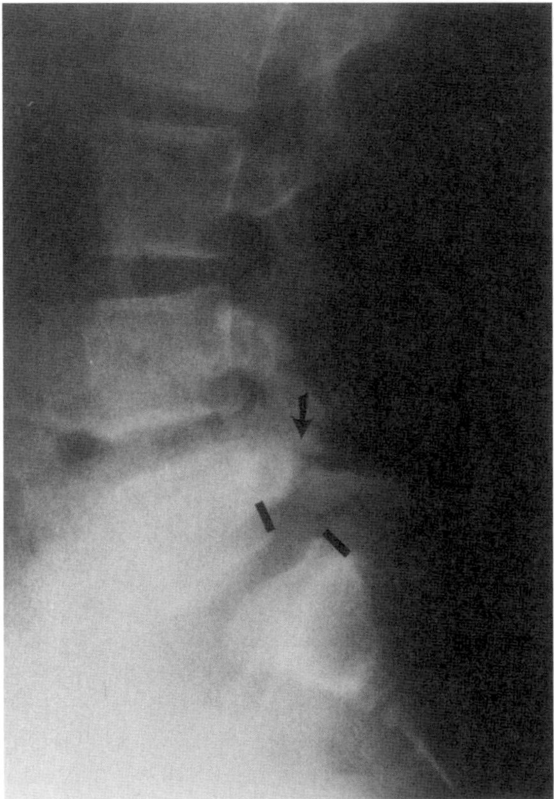

Fig. 46.14 Spondylolisthesis. Lateral view in a 17-year-old male football lineman.

Bone scans or CT scans may be helpful in following the status of a lesion.[138,158,159] A positive bone scan usually indicates that the defect is healing or has the potential to heal; however, a cold scan should not be taken as a contraindication to bracing.[147] Hamstring tightness is also an indicator of the success of treatment. Patients who fail to improve after an appropriate bracing regimen or who are unable to be weaned from the brace may require surgery. Posterolateral in situ fusion of L5–S1 is usually performed for L5 spondylolysis with post-operative bracing until fusion for up to 6 months. For spondylolysis of L4 or above, direct repair of the pars defect with wiring or osteosynthesis can be attempted, maintaining a motion segment and allowing earlier return to activity.[160–162] Management of the spondylolisthesis in the adolescent athlete depends on the degree of slippage and the severity of symptoms. Fortunately, it is rare to see progressive listhesis in the adolescent onset stress fracture pars defect seen in young athletes. For patients who remain symptomatic despite bracing, posterolateral in situ fusion of L5–S1 with post-operative bracing is performed.[150,152,163,164] Fusion should be extended to L4 for slips >50%. A slip of over 50% in the immature spine should be stabilized, even in an asymptomatic individual, because of the high risk of progression.[152,163,164] The asymptomatic athlete with <25% spondylolisthesis should be allowed to participate in all sports, including contact sports, while being followed periodically for progression (Fig. 46.14).[165] Asymptomatic athletes with 25–50% slippage fall into a controversial category. Some advocate observation for progression, some advocate avoidance of contact sports, and some advocate surgical management if the patient wishes to return to competitive sports. It is rare that an individual with high-grade slippage and severe lumbosacral kyphosis may benefit from reduction and fusion as opposed to in situ fusion; however, this is associated with a higher risk of neurologic complications.[166] Decompression in conjunction with fusion is reserved for a clear neurologic deficit and a readily discernible lesion such as the hypertrophied fibrocartilaginous mass at the level of the pars defect, irritating the L5 root. With high-grade slips, the sacral dome may stretch the thecal sac and sacral nerve roots.

Discogenic disorders

Although much less common in adolescents than adults, disc herniation and degenerative disc disease can occur in the young adolescent athlete. The true incidence is unknown, however, it is estimated that between 1 and 4% of all disc herniations occur in the paediatric population and less than 10% of young athletes' back pain is discogenic.[142,167,168–171] The natural history of disc disease in this population is not well understood, although some studies have suggested that these patients continue to have back problems as adults.[172] Acute macrotrauma may result in acute disc herniation as in collision-sport athletes and weightlifters, while repetitive microtrauma may result in degenerative disc disease or insidious herniation as in gymnasts. In contrast to adults with pre-existing degenerative disc changes, disc tissue in adolescents is usually noted to be firm, well hydrated, and solidly attached to the cartilaginous end plate.[171–175] These anatomic differences may predispose to disc herniation into the vertebral body or through an end-plate fracture rather than the classic extruded or sequestered disc through the annulus seen in adults. Disc herniations have been associated with sports with repetitive flexion and axial loading of the lumber spine, such as gymnastics, running, American football, weightlifting, basketball, soccer, and tennis.

The diagnosis can be difficult to determine clinically because the presentation can be quite different from the classic radicular symptomotology of the adult. In the adolescent with a ruptured disc, the most frequent complaint is low back pain with radiation confined to the buttock. There may be a decrease in hamstring flexibility, limited motion, abnormal gait or running pattern, asymmetric paravertebral spasm, or subtle 'sciatic' scoliosis. Neurologic findings of altered reflexes, muscle weakness, and atrophy are rare. In cases of severe pain and systemic symptoms, white blood cell count, sedimentation rate, and bone scan should be performed to rule out occult disc-space infection. Work-up includes lumbosacral spine films which may show end-plate fracture. Disc-space narrowing is unusual. MRI confirms the presence of a neurocompressive lesion (Fig. 46.15). A non-operative approach is the mainstay of management for both disc herniation and discogenic pain. Initial treatment is aimed at resting the back and avoiding sporting activities. Brace treatment with a 15° lumbar lordosis module has been a useful adjunct to the management of adolescent athletes with discogenic pain that does not respond to rest.[155] In our experience, rigid bracing is more effective than use of a soft corset and allows the athlete to return to daily activities and a light training programme. If the athlete is still symptomatic at 8–12 weeks, epidural corticosteroids are considered.[176] For those who fail non-operative management or have evidence of cauda equina syndrome or severe motor loss, discectomy may be necessary. In general, surgical intervention in this age group has good short-term results; however, return to high-level competitive sports may not be possible.[156,167,172,177] In addition, the risk of long-term sequelae such as degenerative changes at the involved level or herniation at a different level is not well understood.

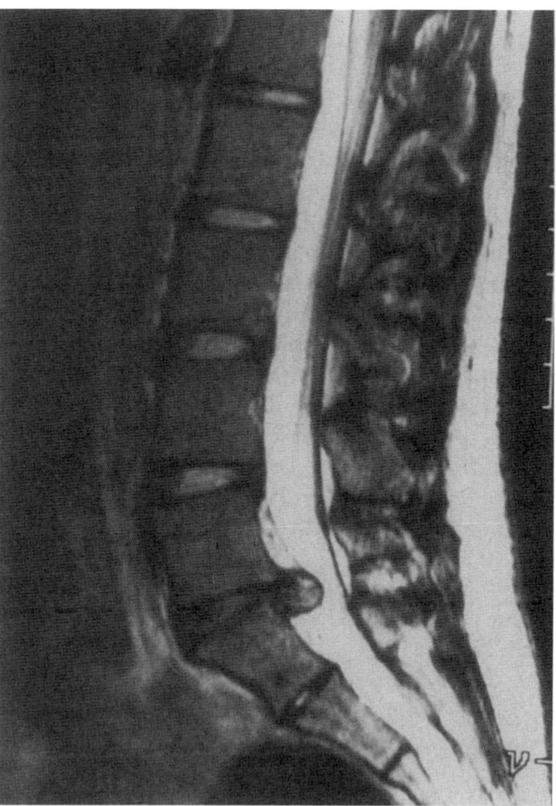

Fig. 46.15 Herniated disc. Sagital MRI in a 17-year-old gymnast.

A condition that is almost indistinguishable from a herniated lumbar disc is a slipped vertebral apophysis or end-plate fracture.[174,178] This condition is often associated with heavy lifting and typically involves displacement of the posterior inferior apophysis of L4 with its disc attachment into the vertebral canal. Patients present with signs of a herniated disc with neurologic findings. X-rays reveal the avulsion fragment and MRI reveals an extradural mass. Treatment consists of excision of both the cartilaginous disc and the bony fragment with relief of symptoms.

Scoliosis

Idiopathic scoliosis generally does not cause pain and does not interfere with sports. Scoliotic curves are often detected by asymmetry noted by parents, coaches, or screening. Forward bending accentuates the deformity by revealing the rotational deformity associated with coronal plane curvature. After a thorough history and examination to rule out associated abnormalities, full-length standing spine X-rays are obtained and the curve measured. Full-time bracing is initiated for progressive curves or, in general, curves over 25° in a child with substantial growth remaining. The braced patient is allowed to participate in sports out of the brace, and there is no evidence that sports participation increases the risk of curve progression. On the contrary, physical activity and strengthening are an essential aspect of brace management of scoliosis. After growth is complete, bracing is discontinued and no restrictions are placed on the adolescent with idiopathic scoliosis. Patients with progressive curves despite bracing or curves over 50°, have a high incidence of progression after maturity and are treated with spinal instrumentation and fusion. Post-operatively, sports are restricted until the fusion mass heals and matures. Following fusion for scoliosis, contact sports and vigorous gymnastics are restricted due to risks of pseudarthrosis, hardware failure, and degenerative changes about the fused levels.[179]

Scheuermann's disease

Scheuermann's disease consists of kyphosis of the thoracic spine with anterior vertebral wedging, Schmorl's nodes, and vertebral end-plate deformity. Radiographic criteria include wedging of 5° or more of three consecutive vertebrae.[180] The aetiology is unknown, although repetitive flexion microtrauma and fatigue failure are implicated. Patients typically present due to deformity without pain. On physical examination, patients have a roundback deformity with increased lumbar lordosis in the standing position. Most are unable to correct this deformity with forced hyperextension. Hamstrings are invariably tight. Treatment of Scheuermann's kyphosis consists of posture training, pelvic control, abdominal strengthening, and flexibility exercises to address the tight hamstrings and lumbodorsal fascia. Progressive kyphosis over 50° in an immature child is an indication for bracing and progression to curves beyond 70° is an indication for spinal fusion. Idiopathic kyphosis without radiographic changes of Scheuermann's disease is seen about the adolescent growth spurt in children with tight lumbodorsal fascia and hamstrings who subsequently compensate for this pelvic tilt with thoracic kyphosis. In general, this is a flexible kyphosis that can be managed with posture, strength, and flexibility training.

Atypical Scheuermann's disease consists of degenerative changes of the disc and vertebral end plates at the thoracolumbar junction. This is seen in adolescent athletes involved in vigorous flexion–extension activity of the spine such as gymnastics, diving, and rowing. Irregularities of the ring apophysis, end-plate wedging, and Schmorl's nodes may be seen on radiographs. These changes are often accompanied by pain and are thought to result from microtrauma with resultant end-plate fractures or disc herniation through the anterior ring apophysis with secondary bony deformation of the vertebrae.[170] Typically, the adolescent with atypical Scheuermann's has a flat back with thoracic hypokyphosis and lumbar hypolordosis. Pain is accentuated by forward flexion and relieved with rest. Our treatment utilizes full-time bracing with a molded thoracolumbar orthosis of 15° extension advanced to 30° if tolerated. Abdominal strengthening, hamstring stretching, and pelvic control are also initiated. The gymnast is often able to slowly return to activity in 3–6 months.

Fractures

Fractures of the thoracolumbar spine in child and adolescent athletes are quite rare. Most reports of spinal injuries with neurologic deficits in children involve the cervical spine.[181,182] It takes considerable force to result in thoracolumbar fracture in the adolescent athlete and the absence of a major force should prompt a search for a pathologic lesion. The classification and stability of compression fractures can be conceptualized in Denis's 3-column model where the anterior column consists of the anterior longitudinal ligament and the anterior half of the vertebral body, the middle column consists of the posterior half of the vertebral body and the posterior longitudinal ligament, and the posterior column consists of the posterior elements and ligamentous structures. Instability is inferred when two columns are disrupted. Evaluation of these injuries includes a thorough history and physical examination, including neurologic, cardiopulmonary, and abdominal assessment. Anteroposterior and lateral X-rays of the spine are obtained and further studies are performed as needed such as CT to define the extent of bony injury and MRI to evaluate neurologic involvement or disc injury. Stable compression fractures of less than 50% can be treated in a molded thoracolumbar orthosis or hyperextension brace for 6–12 weeks, depending on healing and symptoms (Fig. 46.16). Return to sports is allowed when the athlete is pain free and has full strength and flexibility. Unstable fracture dislocations, fractures with neurologic compromise, and fractures with significant deformity may require spinal fusion with possible neurologic decompression.

Apophyseal avulsion injuries resulting from rapid flexion, extension, and torsion are specific to the adolescent. Transverse process fractures may occur with contact sports. Associated intrathoracic, abdominal, and retroperitoneal injuries are the initial concerns. Management of these injuries consists of rest, followed by gradually increased range of motion and strength. Temporary bracing may be helpful. Return to gymnastics and contact sports is allowed when normal flexibility and strength are obtained.

Mechanical back pain

Mechanical back pain secondary to acute or chronic musculoligamentous strains and sprains is rare in the young athlete and should be a diagnosis of exclusion in children with low back pain. Such back pain is thought to represent overuse or stretch injuries of the soft tissues including the muscle–tendon unit, ligaments, joint

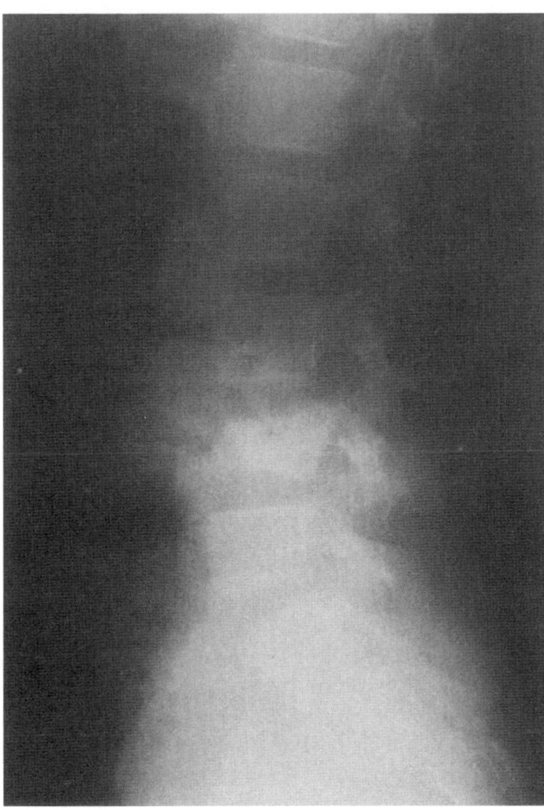

Fig. 46.16 Compression fracture. Lateral view in a 10-year-old female child.

capsules, and facets. This is more commonly seen in the older age group and may be related to the adolescent growth spurt. Young athletes with mechanical back pain may be predisposed to injury due to weak abdominal musculature, tight lumbodorsal fascia, tight hamstrings, limited lumbar motion, and poor training technique.[183] The pain is often nondescriptive, exacerbated by activity, and relieved by rest. Physical examination reveals paraspinal muscle tenderness, decreased flexibility, and limited spinal motion. X-rays are normal. Acutely, treatment consists of rest. Massage, NSAID's, and phonophoresis may be helpful. Once the acute phase has resolved, a rehabilitation programme consisting of posture control, abdominal strengthening, and flexibility is initiated. Return to sport is gradually allowed with resolution of pain and return of strength and flexibility. Proper technique, conditioning, and stretching are emphasized.

Summary

- Children and adolescents are not smaller adults. Injury patterns in children and adolescents are unique to the growing musculoskeletal system.
- Injuries to the trunk and upper extremity are being seen more frequently in recent years due to expanded participation in organized sports, increased training time and competition in this age group. In addition, increased awareness of athletic injuries by physicians and trainers will result in more reporting of these injuries.
- Early recognition of injuries prevent deformity formation and facilitate full return to sports.

References

1. Goldberg B, Rosenthal PP, Nicholas JA (1984). Injuries in youth football. *Phys Sports Med* **12**, 122–32.
2. Olson OC (1979). The Spokane study: high school football injuries. *Phys Sports Med* **7**, 75–82.
3. Consumer Product Safety Commission: Bicycle related injuries: Data from the National Electronic Injury Surveillance System (1987). *JAMA* **257**, 3334–7.
4. Kirburz D, Jacobs R, Reckling F, Mason J (1986). Bicycle accidents and injuries among adult cyclists. *Am J Sports Med* **14**, 416–19.
5. Culpepper MI, Niemann KMW (1983). High school football injuries in Birmingham, Alabama. *S Med J* **76**, 873–8.
6. Kocher MS, Feagin JA Jr (1996). Shoulder injuries during alpine skiing. *Am J Sports Med* **24**, 665–9.
7. Requa R, Garrick JG (1981). Injuries in interscholastic wrestling. *Phys Sports Med* **9**, 44–51.
8. Snook GA (1982). Injuries in intercollegiate wrestling: A 5 year study. *Am J Sports Med* **10**, 142–4.
9. Gainor BM, Piotrowski G, Puhl J, Allen WC, Hagen R (1980). The throw: Biomechanics and acute injury. *Am J Sports Med* **8**, 114–18.
10. Tullos HS, Fain RH (1974). Little league shoulder: Rotational stress fracture of proximal humeral epiphysis. *J Sports Med* **2**, 152–3.
11. Tullos HS, King JW (1972). Lesions of the pitching arm in adolescents. *JAMA* **220**, 264–71.
12. Albright JA, Jokl P, Shaw R, Albright JP (1978). Clinical study of baseball pitchers: Correlation of injury to the throwing arm with method of delivery. *Am J Sports Med* **6**, 15–21.
13. Barnett LS (1985). Little league shoulder syndrome: Proximal humeral epiphysis in adolescent baseball pitchers. *J Bone Joint Surg* **67A**, 495–6.
14. Cahill BR, Tullos HS (1974) Little league shoulder. *Sports Med* **2**, 150–3.
15. Dotter WE (1953). Little leaguer's shoulder: A fracture of the proximal epiphyseal cartilage of the humerus due to baseball pitching. *Guthrie Clinic Bull* **23**, 68–72.
16. Lipscomb AB (1975). Baseball injuries in growing athletes. *J Sports Med* **3**, 25 31.
17. Torg JS, Pollack H, Sweterlitsch P (1972). The effect of competitive pitching on the shoulders and elbows of preadolescent baseball players. *Pediatrics* **49**, 267–72.
18. Priest JD, Nagel DA (1976). Tennis shoulder. *Am J Sports Med* **4**, 28–42.
19. Richardson AB, Jobe FW, Collins HR (1980). The shoulder in competitive swimming. *Am J Sports Med* **8**, 159–63.
20. Fulton NN, Albright JP, El-Khoury GY (1979). Cortical desmoid-like lesion of the proximal humerus and its occurence in gymnasts. *Am J Sports Med* **7**, 57–61.
21. Goldberg MJ (1980). Gymnastic injuries. *Orthop Clin North Am* **11**, 717–32.
22. Snook GA (1979). Injuries in women's gymnastics: A 5 year study. *Am J Sports Med* **7**, 242–4.
23. Brooks AL, Henning GD (1972). Injury to the proximal clavicular epiphysis. *J Bone Joint Surg* **54A**, 1347–51.
24. Denham RH, Dingley AF (1967). Epiphyseal separation of the medial clavicle. *J Bone Joint Surg* **49A**, 1179–83.
25. Lewonowski K, Bassett GS (1992). Complete posterior retrosternal epiphyseal separation: A case report and review of the literature. *Clin Orthop* **281**, 84–8.
26. Winter J, Sterner S, Maurer D, Varecka T, Zarzycki M (1989). Retrosternal epiphyseal disruption of medial clavicle: Case and review in children. *J Emerg Med* 7, 9–13.
27. Destouet JM, Gilula LA, Murphy WA, Sagel SS (1981). Computed tomography of the sternoclavicular joint and sternum. *Radiology* **138**, 123–8.

28. Selesnick FH, Jablon M, Frank C, Post M (1984). Retrosternal dislocation of the clavicle. *J Bone Joint Surg* **66A**, 287–91.
29. Wirth MA, Rockwood CA (1996). Acute and traumatic injuries of the sternoclavicular joint. *J Am Acad Orthop Surg* **4**, 268–78.
30. Clark RL, Milgram JW, Yawn DH (1974). Fatal aortic perforation and cardiac tamponade due to Kirschner wire migrating from the right sternoclavicular joint. *South Med J* **67**, 316–18.
31. Nogi J, Heckman JD, Hakala M, Sweet DE (1975). Non-union of the clavicle in a child: A case report. *Clin Orthop* **110**, 19–21.
32. Nordquist A, Petersson C (1994). The incidence of fractures of the clavicula. *Clin Orthop* **300**, 127–32.
33. Bowen A (1983). Plastic bowing of the clavicle in children: A report of two cases. *J Bone Joint Surg* **65A**, 403–5.
34. Kubiak R, Slongo T (2002). Operative treatment of clavicle fractures in children: A review of 21 years. *J Pediatr Orthop* **22**, 736–9.
35. Howard FM, Shafer SJ (1965). Injury to the clavicle with neurovascular complications: A stufy of fourteen cases. *J Bone Joint Surg* **47A**, 1335–46.
36. Zenni EJ, Krieg JK, Rosen MJ (1981). Open reduction and internal fixation of clavicular fractures. *J Bone Joint Surg* **63A**, 147–51.
37. Black GB, McPherson JA, Reed MH (1991). Traumatic pseudodislocation of the acromioclavicular joint in children. *Am J Sports Med* **19**, 644–66.
38. Eidman DK, Siff SJ, Tullos HS (1981). Acromioclavicular lesions in children. *Am J Sports Med* **9**, 150–4.
39. Falstie-Jensen S, Mikkelsen P (1982). Pseudodislocation of the acromioclavicular joint. *J Bone Joint Surg* **64B**, 368–9.
40. Havranek P (1989). Injuries of the distal clavicular physis in children. *J Pediatr Orthop* **9**, 213–5.
41. Ogden JA (1984). Distal clavicular physeal injury. *Clin Orthop* **188**, 68–73.
42. Rockwood CA (1982). Fractures of outer clavicle in children and adults. *J Bone Joint Surg* **64B**, 642–9.
43. Bjerneld H, Hovelius L, Thorling J (1983). Acromioclavicular separatons treated conservatively. *Acta Orthop Scand* **54**, 743–5.
44. Galpin RD, Hawkins RJ, Grainger RW (1985). A comparative analysis of operative versus nonoperative management of grade III acromioclavicular separattions. *Clin Orthop* **193**, 150–5.
45. Larsen E, Bjerg-Nielsen A, Christensen P (1986). Conservative or surgical treatment of acromioclavicular dislocation. *J Bone Joint Surg* **68A**, 552–5.
46. Cahill BR (1992). Atraumatic osteolysis of the distal clavicle: A review. *Sports Med* **13**, 214–22.
47. Scavenius M, Iversen BF (1992). Nontraumatic clavicular osteolysis in weight lifters. *Am J Sports Med* **20**, 463–7.
48. LarsonRL, SingerKM, Bergstrom R, Thomas S (1976). Little League survey: The Eugene study. *Am J Sports Med* **4**, 201–9.
49. Lyman S, Fleisig G, Andrews JR, Osinski ED (2002). Effect of pitch type, pitch count, and pitching mechanics on risk of elbow and shoulder pain in youth baseball pitchers. *Am J Sports Med* **30**, 463–8.
50. Kohler R, Trillaud JM (1983). Fracture and fracture separation of the proximal humerus in children: Report of 136 cases. *J Pediatr Orthop* **3**, 326–32.
51. Baxter MP, Wiley J (1986). Fractures of the proximal humeral epiphysis: Their influence on humeral growth. *J Bone Joint Surg* **68B**, 570–3.
52. Dameron TB, Reibel DB (1969). Fractures involving the proximal humeral eoiohyseal plate. *J Bone Joint Surg* **51A**, 289–97.
53. Neer CS, Horowitz BS (1965). Fractures of the proximal humeral epiphyseal plate. *Clin Orthop* **41**, 24–31.
54. Nilsson S, Svartholm F (1965). Fracture of the upper end of the humerus in children. *Acta Chir Scand* **130**, 433–9.
55. Sherk H, Probst C (1975). Fractures of the proximal humeral epiphysis. *Orthop Clin North Am* **6**, 401–13.
56. Williams DJ (1981). The mechanisms producing fracture separation of the proximal humeral epiphysis. *J Bone Joint Surg* **63B**, 102–7.
57. Dobbs MB, Luhmann SL, Gordon JE, Strecker WB, Schoenecker PL (2003) Severely displaced proximal humeral epiphyseal fractures. *J Pediatr Orthop* **23**, 208–15.
58. Asher MA (1976). Dislocations of the upper extremity in children. *Orthop Clin North Am* **7**, 583–91.
59. Hovelius L (1987). Anterior dislocation of the shoulder in teenagers and young adults. *J Bone Joint Surg* **69A**, 393–9.
60. Marans HJ, Angel KR, Schemitsch EH, Wedge JH (1992). The fate of traumatic anterior dislocation of the shoulder in children. *J Bone Joint Surg* **74A**, 1242–4.
61. Rowe CR (1963). Anterior dislocation of the shoulder: Prognosis and treatment. *Surg Clin North Am* **43**, 1609–14.
62. Rowe CR (1956). Prognosis in dislocation of the shoulder. *J Bone Joint Surg* **38A**, 957–77.
63. Wagner KT, Lyne ED (1983). Adolescent traumatic dislocations of the shoulder with open epiphysis. *J Pediatr Orthop* **3**, 61–2.
64. Aronen JG, Regan K (1984). Decreasing the incidence of recurrence of first time anterior shoulder dislocation with rehabilitation. *Am J Sports Med* **12**, 283–91.
65. Burkhead WZ, Rockwood CA (1992). Treatment of instability of the shoulder with an exercise program. *J Bone Joint Surg* **74A**, 890–6.
66. Simonet WT, Cofield RH (1984). Prognosis in anterior shoulder dislocation. *Am J Sports Med* **12**, 19–24.
67. Deitch J, Mehlman CT, Foad SL, Obbehat A, Mallory M (2003). Traumatic anterior shoulder dislocation in adolescents. *Am J Sports Med* **31**, 758–63.
68. Jones KJ, Wiesel B, Ganley TJ, Wells L (2007). Functional outcomes of early arthroscopic bankart repair in adolescents aged 11 to 18 years. *J Pediatr Orthop* **27**, 209–13.
69. Carter C, Sweetnam R (1960). Recurrent dislocation of the patella and the shoulder: Their association with familial joint laxity. *J Bone Joint Surg* **42B**, 721–7.
70. Neer CS, Foster DR (1980). Inferior capsular shift for involuntary inferior and multidirectional instability of the shoulder. *J Bone Joint Surg* **62A**: 897–908.
71. Bigliani LU, D'Alessandro DF, Duralde XA, McIlveen SJ (1989). Anterior acromioplasty for subacromial impingement in patients younger than 40 years of age. *Clin Orthop* **246**, 111–6.
72. Hawkins RJ, Kennedy JC (1980). Impingement syndrome in athletes. *Am J Sports Med* **8**, 151–7.
73. Tibone JE (1983). Shoulder problems of adolescence. *Clin Sports Med* **2**, 423–6.
74. Tibone JE, Elrod B, Jobe FW, Kerlan RK, Carter VS, Shields CL jr., Lombardo SJ, Yocum L (1986). Surgical treatment of tears of the rotator cuff in athletes. *J Bone Joint Surg* **68A**, 887–91.
75. Pappas AM (1982). Elbow problems associated with baseball during childhood and adolescence. *Clin Orthop* **164**, 30–41.
76. Aronem JG (1985). Problems of the upper extremity in gymnastics. *Clin Sports Med* **4**, 61–71.
77. Otsuka NY, Kasser JR (1997). Supracondylar fractures of the humerus in children. *J Am Acad Orthop Surg* **5**, 19–26.
78. Skaggs DL (1997). Elbow fractures in children: Diagnosis and Management. *J Am Acad Orthop Surg* **5**, 303–12.
79. Brauer CA, Lee BM, Bae DS, Waters PM, Kocher MS (2007). A systematic review of medial and lateral entry pinning versus lateral entry pinning for supracondylar fractures of the humerus. *J Pediatr Orthop* **27**, 181–6.
80. Kocher MS, Kasser JR, Waters PM, Bae D, Snyder BD, Hresko MT, Hedequist D, Karlin L, Kim YJ, Murray MM, Millis MB, Emans JB, Dichtel L, Matheney T, Lee BM (2007). Lateral entry compared with medial and lateral entry pin fixation for completely displaced supracondylar humeral fractures in children. A randomized clinical trial. *J Bone Joint Surg Am* **89**, 706–12.
81. Davids J, Maguire M, Mubarak S, Wenger DR. (1994). Lateral condylar fracture of the humerus following posttraumatic cubitus varus. *J Pediatr Orthop* **14**, 466–70.
82. Bernstein SM, McKeever P, Bernstein L (1993). Percutaneous reduction of displaced radial neck fractures in children. *J Pediatr Orthop* **13**, 85–8.

83. Gill TJ, Micheli LJ (1996). The immature athlete: Common injuries and overuse syndromes of the elbow and wrist. *Clin Sports Med* **15**, 401–23.
84. Farsetti P, Potenza V, Caterini R, Ippolito E (2001). Long term results of treatment of fractures of the medial humeral epicondyle in children. *J Bone Joint Surg Am* **83**, 1299–1305.
85. Dias J, Johnson G, Hoskinson J, Sulaiman K (1987). Management of severely displaced medial epicondyle fractures. *J Orthop Trauma* **1**, 59–62.
86. Josefsson PO, Danielsson LG (1986). Epicondylar elbow fracture in children: 35 year follow-up of 56 unreduced cases. *Acta Orthop Scand* **57**, 313–5.
87. Woods GW, Tullos HS (1977). Elbow instability and medial epicondyle fractures. *Am J Sports Med* **5**, 23–30.
88. Carlioz H, Abols Y (1984). Posterior dislocation of the elbow in children. *J Pediatr Orthop* **4**, 8–12.
89. Jackson DW, Silvino N, Reiman P (1989). Osteochondritis in the female gymnasts's elbow. *Arthroscopy* **5**, 129–36.
90. Brogdon BG, Crow NE (1960). Little Leaguer's elbow. *Am J Roentgenel* **83**, 671–5.
91. Gugenheim JJ, Stanley RF, Wood GW, Tullos HS (1976). Little League survey: The Houston study. *Am J Sports Med* **4**, 189–200.
92. Hang YS (1982). Little League elbow: A clinical and biomechanical study. *Int Orthop* **3**, 70–8.
93. Slager RF (1977). From Little League to the big league, the weak spot is the arm. *Am J Sports Med* **5**, 37–48.
94. Smith MGH (1964). Osteochondritis of the humeral capitellum. *J Bone Joint Surg* **46B**, 50–4.
95. Tiynon MC, Anzel SH, Waugh TR (1976). Surgical management of osteochondritis dissecans of the capitellum. *Am J Sports Med* **4**, 121–8.
96. Takahara M, Mura N, Sasaki J, Harada M, Ogino T (2007). Classification, treatment, and outcome of osteochondritis dissecans of the humeral capitellum. *J Bone Joint Surg Am* **89**, 1205–14.
97. Chambers RB (1979). Orthopedic injuries in athletes (ages 6 to 17). *Am J Sports Med* **7**, 195–7.
98. Watson AW (1984). Sports injuries during one academic year in 6,799 Irish school children. *Am J Sports Med* **12**, 65–71.
99. Zaricznyj B, Shattuck LJ, Mast TA, Robertson RV, D'Elia G (1980). Sports-related injuries in school-aged children. *Am J Sports Med* **8**, 318–24.
100. Blitzer CM, Johnson RJ, Ettlinger CF, Aggeborn K (1984). Downhill skiing injuries in children. *Am J Sports Med* **12**, 142–7.
101. Garrick JF, Regua RK (1980). Epidemiology of women's gymnastic injuries. *Am J Sports Med* **8**, 261–4.
102. Sullivan JA, Gross RH, Grana WA, Garcia-Mural CA (1980). Evaluation of injuries in youth soccer. *Am J Sports Med* **8**, 325–7.
103. Mann DC, Rajmaira S (1990). Distribution of physeal and non-physeal fractures in 2650 long bone fractures in children aged 0–16 years. *J Pediatr Orthop* **10**, 713–6.
104. Friberg K (1970). Remodeling after distal forearm fractures. *Acta Orthop Scand* **50**, 731–50.
105. Landfried MJ, Stenclik M, Sui JG (1991). Variant of Galeazzi fracture-dislocation in children. *J Pediatr Orthop* **11**, 332–5.
106. Rodriguez-Merchan EC (2005). Pediatric fractures of the forearm. *Clin Orthop* **432**, 65–72.
107. Roy S, Caine D, Singer KM (1985). Stress changes of the distal radius epiphysis in young gymnasts. *Am J Sports Med* **13**, 301–8.
108. Mandelbaum BR, Bartolozzi AR, Davis CA, Teurlings L, Bragonier B (1989). Wrist pain syndrome in the gymnast. *Am J Sports Med* **17**, 305–17.
109. Vender MI, Watson HK (1988) Acquired Madelung-like deformity in a gymnast. *J Hand Surg* **13A**, 19–21.
110. Terry CL, Waters PM (1998). Triangular fibrocartilage injuries in pediatric and adolescent patients. *J Hand Surg* **23A**, 626–34.
111. Fabre O, De boeck H, Haentjens P (2001). Fractures and nonunions of the carpal scaphoid in children. *Acta Orthop Belg* **67**, 121–5.
112. Mintzer CM, Waters PM, Simmons BP (1995). Nonunion of the scaphoid in children treated with Herbet screw fixation and bone grafting. A report of five cases. *J Bone Joint Surg* **77B**, 98–100.
113. Riester JN, Baker BE, Mosher JF, Lowe D (1985). A review of scaphoid fracture healing in competetive athletes. *Am J Sports Med* **13**, 154–161.
114. Southcott R, Rosman MA (1977). Non-union of carpal scaphoid fractures in children. *J Bone Joint Surg* **59B**, 20–3.
115. Hanks GA, Kalenak A, Bowman LS, Sebastianelli WJ (1989). Stress fractures of the carpal scaphoid. A report of four cases. *J Bone Joint Surg* **71A**, 938–41.
116. Manzione M, Pizzutillo PD (1981). Stress fracture of the scaphoid waist. *Am J Sports Med* **9**, 268–9.
117. Burton RI, Eaton RG (1973). Common hand injuries in the athlete. *Orthop Clin North Am* **4**, 809–38.
118. Hastings H, Simmons BP (1984). Hand fractures in children. *Clin Orthop* **188**, 120–30.
119. McCue FC, Baugher WH, Kulund DN, Gieck JH (1979). Hand and wrist injuries in the athlete. *Am J Sports Med* **7**, 275–86.
120. Posner MA (1977). Injuries to the hand and wrist in athletes. *Orthop Clin North Am* **8**, 593–617.
121. Simmons BP, Lovallo JL (1988). Hand and wrist injuries in children. *Clin Sports Med* **7**, 495–512.
122. Leddy JP, Packer JW (1977). Avulsion of the profundus tendon insertion in athletes. *J Hand Surg* **2**, 66–9.
123. Ciullo JV, Jackson DW (1985). Pars interarticularis stress reaction, spondylolysis, and spondylolisthesis in gymnasts. *Clin Sports Med* **4**, 95–110.
124. Ferguson RH, McMaster JF, Stanitski CL (1974). Low back pain in college football linemen. *Am J Sports Med* **2**, 63–9.
125. Hall SJ (1986). Mechanical contribution to lumbar stress injuries in female gymnasts. *Med Sci Sports Exerc* **18**, 599–602.
126. Howell DW (1984). Musculoskeletal profile and incidence of musculoskeletal injuries in lightweight women rowers. *Am J Sports Med* **12**, 278–81.
127. Ireland ML, Micheli LJ (1987). Bilateral stress fracture in the lumbar pedicle in a ballet dancer. *J Bone Joint Surg* **69A**, 140–2.
128. Jackson DW, Wiltse LL, Cirincione RJ (1976). Spondylolysis in the female gymnast. *Clin Orthop* **117**, 68–73.
129. McCarroll JR, Miller JM, Ritter MA (1986). Lumbar spondylolysis and spondylolisthesis in college football players. *Am J Sports Med* **14**, 404–6.
130. Micheli LJ (1983). Back injuries in dancers. *Clin Sports Med* **2**, 473–84.
131. Micheli LJ (1985). Back injuries in gymnastics. *Clin Sports Med* **4**, 85–93.
132. Semen RL, Spengler D (1981). Significance of lumbar spondylolysis in college football players. *Spine* **6**, 172–4.
133. Micheli LJ (1979). Low back pain in the the adolescent: Differential diagnosis. *Am J Sports Med* **7**, 362–4.
134. Rosenberg NJU, Bargar WL, Friedman B (1981). The incidence of spondylolysis and spondylolisthesis in nonambulatory patients. *Spine* **6**, 35–8.
135. O'Neill DB, Micheli LJ (1989). Post-operative radiographic evidence for fatigue fracture as the etiology of spondylolysis. *Spine* **14**, 1342–55.
136. Hoshina H (1980). Spondylolysis in athletes. *Phys Sports Med* **8**, 75–78.
137. Baker DR, McHolick W (1956). Spondylolysis and spondylolisthesis in children. *J Bone Joint Surg* **38A**, 933–4.
138. Collier BD, Johnson RP, Carrera GF, Meyer GA, Schwab JP, Flatley TJ, Isitman AT, Hellman RS, Zielonka JS, Knobel J (1985). Painful spondylolysis or spondylolisthesis studied by radiography or single photon emission computed tomography. *Radiology* **154**, 207–11.
139. LaFond G (1962). Surgical treatment of spondylolisthesis. *Clin Orthop* **22**, 175–9.
140. Hutton WC, Stott JRR, Cyron BM (1977). Is spondylolysis a fatigue fracture? *Spine* **2**, 202–29.

141. Letts M, Smallman T, Afanasiev R, Gouw G (1986). Fracture of the pars interarticularis in adolescent athletes: A clinical-biomechanical analysis. *J Pediat Orthop* **6**, 40–6.

142. Fredrickson BE, Baker D, McHolick, WJ, Yuan HA, Lubicky JPL (1984). The natural history of spondylolysis and spondylolisthesis. *J Bone Joint Surg* **66A**, 699–707.

143. Winney-Davies R, Scott JHS (1979). Inheritance and spondylolisthesis-a radiographic family survey. *J Bone Joint Surg* **61B**, 301–5.

144. Phalen GS, Dickson JA (1961). Spondylolisthesis and tight hamstrings. *J Bone Joint Surg* **43A**, 505–12.

145. Bellah RD, Summerville DA, Treves ST, Micheli LJ (1991). Low-back pain in adolescent athletes: Detection of stress injury to the pars interarticularis with SPECT. *Radiology* **180**, 509–12.

146. Staendert CJ, Herring SA (2000). Spondylolysis: a critical review. *Br J Sports Med* **34**, 415–42.

147. Morita T, Ikata T, Katoh S, Miyake R (1995). Lumbar spondylolysis in children and adolescents. *J Bone Joint Surg* **77B**, 620–5.

148. Campbell RS, Grainger AJ, Hide IG, Papastefanou S, Greenough CG. (2005). Juvenile spondylolysis: A comparative analysis of CT, SPECT, and MRI. *Skeletal Radiol* **34**, 63–73.

149. Saraste H (1984). Prognostic radiologic aspects of spondylolisthesis. *Acta Radiol* **25**, 427–34.

150. Saraste H (1987). Long-term clinical and radiographic follow-up of spondylolysis and spondylolisthesis. *J Pediatr Orthop* **7**, 631–8.

151. Turner R, Bianco A (1971). Spondylolysis and spondylolisthesis in children and teenagers. *J Bone Joint Surg* **53A**, 1298–306.

152. Wiltse LL, Jackson DW (1976). Treatment of spondylolisthesis and spondylolysis in children. *Clin Orthop* **117**, 92–100.

153. Wiltse LL, Widell EH, Jackson DW (1974). Fatigue fracture: The basic lesion in isthmic spondylolisthesis. *J Bone Joint Surg* **57A**, 17–22.

154. Calmels P, Fayolle-Minon I (1996). An update on orthotic devices for the lumbar spine based on a review of the literature. *Rev Rheum (Engl Ed)* **63**, 285–91.

155. Micheli LJ, Hall JE, Miller ME (1980). Use of modified Boston back brace for back injuries in athletes. *Am J Sports Med* **8**, 351–6.

156. Micheli LJ, Steiner ME (1985). Treatment of symptomatic spondylolysis and spondylolisthesis with the modified Boston brace. *Spine* **10**, 937–43.

157. d'Hemecourt PA, Zurakowski D, Kriemler S, Micheli LJ. (2002). Spondylolysis: Returning the athlete to sports participation with brace treatment. *Orthopedics* **25**, 653–7.

158. Congeni J, McCulloch J, Swanson K (1997). Lumbar spondylolysis. A study of natural progression in athletes. *Am J Sports Med* **25**, 248–53.

159. Papanicolaou N, Wilkinson RH, Emans JB, Treves S, Micheli LJ (1985). Bone scintigraphy and radiography in young athletes with low back pain. *Am J Roentgenol* **145**, 1039–44.

160. Bradford DS, Iza J (1985). Repair of the defect in spondylolysis or minimal degress of spondylolisthesis by segmental fixation and bone grafting. *Spine* **10**, 673–9.

161. Buck J (1970). Direct repair of the defect in spondylolisthesis. *J Bone Joint Surg* **52B**, 432–7.

162. Buring K, Fredensborg N (1973). Osteosynthesis of spondylolysis. *Acta Orthop Scand* **44**, 91–7.

163. Boxall D, Bradford D, Winter R, Moe JH (1979). Management of severe spondylolisthesis in children and adolescents. *J Bone Joint Surg* **61A**, 479–95.

164. Hensinger R, Lang J, MacEwen G (1976). Surgical management of spondylolisthesis in children and adolescents. *Spine* **1**, 207–14.

165. Muschik M, Hahnel H, Robinson PN, Perka C, Muschik C (1996). Competitive sports and the progression of spondylolisthesis. *J Pediatr Orthop* **16**, 364–9.

166. Bradford DS (1979). Treatment of severe spondylolisthesis: A combined approach for reduction and stabilization. *Spine* **4**, 423–9.

167. Borgesen SE, Vang PS (1974). Herniation of the lumbar intervertebral disk in children and adolescents. *Acta Orthop Scand* **45**, 540–9.

168. Epstein JA, Epstein NE, Marc J, Rosenthal AD, Lavine LS (1984). Lumbar intervertebral disk herniation in teenage children: Recognition and management of associated anomalies. *Spine* **9**, 427–32.

169. Garrido E, Humphreys RP, Hendrick EB, Hoffman HJ (1978). Lumbar disc disease in children. *Neurosurgery* **2**, 22–6.

170. Swärd L, Hellström M, Jacobsson B, Nyman R, Peterson L (1990). Acute injury of the vertebral ring apophysis and intervertebral disc in adolescent gymnasts. *Spine* **15**, 144–8.

171. Swärd L, Hellström M, JacobssonB, Nyman R, Peterson L (1991). Disc degeneration and associated abnormalities of the spine in elite gymnasts. *Spine* **16**, 437–43.

172. DeOrio JK, Bianco AJ (1982). Lumbar disc excision in children and adolescents. *J Bone Joint Surg* **64A**, 991–5.

173. Kurihara A, Kataoka O (1980). Lumbar disc herniation in children and adolescents. A review of 70 operated cases and their minimum 5 year follow-up studies. *Spine* **5**, 443–51.

174. Lippitt AB (1976). Fracture of a vertebral body end plate and disk protrusion causing subarachnoid block in an adolescent. *Clin Orthop* **116**, 112–5.

175. Resnick D, Niwayama G (1978). Intravertebral disk herniation: Cartilaginous (Schmorl's nodes). *Radiology* **126**, 57–65.

176. Jackson DW, Rettig A, Wiltse LL (1980). Epidural cortisone injections in the young athletic adult. *Am J Sports Med* **8**, 239–43.

177. Day AL, Friedman WA, Indelicato PA (1987). Observations on the treatment of lumbar disck disease in college football players. *Am J Sports Med* **15**, 72–5.

178. Techakapuch S (1981). Rupture of the lumbar cartilage plate into the spinal canal in an adolescent. A case report. *J Bone Joint Surg* **63A**, 481–2.

179. Micheli LJ (1985). Sports following spinal surgery in the young athlete. *Clin Orthop* **198**, 152–7.

180. Sorenson HK (1964). *Scheuermann's juvenile kyphosis.* Munksgaard, Copenhagen.

181. Hubbard DD (1974). Injuries of the spine in children and adolescents. *Clin Orthop* **100**, 56–65.

182. Kewalramani MD, Tori JA (1980). Spinal cord traumain children: Neurological patterns, radiologic features, and pathomechanics of injury. *Spine* **5**, 11–8.

183. Kujala UM, Taimela S, Oksanen A, Salminen JJ (1997). Lumbar mobility and low back pain during adolescece. A longitudinal three-year follow-up study in athletes and controls. *Am J Sports Med* **25**, 363–8.

CHAPTER 47

Lower-limb injuries in sporting children

Umile Giuseppe Longo and Nicola Maffulli

Introduction

Physical activity plays a significant role in the well-being of a child. A well-designed exercise programme enhances the immediate physical, psychomotor, and intellectual attainments of a child.[1] Long-term health benefits depend on continuation of the physical activity, thus enhancing well-being and favouring the balanced development of a child.[1] In the past two decades, competitive sports participation has become an established feature of childhood in Western countries.[2,3] Many of the youngsters in these countries initiate year-round training and specialization in their sports at a very early age.

Concern over possible growth inhibition effects of competitive sports has been and continues to be a source of much scientific debate,[4] but there is no definitive evidence to indicate that training affects either positively or negatively the growth and maturation in young athletes.

Injuries during sport seem to be unavoidable and up to 30–40% of all accidents in children and adolescents occur during sports.[5] Nevertheless, the rate of injury is lower in children than in mature adolescents.[6] Prevention has been implemented, but, given the large number of participants, health care professionals are often confronted by acute and chronic musculoskeletal injuries in young athletes.

The intensity of exercise, the mental and physical readiness for performance, and the type of sports also play a significant role, with swimming, ball sports, and riding and ice skating having low, medium, and high risk prevalence, respectively. Each sport has a typical pattern of injury; for instance, knee contusions are the most common skiing injuries in children.[7]

The lower extremity is under specific biomechanical demands important in the context of the increasing numbers of athletes in soccer, skiing, and running.[5]

The musculoskeletal system in childhood

To understand children's injuries, it is important to have an insight into the peculiarities of the growing musculoskeletal system. Tendons and ligaments are relatively stronger than the epiphyseal plate, and considerably more elastic. Therefore, in severe trauma, the epiphyseal plate, being weaker than the ligaments, gives way. Hence, growth plate damage is more common than ligamentous injuries.[6,8–11]

In children, bones and muscles show increased elasticity[9] and heal faster.[11] Weight bearing is beneficial for the skeleton, but excessive strains may produce serious injuries to joints.[9] Low-intensity training can stimulate bone growth, but high intensity training can inhibit it.[12] There are adaptive changes to sport activity, and up to puberty muscular strength is similar in girls and boys.[13]

Different metabolic and psychological aspects of childhood in sport

Children produce more heat relative to body mass, have a low-sweating capacity, and also tend not to drink enough compared to adults.[13] Therefore, heat prostration and exhaustion, especially in hot climates, is more likely than in adults (see Chapter 23). This may result in an increased number of injuries.[13]

Young competitors may have the same chronological age but not necessarily the same biological age[11] and children need to be more closely matched with the other competitors not just by chronological age but also by biological age[14,15] (and see Chapter 12). It is also possible that parents and coaches push children too hard,[11,16] not appreciating that time is needed to develop high-performance abilities.[17] Children may also develop psychological complications following injuries.[18]

Endogenous risk factors

There are a number of well-established risk factors for paediatric musculoskeletal injury in sport.[19–22] Imbalances in the musculoskeletal system may influence the rate of occurrence of injuries.[11] Common conditions such as pes cavus, pes planus and calcaneus valgus may play a role in the aetiology of some injuries.[11] Anatomical factors have been hypothesized in the aetiology of injuries where overuse is common, such as in patellofemoral stress syndrome, ileotibial band syndrome, medial tibial stress syndrome, and plantar fascitis.[23] Compared to adults, children have decreased strength and endurance,[24–26] which has to be taken into account when planning training and competition.

With growth spurts, there is a decrease in flexibility due to relative bone lengthening. This predisposes to injury in the absence of appropriate stretching exercises, prior to commencing sport. Studies in adults have shown that stretching prior to exercise does not reduce the incidence of injury,[27,28] although it remains to be seen whether this is also the case in children. Training in improper environments or with incorrect footwear equipment can also result in injury. Cross-training and gradual change in training schedules is good practice. Players should ideally be matched with appropriate body protection and supervision. Balanced nutrition is vital: the amenorrhoeic anorexic female with reduced bone mineral density is at higher risk of injury.[29,30] High-resistance training may also predispose children to an increased risk of injury if not properly supervised.[31]

Epidemiology of lower-limb injuries

The actual incidence of injury in children's sports is very difficult, if not impossible, to determine.[32,33] Published studies vary significantly in terms of populations studied, methodology used, and types and severity of injuries reported. In addition, because of the different criteria used to define an injury, comparisons between reports are difficult, and any such comparisons should be interpreted with caution.

Approximately 3%–11% of school children are injured per year while participating in sport. Twice as many boys as girls sustain sports-related injuries,[9,34–36] although some authors report a similar incidence between the genders.[13,37] Boys, however, still sustain more severe injuries, possibly because they are more aggressive. For certain sports, such as horse riding, injuries are four times more common in females.[35] Sports involving contact and jumping have the highest injury levels, with football in particular accounting for the majority of injuries.[37,38] Elite athletes, however, have lower injury rates than the general sporting populations.[39] Using a mixed longitudinal study design, an incidence rate of less than one injury per 1000 h of training in 453 elite young British athletes was reported.[25] In general, the incidence of sports injuries seems to increase with age, approaching the incidence rate of senior players in the older children.

Schmidt and Höllwarth[35] compared the frequency of sport injuries according to their location. They found that 43.8% of all injuries occur in the upper extremity, 16% in the head, and 34.5% in the lower extremity, with a peak at age 12 years. Sprains, contusions, and lacerations account for the majority (60%) of injuries.[40,41]

In the lower extremity, the knee joint is most often involved.[42] In adults, knee injuries are responsible for 20%[43] of all football (soccer) injuries, and 13%[44] of all American football injuries. Ankle injuries are frequent as well and, in a study of gymnastics[45] and tennis,[46] they were even more common than knee injuries.

Traumatic injuries are often typical of a specific sport.[47] The pattern of injury has changed over the years and is related to sporting equipment.[7] Currently, an increased number of overuse injuries are being reported. O'Neill and Micheli[10,48,49] relate this to the fact that, in highly competitive sports, young athletes tend to train exclusively in their chosen sport. Overuse or chronic injuries as a result of repetitive microtrauma manifest as bursitis, tendinopathy, stress fracture, chondromalacia patellae, osteochondritis dissecans (OCD) and traction apophysitis,[9,10,26,48,50,51] and are more common in the lower extremity.[52] Risk factors may include training errors, muscle–tendon imbalance, anatomical alignments, footwear, and nutritional factors.[48] However, a prospective study involving 136 adult subjects could not prove any influence of flexibility, anthropometric characteristics, and malalignment of the lower limb on the total number of injuries.[53]

Injury characteristics and severity

Injuries can either occur acutely, and are associated with a macrotraumatic event, such as fractures and sprains, or arise gradually due to a repetitive microtraumatic event such as stress fracture, OCD, apophysitis, or tendinopathies.[51] Presentation for macrotrauma is invariably not delayed. There is typically a good clear history and mechanism of injury. On examination, there will be pain and, depending on the area of the body, swelling and deformity. This will allow the examiner to determine a likely diagnosis and whether any further investigations are warranted. Luckily, the majority of injuries are minor and require a short period of rest, analgesia, and compression prior to graduated formal rehabilitation. Microtrauma or overuse injuries invariably give a more insidious onset of symptoms that are typically related to activity. These symptoms will obviously depend very much on the anatomical location. In the younger individual, they may present purely with reduced performance or a limp. Exact identification of the anatomical area injured can be difficult. History and examination are vital. The type of sport played may give extra clues to the likely diagnosis, although further investigations may be required to confirm the diagnosis. Management generally requires a period of relative rest, with the child partaking in a different sport to allow healing while maintaining general condition. If this fails, then rest must be absolute, and referral for specialist assessment is advisable. Coaches are appropriately advised to observe attitude, behaviour, and development which may suggest neglect or abuse. This may be evident acutely or present as a chronic injury.

The severity of injuries spans broadly from sprains and contusions to death, and certain types of injury occur more commonly in specific sports. For example, spiral fractures of the tibia are the most common fracture in children with skiing injuries,[7,47] and in basketball ankle injuries are the most common injury seen.[54] Fortunately, the vast majority of sports injuries are minor and do not require medical attention. Very serious sports accidents in youth, such as brain or spinal cord damage, lesions of the heart, or submersions leading to invalidity or death, are exceptional.[38]

Ligament, muscle, and tendon injuries

Ligaments in youth are considerably more elastic than in adults.[11] Sprains are common, especially in lax individuals,[24] and are normally well tolerated.[26] Ankle sprains are more common in patients with weak and deconditioned peroneal muscles and pes cavus varus deformity.[11] In general, they should be managed conservatively with the use of orthotics if the hind foot is in varus. The first-line management in chronic ankle instability should be strengthening and proprioceptive training.[11,55] The prophylactic effect of external stabilization with strapping remains doubtful, and there seems to be no effect of high-top shoes in preventing ankle sprains in 622 college basketball players.[56]

Chronic compartment syndrome occurs even in young athletes[55] and is typical in running.[57] In these patients, compartment pressure monitoring, modification of activity, and fasciotomy should be considered.

Muscle injuries

Quadriceps contusions may produce local muscle bleeds associated with injury.[9,58] As in other muscle injuries, the injury may occur from a direct blow, sudden explosive action, or occasionally from a more trivial action. Management includes rest, ice, compression, elevation, and analgesia. Restriction of sport is essential followed by a graduated return to sport. Healing with fibrous tissue, the area may be prone to further injury. Occasionally a lump is palpable, and, if there are any concerns, magnetic resonance imaging (MRI) is useful to exclude neoplasia.[57,59]

Ligament injuries

Injuries of the knee most often result in physeal injuries because ligaments are stronger than growth plates. In one study, 90% of young athletes over the age of 12 years, with anterior cruciate ligaments (ACL) disruptions, were found to have intrasubstance tears.[60] An MRI scan may be performed to ascertain whether an ACL tear has indeed occurred. Although MRI has a good ability to predict ACL disruption, with a specificity of 95% and a sensitivity of 88%, clinical examination is still paramount.[61,62] Conservative management of ACL rupture leads to severe instability and poor knee function, and carries the risk of sustaining secondary injuries such as meniscal tears.[63–65] However, operative reconstruction of the ACL in skeletally immature patients has the potential to cause growth arrest or result in leg length discrepancy due to physeal damage. Complications such as femoral valgus deformity with arrest of the lateral femoral physis, tibial recurvatum with arrest of the tibial tubercle apophysis, genu valgum without arrest and leg length discrepancy have been reported.[66] As a result, several authors have advised delayed surgery, allowing time for skeletal maturity prior to reconstructing the ACL.[5,67,68]

Several studies have reported on ACL reconstruction in skeletally immature patients. Soft tissue grafts seem to have no influence on epiphyseal growth.[67,69] Smith and Tao[5] recommend hamstring tendon grafts using central tibial tunnel placement. Lo[70] found no leg length discrepancy in five patients, aged between 8 and 14 years, who underwent ACL reconstruction. More recently, in a series of 47 knees that underwent ACL reconstruction with a four strand hamstrings graft, no leg length discrepancy or growth arrest occurred.[63] Leg length discrepancies after ACL reconstruction may represent anatomically normal variants.[71,72] Despite this, it is essential that the risks and benefits of ACL reconstruction be analysed prior to surgery in skeletally immature patients.[66,73]

Medial cruciate ligaments (MCL) and lateral collateral ligament (LCL) injuries are managed non-operatively as in adults. Rarely, children may sustain tears in the posterolateral corner of the knee, and in such situations, surgery is indicated. Injuries of the posterior cruciate ligament, however, can be managed conservatively or operatively after the growth plates have closed.[5]

Tendinopathy

Tendinopathy is a common overuse injury of the lower extremity.[74] Most affected is the site of tendon insertion, the apophysis.[48] In most patients, partial rest and strapping are sufficient. Absolute immobilization leads to musculoskeletal atrophy.[11] Over the past few years, various new therapeutic options have been proposed for the management of tendinopathy. Despite the morbidity associated with tendinopathy, management is far from scientifically based, and many of the therapeutic options described and in common use lack hard scientific background. Physical therapy, rest, training modification, splintage, taping, cryotherapy, electrotherapy, shock-wave therapy, hyperthermia, pharmaceutical agents such as non-steroidal anti-inflammatory drugs and various peri-tendinous injections have been proposed. Most essentially follow the same principles. Managements that have been investigated with randomized controlled trials include non-steroidal anti-inflammatory medication, eccentric exercise, glyceryl trinitrate patches, electrotherapy (microcurrent and microwave), sclerosing injections, and shock-wave treatment. Despite this abundance of therapeutic options, very few randomized prospective, placebo, controlled trials exist to assist in choosing the best evidence-based management in children with tendinopathy.

A brief overview of the most common tendinopathies of the lower limb is given in Table 47.1.

Joint injuries

Hip

Direct forces such as dashboard injuries may dislocate the hip and fracture the acetabulum,[76] and such fracture dislocations are usually posterior.[77] After emergency reduction, patients should be kept in traction for 3–6 weeks. A haematoma can be evacuated.[78] MRI is recommended to exclude soft tissue interposition, and later to identify vascular necrosis of the femoral head.

The long-term consequences of hip dislocations can be serious: 50% of patients develop avascular necrosis of the femoral head, and if the acetabular limbus is torn, the stability of the hip joint can be seriously impaired.[79]

Knee

Patellar subluxation or dislocation occurs in 1 in 1000 children aged between 9 and 15 years[80] (Fig. 47.1). A common cause is a twisting injury, when the femur is twisted medially with the foot planted on the ground, or direct trauma. Patella alta, in which the patella rides high in the femoral groove, predisposes to patellar instability,[9] and may be accompanied by chronic low-grade knee pain due to patellofemoral stress syndrome.[48] Spontaneous reduction is possible, and the patient may present with an effusion at times due to injury of the ACL.[5] Management consists of immediate reduction of the dislocated patella. However, one in six patients will develop recurrent dislocations and will require realignment surgery. Skyline radiographs are recommended to exclude marginal osteochondral fractures which can result in loose bodies.[9]

Giving way of the knee on twisting should be considered of patellar origin until proved otherwise. Although meniscal problems in this age group are unusual and are generally associated with a discoid meniscus with a painless clonking noise before the tear, meniscal lesions in adolescents need to be considered and warrant arthroscopy.[81]

In the case of meniscal injuries, repair of torn menisci is recommended because of the extremely poor long-time results following meniscectomy in children.[80,82]

Haemarthrosis of the knee is often accompanied by severe ligamentous or meniscal injury.[83] In 70 young patients with haemarthrosis after acute trauma, Stanitski[84] found that 47% had ACL tears and 47% a meniscal tear. In adolescents (13–18 years), the

Table 47.1 Common forms of soft tissue injury of the lower limb[11,48,55,75]

Type	Reason	Remarks	Conservative management
Snapping hip	Stenosing tenosynovitis of the ileopsoas tendon	May be subluxation of the hip joint	Exercises to strengthen the hip extensors and abductors
Shin splint syndrome = medial tibial stress syndrome	Overuse of the soleus muscle on its attachment to the tibia	Often in runners	Rest, orthotics to prevent hyperpronation, running on soft surfaces
Posterior tibial tendinopathy	Repetitive excessive traction (with hyperpronation)	Often associated with excessive mid-foot pronation	Orthotics to control excessive pronation, cortisone injection, physiotherapy
Achilles tendinopathy	Excessive eccentric weight loading	Often bilateral and associated with calcaneal apophysitis	Conservative, eccentric exercises, shock-wave therapy
Peroneal tendinopathy	Impingement in the excessively pronated foot	—	Orthotics, cortisone injections
Tibialis anterior tendinopathy	Direct pressure in skates or ski boots	—	Alter footwear, vaseline, pad to reduce friction
Extensor hallucis longus tendinopathy	Tight heel cords with lack of ankle dorsiflexion results in increased activity of the extensor hallucis tendon	—	Heel lifts and orthotics to support the forefoot
Plantar fascitis	Predisposition: pes cavus or pes planus	—	Physiotherapy, orthotics, cortisone injections, alteration of activity, shock-wave therapy

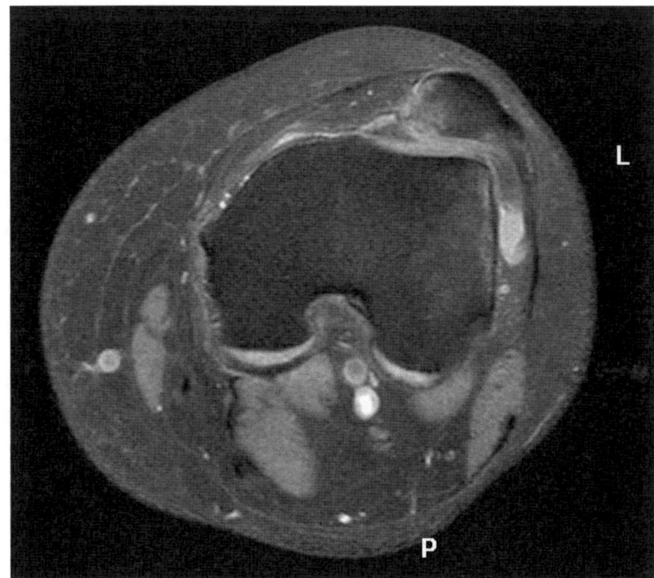

Fig. 47.1 Patellar subluxation

rate was 65% and 45%, respectively. Tightness may be a predisposing factor.[85]

Foot

Pain in the first metatarsal–cuneiform joint is rare and most often relates to hypermobility of the joint due to hind foot or subtalar joint pronation.[75] Orthotics limiting such hypermobility may be successful.

Problems of the first metatarso–phalangeal joint in children differ from those in adults due to the lack of arthritic changes.[86] These can occur in children with pes planus and hallux valgus, when a bunion rubs against the shoe. This appears to be a congenital abnormality rather than the results of poorly fitting shoes.[87] Management consists of orthotics and wider fitting shoes, and if symptoms persist, surgery after the growth plate has closed.[75]

Bone injuries

Epiphyseal injuries

The growing parts of the bone include the physis and the epiphysis. Two types of epiphyses are found in the extremities: traction and pressure.[88] Traction epiphyses (or apophyses) are located at the site of attachment of major muscle tendons to bone and are subjected primarily to tensile forces. The apophyses contribute to bone shape but not to longitudinal growth. As a result, acute or chronic injuries affecting traction growth plates are not generally associated with disruption of longitudinal bone growth.[88]

Pressure epiphyses are situated at the end of long bones and are subjected to compressive forces. The epiphyses of the distal femur and proximal tibia are examples of pressure epiphyses. The growth plate or physis is located between the epiphysis and metaphysis and is the essential mechanism of endochondral ossification.[88,89] By contrast with traction growth plates, injury to pressure epiphyses and their associated growth plates may result in growth disturbance. These are weaker areas, and therefore, predisposed to injury. Injuries of the epiphyseal plates have bee classified into five types.[90]

Type I injuries show a complete separation of the epiphysis from the metaphysis without any bone fracture. The germinal cells of the growth plate remain with the epiphysis, and the calcified layer remains with the metaphysis. In type II, the most common physeal injuries, the line of separation extends along the growth plate, then out through a portion of the metaphysis, producing a triangular-shaped metaphyseal fragment sometimes referred to as the Thurston Holland sign. Type III, which is intra-articular, extends from the joint surface to the weak zone of the growth plate and then extends along the plate to its periphery (Fig. 47.2). In type IV, often involving the distal humerus, a fracture extends from the joint surface through the epiphysis, across the full thickness of the growth plate and through a portion of the metaphysis, thereby producing a complete split. In type V, a relatively uncommon injury, there is compression of the growth plate, thereby extinguishing further growth.

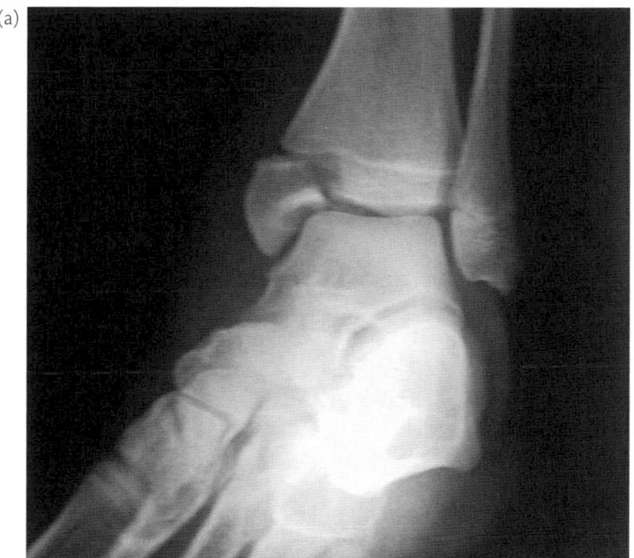

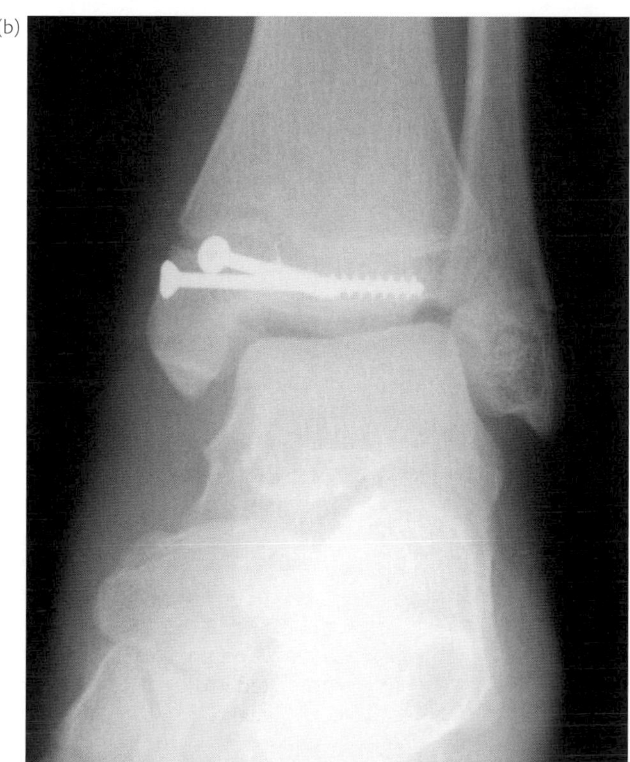

Fig. 47.2 (a) A type III injury of the distal tibia. (b) Open reduction and internal fixation of type III injury of the distal tibia, without damage to the cartilage plate.

Prognosis for types I and II fractures is good if the germinal cells remain with the epiphysis, and circulation is unchanged. However, these injury types are not as innocuous as originally believed, and can be associated with risk of growth impairment.[91,92] Type III injuries have a good prognosis if the blood supply in the separated portion of the epiphysis is still intact and the fracture is not displaced. Surgery can be necessary to restore the joint surface to normal. In type IV injuries, surgery is needed to restore the joint surface to normal and to perfectly align the growth plate. Type IV injuries have a poor prognosis unless the growth plate is completely and accurately realigned. A diagnosis of Salter V injury can be difficult at the time of injury. Growth can be disturbed, and given the nature of the injury, may only become obvious at a later stage. Physeal injuries can be difficult to diagnose by radiographs. Therefore, if clinically suspected, protection of the limb with a cast and repeat radiographs and examination after two weeks are useful.[93]

Fractures

Pelvis, femur, patella, and tibia

Pelvic fractures are mostly found in polytrauma patients and require careful investigation of internal organs and, in most patients, external fixation. In children, they rarely occur in sports. Similarly, physeal fractures of the proximal femur and acetabulum are seldom associated with sports[76,94] and are often a result of high-energy trauma. Open reduction and internal fixation with pins across the epiphysis is recommended. Patients and their families should be counselled regarding the high risk of avascular necrosis of the femoral head and of premature closure of the epiphysis in such injuries.[76] The risk of avascular necrosis varies with the location of the fracture, and it is possible to identify four categories: transepiphyseal fractures carry a 80–100% risk, proximal femoral neck fractures a 50–80% risk, distal femoral neck fractures a 30–50% risk, and intertrochanteric fractures a 10% risk.[78] Pseudarthrosis, also a result of the limited blood supply to the femoral head, carries a 40% risk. Also common is coxa vara, a complication of early closure of the medial epiphysis, with a 25% risk.[78] Anatomical reduction and internal fixation are necessary to avoid these complications.

Slipping of the upper femoral epiphysis occurs mainly in overweight boys with underdeveloped gonads, and in tall thin children during the growth spurt between 10 and 16 years. The child frequently presents after an injury in which the thigh has apparently become suddenly painful. Close questioning often reveals some premonitory discomfort. Knee pain is often the presenting complaint because of the nerve supply of the hip, and many children are referred to an orthopaedic clinic with a painful knee for unknown causes. The physical signs consist of loss of internal rotation or even fixed external rotation and shortening of the leg, with external rotation of the foot while standing. With the child supine on the couch, internal rotation is restricted or impossible. Such physical signs demand a radiograph of the hip. The deformity is much easier to see in the lateral view. Surgical management to prevent further displacement consists of internal fixation of the upper femoral epiphysis in situ without attempting to reduce it. Despite appropriate and prompt management, avascular necrosis and chondrolysis may ensue, putting an end to an athletic career, and the hip at risk of secondary osteoarthritis.[95] Hypothyroidism and renal osteodystrophy may be associated with epiphysiolysis[95] and should be excluded. Operative management is generally performed on an emergency basis and pinning in situ is recommended.[96]

Femoral fractures can often be managed conservatively, especially in younger children. Shaft fractures are often managed with the application of a spica cast after an initial period of traction[97,98] because deviation of the femoral axis will correct spontaneously. In older children and adolescents, however, operative management with external fixation, plating or intramedullary nailing is indicated.[98] Femoral nailing carries a risk of femoral head necrosis; therefore, some authors prefer external fixation or flexible unreamed nails.[78,99,100] In anatomically reduced femoral-shaft fractures, leg length discrepancy is also possible because of the increased blood supply to the fracture area,[78] which results in increased growth of the fractured limb.

Tibial shaft fractures are the most common fractures in skiing.[7,47] Management should be conservative for closed fractures, while for open or complicated fractures, anatomical reposition and stable fixation is necessary[78,101] (Fig. 47.3). Osteochondral fractures around the knee are accompanied mostly by severe haemarthrosis.[83]

Table 47.2 shows an overview of the different pattern and management possibilities of femoral, tibial, and patellar fractures.

Ankle

Symptomatic medial malleolar ossifications should be considered in the differential diagnosis of ankle pain in young athletes. On radiographs, spherical ossicles are visible, and conservative management is appropriate.[84]

Ankle fractures are caused by major violence and, if undisplaced, they do not need internal fixation. Tillaux–Chaput fractures are Salter–Harris type III fracture of the distal tibia, with an epiphyseal fragment connected to the syndesmosis. This fracture occurs in young athletes close to the end of puberty and requires internal fixation.[78]

The most common fractures of the ankle after twisting[87] are type I or II Salter injuries with an open distal fibular epiphysis.[9,91] These fractures often close up, leaving only tenderness over the epiphysis with normal radiographs. Stress radiographs, however, usually reveal the underlying pathology and, according to the age of the patient, internal fixation should be considered.[9,11,98,102,103]

An overview of ankle fractures is given in Table 47.3.

Foot

The most common complaint is heel pain due to Sever's lesion (Table 47.5). Forefoot problems are common, especially after chronic overload. Osteochondroses typically occur around the tarsal and metatarsal bones of the foot. Freiberg's lesion consists of collapse of the articular surface and subchondral bone of the metatarsal head.[87] Most commonly the second metatarsal is affected (68%), but it is also found in the third (27%) or fourth (5%) metatarsal.[104] The collapse is related to reduced blood supply caused by mechanical overload. The main principle of management is to redistribute load, with help from orthotics if necessary.[78,87] Late surgery in adulthood can also be considered for resistant cases.[105,106] Avascular necrosis of the tarsal navicular bone, Köhler's lesion, results in localized pain. It is diagnosed by radiographically increased density of the navicular.[87] Management

(a)

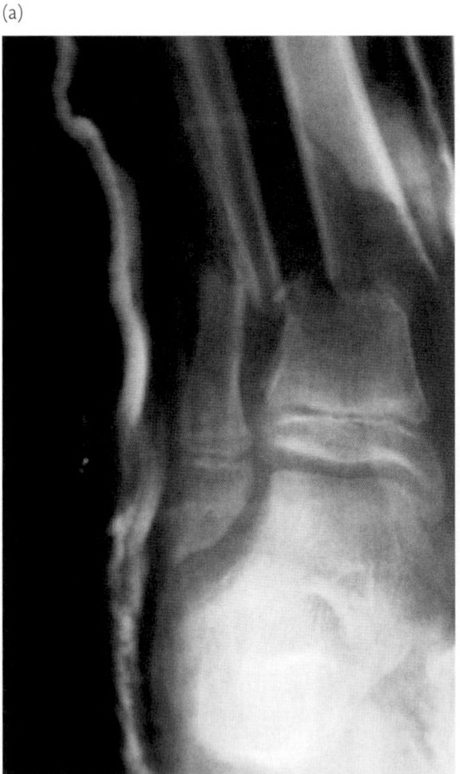

(b)

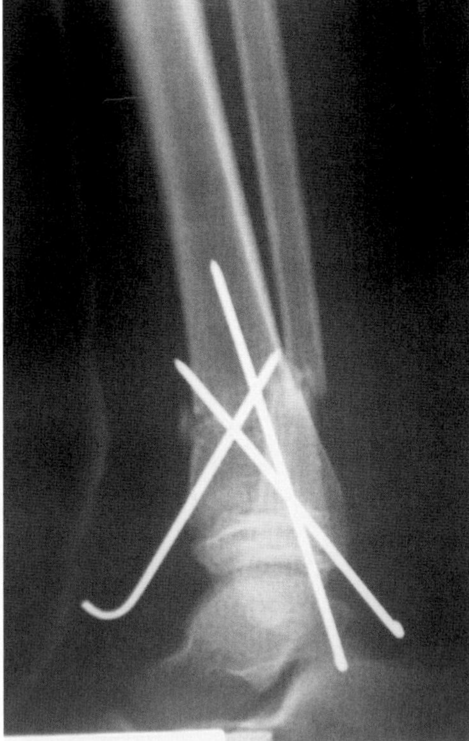

Fig. 47.3 (a) Fracture of the distal diaphysis of tibia and fibula. (b) The surgical management of the fracture of the distal diaphysis of tibia and fibula.

Table 47.2 Common fractures and epiphyseal injuries of femur, patella, and tibia[9,83,97]

Type	Cause	Remarks	Management
Proximal femur fractures	Direct trauma	High risk of femoral head necrosis, pseudarthrosis, and coxa vara	ORIF[a] and non-weight bearing for 3 to 6 months
Femoral stress fractures	Repetitive overload	Rare crescendo painm initial radiographs may be normal	Reduction of activity to a pain-free level
Distal femoral physeal fracture	High-velocity trauma	Uncommon in sports often Salter V fractures with disturbance of leg length growth	ORIF for Salter III and IV
Patellar fractures	Direct trauma or avulsion	—	ORIF in the case of patellar surface disruption
Sleeve fractures of the patella	Periosteum is stripped downwards in continuity with the tendon resulting in double patella appearance	Diagnosis usually missed	Early surgery
Proximal tibia fracture	Direct trauma	Often with an avulsion fracture of the patellar tendon, injury to peroneal nerve possible	ORIF if displaced
Tibial shaft fracture	Direct or twisting trauma		Conservative, if displaced or open: ORIF
Tibial stress fractures	Repetitive overload	Crescendo pain, initial radiographs may be normal	Reduction of activity to a pain-free level for 8 to 12 weeks
Tibial eminence fracture (avulsion of tibial spine)	Direct trauma or forceful hyperextension with rotation	Complication: ACL laxity	ORIF for displaced fractures
Tibial tuberosity fracture	Intensive jumping	Predisposition from Osgood-Schlatter`s lesion	ORIF in displaced fractures

[a]legend: ORIF-open reduction and internal fixation.

Table 47.3 Ankle fractures and epiphyseal injuries[9,11]

Type	Predisposing factors	Conservative management	Operative management
Epiphyseal fracture	Weak and deconditioned tendons Pes cavus Tarsal coalition	Early motion/taping, casting, aircast splint	ORIF for Salter III and IV
Osteochondral fractures	—	Early motion, non-weight bearing	Occasionally but possible, normally undisplaced detached fragment: ORIF
Chronic osteochondral fracture (without displacement):	—	Casting	Failure of nonsurgical management: surgical debridement, forage, grafting
Isolated fibula fracture	Varus deformity of the hind foot	Casting or splint	Displaced: ORIF
Fibular fracture with medial malleolus fracture	—	Casting in anatomical position	Unstable fracture needs ORIF
Ankle mortis fracture without displacement	—	—	Unstable fracture needs ORIF
Triplane fracture of the distal tibia	—	—	ORIF required

is usually conservative with orthotics or a period in plaster.[107,108] Generally, it takes 2–3 years to return to normal.

An overview of the most common bony injuries of the foot is given in Table 47.4.

Avulsion fractures and apophysitis

Avulsion fractures are common. They arise because of sudden intense muscular traction exerted on the immature skeleton. Tendons are relatively stronger than bones and avulsion of growth plates are the result of chronic or acute traction. Osgood–Schlatter lesion, a traction apophysitis of the tibial tubercle,[109] and Sever's lesion (Fig. 47.4), a traction apophysitis of the calcaneal apophysis, are the most common traction apophysitis.[51] They are common in boys around the time of growth spurts.[48] The onset of pain is commonly induced by a higher-than-normal amount of physical activity. Conservative management is normally sufficient.

The anterior inferior iliac spine tends to fail during football when the kicking foot is suddenly blocked, as happens in a tackle (Fig. 47.5). More often, when the foot hits the ground, the anterior inferior iliac spine is pulled off by the reflected head of rectus femoris. In similar circumstances, the psoas muscle can avulse the lesser trochanter. The whole apophyseal plate of the ischium can separate through the powerful pull of the hamstrings. This can happen in cross-country running when the ditch being jumped is wider than expected, and the leading leg is overstretched. More rarely, the anterior superior iliac spine can be avulsed by the action of sartorius in a bad gymnastics vault landing. The whole iliac crest apophysis can also be pulled off by the abdominal muscles, although displacement is uncommon.

Typically, the young athlete gives a history of severe, immediate, and well-localized pain, and the appropriate radiographic views confirm the diagnosis. As the avulsions are deep, cryotherapy is unhelpful, and oral analgesia is the preferred option for pain relief, with rest and gradual return to activity as pain permits. Immediate surgery is not indicated, and late surgery is rarely required despite occasional dramatic radiographic changes.

Table 47.4 Bony foot injuries[9,11,75,83]

Type	Predisposition	Conservative management	Operative management
Sesamoiditis of the first metatarsal	Pes cavus	Orthotics, metatarsal pad	—
Metatarsalgia of the metatarso–phalangeal joints	Morton`s foot with a short first ray	Modified activity, metatarsal pad	—
Freiberg's lesion	Long second metatarsal	Modified activity, insert to unload the metatarsal head, rigid-soled shoes	Late surgery
Fracture of the metatarsal	—	Plaster casting	—
Stress fracture of 2nd to 4th metatarsals	Pes cavus	Decrease activity, modify footwear	—
Navicular stress fracture	Kohler's lesion cricket bowling	Activity reduction, casting for 4–6 weeks	Occasionally screw fixation
Jones fracture of the fifth metatarsal	—	Plaster casting	Surgery for non-union
Painful tarsal coalition	Bony or cartilaginous bar in the hind foot	Physiotherapy, alteration of activity or footwear	Late surgery

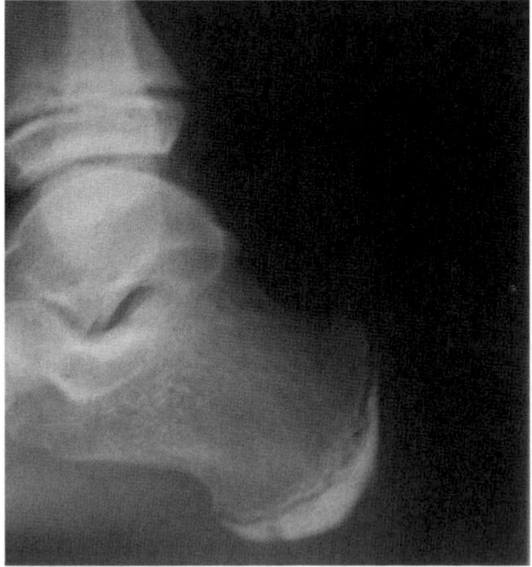
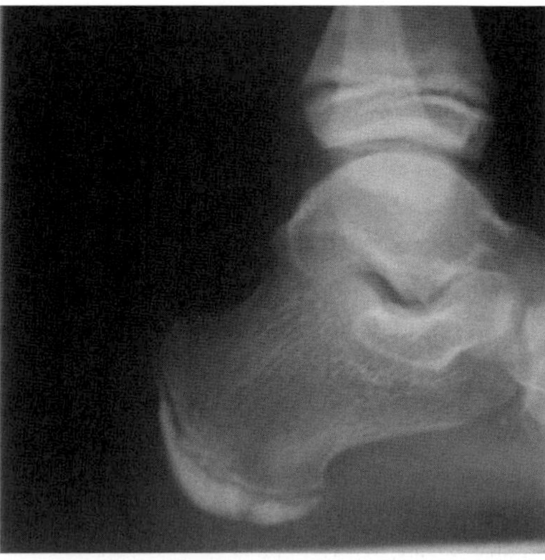

Fig. 47.4 Bilateral Sever's disease.

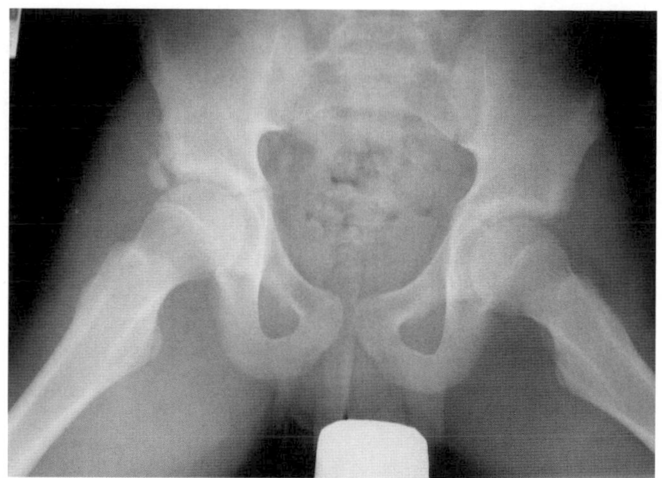

Fig. 47.5 Avulsion of the anterior inferior iliac spine.

Sinding–Larsen–Johansson lesion is a syndrome of tenderness and radiographic fragmentation localized at the inferior pole of the patella. The lesion can be considered a calcific tendinopathy in an avulsed portion of the patellar tendon and is self-limiting.

A mature tibial tubercle forms from ossification centres in the epiphysis. The pulling action of the patellar tendon may cause inflammation and pain, resulting in the clinical entity known as Osgood–Schlatter's lesion. Osgood–Schlatter's lesion occurs in girls between 8 and 13 years of age, and in boys between 10 and 15 years of age. Boys are nearly twice as commonly affected as girls, possibly because of their higher activity levels. The onset of pain is commonly induced by a higher-than-normal amount of physical activity. Conservative management is normally sufficient.

Sever's lesion presents with well-localized, activity-related pain at the tip of the heel and radiographic fragmentation of the calcaneal apophysis. Sever's lesion may result from intensive training and improper footwear.[48] Some authors consider Sever's lesion to be a form of stress fracture, but there is often a similar radiographic appearance of the other asymptomatic side. Severs's lesion is often bilateral.[48] The pain responds to rest and a shock absorber under the heel. Table 47.5 presents an overview.

Osteochondritis dissecans

Osteochondritis dissecans (OCD) can be due to intense physical activity[110] causing repetitive microtrauma.[48,111] This can be shown by the rate of OCD being three times more prevalent in active boys than in girls around puberty, and also in competitive sports involving jumping.[78] OCD usually occurs in the lateral aspect of the medial femoral condyle, femoral head, and middle third of the lateral border of the talus.[78,112,113] The radiographic diagnosis can be confirmed by MRI and, if necessary, definitive management can be performed by arthroscopy. In general, management is conservative in stable lesions and, with larger fragments, arthroscopic removal of intra-articular loose bodies or fixation is recommended. The long-term prognosis associated with excision of the fragment is poor because of an increased risk of osteoarthritis.[114]

Stress fractures

Stress fractures are difficult to diagnose[48] and are often associated with training errors.[10] Endogenous factors such as body size, sex, diet, hormonal status, and anatomical factors are important as well, but difficult to prove.[23] Stress fractures occur more often in women, in particular amenorrhoeic athletes with decreased bone density.[29,30] Stress fractures occur more often in organized sports.[76]

Typical locations are the metatarsals, the middle and proximal tibia, the proximal femur, and the calcaneus.[48,78] A study of 320 stress fractures reported that 49% of them occur in the tibia, 25% in the tarsal bones, and 9% in the metatarsals.[115] Varus alignment seems to play an important role in lower-extremity stress fractures. Stress fractures of the navicular are associated with a short first metatarsal, metatarsal adductus, and limited ankle dorsiflexion and subtalar motion.[116]

Diagnosis may be difficult on plain radiographs taken at the time of onset of pain, and therefore, should be repeated 2–3 weeks later. At this stage, however, the rapid periosteal response can be confused with infections or tumours. MRI[117] or computed tomography (CT)[118,119] may be helpful. If the clinical picture is not typical, a technetium scan is indicated.[120] Primary management consists of immobilization with exercise within the limitations of pain.

Legg–Calve–Perthes disease

Legg–Calve–Perthes disease, a form of avascular necrosis of the femoral head, occurring mainly between 5 and 10 years of age. The condition is probably due to two or more episodes of raised intra-articular pressure,[121] the influence of sports is doubtful.[9] It presents as an irritable hip with sclerosis of the femoral head. In general, the more complete the lesion, the worse the outcome. On the other hand, the earlier its onset, the better the outcome. If Legg–Calve–Perthes disease does occur in a young athlete, a temporary interruption or limitation of sports activities is necessary. In the early phases of Legg–Calve–Perthes disease, plain radiographs may be normal, but bone scanning may show decreased uptake in the femoral head. MRI does provide better evaluation of involvement in the early stages of Legg–Calve–Perthes disease than plain radiography, but its cost-effectiveness needs to be assessed.[122] Management is either conservative or surgical, depending on various indications and the stage of the disease.[123] Despite its benignity, investigations are mandatory to exclude the rare cases of tuberculosis or bone tumour that may present as an irritable hip. A larger joint effusion is generally a sign of sepsis, usually caused by *Staphylococcus aureus*. In this instance, the young athlete will generally present with pyrexia, malaise, and severe fatigue. Bone scanning shows increased uptake at both sides of the joint. If pus is aspirated, the hip should be explored surgically, and antibiotics started.

Tarsal coalitions and sinus tarsi problems

Tarsal coalitions (Fig. 47.6) can cause pain associated with physical activity, and should be suspected after a history of multiple ankle sprains and subtalar stiffness on examination.[87] Most commonly, the subtalar joint is affected, followed by coalition between the calcaneus and navicular.[124] The coalition can be fibrous, cartilaginous, or osseous, and is accompanied by loss of supination. Management consists of casting in the painful stage and surgery for the calcaneal navicular coalition for young children at a later stage.[75]

Table 47.5 Avulsion fractures and apophysitis

Location		Remarks	Management
Pelvis and hip	Anterior inferior iliac spine Lesser trochanter Iliac crest whole ischium	Caused by psoas Caused by psoas Caused by sartorius, abductors, and hamstrings	Conservative: non-weight bearing for 3 weeks Operative: considered when long fragments are displaced
Knee	Osgood Schlatter: traction apophysitis of the tibial tubercle	—	Conservative Operative: when pain persists with excision of intratendinous ossicles
	Sinding–Larsen–Johannson: lower patella pole	—	Conservative
Ankle and foot	Avulsion of a bony fragment of the anterior tibio-fibular ligament from the distal tibial epiphysis	Tillaux fracture	Internal fixation
	Iselin's lesion: apophysitis of the fifth metatarsal	Rare	Conservative
	Sever`s lesion	Excessive tensile loads in tension. Predisposition: tight heel cord, often associated with Achilles tendinopathy, age is usually 8 to 13 years	Conservative (shock absorber), avoid barefoot walking: physiotherapy, stretching and strengthening, and casting, if persistent

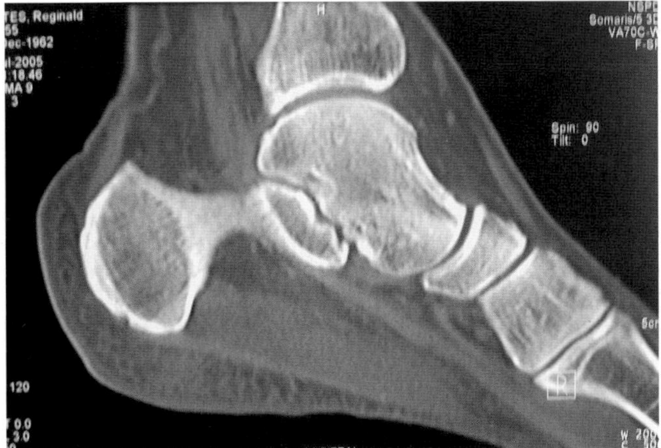

Fig. 47.6 CT scan of a tarsal coalition

Sinus tarsi syndrome often occurs after starting a new activity.[75] Patients show tenderness in the sulcus of the sinus tarsi with swelling, at time. Management should consist of limiting pronation by orthotics[75,87] and, if the pain persists, surgery is indicated.[49]

Navicular problems

Navicular pain in young athletes is common and is often accompanied by irritation of the tibialis posterior tendon insertion. It can also be caused by an accessory navicular bone. Excessive pronation can be limited by the use of orthotics.[75]

Prevention

The epidemiological approach in sports traumatology aims to quantify the occurrence of sports injuries in relation to who is affected by injuries, where and when these injuries have occurred, and what is their outcome (descriptive approach). Efforts are also made to explain why and how such injuries occur, to develop strategies to limit their occurrence, and to prevent them (analytical approach).[125] Preventing sports injuries in young individuals is important to reduce the short- and long-term social and economic consequences.[38] The epidemiological approach implies that injuries do not happen purely by chance.[126]

Most of the preventive measures suggested in the literature have arisen from descriptive research and have not been derived from risk factors that have been substantiated as defensible injury predictors through correlational or experimental research.[125] Not only will children have their own risk factors but so will their particular sports. There has already been widespread involvement in assessing general risks and trends that result in children's injuries.[127,128] Once the analytical evidence points to an association between certain risk factors and injury, thereby establishing a degree of predictability for those participants who are likely to sustain an injury, a method of intervention can be devised for prevention.[129] Intervention can be either therapeutic, using tapes or braces to an injured area resulting in reduction in re-injuries, or preventive, in which an agent or procedure is tried on athletes free from injury and is evaluated by recording the reduction of risk of injury.

Sports-specific studies, for example, skiing, baseball, skating, tennis, or gymnastics, all have similar conclusions regarding safety barriers or run-offs, adequate supervision, appropriate warm-ups, and protective equipment.[13,130–133] Up to approximately one-third of injuries may be preventable. Many of these parallel adult sporting commonsense issues. Perceived insight into injury risk has not been reported. Issues specific to children include more fair matching of size, weight and height, appropriate supervision, properly fitting equipment for young individuals, and limiting external pressure imposed by parents and coaches. This is a difficult balance to achieve.

The value of preparticipation screening is to limit the participation of the most susceptible individuals, and continues to be evaluated.[134,135] Balance, for example, can be used as a predictor of future ankle injury.[134] Prevention is based on defining the fitness and flexibility required as well as the general medical status. These variables need to be measured appropriately and advice given to maintain or improve physical status. Pre-season conditioning works well to reduce early-season injuries.[136] Well-reported successful cases of injury prevention have followed a number of important working parties. Perhaps the most well known include reduction in the rates of quadriplegia following the banning of spearing in American football, the use of appropriate head and face guards in ice hockey, breakaway bases in baseball,[137] appropriate ball selection, limiting repetitive actions, for example, in throwing and bowling sports and appropriate fluid management in hot weather. However, not all such interventions are entirely successful; for example, the use of chest protectors in baseball does give extra protection, but commotio cordis has still been reported.[138]

Conclusions

We have given an overview on sports-related injuries of the lower limb in children with emphasis on the management. Overall, injuries in children are uncommon, and although their incidence increases with age, most are self-limiting and have no long-term effects. Any sport can cause musculoskeletal injuries, and the specific pattern and location of injuries of each sport should be known by health professionals. Training programmes and performance standards should take into account the biological age of the participants, and their physical and psychological immaturity, more than their chronological age. A deep knowledge of the different aspects of training, including duration, intensity, frequency, and recovery, are needed to avoid serious damage to the musculoskeletal system of athletic children.

Physical injury is an inherent risk in sports participation, and to a certain extent, must be considered an inevitable cost of athletic training and competition. However, coaches and parents can minimize the risk of injury by ensuring the proper selection of sporting events, using appropriate equipment, enforcing rules, using safe playing conditions and providing adequate supervision. Although injuries in young athletes are sustained, it is important to balance the negative effects of sports injuries with the many social, psychological, and health benefits that a serious commitment to sport brings.[139–141]

Summary

- Physical activity seems to play a significant role in the well-being of a child, but there is no definitive evidence to indicate that training affects either positively or negatively the growth and maturation in young athletes.
- The actual incidence of injury in children's sports is very difficult, if not impossible, to determine.
- Imbalances in the musculoskeletal system of children may influence the rate of occurrence of injuries. Common conditions such as pes cavus, pes planus, and calcaneus valgus may play a role in the aetiology of some injuries.
- With growth spurts, there is a decrease in flexibility due to relative bone lengthening. This predisposes to injury in the absence of appropriate stretching exercises, prior to commencing sport.
- We give an overview on sports-related injuries of the lower limb in children with emphasis on the management.
- Most injuries in children are self-limiting and have no long-term effects.
- Any sport can cause musculoskeletal injuries, and the specific pattern and location of injuries of each sport should be known by health professionals.
- Training programmes and performance standards should take into account the biological age of the participants, and their physical and psychological immaturity, more than their chronological age. A deep knowledge of the different aspects of training, including duration, intensity, frequency, and recovery, are needed to avoid serious damage to the musculoskeletal system of athletic children.

References

1. Shephard RJ (1984). Physical activity and the child. *Sports Med* **1**, 205–33.
2. Davidson RG, Taunton JE (1987). Achilles tendinitis. *Med Sports Sci* **23**, 71–9.
3. Caine D, Caine C, Maffulli N (2006). Incidence and distribution of pediatric sport-related injuries. *Clin J Sport Med* **16**, 500–13.
4. Maffulli N, Baxter-Jones AD, Grieve A (2005). Long term sport involvement and sport injury rate in elite young athletes. *Arch Dis Child* **90**, 525–7.
5. Smith AD, Tao SS (1995). Knee injuries in young athletes. *Clin Sports Med* **14**, 629–50.
6. Klenerman L (1994). ABC of sports medicine. Musculoskeletal injuries in child athletes. *BMJ* **308**, 1556–9.
7. Deibert MC, Aronsson DD, Johnson RJ, Ettlinger CF, Shealy JE (1998). Skiing injuries in children, adolescents, and adults. *J Bone Joint Surg Am* **80**, 25–32.
8. Kruger-Franke M, Pforringer W (1991). [Epiphyseal injuries of the lower extremity in sports]. *Sportverletz Sportschaden* **5**, 37–41.
9. Maffulli N, Baxter-Jones AD (1995). Common skeletal injuries in young athletes. *Sports Med* **19**, 137–49.
10. Micheli LJ, Fehlandt AF, Jr. (1992). Overuse injuries to tendons and apophyses in children and adolescents. *Clin Sports Med* **11**, 713–26.
11. Stanish WD (1995). Lower leg, foot, and ankle injuries in young athletes. *Clin Sports Med* **14**, 651–68.
12. Tipton CM, Matthes RD, Maynard JA, Carey RA (1975). The influence of physical activity on ligaments and tendons. *Med Sci Sports* **7**, 165–75.
13. Castiglia PT (1995). Sports injuries in children. *J Pediatr Health Care* **9**, 32–3
14. Baxter-Jones AD (1995). Growth and development of young athletes. Should competition levels be age related? *Sports Med* **20**, 59–64.
15. Baxter-Jones AD, Helms P, Maffulli N, Baines-Preece JC, Preece M (1995). Growth and development of male gymnasts, swimmers, soccer and tennis players: A longitudinal study. *Ann Hum Biol* **22**, 381–94.
16. Baxter-Jones AD, Maffulli N (2003). Parental influence on sport participation in elite young athletes. *J Sports Med Phys Fitness* **43**, 250–5.
17. Wojtys EM (1987). Sports injuries in the immature athlete. *Orthop Clin North Am* **18**, 689–708.
18. Pillemer FG, Micheli LJ (1988). Psychological considerations in youth sports. *Clin Sports Med* **7**, 679–89.
19. Wilkins K (1980). The uniqueness of the young athlete: Musculoskeletal injuries. *Am J Sports Med* **8**, 377–82.

20. Micheli LJ, Glassman R, Klein M (2000). The prevention of sports injuries in children. *Clin Sports Med* **19**, 821–34.
21. Purvis JM, Burke RG (2001). Recreational injuries in children: Incidence and prevention. *J Am Acad Orthop Surg* **9**, 365–74.
22. Baxter-Jones AD, Maffulli N (2002). Intensive training in elite young female athletes. Effects of intensive training on growth and maturation are not established. *Br J Sports Med* **36**, 13–15.
23. Krivickas LS (1997). Anatomical factors associated with overuse sports injuries. *Sports Med* **24**, 132–46.
24. Lysens RJ, Ostyn MS, Vanden Auweele Y, Lefevre J, Vuylsteke M, Renson L (1989). The accident-prone and overuse-prone profiles of the young athlete. *Am J Sports Med* **17,** 612–19.
25. Maffulli N, King JB, Helms P (1994). Training in elite young athletes (the Training of Young Athletes (TOYA) Study): Injuries, flexibility and isometric strength. *Br J Sports Med* **28**, 123–36.
26. Stanitski CL (1989). Common injuries in preadolescent and adolescent athletes. Recommendations for prevention. *Sports Med* **7**, 32–41.
27. Pope RP, Herbert RD, Kirwan JD, Graham, BJ (2000). A randomized trial of preexercise stretching for prevention of lower-limb injury. *Med Sci Sports Exerc* **32**, 271–7.
28. Shrier I (2000). Stretching before exercise: An evidence based approach. *Br J Sports Med* **34**, 324–5.
29. Barrow GW, Saha S (1988) Menstrual irregularity and stress fractures in collegiate female distance runners. *Am J Sports Med* **16**, 209–16.
30. Jones BH, Bovee MW, Harris JM 3rd, Cowan DN (1993). Intrinsic risk factors for exercise-related injuries among male and female army trainees. *Am J Sports Med* **21**, 705–10.
31. Faigenbaum AD (2000). Strength training for children and adolescents. *Clin Sports Med* **19,** 593–619.
32. Caine DJ, Maffulli N (2005). Epidemiology of children's individual sports injuries. An important area of medicine and sport science research. *Med Sport Sci* **48**, 1–7.
33. Maffulli N, Caine D (2005). The Epidemiology of Children's Team Sports Injuries. *Med Sport Sci* **49**, 1–8.
34. Crompton B, Tubbs N (1977). A survey of sports injuries in Birmingham. *Br J Sports Med* **11**, 12–15.
35. Schmidt B, Höllwarth ME (1989). Sportunfälle im Kindes- und Jugendalter. *Zeitschrift für Kinderchirurgie* **44**, 357–62.
36. Zaricznyj B, Shattuck LJ, Mast TA, Robertson RV, D'Elia G (1980). Sports-related injuries in school-aged children. *Am J Sports Med* **8**, 318–24.
37. Sahlin Y (1990). Sport accidents in childhood. *Br J Sports Med* **24**, 40–4.
38. Tursz A, Crost M (1986). Sports-related injuries in children. A study of their characteristics, frequency, and severity, with comparison to other types of accidental injuries. *Am J Sports Med* **14**, 294–9.
39. Baxter-Jones A, Maffulli N, Helms P (1993). Low injury rates in elite athletes. *Arch Dis Child* **68**, 130–2.
40. Cotta H, Steinbrück K (1982). *Sportverletzungen und sportschäden im breitensport*, pp. 703–10. Kongreßband Deutscher-Sportärzte-Kongreß Köln.
41. Bridgman SA, Clement D, Downing A, Walley G, Phair I, Maffulli N (2003). Population based epidemiology of ankle sprains attending accident and emergency units in the West Midlands of England, and a survey of UK practice for severe ankle sprains. *Emerg Med J* **20**, 508–10.
42. DeHaven KE, Lintner DM (1986). Athletic injuries: Comparison by age, sport, and gender. *Am J Sports Med* **14**, 218–24.
43. Ekstrand J, Gillquist J (1983). Soccer injuries and their mechanisms: A prospective study. *Med Sci Sports Exerc* **15**, 267–70.
44. Pritchett JW (1982). A statistical study of knee injuries due to football in high-school athletes. *J Bone Joint Surg Am* **64**, 240–2.
45. Lindner KJ, Caine DJ (1990). Injury patterns of female competitive club gymnasts. *Can J Sport Sci* **15**, 254–61.
46. Hutchinson MR, Laprade RF, Burnett QM, 2nd, Moss R, Terpstra J (1995). Injury surveillance at the USTA Boys' Tennis Championships: A 6-yr study. *Med Sci Sports Exerc* **27**, 826–30.
47. Ungerholm S, Gierup J, Lindsjo U, Magnusson A (1985). Skiing injuries in children: Lower leg fractures. *Int J Sports Med* **6**, 292–7.
48. O'Neill DB, Micheli LJ (1988). Overuse injuries in the young athlete. *Clin Sports Med* **7**, 591–610.
49. O'Neill DB, Micheli LJ (1989). Tarsal coalition. A followup of adolescent athletes. *Am J Sports Med* **17**, 544–9.
50. Dalton SE (1992). Overuse injuries in adolescent athletes. *Sports Med* **13**, 58–70.
51. Maffulli N (1990). Intensive training in young athlete. The orthopaedic surgeon's viewpoint. *Sports Med* **9**, 229–43.
52. Larkins PA (1991). The little athlete. *Aust Fam Physician* **20**, 973–4, 976–8.
53. Twellaar M, Verstappen FT, Huson A, van Mechelen W (1997). Physical characteristics as risk factors for sports injuries: A four year prospective study. *Int J Sports Med* **18**, 66–71.
54. Emerson RJ (1993). Basketball knee injuries and the anterior cruciate ligament. *Clin Sports Med* **12**, 317–28.
55. Bernhardt DT, Landry GL (1995). *Sport injuries in young athletes.* Advances in pediatrics, Mosby-Year Book, St Louis.
56. Barrett JR, Tanji JL, Drake C, Fuller D, Kawasaki RI, Fenton RM (1993). High- versus low-top shoes for the prevention of ankle sprains in basketball players. A prospective randomized study. *Am J Sports Med* **21**, 582–5.
57. Blue JM, Matthews LS (1997). Leg injuries. *Clin Sports Med* **16**, 467–78.
58. Maffulli N (1992). The growing child in sport. *Br Med Bul* **148**, 561–8.
59. Bernhardt DT, Landry GL (1995). Sports injuries in young athletes. *Adv Pediatr* **42**, 465–500.
60. Kellenberger R, von Laer L (1990). Nonosseous lesions of the anterior cruciate ligaments in childhood and adolescence. *Prog Pediatr Surg* **25**, 123–31.
61. McDermott MJ, Bathgate B, Gillingham BL, Hennrikus WL (1998). Correlation of MRI and arthroscopic diagnosis of knee pathology in children and adolescents. *J Pediatr Orthop* **18**, 675–8.
62. Lee K, Siegel MJ, Lau DM, Hildebolt CF, Matava MJ (1999). Anterior cruciate ligament tears: MR imaging-based diagnosis in a pediatric population. *Radiology* **213**, 697–704.
63. Aichroth PM, Patel DV, Zorrilla P (2002). The natural history and treatment of rupture of the anterior cruciate ligament in children and adolescents. A prospective review. *J Bone Joint Surg Am* **84B**, 38–41.
64. Shea K, Apel P, Pfeiffer R (2003). Anterior cruciate ligament injury in paediatric and adolescent patients: a review of basic science and clinical research. *Sports Med* **33**, 455–71.
65. Kapoor B, Clement DJ, Kirkley A, Maffulli N (2004). Current practice in the management of anterior cruciate ligament injuries in the United Kingdom. *Br J Sports Med* **38**, 542–4.
66. Kocher MS, Hovis WD, Hawkins RJ (2002). Management and complications of anterior cruciate ligament injuries in skeletally immature patients: A survey of the Herodicus Society and The ACL Study Group. *J Pediatr Orthop* **22**, 452–7.
67. McCarroll JR, Shelbourne KD, Porter DA, Rettig AC, Murray S (1994). Patellar tendon graft reconstruction for midsubstance anterior cruciate ligament rupture in junior high school athletes. An algorithm for management. *Am J Sports Med* **22**, 478–84.
68. Nottage WM, Matsuura PA (1994). Management of complete traumatic anterior cruciate ligament tears in the skeletally immature patient: Current concepts and review of the literature. *Arthroscopy* **10**, 569–73.
69. Parker AW, Drez D Jr, Cooper JL (1994). Anterior cruciate ligament injuries in patients with open physes. *Am J Sports Med* **22**, 44–7.
70. Lo IK, Kirkley A, Fowler PJ, Miniaci A (1997). The outcome of operatively treated anterior cruciate ligament disruptions in the skeletally immature child. *Arthroscopy* **13**, 627–34.

71. Lipscomb AB, Anderson AF (1986). Tears of the anterior cruciate ligament in adolescents. *J Bone Joint Surg Am* **68**, 19–28.
72. Andrews M, Noyes FR, Barber-Westin SD (1994). Anterior cruciate ligament allograft reconstruction in the skeletally immature athlete. *Am J Sports Med* **22**, 48–54.
73. Paletta GA (2003). Special considerations. Anterior cruciate ligament reconstruction in the skeletally immature. *Orthop Clin North Am* **34**, 65–77.
74. Maffulli N, Wong J, Almekinders LC (2003). Types and epidemiology of tendinopathy. *Clin Sports Med* **22**, 675–92.
75. Santopietro FJ (1988). Foot and foot-related injuries in the young athlete. *Clin Sports Med* **7**, 563–89.
76. Walker RN, Green NE, Spindler KP (1996). Stress fractures in skeletally immature patients. *J Pediatr Orthop* **16**, 578–84.
77. Offierski CM (1981). Traumatic dislocation of the hip in children. *J Bone Joint Surg Br* **63**-B,194–7.
78. Niethard FU (1997). *Kinderorthopädie*. Thieme, Stuttgart-New York.
79. Nietosvaara Y, Aalto K, Kallio PE (1994). Acute patellar dislocation in children: incidence and associated osteochondral fractures. *J Pediatr Orthop* **14**, 513–15.
80. Manzione M, Pizzutillo PD, Peoples AB, Schweizer PA (1983). Meniscectomy in children: A long-term follow-up study. *Am J Sports Med* **11**, 111–15.
81. Binfield PM, Maffulli N, Good CJ, King JB (2000). Arthroscopy in sporting and sedentary children and adolescents. *Bull Hosp Jt Dis* **59**, 125–30.
82. Zaman M, Leonard MA (1978). Meniscetomy in children: A study of 59 knees. *J Bone Joint Surg (Br)* **60**, 436–7.
83. Buckley SL (1994). Sports injuries in children. *Curr Opin Pediatr* **6**, 80–4.
84. Stanitski CL, Harvell JC, Fu F (1993). Observations on acute knee hemarthrosis in children and adolescents. *J Pediatr Orthop* **13**, 506–10.
85. Marshall JL, Tischler HM (1981). Screening for sports. *New York J Med* **9**, 68–75.
86. Coughlin M, Mann R (1987). The pathophysiology of the juvenile bunion. In: Griffin P (ed): *Instructional Course Lectures* **26**, 123–36.
87. Griffin LY (1994). Common sports injuries of the foot and ankle seen in children and adolescents. *Orthop Clin North Am* **25**, 83–93.
88. Caine D, DiFiori J, Maffulli N (2006). Physeal injuries in children's and youth sports: Reasons for concern? *Br J Sports Med* **40**, 749–60.
89. Maffulli N (2001). Epiphyseal injuries of the proximal phalanx of the hallux. *Clin J Sport Med* **11**, 121–3.
90. Salter RB, Harris WR (1963). Injuries involving the epiphyseal plate. *J Bone Joint Surg Am* **45**, 587–622.
91. Ogden JA (1982). *Skeletal injury in the child.* Lea & Febinger, Philadelphia.
92. Goldberg VM, Aadalen R (1978). Distal tibial epiphyseal injuries: The role of athletics in 53 cases. *Am J Sports Med* **6**, 263–8.
93. Gregg JR, Das M (1982). Foot and ankle problems in the preadolescent and adolescent athlete. *Clin Sports Med* **1**, 131–47.
94. Larson RL (1973). Epiphyseal injuries in the adolescent athlete. *Orthop Clin North Am* **4**, 839–51.
95. Wolman RL, Harries MG, Fyfe I (1989). Slipped upper femoral epiphysis in an amenorrhoeic athlete. *BMJ* **299**, 720–1.
96. Weinstein SL, Morrissy RT, Crawford AH (1984). Slipped capital femoral epiphysis. In *AAOS Instructional Course Lectures*, vol. 33. pp. 327–49. CV Mosby, St Louis.
97. Albiñana J (1997). Pediatric orthopaedic problems in lower limbs. *Curr Opin Orthop* **8**, 10–15.
98. England SP, Sundberg S (1996). Management of common pediatric fractures. *Ped Clin N Am* **43**, 991–1012.
99. Beaty JH, Austin SM, Warner WC, Canale ST, Nichols L (1994). Interlocking intramedullary nailing of femoral-shaft fractures in adolescents: Preliminary results and complications. *J Pediatr Orthop* **14**, 178–83.
100. O'Malley DE, Mazur JM, Cummings RJ (1995). Femoral head avascular necrosis associated with intramedullary nailing in an adolescent. *J Pediatr Orthop* **15**, 21–3.
101. Siegmeth A, Wruhs O, Vecsei V (1998). External fixation of lower limb fractures in children. *Eur J Pediatr Surg* **8**, 35–41.
102. Ertl JP, Barrack RL, Alexander AH, VanBuecken K (1988). Triplane fracture of the distal tibial epiphysis. Long-term follow-up. *J Bone Joint Surg Am* **70**, 967–76.
103. Maffulli N (2006). Radial overgrowth and deformity after metaphyseal fracture fixation in a child. *Clin Orthop Relat Res* **443**, 350.
104. Binek R, Levinsohn EM, Bersani F, Rubenstein H (1988). Freiberg disease complicating unrelated trauma. *Orthopedics* **11**, 753–7.
105. Gauthier G, Elbaz R (1979). Freiberg's infraction: A subchondral bone fatigue fracture. A new surgical treatment. *Clin Orthop Relat Res* **142**, 93–5.
106. Sproul J, Klaaren H, Mannarino F (1993). Surgical treatment of Freiberg's infraction in athletes. *Am J Sports Med* **21**, 381–4.
107. Ippolito E, Ricciardi Pollini PT, Falez F (1984). Kohler's disease of the tarsal navicular: long-term follow-up of 12 cases. *J Pediatr Orthop* **4**, 416–17.
108. Williams GA, Cowell HR (1981). Kohler's disease of the tarsal navicular. *Clin Orthop Relat Res* **344**, 53–8.
109. Inoue G, Kuboyama K, Shido T (1991). Avulsion fractures of the proximal tibial epiphysis. *Br J Sports Med* **25**, 52–6.
110. Aichroth P (1971). Osteochondritis dissecans of the knee. A clinical survey. *J Bone Joint Surg Br* **53**, 440–7.
111. Canale ST, Belding RH (1980). Osteochondral lesions of the talus. *J Bone Joint Surg Am* **62**, 97–102.
112. Berndt AL, Harty M (1959). Transchondral fractures (osteochondritis dissecans) of the talus. *J Bone Joint Surg Am* **41-A,** 988–1020.
113. Twyman RS, Desai K, Aicroth PM (1991). Osteochondritis dissecans of the knee: A long term study. J *Bone Joint Surg Br* **53**, 440–7.
114. Anderson AF, Pagnani MJ (1997). Osteochondritis dissecans of the femoral condyles. Long-term results of excision of the fragment. *Am J Sports Med* **25**, 830–4.
115. Matheson GO, Clement DB, McKenzie DC, Taunton JE, Lloyd-Smith DR, MacIntyre JG (1987). Stress fractures in athletes. A study of 320 cases. *Am J Sports Med* **15**, 46–58.
116. Torg JS, Pavlov H, Torg E (1987). Overuse injuries in sport: The foot. *Clin Sports Med* **6**, 291–320.
117. Sallis RE, Jones K (1991). Stress fractures in athletes: How to spot this under diagnosed injury. *Postgrad Med* **89**, 185–92.
118. Khan KM, Fuller PJ, Brukner PD, Kearney C, Burry HC (1992). Outcome of conservative and surgical management of navicular stress fracture in athletes. Eighty-six cases proven with computerized tomography. *Am J Sports Med* **20**, 657–66.
119. Kiss ZS, Khan KM, Fuller PJ (1993). Stress fractures of the tarsal navicular bone: CT findings in 55 cases. *AJR Am J Roentgenol* **160**, 111–15.
120. Rosen PR, Micheli LJ, Treves S (1982). Early scintographic diagnosis of bone stress and fractures in athletic adolescents. *Pediatrics* **70**, 11–15.
121. Quain S, Catterall A (1986). Hinge abduction of the hip. Diagnosis and treatment. *J Bone Joint Surg Br* **68**, 61–4.
122. Henderson RC, Renner JB, Sturdivant MC, Greene WB (1990). Evaluation of magnetic resonance imaging in Legg-Perthes disease: a prospective, blinded study. *J Pediatr Orthop* **10**, 289–97.
123. Evans IK, Deluca PA, Gage JR (1988). A comparative study of ambulation-abduction bracing and varus derotation osteotomy in the treatment of severe Legg-Calve-Perthes disease in children over 6 years of age. *J Pediatr Orthop* **8**, 676–82.
124. Harris R, I., Beath T (1948). Etiology of peroneal spatic flat foot. *J Bone Joint Surg Br* **624,** 61–4.
125. Caine CG, Caine DJ, Lindner KJ (1996). *Epidemiology of sports injuries.* Human Kinetics, Champaign IL.

126. Duncan DF (1988). *Epidemiology*. Basis for disease prevention and health promotion. Macmillan, New York.
127. Hackam DJ, Kreller M, Pearl RH (1999). Snow-related recreational injuries in children: Assement of morbidity and management Strategies. *J Pediatr Surg* **34**, 65–9.
128. Helms PJ (1997). Sports injuries in children: Should we be concerned? *Archiv Dis Childhood* **77**, 161–3.
129. Meeuwisse WH (1991). Predictability of sports injuries. What is the epidemiological evidence? *Sports Med* **12**, 8–15.
130. Kocher MS, Waters PM, Micheli LJ (2000). Upper extremity injuries in the paediatric athlete. *Sports Med* **30**, 117–35.
131. Zetaruk MN (2000). The young gymnast. *Clin Sports Med* **19**, 757–80.
132. Stevenson MR, Finch CF, Elliot B, Kresnow M (2000). Sport, age and sex specific incidence of sports injuries in Western Australia. *Br J Sports Med* **34**, 188–94.
133. Coulon L, Lackey G, Mok M, Nile D (2001). A profile of little athletes' injuries and the prevention methods used. *J Sci Med Sport* **4**, 48–58.
134. Metzel JD (2000). The adolescent preparticipation physical examination. Is it helpful. *Clin Sports Med* **19**, 577–92.
135. Reed FE (2001). Improving the preparticipation exam process. *J S C Med Assoc* **97**, 342–6.
136. Heidt RS, Sweeterman LM, Carlonas RL, Traub JA, Tekulve FX (2000). Avoidance of soccer injuries with preseason conditioning. *Am J Sports Med* **28**, 659–62.
137. Janda DH, Bir C, Kedrosle B (2001). A comparison of standard vs. breakaway bases: An analysis of a preventative intervention for softball and baseball for and ankle injuries. *Foot Ankle Int* **22**, 810–16.
138. Viano DC, Bir CA, Cheney AK, Janda DH (2000). Prevention of commotio cordis in baseball: An evaluation of chest protectors. *J Trauma* **49**, 1023–8.
139. Ostrum GA (1993). Sports-related injuries in youth: Prevention is the key-and nurses can help! *Pediatric Nurs* **19**, 333–42.
140. Brady TA, Cahill BR, Bodnar LM (1982). Weight training-related injuries in the high school athlete. *Am J Sports Med* **10**, 1–5.
141. Sewall L, Micheli LJ (1986). Strength training for children. *J Pediatr Orthop* **6**, 143–6.

CHAPTER 48

Injuries to the head and cervical spine

Robert C. Cantu and Robert V. Cantu

Introduction

Today, many parts of the body can be replaced, either by artificial hardware, transplantation, or tissue regeneration. The head and cervical spine are unique in that their contents, the brain and spinal cord, cannot be replaced or transplanted, and are mostly incapable of regeneration. Thus, injury to the head and neck takes on a singular importance. Furthermore, injuries to the head and neck are the most frequent catastrophic athletic injury.[1,2]

With these facts in mind, Table 48.1 contains the most hazardous sports for the head and cervical spine.

Other sports may have an overall risk of serious head and spine injury that is low, but have a certain position or event that is considered high risk. One example of this is soccer, where the goalkeeper is considered a high risk position and another sport is track and field, where pole vaulting is a high risk event. In a review of 32 catastrophic injuries in pole vaulters between 1982 and 1998, it was found that 53% of athletes were seriously injured or died after their body landed on the pad but their head hit the surrounding hard surface. It was recommended to increase the size of the landing pads and to ensure the surrounding ground is a soft material.[3] In youth baseball, the pitcher is more prone to head injury from the batted ball. In 11 of 14 cases of head injury reported from 1982 to 2002, the pitcher was hit by a player using an aluminum bat and in the remaining three cases the type of bat could not be recalled.[4] It has been recommended that the aluminum bat not be used in youth baseball and that pitchers wear head protection. Unsupervised recreational sports, including skiing, skating, and horse riding, have reports of catastrophic head and neck injuries, but full statistics on relative rate of injury are not available.

In many organized youth sports, the risk of serious head and neck injury increases with age. American football is an example of this. There is virtually no death or quadriplegia at the Pop Warner level, but the risk steadily rises in junior high, high school, and college, and is highest by far at the professional level. These differences are primarily due to the fact that at young ages the participants' weight and speed and resulting force of impact are low compared to skeletally mature athletes.

Although the sport of soccer has generally been regarded as safe, except for the goalkeeper, new information from the Netherlands has revealed that all players are at risk for concussion and that chronic traumatic brain injury is not uncommon.[5] Neuropsychologic testing of 53 professional soccer players showed impaired memory, planning, and visuoperceptual processing compared to controls.[6] A direct relationship was also seen between the number of concussions and the frequency of heading the ball. As a soccer ball weighs approximately one pound and can travel up to 100 km·h^{-1} (60 miles·h^{-1}) at the professional level, it is not surprising to realize it can lead to a concussion.

Health professionals responsible for the care of athletes who could sustain head and neck trauma should make certain organizational decisions before the season begins. First, a 'captain' of the medical team responsible for supervising on the field management of the injured athlete should be designated. Although this will usually be the team physician, in certain localities it may be the athletic trainer or an emergency medical technician. Second, all necessary emergency equipment for the head or spine injured athlete should be on the sidelines. At a minimum, this would include equipment for the initiation and maintenance of cardiopulmonary resuscitation (CPR).

Table 48.1 Sports with highest risk for injury to head and cervical spine

1. Auto racing	12. Martial arts
2. Boxing	13. Motorcycling
3. Cheerleading	14. Parachute
4. Cycling	15. Rugby
5. Diving	16. Skating/rollerblading
6. Equestrian sports	17. Skiing
7. Football	18. Sky diving
8. Gymnastics	19. Soccer (goalie)
9. Hang gliding	20. Track (pole vaulting)
10. Ice hockey	21. Trampolining
11. Lacrosse	22. Wrestling

According to statistics from the National Center for Catastrophic Sports Injury Research, the four common school sports with the highest risk of head and cervical spine injury per 100,000 participants are American football, gymnastics, ice hockey, and wrestling. The incidence of injury per 100,000 participants is similar between the four sports and actually slightly higher in cheerleading than in football. Because over 1.5 million youths play football yearly and fewer than 100,000 participate in each of the other sports, the absolute numbers are highest in football.

Types of head injury

The differential diagnosis with a head injury includes: cerebral concussion, intracranial hemorrhage, second impact syndrome or malignant brain oedema, and post-concussion syndrome.

Intracranial haemorrhage

The leading cause of death from athletic head injury is intracranial haemorrhage. There are four types of haemorrhage of which the examining trainer or physician must be aware (see Fig. 48.1). Because all four types of intracranial haemorrhage may be fatal, rapid and accurate initial assessment as well as appropriate follow-up is mandatory after an athletic head injury.

Epidural haematoma

An epidural or extradural haematoma is usually the most rapidly progressing intracranial haematoma. It is frequently associated with a fracture of the temporal bone and results from a tear of the artery supplying the covering (dura) of the brain. The resulting haematoma accumulates inside the skull but outside the covering of the brain. As the bleeding results from a torn artery, it may progress rapidly and reach a fatal size in 30 to 60 min. Classically an initial loss of consciousness, followed by a 'lucid interval', and then further loss of consciousness has been described with epidural haematomas, although this does not always occur. Alternatively, the athlete may not regain consciousness or may remain conscious initially before developing an increasing headache and progressive

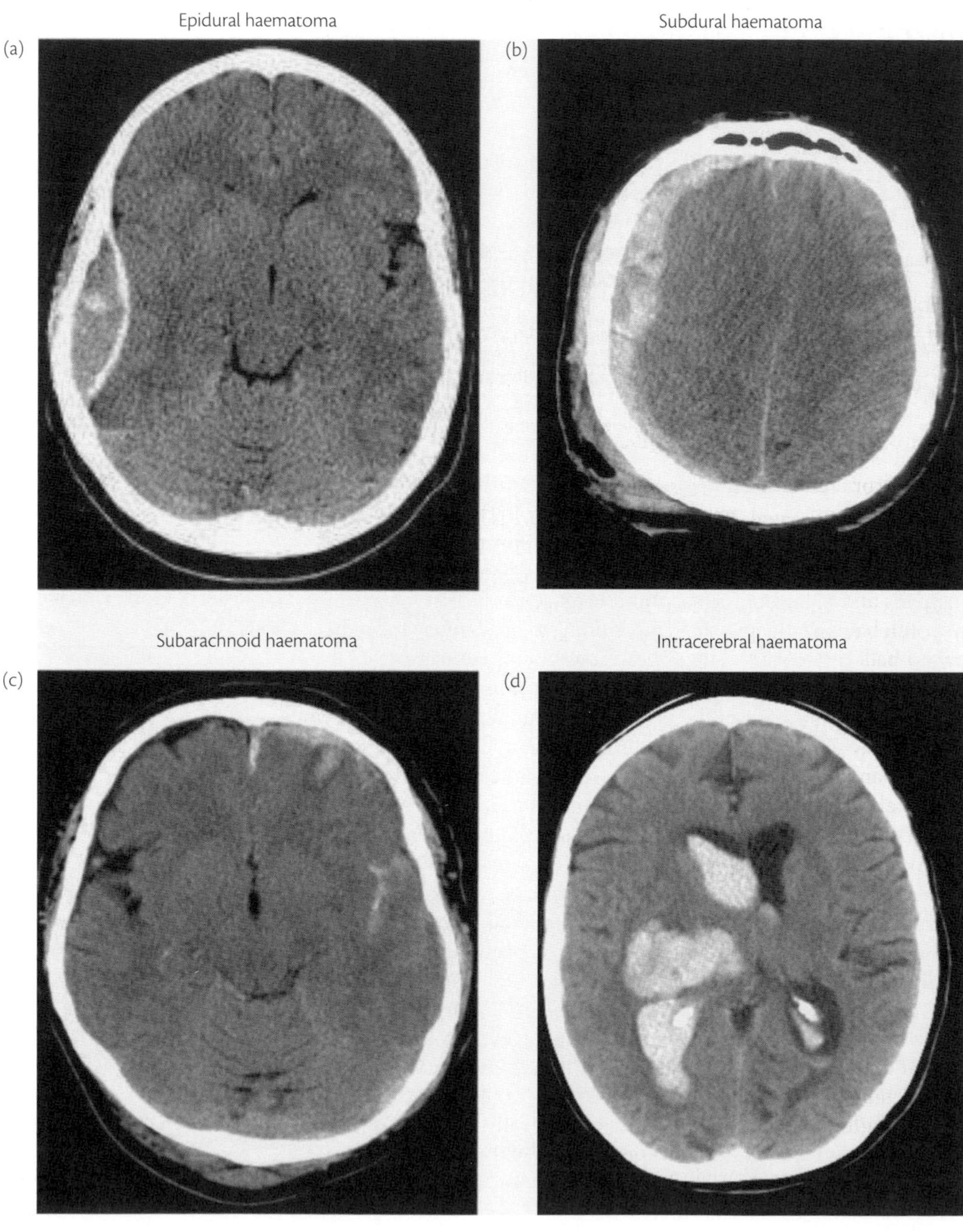

Fig. 48.1 Four types of Intracranial Haemorrhage. (a) Epidural haematoma, (b) Subdural haematoma, (c) Subarachnoid haematoma, (d) Intracerebral haematoma.

loss of consciousness. This deterioration occurs as the clot accumulates and the intracranial pressure increases. This lesion, if present, will almost always declare itself within an hour or two of the time of injury. Often the brain substance is free from direct injury; thus if the clot is promptly removed surgically, full recovery may be expected. Because the lesion is rapidly and almost universally fatal if missed, all athletes receiving a major head injury must be very closely and frequently observed during the ensuing several hours, preferably for 24 hours. This observation should be done at a facility where full neurosurgical services are available.

Subdural haematoma

The subdural haematoma is the most common cause of fatal athletic head injury. A subdural haematoma occurs between the brain surface and the dura, and so is located under the dura and directly on the brain. A subdural haematoma often results from a torn vein running from the surface of the brain to the dura. It may also result from a torn venous sinus or even a small artery on the surface of the brain. With this injury, there is often associated injury to the brain tissue. If a subdural haematoma necessitates surgery in the first 24 hours, the mortality rate is high owing not to the clot itself, but to the associated brain damage from the initial injury. With a subdural haematoma that progresses rapidly, the athlete usually does not regain consciousness and the need for immediate neurosurgical evaluation is obvious. Occasionally, the brain itself is not directly injured and a subdural haematoma develops slowly over a period of days to weeks. This chronic subdural haematoma, although often associated with headache, may initially cause a variety of very mild, almost imperceptible mental, motor, and sensory signs and symptoms. Because its recognition and removal will lead to full recovery, it must always be suspected in an athlete who has previously sustained a head injury and who, days or weeks later, is 'not quite right.' A computerized axial tomography (CAT) scan of the head will show such a lesion.

Intracerebral haematoma

An intracerebral haematoma occurs when there is bleeding into the brain substance itself, usually from a torn artery. It also may result from rupture of a congenital vascular lesion such as an aneurysm or arteriovenous malformation. Intracerebral haematomas are not usually associated with a lucid interval and may be rapidly progressive. Death occasionally occurs before the injured athlete can be transported to a hospital. Because of the intense reaction such a tragic event precipitates among fellow athletes, family, students, and even the community at large, and because of the inevitable rumors that follow, it is imperative to obtain a complete autopsy in such an event to clarify fully the causative factors. Often the autopsy will reveal a congenital lesion, which may indicate that the cause of death was other than presumed and ultimately unavoidable. Only by such full, factual elucidation will appropriate feelings of guilt in fellow athletes, friends, and family be assuaged.

Subarachnoid haemorrhage

In a subarachnoid haemorrhage, the bleeding is confined to the surface of the brain. The bleeding results from disruption of the tiny surface brain vessels and is analogous to a bruise. As with the intracerebral haematoma, there is often brain swelling and such a haemorrhage can also result from a ruptured cerebral aneurysm or arteriovenous malformation. Because bleeding is superficial, surgery is not usually required unless a congenital vascular anomaly is present.

Such a contusion of the brain usually causes headache and often an associated neurologic deficit, depending on the area of the brain involved. The irritative properties of the bleed may also precipitate a seizure. If a seizure occurs it is important to logroll the patient onto his side, so that blood or saliva will roll out of the mouth and the tongue cannot fall back, obstructing the airway. If one has a padded tongue depressor or an oral airway, it can be inserted between the teeth, however under no circumstances should one insert their fingers into the mouth of an athlete who is having a seizure, as amputation can easily result. Usually such a traumatic seizure will last only for a minute or two. The athlete will then relax and transportation to the nearest medical facility can be effected.

Concussion

Concussion is derived from the Latin *concussus*, which means 'to shake violently'.[7] The Committee on Head Injury Nomenclature of the Congress of Neurological Surgeons defines concussion as 'a clinical syndrome characterized by immediate and transient post-traumatic impairment of neural function, such as alteration of consciousness, disturbance of vision, equilibrium, etc, due to brainstem involvement'.[8] As Kelly has stated, a concussion is a 'trauma-induced alteration in mental status that may or may not involve loss of consciousness'.[8] The American Orthopaedic Society for Sports Medicine defines concussion as 'any alteration in cerebral function caused by a direct or indirect (rotation) force transmitted to the head resulting in one or more of the following acute signs and symptoms: a brief loss of consciousness, light-headedness, vertigo, cognitive and memory dysfunction, tinnitus, blurred vision, difficulty concentrating, amnesia, headache, nausea, vomiting, photophobia, or balance disturbance. Delayed signs and symptoms may also include sleep irregularities, fatigue, personality changes, inability to perform usual daily activities, depression, or lethargy'.[8]

Concussion is the most common athletic head injury, with one in five high school American football players suffering one annually. A player who has already sustained one concussion in football is four to six times more likely to sustain a second compared to the athlete who has had none.[9] The rates of concussion in some popular sports are listed in Tables 48.1 and 48.2.[10] The true incidence is difficult to ascertain, as many concussions go unrecognized or

Table 48.2 Evidence based classification schemes for concussion[7]

	Mild: Grade 1	**Moderate: Grade 2**	**Severe: Grade 3**
Cantu	No LOC*, PTA**/PCCS*** less than 30 min	LOC < 1 min, PTA > 30 min but <24 hours, PCCS > 30 min but <7days	LOC > 1 min, PTA > 24 hours, PCSS > 7 days
American Academy of Neurology	Transient confusion; no LOC; symptoms or abnormalities resolve in <15 min	Transient confusion; no LOC; symptoms or abnormalities last >15 min	Any LOC

*Loss of Consciousness.

**Post-traumatic amnesia (PTA:anterograde/retrograde).

***Post-concussion signs/symptoms (PCSS) other than amnesia.

unreported, but estimates at all levels in American football have been as high as 250,000 per year.[11] One survey found that 20% of high school American football players had sustained some form of concussion.[11]

Although it was previously thought that a concussion is a physiologic disturbance without structural damage, animal and human data have shown that neurochemical and structural changes with loss of brain cells can occur. A neurochemical cascade begins within minutes following a concussion and can continue for days.[12] It is during this period that neurons remain in a vulnerable state, susceptible to minor changes in cerebral blood flow, increases in intracranial pressure, and anoxia. Animal studies have shown that during this susceptible period, a decrease in cerebral blood flow that normally would have little consequence can produce extensive neuronal cell death.[12]

Following a concussion or minor traumatic brain injury, disruption of the neuronal cell membrane, stretching of axons, and opening of potassium channels lead to an efflux of potassium out of affected neurons.[13] Depolarization of neurons leads to release of glutamate, which further induces an efflux of potassium. The extracellular potassium leads to a release of excitatory amino acids and further depolarization, both serving to further increase extra-cellular potassium. Increased adenosine triphosphate (ATP) is required to restore the imbalance in potassium and membrane potential. Glucose utilization increases, leading to a state of hyperglycolysis that in rat studies lasts several hours but in humans may last significantly longer. Lactate levels increase, which can cause neuronal damage and lead to increased vulnerability to cell damage.[13]

Several attempts have been made to classify concussions based on their severity, with guidelines for return to play. The most commonly used classifications have three grades, with a type 1 described as mild, type 2 as moderate, and type 3 as severe. The classification schemes vary somewhat, but are all based on clinical presentation of the athlete, and especially with the Cantu Classification, the duration of symptoms (Table 48.2).

The late effects of repeated head trauma of concussive or even subconcussive force lead to anatomical patterns of chronic brain injury with correlating signs and symptoms. Martland first introduced the term 'punch drunk' in 1928 which is more formally now called dementia pugilistica.[14] Although the term originally referred to boxers, the underlying traumatic encephalopathy can occur in anyone subjected to repeated blows to the head from any cause.

The characteristic signs and symptoms of the punch drunk state include the gradual appearance of a euphoric dementia with emotional lability, the victim displaying little insight into his deterioration. Speech and thought become progressively slower and memory deteriorates considerably. Wide mood swings may occur with intense irritability, sometimes leading to uninhibited violent behavior. Simple fatuous cheerfulness is, however, the most common prevailing mood, though sometimes there is depression with paranoia. From the clinical standpoint, the neurologist may encounter almost any combination of pyramidal, extrapyramidal, and cerebellar signs. Tremor and dysarthria are two of the most common findings.

Corsellis *et al.*[15] described the autopsy findings in the brains of men who had been boxers. They described a characteristic pattern of cerebral change that appeared to have resulted from boxing and explained many of the features of the punch drunk syndrome. Changes were seen in the middle of the brain, which in some instances was essentially sheared into two layers. Destruction was seen in the limbic system, a portion of the brain that governs emotion and plays a role in memory and learning. A characteristic loss of cells was seen in the cerebellum, a part of the brain regulating balance and coordination. Microscopic changes were also seen throughout the brain resembling changes seen with Alzheimer's disease. Neurofibrillary tangles but not senile plaques were observed, such that it was thought to be a distinct entity, unique to subjects who had suffered multiple blows to the head.

Recently, a less severe variant of chronic traumatic encephalopathy has been seen and reported in deceased NFL football players. Clinically it consists of cognitive impairment and depression and neuropathologically is characterized by neurofibrillary tangles and neutrophile threads of tau protein deposition.[16,17]

Post-concussion syndrome

Although uncommon, post-concussive symptoms can last more than a month and lead to the post-concussion syndrome. The symptoms typically include headache (especially with exertion), dizziness, fatigue, irritability, and especially impaired memory and concentration. The persistence of these symptoms reflects altered neurotransmitter function and usually correlates with the duration of post-traumatic amnesia.[18] When these symptoms persist, the athlete should be evaluated with magnetic resonance imaging (MRI). Return to competition should be deferred until all symptoms have abated and the diagnostic studies are normal. Once symptoms have resolved, neuropsychiatric testing can be performed and used for future comparison.

Malignant brain oedema syndrome

Malignant brain oedema is seen in paediatric athletes. The syndrome consists of rapid neurological deterioration from an alert conscious state to coma and sometimes death, minutes to several hours after the head trauma.[19,20] Pathology studies show diffuse brain swelling often with little or no direct brain injury.[20] Langfitt and colleagues have shown the cerebral swelling is the result of a hyperaemia or vascular engorgement.[21,22] Prompt recognition is extremely important because there is little initial brain injury and the serious or fatal neurological outcome is secondary to raised intracranial pressure with herniation. Prompt treatment with intubation, hyperventilation, and osmotic agents has helped to reduce mortality.[23,24]

Second impact syndrome

Saunders and Harbaugh coined the term 'second impact syndrome of catastrophic head injury' in 1984, although Schneider first described two cases matching the description in 1973.[25,26] The syndrome occurs when an athlete who sustains a head injury-often a concussion or worse injury such as a cerebral contusion-sustains a second head injury before symptoms associated with the first have cleared.[27–29] The symptoms may include visual, motor, or sensory changes and difficulty with thought and memory. The second head injury may be remarkably minor, perhaps only a blow to the chest that indirectly imparts accelerative forces to the brain. The athlete may appear stunned, but usually does not lose consciousness and often completes the play. The athlete may remain on the field or walk off under his own power.

What separates the second impact syndrome from a concussion or even a subdural haematoma is the ensuing events after the second impact. Usually within seconds to minutes of the second impact, the athlete-conscious yet stunned-quite precipitously collapses to the ground. The athlete quickly becomes unconscious with rapidly dilating pupils, loss of eye movement, and evidence of respiratory failure.

The pathophysiology of second impact syndrome is thought to involve a loss of autoregulation of the brain's blood supply. The loss of autoregulation leads to vascular engorgement within the cranium, which in turn markedly increases intracranial pressure and leads to herniation either of the medial surface (uncus) of the temporal lobe, lobes below the tentorium, or the cerebellar tonsils through the foramen magnum. Animal research has shown that vascular engorgement of the brain after a mild head injury is difficult if not impossible to control.[30,31] The usual time from the second impact to brainstem failure is rapid, taking 2–5 min. Once brain herniation and brain stem compromise occur, ocular involvement and respiratory failure precipitously ensue. Demise occurs far more rapidly than usually seen with an epidural haematoma.

Incidence

Although the exact incidence is not known, second impact syndrome is likely more common than previous reports have suggested. Over a 13 year period (1980–1993), the National Center for Catastrophic Sports Injury Research in Chapel Hill, North Carolina, identified 35 probable cases among American football players alone.[32] Seventeen of these cases were confirmed at the time of surgery or at autopsy, while 18 cases lacked sufficient documentation at autopsy, but most probably represented additional cases. Careful scrutiny excluded the diagnosis in 22 of the 57 cases originally suspected.[32]

Second impact syndrome is not limited to American football. Fekete[33] described a 16-year-old high school hockey player who fell during a game, striking the back of his head on the ice. The boy lost consciousness and afterward complained of unsteadiness and headaches. While playing in the next game 4 days later, he was checked forcibly and fell striking his left temple on the ice. His pupils rapidly became fixed and dilated and he died within 2 hours while in transit to a neurosurgical facility. Autopsy revealed brain contusion of several days duration, an oedematous brain with a thin layer of subdural and subarachnoid haemorrhage, and bilateral herniation of the cerebellar tonsils into the foramen magnum. Though Fekete did not use the label 'second impact syndrome', the clinical course and autopsy findings are consistent with the syndrome.

Other case reports of second impact syndrome exist. McQuillen *et al.*[34] described an 18-year-old downhill skier who suffered the syndrome and remained in a persistent vegetative state. Kelly *et al.*[35] reported on a 17-year-old football player who died as a result of the syndrome. Physicians who cover athletic events, especially those in which head trauma is likely, must understand the second impact syndrome and be prepared to initiate emergency treatment.

Prevention

Since the second impact syndrome has a mortality rate of nearly 50% and a morbidity rate approaching 100%, prevention takes on the utmost importance. An athlete who is symptomatic from a head injury, must not participate in contact or collision sports. Return should be delayed until all cerebral symptoms have subsided, preferably for at least 1 week. Whether it takes days, weeks, or months to reach the asymptomatic state, the athlete should not be allowed to practice or compete while still suffering post-concussion symptoms. Team physicians and trainers must educate coaches, players (and their parents) as to the significance of the problem. Files of the National Center for Catastrophic Sport Injury Research include cases of young athletes who did not report their cerebral symptoms, fearing they would not be allowed to compete. Not knowing they were jeopardizing their lives, they played with post-concussion symptoms and tragically developed the second impact syndrome.

Diffuse axonal injury

This condition results from high energy shearing forces imparted to the brain that literally sever axonal connections without intracranial hematoma. The patient is usually rendered unconscious with a low Glascow coma scale and a negative head computed tomography (CT). Immediate neurosurgical triage for treatment of increased intracranial pressure is indicated.

Management guidelines for the head injured athlete

Immediate treatment

Initial evaluation of any head injured athlete follows the A,B,C's of trauma resuscitation. The first priority of the team physician is ensuring that the athlete is maintaining an adequate airway and is breathing. Next, physical examination should ensure maintenance of circulation. After these critical assessments have been made, attention can be focused on the neurological examination.

Definitive treatment

Definitive treatment of grade 2 and grade 3 concussions, second impact syndrome, intracranial haematomas, and diffuse axonal shear should take place at a medical facility where neurosurgical and neuroradiological capabilities are present. In the case of intracranial haematoma, definitive treatment may require surgical evacuation of the blood clot. For severe concussions, observation is appropriate with careful neurological monitoring.

What tests to order and when

After a grade 1 concussion, observation alone may be all that is indicated. In cases of grade 2 where there has been loss of consciousness and in most all grade 3 concussions, a CT scan or MRI of the brain is recommended. In the case of the second impact syndrome and intracranial haemorrhage, emergent scanning with either a CT scan or MRI is appropriate.

When to refer

All athletes with other than a grade 1 concussion should be referred for a neurological or neurosurgical evaluation following removal from the athletic contest.

When to operate

Close head injuries such as concussion and diffuse axonal shear do not require surgery. Intracranial haematomas, depending on their size and location, may require prompt surgical evacuation. Congenital vascular anomalies, such as aneurysm or arterial venous malformation, may require planned deliberate surgical intervention.

Return to competition

Table 48.3 provides guidelines for return to competition after a cerebral concussion. Other guidelines exist also based on the severity and number of prior concussions.[35–37] While the guidelines have some differences, they do share one common recommendation, that no athlete still symptomatic from a previous injury should return to practice or competition and risk the second impact syndrome.

A final comment on concussions

Following a concussion, a thorough review of the circumstances resulting in the concussion should occur. In our experience as team physicians, athletes who sustained repeated concussions were often using their heads unwisely, illegally, or both. If available, videotapes of the incident should be reviewed by the team physician, trainer, coach, and player to see if improper technique was a factor. Equipment should also be checked to be certain it fits precisely and it has been maintained, especially the air pressure in air helmets. Additionally, neck strength and development should be assessed.

Types of spine injuries

Fracture, concussion, contusion, haemorrhage

The same traumatic lesions that affect the brain may also occur to the cervical spinal cord, namely concussion, contusion, and various types of haemorrhage. Unlike the head, where subdural haematoma is the most common and lethal haemorrhage, in the cervical spine a subdural is quite uncommon, with no reports in the National Center for Catastrophic Sports Injury Research (NCCSIR). In the cervical spine the intraspinal haematoma (within the cord) is the most common and the epidural the next most common haemorrhage. All spinal cord injuries reported in the NCCSIR have been in the cervical spine, with none in the thoracic or lumbar region.

The major concern with a cervical spinal injury is the possibility of an unstable fracture that may produce quadriplegia. In the NCCSIR registry, all cases of quadriplegia in the absence of spinal stenosis, resulted from fracture dislocation of the cervical spine. At the time of injury, on the field, there is no way to determine the presence of an unstable fracture. Diagnosing a fracture requires appropriate radiographic evaluation. At the time of injury there is also no way of differentiating between a fully recoverable and a permanent case of quadriplegia. If the patient is fully conscious, a cervical fracture or cervical cord injury is usually accompanied by rigid cervical muscle spasm and pain that immediately alerts the athlete and physician to the presence of such an injury. It is the unconscious athlete, unable to say his or her neck hurts and unable to produce protective neck muscle spasm, that is most susceptible to further cord injury if caregivers do not assume the presence of such an injury.

With the neck injured or unconscious athlete, it is imperative that no neck manipulation be carried out on the field. The athlete must be transported with the head and neck immobilized to the medical facility. On arrival at the medical facility a detailed neurlogic exam and appropriate radiographic studies are obtained. Either a full cervical spine series or a CT scan should be obtained. As many as 20% of unstable cervical spine injuries may be missed when only a cross table lateral cervical spine radiograph is obtained.[38] In the adolescent, there can normally exist a slight displacement of the second cervical vertebra (1–2 mm) over the third due to the hypermobility of these segments. Failure to recognize this normal 'pseudosubluxation' can lead to over treatment.

One issue that has received attention in the literature is whether to remove the athletic helmet for transport of a spine injured patient. The National Athletic Trainers' Association (NATA) formed the Inter-association Task Force for Appropriate Care of the Spine-Injured Athlete in 1998 and it concluded that helmets and shoulder pads should be left in place to provide support and help maintain alignment for the athlete with a known or suspected cervical spine injury.[39] Multiple studies, both cadaveric and human, support this conclusion.[40–42] As in the head injured athlete, the face mask is removed from the helmet in the event immediate airway access is required. The recommendation applies to sports such as football, hockey, and lacrosse in which the athlete is wearing shoulder pads, but not to automobile racing in which the entire helmet must be removed for airway access.

Table 48.3 Guidelines for return to competition after cerebral concussion

Grade 1	Grade 2	Grade 3
First concussion		
Athlete may return to play that day in select situations if clinical examination results are normal at rest and with exertion, otherwise return to play in one week	Athlete may return to play in 2 weeks if asymptomatic at rest and with exertion for 7 days	Athlete may return to play in 1 month if asymptomatic at rest and exertion for 7 days
Second concussion		
Return to play in 2 weeks if asymptomatic for 1 week	Minimum of 1 month; may return to play then if asymptomatic for 1 week; consider terminating season	Terminate season; may return to play next season if asymptomatic
Third concussion		
Terminate season; may return to play next season if asymptomatic	Terminate season; may return to play next season if asymptomatic	

Stingers

Stingers or burners are terms used by athletes and trainers to describe a set of symptoms that involve pain, burning, or tingling down an arm occasionally accompanied by localized weakness. The symptoms typically abate within seconds or minutes, rarely persisting for days or longer. It has been estimated that 50% of American football players will sustain a stinger at least once during their career.[43]

There are two typical mechanisms by which stingers may occur; traction on the brachial plexus, or nerve root impingement within the cervical neural foramen. The majority of high school stingers are due to the traction type, while most college level and virtually all at the professional ranks result from a pinch phenomenon within the neural foramen.

With either type of stinger, the athlete experiences a shock-like sensation of pain and numbness radiating into the arm and hand. The symptoms are typically purely sensory and most commonly involve the C5 and C6 dermatomes. On occasion, weakness may also be present. The most common muscles involved include the deltoid, biceps, supraspinatus, and infraspinatus.

Stingers are unilateral and virtually never involve the lower extremities. If symptoms are bilateral or involve the legs, then the burning hands syndrome or spinal cord injury must be considered.

When stingers are not associated with any neck pain or limitation of neck movement and all motor and sensory symptoms clear within seconds to minutes, the athlete may safely return to competition. This is especially true if the athlete has previously experienced similar symptoms. If symptoms do not completely resolve or the athlete complains of neck pain, return should be deferred pending further work-up.

On rare occasions a stinger may result in prolonged sensory complaints or weakness. In such a situation, MRI imaging of the cervical spine should be considered to look for a herniated disc or other pathology. If symptoms persist for more than 2 weeks, electromyography should allow for an accurate assessment of the degree and extent of injury.

Some athletes seem predisposed to develop a series of recurrent stingers. It has been suggested that repeated stinger injuries over many years may lead to proximal arm weakness and constant pain. Thus if an athlete suffers two or more stingers, particularly in rapid succession, consideration can be given to the use of high shoulder pads supplemented by a soft cervical roll, which should limit lateral neck flexion and extension. Examining or changing the athlete's blocking and tackling techniques or changing the player's position also may help to prevent recurrences. If stingers repeatedly occur despite these interventions, then cessation of the causative athletic activity may be necessary.

Transient quadriplegia

Transient quadriplegia or bilateral neurologic symptoms after a player takes a hit in a contact sport raises the spectre of spinal cord compromise. In some athletes, spinal stenosis may be a contributing factor. Although radiographic bone measurements can suggest stenosis is present, physicians are cautioned against making the diagnosis with this technique alone. Instead, diagnostic technologies that view the spinal cord itself, such as MRI, or contrast positive CT or myelography, should be employed. These imaging methods can determine if the spinal cord has a normal functional reserve: the space largely filled with a protective cushion of cerebrospinal fluid (CSF) between the cord and the spinal canal's interior walls lined by bone, disc, and ligament. In addition, these techniques determine whether the nerve tissue is deformed by an abnormality such as a disc protrusion, bony osteophyte or posterior buckling of the ligamentum flavum.

Controversy persists as to whether cervical stenosis increases the risk of spinal cord injury. It is the opinion of the senior author that athletes who have had spinal cord symptoms from sports-related injuries and are shown to have true spinal stenosis on MR imaging should not be allowed to return to contact sports. There is a growing body of evidence in the sports medicine, neurology, and radiology fields that indicates spinal stenosis predisposes a patient to spinal cord injury.[44–46]

Several studies have shown the dangers of spinal stenosis. Matsuura *et al.*[47] compared the spinal dimensions of 100 controls with those of 42 patients who had spinal cord injuries. They found that the control group had significantly larger sagittal spinal canal diameters than did the patients who had spinal cord injuries. Furthermore, the National Center for Catastrophic Sports Injury Research has no instance of complete neurologic recovery in spinal stenotic athletes with fracture dislocation of the cervical spine, whereas there are a number of such complete recoveries in athletes with normal size spinal canals. There are also several instances of permanent quadriplegia in athletes with tight spinal stenosis without fracture or demonstrated instability. Based on these findings, the senior author feels strongly that identification of 'functional spinal stenosis' is a contraindication to further participation in contact/collision sports.

The question of spinal stenosis may receive increasing attention, as several professional football teams require detailed investigation of the cervical and lumbar spine (including MR imaging) as part of the draft process. Presently, there are no good guidelines to help physicians advise an athlete with a narrow but asymptomatic cervical spinal canal. When such an abnormality is encountered, management must be individualized according to the patient's symptoms, the degree of canal stenosis, and the perceived risk of permanent neurologic injury.

Vascular injury

A final uncommon but serious neck injury involves the carotid arteries. By either extremes of lateral flexion or extension or a forceful blow by a relatively fixed, narrow object such as a forearm, the inner layer (intima) of the carotid artery may be torn. The intimal tear can lead to clot formation at the site of injury, resulting in emboli to the brain or complete occlusion of the artery causing a major stroke. With a fracture dislocation, injury to the vertebral artery may occur leading to a brainstem stroke.

Return to play

It is recommended that an athlete not return to competition after a neck injury until he or she is free of neck or arm pain, has a full range of neck motion without discomfort or spasm, and neck strength in flexion, extension, and on each side has returned to pre-injury levels. If a pre-injury profile is unknown, strength should at least be symmetrical. MR imaging should not reveal significant disc disease or functional spinal stenosis.

Because of their participation in the Special Olympics, it is important to realize that as high as 4% of children with Down's syndrome may have abnormalities of the cervical spine.[48] The most common abnormality is subluxation at the atlantoaxial (C1–2) joint followed by atlanto-occipital subluxation.[49] It is recommended that cervical spine stability be assessed in all patients with Down's syndrome who wish to participate in athletic activities, especially those involving the head and neck, such as soccer.

Conclusion

Injuries to the head and neck are the most frequent catastrophic sports injury, and head injuries are the most common direct athletic cause of death. Although direct compressive forces may injure the brain, neural tissue is particularly susceptible to injury from shearing stresses, which are most likely to occur when rotational forces are applied to the head.

The most common athletic head injury is concussion, which may vary widely in severity. Intracranial haemorrhage is the leading cause of head injury death in sports, making rapid initial assessment and appropriate follow up mandatory after a head injury. Diffuse cerebral swelling is another serious condition that may be found in the child or adolescent athlete, and the second impact syndrome is a major concern in adult athletes.

Many head and neck injuries are the result of improper playing techniques and can be reduced by teaching proper skills and enforcing safety promoting rules. Improved conditioning (particularly of the neck), protective headgear, and careful medical supervision of athletes will also minimize this type of injury.

Summary

- Four common school sports with highest risk of head and cervical spine injury per 100,000 participants, American football, gymnastics, ice hockey, and wrestling as well as sports with overall low risk but position or event at high risk (pole vault in track) are discussed as regards mechanism of injury and its prevention.
- The differential diagnosis of the most common athletic head injuries including cerebral concussion, intracranial hemorrhage, second impact syndrome or malignant brain oedema syndrome, post-concussion syndrome, are discussed and illustrated.
- Management guidelines are presented for athletic head injuries including immediate treatment, definitive treatment, what tests to order, when to refer, when to operate, and when to return to competition.
- Management and return to play guidelines are presented for athletic spine and spinal cord injuries including spine fractures and spinal cord concussion/contusion and hemorrhage.
- Also covered are the diagnosis and management of:
  - (i) Stingers which may involve injury to the brachial plexus or cervical nerve root.
  - (ii) Vascular injuries of the neck involving either the carotid or vertebral artery.
  - (iii) Special concerns regarding the Down's Syndrome patient and atlantoaxial (C1–2) subluxation.

References

1. Cantu RC (1986). Guidelines for return to contact sports after a cerebral concussion. *Phys Sports Med* **40**, 10–14.
2. Cantu RC (1987). *The exercising adult* (2nd ed.). McMillan Publishing Co, New York.
3. Boden BP, Pasquina P, Johnson J, Mueller FO (2001). Catastrophic injuries in pole-vaulters. *Am J Sports Med* **29**, 50–4.
4. Boden BP, Tacchetti R, Mueller FO (2004). Catastrophic injuries in high school and college baseball players. *Am J Sports Med* **32**, 1189–96.
5. Proctor MR, Cantu RC (2000). Head and neck injuries in young athletes. *Clin Sports Med* **19**(4), 693–715.
6. Matser JT, Kessels AGH, Jordan BD, Lezak MD, Troost J (1998). Chronic traumatic brain injury in professional soccer players. *Neurology* **51**, 791–6.
7. Cantu RC (2003). Recurrent athletic head injury: risks and when to retire. *Clin Sports Med* **22**, 593–603.
8. Cooper MT, McGee KM, Anderson DG (2003). Epidemiology of athletic head and neck injuries. *Clin Sports Med* **22**, 427–43.
9. Zemper E (1994). Analysis of cerebral concussion frequency with the most common models of football helmets. *J Athl Train* **29**, 44–50.
10. Dick RW (1994). A summary of head and neck injuries in collegiate athletes using the NCAA injury surveillance system In: Hoerner EF (ed.), *Head and neck injuries in sports*, pp. 13–19. American Society for Testing and Material, Philadelphia.
11. Gerberich SG, Priest JD, Boen JR, Straub CP, Maxwell RE (1983). Concussion incidences and severity in secondary school varsity football players. *Am J Pub Health* **73**, 1370–5.
12. Echemendia RJ, Cantu RC (2003). Return to play following sports-related mild traumatic brain injury: The role of neuropsychology. *Appl Neuropsychol* **10**, 48–55.
13. Grindel SH (2003). Epidemiology and pathophysiology of minor traumatic brain injury. *Curr Sports Med Rep* **2**, 18–23.
14. Martland HS (1928). Punch drunk. *JAMA* **91**, 1103–7.
15. Corsellis JAN, Bruton CJ, and Freeman-Browne D (1973). The aftermath of boxing. *Psychol Med* **3**, 270–303.
16. Omalu BI, DeKosky ST, Minster RL, Kamboh MI, Wecht CH (2005). Chronic traumatic encephalopathy in a National Football League player. *Neurosurgery* **57**, 128–34.
17. Omalu B, DeKosdy S, Hamilton R, Minster RL, Kamboh MI, Shakir AM, Wecht CH (2006). Chronic traumatic encephalopathy in a National Football League player: Part II. *Neurosurgery* **59**, 1086–93.
18. Guthkelch AN (1979). Post-traumatic amnesia, post-concussional symptoms and accident neurosis. *Acta Neurochir Suppl* **29**, 120–3.
19. Pickles W (1950). Acute general edema of the brain in children with head injuries. *N Engl J Med* **242**, 607–11.
20. Schnitker MT (1949). Syndrome of cerebral concussion in children. *J Pediatr* **35**, 557–60.
21. Langfitt TW, Kassell NF (1968). Cerebral vasodilatation produced by brain-stem stimulation: Neurogenic control vs. autoregulation. *Am J Physiol* **215**, 90–7.
22. Langfitt TW, Tannenbaum HM, and Kassell NF (1966). The etiology of acute brain swelling following experimental head injury. *J Neurosurg* **24**, 47–56.
23. Bowers SA, and Marshall LF (1980). Outcome in 200 consecutive cases of severe head injury treated in San Diego County: A prospective analysis. *Neurosurgery* **6**, 237–42.
24. Bruce DA, Schut L, Bruno LA, Wood JH, Sutton LN (1978). Outcome following severe head injuries in children. *J Neurosurg* **48**, 679–88.
25. Saunders RL, Harbaugh RE (1984). Second impact in catastrophic contact-sports head trauma. *JAMA* **252**, 538–9.
26. Schneider RC (1973). *Head and neck injuries in football*. Williams and Wilkins, Baltimore.
27. Cantu RC (1992). Second impact syndrome: Immediate management. *Phys Sports Med* **20**, 55–66.
28. Cantu RC, Voy R (1995). Second impact syndrome a risk in any contact sport. *Phys Sports Med* **23**, 27–34.
29. McQuillen JB, McWuillen EN, Morrow P (1988). Trauma, sports and malignant cerebral edema. *Am J Forensic Med Pathol* **9**, 12–15.
30. Moody RA, Raumsuke S, Mullan SF (1968). An evaluation of decompression in experimental head injury. *J Neurosurgery* **29**, 586–90.
31. Langfitt TW, Weinstein JD, Kassell NF (1963). Cerebral vasomotor paralysis produced by intracranial hypertension. *Neurology* **13**, 622–41.
32. Cantu RC (1992). Second impact syndrome: Immediate management. *Phys Sports Med* **20**, 55–66.
33. Fekete JF (1968). Severe brain injury and death following rigid hockey accidents. The effectiveness of the "safety helmets" of amateur hockey players. *Can Med Assoc J* **99**, 1234–9.
34. McQuillen JB, McWuillen EN, Morrow P (1988). Trauma, sports and malignant cerebral edema. *AmJ Forensic Med Path* **9**, 12–15.
35. Kelly JP, Nichols JS, Filley CM, Lillehei KO, Rubinstein D, Kleinschmidt-DeMasters BK (1991). Concussion in sports: Guidelines

for the prevention of catastrophic outcome. *JAMA* **266**, 2867–9.

36. Nelson WE, Jane JA, Gieck JH (1984). Minor head injury in sport: A new classification and management. *Phys Sports Med* **12**, 103–7.
37. Torg JA (1991). *Athletic injuries to the head, neck, and face*. Mosby Yearbook, St Louis.
38. Herzog RJ, Wiens JJ, Dillingham MF, Sontag MJ (1991). Normal cervical spine morphometry and cervical spinal stenosis in asymptomatic professional football players: Plain film radiography, multiplanar computed tomography, and magnetic resonance imaging. *Spine* **116**, S178–86.
39. Banerjee R, Palumbo MA, Fadale PD (2004). Catastrophic cervical spine injuries in the collision sport athlete, part 2. *Am J Sports Med* **32**, 1760–4.
40. LaPrade RF, Schnetzler KA, Broxterman RJ, Wentorf F, Gilbert TJ (2000). Cervical spine alignment in the immobilized ice hockey player: A computed tomography analysis of the effects of helmet removal. *Am J Sports Med* **28**, 800–3.
41. Palumbo MA, Hulstyn MJ, Fadale PD, O'Brien T, Shall L (1996). The effect of protective football equipment on alignment of the injured cervical spine: Radiographic analysis in a cadaveric model. *Am J Sports Med* **24**, 446–53.
42. Peris MD, Donaldson WF III, Towers J, Blanc R, Muzzonigro TS (2002). Helmet and shoulder pad removal in suspected cervical spine injury: Human control model. *Spine* **27**, 995–8.
43. Feldick HG, Albright JP (1976). Football survey reveals "missed" neck injuries. *Phys Sports Med* **4**, 77–81.
44. Eismont FJ, Clifford S, Goldberg M, Green B (1984). Cervical sagittal spinal canal size in spine injury. *Spine* **9**, 663–6.
45. Torg JS, Ramsey-Emrhein JA (1997). Management guidelines for participation in collision activities with congenital, developmental, or postinjury lesions involving the cervical spine. *Clin J Sport Med* **7**, 273–91.
46. Dec KL, Cole SL, Dec SL (2007). Screening for catastrophic neck injuries in sports. *Curr Sports Med Rep* **6**, 16–19.
47. Matsuura P, Waters RL, Adkins RH, Rothman S, Gurbani N, Sie L (1989). Comparison of computerized tomography parameters of the cervical spine in normal control subjects and spinal cord-injured patients. *J Bone Joint Surg Am* **71**, 183–8.
48. Cope R, Olson S (1987). Abnormalities of the cervical spine in Down's syndrome: Diagnosis, risks, and review of the literature with particular reference to the Special Olympics. *South Med J* **80**, 33–6.
49. Rosenbaum DM, Blumhagen JD, King HA (1986). Atlanto-occipital subluxation in Down's syndrome. *AJR Am J Roentgen* **146**, 1269–72.

Index